PETERSON'S
NURSING
PROGRAMS
2008

PETERSON'S

A ⓝelnet COMPANY

About Peterson's, a Nelnet company

Peterson's (www.petersons.com) is a leading provider of education information and advice, with books and online resources focusing on education search, test preparation, and financial aid. Its Web site offers searchable databases and interactive tools for contacting educational institutions, online practice tests and instruction, and planning tools for securing financial aid. Peterson's serves 110 million education consumers annually.

For more information, contact Peterson's, 2000 Lenox Drive, Lawrenceville, NJ 08648; 800-338-3282; or find us on the World Wide Web at www.petersons.com/about.

Editor: Linda Seghers; Production Editor: Mark D. Snider; Copy Editors: Bret Bollmann, Michael Haines, Sally Ross, Jill C. Schwartz, Pam Sullivan, Valerie Bolus Vaughan; Research Project Manager: Christine Lucas; Research Associate: Helen Hannan; Programmer: Phyllis Johnson; Manufacturing Manager: Ivona Skibicki; Composition Manager: Linda M. Williams; Client Service Representatives: Mimi Kaufman, Danielle Vreeland

ISSN 1552-7743
ISBN-13: 978-0-7689-2412-1
ISBN-10: 0-7689-2412-X

Printed in the United States of America

10 9 8 7 6 5 4 3 2 1   09 08 07

Thirteenth Edition

CONTENTS

FOREWORD

The American Association of Colleges of Nursing (AACN) is proud to collaborate on *Peterson's Nursing Programs 2008*.

According to the Bureau of Labor Statistics, more than 1 million new and replacement registered nurses will be needed by the year 2012 to fill new positions and vacancies. As registered nurses find employment beyond hospitals in such areas as home care, community health, and long-term care, newly licensed RNs must have the proper education and training to work in these settings. It is vital that those seeking to enter or advance in a nursing career find the appropriate nursing program. This guide allows readers to find the program that best fits their needs, whether beginning a new career in nursing or attempting to advance one.

According to AACN's most recent annual institutional survey, enrollment in entry-level B.S.N. programs continues to climb. Gains were reported in all parts of the country in 2005, with an overall 13 percent increase in enrollments nationwide. Nursing schools are working hard to find creative solutions to expand capacity and recruit new students during this nursing shortage.

Although the health-care environment is complex and dynamic, there continues to be a significant demand for professional-level nurses. The primary route into professional-level nursing is the four-year baccalaureate degree. The professional nurse with a baccalaureate degree is the only basic nursing graduate prepared to practice in all health-care settings, including critical care, public health, primary care, and mental health. In addition, advanced practice nurses (APNs) deliver essential services as nurse practitioners, certified nurse-midwives, clinical nurse specialists, and nurse anesthetists. APNs typically are prepared in master's degree programs, and the demand for their services is expected to increase substantially.

Higher education in nursing expands the gateway to a variety of career opportunities in the health-care field. In addition to providing primary care to patients, graduates can work as case managers for the growing numbers of managed-care companies or can assume administrative or managerial roles in hospitals, clinics, insurance companies, and other diverse settings.

The Nursing School Adviser section of this guide is instructive and invaluable. Whether you are a high school student looking for a four-year program, an RN returning to school, or a professional in another field contemplating a career change, this section will address your concerns. This information presents various nursing perspectives to benefit students from diverse backgrounds.

Peterson's effort in making this guide well organized and convenient to read cannot be overstated. Peterson's has worked with AACN in producing a publication that is comprehensive and user-friendly. Like the previous editions, this edition is a genuine collaborative work, as AACN provided input from start to finish.

AACN's dedication and achievements in advancing the quality of baccalaureate and graduate nursing education are appreciated by Peterson's. We at AACN are fortunate to work with an organization that prides itself on being the leading publisher of education search and selection.

Furthermore, this publication would not be possible without the cooperation of the institutions included in this guide. We acknowledge the time and effort of those who undertook the task of completing and returning the surveys regarding their programs. We certainly appreciate their contribution.

Peterson's Nursing Programs 2008 is the only comprehensive and concise guide to baccalaureate and graduate nursing education programs in the United States and Canada. We hope its contents will serve as the impetus for those looking for a rewarding and satisfying career in health care. AACN is proud to present this publication to the nursing profession and to those who seek to enter it.

—Jeanette Lancaster, Ph.D., RN, FAAN
President, AACN

—Geraldine D. Bednash, Ph.D., RN, FAAN
Executive Director, AACN

A Note from the Peterson's Editors

For more than thirty-five years, Peterson's has given students and parents the most comprehensive, up-to-date information on undergraduate and graduate institutions in the United States, Canada, and abroad.

Peterson's Nursing Programs 2008 provides prospective nursing students with the most comprehensive information on baccalaureate and graduate nursing education in the United States and Canada. Our goal is to help students find the best nursing program for them.

To this end, Peterson's has joined forces with the American Association of Colleges of Nursing (AACN), the national voice for America's baccalaureate- and higher-degree nursing education programs. AACN's educational, research, governmental advocacy, data collection, publications, and other programs work to establish quality standards for bachelor's- and graduate-degree nursing education, assist deans and directors to implement those standards, influence the nursing profession to improve health care, and promote public support of baccalaureate and graduate education, research, and practice in nursing—the nation's largest health-care profession.

For those seeking to enter the nursing profession or to further their nursing careers, *Peterson's Nursing Programs 2008* includes information needed to make important nursing program decisions and to approach the admissions process with knowledge and confidence.

The Nursing School Adviser section contains useful articles to help guide nursing education choices, with information on nursing careers today, selecting a nursing program, financing nursing education, returning to school, and more. There are also listings that provide valuable contact information for financial aid resources and specialty nursing organizations. And if you are one of the many people interested in accelerated nursing programs, there is an article that offers an in-depth look at this increasingly popular approach to nursing education. It is a must-read for those wishing to enter an accelerated baccalaureate or generic master's degree program.

At the end of **The Nursing School Adviser** is the "How to Use This Guide" article, which explains some of the key factors to consider when choosing a nursing program. In addition, it explains how the book is organized and shows you how to maximize your use of *Peterson's Nursing Programs 2008* to its full potential.

If you already have specifics in mind, such as a particular program or location, turn to the **Quick-Reference Chart.** Here you can search through "Nursing Programs At-a-Glance" for particular degree options offered by schools, listed alphabetically by state.

In the **Profiles of Nursing Programs** section you'll find expanded and updated nursing program descriptions, arranged alphabetically by state. Each profile provides all of the need-to-know information about accredited nursing programs in the United States and Canada.

If you are looking for additional information, you can turn to the **Close-Ups of Nursing Programs** section. Here you will find more than 60 two-page narrative descriptions written by admissions deans who chose to provide additional information about their schools and programs.

Finally, turn to the back of the book to find eight **Indexes** listing institutions offering *baccalaureate, master's, concentrations within master's, doctoral, post-doctoral, distance learning,* and *continuing education* programs. The last index lists every college and university contained in the guide along with its corresponding page reference.

Peterson's publishes a full line of resources to help guide you and your family through the college admission process. These publications can be found at your local bookstore, library, and high school guidance office, and you can access us online at www.petersons.com.

We welcome any comments or suggestions you may have about this publication and invite you to complete our online survey at **www.petersons.com/booksurvey.** Or you can fill out the survey at the back of this book, tear it out, and mail it to us at:

Publishing Department
Peterson's, a Nelnet company
2000 Lenox Drive
Lawrenceville, NJ 08648

Your feedback will help us make your educational dreams possible. The editors at Peterson's wish you great success in your nursing program search.

THE NURSING SCHOOL ADVISER

Nursing Fact Sheet

Misconceptions about nursing have contributed to misinformation about the profession. Here are the real facts:

- **Nursing is the nation's largest health-care profession, with more than 2.9 million registered nurses nationwide.** Of all licensed RNs, 2.42 million, or 83.2 percent, are employed in nursing.
- **Nursing students account for more than half of all health professions students in the United States.**
- **Nurses comprise the largest single component of hospital staff, are the primary providers of hospital patient care, and deliver most of the nation's long-term care.**
- **Most health-care services involve some form of care by nurses.** Although 56.2 percent of all employed RNs work in hospitals, many are employed in a wide range of other settings, including private practices, health-maintenance organizations, public health agencies, primary-care clinics, home health care, nursing homes, outpatient surgicenters, nursing school–operated nursing centers, insurance and managed-care companies, schools, mental health agencies, hospices, the military, industry, nursing education, and health-care research.
- **Though often collaborative, nursing does not "assist" medicine or other fields.** Nursing operates independent of, not auxiliary to, medicine and other disciplines. Nurses' roles range from direct patient care and case management to establishing nursing practice standards, developing quality assurance procedures, and directing complex nursing-care systems.
- **With more than four times as many RNs in the United States as physicians,** nursing delivers an extended array of health-care services, including primary and preventive care by advanced nurse practitioners in such areas as pediatrics, family health, women's health, and gerontological care. Nursing's scope also includes services by certified nurse-midwives and nurse anesthetists, as well as care in cardiac, oncology, neonatal, neurological, and obstetric/gynecological nursing and other advanced clinical specialties.
- **The primary pathway to professional nursing, as compared to technical-level practice, is the four-year Bachelor of Science in Nursing (B.S.N.) degree.** Registered nurses are prepared through a baccalaureate program; a two- to three-year associate degree in nursing program; or a three-year hospital training program, receiving a hospital diploma. All take the same state licensing exam—the NCLEX-RN®. *(The number of diploma programs has declined steadily—to less than 10 percent of all basic RN education programs—as nursing education has shifted from hospital-operated instruction into the college and university system.)*
- **With patient care growing more complex, ensuring a sufficient RN workforce isn't merely a matter of how many nurses are needed, but rather an issue of preparing an adequate number of nurses with the right *educational mix* to meet health care demands.** The National Advisory Council on Nurse Education and Practice has urged that at least two thirds of the basic nurse workforce hold baccalaureate or higher degrees in nursing by 2010. Currently, only 47.2 percent do.
- **According to the U.S. Bureau of Labor Statistics, employment for registered nurses will grow faster than for most other occupations through 2014.** Other federal projections indicate that by 2020, the U.S. nursing shortage will grow to more than 800,000 registered nurses. Even as health care continues to shift beyond the hospital to more community-based primary care and other outpatient sites, federal projections say the rising complexity of acute care will see demand for RNs in hospitals climb by 36 percent by the year 2020.

From "Your Nursing Career: A Look at the Facts," updated September 5, 2006. Reprinted with permission from the American Association of Colleges of Nursing.

Counselors of Care in the Modern Health-Care System

Geraldine Bednash, Ph.D., RN, FAAN
Executive Director
American Association of Colleges of Nursing

A Different Era

The nursing profession is alive and reshaping itself. The role of nurses as those who minister exclusively to a patient's basic-care needs has changed. Much of the effectiveness and productivity of the future health-care industry will derive from the training of and services provided by nurses.

Modern nurses take a proactive role in health care by addressing health issues before they develop into problems. They oversee the continued care of patients who have left the health-care facility. Nurses are expected to make complex decisions in areas ranging from patient screening to diagnosis and education. They explore and document the effects of alternative therapies (e.g., guided imagery) and address public health problems, such as teen pregnancy. They explore and understand new technology and how it relates both to patient care and to their own job performance. They work in a variety of settings and are held accountable for their decisions. In today's health-care environment, health-care administrators must recruit nurses with a broad, well-rounded education.

Health-care providers must change the way they administer care. Instead of focusing on the treatment of illness, they must promote wellness. Nurses will oversee patient treatment and medication and must understand the repercussions of these health-care processes for the patient and his or her family.

Cost is the driving force behind this industry-wide transformation. Insurance companies have, for the most part, instigated changes in the way health-care benefits are paid. The old fee-for-service system is no longer the only option. The trend toward managed care, in which a fixed amount of money is allocated for the care of each patient, is changing the way care is provided. It seems that employers of the future will recruit nurses who understand the overall structure of the health-care industry, who possess highly developed critical-thinking skills, and who bring to their positions a well-rounded understanding of the risks and benefits of every health-care decision.

Counselors of Care

Job prospects for graduates of nursing programs are positive. Although many graduates receive associate degrees as registered nurses (RNs), hospital administrators and other employers want applicants with at least a Bachelor of Science in nursing degree.

To practice in a fast-changing health system, entry-level RNs must understand community-based primary care and emphasize health promotion and cost-effective coordinated care—all hallmarks of baccalaureate education. In addition to its broad scientific curriculum and focus on leadership and clinical decision-making skills, a Bachelor of Science in nursing degree education provides specific preparation in community-based care not typically included in associate degree or hospital diploma programs. Moreover, the nurse with a baccalaureate degree is the only basic nursing graduate prepared for all health-care settings—critical care, outpatient care, public health, and mental health—and so has the flexibility to practice in outpatient centers, private homes, and neighborhood clinics where demand is fast expanding as health care moves beyond the hospital to more primary and preventive care throughout the community.

Health-care administrators realize that patients are becoming more sophisticated about the care they receive, requiring an explanation and understanding of their health needs. Nurses will have to be knowledgeable care providers, working with physicians, pharmacists, and public health officials in interdisciplinary settings to satisfy these requirements.

Broader training enables graduates of baccalaureate programs to provide improved and varying types of care, and ensures stability and security in an industry now noted for its instability.

Promising Opportunities

One of the rewards of a baccalaureate education can be a competitive salary. Graduates of four-year degree programs can expect salaries starting around $35,000 per year, a figure that might fluctuate depending on geographic area and, more specifically, by the demand in that area. Obviously, the greater the need for nurses, the higher their salaries.

The baccalaureate degree also serves as a foundation for the pursuit of a master's degree in nursing, which prepares students for the role of advanced practice nurse (APN). Students can earn degrees as clinical nurse specialists in neonatology, oncology, cardiology, and other specialties or as nurse practitioners, nurse-midwives, or nurse anesthetists. Master's-prepared nurses can also enjoy rewarding careers in nursing administration and education.

These programs generally span one to two years. Graduates can expect starting salaries of approximately $50,000 annually in advanced practice nursing settings, and demand for these graduates is expected to be high over the next fifteen years. In some localities, for example, the nurse practitioner may be the sole provider of health care to a family.

Overall Transformation

The nursing field must be transformed to be compatible with the overall changes in the health-care industry. The latest statistics put the average age of nurses at 46.8, with only 16.6 percent of nurses under the age of 35. It is projected that over the next ten years much of the nursing population will retire. Employment is projected to increase 27 percent or more between 2007 and 2014.

The traditional career path of nurses is expected to change. More nurses will enter master's programs directly from baccalaureate programs, and more master's degree graduates will pursue doctoral degrees at a younger age. Since nurses will play a critical role in providing health care, a four-year baccalaureate degree is a crucial first step in preparing nurses to assume increased patient responsibilities within the health-care system.

RNs Returning to School: Choosing a Nursing Program

Marilyn Oermann, Ph.D., RN, FAAN
Professor
College of Nursing
Wayne State University

If you are thinking about returning to school to complete your baccalaureate degree or to pursue a graduate degree in nursing, you are not alone. Registered nurses (RNs) are returning to school in record numbers, many seeking advancement or transition to new roles in nursing. Over the last two decades, the number of RNs prepared initially in diploma and associate degree in nursing programs who have graduated from baccalaureate nursing degree programs has more than doubled, according to the AACN. There are expanded opportunities for nurses with baccalaureate degrees in nursing. Although the decision to return to school means considerable investment of time, financial resources, and effort, the benefits can be overwhelmingly positive.

Higher education in nursing opens doors to many opportunities for career growth not otherwise available. By continuing your education, you can:

- update your knowledge and skills, critical today in light of rapid advances in health care.

- move more easily into a new role within your organization or in other health-care settings.

- pursue a different career path within nursing.

Moreover, returning to school brings personal fulfillment and satisfaction gained through learning more about nursing and the changing health-care system and using that knowledge in the delivery and management of patient care.

More Skills and Flexibility Needed

If you are contemplating returning to school, here are some facts to consider. The health-care system continues to undergo dramatic changes. These changes include hospitalized patients who are more acutely ill; an aging population; technological advances that require highly skilled nursing care; a greater role for nurses in primary care, health promotion, and health education; and the need for nurses to care for patients and families in multiple settings, such as schools, workplaces, homes, clinics, and outpatient facilities, as well as hospitals. With the nursing shortage, nurses are in great demand in hospitals. Moreover, as hospitals continue to become centers for acute and critical care, the nurse's role in both patient care and management of other health-care providers in the hospital has become more complex, requiring advanced knowledge and skills.

Because of the complexity of today's health-care environment, AACN and other leading nursing organizations have called for the baccalaureate degree in nursing as the minimum educational requirement for professional nursing practice. In fact, nurse executives in hospitals have indicated their desire for the majority of nurses on staff to be prepared at least at the baccalaureate level to handle the increasingly complex demands of patient care and management of health-care delivery. The baccalaureate nursing degree is essential for nurses to function in different management roles, move across employment settings, have the flexibility to change positions within nursing, and advance in their career. Baccalaureate nursing degree programs prepare the nurse for a broad role within the health-care system and for practice in hospitals, community settings, home health care, neighborhood clinics, and other outpatient settings where opportunities are expanding. Continuing education provides the means for nurses to prepare themselves for a future role in nursing.

The demand for nurses with baccalaureate and more advanced degrees will continue to grow. There is an excess of nurses prepared at the associate degree level, a mounting shortage of baccalaureate-prepared nurses, and only half as many nurses prepared at master's and doctoral levels as needed. Nurses with baccalaureate nursing degrees are needed in all areas of health care, and the demand for nurses with master's and doctoral preparation for advanced practice, management, teaching, and research will continue.

Identifying Strategies

The decision to return to school marks the beginning of a new phase in your career development. It is essential for you to plan this future carefully. Why are you thinking about returning to school, and what do you want to accomplish by doing so? Understanding why you want to go back to school will help you select the best program for you. Knowing what you want to accomplish will help you to focus on your goals and overcome the obstacles that could prevent you from achieving your full potential.

Even if you decide that additional education will help you reach your professional goals, you may also have a list of reasons why you think you cannot return to school—no time, limited financial resources, fear of failure, and concerns about meeting family responsibilities, among others. If you are concerned about the demands of school combined with existing responsibilities, begin by identifying strategies for incorporating classes and study time into your present schedule or consider taking an online course. Remember, you can start your program with one course and reevaluate your time at the end of the term.

Research and anecdotal evidence from adults returning to college indicate that despite their need to balance school work with a career and, often, family responsibilities, these adult learners experience less stress and manage their lives better than they had thought possible. Many of these adult learners report that the satisfaction gained from their education more than compensates for any added stress. Furthermore, studies of nurses who have returned to school suggest that while their education may create stress for them, most nurses cope effectively with the demands of advanced education.

If costs are of concern, it is best to investigate tuition-reimbursement opportunities where you are employed, scholarships from the nursing program and other nursing organizations, and loans. The financial aid officer at the program you are considering is probably the best available resource to answer your financial assistance questions.

If you are unsure of what to expect when returning to school, remember that such feelings are natural for anyone facing a new situation. If you are motivated and committed to pursuing your degree, you will succeed. Most nursing programs offer resources, such as test-taking skills, study skills, and time-management workshops, as well as assistance with academic problems. You can combine school, work, family, and other responsibilities. Even with these greater demands, the benefits of education outweigh the difficulties.

Clarifying Career Goals

Nursing, unlike many other professions, has a variety of educational paths for nurses returning for advanced education. You should decide if baccalaureate- or graduate-level work is congruent with your career goals. The next step in this process is to reexamine your specific career goals, both immediate and long-term, to determine the level and type of nursing education you will need to meet them. Ask yourself what you want to be doing in the next five to ten years. Discuss your ideas with a counselor in a nursing education program, nurses who are practicing in roles you are considering, and others who are enrolled in a nursing program or who have recently completed a nursing degree.

Baccalaureate degree nursing programs prepare nurses as generalists for practice in all health-care settings. Graduate nursing education occurs at two levels— master's and doctoral. Master's programs vary in length, typically between one and two years. Preparation for roles in advanced practice as nurse practitioners, certified

nurse midwives, clinical nurse specialists, certified registered nurse anesthetists, nursing administrators, and nursing educators requires a master's degree in nursing. Many programs meet the needs of RNs by offering options such as accelerated course work, advanced placement, evening and weekend classes, and distance learning courses.

A trend in education for RNs is accelerated programs that combine the baccalaureate and master's nursing programs. These combined programs are designed for RNs without degrees whose career goals involve advanced nursing practice and other roles requiring a master's degree. Nurses who complete these combined programs may be awarded both a baccalaureate and a master's degree in nursing or a master's degree only.

At the doctoral level, nurses are prepared for a variety of roles, including research and teaching. Doctoral programs generally consist of three years of full-time study beyond the master's degree, although some programs admit baccalaureate graduates and include the master's-level requirements and degree within the doctoral program.

Matching a Program to Your Needs

Once you have defined your career goals and the level of nursing education they will require, the next step is matching your needs with the offerings and characteristics of specific nursing programs. Some of the criteria you may want to consider in evaluating potential schools of nursing include the types of programs offered, the length of the program and its specific requirements, the availability of full- and part-time study and number of credits required for part-time study, the flexibility of the program, if distance education courses are available, and the days, times, and sites at which classes and clinical experiences are offered as they relate to your work schedule. Take into consideration the program's accreditation status; faculty qualifications in terms of research, teaching, and practice; and the resources of the school of nursing and of the college/university, such as library holdings, computer services, and statistical consultants. You should also consider the clinical settings used in the curriculum and their relationship to your career goals, as well as the availability of financial aid for nursing students.

Carefully review the admission criteria, including minimum grade point average; scores required on any admission tests, such as the Graduate Record Examinations (GRE) for master's and doctoral programs; and any requirements in terms of work experience. For students returning for a baccalaureate degree, prior nursing knowledge may be validated through testing, transfer of courses, and other mechanisms. Review these options prior to applying to a program.

While the intrinsic quality and characteristics of the program are important, your own personal goals and needs have to be included in your decision. Consider commuting distance, if courses are offered online, costs in relation to your financial resources, program design, and flexibility of the curriculum in relation to your work, family, and personal responsibilities. While the majority of nursing programs offer part-time study, many programs also schedule classes to accommodate work situations.

Many schools offer nursing courses online, and in some places, the entire baccalaureate and master's programs are available through distance learning. The largest enrollment in nursing distance learning is in baccalaureate programs for RNs. Distance learning allows RNs to further their education no matter where they live. Many nurses prefer online courses because they can learn at times convenient for them, especially considering competing demands associated with their jobs, families, and other commitments.

Ensure Your Success

Once you have made the decision to return to school and have chosen the program that best meets your needs, take an additional step to ensure your success. Identify the support you will need, both academic and personal, to be successful in the nursing program. Academic support is provided by the institution and may include tutoring services, learning resource centers, computer facilities, and other resources to support your learning. You should take advantage of available support services and seek out resources for areas in which you are weak or need review. Academic support services, however, need to be complemented by personal support through family, friends, and peers. With a firm commitment to pursuing advanced education, a clear choice of a nursing program to meet your goals, and support from others, you are certain to find success in returning to school.

BACCALAUREATE PROGRAMS

Linda K. Amos, Ed.D., RN, FAAN
*Former Associate Vice President for Health
    Sciences*
Professor of Nursing
University of Utah

The health-care industry has continued to change dramatically over the past few years, transforming the roles and escalating opportunities for nurses. The current shortage of nurses is caused by an increased number of hospitalized patients who are older and more acutely ill, a growing elderly population with multiple chronic health problems, and expanded opportunities in HMOs, home care, occupational health, surgical centers, and other primary-care settings. Expanding technological advances prolonging life require more highly skilled personnel.

The increasing scope of nursing opportunities will grow immensely as nurses become the frontline providers of health care. They are assuming important roles in the provision of managed care, and they will be responsible for coordinating and continuing the care outside traditional health-care facilities. Nurses will play a big role in educating the public and addressing the social and economic factors that impact quality of care.

Worldwide Standards

The nursing student of the future will receive a wealth of information. Understanding the technology used to manage that information will be essential to their ability to track and assess care. In this area, nurses will be able to provide care over great distances. In some areas, care is being managed by the nurse via tele-home health over the Internet. Use of the Internet and other computer-oriented systems are now an integral part of the tools used by nurses. Nurses of the future, therefore, will have to become aware of worldwide standards of care. Nevertheless, the primary job of a nurse will be making sure that the right person is providing the right care at the right cost.

This goal will be accomplished as the industry turns away from the hospital as the center of operation. Nurses will work in a broad array of locations, such as clinics, outpatient facilities, community centers, schools, and even places of business. Hospitals are now places only for the very sick, and the name itself may be changed to acute-care center.

Much of the emphasis in health care will shift to preventive care and the promotion of health. In this system, nurses will take on a broader and more diverse role than in the past.

Unlimited Opportunities, Expanded Responsibilities

The four-year baccalaureate programs in today's nursing colleges provide the educational and experiential base not only for entry-level professional practice, but also as the platform on which to build a career through graduate-level study for roles as advanced practice nurses, such as nurse practitioners, nurse midwives, clinical specialists, and nurse administrators and educators. Nurses at this level can be expected to specialize in oncology, pediatrics, neonatology, obstetrics and gynecology, critical care, infection control, psychiatry, women's health, community health, and neuroscience. The potential and responsibilities at this level are great. Increasingly, many families use the nurse practitioner for all health-care needs. In almost all states, the nurse practitioner can prescribe medications and provide health care for the management of chronic non-acute illnesses and preventive care.

The health-care system demands a lot from nurses. The education of a nurse must transcend the traditional areas, such as chemistry and anatomy, to include health promotion, disease prevention, screening, genetic counseling, and immunization. Nurses should understand how health problems may have a social cause, such as poverty and environmental contamination, as well as have insight into human psychology, behavior, cultural mores, and values.

The transformation of the health-care system offers unlimited opportunities for nurses at the baccalaureate and graduate levels as care in urban and rural settings becomes more accessible. According to the U.S. Bureau of Labor Statistics, employment of RNs will grow faster than the average for all occupations through 2012, due largely to growing demand in settings such as health maintenance organizations, community health centers, home care, and long-term care. The increased complexity of health problems and increased management of health problems out of the hospitals require highly educated and well-prepared nurses at the baccalaureate and graduate levels. It is an exciting era in nursing, one that holds exceptional promise for nurses with a baccalaureate nursing degree.

The compensation for new nurses is again becoming competitive with that of other industries. Entry-level nurses with baccalaureate degrees in nursing can expect a salary range from about $31,000 to $46,000 per year, depending on geographic location and experience. Five years into their careers, the national average for nurses with four-year degrees is over $50,000 per year, with many earning over $65,000. The current shortage has prompted sign-on bonuses and other incentives to attract and retain staff.

Applying to College

Meeting the school's general entrance requirements is the first step toward a university or college degree in nursing. Admission requirements may vary, but a high school diploma or equivalent is necessary. Most accredited colleges consider SAT scores along with high school grade point average. A strong preparatory class load in science and mathematics is generally preferred among nursing schools. Students may obtain specific admission information by writing to the schools' nursing departments.

To apply to a nursing school, contact the admission offices of the colleges or universities you are interested in and request the appropriate application forms. With limited spaces in nursing schools, programs are competitive and early submission of an application is recommended.

Accreditation

Accreditation of the nursing program is very important, and it should be considered on two levels—the accreditation of the university or college and the accreditation of the nursing program. Accreditation is a voluntary process in which the school or the program asks for an external review of its programs, facilities, and faculty. For nursing programs, the review is performed by peers in nursing education to ensure program quality and integrity.

Baccalaureate nursing programs have two types of regular systematic reviews. First, the school must be approved by the state board of nursing. This approval is necessary to ensure that the graduates of the program may sit for the licensing examinations offered through the National Council of State Boards of Nursing, Inc. The second is accreditation administered by a nursing accreditation agency that is recognized by the U.S. Department of Education.

Although accreditation is a voluntary process, access to federal loans and scholarships requires accreditation of the program, and most graduate schools only accept students who have earned degrees from accredited schools. Further, accreditation ensures an ongoing process of quality improvement that is based on national standards. Canadian nursing school programs are accredited by the Canadian Association of University Schools of Nursing, and the Canadian programs listed in this book must hold this accreditation. There are two recognized accreditation agencies for baccalaureate nursing programs in the United States: the Commission on Collegiate Nursing Education (CCNE) and the National League for Nursing Accrediting Commission (NLNAC).

Focusing Your Education

Academic performance is not the sole basis of acceptance into the upper level of the nursing program.

Admission officers also weigh such factors as student activities, employment, and references. Moreover, many require an interview and/or essay in which the nursing candidate offers a goal statement. This part of the admission process can be completed prior to a student's entrance into the college or university or prior to the student's entrance into the school of nursing itself, depending on the program.

In this interview or essay, students may list career preferences and reasons for their choices. This allows admission officers to assess the goals of students and gain insights into their values, integrity, and honesty. One would expect that a goal statement from a student who is just entering college would be more general than that of a student who has had two years of preprofessional nursing studies. The more experienced student would be likely to have a more focused idea of what is to be gained by an education in nursing; there would be more evidence of the student's values and the ways in which she or he relates them to the knowledge gained from preprofessional nursing classes.

Baccalaureate Curriculum

A standard basic or generic baccalaureate program in nursing is a four-year college or university education that incorporates a variety of liberal arts courses with professional education and training. It is designed for high school graduates with no previous nursing experience.

Currently, there are more than 600 baccalaureate programs in the United States. Of the 583 programs that responded to a fall 2005 survey conducted by the American Association of Colleges of Nursing, total enrollment in all nursing programs leading to a baccalaureate degree was 163,706. A report from the National Advisory Council on Nursing Education recommends that at least two thirds of the nursing workforce hold a baccalaureate degree or higher by 2010, compared to the current 40 percent.

The baccalaureate curriculum is designed to prepare students for work within the growing and changing health-care environment. With nurses taking more of an active role in all facets of health care, they are expected to develop critical-thinking and communication skills in addition to receiving standard nurse training in clinics and hospitals. In a university or college setting, the first two years include classes in the humanities, social sciences, basic sciences, business, psychology, technology, sociology, ethics, and nutrition.

In some programs, nursing classes start in the sophomore year, whereas others have students wait until they are juniors. Many schools require satisfactory grade point averages before students advance into professional nursing classes. On a 4.0 scale, admission into the last two years of the nursing program may require a minimum GPA of 2.5 to 3.0 in preprofessional nursing classes. The national average is about 2.8, but the cutoff level varies with each program.

In the junior and senior years, the curriculum focuses on the nursing sciences and emphasis moves from the classroom to health facilities. This is where students are exposed to clinical skills, nursing theory, and the varied roles nurses play in the health-care system. Courses include nurse leadership, health promotion, family planning, mental health, environmental and occupational health, adult and pediatric care, medical and surgical care, psychiatric care, community health, management, and home health care.

This level of education comes in a variety of settings: community hospitals, clinics, social service agencies, schools, and health-maintenance organizations. Training in diverse settings is the best preparation for becoming a vital player in the growing health care field.

Reentry Programs

Practicing nurses who return to school to earn a baccalaureate degree will have to meet requirements that may include possession of a valid RN license and an associate degree or hospital diploma from an accredited institution. Again, it is best to check with the school's admissions department to determine specifics.

Nurses returning to school will have to consider the rapid rate of change in health care and science. A nurse who passed an undergraduate-level chemistry class ten years ago would probably not receive credit for that class today, due to the growth of knowledge in that and all other scientific fields. The need to reeducate applies not only to practicing nurses returning to school, but also to all nurses throughout their careers.

In the same vein, nurses with diplomas from hospital programs who want to work toward a baccalaureate degree would find themselves in need of meeting the common requirements for more clinical practice as well as developing a deeper understanding of community-based nursing practices, such as health prevention and promotion.

There are colleges and universities available to the RN in search of a baccalaureate that give credit for previous nurse training. These programs are designed to accommodate the needs and career goals of the practicing nurse by providing flexible course schedules and credit for previous experience and education. Some programs lead to a master's-level degree, a process that can take up to three years. Licensed practical nurses (LPNs) can also continue their education through baccalaureate programs.

Nurses thinking of reentering school may also consider other specialized programs. For example, there are programs aimed at enabling a nurse with an A.D.N. degree or an LPN/LVN license to earn a B.S.N. Also, accelerated B.S.N. programs are available for students with degrees in other fields.

RN to Baccalaureate Programs Fact Sheet

More than 600 RN to baccalaureate programs are available nationwide, including 169 programs offered in a more intense, accelerated format. Program length varies between one and two years depending upon the school's requirements, program type, and the student's previous academic achievement.

Concerns about the limited availability of RN to baccalaureate programs are unfounded. In fact, there are more RN to baccalaureate programs available (579) than four-year nursing programs (476) or accelerated bachelor's degree programs for non-nursing college graduates (185). Access to RN to baccalaureate programs is further enhanced since many programs are offered completely online or on-site at various health-care facilities.

Enrollment in RN to baccalaureate programs is increasing in response to calls for a more highly educated nursing workforce. From 2004 to 2005, enrollments increased by 8.3 percent, or by 2,772 students, marking the third year of increases in RN to baccalaureate programs.

Hundreds of articulation agreements between A.D.N. and diploma programs and four-year institutions exist nationwide, including some statewide agreements, to facilitate students seeking baccalaureate-level nursing education. Before enrolling in diploma and A.D.N. programs, students are encouraged to check with school administrators to see what articulation agreements exist with baccalaureate degree–granting schools and to determine which course work will be transferable.

Choosing a Program

With more than 600 baccalaureate programs in the United States, some research will reveal which programs match your needs and career objectives.

If you have no health-care experience, it might be best to gain some insight into the field by volunteering or working part-time in a care facility, such as a hospital or an outpatient clinic. Talking to nurse professionals about their work will also lend insight into how your attributes may apply to the nursing field.

When considering a nursing education, consider your personal needs. Is it best for you to work in a heavily structured environment or one that offers more flexibility in terms of, say, integrating a part-time work schedule into studies? Do you need to stay close to home? Do you prefer to work in a large health-care system, such as a health maintenance organization or a medical center, or do you prefer smaller, community-based operations?

As for nursing programs, it is best to ask the following questions: How involved is the faculty in developing students for today's health-care industry? How strong is the school's affiliation with clinics and hospitals? Is there any assurance that a student will gain an up-to-date educational experience for the current job market? Are a variety of care settings available? How much time in clinics will be needed for graduation? What are the program's resources in terms of computer and science laboratories? Does the school work with hospitals and community-based centers to provide health care? How available is the faculty to oversee a student's curriculum?

What kind of student support is available in terms of study groups and audiovisual aids? Moreover, what kind of counseling from faculty members and administrators is available to help students develop well-rounded, effective progress through the program?

Visiting a school and talking to the program's guidance counselors will give you a better understanding of how a particular program or school will fit your needs. You can get a closer look at the faculty, its members' credentials, and the focus of the program. It's also not too early to consider what each program can offer in terms of job placement.

Master's Programs

Kathleen Dracup, D.N.Sc., RN
Professor and Dean
School of Nursing
University of California, San Francisco

The transformation of the health-care system is taking place as you read this, and it can be seen even today in the most common areas.

- A mother brings her child into a clinic for treatment of an earache. Instead of a physician, a nurse practitioner provides the care.

- A patient is readied for surgery. A variety of specialists move about the surgery room, but it's not a specially trained physician administering the anesthetic—it's a certified nurse anesthetist.

- During the recovery from an acute illness, it's decided that the patient no longer needs to stay in the hospital but isn't well enough to return home. It's decided that the best place to continue the recovery is an intermediate-care facility. Who makes that decision? A clinical nurse specialist. Who oversees the physical and emotional rehabilitation programs at this facility? Another clinical nurse specialist.

These health-care professionals are all advanced practice nurses (APNs). All have graduate-level degrees, and they serve as proof that the demand for nurses with master's and doctoral degrees for advanced practice, clinical specialties, teaching, and research will double the supply.

Another study estimated that the U.S. could save as much as $8.75 billion annually if APNs were used appropriately in place of physicians. As more and more of the restrictions on APNs succumb to legislative or economic forces, the demand for graduate-level nurses is expected to remain high.

Educational Core for APN

A master's degree in nursing is the educational core that allows advanced practice nurses to work as nurse practitioners, certified nurse-midwives, clinical nurse specialists, and certified nurse anesthetists.

Nurse practitioners conduct physical exams, diagnose and treat common acute illnesses and injuries, administer immunizations, manage chronic problems such as high blood pressure and diabetes, and order lab services and X-rays.

Nurse-midwives provide prenatal and gynecological care, deliver babies in hospitals and private settings such as homes, and follow up with postpartum care.

Clinical nurse specialists provide a range of care in specialty areas, such as oncology, pediatrics, and cardiac, neonatal, obstetric/gynecological, neurological, and psychiatric nursing.

Nurse anesthetists administer anesthesia for all types of surgery in operating rooms, dental offices, and outpatient surgical centers.

Master's degrees in nursing administration or nursing education are also available.

There are more than 330 master's degree programs accredited by the Commission on Collegiate Nursing Education (CCNE) or by the National League for Nursing Accrediting Commission (NLNAC). The wide spectrum of programs includes the Master of Science in Nursing (M.S.N.) degree, Master of Nursing (M.N.) degree, Master of Science (M.S.) degree with a major in nursing, or Master of Arts (M.A.) degree with a nursing major. The specific degrees depend on the requirements set by the college or university or by the faculty of the nursing program. There are accelerated programs for RNs, which allow the nurse with a hospital diploma or associate degree to earn both a baccalaureate and a master's degree in a condensed program. Some schools offer accelerated master's degree programs for nurses with non-nursing degrees and for non-nursing college graduates. There are joint-degree programs, such as a master's in nursing combined with a Master of Business Administration, Master of Public Health, or Master of Hospital Administration.

Master's Curriculum

The master's degree builds on the baccalaureate degree to enable the student to develop expertise in one area. That specialty can range from running a hospital to providing care for prematurely born babies, from researching the effectiveness of alternative therapies to tackling social and economic causes of health problems. It is an opportunity for the student who has assessed his or her personal career goals and matched them to individual, community, and industry needs. What students can do with their APN degrees is limited only by their imagination.

Full-time master's programs consist of eighteen to twenty-four months of uninterrupted study. Many graduate school students, however, fit their master's-level studies around their work schedules, which can extend the time it takes to graduate.

Master's-level study incorporates theories and concepts of nursing science and their applications, along with the management of health care. Research is used to provide a foundation for the improvement of health-care techniques. Students also have the opportunity to develop the knowledge, leadership skills, and interpersonal skills that will enable them to improve the health-care system.

Classroom and clinical work are involved throughout the master's program. In class, students spend less time listening to lectures and taking notes and more time participating in student- and faculty-led seminars and roundtable discussions. Extended clinical work is generally required.

Graduate-level education in many programs includes courses in statistics, research management, health economics, health policy, health-care ethics, health promotion, nutrition, family planning, mental health, and the prevention of family and social violence. When students begin to concentrate their study in their clinical areas, any number of courses that support their chosen specialty may be included. For example, a nurse wanting to specialize in pediatrics may take courses in child development.

A clinical nurse specialist can focus on acute care, geriatrics, adult health, community health, critical care, gerontology, rehabilitation, and cardiovascular, surgical, oncology, maternity/newborn, pediatric, mental/psychiatric, and women's health nursing. Areas of specialization in nurse practitioner programs include acute care, adult health, child care, community health, emergency care, geriatric care, neonatal health, occupational health, and primary care.

Admission Requirements

The admission requirements for master's programs in nursing vary a great deal. Generally, a bachelor's degree from a school accredited by the Commission on Collegiate Nursing Education or by the National League for Nursing Accrediting Commission and a state RN license are required. Scores from the Graduate Record Examinations (GRE) or the Miller Analogies Test (MAT), college transcripts, letters of reference, and an essay are typically required. Nonnurses and nurses with nonnursing degrees have special requirements. The profiles and in-depth descriptions of colleges and universities in this publication will give you an idea of each school's specific requirements.

It is important to remember that admissions officers look at a student's transcripts, clinical work, and letters of reference together. A low grade point average is not an automatic knockout—admissions officers are after a composite package. Also, some specialties require specific courses. Students in the nurse anesthetist program, for instance, must have an upper-level college course in biochemistry.

A Master's That's Best for You

Most nurses who think of entering a master's program already have been practicing nursing. They have a good idea what they want to specialize in before they apply for admission. It is crucial to know what you want to study before you enter a master's program.

The best way to ensure success in a master's program is for you to understand your individual strengths and career desires and then find the faculty and college setting that are best suited to help you develop those strengths. Students must make an effort to educate themselves as to the strength of the faculty in each college's master's program. That's the best thing to look for: a strong faculty in one specialty.

This can be tricky. One university's master's program may be rated reasonably high in all fields. Another program might not be rated as high overall, but its cardiovascular program, for example, may be one of the best due to its access to facilities or the fact that its faculty is in the process of developing an innovative new treatment.

This type of information is not hard for the master's candidate to discover; it just takes time. Such information is available from each school's admissions office, which should be more than happy to promote its nursing faculty and support its opinion with proof, such as the research papers that faculty members have published in journals or the number of degrees each faculty member carries.

This type of research is the best way to find a program that meets your needs. The profiles of master's nursing programs in this book should help. If you can, narrow the list to three or four graduate schools and then write each school's admissions department for catalogs and other information. Visit the schools and take time to talk to a guidance counselor from the nursing program.

Other key questions to consider when applying for a master's program are: Does the school offer financial aid, such as loans, scholarships, fellowships, or teaching posts? How much clinical work is needed? Does the clinical work meet your needs, and does the type of clinical work involved match what you understand the health-care system will be using when you graduate? Is the course work flexible? Can you work part-time and still progress toward a master's degree? This is important to know. A majority of master's program students continue to work while they pursue the degree. Therefore, master's degree programs may present a flexible offering of short courses to meet the student's schedule demands.

Some programs require a thesis, whereas others provide another type of culminating experience, such as a comprehensive examination.

The Master's Trends

Today's master's programs have increased the amount of clinical practice that students engage in so that graduates enter the job market ready for certification. There is also a greater emphasis on applying new research findings to methods of patient care. This might involve students' reading literature about new treatments and then incorporating the appropriate changes.

All master's program candidates should consider courses in cost-benefit analysis. As managed-care systems become predominant in the industry, health-care workers will be asked to justify the expense of their treatment as well as its effectiveness. This leads to the crucial issue of quality. There will always be a strong effort to minimize costs in every health-care procedure, but that cannot compromise the quality of care. It's safe to say that discharging a newborn too soon from a hospital due to shortsightedness can be quite costly.

Depending on the specialty, master's candidates entering the job market may be expected to oversee auxiliary-care providers, such as nurse aides or other unlicensed employees. They may work in a team structure, and, in this capacity, the nurse specialist may be expected to manage, motivate, and steer the group. This requires team-building as well as other management techniques.

While everyone in the health-care facility will have a part in ensuring patient satisfaction, nurses, particularly advanced practice nurses, will shoulder a great deal of this load. Developing interpersonal and communication skills, as well as having an understanding of human behavior, will make it easier for the advanced practice nurse to help patients to understand modern health-care procedures, which no doubt will improve their feelings of satisfaction.

Finally, nurses at all levels should be aware of the need for flexibility. Many health-care organizations are reducing the number of beds in hospitals and transferring the care of a growing number of patients to other types of facilities or settings. In light of this trend, it's best for the master's program student to gain experience in a variety of places, such as homes, clinics, and community-based settings.

The demand for high-quality care will continue to grow. Medical innovations and technological advances will continue. The quality and effectiveness of health care will continue to improve, and nurses with graduate degrees will play an active role in this trend.

The Hot Employment Spots

The health-care industry has undergone such radical transformation in the last five years that administrators feel they cannot predict whether any one geographic region will have more hirings than another. Generally, nurses with master's degrees will be in demand in all regions of the country, in both the U.S. and Canada.

Industry trends indicate that along with continuing opportunities in hospitals, more and more nurses will also work outside the hospital in outpatient clinics and community settings and even in businesses. As patients spend less and less time in hospitals, there is a need for nurse specialists to oversee home-care settings and ensure that the quality of care there is high. In this vein, some nurses are taking the initiative and running their own businesses as health-care providers, offering services as they see fit in whatever locations are appropriate.

RN to Master's Degree Programs Fact Sheet

Currently, there are 144 programs available nationwide to transition RNs with diplomas and associate degrees to the master's degree level. These programs prepare nurses to assume positions requiring graduate preparation, including the advanced practice roles of nurse practitioner, clinical nurse specialist, certified nurse-midwife, and certified registered nurse anesthetist. Master's degree-prepared nurses are in high demand as expert clinicians, nurse executives, clinical educators, health policy consultants, and research assistants.

RN to master's degree programs generally take about three years to complete, with specific requirements varying by institution and the student's previous course work. Although the majority of these programs are offered in traditional classroom settings, some RN to master's programs are offered largely online or in a blended classroom/online format.

The baccalaureate-level content missing from diploma and A.D.N. programs is built into the front end of the RN to master's degree program. Mastery of this upper-level basic nursing content is necessary for students to move on to graduate study. Upon completion, programs award both a baccalaureate and a master's degree.

The number of RN to master's degree programs has doubled within the past ten years, from seventy programs in 1994 to 144 programs today. According to AACN's 2005 survey of nursing schools, nineteen new RN to master's degree programs are in the planning stages.

Immediate Rewards

Advanced practice nurses right out of school can expect annual salaries ranging from $60,000 to $90,000, depending on geographic location and previous experience. However, some rural county health clinics start their nurse practitioners at salaries as low as $40,000 per year.

Certified nurse anesthetists and certified nurse-midwives, however, draw larger salaries. Nurse-midwives, for example, can draw first-year salaries as high as $90,000 per year. Areas such as the Northeast and the West Coast tend to have nurses in these fields at the higher end of the salary scale. After five years of practice, the salary range for APNs stretches from $60,000 to $100,000 a year. Again, it depends on location. After five years, nurse-midwives earn salaries ranging from $65,000 to $120,000 annually.

ACCELERATED PROGRAMS

With the Bureau of Labor Statistics projecting the need for more than a million new and replacement registered nurses by the year 2012, nursing schools around the country are exploring creative ways to increase student capacity and reach out to new student populations. The challenge inherent in these efforts is to quickly produce competent nurses while maintaining the integrity and quality of the nursing education provided.

One innovative approach to nursing education that is gaining momentum nationwide is the accelerated degree program for non-nursing graduates. Offered at both the baccalaureate and master's degree levels, these programs build on previous learning experiences and transition individuals with undergraduate degrees in other disciplines into nursing.

Shifts in the economy and the desire of many adults to make a post–September 11 difference in their work have increased interest in the nursing profession among "second-degree" students. For those with a prior degree, accelerated baccalaureate programs offer the quickest route to becoming a registered nurse, with programs generally running 12–18 months long. Generic master's degrees, also accelerated in nature and geared to non-nursing graduates, generally take three years to finish. Students in these programs usually complete baccalaureate-level nursing courses in the first year, followed by two years of graduate study.

Though not new to nursing education, accelerated programs have proliferated over the past fifteen years. In 1990, thirty-one accelerated baccalaureate (B.S.N.) programs and twelve generic master's (M.S.N.) programs were offered around the country.

Today, 187 accelerated baccalaureate nursing programs are operating, and the number of generic master's programs has increased to fifty-nine. According to AACN's database on enrollment and graduations, which is based on responses from 628 of 722 institutions (87 percent), thirty-seven new accelerated B.S.N. programs are now in the planning stages. This number far outpaces all other types of entry-level nursing programs currently being considered at four-year nursing schools. Ten new generic master's programs are also taking shape.

Graduates of accelerated programs are prized by nurse employers who value the many layers of skill and education these graduates bring to the workplace. Employers report that these graduates are more mature, possess strong clinical skills, and are quick studies on the job. Many practice settings are partnering with schools and offering tuition repayment to graduates as a mechanism to recruit highly qualified nurses.

Changing Gears: Second-Degree Students

The typical second-degree nursing student is motivated, older, and has higher academic expectations than high school–entry baccalaureate students. Accelerated students excel in class and are eager to gain clinical experiences. Faculty members find them to be excellent learners who are not afraid to challenge their instructors.

"Our accelerated students are a remarkable group," said Nancy DeBasio, Ph.D., RN, Dean of the Research College of Nursing in Kansas City. "Their mean GPA is 3.3, they come from a wide array of backgrounds, and the experiences they bring with them enrich their nursing." The compressed program format is a key motivator for this group of students. "Our exit surveys indicate that the one-year program completion time is a primary reason for enrollment in our program," Dr. DeBasio explained.

Second-degree students bring new dimensions to nursing and a rich history of prior learning. "We are seeing a steady increase in applicants to our accelerated program this year, and those accepted come with backgrounds that are varied and impressive," said Janet B. Younger, Ph.D., RN, Associate Dean of the School of Nursing at Virginia Commonwealth University. "We welcomed several Ph.D.'s, some M.D.'s from other countries, and a few fine arts majors. These students excel in class and perform very well post-graduation."

Students in accelerated programs are competitive, maintain high grade point averages, and almost always pass the NCLEX-RN licensure exam on the first attempt. "Second-degree candidates are excellent students and are very likely to see the program through to graduation," said Afaf Meleis, Ph.D., RN, FAAN, Dean of the University of Pennsylvania School of Nursing. "These students are committed to their studies, actively engaged in research, and very often involved in university organizations."

Susan M. Di Biase, M.S.N., CRNP, a faculty member at Jacksonville State University in Alabama, knows a thing or two about second-degree students. She was one. "As a nurse educator, I have taught dozens of second-degree students who often distinguish themselves as class leaders," explained Di Biase. "When I was taking classes, I thought the students were strong academically, and many said nursing was harder than their first degree. My first employer made a custom of hiring second-degree students because she thought they were good thinkers and strong patient advocates."

Accelerated Baccalaureate Programs

Accelerated baccalaureate programs accomplish programmatic objectives in a shorter time frame than traditional four-year programs, usually through a combination of bridge courses and core content. Instruction is intense, with courses offered full-time with no breaks between sessions. Students receive the same number of clinical hours as their counterparts in traditional programs. Admission standards are high with programs typically requiring a minimum of a 3.0 GPA and a thorough prescreening process. Typically, students with a prior degree are not required to take the liberal arts content included in a four-year B.S.N. program. Accelerated programs do require prerequisites, many of which may have been completed during the student's initial degree program. "Before students can begin our program, their college transcripts are reviewed to assure that all prerequisites are met," stated Maureen C. Creegan, Ed.D., RN, Nursing Program Director at Dominican College (NY). "Almost all students meet the arts and social sciences requirements; most do not meet the natural sciences requirements, including anatomy and microbiology. To assist students, we offer back-to-back prerequisite courses just prior to the start of the accelerated program."

Accelerated programs require a heavy credit load and intense clinical experiences. Identifying students who will flourish in this environment is a priority for administrators. "Due to the intensity of the program, an interview was added to the admission process to better screen students," explained Maryann Forbes, Ph.D., RN, Accelerated Baccalaureate Program Director at Stony Brook University (NY). "Faculty members feel that the interview and ongoing mentoring are key components to student success. The most successful accelerated students are bright, inquisitive, and sophisticated consumers of higher education who actively pursue learning opportunities," said Harriet Feldman, Ph.D., RN, FAAN, Dean of the Lienhard School of Nursing at Pace University (NY), whose Combined Degree Program (B.S.N./M.S.) has been in existence since 1984. "As adults, these students tend to know what they need and aggressively pursue programs that best meet their needs: fast-tracked, competitive, and well respected. While some students do attend part-time, most are full-time students who want to reach their career objective as quickly and efficiently as possible."

"Our accelerated B.S.N. program attracts second-career seekers who are unable to make the time and financial commitment to a generic master's program," explained Elizabeth McGann, D.N.Sc., RN, CS, Dean of the Department of Nursing at Quinnipiac University (CT). "Our program gives students the option of entering basic nursing practice now with graduate education as a potential future step."

Generic Master's Degree Programs

Having already completed a degree at the baccalaureate or graduate level, many second-degree students are attracted to the generic master's program as the natural next step in their higher education. "Why would a bachelor's-prepared applicant, thinking about a career in health care, want to get a second bachelor's in nursing when they can get a professional master's or doctorate in every other health-care field?," asked Melanie Dreher, Ph.D., RN, FAAN, Dean of the University of Iowa College of Nursing. Recently approved by the state board, Iowa's professional Master's Degree in Nursing and Healthcare Practice may be completed in four semesters including a semester-long clinical internship that occurs five days a week for three months.

"In 1974, Yale University was the first school to open its door to college graduates who were not yet nurses and instituted the Graduate Entry Prespecialty in Nursing (GEPN)," explained Sharon Sanderson, Director of Student Recruitment for Yale's School of Nursing. "We recognized that bright, committed people without a background in nursing could be prepared as advanced practice nurses." At Marquette University in Wisconsin, students admitted into the direct-entry M.S.N. program are high achievers. "Our students are self-motivated, have definite goals, demonstrate good study habits, and succeed," explained Judith Fitzgerald Miller, Ph.D., RN, FAAN, Interim Dean of the College of Nursing.

"Our generic M.S.N. students bring a wonderful expertise to the class," said Arlene Lowenstein Ph.D., RN, Director of the Graduate Program in Nursing at MGH Institute of Health Professions in Boston. "We run the gamut from a 53-year-old male lawyer, students holding Ph.D.'s and master's degrees in other fields, and students fresh out of a liberal arts program. One of my past students was a horticulture major who wrote a paper on therapeutic gardens for health-care settings. As they learn from us, we also learn from them, and they learn from each other. Second-degree students are a challenging, exciting group with the potential to make significant contributions to nursing as well as to their patients, families, and communities."

Interest in generic M.S.N. programs is running high. In Chicago, the DePaul University program grew from 20 students last year to 48 students this fall with a minimal amount of advertising. "With little more than a one-sentence notice about the program on the school's Web site when the program was announced, we received more than 100 inquiries and more than forty applications in short order," said Kathryn Anderson, Ph.D., RN,

Graduate Program Director at the Seattle University School of Nursing. "Based on this initial response, it's obvious that the most effective marketing tool is the program itself."

Many universities offer both accelerated baccalaureate and generic master's programs with opportunities for students to apply credits to both degree programs. New York University, for example, offers a dual-degree program that enables B.S.N. students to take a maximum of 9 credits at the graduate level while completing the bachelor's degree, thus accelerating the completion of an M.S.N.

Education-Practice Setting Partnerships

Nurse employers recognize the value and skills second-degree students bring to the work setting as evidenced by the growing number of partnerships forming to support these graduates. "Our cooperative relationship with Poudre Valley Hospital brings the educational and practice settings closer together with clinical nurses at the hospital serving in faculty roles," explained Sandra Baird, Ed.D., B.S.N., Director of the School of Nursing at the University of North Colorado. The school is working to branch out and establish cooperative relationships with a wider network of health-care settings. "Second-degree students are a very attractive catch for any health-care institution and many are willing to fund them in exchange for work commitments after graduation," said Donna Ayers Snelson, M.S.N., RN, Chair of the Nursing Department at College Misericordia (PA)." Although Creighton University (NE) is a private institution with a significantly higher tuition than public institutions, the reputation of its program led two Omaha health systems and four rural hospitals to offer full-tuition scholarships to accelerated nursing students in exchange for employment commitments. "More than half of the students in the accelerated baccalaureate program accepted tuition scholarships from area hospitals in return for a commitment to work in basic practice prior to going on for a master's degree," added Linda Cronenwett, Ph.D., RN, FAAN, Dean of the School of Nursing at University of North Carolina–Chapel Hill. Research College of Nursing uses both grant-funded initiatives and clinical connections to build student capacity. "Recently we received a $100,000 grant from the Helene Fuld Health Trust to support financial aid for our accelerated students," said Dean Nancy DeBasio. "Fuld had never supported this type of student before, but we were able to demonstrate that these students were economically disadvantaged, not always eligible for traditional undergraduate funding, and unable to work due to the program's intensity." The school also partners with a local health-care system to secure educational debt repayment for accelerated students in exchange for work commitments. It is projected that this arrangement will save the health system more than $3 million in nurse recruitment costs over three years.

Nursing Education in the Fast Lane

Although accelerated programs have proven to produce highly qualified nurses, the programs do present some unique challenges to nursing education. "Teaching accelerated students can be challenging because of their experience, age, and high level of inquiry," said Mary E. Pike, M.S.N., RN, faculty member at Bellarmine University (KY). "Some students struggle with the transition from being a competent, worldly adult to returning to life as an undergraduate student." One key to facilitating this transition and encouraging student success is using experienced faculty members who are comfortable teaching adults. In instances where employers are not repaying educational debt, the cost of an accelerated program can be prohibitive. "I receive many inquiries about our accelerated program, but the lack of financial aid is the major deterrent," said Arlene G. Wiens, Ph.D., RN, Nursing Department Chair at Eastern Mennonite University (VA). Some find the pace of accelerated programs to be too intense and opt for more regularly paced programs offered for second-degree nursing students. "The accelerated format is taxing, and some find it too difficult to assimilate into their daily routines," said Louann Zinsmeister, D.N.Sc., M.S.N., RN, instructor at Messiah College (PA). "These students often transfer into a more traditionally paced two-year B.S.N. program that permits them to continue working and attend to family responsibilities while completing a nursing degree." For students who cannot accommodate full-time study, schools are looking for creative alternatives. "We are opening a part-time evening program so second-degree students and adult learners can obtain a degree while working full-time," added Donna Ayers Snelson of College Misericordia. "Students attend classes two nights a week and are still able to obtain a nursing degree in two years and one semester."

Post-Graduation Success

In addition to nursing skills, second-degree students bring additional layers of education and significant work experience to their role as nurses, which enhance their clinical practice. "Initially when we began our program in 1991, our clinical partners were quite doubtful about what we could produce in one year," explained Dr. DeBasio of the Research College of Nursing. "Now they are at our doorstep each year to snap up students as they graduate." The college has tracked students through their careers and found that accelerated students move into management positions more quickly and generally excel in their roles." Employers of advanced practice nurses (APN) are equally pleased with graduates from both our traditional and generic M.S.N. programs," stated Linda D. Norman, D.S.N., RN, Senior Associate Dean for Academics at Vanderbilt University School of Nursing. Employers rated Vanderbilt's M.S.N. graduates who did not have a nursing background equally high in terms of level of preparation for APN positions as those who entered with a B.S.N. degree. "We know that employers love hiring accelerated graduates because they are bright, have a track record of success, and possess an understanding of the work world not always found in younger students," said Patricia Ladewig, Ph.D., RN, Dean of the School of Health Care Professions at Regis University in Denver. "We have found that second-degree students are readily accepted by employers who understand that these graduates lacked only vacation during their academic program," confirmed Sandra S. Angell, M.L.A., RN, Associate Dean for Academic and Student Support Services at The Johns Hopkins University School of Nursing.

Growing Demand for Accelerated Programs

With a greater number of second-degree students turning to nursing, the demand for accelerated programs is growing. At the University of Pennsylvania, application trends over the past 6 years show a 34 percent increase in applications from 1995 to 2001. "Within two weeks of the program's approval by the state board and without any public announcement, we received more than fifty requests for applications almost immediately," explained Marianne W. Rogers, Ed.D., RN, Chairperson for Nursing at the University of Southern Maine. "Our program is growing very quickly, and we have seen almost a 100 percent increase in applications compared to last year," said Linda A. Bernhard, Ph.D., RN, Associate Dean for Undergraduate Studies at The Ohio State University. The 16-month Second Career/Second Degree program in nursing at Wayne State University in Michigan experienced a 25 percent increase in enrollment from fall 2000 to fall 2001, making it one of the school's most popular degree offerings. Enrollment in the University of Virginia's second-degree program has doubled since it was introduced in 1988. "At this time, we are seeing an enormous increase in the numbers of applicants with bachelor's degrees applying for our new 12-month accelerated pathway to the B.S.N.," reports Christena Langley, Ph.D., RN, Assistant Dean for Undergraduate Programs at the College of Nursing and Health Science at George Mason University (VA). "Many of them are recent college graduates who are looking for the quickest route to the B.S.N. They are confident that they can adapt to the accelerated pace given their past success in college."

Supporting Accelerated Nursing Programs

Second-degree students bring a wealth of knowledge, experience, and energy to the nursing workforce and are highly skilled clinicians. With calls for nursing schools to produce more graduates in response to the nursing shortage, a similar call should go out to employers and legislators to increase support for accelerated nursing programs. Hospitals, health-care systems, and other practice settings are encouraged to form partnerships with schools offering accelerated programs to remove the student's financial burden in exchange for a steady stream of new nurse recruits. Legislators on the state and federal levels are encouraged to increase scholarship and grant funding for these programs that produce entry-level nurses faster than any other basic nursing education program. These programs are ideal career transition vehicles for those segments of the labor force impacted by recent fluctuations in the economy." The overwhelming response to our accelerated programs demonstrates the existence of a deep pool of career changers available to nursing," said Gloria F. Donnelly, Ph.D., RN, FAAN, Dean of the College of Nursing and Health Professions at Drexel University (PA). "We need to do more to remove barriers and attract more second-degree students to the nursing profession."

"Accelerated Programs: The Fast-Track to Careers in Nursing," updated January 2007. Reprinted with permission of the American Association of Colleges of Nursing.

THE NURSE PH.D.: A VITAL PROFESSION NEEDS LEADERS

Carole A. Anderson, Ph.D., RN, FAAN
Vice Provost for Academic Administration
The Ohio State University

There is no doubt that education is the path for a nurse to achieve greater clinical expertise. At the same time, however, the nursing profession needs more nurses educated at the doctoral level to replenish the supply of faculty and researchers. The national shortage of faculty will soon reach critical proportions, having a significant impact on educational programs and their capacity to educate future generations of nursing students.

Although the number of doctorate programs has continued to increase, the total enrollment of students in these programs has remained fairly constant, resulting in a shortage of newly trained Ph.D.'s to renew faculty ranks. As a result, approximately 50 percent of nursing faculty possess the doctorate as a terminal degree. Furthermore, with many advances being made in the treatment of chronic illnesses, there is a continuing need for research that assists patients in living with their illness. This research requires individual investigators who are prepared on the doctoral level.

One reason there is a lack of nurses prepared at the doctoral level is that, compared to other professions, nurses have more interruptions in their careers. Many in the profession are women who work as nurses while fulfilling responsibilities as wives and mothers. As a result, many pursue their education on a part-time basis. Also, the nursing profession traditionally has viewed clinical experience as being a prerequisite to graduate education. This career path results in fewer individuals completing the doctorate at an earlier stage in their career, thereby truncating their productivity as academics, researchers, and administrators. To reverse this trend, many nursing schools have developed programs that admit students into graduate (doctoral and master's) programs directly from their undergraduate or master's programs.

Nursing Research

When nurses do research for their doctorates, many people tend to think that it focuses primarily on nurses and nursing care. In reality, nurses carry out clinical research in a variety of areas, such as diabetes care, cancer care, and eating disorders.

In the last twenty years advances in medicine have involved, for the most part, advancing treatment, not cures. In other words, no cure for the illness has been discovered, but treatment for that illness has improved. However, sometimes the treatment itself causes problems for patients, such as the unwelcome side effects of chemotherapy. Nurses have opportunities to devise solutions to problems like these through research, such as studies on how to manage the illness and its treatment, thereby allowing individuals to lead happy and productive lives.

The Curricula

Doctoral programs in nursing are aimed at preparing students for careers in health administration, education, clinical research, and advanced clinical practice. Basically, doctoral programs prepare nurses to be experts within the profession, prepared to assume leadership roles in a variety of academic and clinical settings, course work, and research. Students are trained as researchers and scholars to tackle complex health-care questions. Program emphasis may vary from a focus on health education to a concentration on policy research. The majority of doctoral programs confer the Doctor of Philosophy (Ph.D.) degree, but some award the Doctor of Nursing Science (D.N.S. or D.N.Sc.), the Doctor of Science in Nursing (D.S.N.), the Nursing Doctorate (N.D.), and the Doctor of Education (Ed.D.).

Doctoral nursing programs traditionally offer courses on the history and philosophy of nursing and the development and testing of nursing and other health-care techniques, as well as the social, economic, political, and ethical issues important to the field. Data management and research methodology are also areas of instruction. Students are expected to work individually on research projects and complete a dissertation.

Doctoral programs allow study on a full- or part-time basis. For graduate students who are employed and therefore seek flexibility in their schedules, many programs offer courses on weekends and in the evenings.

Admission Requirements

Admission requirements for doctoral programs vary. Generally, a master's degree is necessary, but in some schools a master's degree is completed in conjunction with fulfillment of the doctoral degree requirements. Standard requirements include an RN license, Graduate Record Examinations (GRE) scores, college transcripts, letters of recommendation, and an essay. Students applying for doctoral-level study should have a solid foundation in nursing and an interest in research. Programs are usually the equivalent of three to five years of full-time study.

Selecting a Doctoral Program

Selecting a doctoral program comes down to personal choice. Students work closely with professors, and, thus, the support and mentoring you receive while pursuing your degree is as vital as the quality of the facilities. The most important question is whether there is a "match" between your research interest and faculty research. Many of the same questions you would ask about baccalaureate and master's degree programs apply to doctoral programs. However, in a doctoral program, the contact with professors, the use of research equipment and facilities, and the program's flexibility in allowing you to choose your course of study are critical.

Other questions to consider include: Does the university consider research a priority? Does the university have adequate funding for student research? Many nurses with doctoral degrees make the natural transition into an academic career, but there are many other career options available for nurses prepared at this level. For example, nurses prepared at the doctoral level are often hired by large consulting firms to work with others in designing solutions to health-care delivery problems. Others are hired by large hospital chains to manage various divisions, and some nurses with doctoral degrees are hired to manage complex health-care systems at the executive level. On another front, they conduct research and formulate national and international health-care policy. In short, because of the high level of education and a shortage of nurses prepared at this level, there are a number of options.

Salaries are related to the various positions. Faculty salaries vary by the type of institution and by faculty rank, typically ranging from approximately $50,000 at the assistant professor level to over $100,000 at the professor level. Salaries of nurse executives also vary, with the lowest salaries being in small rural hospitals and the highest being in complex university medical centers. In the latter, average salaries are well over $100,000 and often reach close to $200,000 annually. Consultant salaries are wide-ranging but often consist of a base plus some percentage of work contracted. Clinical and research positions vary considerably by the type of institution and the nature of the work. Needless to say, a doctoral education does provide individuals with a wide range of opportunities, with salaries commensurate with the type and level of responsibilities. Are there opportunities to present research findings at professional meetings? Is scholarship of faculty, alumni, and students presented at regional and national nursing meetings and subsequently published? Has the body of research done at a university enhanced the knowledge of nursing and health care?

AACN INDICATORS OF QUALITY IN RESEARCH-FOCUSED DOCTORAL PROGRAMS IN NURSING

Schools of nursing must consider the indicators of quality in evaluating their ability to mount research-focused doctoral programs. High-quality programs require a large number of increasingly scarce resources and a critical mass of faculty members and students. The AACN Indicators of Quality in Research-Focused Doctoral Programs in Nursing represent those indicators that should be present in a research-focused program.

There is considerable consensus within the discipline that while there are differences in the purpose and curricula of Ph.D. and Doctor of Nursing/Doctor of Nursing Science programs, most programs emphasize preparation for research. Therefore, AACN recommends continuing with a single set of quality indicators for research-focused doctoral programs in nursing whether the program leads to a Ph.D. or to a Doctor of Nursing or Doctor of Nursing Science degree.

The following indicators apply to the Doctor of Philosophy (Ph.D.) in nursing, Doctor of Nursing Science (D.N.S. or D.N.Sc.), and Doctor of Nursing (N.D.) degrees.

Faculty

I. Represent and value a diversity of backgrounds and intellectual perspectives.

II. Meet the requirements of the parent institution for graduate research and doctoral education; a substantial proportion of faculty hold earned doctorates in nursing.

III. Conceptualize and implement productive programs of research and scholarship that are developed over time and build upon previous work, are at the cutting edge of the field of inquiry, are congruent with research priorities within nursing and its constituent communities, include a substantial proportion of extramural funding, and attract and engage students.

IV. Create an environment in which mentoring, socialization of students, and the existence of a community of scholars is evident.

V. Assist students in understanding the value of programs of research and scholarship that continue over time and build upon previous work.

VI. Identify, generate, and utilize resources within the university and the broader community to support program goals.

VII. Devote a significant proportion of time to dissertation advisement. Generally, each faculty member should serve as the major adviser/chair for no more than 3 to 5 students during the dissertation phase.

Programs of Study

The emphasis of the program of study is consistent with the mission of the parent institution, the discipline of nursing, and the degree awarded. The faculty's areas of expertise and scholarship determine specific foci in the program of study. Requirements and their sequence for progression in the program are clear and available to students in writing. Common elements of the program of study are outlined below.

I. Core and related course content—the distribution between nursing and supporting content is consistent with the mission and goals of the program, and the student's area of focus and course work are included in:

   A. Historical and philosophical foundations to the development of nursing knowledge

   B. Existing and evolving substantive nursing knowledge

   C. Methods and processes of theory/knowledge development

   D. Research methods and scholarship appropriate to inquiry

   E. Development related to roles in academic, research, practice, or policy environments

II. Elements for formal and informal teaching and learning focus on:

   A. Analytical and leadership strategies for dealing with social, ethical, cultural, economic, and political issues related to nursing, health care, and research

   B. Progressive and guided student scholarship research experiences, including exposure to faculty's interdisciplinary research programs

C. Immersion experiences that foster the student's development as a nursing leader, scholarly practitioner, educator, and/or nurse scientist

D. Socialization opportunities for scholarly development in roles that complement students' career goals

III. Outcome indicators for the programs of study include:

    A. Advancement to candidacy requires faculty's satisfactory evaluation (e.g., comprehensive exam) of the student's basic knowledge of elements I-A through I-E identified above

    B. Dissertations represent original contributions to the scholarship of the field

    C. Systematic evaluation of graduate outcomes is conducted at regular intervals

    D. Within three to five years of completion, graduates have designed and secured funding for a research study, or, within two years of completion, graduates have utilized the research process to address an issue of importance to the discipline of nursing or health care within their employment setting

    E. Employers report satisfaction with graduates' leadership and scholarship at regular intervals

    F. Graduates' scholarship and leadership are recognized through awards, honors, or external funding within three to five years of completion

Resources

I. Sufficient human, financial, and institutional resources are available to accomplish the goals of the unit for doctoral education and faculty research.

    A. The parent institution exhibits the following characteristics:

        1) Research is an explicit component of the mission of the parent institution

        2) An office of research administration

        3) A record of peer-reviewed external funding

        4) Postdoctoral programs

        5) Internal research funds

        6) Mechanisms that value, support, and reward faculty and student scholarship and role preparation

        7) A university environment that fosters interdisciplinary research and collaboration

    B. The nursing doctoral program exhibits the following characteristics:

        1) Research active faculty as well as other faculty experts to mentor students in other role preparations

        2) Provide technical support for:

            (a) Peer review of proposals and manuscripts in their development phases

            (b) Research design expertise

            (c) Data management and analysis support

            (d) Hardware and software availability

            (e) Expertise in grant proposal development and management

        3) Procure space sufficient for:

            (a) Faculty research needs

            (b) Doctoral student study, meeting, and socializing

            (c) Seminars

            (d) Small-group work

    C. Schools of exceptional quality also have:

        1) Centers of research excellence

        2) Endowed professorships

        3) Mechanisms for financial support to allow full-time study

        4) Master teachers capable of preparing graduates for faculty roles

II. State-of-the-art technical and support services are available and accessible to faculty, students, and staff for state-of-the-science information acquisition, communication, and management.

III. Library and database resources are sufficient to support the scholarly endeavors of faculty and students.

Students

I. Students are selected from a pool of highly qualified and motivated applicants who represent diverse populations.

II. Students' research goals and objectives are congruent with faculty research expertise and scholarship and institutional resources.

III. Students are successful in obtaining financial support through competitive intramural and extramural academic and research awards.

IV. Students commit a significant portion of their time to the program and complete the program in a timely fashion.

V. Students establish a pattern of productive scholarship, collaborating with researchers in nursing and other disciplines in scientific endeavors that result in the presentation and publication of scholarly work that continues after graduation.

Evaluation

The evaluation plan:

I. Is systematic, ongoing, comprehensive, and focuses on the university's and program's specific mission and goals.

II. Includes both process and outcome data related to these indicators of quality in research-focused doctoral programs.

III. Adheres to established ethical and process standards for formal program evaluation, e.g., confidentiality and rigorous quantitative and qualitative analyses.

IV. Involves students and graduates in evaluation activities.

V. Includes data from a variety of internal and external constituencies.

VI. Provides for comparison of program processes and outcomes to the standards of its parent graduate school/university and selected peer groups within nursing.

VII. Includes ongoing feedback to program faculty, administrators, and external constituents to promote program improvement.

VIII. Provides comprehensive data in order to determine patterns and trends and recommend future directions at regular intervals.

IX. Is supported with adequate human, financial, and institutional resources.

Approved by AACN Membership, November 2001.

WHAT YOU NEED TO KNOW ABOUT ONLINE LEARNING

Rosalee C. Yeaworth, Ph.D., RN, FAAN
Professor and Dean Emerita
College of Nursing
University of Nebraska Medical Center

Sue Schmidt, M.A. in Education and Human
Development
Designer Web Management
MediaOne

Half a century ago, young women who graduated from high school and chose to enter a nursing program were expected to move into a "nurses' home," which housed not only dormitory-style rooms but also classrooms and faculty offices. Most of the clinical learning was done in apprenticeship style in a single hospital setting. There was no such thing as distance learning.

However, over the course of the past half century, nursing education, like health care and education in general, has changed dramatically, creating a need for educators to implement distance education programs. The demographics of nursing students have changed. Not only is the nursing student far more likely to be a man than fifty years ago, but also the student who once was referred to as "nontraditional" is now becoming the traditional student. These students are mature, employed individuals who have complex family responsibilities and often live or work some distance from the university offering the courses they wish to take. The rapid advances in health-care knowledge and technology have increased the demand for nurses with graduate degrees. All nurses are faced with the need to enhance their knowledge through lifelong education as their roles and expectations change. In addition, a much greater effort is being made to provide education and training to residents in rural settings in the hope that they will continue to live and work in these areas.

Universities are addressing these changing educational needs by using advanced technologies and new communication capabilities. Distance learning offerings are continually enhanced by using new technologies and delivery systems such as the Internet and desktop videoconferencing. These technologies enable universities to reach beyond the boundaries imposed on them by traditional classrooms to deliver educational material to students located in different, noncentralized locations, thus allowing instruction and learning to occur independently of time and place. This model, known as "distributive learning," can be used in combination with traditional classroom-based courses and with traditional distance learning courses, or to create wholly virtual classrooms.

Tools used for distance education include:

E-mail: This is one of the most commonly used communication tools. It allows for a one-to-one exchange of information between the sender and receiver of the e-mail message. Course papers and draft materials may be sent, commented on, and returned as attached documents.

Listservs: This is a one-to-many communication exchange. People subscribe to listservs based on discussion topics that interest them. When a participant on a listserv sends an e-mail to the listserv, the message is copied and sent to all people who have subscribed to it. Listservs are generally free; there is no charge to subscribe.

Discussion Groups: This is a many-to-many communication exchange. E-mail and listservs deliver the messages directly to your electronic mailbox. Discussion groups, on the other hand, are retained in a specified area on the Internet. You must go to the discussion group to post your comments and read and reply to the comments of others. The advantage of a discussion group over e-mail or listservs is that the comments can be viewed easily by all and the sequence of comments and replies posted is readily apparent in its structure.

Chat Rooms: Chat is synchronous communication as the participants are online at the same time talking to each other. E-mail, listservs, and discussion groups, on the other hand, are asynchronous communication. With moderated chat, a moderator views the questions and comments posed by the participants and selects those that will be seen by all participants. After posting the comment or question, the moderator answers it. In a regular chat room, there is no management over what is or is not posted.

Streaming Video: Entire lectures can be delivered using streaming video technology. Even students accessing the material with slower modems can receive clear audio and good video images.

Desktop Videoconferencing: With a small camera mounted on top of the computer, students and faculty members are able to see and talk with each other using desktop videoconferencing software.

Virtual Reality: Student lounges can be constructed visually using virtual reality software. When students want to have a discussion with other students, they literally walk into the lounge as an avatar (a visual image of themselves they have selected) and hold live chat sessions with their fellow classmates.

Web Sites: Components of or the entire course content can be delivered via the Internet through the creation of a Web site. Any or all of the technology tools noted above can be linked through an educational Web site. Among other things, a Web site includes the syllabus, discussion groups, assignments, student lounges, faculty information, resources (including links to Web documents that enrich the course content), lecture notes, and other course components. Traditional distance education tools, such as satellite transmission, videotapes, telephone conferences, correspondence material, and CD-ROM interactive instruction, are also frequently used in conjunction with Web-delivered course material.

The key to using technology successfully is to define your goals and objectives and then decide which technology or combination of technologies will be most effective. Keep in mind that faculty members and students must have the appropriate computer equipment and user knowledge to participate in distance learning. Even though computers today are much more user-friendly, it is important to allot some time for students to become accustomed to using the new technologies necessary for transmitting their course material. Campus information technology services should work closely with the faculty to prepare introductory manuals or self-help materials for students. Information technology specialists should be available to answer technology questions or solve problems so that faculty members can concentrate on the course content questions. Enthusiasm can be dampened if too much time must be devoted to learning the technology or dealing with technology problems.

When deciding to take distance-learning courses, other factors must be considered. What you need to participate in distance learning varies with the sophistication of the tools used by the course instructor. Sending and receiving e-mail, participating in discussion groups, and viewing online syllabi require fairly simple technology. You need a computer with a modem and an Internet service provider (ISP). When selecting an ISP, participants should consider cost, reliability of access, and speed. World Wide Web access provided through your cable provider is generally more expensive but provides significantly faster access to documents. Video streaming and desktop videoconferencing require more sophisticated computer systems. Sometimes, in rural areas, the local telephone company or the Internet or TV provider may be limited in their services. Students may find, for example, that they have to use a teleconference line for sound with desktop videoconferencing. It is important to investigate the technology issues in your area before undertaking a course, because technical limitations can add to the cost and decrease your satisfaction and learning. Access to the campus bookstore and library may be a concern for students who are at considerable distance from the school offering the course. Books and supplies may be ordered online from the bookstore, and journal articles can be made available from the library through electronic reserve. Courses that use electronic reserve usually require a fee to cover copyright costs.

Some advantages of distance learning are:

Student-Centered versus Instructor-Directed Learning: Students take an active role in their own learning experience. They are able to select what material they need to cover more extensively and are given the opportunity for exploration through accessing linked material provided by their instructor. They are also given more opportunity to learn at their own pace and select the time when they are more prepared to effectively view the course material.

Flexibility: Students may work at their own computers on a weekend or the middle of the night, not having to worry about library hours or driving in bad weather. Valuable time can be focused on learning rather than on the logistics of getting to class.

Accessibility: Students who would not be able to attend classes because of geographic proximity or time constraints are now able to participate.

Student Interaction Increases: Interaction increases in a distance learning environment. Students not only listen and take notes, but they also pose ideas to and ask questions of the instructor as well as other students in discussion groups. Interaction is encouraged, and the instructor has a better understanding of what and how the student is learning. In most classroom settings, it is very difficult to get students to discuss a topic. They may ask a question of or make a comment to the instructor, but they seldom interact with classmates about course topics.

Collaboration and Team Problem Solving: Using asynchronous and synchronous communication tools, students can work together on projects much more easily today. It has always been difficult to bring a group together face-to-face to discuss what needs to be done. Through these new communication channels, information can be easily passed among a group, and resources, such as research documents and drafts of works in progress, can be distributed instantly.

Increased Sharing of Knowledge: In the traditional classroom, the instructor is the primary source of information. In distance learning, using tools such as a discussion group, students have a greater opportunity to share their knowledge and experience, allowing the members of the group to learn from each other. In addition, access to the Internet allows students to access the experience and knowledge of others outside their immediate classroom setting.

Immediate Access to Updated Material: Any material or announcements that have been changed can be distributed instantly, reducing distribution costs and providing students with access to the most current information.

Developing Needed Technology Skills: Students are learning technology skills that they can apply later in their work setting.

Some important factors should be considered when deciding if a distance education model is right for you. It has been shown that students can learn course content by distance methods as well as or better than in the traditional classroom setting. Less information is available on socialization issues related to the nurse generalist, specialist, or practitioner roles. Socialization involves internalizing attitudes, values, and norms. The role modeling, mentoring, and collegial friendships may or may not be as adaptable to distance methods. Careful selection of clinical settings for experience, on-site preceptors, requirements for certain on-campus experiences, and group attendance of students and faculty members at regional or national meetings are some methods used to assist socialization.

Distance learning will not suffice for the "college experience" of joining sororities and fraternities and of participating in athletic and social activities that many young undergraduate students desire. On the other hand, for the adult learner with job and family responsibilities, the distance education methodologies can provide the opportunity to participate in educational experiences that might otherwise have been beyond consideration.

When selecting your educational program, you should clearly define your goals for your educational experiences. If you want the opportunity to have clinical experience in a particular setting, to be a research or teaching assistant to a certain person, or to be mentored by a selected expert, then your choice would be an on-site educational environment in a particular setting. However, if you want a degree from a particular institution but do not want to move or travel there, you need to explore the distance learning opportunities offered. You need to remember that it is not an either-or proposition. You may be able to combine traditional classroom-based courses with distance learning for selected courses to optimize your overall educational program.

Distance learning is used by more and more educational institutions to provide both degree and continuing education. Many schools collaborate to offer students a selection of courses taught by different colleges and universities. A recent collaborative effort is the Western Governors University, a virtual university that is a partnership involving eighteen states and approximately 100 participating colleges and universities.

As noted above, the world is changing and so is the way we deliver nursing education. Distance education has opened a world of opportunities to students and faculty members. Students now have the ability to further their education by removing many of the time and access barriers they previously faced. Faculty members are presented with new and exciting challenges as they begin to use innovative technologies in their course delivery. With careful consideration and planning, the outcome will enhance the overall learning experience of both learner and teacher.

THE INTERNATIONAL NURSING STUDENT

For many international students completing baccalaureate, master's, or doctoral nursing programs, their choice of learning institutions is obvious. U.S. and Canadian colleges and universities are considered to offer the finest programs of nursing education available anywhere in the world. U.S. and Canadian nursing programs are renowned for their breadth and flexibility, for the excellence of their basic curriculum structure, and for their commitment to extensive on-site clinical training. Nursing study in the U.S. and Canada also affords students the opportunity for hands-on learning and practice in the world's most technologically advanced health-care systems. For many international nursing students, and especially for students from countries that are medically underserved, these features make U.S. and Canadian nursing programs unsurpassed.

Applying to Nursing School

The application process for international students often involves the completion of two separate written applications. Many colleges screen international candidates with a brief preliminary application requesting basic biographical and educational information. This document helps the admission officer determine whether the student has the minimum credentials for admission before requiring him or her to begin the lengthy process of completing and submitting final application forms.

Final applications to U.S. and Canadian colleges and universities vary widely in length and complexity, just as specific admission requirements vary from institution to institution. However, international nursing students must typically have a satisfactory scholastic record and demonstrated proficiency in English. To be admitted to any postsecondary institution in the United States or Canada, you must have satisfactorily completed a minimum of twelve years of elementary and secondary education. The customary cycle for this education includes a six-year elementary program, a three-year intermediate program, and a three-year postsecondary program, generally referred to as high school in the U.S. In addition, nursing school programs generally require successful completion of several years of high school-level mathematics and science.

The documentation of satisfactory completion of secondary schooling (and university education, in the case of graduate-level applicants) is achieved through submission of school reports, transcripts, and teacher recommendations. Because academic records and systems of evaluation differ widely from one educational system to the next, request that your school include a guide to grading standards. If you have received your secondary education at a school in which English is not the language of instruction, be certain to include official translations of all documents.

International students who have completed some university-level course work in their native country may be eligible to receive credit for equivalent courses at the U.S. or Canadian institution in which they enroll. Under special circumstances, practical nursing experience may also qualify for university credit. Policies regarding the transfer of or qualification for credits based on education or nursing experience outside the U.S. (or Canada for Canadian schools) vary widely, so be certain to inquire about these policies at the universities or colleges that interest you.

Language skills are a key to scholastic success. "The ability to speak, write, and understand English is an important determinant of success," says Joann Weiss, former Director of the Nursing and Latin American Studies dual-degree programs at the University of New Mexico in Albuquerque. Her advice for potential international applicants is simple: "Develop a true command of written and spoken English." English proficiency for students who have not received formal education in English-speaking schools is usually demonstrated via the Test of English as a Foreign Language (TOEFL); minimum test scores of 550 to 580 are commonly required. This policy, as well as the level of proficiency required, varies from school to school, so be sure to investigate each college's policies.

In addition, most universities offer some form of English language instruction for international students, often under the rubric ESL (English as a second language). Students who require additional language study to meet admission requirements or students who wish to deepen their skills in written or verbal English should inquire about ESL program availability.

Many colleges and universities also require that all undergraduate applicants take a standardized test—either the SAT and three SAT Subject Tests or the ACT. Like their U.S. and Canadian counterparts, international applicants to graduate-level nursing programs are required by most institutions to take the standardized Graduate Record Examinations (GRE).

Applicants should also be aware that financial assistance for international students is usually quite limited. To spare international students economic hardship during their schooling in the U.S. or Canada, many colleges and universities require them to demonstrate the availability of sufficient financial resources for tuition and minimum living expenses and supplies. As with so many admission requirements, policies regarding financial aid vary considerably; find out early what the policies are at the colleges that interest you.

Attending School in the U.S. or Canada

Once you are accepted by the college or university of your choice, take full advantage of the academic and personal advising systems offered to international students. Most institutions of higher education in the U.S. and Canada maintain an international student advisory office staffed with trained counselors. In addition to general academic counseling and planning, an international adviser can assist in a broad range of matters ranging from immigration and visa concerns to employment opportunities and health-care issues.

With few exceptions, all university students also obtain specialized academic counseling from an assigned faculty adviser. Faculty advisers monitor academic performance and progress and try to ensure that students meet the institutional requirements for their degree. Faculty advisers are excellent sources of information regarding course selection, and some advisers offer tutorials or special language or educational support to international students.

Although all university students face academic challenges, international students often find life outside the classroom equally demanding. Suddenly introduced into a new culture where the way of life may be dramatically different from that of their native country, international students often face a variety of social, domestic, medical, religious, or emotional concerns. Questions about social conventions, meal preparation, or other personal concerns can often be addressed by your international or faculty adviser.

Lorraine Rudowski, Assistant Professor and International Student Adviser at the College of Nursing and Health Science at George Mason University in Fairfax, Virginia, emphasizes the benefits of a strong relationship with your advisers: "My job as an adviser is to provide comprehensive support to my students—from academic counseling and opportunities for language development to emotional support and guidance to attending parties or other informal social events to ease the sense of social and personal isolation often experienced by foreign students."

Dr. Rudowski says international students would do well to find a sponsor or confidant within the university, someone who understands the conventions of the student's native country. "A culturally sensitive sponsor is better equipped to understand the unique needs of each international student and is much more likely to help students obtain the assistance they need, whether we're talking about religious issues, help with study methods or social skills, or simply knowing how to deal with such everyday chores as cooking and cleaning. All of these matters can be sources of deep concern to international students."

Yet for all the academic, social, and personal challenges facing international nursing students, there is good news. Deans of nursing, professors, and advisers typically praise the motivation and determination of their international students, and international nursing students often boast matriculation rates that match or exceed those of their U.S. and Canadian counterparts.

For more information about the rules and regulations governing international students' entrance to U.S. schools, log on to infoUSA, part of the U.S. Department of State's Web site, at http://usinfo.state.gov/usa/infousa/educ/studyus.htm.

SPECIALTY NURSING ORGANIZATIONS

Academy of Medical-Surgical Nurses
East Holly Avenue
Box 56
Pitman, NJ 08071-0056
866-877-AMSN (toll-free)
E-mail: amsn@ajj.com
www.medsurgnurse.org

Air & Surface Transport Nurses Association
7995 East Prentice Avenue
Suite 100
Greenwood Village, CO 80111
800-897-NFNA (toll-free)
Fax: 303-770-1614
E-mail: astna@gwami.com
www.astna.org

American Academy of Ambulatory Care Nursing
East Holly Avenue
Box 56
Pitman, NJ 08071-0056
856-256-2350
E-mail: aaacn@ajj.com
www.aaacn.org

American Association of Critical-Care Nurses
101 Columbia
Aliso Viejo, CA 92656-4109
949-362-2000
800-899-2226 (toll-free)
Fax: 949-362-2020
E-mail: info@aacn.org
www.aacn.org

American Association of Diabetes Educators
100 West Monroe Street
Suite 400
Chicago, IL 60603
800-338-3633 (toll-free)
Fax: 312-424-2427
E-mail: aade@aadenet.org
www.aadenet.org

The American Association of Legal Nurse Consultants
401 North Michigan Avenue
Chicago, IL 60611
877-402-2562 (toll-free)
Fax: 312-673-6655
E-mail: info@aalnc.org
www.aalnc.org

American Association of Neuroscience Nurses
4700 West Lake Avenue
Glenview, IL 60025
847-375-4733
888-557-2266 (toll-free)
Fax: 877-734-8677
E-mail: info@aann.org
www.aann.org

American Association of Nurse Anesthetists
222 South Prospect Avenue
Park Ridge, IL 60068-4001
847-692-7050
Fax: 847-692-6968
E-mail: info@aana.com
www.aana.com

American Association of Nurse Attorneys
P.O. Box 515
Columbus, OH 43216-0515
877-538-2262 (toll-free)
Fax: 614-221-2335
E-mail: taana@taana.org
www.taana.org

American Association of Occupational Health Nurses, Inc.
2920 Brandywine Road
Suite 100
Atlanta, GA 30341
770-455-7757
Fax: 770-455-7271
E-mail: aaohn@aaohn.org
www.aaohn.org

American Association of Spinal Cord Injury Nurses
75-20 Astoria Boulevard
Jackson Heights, NY 11370
718-803-3782
Fax: 718-803-0414
E-mail: aascin@unitedspinal.org
www.aascin.org

American College of Nurse-Midwives
8403 Colesville Road
Suite 1550
Silver Spring, MD 20910
240-485-1800
Fax: 240-485-1818
www.midwife.org

American College of Nurse Practitioners (ACNP)
1501 Wilson Boulevard
Suite 509
Arlington, VA 22209
703-740-2529
Fax: 703-740-2533
E-mail: acnp@acnpweb.org
www.acnpweb.org

American Holistic Nurses Association
P.O. Box 2130
Flagstaff, AZ 86003-2130
800-278-2462 (toll-free)
E-mail: info@ahna.org
www.ahna.org

American Nephrology Nurses' Association
East Holly Avenue
Box 56
Pitman, NJ 08071-0056
856-256-2320
888-600-ANNA (toll-free)
E-mail: anna@ajj.com
www.annanurse.org

SPECIALTY NURSING ORGANIZATIONS

American Psychiatric Nurses Association
1555 Wilson Boulevard
Suite 602
Arlington, VA 22209
866-243-2443 (toll-free)
Fax: 703-243-3390
E-mail: inform@apna.org
www.apna.org

American Public Health Association
800 I Street, NW
Washington, DC 20001-3710
202-777-APHA
Fax: 202-777-2534
E-mail: comments@apha.org
www.apha.org

American Radiological Nurses Association
7794 Grow Drive
Pensacola, FL 32514
866-486-2762 (toll-free)
Fax: 850-484-8762
E-mail: arna@puetzamc.com
www.arna.net

American Society for Pain Management Nursing
P.O. Box 15473
Lenexa, KS 66285-5473
913-752-4975
Fax: 913-599-5340
E-mail: aspmn@goamp.org
www.aspmn.org

American Society of Ophthalmic Registered Nurses
P.O. Box 193030
San Francisco, CA 94119
415-561-8513
Fax: 415-561-8531
E-mail: asorn@aao.org
http://webeye.ophth.uiowa.edu/asorn

American Society of PeriAnesthesia Nurses
10 Melrose Avenue
Suite 110
Cherry Hill, NJ 08003-3696
877-737-9696 (toll-free)
Fax: 856-616-9601
E-mail: aspan@aspan.org
www.aspan.org

American Society of Plastic Surgical Nurses
7794 Grow Drive
Pensacola, FL 32514
850-473-2443
Fax: 850-484-8762
E-mail: aspsn@puetzamc.com
www.arna.net

Association for Death Education and Counseling
60 Revere Dr.
Suite 500
Northbrook, IL 60062
847-509-0403
Fax: 847-480-9282
E-mail: info@adec.org
www.adec.org

Association for Professionals in Infection Control and Epidemiology
1275 K Street, NW
Suite 1000
Washington, DC 20005-4006
202-789-1890
Fax: 202-789-1899
E-mail: apicinfo@apic.org
www.apic.org

Association of Nurses in AIDS Care
3538 Ridgewood Road
Akron, OH 44333
800-260-6780 (toll-free)
Fax: 330-670-0109
E-mail: anac@anacnet.org
www.anacnet.org

Association of Pediatric Oncology Nurses
4700 West Lake Avenue
Glenview, IL 60025
847-375-4724
Fax: 877-734-8755
E-mail: info@apon.org
www.apon.org

Association of Perioperative Registered Nurses
2170 South Parker Road
Suite 300
Denver, CO 80231
800-755-2676 (toll-free)
E-mail: custserv@aorn.org
www.aorn.org

Association of Rehabilitation Nurses
4700 West Lake Avenue
Glenview, IL 60025
800-229-7530 (toll-free)
E-mail: info@rehabnurse.org
www.rehabnurse.org

Association of Women's Health, Obstetric, and Neonatal Nurses
2000 L Street, NW
Suite 740
Washington, DC 20036
800-673-8499 (toll-free in the U.S.)
800-245-0231 (toll-free in Canada)
Fax: 202-728-0575
www.awhonn.org

Dermatology Nurses' Association
Box 56, East Holly Avenue
Pitman, NJ 08071-0056
800-454-4362 (toll-free)
E-mail: dna@ajj.com
http://dna.inurse.com

Developmental Disabilities Nurses Association
1685 H Street
PMB 1214
Blaine, WA 98230
800-888-6733 (toll-free)
Fax: 360-332-2280
E-mail: contact@ddna.org
www.ddna.org

Emergency Nurses Association
915 Lee Street
Des Plaines, IL 60016-6569
800-900-9659 (toll-free)
Fax: 847-460-4001
E-mail: enainfo@ena.org
www.ena.org

Hospice and Palliative Nurses Association
One Penn Center West
Suite 229
Pittsburgh, PA 15276
412-787-9301
Fax: 412-787-9305
E-mail: hpna@hpna.org
www.hpna.org

Infusion Nurses Society
315 Norwood Park South
Norwood, MA 02062
781-440-9408
Fax: 781-440-9409
www.ins1.org

International Nurses Society on Addictions
2170 S. Parker Rd.
Suite 229
Denver, CO 80231
484-318-6739
Fax: 303-369-0982
E-mail: info@intnsa.org
www.intnsa.org

National Association for Home Care & Hospice
228 Seventh Street, SE
Washington, DC 20003
202-547-7424
Fax: 202-547-3540
E-mail: exec@nahc.org
www.nahc.org

National Association of Clinical Nurse Specialists
2090 Linglestown Road
Suite 107
Harrisburg, PA 17110
717-234-6799
Fax: 717-234-6798
E-mail: info@nacns.org
www.nacns.org

National Association of Directors of Nursing Administration in Long-Term Care
10101 Alliance Road
Suite 140
Cincinnati, OH 45242
800-222-0539 (toll-free)
Fax: 513-791-3699
E-mail: info@nadona.org
www.nadona.org

National Association of Neonatal Nurses
4700 West Lake Avenue
Glenview, IL 60025-1485
800-451-3795 (toll-free)
Fax: 888-477-6266
E-mail: info@nann.org
www.nann.org

National Association of Nurse Practitioners in Women's Health
505 C Street, NE
Washington, DC 20002
202-543-9693
Fax: 202-543-9858
E-mail: info@npwh.org
www.npwh.org

National Association of Orthopaedic Nurses
401 North Michigan Avenue
Suite 2200
Chicago, IL 60611
800-289-6266 (toll-free)
Fax: 312-527-6658
E-mail: naon@smithbucklin.com
www.orthonurse.org

National Association of Pediatric Nurse Practitioners
20 Brace Road
Suite 200
Cherry Hill, NJ 08034-2633
856-857-9700
Fax: 856-857-1600
E-mail: info@napnap.org
www.napnap.org

National Association of School Nurses
8484 Georgia Avenue
Suite 420
Silver Spring, MD 20910
866-627-6767 (toll-free)
Fax: 301-585-1791
E-mail: nasn@nasn.org
www.nasn.org

National Gerontological Nursing Association
7794 Grow Drive
Pensacola, FL 32514
800-723-0560 (toll-free)
Fax: 850-484-8762
E-mail: ngna@puetzamc.com
www.ngna.org

National Organization of Nurse Practitioner Faculties
1522 K Street, NW
Suite 702
Washington, DC 20005
202-289-8044
Fax: 202-289-8046
E-mail: nonpf@nonpf.org
www.nonpf.com

Oncology Nursing Society
125 Enterprise Drive
Pittsburgh, PA 15275
866-257-4ONS (toll-free)
Fax: 877-369-5497
E-mail: customer.service@ons.org
www.ons.org

Preventive Cardiovascular Nurses Association
613 Williamson Street
Suite 205
Madison, WI 53703
608-250-2440
Fax: 608-250-2410
E-mail: info@pcna.net
www.pcna.net

Respiratory Nursing Society
c/o Gina Magnotti
1018 Jamison Ave., SE
Roanoke, VA 24013
540-598-6980
E-mail: customerservice@RespiratoryNursingSociety.org
www.respiratorynursingsociety.org

Society for Vascular Nursing
Primary Contact: Angela Wetherbee
978-744-5005
978-744-5029
www.svnnet.org

Society of Gastroenterology Nurses and Associates
401 North Michigan Avenue
Chicago, IL 60611-4267
800-245-7462 (toll-free)
Fax: 312-527-6658
E-mail: sgna@smithbucklin.com
www.sgna.org

SPECIALTY NURSING ORGANIZATIONS

Society of Otorhinolaryngology and Head-Neck Nurses, Inc.
116 Canal Street
Suite A
New Smyrna Beach, FL 32168
386-428-1695
Fax: 386-423-7566
E-mail: info@sohnnurse.com
www.sohnnurse.com

Society of Urologic Nurses and Associates
East Holly Avenue
Box 56
Pitman, NJ 08071
888-827-7862 (toll-free)
E-mail: suna@ajj.com
www.suna.org

Wound, Ostomy and Continence Nurses Society
15000 Commerce Parkway, Suite C
Mt. Laurel, NJ 08054
888-224-WOCN (toll-free)
Fax: 856-439-0525
E-mail: wocn_info@wocn.org
www.wocn.org

PAYING FOR YOUR NURSING EDUCATION

Whether you are considering a baccalaureate degree in nursing or have completed your undergraduate education and are planning to attend graduate school, finding a way to pay for that education is essential.

The cost to attend college is considerable and is increasing each year at a rate faster than most other products and services. In fact, the cost of a nursing education at a public four-year college can be more than $14,000 per year, including tuition, fees, books, room and board, transportation, and miscellaneous expenses. The cost at a private college or university, at either the graduate or undergraduate level, can be more than $30,000 per year.

This is where financial aid comes in. Financial aid is money made available by the government and other sources to help students who otherwise would be unable to attend college. More than $152 billion in aid is provided to students each year (College Board, Trends in Student Aid, 2006). Most college students in this country receive some form of aid, and all prospective students should investigate what may be available. Most of this aid is given to students because neither they nor their families have sufficient personal resources to pay for college. This type of aid is referred to as need-based aid. Recipients of need-based aid include traditional students just out of high school or college, as well as older, nontraditional students who are returning to college or graduate school.

There is also merit-based aid, which is awarded to students who display a particular ability. Merit scholarships are based primarily on academic merit, but may include other special talents. Many colleges and graduate schools offer merit-based aid in addition to need-based aid to their students.

Types and Sources of Financial Aid

There are three types of aid: scholarships (also known as grants or gift aid), loans, and student employment (including fellowships and assistantships). Scholarships and grants are outright gifts and do not have to be repaid. Loans are borrowed money that must be repaid with interest, usually after graduation. Student employment provides jobs during the academic year for which students are paid. For graduate students, student employment may include fellowships and assistantships in which students work, receive free or reduced tuition, and may be paid a stipend for living expenses.

Federal Financial Aid Programs

Program	Maximum/year
Federal Pell Grants	$4050 (undergraduate students only)
Federal Supplemental Educational Opportunity Grants (FSEOG)	$4000 (undergraduate students only)
Academic Competitivess Grants (must be Pell Grant eligible)	$750 (first-year students) $1300 (second-year students)
SMART Grants (must be Pell Grant eligible)	$4000 (third- and fourth-year students)
Federal Perkins Loans	$4000 (undergraduate students) $6000 (graduate students)
Federal Stafford/Direct Loans (subsidized)	$3500 (first-year students) $4500 (second-year students) $5500 (third- and fourth-year students) $8500 (graduate students)
Federal Stafford/Direct Loans (unsubsidized)	$3500 (first-year students)* $4500 (second-year students)* $5500 (third- and fourth-year students)* $7500 (independent first-year students)* $8500 (independent second-year students)* $10,500 (independent third- and fourth-year students)* $20,500 (graduate students)*
Federal PLUS Loans	Up to cost of attendance (less other financial aid received)
GRADPLUS	For graduate students, up to cost of attendance (less other financial aid received)

These amounts are inclusive of subsidized loans

Most of the aid available to students is need-based and comes from the federal government through eight financial aid programs. Four of these programs are grant-based—Federal Pell Grants, Academic Competitiveness Grants, SMART Grants, and Federal Supplemental Educational Opportunity Grants—and are only available to undergraduate students. Three are loan programs—Federal Perkins Loans, Federal Stafford Loans (subsidized and unsubsidized), Federal PLUS (Parent Loan for Undergraduate Students), and GRADPLUS loans—that are provided to both undergraduate and graduate students.

The final program is a student employment program called the Federal Work-Study Program, which is also awarded to undergraduate and graduate students based on financial need.

The federal government also offers a number of programs especially for nursing students. For example, the U.S. Department of Health and Human Services offers Nursing Student Scholarships, Nursing Student Loans, the Nursing Education Loan Repayment Program, and the Scholarship for Disadvantaged Students (SDS) program. Some of these programs require that one works in a designated nursing shortage area for a period of time. These programs are administered by the nursing school's financial aid office. For more information, log on to http://bhpr.hrsa.gov/dsa.

The second-largest source of aid is from the colleges and universities themselves. Almost all colleges have aid programs from institutional resources, most of which are grants, scholarships, and fellowships. These can be either need- or merit-based.

A third source of aid is from state governments. Nearly every state provides aid for students attending college in their home state, although most only have programs for undergraduates. Most state aid programs are scholarships and grants, but many states now have low-interest loan and work-study programs. Most state grants and scholarships are not "portable," meaning that they cannot be used outside of your home state of residence.

A fourth source of aid is from private sources such as corporations, hospitals, civic associations, unions, fraternal organizations, foundations, and religious groups that give scholarships, grants, and fellowships to students. Most of these are not based on need, although the amount of the scholarship may vary depending upon financial need. The competition for these scholarships can be formidable, but the rewards are well worth the process. Many companies also offer tuition reimbursement to employees and their dependents. Check with the personnel or human resources department at your or your parents' place of employment for benefit and eligibility information.

Eligibility for Financial Aid

Since most of the financial aid that college students receive is need-based, colleges employ a process called "need analysis" to determine student awards. For most applicants, there is one form that the student and parents (if the student is a dependent) fill out on which family income, assets, and household information is reported. This form is the Free Application for Federal Student Aid (FAFSA). The end result of this need analysis is the student's "Expected Family Contribution," or EFC, representing the amount a family should be able to contribute toward educational expenses.

Dependent or Independent

The basic principle of financial aid is that the primary responsibility for paying college expenses resides with the family. In determining your EFC, you will first need to know who makes up your "family." That will tell you whose income is counted when the need analysis is done.

Graduate Students: By definition, all graduate nursing students are considered independent for federal aid purposes. Therefore, only your income and assets (and your spouse's if you are married) count in determining your expected family contribution.

Undergraduate Students: If you are financially dependent upon your parents, then their income and assets, as well as yours, are counted toward the family contribution. But if you are considered independent of your parents, only your income (and your spouse's if you are married) counts in the calculation.

According to the U.S. Department of Education, in order to be considered independent for financial aid for 2007–08, you must meet any ONE of the following:

• You were born before January 1, 1984.

• You are married.

• You are or will be enrolled in a master's or doctoral program (beyond a bachelor's degree) during the 2007–08 school year.

• You have children who receive more than half their support from you.

• You have dependents (other than your children or spouse) who live with you and who receive more than half of their support from you and will continue to receive more than half their support from you through June 30, 2008.

• You are an orphan or ward of the court (or were a ward of the court until age 18).

• You are a veteran of the U.S. Armed Forces. ("Veteran" includes students who attended a U.S. service academy and who were released under a condition other than dishonorable. Also, National Guard and Reserve members who served in combat areas can be classified as independent. Contact your financial aid office for more information.)

If you meet any one of these conditions, you are considered independent and only your income and assets (and your spouse's if you are married) count toward your family contribution. Remember, if you are attending school as a graduate student, you are automatically independent for federal aid consideration.

If there are extraordinary circumstances, the financial aid administrator at the college you will be attending has the authority to make a change to your dependency status. You will need to provide extensive documentation of your family situation.

If you are considered an independent student, take your total family income for the previous year, subtract all state and federal taxes paid (including FICA), subtract another $3000 ($6000 if you are married), and divide the result in half. If your family income is less than $50,000, this is your estimated EFC. If your income is greater than $50,000 or you did not file a 1040A or 1040EZ in 2006, add 20 percent (12 percent if you have children) of your total assets (bank accounts, stocks, etc.). This result is your estimated EFC. If you are dependent, the EFC formula is more complicated. Check out www.petersons.com/finaid/efcsimplecalc.asp to determine your estimated EFC.

Determining Cost and Need

Now that you know approximately how much you and your family will be expected to contribute toward your college expenses, you can subtract the EFC from the total cost of attending a college or graduate school to determine the amount of need-based financial aid for which you will be eligible. The average cost listed assumes that you will be attending nursing school full-time. If you will be attending part-time, you should adjust costs accordingly. For a more accurate estimate of the cost of attendance at a particular college, check the financial aid information usually available on the college's Web site or in its publications.

Applying for Financial Aid

After you have subtracted your EFC from the cost of your education and determined your financial need, you will have a better understanding of how much assistance you will need. Even if you do not demonstrate financial need, you are still encouraged to file the FAFSA, as you may be eligible for assistance that is not based on need. The process for applying for aid can be confusing if you are not familiar with completing these types of applications. If you need assistance, you should contact the financial aid office for help.

Undergraduate and graduate students applying for aid must fill out the FAFSA. This application is available in high school guidance offices, college financial aid offices, state education department offices, and many local libraries. You are strongly encouraged to file the FAFSA online at www.fafsa.ed.gov. If you file online, you will need to have a Personal Identification Number (PIN). The PIN can easily be obtained at www.pin.ed.gov. Dependent students will need a PIN for themselves and one parent. By filing online, your application is processed faster, and you are far less likely to make major errors. The FAFSA, whether you file a paper application or online, becomes available in November or December, almost a year before the fall term in which you will enroll, but you cannot complete it until after January 1.

If you file a paper application, you and your parents (if appropriate) must sign your completed FAFSA and mail it to a processing center in the envelope provided. Do not send any additional materials, but do make copies of everything you filled out.

The processing center enters the data into a computer that runs the federal methodology of need analysis to calculate your EFC. This center then distributes the information to the schools and agencies you listed on the FAFSA. The actual determination of need and the awarding of aid are handled by each college financial aid office.

It is generally recommended that you complete the FAFSA as soon as possible after January 1. You should check with each college to which you are applying to determine its filing deadline. It is important to meet all college deadlines for financial aid, since there is a limited amount of funds available. However, students who procrastinate can still file for federal aid any time during the year.

What Happens After You Submit the FAFSA?

Two to four weeks after you send in your completed FAFSA, you will receive a Student Aid Report (SAR) that shows the information you reported and your official EFC. This is an opportunity for you to make corrections or to have the information sent to any new school you are considering that you did not list on the original FAFSA. The SAR contains instructions on how to make corrections or to designate additional schools. If you provided an e-mail address on the FAFSA, this information will be sent to this address rather than through conventional mail.

At the same time that you receive the SAR, the college(s) you specified also receive the information. The financial aid office at the school may request additional information from you or may ask you to provide documentation verifying the information you reported on the FAFSA. For example, they may ask you for a copy of your (and your parents') income tax return or official forms verifying any untaxed income you or your parents received (e.g., Social Security, disability, or welfare benefits).

Once the financial aid office is satisfied that the information is correct, you will receive a financial aid offer. Many colleges like to make this offer in the spring prior to the fall enrollment so that students have ample opportunity to make their plans. However, some colleges will wait until summer to notify you.

Other Applications

The FAFSA is the required form for applying for federal and most state financial aid programs. Most schools also use the FASFA to determine eligibility for institutional aid; however, some colleges and graduate schools require additional information to determine eligibility for institutional aid. Nearly 500 colleges and universities, plus more than 200 private scholarship programs, employ a form called the Financial Aid PROFILE® from the College Scholarship Service (CSS). While the form is similar to the FAFSA, several additional questions must be answered for colleges that award their own funds. You begin the process in October or November by completing a PROFILE® Registration form on which you designate the schools to which you are applying. A few weeks later, you will receive a customized, individualized application that you complete and send back to CSS, which, in turn, forwards your application information to the schools you selected. There is a fee charged for each school listed on the application.

Financial Aid Offer

If you qualify for need-based aid, a college will typically offer a combination of the three types of assistance—scholarship/grant, loan, and work-study—to meet this need. An offer of aid usually is made after you have been admitted to the college or program. You may accept all or part of the financial aid package. If you will be enrolling part-time (fewer than 12 credits per term), be sure to contact the financial aid office in advance since this may have impact on your overall aid elibility.

If you are awarded Federal Work-Study aid, the amount you are awarded represents your earnings limit for the academic year under the program. In general, schools assume you will earn this money on an hourly basis, so it cannot be used to pay your term bill charges. On most campuses there are many jobs available for students. Not all of these are limited to students in the Federal Work-Study program. Check with your placement office or financial aid office for more information.

Keep in mind that the student budget used to establish eligibility for financial aid is based on averages. It may not reflect your actual expenses. Student budgets usually reflect most expenses for categories of students (for example, single students living in their parents' home, campus-provided housing, or living in an apartment or house near campus, etc.). But if you have unusual expenses that are not included, you should consult with your school's financial aid office regarding a budget adjustment.

If Your Family or Job Situation Changes

Because a family contribution is based on the previous year's income, many nursing students find they do not qualify for need-based aid (or not enough to pay their full expenses). This is particularly true of older students who were working full-time last year but are no longer doing so or who will not work during the academic year. If this is your situation, you should speak to a counselor in the financial aid office about making an adjustment in your family contribution need analysis. Financial aid administrators may make changes to any of the elements that go into the need analysis if there are conditions that merit a change. Contact the financial aid office for more information.

Don't Qualify for Need-Based Aid?

If you don't qualify for need-based aid but feel you do not have the resources necessary to pay for college or graduate school, you still have several options available.

First, there are two student loan programs for which need is not a consideration. These two programs are the Federal Unsubsidized Stafford Loans and the Unsubsidized Direct Loans. There is also a non-need-based loan program for parents of dependent students called the Federal PLUS loan. If you or your parents are interested in borrowing through one of these programs, you should check with the financial aid office for more information. There are also numerous private or alternative loan sources available for parents. For many students, borrowing to pay for a nursing education can be an excellent investment in one's future. At the same time, be sure that you do not overburden yourself when it comes to paying back the loans. Before you accept a student loan, the financial aid office will schedule a counseling session to make certain that you know the terms of the loan and that you understand the ramifications of borrowing. If you can do without, it is often suggested that you postpone student loans until they are absolutely necessary.

For graduate nursing students, there is a new federal loan program named GRADPLUS. Students who are looking into alternative loan programs should be sure to compare any terms and conditions with this new federal program. Students should borrow through the GRADPLUS (or other alternative loan) program only after they have utilized the Federal Stafford Loans or Direct Loans program. You can borrow GRADPLUS and alternative loan funds up to the cost of attendance less any other financial aid received.

A second option if you do not qualify for need-based aid is to search for scholarships. Be wary of scholarship search companies that promise to find you scholarships but require you to pay a fee. There are many resources that provide lists of scholarships, including the annually published *Peterson's Scholarships, Grants & Prizes,* which are available in libraries, counselors' offices, and bookstores. Non-need scholarships require application forms and are extremely competitive; only a handful of students from thousands of applicants receive awards. Check out opportunities on our site, www.petersons.com.

Another option is to work more hours at an existing job or to find a paying position if you do not already have one. The student employment or placement office at your college should be able to help you find a job, either on or off campus. Many colleges have vacancies remaining after they have placed Federal Work-Study eligible students in their jobs.

You should always contact the financial aid office at the school you plan to attend for advice concerning sources of college-based and private aid.

Employer-Paid Financial Aid

Bob Atwater is a certified personnel consultant and certified medical staff recruiter and founder of Atwater Consulting & Recruiting in Lilburn, Georgia, a consulting firm for the employment and recruitment of physician assistants, nurse practitioners, certified nurse midwives, nurses, and nursing managers.

Health-care administrators, Atwater says, have coined a phrase to characterize their efforts to meet the growing demand for nurses with better skills and training: "Grow your own."

"Constant training through the course of a nursing career is the only way to keep pace with the technological and medical advances, but it can be a financial burden on the nurse," Atwater says.

That is why many employers now give qualified employees a benefits package that includes a continuing education allowance.

For the employer, this type of benefits package can help to recruit candidates willing to further their careers through education. Administrators feel it is the best way to build a staff of nurses with up-to-date certifications in all areas.

In a constantly expanding field, nurses should be required to continue and update their education. The nurses get a paid education, can keep their job, and work flexible hours while they are going to school. Inquiries about these allowances should be made during an interview with the company's human resources department. Additional information can be obtained from the nursing school, local hospitals in the area, or from other health-care professionals. There are many attractive options available because of the nationwide shortage of qualified nurses. Check with a number of potential employers before agreeing to any long-term contract.

SOURCES OF FINANCIAL AID FOR NURSING STUDENTS

The largest proportion of financial aid for college expenses comes from the federal government and is given on the basis of financial need. Beyond this federal need-based aid, which should always be the primary source of financial aid that a prospective student investigates and which is given regardless of one's field of study, a sizable amount of scholarship assistance specifically meant to help students in nursing programs is also available from government agencies, associations, civic or fraternal organizations, and corporations. These sources of aid can be particularly attractive for students who may not be eligible for need-based aid. The following list presents some of the major sources of financial aid specifically for nursing students. Not listed are scholarships that are specific to individual colleges and universities or limited to residents of a particular place or to individuals who have relatively unusual qualifications. Students seeking financial aid should investigate all appropriate possibilities, including sources not listed here. A student can find this information in libraries, bookstores, and guidance offices guides, including two of Peterson's annually updated publications: *Peterson's College Money Handbook,* for information about undergraduate awards given by the federal government, state governments, and specific colleges, and *Peterson's Scholarships, Grants & Prizes,* for information about awards from private sources.

Students should also check out the many scholarship search engines available on the Web, especially www. petersons.com/finaid and www.aacn.nche.edu/Education/ Financialaid.htm.

Air Force Institute of Technology
Award Name: Air Force Active Duty Health Professions Loan Repayment Program
Program Description: Program provides up to $30,651 to repay qualified educational loans in exchange for active duty service in the U.S. armed forces.
Application Contact: Air Force Institute of Technology
AFIT/ENEM
2275 D Street
Building 16, Room 120
Wright Patterson AFB, OH 45433-7221
800-543-3490 (toll-free)
E-mail: enem.adhplrp@afit.edu
http://www.afit.edu/adhplrp

American Association of Colleges of Nursing (AACN)
Award Name: Campus RN/AACN Scholarship Fund
Program Description: This scholarship program supports students who are seeking a baccalaureate, master's, or doctoral degree in nursing. Special consideration will be given to students enrolled in a master's or doctoral program with the goal of pursuing a nursing faculty career, completing an RN to baccalaureate program (B.S.N.), or enrolled in an accelerated baccalaureate or master's degree nursing program.
Application Contact: American Association of Colleges of Nursing
One Dupont Circle, NW
Suite 530
Washington, DC 20036
202-463-6930
Fax: 202-785-8320
E-mail: info@campuscareercenter.com
http://aacn.campusrn.com/scholarships/scholarship_rn.asp

American Association of Critical-Care Nurses
Award Name: AACN Educational Advancement Scholarships
Program Description: Nonrenewable scholarships for AACN members who are RNs currently enrolled in undergraduate or graduate NLNAC-accredited programs. The undergraduate award is for use in the junior or senior year. Minimum 3.0 GPA.
Application Contact: American Association of Critical-Care Nurses Scholarships
101 Columbia
Aliso Viejo, CA 92656-4109
800-899-2226 (toll-free)
E-mail: info@aacn.org
www.aacn.org

American Cancer Society
Award Name: Scholarships in Cancer Nursing
Program Description: Renewable awards for graduate students in nursing pursuing advanced preparation in cancer nursing: research, education, administration, or clinical practice. Must be U.S. citizen.
Application Contact: American Cancer Society
Extramural Grants Program
1599 Clifton Road, NE
Atlanta, GA 30329-4251
800-ACS-2345 (toll-free)
E-mail: grants@cancer.org
www.cancer.org

American Health Care Association
Award Name: Durante Nurse Scholarship
Program Description: For students accepted or enrolled in an accredited LPN/RN program and currently employed by an American Health Care Association or National Center for Assisted Living nursing facility.
Application Contact: American Health Care Association
Durante Nurse Scholarship Program
1201 L Street, NW
Washington, DC 20005
202-898-6332
www.ahca.org/about/scholarship.htm

American Holistic Nurses' Association (AHNA)
Award Name: Charlotte McGuire Scholarship Program
Program Description: Open to any licensed nurse or nursing student pursuing holistic education. Experience in holistic health care or alternative health practices is preferred. Must be an AHNA member with a minimum 3.0 GPA.

Application Contact: Charlotte McGuire Scholarships
American Holistic Nurses' Association
P.O. Box 2130
Flagstaff, AZ 86003-2130
800-278-2462 (toll-free)
E-mail: info@ahna.org
www.ahna.org/edu/assist.html

American Indian Graduate Center (AIGC)

Award Name: AIGC Fellowships

Program Description: Graduate fellowships available for American Indian and Alaska Native students from federally recognized U.S. tribes. Applicants must be pursuing a postbaccalaureate graduate or professional degree as a full-time student at an accredited institution in the U.S., demonstrate financial need, and be enrolled in a federally recognized American Indian tribe or Alaska Native group or provide documentation of Indian descent.

Application Contact: American Indian Graduate Center Fellowships
American Indian Graduate Center
4520 Montgomery Boulevard, NE
Suite 1B
Albuquerque, NM 87109
800-628-1920 (toll-free)
E-mail: marveline@aigc.com
www.aigc.com

Association of Perioperative Registered Nurses (AORN)

Award Name: AORN Foundation Scholarships

Program Description: Applicant must be an active RN and a member of AORN for twelve consecutive months prior to application. Reapplication for each period is required. For baccalaureate, master's of nursing, or doctoral degree at an accredited institution. Minimum 3.0 GPA required.

Application Contact: AORN Scholarship Committee
2170 South Parker Road
Suite 300
Denver, CO 80231
800-755-2676 (toll-free)
E-mail: ibendzsa@aorn.org
www.aorn.org/foundation/scholarships.asp

Bethesda Lutheran Homes and Services, Inc.

Award Name: Nursing Scholastic Achievement Scholarship

Program Description: Award for college nursing students with a minimum 3.0 GPA who are Lutheran and have completed their sophomore year of a four-year nursing program or one year of a two-year program. Must be interested in working with people with developmental disabilities.

Application Contact: Bethesda Lutheran Homes and Services, Inc.
Thomas Heuer, Coordinator/NCRC
600 Hoffmann Drive
Watertown, WI 53094
800-369-4636 (toll-free)
E-mail: ncrc@blhs.org
www.blhs.org/youth/scholarships

Foundation of the National Student Nurses' Association, Inc.

Award Names: Scholarship Program

Program Description: One-time awards available to nursing students in various educational situations: enrolled in programs leading to an RN license, RNs enrolled in programs leading to a bachelor's or master's degree in nursing, enrolled in a state-approved school in a specialty area of nursing, and minority students enrolled in nursing or prenursing programs. High school students are not eligible. Funds for graduate study are available only for a first degree in nursing. Based on financial need, academic ability, and health-related nursing and community activities. Application fee of $10. Send self-addressed stamped envelope with two stamps along with application request.

Application Contact: Scholarship Chairperson
Foundation of the National Student Nurses' Association, Inc.
45 Main Street
Suite 606
Brooklyn, NY 11201
718-210-0705
E-mail: nsna@nsna.org
www.nsna.org/foundation

Heart and Stroke Foundation of Canada

Award Name: Nursing Research Fellowships

Program Description: In-training awards for study in an area of cardiovascular or cerebrovascular nursing. Award is directed toward preparing nurses to undertake independent research programs. For master's degree candidates, the programs must include a thesis or project requirement.

Application Contact: Heart and Stroke Foundation of Canada
1402-222 Queen Street
Ottawa, Ontario K1P 5V9
Canada
613-569-4361
E-mail: research@hsf.ca
www.hsf.ca/research/guidelines/strategic.html

International Order of the King's Daughters and Sons, Inc.

Award Name: International Order of King's Daughters and Sons Health Scholarships

Program Description: For study in the health fields. B.A./B.S. students are eligible in junior year. Application must be for at least third year of college. RN students must have completed first year of schooling. Send #10 self-addressed stamped envelope for application and information.

Application Contact: Director
Health Careers Scholarship Department
P.O. Box 1040
Chautauqua, NY 14722-1040
www.iokds.org/scholarship.html

March of Dimes

Award Name: Graduate Scholarships

Program Description: Scholarships for registered nurses enrolled in graduate programs in maternal-child nursing. Must be a member of the Association of Women's Health, Obstetric and Neonatal Nurses; the American College of Nurse-Midwives; or the National Association of Neonatal Nurses (NANN).

Application Contact: Education Services
March of Dimes
1275 Mamaroneck Avenue
White Plains, NY 10605
E-mail: profedu@marchofdimes.com
www.marchofdimes.com

National Alaska Native American Indian Nurses Association (NANAINA)

Award Name: NANAINA Merit Awards

Program Description: Annual $500 awards presented to NANAINA members who are enrolled in a U.S. federally or state-recognized tribe and are enrolled as a full-time undergraduate or graduate nursing student in an accredited or state-approved school of nursing.

Application Contact: Dr. Better Keltner
NANAINA Treasurer
3700 Reservoir Road, NW
Washington DC 20057-1107
888-566-8773 (toll-free)
www.nanainanurses.org

National Association of Hispanic Nurses (NAHN)

Award Name: National Scholarship Awards

Program Description: One-time award to an outstanding Hispanic nursing student. Must have at least a 3.0 GPA and be a member of

NAHN. Based on academic merit, potential contribution to nursing, and financial need.

Application Contact: Miriam Gonzales
Awards/Scholarship Committee Chair
1501 16th Street, NW
Washington, DC 20036
202-387-2477
E-mail: info@thehispanicnurses.org
www.thehispanicnurses.org

National Black Nurses Association, Inc. (NBNA)

Award Names: NBNA Scholarships
Program Description: Scholarships available to nursing students who are members of NBNA and are enrolled in an accredited school of nursing. Must demonstrate involvement in African-American community and present letter of recommendation from local chapter of NBNA.
Application Contact: National Black Nurses Association, Inc.
8630 Fenton Street, Suite 330
Silver Spring, MD 20910-3803
800-575-6298 (toll-free)
E-mail: nbna@erols.com
www.nbna.org/scholarship.htm

National Student Nurses' Association (NSNA)

Award Name: Educational Advancement Scholarships
Program Description: Scholarships are awarded based on academic achievement and demonstrated commitment to nursing through involvement in student organizations and school and community activities related to health care.
Application Contact: National Student Nurses' Association Foundation
45 Main Street
Suite 606
Brooklyn, NY 11201
718-210-0705
E-mail: nsna@nsna.org
www.nsna.org

Nurses' Educational Funds, Inc.

Award Name: Nurses' Educational Fund Scholarships
Program Description: Awards for full-time students at master's level, full-time or part-time at doctoral level, or RNs who are U.S. citizens and members of a national professional nursing association. Application fee: $10.
Application Contact: Nurses' Educational Funds, Inc.
304 Park Avenue South
11th Floor
New York, NY 10010
212-590-2443
E-mail: info@n-e-f.org
www.n-e-f.org

Oncology Nursing Society

Award Name: Scholarships
Program Description: ONF offers nearly a dozen one-time scholarships and awards at all levels of study, with various requirements and purposes, to nursing students who are interested in pursuing oncology nursing. Contact the foundation for details about appropriate awards. Application fee: $5.
Application Contact: Oncology Nursing Society
Development Coordinator
125 Enterprise Drive
RIDC Park West
Pittsburgh, PA 15275-1214
866-257-4667 (toll-free)
E-mail: customer.service@ons.org
www.ons.org/awards

United States Air Force Reserve Officer Training Corps

Award Name: Air Force ROTC Nursing Scholarships
Program Description: One- to four-year programs available to students of nursing and high school seniors. Nursing graduates agree to accept a commission in the Air Force Nurse Corps and serve four years on active duty after successfully completing their licensing examination. Must have at least a 2.5 GPA for one- and four-year scholarships or at least a 2.65 GPA for two- and three-year scholarships. Two exam failures result in a four-year assignment as an Air Force line officer.
Application Contact: Air Force ROTC
551 East Maxwell Boulevard
Maxwell AFB, AL 36112-6106
866-423-7682 (toll-free)
www.afrotc.com/scholarships/index.htm

United States Army Reserve Officers' Training Corps

Award Name: Army ROTC Nursing Scholarships
Program Description: Two- to four-year programs available to students of nursing and high school seniors. Nursing graduates agree to accept a commission in the Army Nurse Corps and serve in the military for a period of eight years. This may be fulfilled by serving on active duty for two to four years, followed by service in the Army National Guard or the United States Army Reserve or in the Inactive Ready Reserve for the remainder of the eight-year obligation.
Application Contact: Army ROTC Cadet Command
Army ROTC Scholarship
Fort Monroe, VA 23651-1052
800-USA-ROTC (toll-free)
www.goarmy.com/rotc/scholarships.jsp

United States Department of Health and Human Services, Bureau of Health Professions

Award Names: Nursing Scholarship
Program Description: Awards for U.S. citizens enrolled or accepted for enrollment as a full- or part-time student in an accredited school of nursing in a professional registered nurse program (baccalaureate, graduate, associate degree, or diploma)
Application Contact: Division of Nursing
U.S. Dept. of Health and Human Services
5600 Fishers Lane, Room 9-35
Parklawn Building
Rockville, MD 20857
301-443-5688
www.bhpr.hrsa.gov/dsa

SEARCHING FOR NURSING SCHOOLS ONLINE

The Internet can be a great tool for students and parents gathering information about nursing programs. There are many worthwhile sites to help guide you through the various aspects of the selection process, including Peterson's Nursing Programs Search at www.petersons.com/nursing.

The majority of nursing programs maintain Web sites, which often provide vast amounts of admissions information. As you surf the Web for information, keep in mind that Web sites can vary greatly in appearance and quality. While some sites are attractive, easy to navigate, and home to large amounts of useful information, others are unimaginative and complex. Upon arriving at a site, determine the source. Who created the site and why? Is the site user-friendly? Can you find the information you need?

How Peterson's Nursing Programs Search Can Help

Nursing school is a serious commitment of time and resources. Therefore, it is important to have the most up-to-date information about prospective schools at your fingertips. That is why Peterson's Nursing Programs Search is a great place to start your nursing program search and selection process.

Peterson's Nursing Programs Search is a comprehensive information resource that will help you make sense of the nursing school admissions process. It offers visitors enhanced search criteria and an easily navigable interface. The site is organized into various sections that make finding a program easy and fun. You can search for nursing programs based on:

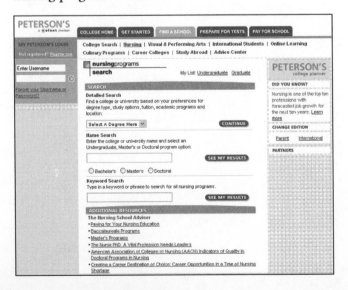

- *Degree type*
- *Institution name*
- *Study options (full-time, part-time)*
- *Tuition*
- *Academic content*
- *Location*
- *Keyword*

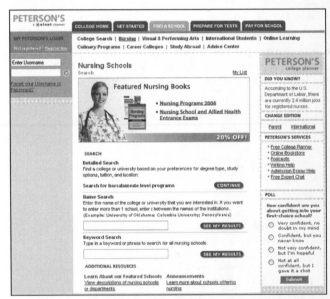

Once you have found the school of your choice, simply click on one of the tabs at the top of the profile to get general information about the institution as a whole and information specific to the nursing program. Tabs include:

- *Students & Faculty*
- *Nursing Program*
- *Campus Life*
- *Financial Aid & Costs*
- *Contact*
- *Inside Scoop*

Resources

View Descriptions

If the schools you are interested in have provided Peterson's with a **Close-Up,** you can do a keyword search on that Close-Up or click the "Inside Scoop" tab. Here, schools are given the opportunity to communicate unique features of their nursing programs to prospective students.

View Announcements

If the schools you are interested in have provided Peterson's with an **Announcement,** you can click on "Announcements" in the "Additional Resources" section of the site, and you will be directed to an alphabetical listing of those schools that provided additional information about their program.

Visit Web Sites

For institutions that have provided information about their Web sites, simply click on the "Visit School Site" button and be taken directly to that institution's Web page. Once you arrive at the school's Web site, look around and get a feel for the place. Often, schools offer virtual tours of the campus, complete with photos and commentary. If you have any questions about the school, a visit to a school's Web site will often answer these questions.

Receive More Information

If, after looking at the information provided on Peterson's Nursing Programs Search and on the school's Web page, you still have questions, you can send an e-mail directly to the admissions department of the school from Peterson's Web site. Just click on the "Get Free Info" button, and type in your contact information and your question or request for additional information. Your message will be received by the school within seconds.

Add to My List

If you've already narrowed your choices down to one or two schools, or you're just starting from scratch, you'll find the tools you need at My List. Here you can:

- Save the list of schools you're interested in, which you can then revisit at any time.
- Access all the features of the site.
- Be reminded of important dates and receive notifications when we add new features to the site.

Use the Tools to Your Advantage

Choosing a school is an involved and complicated process. The tools available to you at www.petersons.com/nursing can help you to be more productive in this process. So, what are you waiting for? Log on. Your future alma mater may be just a click of the mouse away.

HOW TO USE THIS GUIDE

The following includes an overview of the various components of *Peterson's Nursing Programs 2008,* along with background information on the criteria used for including institutions and nursing programs in the guide, and explanatory material to help users interpret details presented within the guide.

Profiles of Nursing Programs

The **Profiles of Nursing Programs** section contains detailed profiles of schools that responded to our online survey and the nursing programs they offer. This section is organized geographically; U.S. schools are listed alphabetically by state or territory, followed by Canadian schools listed alphabetically by province.

The profiles contain basic information about the colleges and universities, along with details specific to the nursing school or department, the nursing student body, and the nursing programs offered.

Schools that are members of a consortium appear with an abbreviated profile. The abbreviated profile lists only the school heading and the specific college or university information, followed by a reference line that refers readers to the consortium profile, which contains detailed program information.

An outline of the profile follows. The items of information found under each section heading are defined and displayed. Any item discussed below that is omitted from an individual profile either does not apply to that particular college or university or is one for which no information was supplied. Each profile begins with a heading with the name of the institution (the college or university), the nursing college or unit, the location of the nursing facilities, the school's Web address, and the institution's founding date, specifically the year in which it was chartered or the year when instruction actually began, whichever date is earlier. In most cases, the location is identical to the main campus of the institution. However, in a few instances, the nursing facilities are not located in the same city or state as the main campus of the college or university.

Basic information about the college follows:

Nursing Program Faculty: The total number of full-time and part-time faculty members, followed by, if provided, the percentage of faculty members holding doctoral degrees.

Baccalaureate Enrollment: The total number of matriculated full-time and part-time baccalaureate program students as of fall 2006 is given. This snapshot of the nursing student body indicates the total number of matriculated students, both full-time and part-time, in the baccalaureate-level nursing program; the school's esti-mate of the percentage of nursing students in each of the following categories is provided, if applicable: women, men, minority, international, and part-time.

Graduate Enrollment: The total number of matriculated full-time and part-time students in graduate programs in fall 2006 and the percentages of women, men, minority, international, and part-time students are given.

Nursing Student Activities: This section lists organizations open only to nursing students, including nursing clubs, Sigma Theta Tau (the international honor society for nursing), recruiter clubs, and Student Nurses' Association.

Nursing Student Resources: This section lists special learning resources available for nursing students within the nursing school's (or unit's) facilities.

Library Facilities: Figures are provided for the total number of bound volumes held by the college or university, the number of those volumes in health-related subjects, and the number in nursing and the number of periodical subscriptions held and the number of those in health-related subjects.

BACCALAUREATE PROGRAMS

Degree: Baccalaureate degree or degrees awarded are specified.

Available Programs: If, in addition to a generic baccalaureate program in nursing, a school has other baccalaureate nursing programs (e.g., accelerated pro-grams or programs for RNs, LPNs, or college graduates with non-nursing degrees) they are specified here.

Site Options: Locations other than the nursing program's main campus at which baccalaureate programs may be taken, including distance learning, are listed. Off-campus classes generally are held in health-care facilities or other educational facilities that are part of or affiliated with the college or nursing school.

Study Options: Lists full-time and part-time options.

Program Entrance Requirements: Lists special require-ments typically required to enter a program of nursing leading to a baccalaureate degree, including completion of a specific program of prerequisite courses, sometimes called prenursing courses. These are specific course credits that must be earned by students who wish to enter the generic baccalaureate program. Students entering into other tracks may be required to prove that they have completed analogous courses. Often the minimum GPA requirement for prerequisite courses differs from that expected for general college courses.

Other requirements are generally self-explanatory. This paragraph also indicates if transfer students are accepted into the program and which **Standardized Test** scores the student must have submitted to the institution. These are noted as required, recommended, and required for some. Tests may include American College Testing, Inc.'s ACT; the College Board's SAT or SAT Subject Tests; and the Test of English as a Foreign Language (TOEFL) for nonnative speakers of English. Special tracks will require appropriate proof of experience, diplomas, or other credentials. Finally, **Application** deadlines and fees are given.

Advanced Placement: This entry indicates that program credits may be granted on the basis of examinations or evaluations of earned credits at other facilities by the program's faculty and administrators.

Expenses: In this section, figures are provided for tuition, mandatory and other fees, and room and board, as well as an estimate of costs for books and supplies, based on the 2006–07 academic year. If a school did not return a survey, expenses for the 2004–05 or 2005–06 academic year are listed. Unless otherwise indicated, tuition is for one full academic year. If applicable, distinct tuition figures are given for state residents and nonresidents. Part-time, summer, and evening tuition is expressed in terms of the per-unit rate (per credit, per semester hour, etc.) specified by the institution. The tuition structure at some institutions is very complex, with different rates for freshmen and sophomores than for juniors and seniors or with part-time tuition prorated on a sliding scale according to the number of credit hours taken. Mandatory fees include such items as activity fees, health insurance, and malpractice insurance.

Financial Aid: Provides information on college-administered aid for baccalaureate-level nursing students, including the percentage of undergraduate nursing students receiving financial aid, all types of aid offered, and application deadlines. Financial aid programs are organized into four categories: gift aid (need-based), awards based on a student's formally designated inability to pay some or all of the cost of education; gift aid (non-need-based), scholarships given on the basis of a student's special achievements, abilities, or personal characteristics; loans, subsidized low-interest student loans that can be need-based or not; and work-study, a need-based program of part-time work offered to help pay educational expenditures. The application deadline is the deadline by which application forms and need calculations, such as the FAFSA, must be submitted to the institution in order to qualify for need-based and institutional aid.

Contact: This section lists the name, title, mailing address, telephone number, and, if available, fax number and e-mail address of the person to contact for admission information about the baccalaureate program.

GRADUATE PROGRAMS

The first three paragraphs provide information that is common to the college's graduate programs in nursing.

Expenses: In this section, figures are provided for tuition, room and board, and required fees based on the 2006–07 academic year. If a school did not return a survey, expenses for the 2004–05 or 2005–06 academic year are listed. Unless otherwise indicated, tuition is for one full academic year. If applicable, distinct tuition figures are given for state residents and nonresidents. Part-time, summer, and evening tuition is expressed in terms of the per-unit rate (per credit, per semester hour, etc.) specified by the institution.

Financial Aid: Provides information on college-administered aid includes the percentage of graduate nursing students receiving financial aid, all types of aid offered, and application deadlines. The major kinds of aid available are listed, including traineeships, low-interest student loans, fellowships, research assistantships, teaching assistantships, and full and partial tuition waivers. If aid is available to part-time students, this is indicated. The application deadline is the deadline by which application forms must be submitted to the college's financial aid office.

Contact: Lists the name, title, mailing address, telephone number, and, if available, fax number and e-mail address of the person to contact for admission information about graduate programs.

MASTER'S DEGREE PROGRAM

Degree(s): Master's degree or degrees awarded are specified. Joint degrees specify which two degrees are given, e.g., M.S.N./M.B.A., M.S./M.H.A., M.S.N./M.P.H., in programs that combine a master's degree (or doctorate) in nursing with a master's degree in another discipline, such as business administration, hospital administration, or public health.

Available Programs: If a college has special tracks that give credit, accelerated programs, or advanced courses designed for students with previous nursing experience or higher education credentials that enable students to complete programs in less time than regularly required, these are specified here in three categories:

For RNs—programs that admit registered nurses with associate degrees or diplomas in nursing and award a master's degree. These include RN-to-master's programs that combine the baccalaureate and master's degrees into one program for nurses· who are graduates of associate or hospital diploma programs and programs that admit registered nurses with non-nursing baccalaureate degrees.

For LPNs—programs that admit licensed practical nurses and award a master's degree.

For College Graduates with Non-Nursing Degrees—programs that admit students with baccalaureate or master's degrees in areas other than nursing and award a master's degree in nursing.

Concentrations Available: Specific areas of study and concentrations offered by the school are listed. Areas of specialization in case management, health-care administration, nurse anesthesia, nurse midwifery, nursing administration, nursing education, and nursing informatics are noted. Clinical nurse specialist and nurse practitioner programs and areas of specialization within them are noted.

Site Options: Locations other than the nursing program's main campus at which the master's degree programs are offered, including distance learning, are listed. Off-campus classes generally are held in health-care facilities or other educational facilities that are part of or affiliated with the nursing school.

Study Options: Lists full-time and part-time options.

Program Entrance Requirements: Lists generally self-explanatory requirements.

Advanced Placement: Indicates that program credits may be granted on the basis of examinations or evaluations of earned credits at other facilities by the program's faculty and administrators.

Degree Requirements: Indicates the number of master's program credit hours required to earn the master's degree and the need for a thesis or qualifying score on a comprehensive examination.

POST-MASTER'S PROGRAM

Listed here are the specific areas of clinical nurse specialist programs, nurse practitioner programs, and other specializations offered as post-master's programs.

DOCTORAL DEGREE PROGRAM

Degree: Doctoral degree awarded is specified.

Areas of Study: Lists specific areas of study and concentration offered by the school.

Program Entrance Requirements: Lists generally self-explanatory requirements.

Degree Requirements: Indicates the number of program credit hours required to earn the doctorate and the need for a dissertation, oral examination, written examination, or residency.

POSTDOCTORAL PROGRAM

Areas of Study: Lists areas of study currently reported. These may change, dependent upon the individuals in the program.

Postdoctoral Program Contact: Lists the name, title, mailing address, telephone number, and, if available, fax number and e-mail address of the person to contact for information about postdoctoral programs.

CONTINUING EDUCATION PROGRAM

The appearance of this heading indicates that the nursing school has a program of continuing education. If provided, the name, title, mailing address, telephone number, fax number, and e-mail address of the person to contact regarding the program are given.

Announcements

Announcements, which appear within some institutions' profiles, have been written by those colleges or universities that wished to supplement the profile data with timely or important information about their institutions or nursing programs. Some chose to mention degree programs that are not yet accredited.

Close-Ups of Nursing Programs

The **Close-Ups of Nursing Programs** section is an open forum for nursing schools to communicate their particular message to prospective students. The absence of any college or university from this section does not constitute an editorial decision on the part of Peterson's. Those who have chosen to write these inclusions are responsible for the accuracy of the content. Statements regarding a school's objectives and accomplishments represent its own beliefs and are not the opinions of the editors. The **Close-Ups of Nursing Programs** are arranged alphabetically by the official institution name.

Indexes

Indexes at the back of the book provide references to profiles by baccalaureate, master's, doctoral, post-doctoral, distance learning, and continuing education programs offered; for master's-level programs, by area of study or concentration; and by institution name.

Abbreviations Used in This Guide

AACN	American Association of Colleges of Nursing
AACSB	AACSB International—The Association to Advance Collegiate Schools of Business
AAHC	Association of Academic Health Centers
AAS	Associate in Applied Science
ABSN	Accelerated Bachelor of Science in Nursing
ACT	American College Testing, Inc.
ACT ASSET	American College Testing Assessment of Skills for Successful Entry and Transfer
ACT COMP	American College Testing College Outcomes Measures Program
ACT PEP	American College Testing Proficiency Examination Program
AD	Associate Degree
ADN	Associate Degree in Nursing

AHNP	Adult Health Nurse Practitioner
ALE	American Language Exam
AMEDD	Army Medical Department
ANA	American Nurses Association
ANP	Adult Nurse Practitioner
APN	Advanced Practice Nurse
ARNP	Advanced Registered Nurse Practitioner
AS	Associate of Science
ASN	Associate of Science in Nursing
BA	Bachelor of Arts
BAA	Bachelor of Applied Arts
BN	Bachelor of Nursing
BNSc	Bachelor of Nursing Science
BRN	Baccalaureate for the Registered Nurse
BS	Bachelor of Science
BScMH	Bachelor of Science in Mental Health
BScN	Bachelor of Science in Nursing
BSEd	Bachelor of Science in Education
BSN	Bachelor of Science in Nursing
CAI	computer-assisted instruction
CAUSN	Canadian Association of University Schools of Nursing
CCNE	Commission on Collegiate Nursing Education
CCRN	Critical-Care Registered Nurse
CFNP	Certified Family Nurse Practitioner
CGFNS	Commission on Graduates of Foreign Nursing Schools
CINAHL	Cumulative Index to Nursing and Allied Health Literature
CLAST	College-Level Academic Skills Test
CLEP	College-Level Examination Program
CNA	Certified Nurse Assistant, Certified Nursing Assistant, Certified Nurses' Aide
CNAT	Canadian Nurses Association Testing
CNM	Certified Nurse-Midwife
CNS	Clinical Nurse Specialist
CODEC	coder/decoder
CPR	cardiopulmonary resuscitation
CRNA	Certified Registered Nurse Anesthetist
CS	Certified Specialist
CSS	College Scholarship Service
DNP	Doctor of Nursing Practice
DNS	Doctor of Nursing Science
DNSc	Doctor of Nursing Science
DOE	U.S. Department of Education
DrPH	Doctor of Public Health
DSN	Doctor of Science in Nursing
EdD	Doctor of Education
EFC	expected family contribution
ERIC	Educational Resources Information Center
ESL	English as a second language
ETN	Enterostomal Nurse
FAAN	Fellow in the American Academy of Nursing
FAF	Financial Aid Form
FAFSA	Free Application for Federal Student Aid
FC	family contribution
FNP	Family Nurse Practitioner
FSEOG	Federal Supplemental Educational Opportunity Grants
GED	General Educational Development test
GMAT	Graduate Management Admission Test
GPA	grade point average
GPO	Government Printing Office
GRE	Graduate Record Examinations
Gyn	gynecology
HIV	human immunodeficiency virus
HMO	health maintenance organization
ICEOP	Illinois Consortium for Educational Opportunities Program
ICU	intensive care unit
ISP	Internet service provider
ITV	interactive television
LD	Licensed Dietician
LPN	Licensed Practical Nurse
LVN	Licensed Vocational Nurse
MA	Master of Arts
MAEd	Master of Arts in Education
MAT	Miller Analogies Test
MBA	Master of Business Administration
MCSc	Master of Clinical Science
MDiv	Master of Divinity
MEd	Master of Education
MEDLINE	MEDLARS On-Line
MELAB	Michigan English Language Assessment Battery
MHA	Master of Hospital Administration Master of Health Administration
MHD	Master of Human Development
MHSA	Master of Health Services Administration
MN	Master of Nursing
MNSc	Master of Nursing Science
MOM	Master of Organizational Management
MPA	Master of Public Affairs
MPH	Master of Public Health
MPS	Master of Public Service
MS	Master of Science
MSBA	Master of Science in Business Administration
M Sc	Master of Science
MSc(A)	Master of Science (Applied)
MScN	Master of Science in Nursing
MSEd	Master of Science in Education
MSN	Master of Science in Nursing
MSOB	Master of Science in Organizational Behavior
NCAA	National Collegiate Athletic Association
NCLEX-RN	National Council Licensure Examination for Registered Nurses
ND	Doctor of Nursing
NLN	National League for Nursing
NNP	Neonatal Nurse Practitioner
NP	Nurse Practitioner
NSNA	National Student Nurses' Association
OB	Organizational Behavior
OB/GYN	obstetrics/gynecology
OCLC	Online Computer Library Center
OM	Organizational Management
PEP	Proficiency Examination Program
PhD	Doctor of Philosophy
PHEAA	Pennsylvania Higher Education Assistance Agency
PHS	Public Health Service
PLUS	Parents' Loan for Undergraduate Students
PNNP	Perinatal Nurse Practitioner
PNP	Pediatric Nurse Practitioner
PSAT	Preliminary SAT
RD	Registered Dietician
RN	Registered Nurse
RN, C	Registered Nurse, Certified
RN, CAN	Registered Nurse, Certified in Nursing Administration
RN, CNAA	Registered Nurse, Certified in Nursing Administration, Advanced
RN, CS	Registered Nurse, Certified Specialist

ROTC	Reserve Officers' Training Corps
RPN	Registered Psychiatric Nurse
SAR	Student Aid Report
SAT	SAT and SAT Subject Tests
SLS	Supplemental Loans to Students
SNA	Student Nurses' Association
SNAP	Student Nurses Acting for Progress
SNO	Student Nurses Organization
SUNY	State University of New York
TAP	Tuition Assistance Program
TB	tuberculosis
TOEFL	Test of English as a Foreign Language
TSE	Test of Spoken English
TWE	Test of Written English
USIS	United States Information Service
WHNP	Women's Health Nurse Practitioner

Data Collection Procedures

The data contained in the preponderant number of nursing college profiles, as well as in the indexes to them, were collected through *Peterson's Survey of Nursing Programs* during winter 2006-07. Questionnaires were posted online for more than 700 colleges and universities with baccalaureate and graduate programs in nursing. With minor exceptions, data for those colleges or schools of nursing that responded to the questionnaires were submitted by officials at the schools themselves. All usable information received in time for publication has been included. The omission of a particular item from a profile means that it is either not applicable to that institution or was not available or usable. In the handful of instances in which no information regarding an eligible nursing program was submitted and research of reliable secondary sources was unable to elicit the desired information, the name, location, and some general information regarding the nursing program appear in the profile section to indicate the existence of the program. Because of the extensive system of checks performed on the data collected by Peterson's, we believe that the information presented in this guide is accurate. Nonetheless, errors and omissions are possible in a data collection and processing endeavor of this scope. Also, facts and figures, such as tuition and fees, can suddenly change. Therefore, students should check with a specific college or university at the time of application to verify all pertinent information.

Criteria for Inclusion in This Book

Peterson's Nursing Programs 2008 covers accredited institutions in the U.S., U.S. territories, and Canada that grant baccalaureate and graduate degrees. The institutions that sponsor the nursing programs must be accredited by accrediting agencies approved by the U.S. Department of Education (USDE) or the Council for Higher Education Accreditation (CHEA) or be candidates for accreditation with an agency recognized by the USDE for its preaccreditation category. Canadian schools may be provincially chartered instead of accredited.

Baccalaureate-level and master's-level nursing programs represented by a profile within the guide are accredited by the National League for Nursing Accrediting Commission (NLNAC) or the Commission on Collegiate Nursing Education (CCNE). Canadian nursing schools are members of the Canadian Association of University Schools of Nursing (CAUSN).

Doctoral, postdoctoral, continuing education, and other nursing programs included in the profiles are offered by nursing schools or departments affiliated with colleges or universities that meet the criteria outlined above.

QUICK-REFERENCE CHART

NURSING PROGRAMS AT-A-GLANCE

	Baccalaureate	Master's	Accelerated	Joint Degree	Post-Master's	Doctoral	Postdoctoral	Continuing Education
U.S. AND U.S. TERRITORIES								
Alabama								
Auburn University	•	•	B					
Auburn University Montgomery	•	•						
Jacksonville State University	•	•						•
Oakwood College	•							
Samford University	•	•		•	•			•
Spring Hill College	•	•	M					
Troy University	•	•			•			
Tuskegee University	•							
The University of Alabama	•	•			•	•		•
The University of Alabama at Birmingham	•	•	B,M	•	•	•	•	
The University of Alabama in Huntsville	•	•			•			•
University of Mobile	•	•						•
University of North Alabama	•							•
University of South Alabama	•	•	B,M		•			
Alaska								
University of Alaska Anchorage	•	•						
Arizona								
Arizona State University at the Downtown Phoenix Campus	•	•	B	•	•	•		•
Grand Canyon University	•	•	B	•	•			•
Northern Arizona University	•	•	B		•			
The University of Arizona	•	•	B		•	•	•	
University of Phoenix Online Campus	•	•	B	•	•			
University of Phoenix-Phoenix Campus	•	•	B		•			•
University of Phoenix-Southern Arizona Campus	•	•	B		•			
Arkansas								
Arkansas State University	•	•						
Arkansas Tech University	•							
Harding University	•							•
Henderson State University	•							
Southern Arkansas University-Magnolia	•							
University of Arkansas	•	•						•
University of Arkansas at Fort Smith	•							
University of Arkansas at Monticello	•							
University of Arkansas at Pine Bluff	•							
University of Arkansas for Medical Sciences	•		B			•	•	•
University of Central Arkansas	•	•			•			
California								
Azusa Pacific University	•	•	B,M		•	•		•
Biola University	•							•
California State University, Bakersfield	•	•	B		•			
California State University, Chico	•	•			•			•
California State University, Dominguez Hills	•	•			•			•
California State University, East Bay	•							
California State University, Fresno	•	•			•			•

B = Baccalaureate; M = Master's

	Baccalaureate	Master's	Accelerated	Joint Degree	Post-Master's	Doctoral	Postdoctoral	Continuing Education
California State University, Fullerton	●	●	M					●
California State University, Long Beach	●	●	M	●	●			
California State University, Los Angeles	●	●	M		●			
California State University, Northridge	●							
California State University, Sacramento	●	●						●
California State University, San Bernardino	●	●						
California State University, Stanislaus	●							
Dominican University of California	●	●						●
Holy Names University	●	●		●	●			
Humboldt State University	●							
Loma Linda University	●	●	B	●	●	●		
Mount St. Mary's College	●	●	B					
National University	●		B					
Pacific Union College	●							●
Point Loma Nazarene University	●	●						●
Samuel Merritt College	●	●	B		●			
San Diego State University	●	●			●			●
San Francisco State University	●	●	B,M		●			●
San Jose State University	●	●						
Sonoma State University	●	●			●			
University of California, Los Angeles	●	●		●	●	●	●	●
University of California, San Francisco		●			●	●	●	
University of Phoenix–Bay Area Campus	●	●	B	●				
University of Phoenix–Central Valley Campus	●	●						
University of Phoenix–Sacramento Valley Campus	●	●	B		●			
University of Phoenix–San Diego Campus	●	●	B					
University of Phoenix–Southern California Campus	●	●	B	●	●			
University of San Diego	●	●	M	●	●	●		
University of San Francisco	●	●	M					●
Western University of Health Sciences		●	M		●			
Colorado								
Colorado State University-Pueblo	●	●	B		●			
Mesa State College	●							
Metropolitan State College of Denver	●							
Regis University	●	●	B					
University of Colorado at Colorado Springs	●	●	B		●	●		●
University of Colorado at Denver and Health Sciences Center	●	●		●	●	●	●	●
University of Northern Colorado	●	●	B		●	●		
University of Phoenix–Denver Campus	●	●	B					
University of Phoenix–Southern Colorado Campus	●	●	B					
Connecticut								
Central Connecticut State University	●							
Fairfield University	●	●	B		●			
Quinnipiac University	●	●	B		●			●
Sacred Heart University	●	●	M	●	●			●
Saint Joseph College	●	●	B,M		●			
Southern Connecticut State University	●	●			●			
University of Connecticut	●	●		●	●	●		●
University of Hartford	●	●		●	●			●
Western Connecticut State University	●	●			●			
Yale University		●		●	●	●	●	

B = Baccalaureate; M = Master's

	Baccalaureate	Master's	Accelerated	Joint Degree	Post-Master's	Doctoral	Postdoctoral	Continuing Education
Delaware								
Delaware State University	•							
University of Delaware	•	•	B		•			
Wesley College	•	•	M		•			•
Wilmington College	•	•	B	•	•			
District of Columbia								
The Catholic University of America	•	•	B	•	•	•		
Georgetown University	•	•	B		•			•
Howard University	•	•	B		•			
University of the District of Columbia	•							
Florida								
Barry University	•	•	B	•	•	•		
Bethune-Cookman College	•							
Florida Agricultural and Mechanical University	•	•			•	•		•
Florida Atlantic University	•	•	B	•	•	•		•
Florida Gulf Coast University	•	•	B,M		•			•
Florida Hospital College of Health Sciences	•							
Florida International University	•	•	B		•	•		
Florida Southern College	•	•	M		•			•
Florida State University	•	•			•			•
Jacksonville University	•	•	B,M	•				
Nova Southeastern University	•	•		•				
St. Petersburg College	•							•
South University	•							
University of Central Florida	•	•	B		•	•		
University of Florida	•	•	B		•	•		
University of Miami	•	•	B,M		•	•		•
University of North Florida	•	•	B		•			
University of Phoenix–Central Florida Campus	•	•	B	•				
University of Phoenix–North Florida Campus	•	•	B					
University of Phoenix–South Florida Campus	•	•		•				
University of Phoenix–West Florida Campus	•	•	B	•				
University of South Florida	•	•	B	•	•	•		•
The University of Tampa	•	•	M		•			
University of West Florida	•							
Georgia								
Albany State University	•	•	B,M		•			
Armstrong Atlantic State University	•	•		•	•			
Brenau University	•	•			•			•
Clayton State University	•							
Columbus State University	•		B					
Emory University	•	•		•	•	•		
Georgia Baptist College of Nursing of Mercer University	•	•			•			•
Georgia College & State University	•	•		•	•			
Georgia Southern University	•	•			•			
Georgia Southwestern State University	•							•
Georgia State University	•	•	B		•	•		
Kennesaw State University	•	•	B					•
LaGrange College	•							
Macon State College	•							

B = Baccalaureate; M = Master's

	Baccalaureate	Master's	Accelerated	Joint Degree	Post-Master's	Doctoral	Postdoctoral	Continuing Education
Medical College of Georgia	•	•	M		•	•		
North Georgia College & State University	•	•			•			
Piedmont College	•							
Thomas University	•	•			•			
University of Phoenix–Atlanta Campus	•	•	B,M					
University of West Georgia	•	•			•			
Valdosta State University	•	•						•
Guam								
University of Guam	•							
Hawaii								
Hawai'i Pacific University	•	•	B	•	•			
University of Hawaii at Hilo	•							
University of Hawaii at Manoa	•	•			•	•		
University of Phoenix–Hawaii Campus	•	•	B		•			
Idaho								
Boise State University	•	•						
Idaho State University	•	•	B,M		•			
Lewis-Clark State College	•							•
Northwest Nazarene University	•							
Illinois								
Aurora University	•							
Benedictine University	•		B					
Blessing–Rieman College of Nursing	•		B					
Bradley University	•	•	M					
Chicago State University	•							
DePaul University	•	•	B		•			
Elmhurst College	•							
Governors State University	•	•			•			
Illinois State University	•	•	B		•			
Illinois Wesleyan University	•							
Lakeview College of Nursing	•		B					
Lewis University	•	•	B,M	•	•			•
Loyola University Chicago	•	•	B	•		•		
MacMurray College	•							
McKendree College	•	•						
Millikin University	•		B					
Northern Illinois University	•	•		•	•			
North Park University	•	•		•	•			
Olivet Nazarene University	•	•	B					
Rockford College	•							
Rush University	•	•	B,M		•	•	•	•
Saint Anthony College of Nursing	•	•			•			
Saint Francis Medical Center College of Nursing	•	•						
St. John's College	•							
Saint Xavier University	•	•		•	•			•
Southern Illinois University Edwardsville	•	•	B		•			•
Trinity Christian College	•							
Trinity College of Nursing and Health Sciences	•							
University of Illinois at Chicago	•	•		•	•	•	•	
University of St. Francis	•	•	B					

B = Baccalaureate; M = Master's

Illinois *(continued)*	Baccalaureate	Master's	Accelerated	Joint Degree	Post-Master's	Doctoral	Postdoctoral	Continuing Education
West Suburban College of Nursing	•	•	B,M		•			
Indiana								
Ball State University	•	•	B		•			
Bethel College	•	•			•			
Goshen College	•							
Indiana State University	•	•			•			•
Indiana University Bloomington	•							
Indiana University East	•							
Indiana University Kokomo	•		B					•
Indiana University Northwest	•							
Indiana University–Purdue University Fort Wayne	•	•						•
Indiana University–Purdue University Indianapolis	•	•	B	•	•	•	•	•
Indiana University South Bend	•		B					
Indiana University Southeast	•							
Indiana Wesleyan University	•	•	B		•			
Marian College	•		B					
Purdue University	•	•			•	•		•
Purdue University Calumet	•	•	M		•			
Purdue University North Central	•							
Saint Mary's College	•		B					
University of Evansville	•							
University of Indianapolis	•	•	B	•	•			
University of Saint Francis	•	•	M		•			
University of Southern Indiana	•	•			•			•
Valparaiso University	•	•	B	•	•			•
Iowa								
Allen College	•	•	B		•			•
Briar Cliff University	•	•						•
Clarke College	•	•			•			•
Coe College	•							
Grand View College	•							•
Iowa Wesleyan College	•							•
Luther College	•							•
Mercy College of Health Sciences	•		B					
Morningside College	•							
Mount Mercy College	•		B					•
St. Ambrose University	•							
The University of Iowa	•	•	M	•	•	•	•	•
Kansas								
Baker University	•							
Bethel College	•							
Emporia State University	•							
Fort Hays State University	•	•			•			
Kansas Wesleyan University	•							
MidAmerica Nazarene University	•		B					•
Newman University	•							
Pittsburg State University	•	•			•			•
Southwestern College	•							
Tabor College	•		B					
University of Kansas	•	•	M		•	•		•
Washburn University	•	•			•			•

B = Baccalaureate; M = Master's

	Baccalaureate	Master's	Accelerated	Joint Degree	Post-Master's	Doctoral	Postdoctoral	Continuing Education
Wichita State University	•	•		•	•	•		
Kentucky								
Bellarmine University	•	•	B	•				•
Berea College	•							•
Eastern Kentucky University	•	•						
Kentucky Christian University	•							•
Kentucky State University	•							
Midway College	•		B					•
Morehead State University	•							
Murray State University	•				•			•
Northern Kentucky University	•	•	B		•			
Spalding University	•	•	B,M		•			•
Thomas More College	•							
University of Kentucky	•	•			•	•		•
University of Louisville	•	•	B		•	•		
Western Kentucky University	•	•			•			•
Louisiana								
Dillard University	•							
Grambling State University	•	•			•			
Louisiana College	•							
Louisiana State University Health Sciences Center	•	•				•		•
Loyola University New Orleans	•	•			•			
McNeese State University	•	•	B					•
Nicholls State University	•							•
Northwestern State University of Louisiana	•	•			•			•
Our Lady of Holy Cross College	•							
Our Lady of the Lake College	•	•						•
Southeastern Louisiana University	•	•	B					
Southern University and Agricultural and Mechanical College	•	•			•	•		
University of Louisiana at Lafayette	•	•	B		•			•
University of Louisiana at Monroe	•		B					•
University of Phoenix–Louisiana Campus	•	•	B	•				
Maine								
Husson College	•	•			•			
Saint Joseph's College of Maine	•	•						•
University of Maine	•	•						
University of Maine at Fort Kent	•		B					
University of New England	•							•
University of Southern Maine	•	•	B	•	•			•
Maryland								
Bowie State University	•	•						
College of Notre Dame of Maryland	•		B					
Columbia Union College	•		B					
Coppin State University	•	•	B		•			
The Johns Hopkins University	•	•	B	•	•	•	•	•
Salisbury University	•	•	B		•			
Towson University	•	•						
University of Maryland, Baltimore	•	•	M	•	•	•		•
Villa Julie College	•		B					

B = Baccalaureate; M = Master's

	Baccalaureate	Master's	Accelerated	Joint Degree	Post-Master's	Doctoral	Postdoctoral	Continuing Education
Massachusetts								
American International College	•	•						
Anna Maria College	•							
Atlantic Union College	•							
Boston College	•	•	M	•	•	•		•
Curry College	•		B					
Elms College	•							
Emmanuel College	•							
Endicott College	•							•
Fitchburg State College	•	•						
Framingham State College	•							
MGH Institute of Health Professions		•			•			•
Northeastern University	•	•	M	•	•			•
Regis College	•	•	B,M		•	•		•
Salem State College	•	•	B,M	•				•
Simmons College	•	•	B,M		•			•
University of Massachusetts Amherst	•	•	B			•		•
University of Massachusetts Boston	•	•			•	•		•
University of Massachusetts Dartmouth	•	•			•			•
University of Massachusetts Lowell	•	•	M			•		
University of Massachusetts Worcester		•			•	•		•
Worcester State College	•	•	B					
Michigan								
Andrews University	•	•			•			
Calvin College	•							
Eastern Michigan University	•	•						
Ferris State University	•	•	B	•				
Grand Valley State University	•	•	B	•	•			•
Hope College	•							
Lake Superior State University	•							
Madonna University	•	•	M	•	•			•
Michigan State University	•	•	B		•	•	•	•
Northern Michigan University	•	•	B		•			•
Oakland University	•	•			•			•
Saginaw Valley State University	•	•	B		•			•
Spring Arbor University	•							
University of Detroit Mercy	•	•	M		•			
University of Michigan	•	•	B,M	•	•	•	•	
University of Michigan–Flint	•	•						•
University of Phoenix–Metro Detroit Campus	•	•	B	•				
University of Phoenix–West Michigan Campus	•	•	B					
Wayne State University	•	•	B,M		•	•	•	•
Western Michigan University	•							
Minnesota								
Augsburg College	•	•						
Bemidji State University	•							•
Bethel University	•	•						•
College of Saint Benedict	•							
College of St. Catherine	•	•			•			
The College of St. Scholastica	•	•	B		•			
Concordia College	•	•	B					

B = Baccalaureate; M = Master's

Peterson's Nursing Programs 2008	Baccalaureate	Master's	Accelerated	Joint Degree	Post-Master's	Doctoral	Postdoctoral	Continuing Education
Gustavus Adolphus College	•							
Metropolitan State University	•	•			•			
Minnesota Intercollegiate Nursing Consortium	•							
Minnesota State University Mankato	•	•	B		•			•
Minnesota State University Moorhead	•	•						
St. Cloud State University	•							
St. Olaf College	•							
University of Minnesota, Twin Cities Campus	•	•		•		•		•
Winona State University	•	•			•			
Mississippi								
Alcorn State University	•	•			•			
Delta State University	•	•	M		•			
Mississippi College	•							
Mississippi University for Women	•	•			•			
University of Mississippi Medical Center	•	•	B,M		•	•		•
University of Southern Mississippi	•	•			•	•		
William Carey College	•	•						
Missouri								
Avila University	•							
Barnes-Jewish College of Nursing and Allied Health	•	•			•			
Chamberlain College of Nursing	•							
Cox College of Nursing and Health Sciences	•		B					•
Graceland University	•	•	B		•			
Lincoln University	•							
Maryville University of Saint Louis	•	•	B,M					
Missouri Southern State University	•							
Missouri State University	•	•	M		•			•
Missouri Western State University	•							
Research College of Nursing	•	•	B					
Saint Louis University	•	•	B	•	•	•		•
Saint Luke's College	•							
Southeast Missouri State University	•	•			•			
Southwest Baptist University	•							
Truman State University	•							
University of Central Missouri	•	•			•			
University of Missouri–Columbia	•	•	B		•	•		•
University of Missouri–Kansas City	•	•			•	•		
University of Missouri–St. Louis	•	•	B			•		
Webster University	•	•						
William Jewell College	•		B					
Montana								
Carroll College	•							•
Montana State University	•	•			•			
Montana State University–Northern	•							
Salish Kootenai College	•							
Nebraska								
Clarkson College	•	•	B		•			•
College of Saint Mary	•							
Creighton University	•	•	B		•			
Midland Lutheran College	•							•

B = Baccalaureate; M = Master's

	Baccalaureate	Master's	Accelerated	Joint Degree	Post-Master's	Doctoral	Postdoctoral	Continuing Education
Nebraska *(continued)*								
Nebraska Methodist College	•	•	B		•			•
Nebraska Wesleyan University	•	•	B,M		•			
Union College	•							
University of Nebraska Medical Center	•	•	B		•	•	•	•
Nevada								
Nevada State College at Henderson	•							
University of Nevada, Las Vegas	•	•			•	•		•
University of Nevada, Reno	•	•	B	•	•			
New Hampshire								
Colby-Sawyer College	•							
Rivier College	•	•		•	•			
Saint Anselm College	•							•
University of New Hampshire	•	•			•			
New Jersey								
Bloomfield College	•							
The College of New Jersey	•	•			•			
College of Saint Elizabeth	•		B					•
Fairleigh Dickinson University, Metropolitan Campus	•	•	B,M		•	•		
Felician College	•	•	B	•	•			
Kean University	•	•	M	•				•
Monmouth University	•	•			•			•
New Jersey City University	•	•						
The Richard Stockton College of New Jersey	•	•						
Rutgers, The State University of New Jersey, Camden College of Arts and Sciences	•	•	B					
Rutgers, The State University of New Jersey, College of Nursing	•	•	B	•	•	•		•
Saint Peter's College	•	•			•			
Seton Hall University	•	•	B	•	•	•		•
Thomas Edison State College	•	•						
University of Medicine and Dentistry of New Jersey	•	•	B		•			•
William Paterson University of New Jersey	•	•	B		•			
New Mexico								
Eastern New Mexico University	•							
New Mexico State University	•	•	B					•
University of New Mexico	•	•	B	•	•	•		
University of Phoenix–New Mexico Campus	•	•	B	•				
New York								
Adelphi University	•	•	B	•	•	•		
College of Mount Saint Vincent	•	•			•			
The College of New Rochelle	•	•	B		•			
College of Staten Island of the City University of New York	•	•			•			
Columbia University	•	•	B,M	•	•	•		•
Daemen College	•	•	B,M		•			
Dominican College	•		B					
D'Youville College	•	•	M		•			
Elmira College	•							•
Excelsior College	•	•						
Hartwick College	•		B					
Hunter College of the City University of New York	•	•		•	•			•
Keuka College	•		B					

	Baccalaureate	Master's	Accelerated	Joint Degree	Post-Master's	Doctoral	Postdoctoral	Continuing Education
Lehman College of the City University of New York	•	•						
Long Island University, Brooklyn Campus	•	•			•			
Long Island University, C.W. Post Campus	•	•			•			
Medgar Evers College of the City University of New York	•		B					
Mercy College	•	•	B,M		•			•
Molloy College	•	•	B		•			•
Mount Saint Mary College	•	•	B		•			
Nazareth College of Rochester	•	•			•			•
New York University	•	•	B	•	•		•	•
Pace University	•	•	B,M		•			•
Roberts Wesleyan College	•		B,M					•
The Sage Colleges	•	•		•	•			
St. Francis College	•							
St. John Fisher College	•	•			•			
St. Joseph's College, New York	•	•						
State University of New York at Binghamton	•	•	B		•	•		•
State University of New York at New Paltz	•	•						
State University of New York at Plattsburgh	•							•
State University of New York College at Brockport	•							
State University of New York Downstate Medical Center	•	•	B	•	•			•
State University of New York Institute of Technology	•	•	B,M		•			•
State University of New York Upstate Medical University	•	•			•			•
Stony Brook University, State University of New York	•	•	B		•			•
Teachers College Columbia University						•		
University at Buffalo, the State University of New York	•	•	B		•	•		
University of Rochester	•	•	B,M		•	•	•	•
Utica College	•							•
Wagner College	•	•			•			
York College of the City University of New York	•							
North Carolina								
Barton College	•							
Cabarrus College of Health Sciences	•							
Duke University	•	•	B	•	•	•		
East Carolina University	•	•	B		•	•		
Fayetteville State University	•							
Gardner-Webb University	•	•		•				
Lees-McRae College	•							
Lenoir-Rhyne College	•							
North Carolina Agricultural and Technical State University	•							
North Carolina Central University	•							
Queens University of Charlotte	•	•	M	•	•			
The University of North Carolina at Chapel Hill	•	•	B		•	•	•	•
The University of North Carolina at Charlotte	•	•			•			•
The University of North Carolina at Greensboro	•	•		•	•	•		
The University of North Carolina at Pembroke	•							
The University of North Carolina Wilmington	•	•						
Western Carolina University	•	•			•			
Winston-Salem State University	•	•	B					•
North Dakota								
Dickinson State University	•							
Jamestown College	•							

B = Baccalaureate; M = Master's

North Dakota *(continued)*	Baccalaureate	Master's	Accelerated	Joint Degree	Post-Master's	Doctoral	Postdoctoral	Continuing Education
Medcenter One College of Nursing	•							
Minot State University	•							
North Dakota State University	•	•				•		
University of Mary	•	•						
University of North Dakota	•	•			•	•		
Ohio								
Ashland University	•		B					
Capital University	•	•	B	•	•			•
Case Western Reserve University	•	•	M	•	•	•	•	•
Cedarville University	•							
Cleveland State University	•	•	B	•				•
College of Mount St. Joseph	•	•	B,M					
Franciscan University of Steubenville	•	•						
Kent State University	•	•	B,M	•	•	•		•
Kettering College of Medical Arts	•							
Lourdes College	•							
Malone College	•	•						•
MedCentral College of Nursing	•		B					
Mercy College of Northwest Ohio	•							
Miami University	•							
Mount Carmel College of Nursing	•	•	B		•			
The Ohio State University	•	•	B,M		•	•		
Ohio University	•	•						
Otterbein College	•	•	B		•			•
Shawnee State University	•							•
The University of Akron	•	•	B		•	•		•
University of Cincinnati	•	•	M	•	•	•		•
University of Phoenix–Cleveland Campus	•	•	B	•				
The University of Toledo	•	•			•			•
Ursuline College	•	•	B,M		•			
Walsh University	•		B					
Wright State University	•	•	B	•	•			•
Xavier University	•	•		•				
Youngstown State University	•	•						
Oklahoma								
Bacone College	•		B					
East Central University	•							
Langston University	•							
Northeastern State University	•		B					
Northwestern Oklahoma State University	•							
Oklahoma Baptist University	•							
Oklahoma City University	•	•	B	•				•
Oklahoma Panhandle State University	•							
Oklahoma Wesleyan University	•		B					
Oral Roberts University	•							
Southern Nazarene University	•	•	M					
Southwestern Oklahoma State University	•							
University of Central Oklahoma	•							
University of Oklahoma Health Sciences Center	•	•	B		•			•
University of Phoenix–Oklahoma City Campus	•	•	B					
University of Phoenix–Tulsa Campus								

B = Baccalaureate; M = Master's

	Baccalaureate	Master's	Accelerated	Joint Degree	Post-Master's	Doctoral	Postdoctoral	Continuing Education
University of Tulsa	•							
Oregon								
Linfield College	•		B					•
Oregon Health & Science University	•	•	B,M	•	•	•	•	•
University of Portland	•	•						
Pennsylvania								
Alvernia College	•							•
Bloomsburg University of Pennsylvania	•	•		•	•			
California University of Pennsylvania	•							
Carlow University	•	•	B,M		•			•
Cedar Crest College	•							
Clarion University of Pennsylvania	•	•	M		•			
College Misericordia	•	•	B,M		•			
DeSales University	•	•	B,M	•	•			•
Drexel University	•	•	B		•	•		•
Duquesne University	•	•	B		•	•		•
Eastern University	•		B					•
East Stroudsburg University of Pennsylvania	•							
Edinboro University of Pennsylvania	•		B					
Gannon University	•	•			•			
Gwynedd-Mercy College	•	•	B		•			
Holy Family University	•	•	B					•
Immaculata University	•	•	B					
Indiana University of Pennsylvania	•	•						
Kutztown University of Pennsylvania	•							
La Roche College	•	•	B					•
La Salle University	•	•		•	•			•
Mansfield University of Pennsylvania	•	•						
Marywood University	•	•		•				•
Messiah College	•							
Millersville University of Pennsylvania	•	•			•			•
Moravian College	•							•
Mount Aloysius College	•		B					•
Neumann College	•	•			•			
Penn State University Park	•	•			•	•	•	•
Pennsylvania College of Technology	•							
Robert Morris University	•	•						
Saint Francis University	•							
Slippery Rock University of Pennsylvania	•	•			•			
Temple University	•	•	B		•			
Thomas Jefferson University	•	•	B,M		•	•		•
University of Pennsylvania	•	•	B,M	•	•	•	•	•
University of Pittsburgh	•	•	B		•	•	•	•
University of Pittsburgh at Bradford	•							
The University of Scranton	•	•	B,M		•			
Villanova University	•	•	B,M		•	•		•
Waynesburg College	•	•	B,M	•		•		
West Chester University of Pennsylvania	•	•	B					
Widener University	•	•	M		•	•		
Wilkes University	•	•	B,M		•			•
York College of Pennsylvania	•	•						

B = Baccalaureate; M = Master's

	Baccalaureate	Master's	Accelerated	Joint Degree	Post-Master's	Doctoral	Postdoctoral	Continuing Education
Puerto Rico								
Inter American University of Puerto Rico, Metropolitan Campus	•		B					
Pontifical Catholic University of Puerto Rico	•							
Universidad Adventista de las Antillas	•							•
Universidad del Turabo	•							
Universidad Metropolitana	•							
University of Puerto Rico at Arecibo	•							
University of Puerto Rico at Humacao	•							
University of Puerto Rico, Mayagüez Campus	•							•
University of Puerto Rico, Medical Sciences Campus	•	•						•
University of the Sacred Heart	•	•						
Rhode Island								
Rhode Island College	•							
Salve Regina University	•							•
University of Rhode Island	•	•			•	•		
South Carolina								
Charleston Southern University	•							
Clemson University	•	•			•			•
Francis Marion University	•							
Lander University	•		B					
Medical University of South Carolina	•	•	B,M		•	•		•
South Carolina State University	•							
University of South Carolina	•	•		•	•	•		
University of South Carolina Aiken	•							•
University of South Carolina Upstate	•		B					
South Dakota								
Augustana College	•	•			•			
Mount Marty College	•							
Presentation College	•							
South Dakota State University	•	•	B		•	•		•
Tennessee								
Aquinas College	•							
Austin Peay State University	•							
Baptist College of Health Sciences	•							
Belmont University	•	•	B		•			
Carson-Newman College	•	•	B		•			
Cumberland University	•		B					
East Tennessee State University	•	•	B		•	•		
King College	•		B	•				
Lincoln Memorial University	•							
Middle Tennessee State University	•							•
Milligan College	•							
South College	•							
Southern Adventist University	•	•	M	•				•
Tennessee State University	•	•			•			
Tennessee Technological University	•	•						
Tennessee Wesleyan College	•							
Union University	•	•	B		•			•
University of Memphis	•	•	B,M					
The University of Tennessee	•	•	B,M		•	•		•

B = Baccalaureate; M = Master's

	Baccalaureate	Master's	Accelerated	Joint Degree	Post-Master's	Doctoral	Postdoctoral	Continuing Education
The University of Tennessee at Chattanooga	•	•			•			•
The University of Tennessee at Martin	•		B					•
The University of Tennessee Health Science Center	•	•	B		•	•		•
Vanderbilt University		•	M	•	•	•	•	•
Texas								
Angelo State University	•	•						
Baylor University	•	•			•			
East Texas Baptist University	•							
Houston Baptist University	•							
Lamar University	•	•		•				•
Lubbock Christian University	•							
Midwestern State University	•	•			•			•
Patty Hanks Shelton School of Nursing	•	•			•			•
Prairie View A&M University	•	•						
Southwestern Adventist University	•							•
Stephen F. Austin State University	•							
Tarleton State University	•							•
Texas A&M International University	•	•						•
Texas A&M University–Corpus Christi	•	•	B,M		•			•
Texas A&M University–Texarkana	•							
Texas Christian University	•	•	B					•
Texas Tech University Health Sciences Center	•	•	B		•			•
Texas Woman's University	•	•			•	•		
University of Mary Hardin-Baylor	•							•
The University of Texas at Arlington	•	•		•	•	•		•
The University of Texas at Austin	•	•		•	•	•	•	
The University of Texas at Brownsville	•	•						
The University of Texas at El Paso	•	•	B		•	•		
The University of Texas at Tyler	•	•	B,M	•	•	•		•
The University of Texas Health Science Center at Houston	•	•	B,M	•	•	•		•
The University of Texas Health Science Center at San Antonio	•	•		•	•	•		•
The University of Texas Medical Branch	•	•	B		•	•		•
The University of Texas–Pan American	•	•			•			
University of the Incarnate Word	•	•		•				
West Texas A&M University	•	•			•			
Utah								
Brigham Young University	•	•			•			
Southern Utah University	•							
University of Phoenix–Utah Campus	•	•	B					
University of Utah	•	•			•	•	•	
Utah Valley State College	•							
Weber State University	•							
Westminster College	•	•			•			
Vermont								
Norwich University	•							
Southern Vermont College	•							
University of Vermont	•	•	B		•			
Virgin Islands								
University of the Virgin Islands	•							•

B = Baccalaureate; M = Master's

	Baccalaureate	Master's	Accelerated	Joint Degree	Post-Master's	Doctoral	Postdoctoral	Continuing Education
Virginia								
Eastern Mennonite University	•							
George Mason University	•	•	B	•	•	•		•
Hampton University	•	•	B		•	•		
James Madison University	•	•	B,M		•			
Jefferson College of Health Sciences	•	•						•
Liberty University	•	•						
Lynchburg College	•							
Marymount University	•	•	B		•			
Norfolk State University	•		B					
Old Dominion University	•	•	B		•			•
Radford University	•	•	M		•			
Shenandoah University	•	•	B		•			•
University of Virginia	•	•	M	•	•	•	•	
The University of Virginia's College at Wise	•							
Virginia Commonwealth University	•	•	B,M	•	•	•		
Washington								
Gonzaga University	•	•	M		•			•
Intercollegiate College of Nursing/Washington State University	•	•	M		•			•
Northwest University	•							
Pacific Lutheran University	•	•	M					•
Seattle Pacific University	•	•			•			
Seattle University	•	•	M		•			
University of Washington	•	•		•	•	•		•
Walla Walla College	•							
West Virginia								
Alderson-Broaddus College	•							
Bluefield State College	•							
Fairmont State University	•							•
Marshall University	•	•	B		•			
Mountain State University	•	•			•			
Shepherd University	•							•
University of Charleston	•							
West Liberty State College	•		B					
West Virginia University	•	•	B		•	•		
West Virginia Wesleyan College	•							•
Wheeling Jesuit University	•	•						
Wisconsin								
Alverno College	•	•						•
Bellin College of Nursing	•	•	B					
Cardinal Stritch University	•	•	B,M					
Carroll College	•							
Columbia College of Nursing/Mount Mary College Nursing Program	•							
Concordia University Wisconsin	•	•						
Edgewood College	•	•						
Marian College of Fond du Lac	•	•			•			
Marquette University	•	•	M	•	•	•		•
Milwaukee School of Engineering	•							
University of Wisconsin-Eau Claire	•	•	B					•
University of Wisconsin–Green Bay	•							

B = Baccalaureate; M = Master's

	Baccalaureate	Master's	Accelerated	Joint Degree	Post-Master's	Doctoral	Postdoctoral	Continuing Education
University of Wisconsin–Madison	•	•	B,M	•	•	•	•	•
University of Wisconsin–Milwaukee	•	•	M	•	•	•		•
University of Wisconsin–Oshkosh	•	•	B		•			•
Viterbo University	•	•			•			•
Wyoming								
University of Wyoming	•	•	B		•			
CANADA								
Alberta								
Athabasca University	•							
University of Alberta	•	•			•	•		
University of Calgary	•	•	B		•	•		
University of Lethbridge	•	•						
British Columbia								
British Columbia Institute of Technology	•							•
Kwantlen University College	•							
Malaspina University-College	•							
Thompson Rivers University	•							•
Trinity Western University	•							
The University of British Columbia	•	•	B			•	•	
The University of British Columbia–Okanagan	•							
University of Northern British Columbia	•							
University of Victoria	•	•				•		
Manitoba								
Brandon University	•							
University of Manitoba	•	•				•		•
New Brunswick								
Université de Moncton	•							•
University of New Brunswick Fredericton	•	•						•
Newfoundland and Labrador								
Memorial University of Newfoundland	•	•	B					
Nova Scotia								
Dalhousie University	•	•	B		•	•		
St. Francis Xavier University	•		B					•
Ontario								
Brock University	•							
Lakehead University	•							
Laurentian University	•							•
McMaster University	•	•				•		
Nipissing University	•							
Queen's University at Kingston	•	•	B					
Ryerson University	•	•						•
Trent University	•		B					
University of Ottawa	•					•	•	
University of Toronto	•	•	B		•	•		
The University of Western Ontario	•		B			•	•	
University of Windsor	•	•						•

B = Baccalaureate; M = Master's

	Baccalaureate	Master's	Accelerated	Joint Degree	Post-Master's	Doctoral	Postdoctoral	Continuing Education
Ontario *(continued)*								
York University	•							•
Prince Edward Island								
University of Prince Edward Island	•							
Quebec								
McGill University	•	•				•	•	
Université de Montréal	•	•				•		
Université de Sherbrooke	•	•				•	•	
Université du Québec à Chicoutimi	•	•	B,M					
Université du Québec à Rimouski	•							•
Université du Québec à Trois-Rivières	•	•						
Université du Québec en Abitibi-Témiscamingue	•							
Université du Québec en Outaouais	•							
Université Laval	•	•				•		•
Saskatchewan								
University of Saskatchewan	•	•	B					•

B = Baccalaureate; M = Master's

PROFILES OF NURSING PROGRAMS

U.S. AND U.S. TERRITORIES

ALABAMA

Auburn University
School of Nursing
Auburn University, Alabama

http://www.auburn.edu/academic/nursing/au_nursing.html
Founded in 1856
DEGREES • BSN • MSN

Nursing Program Faculty 15 (75% with doctorates).
Baccalaureate Enrollment 181
Women 90% **Men** 10% **Minority** 3%
Nursing Student Activities Nursing Honor Society, Sigma Theta Tau, Student Nurses' Association, nursing club.
Nursing Student Resources Academic advising; academic or career counseling; assistance for students with disabilities; bookstore; campus computer network; career placement assistance; computer lab; computer-assisted instruction; e-mail services; employment services for current students; interactive nursing skills videos; Internet; library services; nursing audiovisuals; placement services for program completers; remedial services; resume preparation assistance; skills, simulation, or other laboratory; tutoring.
Library Facilities 3.7 million volumes; 29,355 periodical subscriptions.

BACCALAUREATE PROGRAMS
Degree BSN

Available Programs Accelerated Baccalaureate for Second Degree; Generic Baccalaureate.
Study Options Full-time.
Program Entrance Requirements Minimum overall college GPA of 2.5, transcript of college record, CPR certification, health exam, health insurance, immunizations, minimum GPA in nursing prerequisites of 2.5, professional liability insurance/malpractice insurance, prerequisite course work. Transfer students are accepted. **Standardized tests** *Required:* SAT or ACT, TOEFL for international students. **Application** *Deadline:* 8/1 (freshmen), rolling (transfer). *Notification:* continuous (freshmen). *Application fee:* $25.
Expenses (2006–07) *Tuition, area resident:* full-time $5000. *Tuition, nonresident:* full-time $15,000.
Financial Aid 60% of baccalaureate students in nursing programs received some form of financial aid in 2005–06.
Contact Pam Hennessey, Academic Advisor, School of Nursing, Auburn University, 118 Miller Hall, Auburn University, AL 36849. *Telephone:* 334-844-6754. *Fax:* 334-844-4177. *E-mail:* hennepp@auburn.edu.

GRADUATE PROGRAMS
Contact Dr. Jenny Hamner, Assistant Dean of Nursing, School of Nursing, Auburn University, 118 Miller Hall, Auburn University, AL 36849. *Telephone:* 334-844-5665. *E-mail:* hamnejb@auburn.edu.

MASTER'S DEGREE PROGRAM
Degree MSN

Available Programs Master's.
Concentrations Available Nursing education. *Clinical nurse specialist programs in:* adult health, gerontology, pediatric.
Study Options Full-time and part-time.

Program Entrance Requirements Minimum overall college GPA of 3.0, transcript of college record, nursing research course, statistics course.
Degree Requirements 51 total credit hours, thesis or project.

Auburn University Montgomery
School of Nursing
Montgomery, Alabama

http://www.aum.edu
Founded in 1967
DEGREES • BSN • MSN

Nursing Program Faculty 20 (30% with doctorates).
Baccalaureate Enrollment 350
Women 80% **Men** 20% **Minority** 33% **International** 1% **Part-time** 20%
Graduate Enrollment 6
Nursing Student Activities Nursing Honor Society, Sigma Theta Tau, Student Nurses' Association.
Nursing Student Resources Academic advising; academic or career counseling; assistance for students with disabilities; bookstore; campus computer network; career placement assistance; computer lab; computer-assisted instruction; daycare for children of students; e-mail services; housing assistance; interactive nursing skills videos; Internet; learning resource lab; library services; nursing audiovisuals; remedial services; resume preparation assistance; skills, simulation, or other laboratory; tutoring.
Library Facilities 347,044 volumes (9,568 in nursing); 2,303 periodical subscriptions (273 health-care related).

BACCALAUREATE PROGRAMS
Degree BSN

Available Programs Generic Baccalaureate; RN Baccalaureate.
Study Options Full-time and part-time.
Program Entrance Requirements Transcript of college record, CPR certification, health exam, high school transcript, immunizations, minimum GPA in nursing prerequisites of 2.5, professional liability insurance/malpractice insurance, prerequisite course work. Transfer students are accepted. **Standardized tests** *Required:* SAT or ACT, TOEFL for international students. **Application** *Deadline:* rolling (freshmen), rolling (transfer). *Notification:* continuous (freshmen). *Application fee:* $25.
Advanced Placement Credit by examination available.
Expenses (2006–07) *Tuition, state resident:* full-time $4368; part-time $156 per credit hour. *Tuition, nonresident:* full-time $12,768; part-time $456 per credit hour. *International tuition:* $12,768 full-time. *Room and board:* room only: $2200 per academic year. *Required fees:* full-time $40; part-time $40 per term.
Financial Aid 75% of baccalaureate students in nursing programs received some form of financial aid in 2005–06.
Contact Mrs. Lorinda Brewer Stutheit, Coordinator, Advising and Recruiting, School of Nursing, Auburn University Montgomery, PO Box 244023, Montgomery, AL 36124-4023. *Telephone:* 334-244-3863. *Fax:* 334-244-3243. *E-mail:* lorinda.stutheit@mail.aum.edu.

GRADUATE PROGRAMS
Expenses (2006–07) *Tuition, state resident:* full-time $2500; part-time $43 per credit hour. *Tuition, nonresident:* full-time $7500; part-time $129 per credit hour. *Room and board:* $2100 per academic year. *Required fees:* full-time $285.
Financial Aid 20% of graduate students in nursing programs received some form of financial aid in 2005–06.

Contact Dr. Anita C. All, Professor and Director, School of Nursing, Auburn University Montgomery, 213 Miller Hall, Auburn University, AL 36849-5055. *Telephone:* 334-844-5613. *Fax:* 334-844-4177. *E-mail:* msnnurse@auburn.edu.

MASTER'S DEGREE PROGRAM

Degree MSN

Available Programs Master's.

Concentrations Available Nursing education. *Clinical nurse specialist programs in:* adult health, gerontology, pediatric.

Study Options Full-time and part-time.

Program Entrance Requirements Clinical experience, minimum overall college GPA of 3.0, written essay, 3 letters of recommendation, resume, statistics course.

Degree Requirements 43 total credit hours.

Jacksonville State University
College of Nursing and Health Sciences
Jacksonville, Alabama

http://www.jsu.edu/depart/nursing

Founded in 1883

DEGREES • BSN • MSN

Nursing Program Faculty 25 (28% with doctorates).

Baccalaureate Enrollment 341
Women 86% **Men** 14% **Minority** 18% **International** 4% **Part-time** 25%

Graduate Enrollment 44
Women 91% **Men** 9% **Minority** 16% **Part-time** 59%

Nursing Student Activities Sigma Theta Tau, Student Nurses' Association.

Nursing Student Resources Academic advising; academic or career counseling; campus computer network; computer lab; computer-assisted instruction; e-mail services; Internet; learning resource lab; nursing audiovisuals; remedial services; skills, simulation, or other laboratory; tutoring.

Library Facilities 685,991 volumes (52,402 in health, 1,672 in nursing); 14,376 periodical subscriptions (825 health-care related).

BACCALAUREATE PROGRAMS

Degree BSN

Available Programs Generic Baccalaureate; RN Baccalaureate.

Study Options Full-time and part-time.

Program Entrance Requirements Transcript of college record, CPR certification, health exam, health insurance, high school transcript, immunizations, minimum GPA in nursing prerequisites, professional liability insurance/malpractice insurance, prerequisite course work. Transfer students are accepted. **Standardized tests** *Required:* SAT or ACT, TOEFL for international students. **Application** *Deadline:* rolling (freshmen), rolling (out-of-state freshmen), rolling (transfer). *Notification:* continuous (freshmen), continuous (out-of-state freshmen). *Application fee:* $20.

Expenses (2006–07) *Tuition, state resident:* full-time $4056; part-time $169 per credit hour. *Tuition, nonresident:* full-time $8112; part-time $338 per credit hour. *International tuition:* $8112 full-time. *Room and board:* $3258; room only: $2880 per academic year.

Financial Aid 70% of baccalaureate students in nursing programs received some form of financial aid in 2005–06.

Contact Mr. David Hofland, Student Services Coordinator, College of Nursing and Health Sciences, Jacksonville State University, 700 Pelham Road North, Jacksonville, AL 36265-1602. *Telephone:* 256-782-5276. *Fax:* 256-782-5406. *E-mail:* hofland@jsu.edu.

GRADUATE PROGRAMS

Expenses (2006–07) *Tuition, area resident:* full-time $4050; part-time $225 per credit hour. *Tuition, state resident:* full-time $405; part-time $225 per credit hour. *Tuition, nonresident:* full-time $4050; part-time $225 per credit hour. *International tuition:* $4050 full-time. *Room and board:* $3258; room only: $2880 per academic year.

Financial Aid 60% of graduate students in nursing programs received some form of financial aid in 2005–06.

Contact Dr. Beth Hembree, Director, Graduate Studies, College of Nursing and Health Sciences, Jacksonville State University, 700 Pelham Road North, Jacksonville, AL 36265-1602. *Telephone:* 256-782-5431. *Fax:* 256-782-5406. *E-mail:* bhembree@jsu.edu.

MASTER'S DEGREE PROGRAM

Degree MSN

Available Programs Master's.

Concentrations Available *Clinical nurse specialist programs in:* community health.

Study Options Full-time and part-time.

Program Entrance Requirements Minimum overall college GPA of 3.0, transcript of college record, written essay, interview, 3 letters of recommendation, nursing research course, physical assessment course, statistics course.

Advanced Placement Credit given for nursing courses completed elsewhere dependent upon specific evaluations.

Degree Requirements 36 total credit hours, thesis or project, comprehensive exam.

CONTINUING EDUCATION PROGRAM

Contact Mr. David Hofland, Student Services Coordinator, College of Nursing and Health Sciences, Jacksonville State University, 700 Pelham Road North, Jacksonville, AL 36265-1602. *Telephone:* 256-782-5276. *Fax:* 256-782-5406. *E-mail:* hofland@jsu.edu.

Oakwood College
Department of Nursing
Huntsville, Alabama

Founded in 1896

DEGREE • BS

Library Facilities 128,000 volumes; 610 periodical subscriptions.

BACCALAUREATE PROGRAMS

Degree BS

Available Programs Generic Baccalaureate.

Program Entrance Requirements Standardized tests *Required:* SAT or ACT, TOEFL for international students. **Application** *Deadline:* rolling (freshmen), rolling (transfer). *Early decision:* 3/30. *Notification:* 4/15 (early action). *Application fee:* $20.

Contact Secretary, Department of Nursing, Oakwood College, 7000 Adventist Boulevard, Huntsville, AL 35896. *Telephone:* 256-726-7287. *Fax:* 256-726-8338. *E-mail:* dwilliams@oakwood.edu.

Samford University
Ida V. Moffett School of Nursing
Birmingham, Alabama

http://www.samford.edu

Founded in 1841

DEGREES • BSN • MSN • MSN/MBA

Nursing Program Faculty 30 (54% with doctorates).

Baccalaureate Enrollment 300
Women 97% **Men** 3% **Minority** 5% **International** 2% **Part-time** 10%

Graduate Enrollment 65
Women 88% **Men** 12% **Minority** 32% **Part-time** 5%

Nursing Student Activities Sigma Theta Tau, Student Nurses' Association, nursing club.

Nursing Student Resources Academic advising; academic or career counseling; assistance for students with disabilities; bookstore; campus computer network; career placement assistance; computer lab; computer-assisted instruction; e-mail services; externships; interactive nursing skills videos; Internet; learning resource lab; library services; nursing audiovi-

Peterson's Nursing Programs 2008 *www.petersons.com* **69**

Samford University (continued)

suals; paid internships; placement services for program completers; remedial services; resume preparation assistance; skills, simulation, or other laboratory; tutoring; unpaid internships.

Library Facilities 439,760 volumes (7,000 in health, 2,500 in nursing); 3,724 periodical subscriptions (100 health-care related).

BACCALAUREATE PROGRAMS

Degree BSN

Available Programs Baccalaureate for Second Degree; Generic Baccalaureate; RN Baccalaureate.

Study Options Full-time and part-time.

Program Entrance Requirements Minimum overall college GPA of 2.5, transcript of college record, CPR certification, written essay, health exam, health insurance, high school biology, high school chemistry, 2 years high school math, high school transcript, immunizations, minimum high school GPA of 2.5, minimum GPA in nursing prerequisites of 2.0, professional liability insurance/malpractice insurance, prerequisite course work. Transfer students are accepted. **Standardized tests** *Required:* SAT or ACT, TOEFL for international students. **Application** *Deadline:* 12/15 (freshmen), 8/15 (transfer). *Notification:* continuous (freshmen). *Application fee:* $35.

Advanced Placement Credit given for nursing courses completed elsewhere dependent upon specific evaluations.

Contact *Telephone:* 205-726-2872 Ext. 2746. *Fax:* 205-726-2219.

GRADUATE PROGRAMS

Contact *Telephone:* 205-726-2047. *Fax:* 205-726-2219.

MASTER'S DEGREE PROGRAM

Degrees MSN; MSN/MBA

Available Programs Master's; RN to Master's.

Concentrations Available Nurse anesthesia; nursing administration; nursing education. *Clinical nurse specialist programs in:* acute care, adult health, cardiovascular, community health. *Nurse practitioner programs in:* family health, primary care.

Study Options Full-time and part-time.

Program Entrance Requirements Clinical experience, computer literacy, minimum overall college GPA of 3.0, transcript of college record, CPR certification, immunizations, interview, 3 letters of recommendation, nursing research course, physical assessment course, professional liability insurance/malpractice insurance, prerequisite course work, statistics course, GRE General Test or MAT. *Application deadline:* For spring admission, 1/2. Applications are processed on a rolling basis. *Application fee:* $25.

Advanced Placement Credit given for nursing courses completed elsewhere dependent upon specific evaluations.

Degree Requirements 38 total credit hours.

POST-MASTER'S PROGRAM

Areas of Study Nurse anesthesia; nursing administration; nursing education. *Clinical nurse specialist programs in:* acute care, adult health, cardiovascular, community health. *Nurse practitioner programs in:* family health, primary care.

CONTINUING EDUCATION PROGRAM

Contact *Telephone:* 205-726-2626. *Fax:* 205-726-2219.

Spring Hill College
Division of Nursing
Mobile, Alabama

http://faculty.shc.edu/nursing

Founded in 1830

DEGREES • BSN • MSN

Nursing Program Faculty 8 (84% with doctorates).

Baccalaureate Enrollment 124

Women 86% **Men** 14% **Minority** 12%

Graduate Enrollment 42

Women 95% **Men** 5% **Minority** 45% **Part-time** 40%

Nursing Student Activities Nursing Honor Society, Student Nurses' Association.

Nursing Student Resources Academic advising; academic or career counseling; assistance for students with disabilities; bookstore; campus computer network; career placement assistance; computer lab; computer-assisted instruction; e-mail services; employment services for current students; externships; interactive nursing skills videos; Internet; learning resource lab; library services; nursing audiovisuals; placement services for program completers; resume preparation assistance; skills, simulation, or other laboratory; tutoring; unpaid internships.

Library Facilities 185,868 volumes (330 in health, 300 in nursing); 2,200 periodical subscriptions (58 health-care related).

BACCALAUREATE PROGRAMS

Degree BSN

Available Programs Baccalaureate for Second Degree; Generic Baccalaureate.

Study Options Full-time.

Program Entrance Requirements Minimum overall college GPA of 2.75, transcript of college record, CPR certification, written essay, health exam, health insurance, high school transcript, immunizations, 2 letters of recommendation, minimum GPA in nursing prerequisites of 2.75, professional liability insurance/malpractice insurance, prerequisite course work. Transfer students are accepted. **Standardized tests** *Required:* SAT or ACT, TOEFL for international students. **Application** *Deadline:* 7/15 (freshmen), 7/15 (out-of-state freshmen), rolling (transfer). *Notification:* continuous (freshmen), continuous (out-of-state freshmen). *Application fee:* $25.

Advanced Placement Credit by examination available.

Expenses (2006–07) *Tuition:* full-time $20,700; part-time $773 per credit hour. *Room and board:* $8780; room only: $4860 per academic year. *Required fees:* full-time $1350; part-time $44 per credit; part-time $675 per term.

Financial Aid 80% of baccalaureate students in nursing programs received some form of financial aid in 2005–06. *Gift aid (need-based):* Federal Pell, FSEOG, state, private, college/university gift aid from institutional funds. *Loans:* FFEL (Subsidized and Unsubsidized Stafford PLUS), Alternative loans (i.e., Citiassist, Signature, etc.). *Work-Study:* Federal Work-Study, part-time campus jobs. *Application deadline (priority):* 3/1.

Contact Dr. Carol Harrison, Chair/Professor, Division of Nursing, Spring Hill College, 4000 Dauphin Street, Mobile, AL 36608. *Telephone:* 334-380-4492. *Fax:* 334-380-4495. *E-mail:* charrison@shc.edu.

GRADUATE PROGRAMS

Expenses (2006–07) *Tuition:* full-time $7200; part-time $400 per credit hour. *Required fees:* full-time $100; part-time $50 per term.

Financial Aid 25% of graduate students in nursing programs received some form of financial aid in 2005–06.

Contact Ms. Donna Tarasavage, Director of Marketing and Recruiting, Division of Nursing, Spring Hill College, Division of Graduate Studies, 4000 Dauphin Street, Mobile, AL 36608. *Telephone:* 251-380-3067. *Fax:* 251-460-2190. *E-mail:* dtarasavage@shc.edu.

MASTER'S DEGREE PROGRAM

Degree MSN

Available Programs Accelerated AD/RN to Master's; Master's.

Concentrations Available Clinical nurse leader.

Study Options Full-time and part-time.

Program Entrance Requirements Clinical experience, minimum overall college GPA of 3.0, transcript of college record, immunizations, professional liability insurance/malpractice insurance, prerequisite course work, resume.

Advanced Placement Credit by examination available.

Degree Requirements 36 total credit hours, thesis or project.

Troy University
School of Nursing
Troy, Alabama

Founded in 1887

DEGREES • BSN • MSN

Nursing Program Faculty 40 (47% with doctorates).

Baccalaureate Enrollment 550
Women 88% **Men** 12% **Minority** 35% **International** 4% **Part-time** 10%

Graduate Enrollment 120
Women 97% **Men** 3% **Minority** 23% **Part-time** 29%

Nursing Student Activities Sigma Theta Tau, Student Nurses' Association.

Nursing Student Resources Academic advising; academic or career counseling; assistance for students with disabilities; bookstore; campus computer network; career placement assistance; computer lab; computer-assisted instruction; daycare for children of students; e-mail services; employment services for current students; externships; housing assistance; interactive nursing skills videos; Internet; learning resource lab; library services; nursing audiovisuals; placement services for program completers; remedial services; resume preparation assistance; skills, simulation, or other laboratory; tutoring; unpaid internships.

Library Facilities 443,415 volumes (45,006 in health, 3,843 in nursing); 1,397 periodical subscriptions (703 health-care related).

BACCALAUREATE PROGRAMS

Degree BSN

Available Programs ADN to Baccalaureate; Generic Baccalaureate.
Site Options *Distance Learning:* Phenix City, AL; Montgomery, AL.
Study Options Full-time and part-time.
Program Entrance Requirements Minimum overall college GPA of 2.5, transcript of college record, CPR certification, health exam, health insurance, high school transcript, immunizations, professional liability insurance/malpractice insurance, prerequisite course work. Transfer students are accepted. **Standardized tests** *Recommended:* TOEFL for international students. **Application** *Deadline:* rolling (freshmen), rolling (transfer). *Application fee:* $20.
Advanced Placement Credit by examination available. Credit given for nursing courses completed elsewhere dependent upon specific evaluations.
Financial Aid 90% of baccalaureate students in nursing programs received some form of financial aid in 2005–06.
Contact Ms. Allison Oakes, Departmental Secretary II, School of Nursing, Troy University, 400 Pell Avenue, Troy, AL 36082. *Telephone:* 334-670-3428. *Fax:* 334-670-3744. *E-mail:* aoakes@troy.edu.

GRADUATE PROGRAMS

Financial Aid 40% of graduate students in nursing programs received some form of financial aid in 2005–06.
Contact Dr. Geraldine Allen, Director, MSN Program, School of Nursing, Troy University, 340 Montgomery Street, Montgomery, AL 36104. *Telephone:* 334-834-2320. *Fax:* 334-241-8627. *E-mail:* gallen@troy.edu.

MASTER'S DEGREE PROGRAM

Degree MSN

Available Programs Master's; RN to Master's.
Concentrations Available Nursing administration; nursing education; nursing informatics. *Clinical nurse specialist programs in:* adult health, maternity-newborn. *Nurse practitioner programs in:* family health.
Site Options *Distance Learning:* Phenix City, AL; Montgomery, AL.
Study Options Full-time and part-time.
Program Entrance Requirements Minimum overall college GPA of 3.0, transcript of college record, CPR certification, immunizations, 3 letters of recommendation, physical assessment course, professional liability insurance/malpractice insurance.
Advanced Placement Credit given for nursing courses completed elsewhere dependent upon specific evaluations.
Degree Requirements 39 total credit hours, thesis or project, comprehensive exam.

POST-MASTER'S PROGRAM

Areas of Study *Nurse practitioner programs in:* family health.

Tuskegee University
Program in Nursing
Tuskegee, Alabama

http://www.tusk.edu
Founded in 1881
DEGREE • BSN

Nursing Program Faculty 9 (33% with doctorates).
Baccalaureate Enrollment 156
Women 97% **Men** 3% **Minority** 99%

Nursing Student Activities Nursing Honor Society, Student Nurses' Association.

Nursing Student Resources Academic advising; academic or career counseling; assistance for students with disabilities; bookstore; campus computer network; career placement assistance; computer lab; computer-assisted instruction; e-mail services; externships; interactive nursing skills videos; Internet; learning resource lab; library services; nursing audiovisuals; placement services for program completers; remedial services; resume preparation assistance; skills, simulation, or other laboratory; tutoring.

Library Facilities 623,824 volumes (2,200 in health, 1,279 in nursing); 81,157 periodical subscriptions (250 health-care related).

BACCALAUREATE PROGRAMS

Degree BSN

Available Programs ADN to Baccalaureate; Generic Baccalaureate; RN Baccalaureate.
Study Options Full-time.
Program Entrance Requirements Minimum overall college GPA of 2.5, transcript of college record, CPR certification, written essay, health exam, health insurance, high school biology, high school chemistry, 2 years high school math, 1 year of high school science, high school transcript, immunizations, interview, minimum high school GPA of 2.85, minimum GPA in nursing prerequisites of 2.5, professional liability insurance/malpractice insurance. Transfer students are accepted. **Standardized tests** *Required:* SAT or ACT, TOEFL for international students. **Application** *Deadline:* 4/15 (freshmen), 4/15 (transfer). *Application fee:* $25.
Advanced Placement Credit given for nursing courses completed elsewhere dependent upon specific evaluations.
Expenses (2006–07) *Tuition:* full-time $6700; part-time $2050 per credit hour. *International tuition:* $6700 full-time. *Room and board:* $4090; room only: $4090 per academic year. *Required fees:* full-time $1000.
Financial Aid 95% of baccalaureate students in nursing programs received some form of financial aid in 2005–06.
Contact Dr. Doris S. Holeman, Associate Dean and Director, Program in Nursing, Tuskegee University, 209 Basil O'Connor Hall, Tuskegee, AL 36083. *Telephone:* 334-727-8382. *Fax:* 334-727-5461. *E-mail:* dholeman@tuskegee.edu.

The University of Alabama
Capstone College of Nursing
Tuscaloosa, Alabama

http://nursing.ua.edu
Founded in 1831
DEGREES • BSN • EDD • MSN • MSN/MA

Nursing Program Faculty 31 (61% with doctorates).
Baccalaureate Enrollment 990
Women 88% **Men** 12% **Minority** 20% **International** .4% **Part-time** 9%
Graduate Enrollment 58
Women 95% **Men** 5% **Minority** 25% **Part-time** 75%
Nursing Student Activities Sigma Theta Tau, Student Nurses' Association.

The University of Alabama (continued)

Nursing Student Resources Academic advising; academic or career counseling; assistance for students with disabilities; bookstore; campus computer network; career placement assistance; computer lab; computer-assisted instruction; e-mail services; employment services for current students; interactive nursing skills videos; Internet; learning resource lab; library services; nursing audiovisuals; paid internships; placement services for program completers; resume preparation assistance; skills, simulation, or other laboratory; tutoring; unpaid internships.

Library Facilities 2.6 million volumes (25,000 in health, 98 in nursing); 34,461 periodical subscriptions (1,500 health-care related).

BACCALAUREATE PROGRAMS

Degree BSN

Available Programs Baccalaureate for Second Degree; Generic Baccalaureate; RN Baccalaureate.

Study Options Full-time and part-time.

Program Entrance Requirements Minimum overall college GPA of 2.5, transcript of college record, CPR certification, health exam, health insurance, 4 years high school math, 4 years high school science, high school transcript, immunizations, minimum high school GPA of 2.5, minimum GPA in nursing prerequisites of 2.5, professional liability insurance/malpractice insurance, prerequisite course work. Transfer students are accepted. **Standardized tests** *Required:* SAT or ACT, TOEFL for international students. **Application** *Application fee:* $35.

Advanced Placement Credit by examination available.

Expenses (2006–07) *Tuition, area resident:* full-time $5278; part-time $2639 per semester. *Tuition, nonresident:* full-time $15,294; part-time $7647 per semester. *Room and board:* $5380; room only: $3400 per academic year. *Required fees:* full-time $200.

Financial Aid 50% of baccalaureate students in nursing programs received some form of financial aid in 2005–06.

Contact Ms. Beth Sacksteder Mann, Director of Student Services, Capstone College of Nursing, The University of Alabama, Box 870358, Tuscaloosa, AL 35487-0358. *Telephone:* 205-348-6639. *Fax:* 205-348-5559. *E-mail:* bmann@bama.ua.edu.

GRADUATE PROGRAMS

Expenses (2006–07) *Tuition, state resident:* full-time $5278; part-time $415 per credit hour. *Tuition, nonresident:* full-time $15,294; part-time $901 per credit hour.

Financial Aid 50% of graduate students in nursing programs received some form of financial aid in 2005–06.

Contact Mrs. Pat McCullar, Coordinator of Nursing Student Recruitment, Capstone College of Nursing, The University of Alabama, Box 870358, Tuscaloosa, AL 35487-0358. *Telephone:* 205-348-6640. *Fax:* 205-348-5559. *E-mail:* pmcculla@bama.ua.edu.

MASTER'S DEGREE PROGRAM

Degrees MSN; MSN/MA

Available Programs Master's; RN to Master's.

Concentrations Available Nurse case management.

Study Options Full-time and part-time.

Program Entrance Requirements Clinical experience, computer literacy, minimum overall college GPA of 3.0, transcript of college record, CPR certification, written essay, immunizations, 3 letters of recommendation, nursing research course, professional liability insurance/malpractice insurance, statistics course.

Advanced Placement Credit given for nursing courses completed elsewhere dependent upon specific evaluations.

Degree Requirements 35 total credit hours.

POST-MASTER'S PROGRAM

Areas of Study Nurse case management.

DOCTORAL DEGREE PROGRAM

Degree EdD

Available Programs Doctorate.

Areas of Study Nursing education.

Program Entrance Requirements Minimum overall college GPA of 3.0, letters of recommendation, MSN or equivalent, vita, writing sample.

Degree Requirements Dissertation, written exam, residency.

CONTINUING EDUCATION PROGRAM

Contact Dr. Carolyn C. Dahl, Dean, College of Continuing Studies, Capstone College of Nursing, The University of Alabama, Box 870388, Tuscaloosa, AL 35487-0388. *Telephone:* 205-348-6331. *Fax:* 205-348-9137. *E-mail:* cdahl@ccs.ua.edu.

The University of Alabama at Birmingham
School of Nursing
Birmingham, Alabama

http://www.uab.edu/son/

Founded in 1969

DEGREES • BSN • MSN • MSN/MPH • PHD

Nursing Program Faculty 48 (100% with doctorates).

Baccalaureate Enrollment 288
Women 89% **Men** 11% **Minority** 21% **International** 2% **Part-time** 16%

Graduate Enrollment 281
Women 93% **Men** 7% **Minority** 27% **International** 4% **Part-time** 73%

Nursing Student Activities Nursing Honor Society, Sigma Theta Tau, Student Nurses' Association, nursing club.

Nursing Student Resources Academic advising; academic or career counseling; assistance for students with disabilities; bookstore; campus computer network; career placement assistance; computer lab; computer-assisted instruction; e-mail services; housing assistance; interactive nursing skills videos; Internet; learning resource lab; library services; nursing audiovisuals; paid internships; placement services for program completers; resume preparation assistance; skills, simulation, or other laboratory.

Library Facilities 853,445 volumes (318,000 in health); 3,934 periodical subscriptions (2,566 health-care related).

BACCALAUREATE PROGRAMS

Degree BSN

Available Programs Accelerated RN Baccalaureate; Baccalaureate for Second Degree; Generic Baccalaureate; RN Baccalaureate.

Study Options Full-time and part-time.

Program Entrance Requirements Minimum overall college GPA of 2.5, transcript of college record, CPR certification, written essay, health exam, health insurance, high school transcript, immunizations, minimum high school GPA of 2.0, minimum GPA in nursing prerequisites of 2.5, prerequisite course work. Transfer students are accepted. **Standardized tests** *Required:* SAT or ACT, TOEFL for international students. **Application** *Deadline:* 3/1 (freshmen), 5/1 (transfer). *Notification:* continuous (freshmen). *Application fee:* $30.

Advanced Placement Credit by examination available. Credit given for nursing courses completed elsewhere dependent upon specific evaluations.

Contact *Telephone:* 205-975-7529. *Fax:* 205-975-6142.

GRADUATE PROGRAMS

Contact *Telephone:* 205-934-6787. *Fax:* 205-975-6142.

MASTER'S DEGREE PROGRAM

Degrees MSN; MSN/MPH

Available Programs Accelerated RN to Master's; Master's; RN to Master's.

Concentrations Available Health-care administration; nurse case management; nursing administration. *Clinical nurse specialist programs in:* adult health. *Nurse practitioner programs in:* acute care, adult health, family health, neonatal health, occupational health, pediatric, primary care, women's health.

Study Options Full-time and part-time.

Program Entrance Requirements Clinical experience, minimum overall college GPA of 3.0, transcript of college record, CPR certification, written essay, immunizations, interview, 2 letters of recommendation, nursing research course, physical assessment course, prerequisite course work, statistics course, GRE General Test. *Application deadline:* Applications are processed on a rolling basis. *Application fee:* $35 ($60 for international students).

Advanced Placement Credit given for nursing courses completed elsewhere dependent upon specific evaluations.

Degree Requirements 43 total credit hours, thesis or project.

POST-MASTER'S PROGRAM

Areas of Study *Nurse practitioner programs in:* acute care, adult health, family health, neonatal health, pediatric.

DOCTORAL DEGREE PROGRAM

Degree PhD

Available Programs Doctorate; Post-Baccalaureate Doctorate.

Areas of Study Family health, health promotion/disease prevention, nursing research, nursing science.

Program Entrance Requirements Clinical experience, minimum overall college GPA of 3.0, interview by faculty committee, interview, 3 letters of recommendation, MSN or equivalent, scholarly papers, statistics course, vita, writing sample, GRE General Test. *Application deadline:* Applications are processed on a rolling basis. *Application fee:* $35 ($60 for international students).

Degree Requirements 74 total credit hours, dissertation, oral exam, written exam, residency.

POSTDOCTORAL PROGRAM

Areas of Study Community health, family health.

Postdoctoral Program Contact *Telephone:* 205-934-6852. *Fax:* 205-975-6142.

The University of Alabama in Huntsville
College of Nursing
Huntsville, Alabama

---

http://www.uah.edu/nursing

Founded in 1950

DEGREES • BSN • MSN

Nursing Program Faculty 46 (30% with doctorates).

Baccalaureate Enrollment 625
Women 90% **Men** 10% **Minority** 20% **International** 1% **Part-time** 18%

Graduate Enrollment 175
Women 88% **Men** 12% **Minority** 18% **International** 1% **Part-time** 58%

Nursing Student Activities Sigma Theta Tau, Student Nurses' Association.

Nursing Student Resources Academic advising; academic or career counseling; assistance for students with disabilities; campus computer network; career placement assistance; computer lab; computer-assisted instruction; e-mail services; employment services for current students; housing assistance; interactive nursing skills videos; Internet; learning resource lab; library services; nursing audiovisuals; placement services for program completers; remedial services; resume preparation assistance; skills, simulation, or other laboratory; tutoring.

Library Facilities 334,684 volumes (15,000 in health, 11,562 in nursing); 926 periodical subscriptions (650 health-care related).

BACCALAUREATE PROGRAMS

Degree BSN

Available Programs Baccalaureate for Second Degree; Generic Baccalaureate; RN Baccalaureate.

Study Options Full-time and part-time.

Program Entrance Requirements Minimum overall college GPA of 2.0, transcript of college record, CPR certification, health exam, health insurance, immunizations, minimum GPA in nursing prerequisites of 2.0, professional liability insurance/malpractice insurance, prerequisite course work. Transfer students are accepted. **Standardized tests** *Required:* SAT or ACT, TOEFL for international students. **Application** *Deadline:* 8/15 (freshmen). *Notification:* continuous (freshmen). *Application fee:* $30.

Advanced Placement Credit by examination available. Credit given for nursing courses completed elsewhere dependent upon specific evaluations.

Expenses (2006–07) *Tuition, state resident:* full-time $5300. *Tuition, nonresident:* full-time $11,090. *Room and board:* $5690; room only: $3940 per academic year. *Required fees:* full-time $1800.

Financial Aid 75% of baccalaureate students in nursing programs received some form of financial aid in 2005–06.

Contact Ms. Laura Mann, Director of Nursing Student Affairs, College of Nursing, The University of Alabama in Huntsville, 301 Sparkman Drive, Huntsville, AL 35899. *Telephone:* 256-824-6742. *Fax:* 256-824-6026. *E-mail:* mannl@uah.edu.

GRADUATE PROGRAMS

Expenses (2006–07) *Tuition, state resident:* full-time $6072; part-time $1722 per semester. *Tuition, nonresident:* full-time $12,476; part-time $3520 per semester. *Room and board:* room only: $3550 per academic year. *Required fees:* full-time $2400.

Financial Aid 65% of graduate students in nursing programs received some form of financial aid in 2005–06. 45 fellowships with full and partial tuition reimbursements available (averaging $1,420 per year), 4 teaching assistantships with full and partial tuition reimbursements available (averaging $8,556 per year) were awarded; research assistantships, career-related internships or fieldwork, Federal Work-Study, institutionally sponsored loans, scholarships, traineeships, tuition waivers (full and partial), and unspecified assistantships also available. Aid available to part-time students. *Financial aid application deadline:* 4/1.

Contact Ms. Laura Mann, Director of Nursing Student Affairs, College of Nursing, The University of Alabama in Huntsville, Huntsville, AL 35899. *Telephone:* 256-824-6742. *Fax:* 256-824-6026. *E-mail:* mannl@uah.edu.

MASTER'S DEGREE PROGRAM

Degree MSN

Available Programs Master's; RN to Master's.

Concentrations Available Health-care administration. *Clinical nurse specialist programs in:* adult health. *Nurse practitioner programs in:* acute care, family health.

Study Options Full-time and part-time.

Program Entrance Requirements Minimum overall college GPA of 3.0, transcript of college record, CPR certification, written essay, immunizations, 3 letters of recommendation, professional liability insurance/malpractice insurance, prerequisite course work, statistics course, MAT or GRE. *Application deadline:* For fall admission, 5/30 (priority date); for spring admission, 10/10 (priority date). Applications are processed on a rolling basis. *Application fee:* $40.

Advanced Placement Credit given for nursing courses completed elsewhere dependent upon specific evaluations.

Degree Requirements 42 total credit hours, thesis or project, comprehensive exam.

POST-MASTER'S PROGRAM

Areas of Study Nursing education. *Nurse practitioner programs in:* family health.

CONTINUING EDUCATION PROGRAM

Contact Ms. Ina Warboys, Director of Continuing Education, College of Nursing, The University of Alabama in Huntsville, Huntsville, AL 35899. *Telephone:* 256-824-2456. *Fax:* 256-824-6026. *E-mail:* warboysi@uah.edu.

See full description on page 538.

University of Mobile
School of Nursing
Mobile, Alabama

http://www.umobile.edu/main/nursing1.html

Founded in 1961

DEGREES • BSN • MSN

Nursing Program Faculty 17 (29% with doctorates).

Baccalaureate Enrollment 89
Women 88% **Men** 12% **Minority** 25%

Graduate Enrollment 24
Women 87% **Men** 13% **Minority** 46% **Part-time** 50%

Nursing Student Activities Sigma Theta Tau, Student Nurses' Association.

Nursing Student Resources Academic advising; academic or career counseling; assistance for students with disabilities; bookstore; campus computer network; computer lab; computer-assisted instruction; e-mail services; Internet; learning resource lab; library services; nursing audiovisuals; remedial services; resume preparation assistance; skills, simulation, or other laboratory; tutoring; unpaid internships.

Library Facilities 100,250 volumes (7,846 in health, 6,500 in nursing); 1,043 periodical subscriptions (109 health-care related).

BACCALAUREATE PROGRAMS

Degree BSN

Available Programs Generic Baccalaureate; RN Baccalaureate.
Study Options Full-time.
Program Entrance Requirements Minimum overall college GPA of 2.75, transcript of college record, CPR certification, health exam, health insurance, high school transcript, immunizations, prerequisite course work. Transfer students are accepted. **Standardized tests** *Required:* SAT or ACT, TOEFL for international students. **Application** *Deadline:* rolling (freshmen), rolling (transfer). *Notification:* continuous (freshmen). *Application fee:* $30.
Expenses (2006–07) *Tuition:* full-time $12,000. *Room and board:* $6000; room only: $3300 per academic year. *Required fees:* full-time $1760; part-time $880 per term.
Financial Aid 96% of baccalaureate students in nursing programs received some form of financial aid in 2005–06.
Contact Mrs. Mattie Easter, Assistant Professor, School of Nursing, University of Mobile, 5735 College Parkway, Mobile, AL 36613-2842. *Telephone:* 251-442-2337. *Fax:* 251-442-2520. *E-mail:* measter@mail.umobile.edu.

GRADUATE PROGRAMS

Expenses (2006–07) *Tuition:* full-time $5400; part-time $300 per credit hour. *Required fees:* full-time $70.
Financial Aid 50% of graduate students in nursing programs received some form of financial aid in 2005–06.
Contact Dr. Jan C. Wood, Department Chair, School of Nursing, University of Mobile, 5735 College Parkway, Mobile, AL 36613-2842. *Telephone:* 251-442-2446. *Fax:* 251-442-2520. *E-mail:* jwood@mail.umobile.edu.

MASTER'S DEGREE PROGRAM

Degree MSN

Available Programs Master's.
Concentrations Available Nursing administration; nursing education.
Study Options Full-time and part-time.
Program Entrance Requirements Minimum overall college GPA of 3.0, transcript of college record, CPR certification, immunizations, 3 letters of recommendation, statistics course.
Advanced Placement Credit given for nursing courses completed elsewhere dependent upon specific evaluations.
Degree Requirements 39 total credit hours, thesis or project, comprehensive exam.

CONTINUING EDUCATION PROGRAM
Contact Dr. Elizabeth M. Flanagan, Dean, School of Nursing, University of Mobile, 5735 College Parkway, Mobile, AL 36613. *Telephone:* 251-442-2227. *Fax:* 251-442-2520. *E-mail:* lflanagan@mail.umobile.edu.

University of North Alabama
College of Nursing and Allied Health
Florence, Alabama

http://www2.una.edu/nursing/

Founded in 1830

DEGREE • BSN

Nursing Program Faculty 22 (29% with doctorates).

Baccalaureate Enrollment 180
Women 90% **Men** 10% **Minority** 10% **International** 2%

Library Facilities 380,361 volumes (343,468 in health, 8,476 in nursing); 3,760 periodical subscriptions (493 health-care related).

BACCALAUREATE PROGRAMS

Degree BSN

Available Programs Generic Baccalaureate; RN Baccalaureate.
Program Entrance Requirements Transfer students are accepted.
Standardized tests *Required:* SAT or ACT, TOEFL for international students. **Application** *Deadline:* rolling (freshmen), rolling (transfer). *Application fee:* $25.
Contact *Telephone:* 256-765-4311. *Fax:* 256-765-4935.

CONTINUING EDUCATION PROGRAM
Contact *Telephone:* 256-765-4311. *Fax:* 256-765-4935.

University of South Alabama
College of Nursing
Mobile, Alabama

http://www.southalabama.edu/nursing/

Founded in 1963

DEGREES • BSN • MSN

Nursing Program Faculty 57 (30% with doctorates).

Baccalaureate Enrollment 316
Women 82% **Men** 18% **Minority** 24% **International** 3% **Part-time** 11%

Graduate Enrollment 368
Women 86% **Men** 14% **Minority** 19% **Part-time** 22%

Nursing Student Activities Sigma Theta Tau, Student Nurses' Association.

Nursing Student Resources Academic advising; academic or career counseling; assistance for students with disabilities; bookstore; campus computer network; career placement assistance; computer lab; learning resource lab; library services; nursing audiovisuals; resume preparation assistance.

Library Facilities 1.1 million volumes (2,406 in health, 2,300 in nursing); 7,344 periodical subscriptions (299 health-care related).

BACCALAUREATE PROGRAMS

Degree BSN

Available Programs ADN to Baccalaureate; Accelerated Baccalaureate; Generic Baccalaureate; RN Baccalaureate.
Site Options Fairhope, AL.
Study Options Full-time and part-time.
Program Entrance Requirements Minimum overall college GPA of 2.5, transcript of college record, CPR certification, health exam, health insurance, immunizations, minimum GPA in nursing prerequisites of 2.5, professional liability insurance/malpractice insurance, prerequisite course

work. Transfer students are accepted. **Standardized tests** *Required:* SAT or ACT, TOEFL for international students. **Application** *Deadline:* 7/15 (freshmen), 8/10 (transfer). *Notification:* continuous until 8/10 (freshmen). *Application fee:* $25.

Advanced Placement Credit given for nursing courses completed elsewhere dependent upon specific evaluations.

Contact *Telephone:* 251-434-3410. *Fax:* 251-434-3413.

GRADUATE PROGRAMS

Contact *Telephone:* 251-434-3410. *Fax:* 251-434-3413.

MASTER'S DEGREE PROGRAM

Degree MSN

Available Programs Accelerated Master's; Master's; Master's for Nurses with Non-Nursing Degrees.

Concentrations Available Nursing administration; nursing education. *Clinical nurse specialist programs in:* acute care, community health, family health, gerontology, maternity-newborn, pediatric, psychiatric/mental health, women's health. *Nurse practitioner programs in:* acute care, family health, gerontology, neonatal health, pediatric, psychiatric/mental health, women's health.

Study Options Full-time and part-time.

Program Entrance Requirements Computer literacy, minimum overall college GPA of 3.0, transcript of college record, immunizations, nursing research course, physical assessment course, resume. *Application deadline:* For fall admission, 8/1 (priority date); for winter admission, 11/1 (priority date); for spring admission, 5/1 (priority date). Applications are processed on a rolling basis. *Application fee:* $25.

Advanced Placement Credit given for nursing courses completed elsewhere dependent upon specific evaluations.

Degree Requirements 30 total credit hours, thesis or project.

POST-MASTER'S PROGRAM

Areas of Study Nursing administration; nursing education. *Clinical nurse specialist programs in:* acute care, community health, family health, gerontology, maternity-newborn, pediatric, psychiatric/mental health, women's health. *Nurse practitioner programs in:* acute care, family health, gerontology, neonatal health, pediatric, psychiatric/mental health, women's health.

ALASKA

University of Alaska Anchorage
School of Nursing
Anchorage, Alaska

http://www.son.uaa.alaska.edu

Founded in 1954

DEGREES • BS • MS

Nursing Program Faculty 26 (42% with doctorates).

Baccalaureate Enrollment 224
Women 80% **Men** 20% **Minority** 31% **International** 3% **Part-time** 18%

Graduate Enrollment 60
Women 94% **Men** 6% **Minority** 9% **Part-time** 12%

Nursing Student Activities Sigma Theta Tau, Student Nurses' Association.

Nursing Student Resources Academic advising; academic or career counseling; assistance for students with disabilities; bookstore; campus computer network; career placement assistance; computer lab; computer-assisted instruction; daycare for children of students; e-mail services; interactive nursing skills videos; Internet; learning resource lab; library services; nursing audiovisuals; placement services for program completers; remedial services; resume preparation assistance; skills, simulation, or other laboratory; tutoring.

Library Facilities 894,080 volumes (23,000 in health, 150 in nursing); 3,833 periodical subscriptions (780 health-care related).

BACCALAUREATE PROGRAMS

Degree BS

Available Programs Generic Baccalaureate; RN Baccalaureate.

Study Options Full-time and part-time.

Program Entrance Requirements Minimum overall college GPA of 2.7, transcript of college record, CPR certification, written essay, immunizations, 3 letters of recommendation, minimum GPA in nursing prerequisites of 2.7, professional liability insurance/malpractice insurance, prerequisite course work. Transfer students are accepted. **Standardized tests** *Required:* SAT or ACT, TOEFL for international students. **Application** *Deadline:* 7/1 (freshmen). *Application fee:* $40.

Advanced Placement Credit given for nursing courses completed elsewhere dependent upon specific evaluations.

Expenses (2005–06) *Tuition, state resident:* part-time $123 per credit. *Tuition, nonresident:* part-time $377 per credit. *Room and board:* $3650; room only: $2065 per academic year. *Required fees:* full-time $250; part-time $124 per term.

Financial Aid 90% of baccalaureate students in nursing programs received some form of financial aid in 2004–05. *Gift aid (need-based):* Federal Pell, FSEOG, state, private, college/university gift aid from institutional funds. *Loans:* FFEL (Subsidized and Unsubsidized Stafford PLUS), state. *Work-Study:* Federal Work-Study. *Application deadline:* 8/1 (priority: 4/1).

Contact Ms. Marie Samson, Coordinator of Student Affairs, School of Nursing, School of Nursing, University of Alaska Anchorage, 3211 Providence Drive, Anchorage, AK 99508-8030. *Telephone:* 907-786-4550. *Fax:* 907-786-4558. *E-mail:* anms@uaa.alaska.edu.

GRADUATE PROGRAMS

Expenses (2005–06) *Tuition, state resident:* part-time $244 per credit. *Tuition, nonresident:* part-time $498 per credit. *International tuition:* $730 full-time. *Required fees:* full-time $250; part-time $124 per term.

Financial Aid 30% of graduate students in nursing programs received some form of financial aid in 2004–05. Teaching assistantships, career-related internships or fieldwork and Federal Work-Study available. Aid available to part-time students. *Financial aid application deadline:* 4/1.

Contact Dr. Jill R. Janke, Chair, School of Nursing, University of Alaska Anchorage, 3211 Providence Drive, Anchorage, AK 99508-8030. *Telephone:* 907-786-4570. *Fax:* 907-786-4559. *E-mail:* afjrj@uaa.alaska.edu.

MASTER'S DEGREE PROGRAM

Degree MS

Available Programs Master's.

Concentrations Available Health-care administration; nursing education. *Clinical nurse specialist programs in:* community health, psychiatric/mental health. *Nurse practitioner programs in:* family health, psychiatric/mental health.

Study Options Full-time and part-time.

Program Entrance Requirements Clinical experience, minimum overall college GPA of 3.0, transcript of college record, written essay, 3 letters of recommendation, nursing research course, prerequisite course work, statistics course, GRE or MAT. *Application deadline:* For fall admission, 3/1; for spring admission, 11/1. *Application fee:* $45.

Advanced Placement Credit given for nursing courses completed elsewhere dependent upon specific evaluations.

Degree Requirements 50 total credit hours, thesis or project.

ARIZONA

Arizona State University at the Downtown Phoenix Campus
College of Nursing
Phoenix, Arizona

http://nursing.asu.edu

Founded in 2006

Arizona State University at the Downtown Phoenix Campus (continued)

DEGREES • BSN • DNS • MS • MS/MPH

Nursing Program Faculty 119 (44% with doctorates).

Baccalaureate Enrollment 1,308
Women 91% **Men** 9% **Minority** 26% **International** 1% **Part-time** 18%

Graduate Enrollment 130
Women 95% **Men** 5% **Minority** 12% **Part-time** 39%

Nursing Student Activities Nursing Honor Society, Sigma Theta Tau, Student Nurses' Association, nursing club.

Nursing Student Resources Academic advising; academic or career counseling; assistance for students with disabilities; bookstore; campus computer network; career placement assistance; computer lab; computer-assisted instruction; daycare for children of students; e-mail services; employment services for current students; housing assistance; interactive nursing skills videos; Internet; learning resource lab; library services; nursing audiovisuals; paid internships; placement services for program completers; remedial services; resume preparation assistance; skills, simulation, or other laboratory; tutoring; unpaid internships.

Library Facilities 77,814 volumes in health, 7,501 volumes in nursing; 755 periodical subscriptions health-care related.

BACCALAUREATE PROGRAMS

Degree BSN

Available Programs Accelerated Baccalaureate; Accelerated Baccalaureate for Second Degree; Accelerated RN Baccalaureate; Baccalaureate for Second Degree; Generic Baccalaureate.

Site Options Phoenix, AZ; Scottsdale, AZ; Mesa, AZ.

Study Options Full-time and part-time.

Program Entrance Requirements Minimum overall college GPA of 2.75, transcript of college record, CPR certification, high school chemistry, high school foreign language, 4 years high school math, 3 years high school science, high school transcript, immunizations, minimum high school GPA of 3.0, minimum high school rank 25%, minimum GPA in nursing prerequisites of 2.75, prerequisite course work. Transfer students are accepted.

Advanced Placement Credit by examination available. Credit given for nursing courses completed elsewhere dependent upon specific evaluations.

Contact *Telephone:* 480-965-2987. *Fax:* 480-965-8468.

GRADUATE PROGRAMS

Contact *Telephone:* 480-965-2987. *Fax:* 480-965-8468.

MASTER'S DEGREE PROGRAM

Degrees MS; MS/MPH

Available Programs Master's.

Concentrations Available *Clinical nurse specialist programs in:* acute care, adult health, community health, pediatric, psychiatric/mental health. *Nurse practitioner programs in:* acute care, adult health, family health, neonatal health, pediatric, psychiatric/mental health, women's health.

Site Options Phoenix, AZ.

Study Options Full-time and part-time.

Program Entrance Requirements Clinical experience, minimum overall college GPA of 3.0, transcript of college record, immunizations, interview, 3 letters of recommendation, physical assessment course, prerequisite course work, resume, statistics course, GRE. *Application fee:* $50.

Advanced Placement Credit given for nursing courses completed elsewhere dependent upon specific evaluations.

Degree Requirements 40 total credit hours, thesis or project.

POST-MASTER'S PROGRAM

Areas of Study *Clinical nurse specialist programs in:* acute care, adult health, community health, pediatric, psychiatric/mental health. *Nurse practitioner programs in:* acute care, adult health, family health, neonatal health, pediatric, psychiatric/mental health, women's health.

DOCTORAL DEGREE PROGRAM

Degree DNS

CONTINUING EDUCATION PROGRAM

Contact *Telephone:* 480-965-7431. *Fax:* 480-965-0619.

Grand Canyon University
College of Nursing
Phoenix, Arizona

Founded in 1949

DEGREES • BSN • MSN • MSN/MBA

Nursing Program Faculty 122 (3% with doctorates).

Baccalaureate Enrollment 767
Women 90% **Men** 10% **International** .01% **Part-time** 58%

Graduate Enrollment 227
Women 93% **Men** 7% **Part-time** 89%

Nursing Student Activities Sigma Theta Tau, Student Nurses' Association.

Nursing Student Resources Academic advising; academic or career counseling; assistance for students with disabilities; bookstore; campus computer network; career placement assistance; computer lab; computer-assisted instruction; e-mail services; housing assistance; Internet; learning resource lab; library services; nursing audiovisuals; other; remedial services; resume preparation assistance; skills, simulation, or other laboratory; tutoring.

Library Facilities 75,905 volumes (9,663 in health); 1,174 periodical subscriptions (177 health-care related).

BACCALAUREATE PROGRAMS

Degree BSN

Available Programs ADN to Baccalaureate; Accelerated Baccalaureate; Accelerated Baccalaureate for Second Degree; Generic Baccalaureate; RN Baccalaureate.

Site Options *Distance Learning:* Phoenix, AZ; Tucson, AZ.

Study Options Full-time.

Program Entrance Requirements Minimum overall college GPA of 3.0, transcript of college record, CPR certification, health exam, health insurance, high school transcript, immunizations, minimum GPA in nursing prerequisites of 3.0, prerequisite course work. Transfer students are accepted. **Standardized tests** *Required:* SAT or ACT, TOEFL for international students. **Application** *Deadline:* rolling (freshmen), rolling (transfer). *Notification:* continuous until 9/1 (freshmen). *Application fee:* $50.

Advanced Placement Credit given for nursing courses completed elsewhere dependent upon specific evaluations.

Expenses (2006–07) *Tuition:* full-time $6000. *Room and board:* $7000 per academic year. *Required fees:* part-time $250 per term.

Financial Aid 87% of baccalaureate students in nursing programs received some form of financial aid in 2005–06.

Contact Denise Tolitsky, Business Development Representative/Healthcare Specialist, College of Nursing, Grand Canyon University, 3300 West Camelback Road, Phoenix, AZ 85017. *Telephone:* 602-639-6478. *E-mail:* dtolitsky@gcu.edu.

GRADUATE PROGRAMS

Expenses (2006–07) *Tuition:* part-time $475 per credit hour.

Financial Aid 75% of graduate students in nursing programs received some form of financial aid in 2005–06.

Contact Denise Tolitsky, Business Development Representative/Healthcare Specialist, College of Nursing, Grand Canyon University, 3300 West Camelback Road, Phoenix, AZ 85017. *Telephone:* 602-639-6478. *E-mail:* dtolitsky@gcu.edu.

MASTER'S DEGREE PROGRAM

Degrees MSN; MSN/MBA

Available Programs Master's; RN to Master's.

Concentrations Available Health-care administration; nursing education. *Clinical nurse specialist programs in:* acute care, adult health. *Nurse practitioner programs in:* family health.

Site Options *Distance Learning:* Phoenix, AZ.

Study Options Full-time and part-time.

Program Entrance Requirements Computer literacy, minimum overall college GPA of 3.0, transcript of college record, CPR certification, immunizations, nursing research course, physical assessment course, professional liability insurance/malpractice insurance, statistics course.

Advanced Placement Credit given for nursing courses completed elsewhere dependent upon specific evaluations.

Degree Requirements 52 total credit hours, thesis or project.

POST-MASTER'S PROGRAM

Areas of Study Nursing education. *Clinical nurse specialist programs in:* acute care, adult health. *Nurse practitioner programs in:* family health.

CONTINUING EDUCATION PROGRAM

Contact Mrs. Tracy Schreiner, RN, Assistant Dean of Continuing Education, College of Nursing, Grand Canyon University, 3300 West Camelback Road, Phoenix, AZ 85017. *Telephone:* 623-639-6164. *Fax:* 602-639-7816. *E-mail:* tschreiner@gcu.edu.

See full description on page 490.

Northern Arizona University
School of Nursing
Flagstaff, Arizona

http://www.nau.edu/hp/dept/nurse

Founded in 1899

DEGREES • BSN • MS

Nursing Program Faculty 57 (30% with doctorates).

Baccalaureate Enrollment 376
Women 89% **Men** 11% **Minority** 18% **International** 2% **Part-time** 17%

Graduate Enrollment 47
Women 98% **Men** 2% **Minority** 21% **Part-time** 49%

Nursing Student Activities Nursing Honor Society, Sigma Theta Tau, Student Nurses' Association.

Nursing Student Resources Academic advising; academic or career counseling; bookstore; campus computer network; computer lab; computer-assisted instruction; e-mail services; externships; interactive nursing skills videos; Internet; learning resource lab; library services; nursing audiovisuals; paid internships; remedial services; skills, simulation, or other laboratory; tutoring.

Library Facilities 687,456 volumes; 29,526 periodical subscriptions.

BACCALAUREATE PROGRAMS

Degree BSN

Available Programs ADN to Baccalaureate; Accelerated Baccalaureate; Accelerated Baccalaureate for Second Degree; Generic Baccalaureate; RN Baccalaureate.

Site Options *Distance Learning:* Yuma, AZ; Ganado/Chinle, AZ; Tucson, AZ.

Study Options Full-time and part-time.

Program Entrance Requirements Transcript of college record, CPR certification, written essay, health exam, health insurance, high school transcript, immunizations, 2 letters of recommendation, minimum GPA in nursing prerequisites of 2.75, professional liability insurance/malpractice insurance, prerequisite course work. Transfer students are accepted. **Standardized tests** *Required:* SAT or ACT, TOEFL for international students. **Application** *Deadline:* rolling (freshmen), rolling (transfer). *Notification:* continuous (freshmen). *Application fee:* $25.

Advanced Placement Credit given for nursing courses completed elsewhere dependent upon specific evaluations.

Expenses (2006–07) *Tuition, area resident:* full-time $4550; part-time $270 per credit. *Tuition, nonresident:* full-time $13,490; part-time $596 per credit. *Room and board:* room only: $3488 per academic year. *Required fees:* full-time $300.

Financial Aid 75% of baccalaureate students in nursing programs received some form of financial aid in 2005–06.

Contact Mr. Gregg Schneider, Senior Academic Advisor, School of Nursing, Northern Arizona University, Box 15035, Flagstaff, AZ 86011. *Telephone:* 928-523-6717. *Fax:* 928-523-7171. *E-mail:* gregg.schneider@nau.edu.

GRADUATE PROGRAMS

Expenses (2006–07) *Tuition, state resident:* full-time $4890; part-time $289 per credit. *Tuition, nonresident:* full-time $10,430; part-time $611 per credit. *Required fees:* full-time $150.

Financial Aid 75% of graduate students in nursing programs received some form of financial aid in 2005–06. 1 research assistantship was awarded.

Contact Mr. Gregg Schneider, Senior Academic Advisor, School of Nursing, Northern Arizona University, Box 15035, Flagstaff, AZ 86011. *Telephone:* 928-523-6717. *Fax:* 928-523-7171. *E-mail:* gregg.schneider@nau.edu.

MASTER'S DEGREE PROGRAM

Degree MS

Available Programs Master's.

Concentrations Available Nurse case management; nursing education. *Clinical nurse specialist programs in:* medical-surgical, public health. *Nurse practitioner programs in:* family health.

Site Options *Distance Learning:* Yuma, AZ.

Study Options Full-time and part-time.

Program Entrance Requirements Clinical experience, minimum overall college GPA of 3.0, transcript of college record, CPR certification, written essay, immunizations, interview, 3 letters of recommendation, nursing research course, physical assessment course, professional liability insurance/malpractice insurance, prerequisite course work, resume, statistics course, GRE General Test. *Application deadline:* For fall admission, 2/15 (priority date). *Application fee:* $50.

Degree Requirements 37 total credit hours, thesis or project.

POST-MASTER'S PROGRAM

Areas of Study *Clinical nurse specialist programs in:* medical-surgical.

The University of Arizona
College of Nursing
Tucson, Arizona

http://www.nursing.arizona.edu

Founded in 1885

DEGREES • BSN • MS • PHD

Nursing Program Faculty 58 (55% with doctorates).

Baccalaureate Enrollment 304
Women 92% **Men** 8% **Minority** 25% **International** 1% **Part-time** 14%

Graduate Enrollment 166
Women 94% **Men** 6% **Minority** 21% **International** 3% **Part-time** 54%

Nursing Student Activities Nursing Honor Society, Sigma Theta Tau, Student Nurses' Association.

Nursing Student Resources Academic advising; academic or career counseling; assistance for students with disabilities; bookstore; campus computer network; career placement assistance; computer lab; computer-assisted instruction; e-mail services; externships; housing assistance; interactive nursing skills videos; Internet; learning resource lab; library services; nursing audiovisuals; other; placement services for program completers; skills, simulation, or other laboratory; tutoring.

Library Facilities 4.4 million volumes (215,000 in health, 30,000 in nursing); 23,790 periodical subscriptions (2,000 health-care related).

BACCALAUREATE PROGRAMS

Degree BSN

Available Programs Accelerated Baccalaureate for Second Degree; Generic Baccalaureate.

Study Options Full-time.

The University of Arizona (continued)

Program Entrance Requirements Minimum overall college GPA of 2.75, transcript of college record, CPR certification, written essay, high school foreign language, 4 years high school math, 3 years high school science, immunizations, 2 letters of recommendation, minimum high school GPA of 2.5, minimum GPA in nursing prerequisites of 2.75, prerequisite course work. Transfer students are accepted. **Standardized tests** *Required:* TOEFL for international students. *Recommended:* SAT or ACT. **Application** *Deadline:* 4/1 (freshmen), 6/1 (transfer). *Notification:* continuous (freshmen). *Application fee:* $25.

Advanced Placement Credit by examination available. Credit given for nursing courses completed elsewhere dependent upon specific evaluations.

Expenses (2005–06) *Tuition, state resident:* full-time $4497; part-time $230 per unit. *Tuition, nonresident:* full-time $13,681; part-time $582 per unit. *International tuition:* $13,681 full-time. *Room and board:* $7460 per academic year.

Financial Aid 60% of baccalaureate students in nursing programs received some form of financial aid in 2004–05.

Contact Ms. Vickie Radoye, Assistant Dean for Student Affairs, College of Nursing, The University of Arizona, 1305 North Martin, PO Box 210203, Tucson, AZ 85721-0203. *Telephone:* 520-626-3808. *Fax:* 520-626-6424. *E-mail:* vradoye@nursing.arizona.edu.

GRADUATE PROGRAMS

Expenses (2005–06) *Tuition, state resident:* full-time $8951; part-time $491 per unit. *Tuition, nonresident:* full-time $17,931; part-time $814 per unit. *International tuition:* $17,931 full-time. *Room and board:* $7460 per academic year.

Financial Aid 52% of graduate students in nursing programs received some form of financial aid in 2004–05. 22 fellowships (averaging $1,136 per year), 16 research assistantships with partial tuition reimbursements available (averaging $15,000 per year), 2 teaching assistantships with partial tuition reimbursements available (averaging $15,000 per year) were awarded; career-related internships or fieldwork, institutionally sponsored loans, scholarships, traineeships, and tuition waivers (full) also available. *Financial aid application deadline:* 6/1.

Contact Nancy Banks, Senior Academic Advisor, College of Nursing, The University of Arizona, 1305 North Martin, PO Box 210203, Tucson, AZ 85721-0203. *Telephone:* 520-626-3808. *Fax:* 520-626-6424. *E-mail:* nbanks@nursing.arizona.edu.

MASTER'S DEGREE PROGRAM

Degree MS

Available Programs Master's.

Concentrations Available *Nurse practitioner programs in:* acute care, adult health, family health, psychiatric/mental health.

Site Options *Distance Learning:* Tucson, AZ.

Study Options Full-time and part-time.

Program Entrance Requirements Computer literacy, minimum overall college GPA of 3.0, transcript of college record, CPR certification, written essay, immunizations, 3 letters of recommendation, nursing research course, physical assessment course, resume, statistics course, GRE General Test. *Application deadline:* For fall admission, 1/14. *Application fee:* $50.

Advanced Placement Credit given for nursing courses completed elsewhere dependent upon specific evaluations.

Degree Requirements 44 total credit hours, thesis or project.

POST-MASTER'S PROGRAM

Areas of Study Nursing informatics. *Nurse practitioner programs in:* acute care, adult health, family health, psychiatric/mental health.

DOCTORAL DEGREE PROGRAM

Degree PhD

Available Programs Doctorate; Post-Baccalaureate Doctorate.

Areas of Study Aging, bio-behavioral research, biology of health and illness, gerontology, health-care systems, information systems, nursing research, nursing science.

Site Options *Distance Learning:* Tucson, AZ.

Program Entrance Requirements Minimum overall college GPA of 3.0, interview by faculty committee, interview, 3 letters of recommendation, statistics course, vita, GRE General Test (not required for applicants with a master's degree). *Application deadline:* For fall admission, 1/14. *Application fee:* $50.

Degree Requirements 75 total credit hours, dissertation, oral exam, written exam, residency.

POSTDOCTORAL PROGRAM

Areas of Study Nursing research.

Postdoctoral Program Contact Ms. Vickie Radoye, Assistant Dean for Student Affairs, College of Nursing, The University of Arizona, 1305 North Martin, PO Box 210203, Tucson, AZ 85721-0203. *Telephone:* 520-626-3808. *Fax:* 520-626-6424. *E-mail:* vradoye@nursing.arizona.edu.

University of Phoenix Online Campus
College of Health and Human Services
Phoenix, Arizona

http://www.uopxonline.com/

Founded in 1989

DEGREES • BSN • MSN • MSN/MBA

Nursing Program Faculty 1446 (32% with doctorates).

Baccalaureate Enrollment 4,813
Women 92.4% **Men** 7.6% **Minority** 9.77%

Graduate Enrollment 7,228
Women 87.15% **Men** 12.85% **Minority** 18.01%

Nursing Student Activities Sigma Theta Tau.

Nursing Student Resources Academic advising; academic or career counseling; bookstore; library services.

Library Facilities 444 volumes; 666 periodical subscriptions.

BACCALAUREATE PROGRAMS

Degree BSN

Available Programs Accelerated Baccalaureate; LPN to Baccalaureate.

Study Options Full-time.

Program Entrance Requirements Transcript of college record, 1 letter of recommendation, RN licensure. Transfer students are accepted. **Application** *Deadline:* rolling (freshmen), rolling (transfer). *Application fee:* $110.

Advanced Placement Credit by examination available. Credit given for nursing courses completed elsewhere dependent upon specific evaluations.

Expenses (2006–07) *Tuition:* full-time $14,180. *International tuition:* $14,180 full-time. *Required fees:* full-time $750.

Contact Program Chair, Healthcare, College of Health and Human Services, University of Phoenix Online Campus, CF-A101, 3157 East Elwood Street, Phoenix, AZ 85034-7209. *Telephone:* 602-387-7000.

GRADUATE PROGRAMS

Expenses (2006–07) *Tuition:* full-time $12,664. *International tuition:* $12,664 full-time. *Required fees:* full-time $760.

Contact Program Chair, Healthcare. *Telephone:* 602-387-7000.

MASTER'S DEGREE PROGRAM

Degrees MSN; MSN/MBA

Available Programs Master's; Master's for Nurses with Non-Nursing Degrees.

Concentrations Available Health-care administration; nursing administration; nursing education. *Nurse practitioner programs in:* family health.

Study Options Full-time.

Program Entrance Requirements Clinical experience, computer literacy, minimum overall college GPA of 2.5, transcript of college record. *Application deadline:* Applications are processed on a rolling basis. *Application fee:* $110.

Advanced Placement Credit given for nursing courses completed elsewhere dependent upon specific evaluations.

Degree Requirements 39 total credit hours, thesis or project.

POST-MASTER'S PROGRAM

Areas of Study *Nurse practitioner programs in:* family health.

See full description on page 552.

University of Phoenix–Phoenix Campus
College of Health and Human Services
Phoenix, Arizona

Founded in 1976

DEGREES • BSN • MSN

Nursing Program Faculty 311 (33% with doctorates).

Baccalaureate Enrollment 123
Women 88.62% **Men** 11.38% **Minority** 4.07%

Graduate Enrollment 243
Women 90.61% **Men** 9.39% **Minority** 10.61%

Nursing Student Activities Sigma Theta Tau.

Nursing Student Resources Academic advising; academic or career counseling; assistance for students with disabilities; bookstore; computer lab; library services.

Library Facilities 442 volumes; 666 periodical subscriptions.

BACCALAUREATE PROGRAMS

Degree BSN

Available Programs Accelerated Baccalaureate; LPN to Baccalaureate.

Site Options Mesa, AZ; Chandler, AZ.

Study Options Full-time.

Program Entrance Requirements Transcript of college record, 1 letter of recommendation, RN licensure. Transfer students are accepted.

Standardized tests *Required:* TOEFL for international students. **Application** *Deadline:* rolling (freshmen), rolling (transfer). *Application fee:* $110.

Advanced Placement Credit by examination available. Credit given for nursing courses completed elsewhere dependent upon specific evaluations.

Expenses (2006–07) *Tuition:* full-time $9990. *International tuition:* $9990 full-time. *Required fees:* full-time $750.

Contact Campus College Chair, Nursing, College of Health and Human Services, University of Phoenix–Phoenix Campus, 4635 East Elwood Street, Phoenix, AZ 85040-1958. *Telephone:* 480-804-7600.

GRADUATE PROGRAMS

Expenses (2006–07) *Tuition:* full-time $8880. *International tuition:* $8880 full-time. *Required fees:* full-time $760.

Contact Campus College Chair, Nursing, College of Health and Human Services, University of Phoenix–Phoenix Campus, 4635 East Elwood Street, Phoenix, AZ 85040-1958. *Telephone:* 480-804-7600.

MASTER'S DEGREE PROGRAM

Degree MSN

Available Programs Master's.

Concentrations Available Health-care administration; nursing administration; nursing education. *Nurse practitioner programs in:* family health.

Site Options Mesa, AZ; Chandler, AZ.

Study Options Full-time.

Program Entrance Requirements Clinical experience, computer literacy, minimum overall college GPA of 2.5, transcript of college record. *Application deadline:* Applications are processed on a rolling basis. *Application fee:* $110.

Advanced Placement Credit given for nursing courses completed elsewhere dependent upon specific evaluations.

Degree Requirements 39 total credit hours, thesis or project.

POST-MASTER'S PROGRAM

Areas of Study *Nurse practitioner programs in:* family health.

CONTINUING EDUCATION PROGRAM

Contact Campus College Chair, Nursing, College of Health and Human Services, University of Phoenix–Phoenix Campus, Mail Stop CJ A101, 4635 East Elwood Street, Phoenix, AZ 85040-1958. *Telephone:* 480-557-2279. *Fax:* 480-557-2338.

University of Phoenix–Southern Arizona Campus
College of Health and Human Services
Tucson, Arizona

Founded in 1979

DEGREES • BSN • MSN

Nursing Program Faculty 121 (34% with doctorates).

Baccalaureate Enrollment 27
Women 88.89% **Men** 11.11% **Minority** 7.41%

Graduate Enrollment 74
Women 86.49% **Men** 13.51% **Minority** 5.05%

Nursing Student Activities Sigma Theta Tau.

Nursing Student Resources Academic advising; academic or career counseling; assistance for students with disabilities; bookstore; computer lab; library services.

Library Facilities 444 volumes; 666 periodical subscriptions.

BACCALAUREATE PROGRAMS

Degree BSN

Available Programs Accelerated Baccalaureate; LPN to RN Baccalaureate.

Site Options Yuma, AZ; Nogales, AZ; Sierra Vista, AZ.

Study Options Full-time.

Program Entrance Requirements Transcript of college record, 1 letter of recommendation, RN licensure. Transfer students are accepted.

Standardized tests *Required:* TOEFL for international students. **Application** *Deadline:* rolling (freshmen), rolling (transfer). *Application fee:* $110.

Advanced Placement Credit by examination available. Credit given for nursing courses completed elsewhere dependent upon specific evaluations.

Expenses (2006–07) *Tuition:* full-time $9990. *International tuition:* $9990 full-time. *Required fees:* full-time $750.

Contact Campus College Chair, Nursing, College of Health and Human Services, University of Phoenix–Southern Arizona Campus, 5099 East Grant Road, #120, Tucson, AZ 85712-2732. *Telephone:* 520-881-6512.

GRADUATE PROGRAMS

Expenses (2006–07) *Tuition:* full-time $9576. *International tuition:* $9576 full-time. *Required fees:* full-time $760.

Contact Campus College Chair, Nursing, College of Health and Human Services, University of Phoenix–Southern Arizona Campus, 5099 East Grant Road, Tucson, AZ 85712-2732. *Telephone:* 520-881-6512.

MASTER'S DEGREE PROGRAM

Degree MSN

Available Programs Master's.

Concentrations Available Health-care administration; nursing administration; nursing education. *Nurse practitioner programs in:* family health.

Site Options Yuma, AZ; Nogales, AZ; Sierra Vista, AZ.

Study Options Full-time.

Program Entrance Requirements Clinical experience, computer literacy, minimum overall college GPA of 2.5, transcript of college record. *Application deadline:* Applications are processed on a rolling basis. *Application fee:* $110.

Advanced Placement Credit given for nursing courses completed elsewhere dependent upon specific evaluations.

University of Phoenix–Southern Arizona Campus (continued)
Degree Requirements 39 total credit hours, thesis or project.

POST-MASTER'S PROGRAM
Areas of Study *Nurse practitioner programs in:* family health.

ARKANSAS

Arkansas State University
Department of Nursing
Jonesboro, State University, Arkansas

http://www.conhp.astate.edu/Nursing/
Founded in 1909
DEGREES • BSN • MSN

Nursing Program Faculty 35 (20% with doctorates).
Baccalaureate Enrollment 245
Graduate Enrollment 91
Nursing Student Activities Nursing Honor Society, Sigma Theta Tau.
Library Facilities 604,568 volumes; 1,712 periodical subscriptions.

BACCALAUREATE PROGRAMS
Degree BSN
Available Programs Generic Baccalaureate; LPN to Baccalaureate; RN Baccalaureate.
Site Options Mountain Home, AR; Melbourne, AR; Beebe, AR.
Study Options Full-time.
Program Entrance Requirements Minimum overall college GPA of 2.5, transcript of college record, CPR certification, health exam, immunizations, minimum GPA in nursing prerequisites of 3.5, prerequisite course work. Transfer students are accepted. **Standardized tests** *Required:* SAT or ACT. *Recommended:* ACT. *Required for some:* ACT ASSET or ACT COMPASS. **Application** *Deadline:* rolling (freshmen), rolling (transfer). *Notification:* continuous (freshmen). *Application fee:* $15.
Advanced Placement Credit given for nursing courses completed elsewhere dependent upon specific evaluations.
Contact *Telephone:* 870-972-3074. *Fax:* 870-972-2954.

GRADUATE PROGRAMS
Contact *Telephone:* 870-972-3074. *Fax:* 870-972-2954.

MASTER'S DEGREE PROGRAM
Degree MSN
Available Programs Master's.
Concentrations Available Nurse anesthesia; nursing education. *Clinical nurse specialist programs in:* adult health. *Nurse practitioner programs in:* primary care.
Site Options Mountain Home, AR; Melbourne, AR; Beebe, AR.
Study Options Full-time and part-time.
Program Entrance Requirements Clinical experience, minimum overall college GPA of 2.75, transcript of college record, CPR certification, written essay, immunizations, interview, letters of recommendation, physical assessment course, professional liability insurance/malpractice insurance, statistics course.
Degree Requirements 39 total credit hours, thesis or project, comprehensive exam.

Arkansas Tech University
Program in Nursing
Russellville, Arkansas

http://nursing.atu.edu
Founded in 1909

DEGREE • BSN
Nursing Program Faculty 22 (14% with doctorates).
Baccalaureate Enrollment 429
Women 86% **Men** 14% **Minority** 5% **International** .5% **Part-time** 17%
Nursing Student Activities Nursing Honor Society, Sigma Theta Tau, Student Nurses' Association.
Nursing Student Resources Academic advising; academic or career counseling; assistance for students with disabilities; bookstore; campus computer network; career placement assistance; computer lab; computer-assisted instruction; e-mail services; employment services for current students; housing assistance; interactive nursing skills videos; Internet; learning resource lab; library services; nursing audiovisuals; other; paid internships; placement services for program completers; remedial services; resume preparation assistance; skills, simulation, or other laboratory; tutoring.
Library Facilities 259,372 volumes (16,900 in health, 2,100 in nursing); 1,054 periodical subscriptions (130 health-care related).

BACCALAUREATE PROGRAMS
Degree BSN
Available Programs ADN to Baccalaureate; Generic Baccalaureate; LPN to Baccalaureate; RN Baccalaureate.
Site Options *Distance Learning:* Hot Springs, AR; Harrison, AR; Fort Smith, AR.
Study Options Full-time and part-time.
Program Entrance Requirements Transcript of college record, CPR certification, health exam, immunizations, minimum GPA in nursing prerequisites of 2.75, professional liability insurance/malpractice insurance, prerequisite course work. Transfer students are accepted. **Standardized tests** *Required:* SAT or ACT, TOEFL for international students. **Application** *Notification:* continuous (freshmen).
Advanced Placement Credit by examination available. Credit given for nursing courses completed elsewhere dependent upon specific evaluations.
Expenses (2006–07) *Tuition, state resident:* full-time $4470; part-time $149 per credit hour. *Tuition, nonresident:* full-time $8940; part-time $298 per credit. *International tuition:* $8940 full-time. *Room and board:* $4360; room only: $2460 per academic year. *Required fees:* full-time $410; part-time $4 per credit; part-time $240 per term.
Financial Aid 80% of baccalaureate students in nursing programs received some form of financial aid in 2005–06.
Contact Dr. Rebecca Frances Burris, Professor and Department Chair, Program in Nursing, Arkansas Tech University, 402 West O Street, Russellville, AR 72801. *Telephone:* 479-968-0383. *Fax:* 479-968-0219. *E-mail:* rebecca.burris@atu.edu.

Harding University
College of Nursing
Searcy, Arkansas

http://www.harding.edu
Founded in 1924

DEGREE • BSN
Nursing Program Faculty 26 (29% with doctorates).
Baccalaureate Enrollment 111
Women 85% **Men** 15% **Minority** 2% **International** 4% **Part-time** 10%
Nursing Student Activities Nursing Honor Society, Sigma Theta Tau, Student Nurses' Association.
Nursing Student Resources Academic advising; academic or career counseling; assistance for students with disabilities; bookstore; campus computer network; career placement assistance; computer lab; computer-assisted instruction; e-mail services; employment services for current students; externships; housing assistance; interactive nursing skills videos; Internet; learning resource lab; library services; nursing audiovisuals; placement services for program completers; remedial services; resume preparation assistance; skills, simulation, or other laboratory; tutoring.
Library Facilities 230,499 volumes (5,000 in health, 1,729 in nursing); 16,582 periodical subscriptions (120 health-care related).

BACCALAUREATE PROGRAMS

Degree BSN

Available Programs ADN to Baccalaureate; Generic Baccalaureate; LPN to Baccalaureate; LPN to RN Baccalaureate; RN Baccalaureate.

Site Options Searcy, AR.

Study Options Full-time and part-time.

Program Entrance Requirements Minimum overall college GPA of 2.0, transcript of college record, CPR certification, health exam, high school transcript, immunizations, 3 letters of recommendation, minimum GPA in nursing prerequisites of 2.5, prerequisite course work. Transfer students are accepted. **Standardized tests** *Required:* SAT or ACT, TOEFL for international students. **Application** *Deadline:* 6/1 (freshmen), 6/1 (transfer). *Notification:* continuous (freshmen). *Application fee:* $35.

Advanced Placement Credit by examination available. Credit given for nursing courses completed elsewhere dependent upon specific evaluations.

Expenses (2006–07) *Tuition:* full-time $11,250; part-time $375 per hour. *Room and board:* $5442; room only: $2700 per academic year. *Required fees:* full-time $400.

Financial Aid 95% of baccalaureate students in nursing programs received some form of financial aid in 2005–06. *Gift aid (need-based):* Federal Pell, FSEOG, state, private, college/university gift aid from institutional funds. *Loans:* Federal Nursing Student Loans, FFEL (Subsidized and Unsubsidized Stafford PLUS), Perkins, state, college/university. *Work-Study:* Federal Work-Study, part-time campus jobs. *Application deadline:* Continuous.

Contact Ms. Jeanne L. Castleberry, Assistant to the Dean, College of Nursing, Harding University, 915 East Market Avenue, Box 12265, Searcy, AR 72149-2265. *Telephone:* 501-279-4682. *Fax:* 501-305-8902. *E-mail:* nursing@harding.edu.

CONTINUING EDUCATION PROGRAM

Contact Dr. Cathleen M. Shultz, Dean and Professor, College of Nursing, Harding University, Box 12265, Searcy, AR 72149. *Telephone:* 501-279-4476. *Fax:* 501-279-4669. *E-mail:* shultz@harding.edu.

Henderson State University
Department of Nursing
Arkadelphia, Arkansas

http://www.hsu.edu/dept/nsg/index.html

Founded in 1890

DEGREE • BSN

Nursing Program Faculty 7 (14% with doctorates).

Baccalaureate Enrollment 170
Women 98% **Men** 2% **Minority** 35% **International** 2%

Nursing Student Activities Student Nurses' Association.

Nursing Student Resources Academic advising; academic or career counseling; assistance for students with disabilities; bookstore; campus computer network; career placement assistance; computer lab; computer-assisted instruction; e-mail services; interactive nursing skills videos; Internet; learning resource lab; library services; nursing audiovisuals; remedial services; resume preparation assistance; skills, simulation, or other laboratory; tutoring.

Library Facilities 262,572 volumes (1,000 in health, 200 in nursing); 1,516 periodical subscriptions (40 health-care related).

BACCALAUREATE PROGRAMS

Degree BSN

Available Programs ADN to Baccalaureate; Generic Baccalaureate.

Study Options Full-time and part-time.

Program Entrance Requirements Minimum overall college GPA of 2.5, transcript of college record, CPR certification, immunizations, prerequisite course work. Transfer students are accepted. **Standardized tests** *Required:* SAT or ACT, TOEFL for international students. *Recommended:* ACT. **Application** *Deadline:* 7/15 (freshmen), rolling (transfer). *Notification:* continuous (freshmen).

Advanced Placement Credit given for nursing courses completed elsewhere dependent upon specific evaluations.

Contact Dr. Barbara J. Landrum, DNS, Professor and Department Chair, Department of Nursing, Henderson State University, Box 7803, 1100 Henderson Street, Arkadelphia, AR 71999-0001. *Telephone:* 870-230-5508. *Fax:* 870-230-5390. *E-mail:* landrub@hsu.edu.

Southern Arkansas University–Magnolia
Department of Nursing
Magnolia, Arkansas

Founded in 1909

DEGREE • BSN

Nursing Program Faculty 13 (8% with doctorates).

Nursing Student Resources Academic advising; bookstore; computer lab; Internet; library services.

Library Facilities 151,166 volumes; 1,065 periodical subscriptions.

BACCALAUREATE PROGRAMS

Degree BSN

Available Programs RN Baccalaureate.

Study Options Full-time and part-time.

Program Entrance Requirements Transcript of college record, CPR certification, immunizations, prerequisite course work, RN licensure. Transfer students are accepted. **Standardized tests** *Required:* SAT or ACT, TOEFL for international students. *Recommended:* ACT. **Application** *Deadline:* 8/27 (freshmen), 8/27 (transfer).

Expenses (2006–07) *Tuition, area resident:* full-time $4260; part-time $142 per hour. *Tuition, nonresident:* full-time $6450; part-time $215 per hour. *Required fees:* full-time $180.

Contact Ms. Becky Parnell, RN-BSN Online Completion Student Advisor, Department of Nursing, Southern Arkansas University–Magnolia, 100 East University, Magnolia, AR 71753-5000. *Telephone:* 870-235-4331. *Fax:* 870-235-5058. *E-mail:* bbparnell@saumag.edu.

University of Arkansas
Eleanor Mann School of Nursing
Fayetteville, Arkansas

http://www.uark.edu/coehp

Founded in 1871

DEGREES • BSN • MSN

Nursing Program Faculty 19 (26% with doctorates).

Baccalaureate Enrollment 115
Women 95% **Men** 5% **Minority** 7%

Nursing Student Activities Sigma Theta Tau, Student Nurses' Association.

Nursing Student Resources Academic advising; academic or career counseling; assistance for students with disabilities; bookstore; campus computer network; career placement assistance; computer lab; computer-assisted instruction; e-mail services; employment services for current students; housing assistance; interactive nursing skills videos; Internet; learning resource lab; library services; nursing audiovisuals; other; placement services for program completers; remedial services; resume preparation assistance; skills, simulation, or other laboratory; tutoring.

Library Facilities 1.8 million volumes (60,000 in health, 20,000 in nursing); 18,173 periodical subscriptions (130,000 health-care related).

BACCALAUREATE PROGRAMS

Degree BSN

Available Programs Baccalaureate for Second Degree; Generic Baccalaureate; LPN to Baccalaureate; LPN to RN Baccalaureate; RN Baccalaureate.

University of Arkansas (continued)

Study Options Full-time.

Program Entrance Requirements Minimum overall college GPA of 2.75, transcript of college record, CPR certification, health insurance, immunizations, minimum GPA in nursing prerequisites of 2.75, professional liability insurance/malpractice insurance, prerequisite course work. Transfer students are accepted. **Standardized tests** *Required:* SAT or ACT, TOEFL for international students. **Application** *Deadline:* 8/15 (freshmen), 8/15 (transfer). *Early decision:* 11/15. *Notification:* 10/1 (freshmen), 12/15 (early action). *Application fee:* $40.

Advanced Placement Credit by examination available. Credit given for nursing courses completed elsewhere dependent upon specific evaluations.

Contact *Telephone:* 479-575-3907. *Fax:* 479-575-3218.

GRADUATE PROGRAMS

Contact *Telephone:* 479-575-3907. *Fax:* 479-575-3218.

MASTER'S DEGREE PROGRAM

Degree MSN

Available Programs Master's.

Concentrations Available Nursing education. *Clinical nurse specialist programs in:* acute care, medical-surgical.

Study Options Part-time.

Degree Requirements 42 total credit hours, thesis or project.

CONTINUING EDUCATION PROGRAM

Contact *Telephone:* 479-575-3907. *Fax:* 479-575-3218.

University of Arkansas at Fort Smith

Carol McKelvey Moore School of Nursing
Fort Smith, Arkansas

Founded in 1928

DEGREE • BSN

Nursing Program Faculty 16 (6% with doctorates).

Nursing Student Activities Nursing club.

Nursing Student Resources Academic advising; academic or career counseling; assistance for students with disabilities; bookstore; career placement assistance; computer lab; e-mail services; library services.

Library Facilities 85,358 volumes; 1,750 periodical subscriptions.

BACCALAUREATE PROGRAMS

Degree BSN

Available Programs Generic Baccalaureate; RN Baccalaureate.

Study Options Full-time.

Program Entrance Requirements Transcript of college record, CPR certification, high school biology, high school chemistry, 2 years high school math, immunizations, prerequisite course work, RN licensure. Transfer students are accepted. **Standardized tests** *Required:* ACT, TOEFL for international students. **Application** *Deadline:* rolling (freshmen), rolling (transfer).

Expenses (2006–07) *Tuition, state resident:* full-time $17,846. *Tuition, nonresident:* full-time $37,432.

Contact Dr. Carolyn Mosley, Associate Dean/BSN Program Director, Carol McKelvey Moore School of Nursing, University of Arkansas at Fort Smith, 5210 Grand Avenue, PO Box 3649, Fort Smith, AR 72913-3649. *Telephone:* 479-788-7383. *E-mail:* cmosley@uafortsmith.edu.

University of Arkansas at Monticello

Division of Nursing
Monticello, Arkansas

http://www.uamont.edu/Nursing/

Founded in 1909

DEGREE • BSN

Nursing Program Faculty 7 (14% with doctorates).

Baccalaureate Enrollment 44
Women 95% **Men** 5% **Minority** 27%

Library Facilities 126,229 volumes (441 in health); 862 periodical subscriptions (44 health-care related).

BACCALAUREATE PROGRAMS

Degree BSN

Available Programs ADN to Baccalaureate; LPN to Baccalaureate; RN Baccalaureate.

Study Options Full-time.

Program Entrance Requirements Transcript of college record, CPR certification, written essay, health exam, immunizations, interview, minimum GPA in nursing prerequisites of 2.5, professional liability insurance/malpractice insurance, prerequisite course work. Transfer students are accepted. **Standardized tests** *Required:* TOEFL for international students. *Placement: Required:* SAT or ACT. *Recommended:* ACT. **Application** *Deadline:* 8/1 (freshmen), 8/1 (transfer).

Advanced Placement Credit by examination available. Credit given for nursing courses completed elsewhere dependent upon specific evaluations.

Contact *Telephone:* 870-460-1069. *Fax:* 870-460-1969.

University of Arkansas at Pine Bluff

Department of Nursing
Pine Bluff, Arkansas

http://www.uapb.com

Founded in 1873

DEGREE • BSN

Nursing Program Faculty 7.

Baccalaureate Enrollment 51
Women 94% **Men** 6% **Minority** 96%

Nursing Student Activities Student Nurses' Association.

Nursing Student Resources Academic advising; academic or career counseling; assistance for students with disabilities; bookstore; campus computer network; career placement assistance; computer lab; computer-assisted instruction; e-mail services; housing assistance; interactive nursing skills videos; Internet; learning resource lab; library services; nursing audiovisuals; remedial services; resume preparation assistance; skills, simulation, or other laboratory; tutoring.

Library Facilities 287,857 volumes (2,600 in health, 1,550 in nursing); 3,041 periodical subscriptions (60 health-care related).

BACCALAUREATE PROGRAMS

Degree BSN

Available Programs Generic Baccalaureate.

Study Options Full-time and part-time.

Program Entrance Requirements Minimum overall college GPA of 2.5, transcript of college record, CPR certification, written essay, health exam, immunizations, 3 letters of recommendation, minimum GPA in nursing prerequisites of 2.5, professional liability insurance/malpractice insurance, prerequisite course work. Transfer students are accepted. **Standardized tests** *Required:* TOEFL for international students. **Placement:** *Required:* SAT or ACT. **Application** *Deadline:* rolling (freshmen). *Notification:* continuous (freshmen).

Advanced Placement Credit by examination available. Credit given for nursing courses completed elsewhere dependent upon specific evaluations.

Contact *Telephone:* 870-575-8220. *Fax:* 870-575-8229.

University of Arkansas for Medical Sciences
College of Nursing
Little Rock, Arkansas

http://www.nursing.uams.edu
Founded in 1879
DEGREES • BSN • M SC N • PHD

Nursing Program Faculty 85 (38% with doctorates).

Baccalaureate Enrollment 299

Graduate Enrollment 217

Nursing Student Activities Nursing Honor Society, Sigma Theta Tau, Student Nurses' Association.

Nursing Student Resources Academic advising; academic or career counseling; assistance for students with disabilities; bookstore; campus computer network; computer lab; computer-assisted instruction; e-mail services; externships; interactive nursing skills videos; Internet; learning resource lab; library services; nursing audiovisuals; remedial services; skills, simulation, or other laboratory; tutoring.

Library Facilities 183,975 volumes (183,975 in health); 1,567 periodical subscriptions (1,567 health-care related).

BACCALAUREATE PROGRAMS
Degree BSN

Available Programs ADN to Baccalaureate; Accelerated Baccalaureate for Second Degree; Accelerated RN Baccalaureate; Baccalaureate for Second Degree; Generic Baccalaureate; LPN to Baccalaureate; RN Baccalaureate.

Site Options *Distance Learning:* Texarkana, AR; Helena, AR; Jonesboro, AR; Hope, AR; Fayetteville, AR; El Dorado, AR.

Study Options Full-time.

Program Entrance Requirements Minimum overall college GPA of 2.5, transcript of college record, CPR certification, health exam, health insurance, high school biology, high school chemistry, high school transcript, immunizations, minimum high school GPA of 2.5, professional liability insurance/malpractice insurance, prerequisite course work. Transfer students are accepted.

Advanced Placement Credit by examination available. Credit given for nursing courses completed elsewhere dependent upon specific evaluations.

Expenses (2006–07) *Tuition, area resident:* full-time $2136; part-time $178 per hour. *Tuition, nonresident:* full-time $5328; part-time $444 per hour. *Room and board:* room only: $2700 per academic year. *Required fees:* full-time $915.

Contact Dr. Patricia E. Thompson, Associate Dean for Academic Programs, College of Nursing, University of Arkansas for Medical Sciences, 4301 West Markham, #529, Little Rock, AR 72205-7199. *Telephone:* 501-686-5374. *Fax:* 501-686-8350. *E-mail:* ThompsonPatriciaE@uams.edu.

GRADUATE PROGRAMS
Expenses (2006–07) *Tuition, state resident:* full-time $2520; part-time $252 per hour. *Tuition, nonresident:* full-time $5400; part-time $540 per hour. *Room and board:* room only: $2700 per academic year. *Required fees:* full-time $1135.

Financial Aid Career-related internships or fieldwork and traineeships available.

Contact Dr. Patricia E. Thompson, Associate Dean for Academic Programs, College of Nursing, University of Arkansas for Medical Sciences, 4301 West Markham, #529, Little Rock, AR 72205-7199. *Telephone:* 501-686-5374. *Fax:* 501-686-8350. *E-mail:* ThompsonPatriciaE@uams.edu.

MASTER'S DEGREE PROGRAM
Degree M Sc N

Available Programs Master's; RN to Master's.

Concentrations Available Nursing administration; nursing education. *Clinical nurse specialist programs in:* acute care, adult health, pediatric. *Nurse practitioner programs in:* acute care, family health, gerontology, pediatric, psychiatric/mental health, women's health.

Site Options *Distance Learning:* Texarkana, AR; Helena, AR; Jonesboro, AR; Fayetteville, AR; El Dorado, AR.

Study Options Full-time and part-time.

Program Entrance Requirements Clinical experience, minimum overall college GPA of 2.85, transcript of college record, CPR certification, immunizations, physical assessment course, professional liability insurance/malpractice insurance, statistics course, MAT.

Advanced Placement Credit given for nursing courses completed elsewhere dependent upon specific evaluations.

Degree Requirements 39 total credit hours, thesis or project, comprehensive exam.

DOCTORAL DEGREE PROGRAM
Degree PhD

Available Programs Doctorate; Doctorate for Nurses with Non-Nursing Degrees; Post-Baccalaureate Doctorate.

Areas of Study Advanced practice nursing, clinical practice, forensic nursing, gerontology, health-care systems, nursing administration, nursing education, nursing research, nursing science, oncology, women's health.

Program Entrance Requirements Minimum overall college GPA of 3.65, interview by faculty committee, interview, 4 letters of recommendation, MSN or equivalent, scholarly papers, statistics course, writing sample.

Degree Requirements 60 total credit hours, dissertation, oral exam, written exam.

POSTDOCTORAL PROGRAM
Areas of Study Aging, cancer care, gerontology, nursing research, nursing science.

Postdoctoral Program Contact Dr. Patricia E. Thompson, Associate Dean for Academic Programs, College of Nursing, University of Arkansas for Medical Sciences, 4301 West Markham, #529, Little Rock, AR 72205-7199. *Telephone:* 501-686-5374. *Fax:* 501-686-8350. *E-mail:* ThompsonPatriciaE@uams.edu.

CONTINUING EDUCATION PROGRAM
Contact Dr. Claudia P. Barone, Dean and Professor, College of Nursing, University of Arkansas for Medical Sciences, 4301 West Markham, Slot 529, Little Rock, AR 72205-7199. *Telephone:* 501-686-5374. *Fax:* 501-686-8350. *E-mail:* BaroneClaudiaP@uams.edu.

University of Central Arkansas
Department of Nursing
Conway, Arkansas

http://www.uca.edu/divisions/academic/nursing/
Founded in 1907
DEGREES • BSN • MSN

Nursing Program Faculty 16 (33% with doctorates).

Baccalaureate Enrollment 53
Women 88% **Men** 12% **Minority** 13% **International** 2%

Graduate Enrollment 53
Women 94% **Men** 6% **Minority** 8%

Nursing Student Activities Sigma Theta Tau, Student Nurses' Association.

University of Central Arkansas (continued)

Nursing Student Resources Academic advising; academic or career counseling; assistance for students with disabilities; bookstore; campus computer network; career placement assistance; computer lab; computer-assisted instruction; e-mail services; employment services for current students; externships; housing assistance; interactive nursing skills videos; Internet; learning resource lab; library services; nursing audiovisuals; paid internships; placement services for program completers; remedial services; resume preparation assistance; skills, simulation, or other laboratory; tutoring; unpaid internships.

Library Facilities 505,000 volumes (11,500 in health, 4,500 in nursing); 2,000 periodical subscriptions (80 health-care related).

BACCALAUREATE PROGRAMS

Degree BSN

Available Programs ADN to Baccalaureate; Generic Baccalaureate; LPN to Baccalaureate; LPN to RN Baccalaureate; RN Baccalaureate.

Study Options Full-time and part-time.

Program Entrance Requirements Minimum overall college GPA of 2.5, transcript of college record, written essay, minimum GPA in nursing prerequisites, prerequisite course work. **Standardized tests** *Required:* SAT or ACT, TOEFL for international students. **Application** *Deadline:* rolling (freshmen), rolling (transfer). *Notification:* continuous (freshmen).

Expenses (2005–06) *Tuition, state resident:* full-time $4500. *Tuition, nonresident:* full-time $4500. *International tuition:* $4500 full-time. *Room and board:* $2380; room only: $1800 per academic year. *Required fees:* full-time $1260.

Financial Aid 85% of baccalaureate students in nursing programs received some form of financial aid in 2004–05.

Contact Ann Mattison, Program Coordinator, Department of Nursing, University of Central Arkansas, Doyne Health Science Center, 201 South Donaghey Avenue, Conway, AR 72035. *Telephone:* 501-450-3119. *Fax:* 501-450-5503. *E-mail:* annm@mail.uca.edu.

GRADUATE PROGRAMS

Expenses (2005–06) *Tuition, state resident:* part-time $190 per credit hour. *Tuition, nonresident:* part-time $190 per credit hour. *Required fees:* full-time $1254.

Financial Aid Fellowships, research assistantships, Federal Work-Study, traineeships, and unspecified assistantships available.

Contact Dr. Rebecca Lancaster, RN, Director of Graduate Program, Department of Nursing, University of Central Arkansas, Doyne Health Science Center, 201 South Donaghey Avenue, Conway, AR 72035. *Telephone:* 501-450-3119. *Fax:* 501-450-5560. *E-mail:* BeckyL@uca.edu.

MASTER'S DEGREE PROGRAM

Degree MSN

Available Programs Master's; RN to Master's.

Concentrations Available Nursing education. *Clinical nurse specialist programs in:* community health, family health, medical-surgical, psychiatric/mental health. *Nurse practitioner programs in:* adult health, family health, psychiatric/mental health.

Site Options *Distance Learning:* Russellville, AR; Pine Bluff, AR; Fort Smith, AR.

Study Options Full-time and part-time.

Program Entrance Requirements Clinical experience, minimum overall college GPA of 2.7, transcript of college record, CPR certification, immunizations, professional liability insurance/malpractice insurance, resume, statistics course, GRE General Test. *Application deadline:* For fall admission, 3/1 (priority date); for spring admission, 10/1. Applications are processed on a rolling basis. *Application fee:* $25 ($40 for international students).

Degree Requirements Comprehensive exam.

POST-MASTER'S PROGRAM

Areas of Study Nursing education. *Clinical nurse specialist programs in:* community health, family health, medical-surgical, psychiatric/mental health. *Nurse practitioner programs in:* adult health, family health, psychiatric/mental health.

CALIFORNIA

Azusa Pacific University
School of Nursing
Azusa, California

http://www.apu.edu/nursing/grad

Founded in 1899

DEGREES • BSN • MSN • PHD

Nursing Program Faculty 77 (22% with doctorates).

Baccalaureate Enrollment 236
Women 90% **Men** 10% **Minority** 44% **International** 11% **Part-time** 2%

Graduate Enrollment 110
Women 89% **Men** 11% **Minority** 37%

Nursing Student Activities Sigma Theta Tau, Student Nurses' Association, nursing club.

Nursing Student Resources Academic advising; academic or career counseling; bookstore; campus computer network; career placement assistance; computer lab; computer-assisted instruction; e-mail services; employment services for current students; housing assistance; interactive nursing skills videos; Internet; learning resource lab; library services; nursing audiovisuals; remedial services; resume preparation assistance; skills, simulation, or other laboratory; tutoring.

Library Facilities 185,708 volumes (14,206 in health, 4,712 in nursing); 14,031 periodical subscriptions (432 health-care related).

BACCALAUREATE PROGRAMS

Degree BSN

Available Programs ADN to Baccalaureate; Accelerated Baccalaureate; Accelerated RN Baccalaureate; Generic Baccalaureate.

Study Options Full-time and part-time.

Program Entrance Requirements Minimum overall college GPA of 3.0, transcript of college record, CPR certification, written essay, health exam, high school biology, high school chemistry, 2 years high school math, high school transcript, immunizations, 3 letters of recommendation, minimum high school GPA of 3.0, minimum GPA in nursing prerequisites of 3.0. Transfer students are accepted. **Standardized tests** *Required:* SAT or ACT, TOEFL for international students. **Application** *Deadline:* 6/1 (freshmen), 6/1 (transfer). *Early decision:* 12/1. *Notification:* continuous (freshmen), 1/15 (early action). *Application fee:* $45.

Advanced Placement Credit by examination available. Credit given for nursing courses completed elsewhere dependent upon specific evaluations.

Expenses (2005–06) *Tuition:* full-time $21,550; part-time $900 per unit. *International tuition:* $22,210 full-time. *Room and board:* $5788; room only: $3510 per academic year. *Required fees:* full-time $1030; part-time $620 per term.

Financial Aid 75% of baccalaureate students in nursing programs received some form of financial aid in 2004–05.

Contact Mrs. Barbara Wiltsey, Administrative Assistant for Admissions, School of Nursing, Azusa Pacific University, 901 East Alosta Avenue, Azusa, CA 91702-7000. *Telephone:* 626-815-6000 Ext. 5501. *Fax:* 626-815-5414. *E-mail:* bwiltsey@apu.edu.

GRADUATE PROGRAMS

Expenses (2005–06) *Tuition:* part-time $450 per unit.

Financial Aid 50% of graduate students in nursing programs received some form of financial aid in 2004–05. Teaching assistantships, scholarships, traineeships, and unspecified assistantships available. Aid available to part-time students. *Financial aid application deadline:* 10/15.

Contact Mrs. Barb Barthelmess, Graduate Program Coordinator, School of Nursing, Azusa Pacific University, 901 East Alosta Avenue, Azusa, CA 91702. *Telephone:* 626-815-5386. *Fax:* 626-815-5414. *E-mail:* bbarthelmess@apu.edu.

MASTER'S DEGREE PROGRAM

Degree MSN

Available Programs Accelerated Master's for Non-Nursing College Graduates; Accelerated Master's for Nurses with Non-Nursing Degrees; Master's.

Concentrations Available Nursing administration; nursing education. *Clinical nurse specialist programs in:* adult health, medical-surgical, parent-child, pediatric, school health. *Nurse practitioner programs in:* adult health, family health, pediatric, primary care.

Site Options *Distance Learning:* San Diego, CA.

Study Options Full-time and part-time.

Program Entrance Requirements Clinical experience, computer literacy, minimum overall college GPA of 3.0, transcript of college record, CPR certification, written essay, immunizations, 3 letters of recommendation, nursing research course, physical assessment course, professional liability insurance/malpractice insurance, prerequisite course work, resume, statistics course. *Application deadline:* Applications are processed on a rolling basis. *Application fee:* $45 ($65 for international students).

Advanced Placement Credit by examination available. Credit given for nursing courses completed elsewhere dependent upon specific evaluations.

Degree Requirements 42 total credit hours, thesis or project, comprehensive exam.

POST-MASTER'S PROGRAM

Areas of Study Nursing administration; nursing education. *Clinical nurse specialist programs in:* adult health, medical-surgical, parent-child, pediatric, school health. *Nurse practitioner programs in:* adult health, family health, pediatric, primary care.

DOCTORAL DEGREE PROGRAM

Degree PhD

Available Programs Doctorate.

Areas of Study Community health, family health, nursing education.

Program Entrance Requirements Clinical experience, minimum overall college GPA of 3.5, interview by faculty committee, interview, 3 letters of recommendation, MSN or equivalent, scholarly papers, statistics course, vita, writing sample. *Application deadline:* Applications are processed on a rolling basis. *Application fee:* $45 ($65 for international students).

Degree Requirements 64 total credit hours, dissertation, oral exam, written exam.

CONTINUING EDUCATION PROGRAM

Contact Mrs. Kathryn Speck, Projects Coordinator, School of Nursing, Azusa Pacific University, 901 East Alosta Avenue, Azusa, CA 91702. *Telephone:* 626-815-5385. *Fax:* 626-815-5414. *E-mail:* Kspeck@apu.edu.

Biola University
Department of Nursing
La Mirada, California

Founded in 1908

DEGREE • BSN

Nursing Program Faculty 13 (30% with doctorates).

Baccalaureate Enrollment 220
Women 95% **Men** 5% **Minority** 15% **International** 5% **Part-time** 1%

Nursing Student Activities Student Nurses' Association.

Nursing Student Resources Academic advising; academic or career counseling; assistance for students with disabilities; bookstore; campus computer network; career placement assistance; computer lab; computer-assisted instruction; e-mail services; employment services for current students; housing assistance; Internet; learning resource lab; library services; nursing audiovisuals; placement services for program completers; remedial services; resume preparation assistance; skills, simulation, or other laboratory; tutoring.

Library Facilities 301,956 volumes (20,000 in health, 10,000 in nursing); 17,876 periodical subscriptions (500 health-care related).

BACCALAUREATE PROGRAMS

Degree BSN

Available Programs ADN to Baccalaureate; Baccalaureate for Second Degree; Generic Baccalaureate; LPN to Baccalaureate; RN Baccalaureate.

Study Options Full-time.

Program Entrance Requirements Minimum overall college GPA of 3.0, transcript of college record, CPR certification, written essay, health exam, health insurance, high school biology, high school chemistry, high school foreign language, 2 years high school math, high school transcript, immunizations, interview, 2 letters of recommendation, minimum high school GPA of 3.5, minimum GPA in nursing prerequisites of 2.0, professional liability insurance/malpractice insurance, prerequisite course work. Transfer students are accepted. **Standardized tests** *Required:* SAT or ACT, TOEFL for international students. **Application** *Deadline:* 3/1 (freshmen), 3/1 (transfer). *Early decision:* 12/1. *Notification:* 4/1 (freshmen), 1/15 (early action). *Application fee:* $45.

Advanced Placement Credit by examination available. Credit given for nursing courses completed elsewhere dependent upon specific evaluations.

Expenses (2006–07) *Tuition:* full-time $23,782; part-time $991 per unit. *International tuition:* $23,782 full-time. *Room and board:* $7410; room only: $3580 per academic year. *Required fees:* full-time $1000.

Financial Aid 95% of baccalaureate students in nursing programs received some form of financial aid in 2005–06.

Contact Dr. Anne L. Gewe, Associate Chair/Associate Professor, Department of Nursing, Biola University, 13800 Biola Avenue, La Mirada, CA 90639. *Telephone:* 562-903-4850. *Fax:* 562-903-4803. *E-mail:* anne.gewe@biola.edu.

CONTINUING EDUCATION PROGRAM

Contact Dr. Anne L. Gewe, Associate Chair/Associate Professor, Department of Nursing, Biola University, 13800 Biola Avenue, La Mirada, CA 90639. *Telephone:* 562-903-4850. *Fax:* 562-903-4803. *E-mail:* anne.gewe@biola.edu.

California State University, Bakersfield
Program in Nursing
Bakersfield, California

http://www.csubak.edu

Founded in 1970

DEGREES • BSN • MSN

Nursing Program Faculty 35 (20% with doctorates).

Baccalaureate Enrollment 237
Women 90% **Men** 10% **Minority** 50% **International** 9% **Part-time** 5%

Graduate Enrollment 50
Women 80% **Men** 20% **Minority** 46% **International** 10% **Part-time** 34%

Nursing Student Activities Sigma Theta Tau, Student Nurses' Association.

Nursing Student Resources Academic advising; academic or career counseling; assistance for students with disabilities; bookstore; campus computer network; career placement assistance; computer lab; computer-assisted instruction; daycare for children of students; e-mail services; employment services for current students; externships; housing assistance; interactive nursing skills videos; Internet; learning resource lab; library services; nursing audiovisuals; paid internships; remedial services; skills, simulation, or other laboratory; tutoring; unpaid internships.

Library Facilities 354,016 volumes (20,000 in health, 1,850 in nursing); 2,260 periodical subscriptions (90 health-care related).

BACCALAUREATE PROGRAMS

Degree BSN

Available Programs Accelerated Baccalaureate for Second Degree; Generic Baccalaureate; RN Baccalaureate.

Site Options *Distance Learning:* Visalia, CA; Lancaster, CA.

Study Options Full-time.

California State University, Bakersfield (continued)

Program Entrance Requirements Minimum overall college GPA of 2.0, transcript of college record, CPR certification, health exam, health insurance, high school transcript, immunizations, minimum GPA in nursing prerequisites of 2.8, professional liability insurance/malpractice insurance, prerequisite course work. Transfer students are accepted. **Standardized tests** *Required:* SAT or ACT, TOEFL for international students. *Recommended:* SAT Subject Tests. **Application** *Deadline:* 9/23 (freshmen), 9/23 (transfer). *Notification:* continuous (freshmen). *Application fee:* $55.

Advanced Placement Credit by examination available. Credit given for nursing courses completed elsewhere dependent upon specific evaluations.

Expenses (2006–07) *Tuition, state resident:* full-time $3387; part-time $777 per quarter. *Tuition, nonresident:* full-time $10,170; part-time $226 per unit. *International tuition:* $10,170 full-time. *Room and board:* $5367 per academic year.

Financial Aid 78% of baccalaureate students in nursing programs received some form of financial aid in 2005–06.

Contact Ms. Cheryl Moore, Administrative Coordinator, Program in Nursing, California State University, Bakersfield, Romberg Nursing Education Building, 9001 Stockdale Highway, Bakersfield, CA 93311-1022. *Telephone:* 661-654-2506. *Fax:* 661-654-6003. *E-mail:* cmoore@csub.edu.

GRADUATE PROGRAMS

Expenses (2006–07) *Tuition, state resident:* full-time $3969; part-time $889 per quarter. *Tuition, nonresident:* full-time $10,170; part-time $226 per unit. *International tuition:* $10,170 full-time. *Room and board:* $5367 per academic year.

Financial Aid 80% of graduate students in nursing programs received some form of financial aid in 2005–06. Scholarships and traineeships available.

Contact Dr. Candace Meares, Graduate Coordinator, Program in Nursing, California State University, Bakersfield, 9001 Stockdale Highway, Bakersfield, CA 93311-1022. *Telephone:* 661-654-2093. *Fax:* 661-654-6347. *E-mail:* cmeares@csub.edu.

MASTER'S DEGREE PROGRAM

Degree MSN

Available Programs Master's.

Concentrations Available Clinical nurse leader. *Clinical nurse specialist programs in:* school health. *Nurse practitioner programs in:* family health.

Study Options Full-time and part-time.

Program Entrance Requirements Clinical experience, minimum overall college GPA of 2.5, transcript of college record, CPR certification, written essay, immunizations, 3 letters of recommendation, nursing research course, physical assessment course, professional liability insurance/malpractice insurance, prerequisite course work, resume, statistics course, MAT. *Application deadline:* Applications are processed on a rolling basis. *Application fee:* $55.

Advanced Placement Credit given for nursing courses completed elsewhere dependent upon specific evaluations.

Degree Requirements 67 total credit hours, thesis or project.

POST-MASTER'S PROGRAM

Areas of Study *Clinical nurse specialist programs in:* school health. *Nurse practitioner programs in:* family health.

California State University, Chico
School of Nursing
Chico, California

http://www.csuchico.edu/nurs/nurs.html

Founded in 1887

DEGREES • BSN • MSN

Nursing Program Faculty 29 (28% with doctorates).

Baccalaureate Enrollment 235

Women 89% **Men** 11% **Minority** 23% **Part-time** 1%

Graduate Enrollment 30

Women 90% **Men** 10% **Minority** 10% **Part-time** 100%

Nursing Student Activities Sigma Theta Tau, Student Nurses' Association, nursing club.

Nursing Student Resources Academic advising; academic or career counseling; assistance for students with disabilities; bookstore; campus computer network; career placement assistance; computer lab; computer-assisted instruction; daycare for children of students; e-mail services; employment services for current students; externships; housing assistance; interactive nursing skills videos; Internet; learning resource lab; library services; nursing audiovisuals; paid internships; placement services for program completers; remedial services; resume preparation assistance; skills, simulation, or other laboratory; tutoring; unpaid internships.

Library Facilities 957,181 volumes (17,727 in health, 1,467 in nursing); 24,244 periodical subscriptions (133 health-care related).

BACCALAUREATE PROGRAMS

Degree BSN

Available Programs ADN to Baccalaureate; Baccalaureate for Second Degree; Generic Baccalaureate; LPN to Baccalaureate; RN Baccalaureate.

Study Options Full-time.

Program Entrance Requirements Minimum overall college GPA of 2.5, transcript of college record, CPR certification, health exam, health insurance, immunizations, minimum GPA in nursing prerequisites of 2.0, professional liability insurance/malpractice insurance, prerequisite course work. Transfer students are accepted. **Standardized tests** *Required:* SAT or ACT, TOEFL for international students. **Application** *Deadline:* 11/30 (freshmen), 11/30 (transfer). *Notification:* 3/1 (freshmen). *Application fee:* $55.

Advanced Placement Credit given for nursing courses completed elsewhere dependent upon specific evaluations.

Expenses (2006–07) *Tuition, state resident:* full-time $3412; part-time $1178 per semester. *Tuition, nonresident:* full-time $11,548; part-time $3212 per semester. *Room and board:* $8314; room only: $5478 per academic year. *Required fees:* full-time $200.

Financial Aid 75% of baccalaureate students in nursing programs received some form of financial aid in 2005–06. *Gift aid (need-based):* Federal Pell, FSEOG, state, private, college/university gift aid from institutional funds, United Negro College Fund. *Loans:* Federal Direct (Subsidized and Unsubsidized Stafford PLUS), Perkins, college/university. *Work-Study:* Federal Work-Study. *Application deadline:* Continuous.

Contact Sherry D. Fox, Director, School of Nursing, California State University, Chico, Holt Hall 369, Chico, CA 95929-0200. *Telephone:* 530-898-5891. *Fax:* 530-898-4363. *E-mail:* sdfox@csuchico.edu.

GRADUATE PROGRAMS

Expenses (2006–07) *Tuition, state resident:* full-time $3994; part-time $1346 per semester. *Tuition, nonresident:* full-time $8062; part-time $3380 per semester. *International tuition:* $8062 full-time. *Room and board:* $8314; room only: $5478 per academic year.

Financial Aid 25% of graduate students in nursing programs received some form of financial aid in 2005–06. Career-related internships or fieldwork available.

Contact Irene Morgan, Graduate Coordinator, School of Nursing, California State University, Chico, 400 West 1st Street, Chico, CA 95929-0200. *Telephone:* 530-898-5891. *Fax:* 530-898-4363. *E-mail:* imorgan@csuchico.edu.

MASTER'S DEGREE PROGRAM

Degree MSN

Available Programs Master's.

Concentrations Available Nursing education. *Clinical nurse specialist programs in:* adult health.

Site Options *Distance Learning:* Chico, CA.

Study Options Part-time.

Program Entrance Requirements Clinical experience, minimum overall college GPA of 3.0, transcript of college record, CPR certification, written essay, immunizations, physical assessment course, professional liability insurance/malpractice insurance, statistics course, GRE or MAT. *Application deadline:* For fall admission, 3/1. Applications are processed on a rolling basis. *Application fee:* $55.

Advanced Placement Credit given for nursing courses completed elsewhere dependent upon specific evaluations.

Degree Requirements 30 total credit hours, thesis or project.

POST-MASTER'S PROGRAM
Areas of Study Nursing education.

CONTINUING EDUCATION PROGRAM
Contact Ms. Clare Robe, School of Nursing, California State University, Chico, 400 West 1st Street, Chico, CA 95929-0250. *Telephone:* 530-898-6105. *E-mail:* rce@csuchico.edu.

California State University, Dominguez Hills
Program in Nursing
Carson, California

http://www.csudh.edu/soh/don/index.htm

Founded in 1960

DEGREES • BSN • MSN

Nursing Program Faculty 65 (80% with doctorates).
Baccalaureate Enrollment 641
Women 92% **Men** 8% **Minority** 63% **Part-time** 91%
Graduate Enrollment 387
Women 92% **Men** 8% **Minority** 55% **Part-time** 80%
Nursing Student Activities Nursing Honor Society, Sigma Theta Tau, Student Nurses' Association.

Nursing Student Resources Academic advising; academic or career counseling; assistance for students with disabilities; bookstore; campus computer network; career placement assistance; computer lab; computer-assisted instruction; daycare for children of students; e-mail services; externships; interactive nursing skills videos; Internet; learning resource lab; library services; nursing audiovisuals; remedial services; skills, simulation, or other laboratory; tutoring.

Library Facilities 428,840 volumes (10,000 in nursing); 49,130 periodical subscriptions (215 health-care related).

BACCALAUREATE PROGRAMS
Degree BSN
Available Programs Baccalaureate for Second Degree; RN Baccalaureate.
Site Options *Distance Learning:* Whittier, CA; Apple Valley, CA; Salinas, CA.
Study Options Full-time and part-time.
Program Entrance Requirements Minimum overall college GPA of 2.0, transcript of college record, minimum GPA in nursing prerequisites of 2.0, prerequisite course work, RN licensure. Transfer students are accepted.
Standardized tests *Required:* SAT or ACT, TOEFL for international students. **Application** *Deadline:* rolling (freshmen), rolling (transfer). *Notification:* continuous (freshmen). *Application fee:* $55.
Advanced Placement Credit by examination available. Credit given for nursing courses completed elsewhere dependent upon specific evaluations.
Expenses (2006–07) *Required fees:* full-time $2752; part-time $848 per term.
Financial Aid 95% of baccalaureate students in nursing programs received some form of financial aid in 2005–06. *Gift aid (need-based):* Federal Pell, FSEOG, state, private, college/university gift aid from institutional funds. *Loans:* Federal Direct (Subsidized and Unsubsidized Stafford), FFEL, Perkins. *Work-Study:* Federal Work-Study. *Application deadline:* 4/15 (priority: 3/2).
Contact Dr. Laura M. Inouye, EdD, BSN Coordinator, Program in Nursing, California State University, Dominguez Hills, 1000 East Victoria Street, WH A320, Carson, CA 90747. *Telephone:* 310-243-2005. *Fax:* 310-516-3542. *E-mail:* linouye@csudh.edu.

GRADUATE PROGRAMS
Expenses (2006–07) *Required fees:* full-time $3334; part-time $1016 per term.
Financial Aid 95% of graduate students in nursing programs received some form of financial aid in 2005–06.

Contact Dr. Rose Aguilar Welch, EdD, MSN Coordinator, Program in Nursing, California State University, Dominguez Hills, 1000 East Victoria Street, WH A320, Carson, CA 90747. *Telephone:* 310-243-2112. *Fax:* 310-516-3542. *E-mail:* rwelch@csudh.edu.

MASTER'S DEGREE PROGRAM
Degree MSN
Available Programs Master's; Master's for Nurses with Non-Nursing Degrees.
Concentrations Available Nursing administration; nursing education. *Clinical nurse specialist programs in:* gerontology, parent-child. *Nurse practitioner programs in:* family health.
Site Options *Distance Learning:* Whittier, CA; Salinas, CA.
Study Options Full-time and part-time.
Program Entrance Requirements Clinical experience, minimum overall college GPA of 3.0, transcript of college record, written essay, nursing research course, physical assessment course, prerequisite course work, resume, statistics course. *Application deadline:* For fall admission, 6/1. *Application fee:* $55.
Advanced Placement Credit given for nursing courses completed elsewhere dependent upon specific evaluations.
Degree Requirements 45 total credit hours, comprehensive exam.

POST-MASTER'S PROGRAM
Areas of Study Nursing administration; nursing education. *Clinical nurse specialist programs in:* gerontology, parent-child. *Nurse practitioner programs in:* family health.

CONTINUING EDUCATION PROGRAM
Contact Student Services Center, Program in Nursing, California State University, Dominguez Hills, Student Services Center, 1000 East Victoria Street, Carson, CA 90747. *Telephone:* 800-344-5484. *Fax:* 310-516-3542. *E-mail:* sohadvising@csudh.edu.

California State University, East Bay
Department of Nursing and Health Sciences
Hayward, California

Founded in 1957

DEGREE • BS

Nursing Student Activities Sigma Theta Tau, Student Nurses' Association.

Nursing Student Resources Academic advising; academic or career counseling; assistance for students with disabilities; bookstore; campus computer network; career placement assistance; computer lab; computer-assisted instruction; daycare for children of students; e-mail services; employment services for current students; Internet; learning resource lab; library services; nursing audiovisuals; remedial services; resume preparation assistance; skills, simulation, or other laboratory; tutoring; unpaid internships.

Library Facilities 908,577 volumes; 2,210 periodical subscriptions.

BACCALAUREATE PROGRAMS
Degree BS
Available Programs Generic Baccalaureate; RN Baccalaureate.
Site Options Concord, CA.
Study Options Full-time and part-time.
Program Entrance Requirements Minimum overall college GPA of 2.0, transcript of college record, health exam, minimum GPA in nursing prerequisites of 2.4, prerequisite course work. Transfer students are accepted. **Standardized tests** *Required:* TOEFL for international students. *Required for some:* SAT or ACT. **Application** *Deadline:* 8/31 (freshmen), 8/31 (transfer). *Notification:* continuous (freshmen). *Application fee:* $55.
Advanced Placement Credit given for nursing courses completed elsewhere dependent upon specific evaluations.

California State University, East Bay (continued)

Contact   Lynn Condit, Administrative Assistant, Department of Nursing and Health Sciences, California State University, East Bay, 25800 Carlos Bee Boulevard, Hayward, CA 94542. *Telephone:* 510-885-3481. *Fax:* 510-885-2156. *E-mail:* lcondit@csuhayward.edu.

California State University, Fresno
Department of Nursing
Fresno, California

http://www.csufresno.edu/nursing/

Founded in 1911

DEGREES • BSN • MSN

Nursing Program Faculty 55 (20% with doctorates).

Baccalaureate Enrollment 360
Women 84% **Men** 16% **Minority** 54% **International** 10% **Part-time** 20%

Graduate Enrollment 113
Women 83% **Men** 17% **Minority** 40% **International** 5% **Part-time** 40%

Nursing Student Activities Sigma Theta Tau, Student Nurses' Association.

Nursing Student Resources Academic advising; academic or career counseling; assistance for students with disabilities; bookstore; campus computer network; career placement assistance; computer lab; computer-assisted instruction; daycare for children of students; e-mail services; externships; housing assistance; interactive nursing skills videos; Internet; learning resource lab; library services; nursing audiovisuals; paid internships; placement services for program completers; remedial services; skills, simulation, or other laboratory; tutoring.

Library Facilities 23,961 volumes in health, 1,287 volumes in nursing; 2,617 periodical subscriptions (1,260 health-care related).

BACCALAUREATE PROGRAMS

Degree BSN

Available Programs ADN to Baccalaureate; Baccalaureate for Second Degree; Generic Baccalaureate.

Study Options Full-time.

Program Entrance Requirements Transcript of college record, CPR certification, health exam, immunizations, minimum GPA in nursing prerequisites of 3.0, professional liability insurance/malpractice insurance, prerequisite course work. Transfer students are accepted. **Standardized tests** *Required:* SAT or ACT, TOEFL for international students. **Application Deadline:** 4/1 (freshmen), 4/1 (transfer). *Application fee:* $55.

Advanced Placement Credit by examination available. Credit given for nursing courses completed elsewhere dependent upon specific evaluations.

Expenses (2006–07) *Tuition, state resident:* full-time $3038; part-time $1518 per semester. *Tuition, nonresident:* full-time $8136; part-time $339 per unit. *International tuition:* $8136 full-time. *Room and board:* $7344 per academic year. *Required fees:* full-time $400; part-time $200 per term.

Financial Aid 65% of baccalaureate students in nursing programs received some form of financial aid in 2005–06. *Gift aid (need-based):* Federal Pell, FSEOG, state, private, college/university gift aid from institutional funds. *Loans:* Federal Nursing Student Loans, FFEL (Subsidized and Unsubsidized Stafford PLUS), Perkins, college/university. *Work-Study:* Federal Work-Study. *Application deadline (priority):* 3/1.

Contact   Dr. Michael F. Russler, EdD, Chair, Department of Nursing, California State University, Fresno, 2345 East San Ramon Avenue, MH25, Fresno, CA 93740-8031. *Telephone:* 559-278-2429. *Fax:* 559-278-6360. *E-mail:* michaelr@csufresno.edu.

GRADUATE PROGRAMS

Expenses (2006–07) *Tuition, state resident:* full-time $3620; part-time $1158 per semester. *Tuition, nonresident:* full-time $8136; part-time $339 per unit. *International tuition:* $8136 full-time. *Required fees:* full-time $400; part-time $200 per term.

Financial Aid 30% of graduate students in nursing programs received some form of financial aid in 2005–06. 2 teaching assistantships were awarded; career-related internships or fieldwork, Federal Work-Study, scholarships, and traineeships also available. Aid available to part-time students. *Financial aid application deadline:* 3/1.

Contact   Dr. Keitha Mountcastle, EdD, Graduate Coordinator, Department of Nursing, California State University, Fresno, 2345 East San Ramon Avenue, MH25, Fresno, CA 93740-8031. *Telephone:* 559-278-4691. *Fax:* 559-278-6360. *E-mail:* keitha@csufresno.edu.

MASTER'S DEGREE PROGRAM

Degree MSN

Available Programs Master's; Master's for Nurses with Non-Nursing Degrees.

Concentrations Available Nursing education. *Clinical nurse specialist programs in:* acute care, community health, critical care, pediatric, psychiatric/mental health, public health. *Nurse practitioner programs in:* family health, pediatric.

Study Options Full-time and part-time.

Program Entrance Requirements Clinical experience, computer literacy, minimum overall college GPA of 3.0, transcript of college record, CPR certification, written essay, 3 letters of recommendation, nursing research course, physical assessment course, professional liability insurance/malpractice insurance, prerequisite course work, resume, statistics course, GRE General Test. *Application deadline:* For fall admission, 5/1; for spring admission, 10/1. Applications are processed on a rolling basis. *Application fee:* $55.

Advanced Placement Credit given for nursing courses completed elsewhere dependent upon specific evaluations.

Degree Requirements 38 total credit hours, thesis or project, comprehensive exam.

POST-MASTER'S PROGRAM

Areas of Study *Nurse practitioner programs in:* family health, pediatric.

CONTINUING EDUCATION PROGRAM

Contact   Dr. Berta Gonzalez, EdD, Associate Vice President, Department of Nursing, California State University, Fresno, 5005 North Maple Avenue, ED76, Fresno, CA 93740-0076. *Telephone:* 559-278-0333. *Fax:* 559-278-0395. *E-mail:* bertag@csufresno.edu.

California State University, Fullerton
Department of Nursing
Fullerton, California

http://nursing.fullerton.edu/

Founded in 1957

DEGREES • BSN • MSN

Nursing Program Faculty 61 (20% with doctorates).

Baccalaureate Enrollment 558
Women 87% **Men** 13% **Minority** 61% **International** 1% **Part-time** 92%

Graduate Enrollment 186
Women 79% **Men** 21% **Minority** 41% **International** 1% **Part-time** 51%

Nursing Student Activities Nursing Honor Society, Sigma Theta Tau, Student Nurses' Association.

Nursing Student Resources Academic advising; academic or career counseling; assistance for students with disabilities; bookstore; campus computer network; computer lab; daycare for children of students; e-mail services; housing assistance; Internet; library services; resume preparation assistance; skills, simulation, or other laboratory; tutoring.

Library Facilities 1.2 million volumes (16,982 in health, 905 in nursing); 29,888 periodical subscriptions (5,817 health-care related).

BACCALAUREATE PROGRAMS

Degree BSN

Available Programs ADN to Baccalaureate; Baccalaureate for Second Degree.

Site Options *Distance Learning:* Sacramento, CA; Riverside, CA.

Study Options Full-time and part-time.

Program Entrance Requirements Transcript of college record, CPR certification, immunizations, 2 letters of recommendation, minimum GPA in nursing prerequisites of 2.0, professional liability insurance/malpractice insurance, prerequisite course work, RN licensure. Transfer students are accepted. **Standardized tests** *Required:* SAT or ACT, TOEFL for international students. **Application** *Deadline:* 11/30 (freshmen), rolling (transfer). *Notification:* continuous (freshmen). *Application fee:* $55.

Advanced Placement Credit given for nursing courses completed elsewhere dependent upon specific evaluations.

Financial Aid *Gift aid (need-based):* Federal Pell, FSEOG, state, private, college/university gift aid from institutional funds. *Loans:* FFEL (Subsidized and Unsubsidized Stafford PLUS), Perkins, college/university. *Work-Study:* Federal Work-Study. *Application deadline (priority):* 3/2.

Contact Nursing Program, Department of Nursing, California State University, Fullerton, EC-199, PO Box 6868, Fullerton, CA 92834-6868. *Telephone:* 714-278-3336. *Fax:* 714-278-3338. *E-mail:* nursing@fullerton. edu.

GRADUATE PROGRAMS

Financial Aid 30% of graduate students in nursing programs received some form of financial aid in 2005–06.

Contact Ms. Mary Lehn-Mooney, Department of Nursing, California State University, Fullerton, EC-199, PO Box 6868, Fullerton, CA 92834-6868. *Telephone:* 714-278-3336. *Fax:* 714-278-3338. *E-mail:* nursing@fullerton. edu.

MASTER'S DEGREE PROGRAM

Degree MSN

Available Programs Accelerated AD/RN to Master's; Master's.

Concentrations Available Nurse anesthesia; nurse-midwifery; nursing administration. *Clinical nurse specialist programs in:* school health. *Nurse practitioner programs in:* family health, women's health.

Site Options Pasadena, CA.

Study Options Full-time and part-time.

Program Entrance Requirements Clinical experience, minimum overall college GPA of 3.0, transcript of college record, CPR certification, written essay, immunizations, interview, 3 letters of recommendation, nursing research course, professional liability insurance/malpractice insurance, statistics course.

Advanced Placement Credit given for nursing courses completed elsewhere dependent upon specific evaluations.

Degree Requirements 71 total credit hours, thesis or project, comprehensive exam.

CONTINUING EDUCATION PROGRAM

Contact Ms. Debra Day, RN, Department of Nursing, California State University, Fullerton, 800 North State College Boulevard, Extended Ed CP-920, Fullerton, CA 92834-9480. *Telephone:* 714-278-4280. *E-mail:* dday@ fullerton.edu.

California State University, Long Beach
Department of Nursing
Long Beach, California

http://www.csulb.edu/depts/nursing/

Founded in 1949

DEGREES • BSN • MSN • MSN/MPH

Nursing Program Faculty 82 (25% with doctorates).

Baccalaureate Enrollment 521
Women 84.5% **Men** 15.5% **Minority** 63.3% **International** .01%

Graduate Enrollment 299
Women 92.6% **Men** 7.4% **Minority** 59.8% **International** .01% **Part-time** 76.5%

Nursing Student Activities Nursing Honor Society, Sigma Theta Tau, Student Nurses' Association.

Nursing Student Resources Academic advising; Internet; library services; skills, simulation, or other laboratory; tutoring.

Library Facilities 1.5 million volumes; 18,749 periodical subscriptions.

BACCALAUREATE PROGRAMS

Degree BSN

Available Programs ADN to Baccalaureate; Generic Baccalaureate; LPN to Baccalaureate.

Site Options Long Beach, CA.

Study Options Full-time.

Program Entrance Requirements Transcript of college record, CPR certification, health exam, health insurance, immunizations, minimum GPA in nursing prerequisites of 2.5, professional liability insurance/malpractice insurance, prerequisite course work. Transfer students are accepted. **Standardized tests** *Required:* SAT or ACT, TOEFL for international students. **Application** *Deadline:* 11/30 (freshmen), 11/30 (transfer). *Notification:* continuous (freshmen). *Application fee:* $55.

Advanced Placement Credit given for nursing courses completed elsewhere dependent upon specific evaluations.

Expenses (2006–07) *Tuition, state resident:* full-time $2866. *Tuition, nonresident:* full-time $8136. *International tuition:* $8136 full-time.

Contact Dr. Beth R. Keely, Assistant Director, Undergraduate Nursing Programs, Department of Nursing, California State University, Long Beach, 1250 Bellflower Boulevard, Long Beach, CA 90840-0301. *Telephone:* 562-985-4478. *Fax:* 562-985-2382. *E-mail:* bkeely@csulb.edu.

GRADUATE PROGRAMS

Expenses (2006–07) *Tuition, state resident:* full-time $3650. *Tuition, nonresident:* full-time $8100. *International tuition:* $8100 full-time.

Financial Aid Federal Work-Study, institutionally sponsored loans, and scholarships available.

Contact Alison Kliachko-Trafas, Administrative Assistant, Department of Nursing, California State University, Long Beach, 1250 Bellflower Boulevard, Long Beach, CA 90840-0119. *Telephone:* 562-985-4473. *Fax:* 562-985-2382. *E-mail:* akliachk@csulb.edu.

MASTER'S DEGREE PROGRAM

Degrees MSN; MSN/MPH

Available Programs Accelerated Master's for Non-Nursing College Graduates; Master's.

Concentrations Available Health-care administration; nursing education. *Clinical nurse specialist programs in:* adult health. *Nurse practitioner programs in:* adult health, family health, gerontology, pediatric, psychiatric/mental health, women's health.

Study Options Full-time and part-time.

Program Entrance Requirements Clinical experience, minimum overall college GPA of 2.75, transcript of college record, written essay, 3 letters of recommendation, physical assessment course, prerequisite course work, resume, statistics course. *Application deadline:* For fall admission, 7/1; for spring admission, 12/1. Applications are processed on a rolling basis. *Application fee:* $55.

Degree Requirements 37 total credit hours, thesis or project, comprehensive exam.

POST-MASTER'S PROGRAM

Areas of Study *Clinical nurse specialist programs in:* adult health. *Nurse practitioner programs in:* adult health, family health, gerontology, pediatric, school health.

California State University, Los Angeles
School of Nursing
Los Angeles, California

http://www.calstatela.edu/dept/nursing/

Founded in 1947

DEGREES • BS • MS

Nursing Program Faculty 31 (39% with doctorates).

Baccalaureate Enrollment 300

Graduate Enrollment 100

California State University, Los Angeles (continued)
Nursing Student Resources Academic advising.
Library Facilities 1.2 million volumes; 31,366 periodical subscriptions.

BACCALAUREATE PROGRAMS

Degree BS

Available Programs Generic Baccalaureate; RN Baccalaureate.

Program Entrance Requirements Standardized tests *Required:* TOEFL for international students. *Required for some:* SAT or ACT. **Application** *Deadline:* 6/15 (freshmen), 6/15 (transfer). *Application fee:* $55.
Contact *Telephone:* 323-343-4703. *Fax:* 323-343-6454.

GRADUATE PROGRAMS

Contact *Telephone:* 323-343-4700. *Fax:* 323-343-6454.

MASTER'S DEGREE PROGRAM

Degree MS

Available Programs Accelerated Master's for Nurses with Non-Nursing Degrees; Accelerated RN to Master's; Master's.

Concentrations Available Nurse case management; nursing administration; nursing education. *Clinical nurse specialist programs in:* psychiatric/mental health. *Nurse practitioner programs in:* acute care, adult health, family health, pediatric, primary care, women's health.

Program Entrance Requirements Minimum overall college GPA of 3.0, nursing research course, professional liability insurance/malpractice insurance, statistics course. *Application deadline:* For fall admission, 6/30; for spring admission, 2/1. Applications are processed on a rolling basis. *Application fee:* $55.

POST-MASTER'S PROGRAM

Areas of Study *Nurse practitioner programs in:* acute care, adult health, family health, pediatric, primary care.

California State University, Northridge
Nursing Program
Northridge, California

http://www.csun.edu/~nursing/
Founded in 1958
DEGREE • BSN

Nursing Program Faculty 8 (75% with doctorates).

Baccalaureate Enrollment 70
Women 88% **Men** 12% **Minority** 60% **International** 12% **Part-time** 90%
Nursing Student Activities Nursing Honor Society, nursing club.

Nursing Student Resources Academic advising; academic or career counseling; assistance for students with disabilities; bookstore; campus computer network; career placement assistance; computer lab; computer-assisted instruction; daycare for children of students; e-mail services; housing assistance; Internet; learning resource lab; library services; nursing audiovisuals; remedial services; resume preparation assistance; skills, simulation, or other laboratory; tutoring.

Library Facilities 1.2 million volumes (61,848 in health, 1,401 in nursing); 2,754 periodical subscriptions (303 health-care related).

BACCALAUREATE PROGRAMS

Degree BSN

Available Programs ADN to Baccalaureate; RN Baccalaureate.
Study Options Full-time.
Program Entrance Requirements Minimum overall college GPA of 2.5, transcript of college record, CPR certification, written essay, health exam, health insurance, immunizations, interview, 3 letters of recommendation, minimum GPA in nursing prerequisites of 2.5, professional liability insurance/malpractice insurance, prerequisite course work, RN licensure. Transfer students are accepted. **Standardized tests** *Required:*

TOEFL for international students. *Recommended:* SAT or ACT. **Application** *Deadline:* 11/30 (freshmen), rolling (transfer). *Early decision:* 8/30. *Notification:* continuous (freshmen), 9/30 (early action). *Application fee:* $55.
Advanced Placement Credit by examination available. Credit given for nursing courses completed elsewhere dependent upon specific evaluations.

Financial Aid 20% of baccalaureate students in nursing programs received some form of financial aid in 2005–06.

Contact Dr. Martha Highfield, RN, Professor and Program Director, Nursing Program, California State University, Northridge, Health Sciences Department, 18111 Nordhoff Street, Northridge, CA 91330-8285. *Telephone:* 818-677-3649. *Fax:* 818-677-2045. *E-mail:* martha.highfield@csun.edu.

California State University, Sacramento
Division of Nursing
Sacramento, California

http://www.hhs.csus.edu/nrs
Founded in 1947
DEGREES • BSN • MS

Nursing Program Faculty 50 (38% with doctorates).

Baccalaureate Enrollment 300

Graduate Enrollment 180

Nursing Student Activities Sigma Theta Tau, Student Nurses' Association.

Nursing Student Resources Academic advising; academic or career counseling; assistance for students with disabilities; bookstore; campus computer network; computer lab; computer-assisted instruction; daycare for children of students; e-mail services; externships; housing assistance; interactive nursing skills videos; Internet; learning resource lab; library services; nursing audiovisuals; placement services for program completers; remedial services; resume preparation assistance; skills, simulation, or other laboratory; tutoring.

Library Facilities 1.3 million volumes (33,000 in health); 3,761 periodical subscriptions (327 health-care related).

BACCALAUREATE PROGRAMS

Degree BSN

Available Programs ADN to Baccalaureate; Generic Baccalaureate; LPN to RN Baccalaureate; RN Baccalaureate.
Study Options Full-time.
Program Entrance Requirements Minimum overall college GPA of 2.75, transcript of college record, CPR certification, health exam, health insurance, high school biology, high school chemistry, high school foreign language, high school math, immunizations, minimum GPA in nursing prerequisites of 2.75, professional liability insurance/malpractice insurance, prerequisite course work. Transfer students are accepted. **Standardized tests** *Required:* TOEFL for international students. *Required for some:* SAT or ACT. **Application** *Deadline:* 8/1 (freshmen), 7/1 (transfer). *Early decision:* 11/30. *Notification:* 11/1 (freshmen), 11/1 (early action). *Application fee:* $55.
Advanced Placement Credit by examination available.
Contact *Telephone:* 916-278-6525.

GRADUATE PROGRAMS

Contact *Telephone:* 916-278-7298. *Fax:* 916-278-6311.

MASTER'S DEGREE PROGRAM

Degree MS

Available Programs Master's; Master's for Nurses with Non-Nursing Degrees.

Concentrations Available Nursing administration; nursing education. *Clinical nurse specialist programs in:* adult health, community health, family health, gerontology, medical-surgical, parent-child, perinatal, psychiatric/mental health, school health. *Nurse practitioner programs in:* family health, primary care.

Study Options Part-time.

Program Entrance Requirements Clinical experience, minimum overall college GPA of 3.0, transcript of college record, CPR certification, written essay, immunizations, 3 letters of recommendation, nursing research course, professional liability insurance/malpractice insurance, prerequisite course work, statistics course, GRE. *Application deadline:* Applications are processed on a rolling basis. *Application fee:* $55.

Advanced Placement Credit by examination available. Credit given for nursing courses completed elsewhere dependent upon specific evaluations.

Degree Requirements 39 total credit hours, thesis or project.

CONTINUING EDUCATION PROGRAM

Contact *Telephone:* 916-278-6525. *Fax:* 916-278-6311.

California State University, San Bernardino
Department of Nursing
San Bernardino, California

http://nursing.csusb.edu
Founded in 1965
DEGREES • BSN • MSN

Nursing Program Faculty 30 (10% with doctorates).

Baccalaureate Enrollment 210
Women 88% **Men** 12% **Minority** 49%

Graduate Enrollment 36
Women 92% **Men** 8% **Minority** 42%

Nursing Student Activities Nursing Honor Society, Sigma Theta Tau, Student Nurses' Association.

Nursing Student Resources Academic advising; academic or career counseling; assistance for students with disabilities; bookstore; campus computer network; computer lab; computer-assisted instruction; externships; Internet; library services; nursing audiovisuals; remedial services; skills, simulation, or other laboratory.

Library Facilities 731,259 volumes (1,500 in health, 1,000 in nursing); 2,028 periodical subscriptions (5,000 health-care related).

BACCALAUREATE PROGRAMS
Degree BSN

Available Programs ADN to Baccalaureate; RN Baccalaureate.
Study Options Full-time.

Program Entrance Requirements Transcript of college record, CPR certification, written essay, health exam, health insurance, immunizations, minimum GPA in nursing prerequisites of 3.0, professional liability insurance/malpractice insurance, prerequisite course work. Transfer students are accepted. **Standardized tests** *Required:* SAT or ACT, TOEFL for international students. **Application** *Deadline:* rolling (freshmen), rolling (transfer). *Notification:* continuous (freshmen). *Application fee:* $55.

Advanced Placement Credit by examination available. Credit given for nursing courses completed elsewhere dependent upon specific evaluations.

Financial Aid 80% of baccalaureate students in nursing programs received some form of financial aid in 2004–05.

Contact Ms. Anna Wilson, Lecturer/Recruiter, Department of Nursing, California State University, San Bernardino, 5500 University Parkway, San Bernadino, CA 92407. *Telephone:* 909-880-5384. *Fax:* 909-880-7089. *E-mail:* amwilson@csusb.edu.

GRADUATE PROGRAMS

Financial Aid 60% of graduate students in nursing programs received some form of financial aid in 2004–05.

Contact Dr. Susan Lloyd, Director, Master's Program, Department of Nursing, California State University, San Bernardino, 5500 University Parkway, San Bernardino, CA 92407. *Telephone:* 909-880-5380. *Fax:* 909-880-7089. *E-mail:* slloyd@csusb.edu.

MASTER'S DEGREE PROGRAM

Degree MSN

Available Programs Master's.
Concentrations Available Nurse case management; nursing education. *Clinical nurse specialist programs in:* community health, home health care, school health.
Study Options Full-time and part-time.

Program Entrance Requirements Clinical experience, minimum overall college GPA of 3.0, transcript of college record, prerequisite course work, statistics course.

Advanced Placement Credit given for nursing courses completed elsewhere dependent upon specific evaluations.

Degree Requirements 65 total credit hours, thesis or project.

California State University, Stanislaus
Department of Nursing
Turlock, California

http://www.csustan.edu/Nursing/index.htm
Founded in 1957
DEGREE • BSN

Nursing Program Faculty 17 (24% with doctorates).

Baccalaureate Enrollment 164
Women 88% **Men** 12% **Minority** 42% **Part-time** 30%

Nursing Student Activities Sigma Theta Tau, Student Nurses' Association.

Nursing Student Resources Academic advising; academic or career counseling; assistance for students with disabilities; bookstore; campus computer network; career placement assistance; computer lab; computer-assisted instruction; daycare for children of students; e-mail services; employment services for current students; externships; interactive nursing skills videos; Internet; learning resource lab; library services; nursing audiovisuals; resume preparation assistance; skills, simulation, or other laboratory; tutoring.

Library Facilities 369,047 volumes (12,642 in health, 1,338 in nursing); 17,612 periodical subscriptions (93 health-care related).

BACCALAUREATE PROGRAMS
Degree BSN

Available Programs ADN to Baccalaureate; Generic Baccalaureate; LPN to Baccalaureate.
Site Options *Distance Learning:* Stockton, CA.
Study Options Full-time.

Program Entrance Requirements Minimum overall college GPA of 3.0, transcript of college record, CPR certification, health exam, immunizations, minimum GPA in nursing prerequisites of 3.0, professional liability insurance/malpractice insurance, prerequisite course work. Transfer students are accepted. **Standardized tests** *Required:* TOEFL for international students. *Required for some:* SAT or ACT, ELM/EPT, TOEFL. **Application** *Deadline:* 7/1 (freshmen), 7/1 (transfer). *Notification:* continuous (early decision). *Application fee:* $55.

Advanced Placement Credit given for nursing courses completed elsewhere dependent upon specific evaluations.

Expenses (2006–07) *Tuition, state resident:* full-time $2520; part-time $619 per semester. *Tuition, nonresident:* full-time $10,317; part-time $462 per unit. *Room and board:* $10,418; room only: $7178 per academic year. *Required fees:* full-time $600.

Financial Aid 71% of baccalaureate students in nursing programs received some form of financial aid in 2005–06. *Gift aid (need-based):* Federal Pell, FSEOG, state, private, college/university gift aid from institutional funds. *Loans:* FFEL (Subsidized and Unsubsidized Stafford PLUS), Perkins, college/university. *Work-Study:* Federal Work-Study, part-time campus jobs. *Application deadline (priority):* 3/2.

California State University, Stanislaus (continued)

Contact Mrs. Ilene M. Worthington, Administrative Coordinator, Department of Nursing, California State University, Stanislaus, 801 West Monte Vista Avenue, Turlock, CA 95382. *Telephone:* 209-667-3141. *Fax:* 209-667-3690. *E-mail:* iworthington@csustan.edu.

Dominican University of California
Program in Nursing
San Rafael, California

Founded in 1890

DEGREES • BSN • MSN

Nursing Program Faculty 34 (15% with doctorates).

Baccalaureate Enrollment 361
Women 93% **Men** 7% **Minority** 54% **International** 2% **Part-time** 12%

Graduate Enrollment 32
Women 95% **Men** 5% **Minority** 21% **Part-time** 21%

Nursing Student Activities Nursing Honor Society, Sigma Theta Tau, Student Nurses' Association, nursing club.

Nursing Student Resources Academic advising; academic or career counseling; assistance for students with disabilities; bookstore; campus computer network; career placement assistance; computer lab; computer-assisted instruction; e-mail services; housing assistance; interactive nursing skills videos; Internet; learning resource lab; library services; nursing audiovisuals; resume preparation assistance; skills, simulation, or other laboratory; tutoring.

Library Facilities 95,000 volumes (1,200 in health, 1,000 in nursing); 508 periodical subscriptions (1,300 health-care related).

BACCALAUREATE PROGRAMS

Degree BSN

Available Programs Baccalaureate for Second Degree; Generic Baccalaureate; LPN to Baccalaureate; LPN to RN Baccalaureate; RN Baccalaureate.

Study Options Full-time and part-time.

Program Entrance Requirements Minimum overall college GPA of 2.5, transcript of college record, CPR certification, written essay, health exam, health insurance, high school biology, high school chemistry, 2 years high school math, high school transcript, immunizations, 1 letter of recommendation, minimum high school GPA of 2.7, minimum GPA in nursing prerequisites of 3.0, prerequisite course work. Transfer students are accepted. **Standardized tests** *Required:* SAT or ACT, TOEFL for international students. *Recommended:* SAT Subject Tests. **Application** *Deadline:* 8/1 (freshmen), rolling (transfer). *Notification:* continuous until 9/1 (freshmen). *Application fee:* $40.

Advanced Placement Credit given for nursing courses completed elsewhere dependent upon specific evaluations.

Financial Aid 97% of baccalaureate students in nursing programs received some form of financial aid in 2005–06. *Gift aid (need-based):* Federal Pell, FSEOG, state, private, college/university gift aid from institutional funds, Federal Nursing. *Loans:* FFEL (Subsidized and Unsubsidized Stafford PLUS), Perkins, Private loans. *Work-Study:* Federal Work-Study, part-time campus jobs. *Application deadline (priority):* 3/2.

Contact Art Criss, Director of Admissions, Program in Nursing, Dominican University of California, 50 Acacia Avenue, San Rafael, CA 94901-2298. *Telephone:* 415-257-1376. *Fax:* 415-485-3214. *E-mail:* acriss@dominican.edu.

GRADUATE PROGRAMS

Expenses (2006–07) *Tuition:* part-time $720 per unit.

Financial Aid 65% of graduate students in nursing programs received some form of financial aid in 2005–06. Fellowships, career-related internships or fieldwork, Federal Work-Study, scholarships, and tuition waivers (partial) available. Aid available to part-time students.

Contact Dr. Barbara Ganley, RN, Director of Graduate Nursing, Program in Nursing, Dominican University of California, 50 Acacia Avenue, San Rafael, CA 94901-2298. *Telephone:* 415-482-1829. *Fax:* 415-482-1829. *E-mail:* bganley@dominican.edu.

MASTER'S DEGREE PROGRAM

Degree MSN

Available Programs Master's; Master's for Nurses with Non-Nursing Degrees.

Concentrations Available Nursing education. *Clinical nurse specialist programs in:* gerontology.

Study Options Full-time and part-time.

Program Entrance Requirements Clinical experience, minimum overall college GPA of 3.0, transcript of college record, CPR certification, written essay, interview, 2 letters of recommendation, nursing research course, prerequisite course work, statistics course. *Application deadline:* Applications are processed on a rolling basis. *Application fee:* $40.

Advanced Placement Credit given for nursing courses completed elsewhere dependent upon specific evaluations.

Degree Requirements 45 total credit hours, thesis or project.

CONTINUING EDUCATION PROGRAM

Contact Ms. Sandy Baker, Director of Adult and Extended Education, Program in Nursing, Dominican University of California, 50 Acacia Avenue, San Rafael, CA 94901-2298. *Telephone:* 415-458-3255. *Fax:* 415-482-3575. *E-mail:* sbaker@dominican.edu.

See full description on page 468.

Holy Names University
Department of Nursing
Oakland, California

Founded in 1868

DEGREES • BSN • MSN • MSN/MBA

Nursing Program Faculty 44.

Baccalaureate Enrollment 150

Graduate Enrollment 45

Nursing Student Activities Nursing Honor Society, Sigma Theta Tau.

Library Facilities 109,297 volumes; 8,003 periodical subscriptions.

BACCALAUREATE PROGRAMS

Degree BSN

Available Programs RN Baccalaureate.

Program Entrance Requirements RN licensure. **Standardized tests** *Required:* SAT or ACT, TOEFL for international students. **Application** *Deadline:* 8/1 (freshmen), 8/1 (transfer). *Notification:* continuous (freshmen). *Application fee:* $50.

Contact *Telephone:* 510-436-1024. *Fax:* 510-436-1376.

GRADUATE PROGRAMS

Contact *Telephone:* 510-436-1024. *Fax:* 510-436-1376.

MASTER'S DEGREE PROGRAM

Degrees MSN; MSN/MBA

Available Programs Master's.

Concentrations Available Nursing administration. *Nurse practitioner programs in:* family health.

Program Entrance Requirements *Application deadline:* For fall admission, 8/1 (priority date); for spring admission, 12/1 (priority date). Applications are processed on a rolling basis. *Application fee:* $50.

POST-MASTER'S PROGRAM

Areas of Study Nursing administration. *Nurse practitioner programs in:* family health.

Humboldt State University

Department of Nursing
Arcata, California

http://www.humboldt.edu/~nurs

Founded in 1913

DEGREE • BSN

Nursing Program Faculty 12 (25% with doctorates).

Baccalaureate Enrollment 129
Women 85% **Men** 15% **Minority** 21%

Nursing Student Activities Sigma Theta Tau, Student Nurses' Association.

Nursing Student Resources Academic advising; academic or career counseling; assistance for students with disabilities; bookstore; campus computer network; career placement assistance; computer lab; computer-assisted instruction; daycare for children of students; e-mail services; employment services for current students; housing assistance; interactive nursing skills videos; Internet; learning resource lab; library services; nursing audiovisuals; placement services for program completers; remedial services; resume preparation assistance; skills, simulation, or other laboratory; tutoring; unpaid internships.

Library Facilities 1 million volumes (16,000 in health, 750 in nursing); 1,737 periodical subscriptions (152 health-care related).

BACCALAUREATE PROGRAMS

Degree BSN

Available Programs ADN to Baccalaureate; Baccalaureate for Second Degree; Generic Baccalaureate; International Nurse to Baccalaureate; LPN to Baccalaureate; RN Baccalaureate.

Study Options Full-time.

Program Entrance Requirements Minimum overall college GPA of 2.5, transcript of college record, CPR certification, health exam, high school foreign language, 2 years high school math, 1 year of high school science, high school transcript, immunizations, minimum GPA in nursing prerequisites of 2.5, professional liability insurance/malpractice insurance, prerequisite course work. Transfer students are accepted. **Standardized tests** *Required:* TOEFL for international students. *Required for some:* SAT or ACT. **Application** *Deadline:* 11/30 (freshmen), 11/30 (transfer). *Notification:* continuous (freshmen). *Application fee:* $55.

Advanced Placement Credit given for nursing courses completed elsewhere dependent upon specific evaluations.

Expenses (2006–07) *Tuition, state resident:* full-time $3178. *Tuition, nonresident:* full-time $10,170. *Room and board:* $8524 per academic year. *Required fees:* full-time $100.

Financial Aid 70% of baccalaureate students in nursing programs received some form of financial aid in 2005–06.

Contact Dr. Diane S. Benson, EdD, Associate Professor/Chair of Nursing, Department of Nursing, Humboldt State University, 1 Harpst Street, Arcata, CA 95521-8299. *Telephone:* 707-826-3215. *Fax:* 707-826-5141. *E-mail:* nurs@humboldt.edu.

Loma Linda University

School of Nursing
Loma Linda, California

http://www.llu.edu/llu/nursing/

Founded in 1905

DEGREES • BS • MS • MSN/MA • MSN/MPH • PHD

Nursing Program Faculty 40 (50% with doctorates).

Baccalaureate Enrollment 350
Women 78% **Men** 22% **Minority** 68% **International** 19% **Part-time** 22%

Graduate Enrollment 53
Women 96% **Men** 4% **Minority** 40% **International** 8% **Part-time** 82%

Nursing Student Activities Nursing Honor Society, Sigma Theta Tau, Student Nurses' Association, nursing club.

Nursing Student Resources Academic advising; academic or career counseling; assistance for students with disabilities; bookstore; campus computer network; computer lab; computer-assisted instruction; e-mail services; employment services for current students; housing assistance; interactive nursing skills videos; Internet; learning resource lab; library services; nursing audiovisuals; paid internships; resume preparation assistance; skills, simulation, or other laboratory; tutoring.

Library Facilities 322,657 volumes (158,000 in health, 3,916 in nursing); 1,394 periodical subscriptions (2,152 health-care related).

BACCALAUREATE PROGRAMS

Degree BS

Available Programs ADN to Baccalaureate; Accelerated Baccalaureate; Accelerated Baccalaureate for Second Degree; Accelerated LPN to Baccalaureate; Accelerated RN Baccalaureate; Baccalaureate for Second Degree; Generic Baccalaureate; LPN to Baccalaureate; LPN to RN Baccalaureate; RN Baccalaureate.

Study Options Full-time and part-time.

Program Entrance Requirements Minimum overall college GPA of 3.0, transcript of college record, CPR certification, written essay, health exam, high school transcript, immunizations, interview, 3 letters of recommendation, minimum GPA in nursing prerequisites of 3.0, prerequisite course work. Transfer students are accepted. **Standardized tests** *Required:* TOEFL for international students. **Application** *Deadline:* 4/15 (freshmen). *Application fee:* $60.

Advanced Placement Credit by examination available. Credit given for nursing courses completed elsewhere dependent upon specific evaluations.

Financial Aid 95% of baccalaureate students in nursing programs received some form of financial aid in 2005–06.

Contact Mrs. Stephanie Larsen, Director of Admissions, Marketing, and Recruiting, School of Nursing, Loma Linda University, Loma Linda, CA 92350. *Telephone:* 909-558-4923. *Fax:* 909-558-0175. *E-mail:* sllarsen@llu.edu.

GRADUATE PROGRAMS

Financial Aid 26% of graduate students in nursing programs received some form of financial aid in 2005–06.

Contact Ms. Connie Phillips, Administrative Assistant, School of Nursing, Loma Linda University, Loma Linda, CA 92350. *Telephone:* 909-558-8061. *Fax:* 909-558-4134. *E-mail:* nursing@llu.edu.

MASTER'S DEGREE PROGRAM

Degrees MS; MSN/MA; MSN/MPH

Available Programs Master's; RN to Master's.

Concentrations Available Nursing administration; nursing education. *Clinical nurse specialist programs in:* adult health, family health, parent-child, public health. *Nurse practitioner programs in:* adult health, family health, neonatal health, pediatric, primary care.

Study Options Full-time and part-time.

Program Entrance Requirements Clinical experience, minimum overall college GPA of 3.0, transcript of college record, written essay, immunizations, interview, 3 letters of recommendation, nursing research course, prerequisite course work, statistics course.

Degree Requirements Comprehensive exam.

POST-MASTER'S PROGRAM

Areas of Study *Clinical nurse specialist programs in:* public health. *Nurse practitioner programs in:* adult health, family health, neonatal health, pediatric, primary care.

DOCTORAL DEGREE PROGRAM

Degree PhD

Available Programs Doctorate.

Areas of Study Ethics, faculty preparation, health policy, human health and illness, individualized study, nursing education, nursing research, nursing science.

Program Entrance Requirements Clinical experience, minimum overall college GPA of 3.5, interview by faculty committee, interview, 3 letters of recommendation, MSN or equivalent, scholarly papers, statistics course, vita, writing sample.

Loma Linda University (continued)
Degree Requirements 95 total credit hours, dissertation, oral exam, written exam, residency.

See full description on page 504.

Mount St. Mary's College
Department of Nursing
Los Angeles, California

http://www.msmc.la.edu/nursing/
Founded in 1925
DEGREES • BSN • MSN

Nursing Program Faculty 15 (27% with doctorates).

Nursing Student Activities Nursing Honor Society, nursing club.

Nursing Student Resources Academic advising; academic or career counseling; assistance for students with disabilities; bookstore; campus computer network; career placement assistance; computer lab; computer-assisted instruction; daycare for children of students; e-mail services; employment services for current students; housing assistance; interactive nursing skills videos; Internet; learning resource lab; library services; nursing audiovisuals; remedial services; resume preparation assistance; skills, simulation, or other laboratory; tutoring.

Library Facilities 140,000 volumes (4,000 in health, 1,000 in nursing); 750 periodical subscriptions (150 health-care related).

BACCALAUREATE PROGRAMS
Degree BSN

Available Programs ADN to Baccalaureate; Accelerated Baccalaureate; Generic Baccalaureate.

Study Options Full-time.

Program Entrance Requirements Minimum overall college GPA of 2.7, transcript of college record, CPR certification, written essay, health exam, high school chemistry, high school transcript, immunizations, 1 letter of recommendation, minimum GPA in nursing prerequisites of 2.5, professional liability insurance/malpractice insurance, prerequisite course work. Transfer students are accepted. **Standardized tests** *Required:* SAT or ACT, TOEFL for international students. *Recommended:* SAT. **Application** *Deadline:* 2/15 (freshmen), 3/15 (transfer). *Early decision:* 12/1. *Notification:* continuous (freshmen), 1/1 (early action). *Application fee:* $40.

Advanced Placement Credit by examination available. Credit given for nursing courses completed elsewhere dependent upon specific evaluations.

Expenses (2005–06) *Tuition:* full-time $22,824; part-time $840 per unit. *Room and board:* $8895 per academic year. *Required fees:* full-time $960.

Contact Admissions Officer, Department of Nursing, Mount St. Mary's College, 12001 Chalon Road, Los Angeles, CA 90049-1599. *Telephone:* 800-999-9893. *E-mail:* admissions@msmc.la.edu.

GRADUATE PROGRAMS
Expenses (2005–06) *Tuition:* part-time $594 per unit. *Required fees:* full-time $1188.

Contact Graduate Program, Department of Nursing, Mount St. Mary's College, 10 Chester Place, Los Angeles, CA 90007. *Telephone:* 213-477-2676.

MASTER'S DEGREE PROGRAM
Degree MSN

Available Programs Master's.

Concentrations Available Nursing education.

Study Options Part-time.

Program Entrance Requirements Minimum overall college GPA of 3.0, transcript of college record, CPR certification, written essay, immunizations, professional liability insurance/malpractice insurance.

Advanced Placement Credit given for nursing courses completed elsewhere dependent upon specific evaluations.

Degree Requirements 37 total credit hours, thesis or project.

National University
Department of Nursing
La Jolla, California

http://www.nu.edu/nursing-handbook
Founded in 1971
DEGREE • BSN

Nursing Program Faculty 52 (15% with doctorates).

Baccalaureate Enrollment 159
Women 84% **Men** 16% **Minority** 41% **International** 2%

Nursing Student Activities Student Nurses' Association.

Nursing Student Resources Academic advising; academic or career counseling; assistance for students with disabilities; bookstore; campus computer network; computer lab; Internet; library services; nursing audiovisuals; other; remedial services; resume preparation assistance; tutoring.

Library Facilities 250,000 volumes (14,446 in health, 1,167 in nursing); 18,889 periodical subscriptions (2,047 health-care related).

BACCALAUREATE PROGRAMS
Degree BSN

Available Programs Accelerated Baccalaureate; Generic Baccalaureate; LPN to Baccalaureate; RN Baccalaureate.

Study Options Full-time.

Program Entrance Requirements Minimum overall college GPA of 2.0, transcript of college record, CPR certification, written essay, health insurance, immunizations, minimum GPA in nursing prerequisites of 2.75, professional liability insurance/malpractice insurance, prerequisite course work. Transfer students are accepted. **Standardized tests** *Required:* TOEFL for international students. **Application** *Deadline:* rolling (freshmen), rolling (transfer). *Notification:* continuous (freshmen). *Application fee:* $60.

Advanced Placement Credit given for nursing courses completed elsewhere dependent upon specific evaluations.

Expenses (2006–07) *Tuition:* full-time $15,108; part-time $252 per quarter hour. *International tuition:* $15,108 full-time. *Required fees:* full-time $1500.

Financial Aid 89% of baccalaureate students in nursing programs received some form of financial aid in 2005–06.

Contact Mr. Joel Sedano, Admissions Counselor, Department of Nursing, National University, 11255 North Torrey Pines Road, La Jolla, CA 92037. *Telephone:* 800-628-8648 Ext. 8211. *Fax:* 858-642-8709. *E-mail:* jsedano@nu.edu.

Pacific Union College
Department of Nursing
Angwin, California

Founded in 1882
DEGREE • BSN

Nursing Program Faculty 9 (33% with doctorates).

Baccalaureate Enrollment 40
Women 94% **Men** 6% **Minority** 39% **Part-time** 56%

Nursing Student Activities Student Nurses' Association.

Nursing Student Resources Academic advising; academic or career counseling; assistance for students with disabilities; bookstore; campus computer network; career placement assistance; computer lab; e-mail services; externships; housing assistance; Internet; learning resource lab; library services; nursing audiovisuals; skills, simulation, or other laboratory; tutoring.

Library Facilities 173,839 volumes; 812 periodical subscriptions (109 health-care related).

BACCALAUREATE PROGRAMS
Degree BSN

Available Programs ADN to Baccalaureate.

Site Options Fairfield, CA.

Study Options Full-time and part-time.

Program Entrance Requirements Transcript of college record, CPR certification, health exam, health insurance, immunizations, interview, 2 letters of recommendation, minimum GPA in nursing prerequisites of 2.0, professional liability insurance/malpractice insurance, prerequisite course work, RN licensure. Transfer students are accepted. **Standardized tests** *Required:* SAT or ACT, TOEFL for international students. **Application** *Deadline:* rolling (freshmen), rolling (transfer). *Application fee:* $30.

Advanced Placement Credit given for nursing courses completed elsewhere dependent upon specific evaluations.

Expenses (2005–06) *Tuition:* full-time $17,934; part-time $3550 per quarter.

Financial Aid 93% of baccalaureate students in nursing programs received some form of financial aid in 2004–05. *Gift aid (need-based):* Federal Pell, FSEOG, state, private, college/university gift aid from institutional funds. *Loans:* FFEL (Subsidized and Unsubsidized Stafford PLUS), Perkins, college/university. *Work-Study:* Federal Work-Study. *Application deadline (priority):* 3/2.

Contact Mrs. Carol Williams, RN, Coordinator, BSN Program, Department of Nursing, Pacific Union College, One Angwin Avenue, Angwin, CA 94508. *Telephone:* 707-965-7619. *Fax:* 707-965-6499. *E-mail:* cwilliams@puc.edu.

CONTINUING EDUCATION PROGRAM

Contact Dr. Nancy L. Tucker, Chair, Department of Nursing, Pacific Union College, One Angwin Avenue, Angwin, CA 94508. *Telephone:* 707-965-7262. *Fax:* 707-965-6499. *E-mail:* ntucker@puc.edu.

Point Loma Nazarene University
School of Nursing
San Diego, California

http://www.ptloma.edu/nursing

Founded in 1902

DEGREES • BSN • MSN

Nursing Program Faculty 22 (25% with doctorates).

Baccalaureate Enrollment 162
Women 90% **Men** 10% **Minority** 23% **Part-time** 2%

Graduate Enrollment 32
Women 100% **Minority** 25% **Part-time** 5%

Nursing Student Activities Sigma Theta Tau, Student Nurses' Association.

Nursing Student Resources Academic advising; academic or career counseling; bookstore; campus computer network; computer lab; computer-assisted instruction; daycare for children of students; e-mail services; employment services for current students; externships; housing assistance; interactive nursing skills videos; Internet; learning resource lab; library services; nursing audiovisuals; paid internships; resume preparation assistance; skills, simulation, or other laboratory; tutoring; unpaid internships.

Library Facilities 152,377 volumes; 25,505 periodical subscriptions.

BACCALAUREATE PROGRAMS

Degree BSN

Available Programs ADN to Baccalaureate; Baccalaureate for Second Degree; Generic Baccalaureate; LPN to RN Baccalaureate; RN Baccalaureate.

Study Options Full-time.

Program Entrance Requirements Minimum overall college GPA of 2.7, transcript of college record, CPR certification, written essay, health exam, health insurance, high school chemistry, high school foreign language, 2 years high school math, 1 year of high school science, high school transcript, immunizations, interview, 3 letters of recommendation, minimum GPA in nursing prerequisites of 2.3, prerequisite course work. Transfer students are accepted. **Standardized tests** *Required:* SAT or ACT, TOEFL for international students. *Recommended:* SAT. **Application** *Deadline:* 3/1 (freshmen), rolling (transfer). *Early decision:* 12/1. *Notification:* continuous (freshmen), 1/15 (early action). *Application fee:* $50.

Advanced Placement Credit by examination available. Credit given for nursing courses completed elsewhere dependent upon specific evaluations.

Expenses (2005–06) *Tuition:* full-time $20,200; part-time $842 per credit. *International tuition:* $20,200 full-time. *Room and board:* $6880 per academic year. *Required fees:* full-time $800; part-time $45 per term.

Financial Aid 90% of baccalaureate students in nursing programs received some form of financial aid in 2004–05.

Contact Ms. Marsha Reece, Undergraduate Program Assistant, School of Nursing, Point Loma Nazarene University, 3900 Lomaland Drive, San Diego, CA 92106-2899. *Telephone:* 619-849-2425. *Fax:* 619-849-2672. *E-mail:* mreece@ptloma.edu.

GRADUATE PROGRAMS

Expenses (2005–06) *Tuition:* full-time $10,400; part-time $520 per credit. *International tuition:* $10,400 full-time.

Financial Aid 80% of graduate students in nursing programs received some form of financial aid in 2004–05.

Contact Prof. Barbara Taylor, MSN Director/Associate Dean, School of Nursing, Point Loma Nazarene University, 3900 Lomaland Drive, San Diego, CA 92106-2899. *Telephone:* 619-849-2425. *E-mail:* bataylor@ptloma.edu.

MASTER'S DEGREE PROGRAM

Degree MSN

Available Programs Master's.

Concentrations Available Nursing education. *Clinical nurse specialist programs in:* family health, gerontology, medical-surgical, psychiatric/mental health.

Site Options San Diego, CA.

Study Options Full-time and part-time.

Program Entrance Requirements Computer literacy, minimum overall college GPA of 3.0, transcript of college record, CPR certification, written essay, immunizations, interview, 3 letters of recommendation, nursing research course, physical assessment course, professional liability insurance/malpractice insurance, statistics course.

Advanced Placement Credit given for nursing courses completed elsewhere dependent upon specific evaluations.

Degree Requirements 43 total credit hours, thesis or project.

CONTINUING EDUCATION PROGRAM

Contact Ms. Marsha Reece, Program Assistant, School of Nursing, Point Loma Nazarene University, 3900 Lomaland Drive, San Diego, CA 92106-2899. *Telephone:* 619-849-7055. *Fax:* 619-849-2672. *E-mail:* mreece@ptloma.edu.

Samuel Merritt College
School of Nursing
Oakland, California

Founded in 1909

DEGREES • BSN • MSN

Nursing Program Faculty 105 (19% with doctorates).

Baccalaureate Enrollment 320
Women 87% **Men** 13% **Minority** 51% **International** .3% **Part-time** 6%

Graduate Enrollment 343
Women 85% **Men** 15% **Minority** 43% **International** .3% **Part-time** 29%

Nursing Student Activities Sigma Theta Tau, Student Nurses' Association.

Nursing Student Resources Academic advising; academic or career counseling; assistance for students with disabilities; bookstore; campus computer network; computer lab; computer-assisted instruction; e-mail services; housing assistance; interactive nursing skills videos; Internet; learning resource lab; library services; nursing audiovisuals; remedial services; skills, simulation, or other laboratory; tutoring; unpaid internships.

Library Facilities 36,995 volumes (13,329 in health, 2,387 in nursing); 2,970 periodical subscriptions (2,850 health-care related).

Samuel Merritt College (continued)

BACCALAUREATE PROGRAMS

Degree BSN

Available Programs Accelerated Baccalaureate; Generic Baccalaureate.

Site Options San Francisco, CA.

Study Options Full-time and part-time.

Program Entrance Requirements Minimum overall college GPA of 3.0, transcript of college record, health exam, high school biology, high school chemistry, high school foreign language, 2 years high school math, 3 years high school science, high school transcript, immunizations, 1 letter of recommendation, minimum high school GPA of 2.5, minimum GPA in nursing prerequisites of 3.0, prerequisite course work. Transfer students are accepted. **Standardized tests** *Required:* TOEFL for international students. **Application** *Deadline:* 3/1 (transfer). *Notification:* continuous (freshmen). *Application fee:* $35.

Advanced Placement Credit by examination available. Credit given for nursing courses completed elsewhere dependent upon specific evaluations.

Expenses (2006–07) *Tuition:* full-time $29,220; part-time $1214 per unit. *International tuition:* $29,220 full-time. *Room and board:* room only: $4427 per academic year. *Required fees:* full-time $791.

Financial Aid 85% of baccalaureate students in nursing programs received some form of financial aid in 2005–06.

Contact Ms. Anne E. Seed, Director of Admissions, School of Nursing, Samuel Merritt College, Office of Admissions, 370 Hawthorne Avenue, Oakland, CA 94609. *Telephone:* 510-869-6610. *Fax:* 510-869-6525. *E-mail:* admission@samuelmerritt.edu.

GRADUATE PROGRAMS

Expenses (2006–07) *Tuition:* full-time $22,572; part-time $836 per unit. *International tuition:* $22,572 full-time. *Room and board:* room only: $5904 per academic year. *Required fees:* full-time $691.

Financial Aid 87% of graduate students in nursing programs received some form of financial aid in 2005–06. Career-related internships or fieldwork, Federal Work-Study, scholarships, and traineeships available. Aid available to part-time students. *Financial aid application deadline:* 3/2.

Contact Ms. Anne E. Seed, Director of Admissions, School of Nursing, Samuel Merritt College, Office of Admissions, 370 Hawthorne Avenue, Oakland, CA 94609. *Telephone:* 510-869-6610. *Fax:* 510-869-6525. *E-mail:* aseed@samuelmerritt.edu.

MASTER'S DEGREE PROGRAM

Degree MSN

Available Programs Master's; Master's for Non-Nursing College Graduates; Master's for Nurses with Non-Nursing Degrees.

Concentrations Available Nurse anesthesia; nurse case management. *Nurse practitioner programs in:* family health.

Site Options Sacramento, CA.

Study Options Full-time and part-time.

Program Entrance Requirements Clinical experience, computer literacy, minimum overall college GPA of 3.0, transcript of college record, CPR certification, written essay, immunizations, interview, 2 letters of recommendation, prerequisite course work, statistics course. *Application deadline:* For fall admission, 1/15 (priority date). Applications are processed on a rolling basis. *Application fee:* $50.

Advanced Placement Credit by examination available. Credit given for nursing courses completed elsewhere dependent upon specific evaluations.

Degree Requirements 49 total credit hours, thesis or project, comprehensive exam.

POST-MASTER'S PROGRAM

Areas of Study Nurse anesthesia; nurse case management. *Nurse practitioner programs in:* family health.

San Diego State University

School of Nursing
San Diego, California

http://nursing.sdsu.edu

Founded in 1897

DEGREES • BSN • MSN

Nursing Program Faculty 66 (36% with doctorates).

Baccalaureate Enrollment 540

Nursing Student Activities Sigma Theta Tau, Student Nurses' Association.

Nursing Student Resources Academic advising; bookstore; campus computer network; computer lab; daycare for children of students; e-mail services; Internet; library services; nursing audiovisuals; skills, simulation, or other laboratory.

Library Facilities 1.3 million volumes (36,000 in health, 14,000 in nursing); 8,245 periodical subscriptions (335 health-care related).

BACCALAUREATE PROGRAMS

Degree BSN

Available Programs Generic Baccalaureate; RN Baccalaureate.

Study Options Full-time.

Program Entrance Requirements Minimum overall college GPA of 3.0, transcript of college record, CPR certification, written essay, health exam, high school foreign language, high school math, high school transcript, immunizations, minimum high school GPA of 2.5, minimum GPA in nursing prerequisites of 2.5, professional liability insurance/malpractice insurance, prerequisite course work. Transfer students are accepted. **Standardized tests** *Required:* SAT or ACT, TOEFL for international students. **Application** *Deadline:* 11/30 (freshmen), 11/30 (transfer). *Notification:* 3/1 (freshmen). *Application fee:* $55.

Advanced Placement Credit given for nursing courses completed elsewhere dependent upon specific evaluations.

Expenses (2005–06) *Tuition, state resident:* full-time $3466; part-time $1033 per semester. *Tuition, nonresident:* full-time $10,170. *International tuition:* $10,170 full-time. *Room and board:* room only: $11,572 per academic year.

Contact Nursing, School of Nursing, San Diego State University, 5500 Campanile Drive, San Diego, CA 92182-0254. *Telephone:* 619-594-2540. *Fax:* 619-594-2765. *E-mail:* nursing@mail.sdsu.edu.

GRADUATE PROGRAMS

Expenses (2005–06) *Tuition, area resident:* full-time $2402; part-time $1852 per semester. *Tuition, state resident:* full-time $2410; part-time $339 per unit. *Tuition, nonresident:* full-time $10,170; part-time $339 per unit. *International tuition:* $10,170 full-time. *Room and board:* room only: $11,572 per academic year.

Financial Aid Career-related internships or fieldwork, scholarships, traineeships, and unspecified assistantships available.

Contact Associate Professor and Graduate Adviser, School of Nursing, San Diego State University, 5500 Campanile Drive, San Diego, CA 92182-0254. *Telephone:* 619-594-2770. *Fax:* 619-594-2765.

MASTER'S DEGREE PROGRAM

Degree MSN

Available Programs Master's.

Concentrations Available Nurse-midwifery. *Clinical nurse specialist programs in:* adult health, community health, gerontology, school health. *Nurse practitioner programs in:* acute care, adult health, family health, gerontology.

Site Options La Jolla, CA.

Study Options Full-time and part-time.

Program Entrance Requirements Clinical experience, minimum overall college GPA of 3.0, transcript of college record, written essay, 3 letters of recommendation, nursing research course, physical assessment course, professional liability insurance/malpractice insurance, statistics course, GRE General Test. *Application deadline:* For fall admission, 1/15; for spring admission, 11/1. Applications are processed on a rolling basis. *Application fee:* $55.

Advanced Placement Credit by examination available. Credit given for nursing courses completed elsewhere dependent upon specific evaluations.

Degree Requirements 39 total credit hours, thesis or project, comprehensive exam.

POST-MASTER'S PROGRAM

Areas of Study Nurse-midwifery.

CONTINUING EDUCATION PROGRAM

Contact Nursing, School of Nursing, San Diego State University, 5500 Campanile Drive, San Diego, CA 92182-0254. *Telephone:* 619-594-5357. *Fax:* 619-594-2765.

San Francisco State University
School of Nursing
San Francisco, California

Founded in 1899

DEGREES • BSN • MSN

Nursing Program Faculty 40 (50% with doctorates).

Baccalaureate Enrollment 250
Women 88% **Men** 12% **Minority** 53% **International** 2% **Part-time** 5%

Graduate Enrollment 180
Women 80% **Men** 20% **Minority** 80% **International** 10% **Part-time** 20%

Nursing Student Activities Sigma Theta Tau, Student Nurses' Association.

Nursing Student Resources Academic advising; academic or career counseling; assistance for students with disabilities; bookstore; campus computer network; career placement assistance; computer lab; computer-assisted instruction; daycare for children of students; e-mail services; employment services for current students; externships; housing assistance; interactive nursing skills videos; Internet; learning resource lab; library services; nursing audiovisuals; other; placement services for program completers; remedial services; resume preparation assistance; skills, simulation, or other laboratory; tutoring.

Library Facilities 1.2 million volumes (11,000 in health, 1,500 in nursing); 15,644 periodical subscriptions (200 health-care related).

BACCALAUREATE PROGRAMS

Degree BSN

Available Programs ADN to Baccalaureate; Accelerated LPN to Baccalaureate; Generic Baccalaureate; RN Baccalaureate.

Study Options Full-time.

Program Entrance Requirements Minimum overall college GPA of 2.5, transcript of college record, CPR certification, health exam, health insurance, immunizations, minimum GPA in nursing prerequisites of 2.5, professional liability insurance/malpractice insurance, prerequisite course work. Transfer students are accepted. **Standardized tests** *Required:* TOEFL for international students. *Required for some:* SAT or ACT. **Application** *Deadline:* rolling (freshmen). *Notification:* continuous (freshmen). *Application fee:* $55.

Advanced Placement Credit by examination available. Credit given for nursing courses completed elsewhere dependent upon specific evaluations.

Contact *Telephone:* 415-338-2315 Ext. 1. *Fax:* 415-338-0555.

GRADUATE PROGRAMS

Contact *Telephone:* 415-338-1802. *Fax:* 415-338-0555.

MASTER'S DEGREE PROGRAM

Degree MSN

Available Programs Accelerated Master's for Non-Nursing College Graduates; Accelerated Master's for Nurses with Non-Nursing Degrees; Master's; Master's for Non-Nursing College Graduates; Master's for Nurses with Non-Nursing Degrees.

Concentrations Available Nurse case management; nursing administration. *Clinical nurse specialist programs in:* adult health, perinatal, public health. *Nurse practitioner programs in:* family health.

Study Options Full-time and part-time.

Program Entrance Requirements Minimum overall college GPA of 3.0, transcript of college record, CPR certification, written essay, immunizations, 3 letters of recommendation, nursing research course, professional liability insurance/malpractice insurance, resume, statistics course. *Application deadline:* For fall admission, 11/30 (priority date); for spring admission, 5/31. Applications are processed on a rolling basis. *Application fee:* $55.

Advanced Placement Credit by examination available. Credit given for nursing courses completed elsewhere dependent upon specific evaluations.

Degree Requirements 36 total credit hours, thesis or project.

POST-MASTER'S PROGRAM

Areas of Study Nursing administration. *Nurse practitioner programs in:* family health.

CONTINUING EDUCATION PROGRAM

Contact *Telephone:* 415-405-3660. *Fax:* 415-338-0555.

San Jose State University
School of Nursing
San Jose, California

Founded in 1857

DEGREES • BS • MS

Nursing Program Faculty 55 (52% with doctorates).

Baccalaureate Enrollment 550
Women 92% **Men** 8% **Minority** 76% **Part-time** 20%

Graduate Enrollment 101
Women 92% **Men** 8% **Minority** 46% **Part-time** 83%

Nursing Student Activities Sigma Theta Tau, Student Nurses' Association, nursing club.

Nursing Student Resources Academic advising; academic or career counseling; assistance for students with disabilities; bookstore; career placement assistance; computer lab; computer-assisted instruction; housing assistance; interactive nursing skills videos; Internet; learning resource lab; library services; nursing audiovisuals; skills, simulation, or other laboratory; tutoring.

Library Facilities 1.8 million volumes (280 in health, 250 in nursing); 35,390 periodical subscriptions (80 health-care related).

BACCALAUREATE PROGRAMS

Degree BS

Available Programs Generic Baccalaureate; RPN to Baccalaureate.

Site Options Salinas, CA; Gilroy, CA.

Study Options Full-time and part-time.

Program Entrance Requirements Transcript of college record, health insurance, 3 years high school math, minimum high school GPA of 2.0, minimum GPA in nursing prerequisites of 2.0, professional liability insurance/malpractice insurance, prerequisite course work. Transfer students are accepted. **Standardized tests** *Required:* TOEFL for international students. *Required for some:* SAT or ACT. **Application** *Deadline:* 11/30 (freshmen), rolling (transfer). *Notification:* continuous (freshmen). *Application fee:* $55.

Advanced Placement Credit by examination available. Credit given for nursing courses completed elsewhere dependent upon specific evaluations.

Contact *Telephone:* 408-924-3131. *Fax:* 408-924-3135.

GRADUATE PROGRAMS

Contact *Telephone:* 408-924-3144. *Fax:* 408-924-3135.

MASTER'S DEGREE PROGRAM

Degree MS

Available Programs Master's.

San Jose State University (continued)

Concentrations Available Nursing administration; nursing education. *Clinical nurse specialist programs in:* gerontology, school health. *Nurse practitioner programs in:* family health.

Study Options Full-time and part-time.

Program Entrance Requirements Minimum overall college GPA of 3.0, transcript of college record, CPR certification, written essay, immunizations, 3 letters of recommendation, nursing research course, physical assessment course, professional liability insurance/malpractice insurance, resume, statistics course.

Degree Requirements 36 total credit hours, thesis or project.

Sonoma State University
Department of Nursing
Rohnert Park, California

http://www.sonoma.edu/nursing

Founded in 1960

DEGREES • BSN • MSN

Nursing Program Faculty 32 (28% with doctorates).

Baccalaureate Enrollment 140
Women 89% **Men** 11% **Minority** 26% **International** 2% **Part-time** 15%

Graduate Enrollment 109
Women 94% **Men** 6% **Minority** 25% **Part-time** 34%

Nursing Student Activities Nursing Honor Society, Sigma Theta Tau, Student Nurses' Association, nursing club.

Nursing Student Resources Academic advising; academic or career counseling; assistance for students with disabilities; bookstore; campus computer network; career placement assistance; computer lab; computer-assisted instruction; daycare for children of students; e-mail services; employment services for current students; externships; housing assistance; interactive nursing skills videos; Internet; learning resource lab; library services; nursing audiovisuals; remedial services; resume preparation assistance; skills, simulation, or other laboratory; tutoring; unpaid internships.

Library Facilities 636,613 volumes (26,700 in health, 1,400 in nursing); 21,115 periodical subscriptions (64 health-care related).

BACCALAUREATE PROGRAMS

Degree BSN

Available Programs ADN to Baccalaureate; Baccalaureate for Second Degree; Generic Baccalaureate; LPN to Baccalaureate; LPN to RN Baccalaureate; RN Baccalaureate.

Study Options Full-time.

Program Entrance Requirements Minimum overall college GPA of 3.0, transcript of college record, CPR certification, written essay, health exam, health insurance, high school biology, high school chemistry, high school foreign language, 3 years high school math, 2 years high school science, high school transcript, immunizations, 2 letters of recommendation, minimum high school GPA of 3.0, minimum GPA in nursing prerequisites of 3.0, professional liability insurance/malpractice insurance, prerequisite course work. Transfer students are accepted. **Standardized tests** *Required:* SAT or ACT, TOEFL for international students. **Application Deadline:** rolling (freshmen), rolling (transfer). *Notification:* continuous (freshmen). *Application fee:* $55.

Expenses (2006–07) *Tuition, state resident:* full-time $3648; part-time $1296 per semester. *Tuition, nonresident:* full-time $13,818; part-time $3330 per semester. *International tuition:* $13,818 full-time. *Room and board:* $8465; room only: $6102 per academic year. *Required fees:* full-time $60; part-time $30 per term.

Financial Aid 53% of baccalaureate students in nursing programs received some form of financial aid in 2005–06.

Contact Ms. Becky S. Cohen, Administrative Coordinator, Department of Nursing, Sonoma State University, 1801 East Cotati Avenue, Rohnert Park, CA 94928. *Telephone:* 707-664-2465. *Fax:* 707-664-2653. *E-mail:* nursing@sonoma.edu.

GRADUATE PROGRAMS

Expenses (2006–07) *Tuition, state resident:* full-time $4230; part-time $1464 per semester. *Tuition, nonresident:* full-time $12,366; part-time $3498 per semester. *International tuition:* $12,366 full-time. *Room and board:* $10,000; room only: $7652 per academic year. *Required fees:* full-time $40; part-time $20 per term.

Financial Aid 70% of graduate students in nursing programs received some form of financial aid in 2005–06.

Contact Ms. Becky S. Cohen, Administrative Coordinator, Department of Nursing, Sonoma State University, 1801 East Cotati Avenue, Rohnert Park, CA 94928. *Telephone:* 707-664-2465. *Fax:* 707-664-2653. *E-mail:* nursing@sonoma.edu.

MASTER'S DEGREE PROGRAM

Degree MSN

Available Programs Master's.

Concentrations Available Nursing administration; nursing education. *Nurse practitioner programs in:* family health.

Site Options *Distance Learning:* Turlock, CA; Chico, CA.

Study Options Full-time.

Program Entrance Requirements Clinical experience, computer literacy, minimum overall college GPA of 3.0, transcript of college record, CPR certification, written essay, immunizations, 3 letters of recommendation, physical assessment course, professional liability insurance/malpractice insurance, prerequisite course work, statistics course.

Advanced Placement Credit given for nursing courses completed elsewhere dependent upon specific evaluations.

Degree Requirements 32 total credit hours, thesis or project, comprehensive exam.

POST-MASTER'S PROGRAM

Areas of Study *Nurse practitioner programs in:* family health.

University of California, Los Angeles
School of Nursing
Los Angeles, California

http://www.nursing.ucla.edu

Founded in 1919

DEGREES • BS • MSN • MSN/MBA • PHD

Nursing Program Faculty 51 (70% with doctorates).

Baccalaureate Enrollment 80
Women 93% **Men** 7% **Minority** 68% **International** 1%

Graduate Enrollment 330
Women 90% **Men** 10% **Minority** 56% **International** 2%

Nursing Student Activities Nursing Honor Society, Sigma Theta Tau, Student Nurses' Association, nursing club.

Nursing Student Resources Academic advising; assistance for students with disabilities; bookstore; campus computer network; computer lab; daycare for children of students; e-mail services; housing assistance; Internet; library services; nursing audiovisuals.

Library Facilities 7.6 million volumes (760,000 in health, 8,000 in nursing); 94,801 periodical subscriptions (600,000 health-care related).

BACCALAUREATE PROGRAMS

Degree BS

Available Programs ADN to Baccalaureate; Generic Baccalaureate.

Study Options Full-time.

Program Entrance Requirements Transcript of college record, written essay, high school transcript, 2 letters of recommendation. **Standardized tests** *Required:* SAT or ACT, SAT Subject Tests, TOEFL for international students. **Application** *Deadline:* 11/30 (freshmen), 11/30 (transfer). *Notification:* 3/15 (freshmen). *Application fee:* $60.

Expenses (2006–07) *Tuition, state resident:* full-time $7143. *Tuition, nonresident:* full-time $25,827. *International tuition:* $25,827 full-time. *Room and board:* $11,709 per academic year.

Financial Aid 61% of baccalaureate students in nursing programs received some form of financial aid in 2005–06. *Gift aid (need-based):* Federal Pell, FSEOG, state, private, college/university gift aid from institutional funds, United Negro College Fund, Federal Nursing, National Merit. *Loans:* Federal Nursing Student Loans, FFEL (Subsidized and Unsubsidized Stafford PLUS), Perkins, state, college/university. *Work-Study:* Federal Work-Study, part-time campus jobs. *Application deadline (priority):* 3/2.

Contact Ms. Teresa Valenzuela, Undergraduate Student Services Coordinator, School of Nursing, University of California, Los Angeles, Box 951702, Los Angeles, CA 90095-1702. *Telephone:* 310-825-7181. *Fax:* 310-206-7433. *E-mail:* sonsaff@sonnet.ucla.edu.

GRADUATE PROGRAMS

Expenses (2006–07) *Tuition, state resident:* full-time $11,748. *Tuition, nonresident:* full-time $23,993. *International tuition:* $23,993 full-time. *Room and board:* room only: $910 per academic year.

Financial Aid 80% of graduate students in nursing programs received some form of financial aid in 2005–06. 195 fellowships, 4 research assistantships, 2 teaching assistantships were awarded; Federal Work-Study, institutionally sponsored loans, scholarships, and tuition waivers (full and partial) also available. *Financial aid application deadline:* 3/1.

Contact Ms. Kathy Scrivner, Student Affairs Officer, School of Nursing, University of California, Los Angeles, Box 951702, Los Angeles, CA 90095-1702. *Telephone:* 310-825-7181. *Fax:* 310-267-0330. *E-mail:* sonsaff@ucla.edu.

MASTER'S DEGREE PROGRAM

Degrees MSN; MSN/MBA

Available Programs Master's; Master's for Non-Nursing College Graduates.

Concentrations Available Nursing administration. *Clinical nurse specialist programs in:* acute care, gerontology, oncology, pediatric. *Nurse practitioner programs in:* acute care, family health, gerontology, occupational health, oncology, pediatric.

Study Options Full-time.

Program Entrance Requirements Minimum overall college GPA of 3.0, transcript of college record, written essay, 3 letters of recommendation, nursing research course, physical assessment course, prerequisite course work, statistics course, Commission on Graduates of Foreign Nursing Schools Exam. *Application deadline:* For fall admission, 2/1. *Application fee:* $60.

Degree Requirements 72 total credit hours, comprehensive exam.

POST-MASTER'S PROGRAM

Areas of Study Nursing administration. *Nurse practitioner programs in:* acute care, family health, gerontology, oncology, pediatric.

DOCTORAL DEGREE PROGRAM

Degree PhD

Available Programs Doctorate.

Areas of Study Addiction/substance abuse, advanced practice nursing, aging, bio-behavioral research, biology of health and illness, clinical practice, community health, critical care, family health, gerontology, health policy, health promotion/disease prevention, health-care systems, human health and illness, illness and transition, neuro-behavior, nursing administration, nursing research, nursing science, oncology, women's health.

Program Entrance Requirements Minimum overall college GPA of 3.5, 4 letters of recommendation, MSN or equivalent, scholarly papers, statistics course, vita, writing sample, GRE General Test, Commission on Graduates of Foreign Nursing Schools exam. *Application deadline:* For fall admission, 2/1. *Application fee:* $60.

Degree Requirements 127 total credit hours, dissertation, oral exam, written exam, residency.

POSTDOCTORAL PROGRAM

Areas of Study Addiction/substance abuse, adolescent health, aging, cancer care, gerontology, health promotion/disease prevention, nursing research, vulnerable population, women's health.

Postdoctoral Program Contact Dr. Adeline Nyamathi, Associate Dean for Academic Affairs, School of Nursing, University of California, Los Angeles, Box 951702, Los Angeles, CA 90095-1702. *Telephone:* 310-825-8405. *Fax:* 310-206-7433. *E-mail:* anyamath@sonnet.ucla.edu.

CONTINUING EDUCATION PROGRAM

Contact Ms. Salpy Akaragian, Education Specialist, School of Nursing, University of California, Los Angeles, Box 951701, Los Angeles, CA 90095-1701. *Telephone:* 310-206-9581. *E-mail:* nssa@mednet.ucla.edu.

University of California, San Francisco
School of Nursing
San Francisco, California

http://www.nurseweb.ucsf.edu

Founded in 1864

DEGREES • MS • PHD

Nursing Program Faculty 150 (70% with doctorates).

Graduate Enrollment 579

Women 88% **Men** 12% **Minority** 29% **International** 4% **Part-time** 1%

Nursing Student Activities Nursing Honor Society, Sigma Theta Tau, Student Nurses' Association, nursing club.

Nursing Student Resources Academic advising; academic or career counseling; assistance for students with disabilities; bookstore; campus computer network; career placement assistance; computer lab; computer-assisted instruction; daycare for children of students; e-mail services; employment services for current students; housing assistance; interactive nursing skills videos; Internet; learning resource lab; library services; nursing audiovisuals; other; paid internships; placement services for program completers; remedial services; resume preparation assistance; skills, simulation, or other laboratory; tutoring; unpaid internships.

Library Facilities 856,169 volumes in health, 131,046 volumes in nursing; 3,270 periodical subscriptions health-care related.

GRADUATE PROGRAMS

Expenses (2006–07) *Tuition, state resident:* full-time $12,374; part-time $8000 per quarter. *Tuition, nonresident:* full-time $27,411; part-time $8000 per quarter. *International tuition:* $27,411 full-time. *Room and board:* room only: $12,000 per academic year.

Financial Aid 65% of graduate students in nursing programs received some form of financial aid in 2005–06. Fellowships, career-related internships or fieldwork and Federal Work-Study available. Aid available to part-time students.

Contact Mr. Terry Linton, Admissions and Progression Officer, School of Nursing, University of California, San Francisco, Room N319X, 2 Koret Way, San Francisco, CA 94143-0602. *Telephone:* 415-476-1435. *Fax:* 415-476-9707. *E-mail:* terry.linton@nursing.ucsf.edu.

MASTER'S DEGREE PROGRAM

Degree MS

Available Programs Master's; Master's for Non-Nursing College Graduates; Master's for Nurses with Non-Nursing Degrees.

Concentrations Available Nurse-midwifery; nursing administration. *Clinical nurse specialist programs in:* cardiovascular, community health, critical care, gerontology, occupational health, oncology, pediatric, perinatal, psychiatric/mental health. *Nurse practitioner programs in:* acute care, adult health, community health, family health, gerontology, neonatal health, occupational health, oncology, pediatric, psychiatric/mental health.

Study Options Full-time.

Program Entrance Requirements Clinical experience, computer literacy, minimum overall college GPA of 3.0, transcript of college record, CPR certification, written essay, immunizations, 4 letters of recommendation, prerequisite course work, statistics course, GRE General Test. *Application deadline:* For fall admission, 3/1. *Application fee:* $40.

Advanced Placement Credit given for nursing courses completed elsewhere dependent upon specific evaluations.

Degree Requirements 36 total credit hours, comprehensive exam.

POST-MASTER'S PROGRAM

Areas of Study *Nurse practitioner programs in:* adult health, family health, gerontology, neonatal health, pediatric, psychiatric/mental health.

University of California, San Francisco (continued)
DOCTORAL DEGREE PROGRAM
Degree PhD

Available Programs Doctorate; Post-Baccalaureate Doctorate.

Areas of Study Addiction/substance abuse, aging, bio-behavioral research, biology of health and illness, community health, critical care, ethics, family health, gerontology, health policy, health promotion/disease prevention, health-care systems, human health and illness, illness and transition, individualized study, information systems, maternity-newborn, nursing administration, nursing policy, nursing research, nursing science, oncology, urban health, women's health.

Program Entrance Requirements Minimum overall college GPA of 3.0, 4 letters of recommendation, statistics course, writing sample, GRE General Test. *Application deadline:* For fall admission, 3/1. *Application fee:* $40.

Degree Requirements Dissertation, oral exam, written exam, residency.

POSTDOCTORAL PROGRAM
Areas of Study Individualized study.

Postdoctoral Program Contact Mr. Jeff Kilmer, Director, Office of Student and Curricular Affairs, School of Nursing, University of California, San Francisco, Room N319X, 2 Koret Way, San Francisco, CA 94143-0602. *Telephone:* 415-476-1435. *Fax:* 415-476-9707. *E-mail:* jeff.kilmer@nursing.ucsf.edu.

University of Phoenix–Bay Area Campus
College of Health and Human Services
Pleasanton, California

DEGREES • BSN • MSN • MSN/MBA • MSN/MHA

Nursing Program Faculty 101 (28% with doctorates).

Baccalaureate Enrollment 50
Women 94% **Men** 6% **Minority** 40%

Graduate Enrollment 58
Women 87.93% **Men** 12.07% **Minority** 31%

Nursing Student Activities Sigma Theta Tau.

Nursing Student Resources Academic advising; academic or career counseling; assistance for students with disabilities; bookstore; computer lab; library services.

Library Facilities 444 volumes; 666 periodical subscriptions.

BACCALAUREATE PROGRAMS
Degree BSN

Available Programs Accelerated Baccalaureate.

Site Options Novato, CA; Oakland, CA; San Francisco, CA.

Study Options Full-time.

Program Entrance Requirements Transcript of college record, 1 letter of recommendation, RN licensure. Transfer students are accepted. **Standardized tests** *Required:* TOEFL for international students. **Application** *Deadline:* rolling (freshmen), rolling (transfer). *Application fee:* $110.

Advanced Placement Credit by examination available.

Expenses (2006–07) *Tuition:* full-time $12,750. *International tuition:* $12,750 full-time. *Required fees:* full-time $750.

Contact Campus College Chair, Nursing, College of Health and Human Services, University of Phoenix–Bay Area Campus, 7901 Stoneridge Drive, Suite #130, Pleasanton, CA 94588-3677. *Telephone:* 877-416-4100.

GRADUATE PROGRAMS
Expenses (2006–07) *Tuition:* full-time $10,968. *International tuition:* $10,968 full-time. *Required fees:* full-time $760.

Contact Campus College Chair, Nursing, College of Health and Human Services, University of Phoenix–Bay Area Campus, 7901 Stoneridge Drive, Suite #130, Pleasanton, CA 94588-3677. *Telephone:* 877-416-4100.

MASTER'S DEGREE PROGRAM
Degrees MSN; MSN/MBA; MSN/MHA

Available Programs Master's.

Concentrations Available Health-care administration; nursing administration; nursing education.

Site Options Novato, CA; Oakland, CA; San Francisco, CA.

Study Options Full-time.

Program Entrance Requirements Clinical experience, computer literacy, minimum overall college GPA of 2.5, transcript of college record. *Application deadline:* Applications are processed on a rolling basis. *Application fee:* $110.

Advanced Placement Credit given for nursing courses completed elsewhere dependent upon specific evaluations.

Degree Requirements 39 total credit hours, thesis or project.

University of Phoenix–Central Valley Campus
College of Health and Human Services
Fresno, California

Founded in 2004

DEGREES • BSN • MSN

Nursing Program Faculty 50 (32% with doctorates).

Baccalaureate Enrollment 20
Women 75% **Men** 25%

Graduate Enrollment 9
Women 44.44% **Men** 55.56% **Minority** 22.22%

Nursing Student Activities Sigma Theta Tau.

Nursing Student Resources Academic advising; academic or career counseling; bookstore; computer lab; library services.

Library Facilities 444 volumes; 666 periodical subscriptions.

BACCALAUREATE PROGRAMS
Degree BSN

Available Programs RN Baccalaureate.

Site Options Bakersfield, CA; Fresno, CA.

Study Options Full-time.

Program Entrance Requirements Transcript of college record, RN licensure. Transfer students are accepted. **Application** *Deadline:* rolling (freshmen), rolling (transfer). *Application fee:* $110.

Advanced Placement Credit by examination available. Credit given for nursing courses completed elsewhere dependent upon specific evaluations.

Contact Campus College Chair, Nursing, College of Health and Human Services, University of Phoenix–Central Valley Campus, 4900 California Avenue, Tower A, Suite 300, Bakersfield, CA 93309-7018. *Telephone:* 661-663-0300. *Fax:* 661-633-2711.

GRADUATE PROGRAMS
Contact Campus College Chair, Nursing, College of Health and Human Services, University of Phoenix–Central Valley Campus, 4900 California Avenue, Tower A, Suite 300, Bakersfield, CA 93309-7018. *Telephone:* 661-663-0300. *Fax:* 661-633-2711.

MASTER'S DEGREE PROGRAM
Degree MSN

Available Programs Master's.

Concentrations Available Health-care administration; nursing administration.

Site Options Bakersfield, CA; Fresno, CA.

Study Options Full-time.

Program Entrance Requirements Minimum overall college GPA of 2.5, transcript of college record, 1 letter of recommendation.

Advanced Placement Credit given for nursing courses completed elsewhere dependent upon specific evaluations.

Degree Requirements 39 total credit hours, thesis or project.

University of Phoenix–Sacramento Valley Campus
College of Health and Human Services
Sacramento, California

Founded in 1993
DEGREES • BSN • MSN

Nursing Program Faculty 122 (13% with doctorates).
Baccalaureate Enrollment 67
Women 89.55% **Men** 10.45% **Minority** 19.4%
Graduate Enrollment 83
Women 83.13% **Men** 16.87% **Minority** 15.66%
Nursing Student Activities Sigma Theta Tau.
Nursing Student Resources Academic advising; academic or career counseling; assistance for students with disabilities; bookstore; computer lab; library services.
Library Facilities 444 volumes; 666 periodical subscriptions.

BACCALAUREATE PROGRAMS
Degree BSN

Available Programs Accelerated Baccalaureate.
Site Options Modesto, CA; Lathrop, CA; Fairfield, CA.
Study Options Full-time.
Program Entrance Requirements Transcript of college record, 1 letter of recommendation, RN licensure. Transfer students are accepted.
Standardized tests *Required:* TOEFL for international students. **Application** *Deadline:* rolling (freshmen), rolling (transfer). *Application fee:* $110.
Advanced Placement Credit by examination available. Credit given for nursing courses completed elsewhere dependent upon specific evaluations.
Expenses (2006–07) *Tuition:* full-time $12,900. *International tuition:* $12,900 full-time. *Required fees:* full-time $750.
Contact Campus College Chair, Nursing, College of Health and Human Services, University of Phoenix–Sacramento Valley Campus, 1760 Creekside Oaks Drive, #100, Sacramento, CA 95833-3632. *Telephone:* 800-266-2107.

GRADUATE PROGRAMS
Expenses (2006–07) *Tuition:* full-time $12,024. *International tuition:* $12,024 full-time. *Required fees:* full-time $760.
Contact Campus College Chair, Nursing, College of Health and Human Services, University of Phoenix–Sacramento Valley Campus, 1760 Creekside Oaks Drive, #100, Sacramento, CA 95833-3632. *Telephone:* 800-266-2107.

MASTER'S DEGREE PROGRAM
Degree MSN

Available Programs Master's.
Concentrations Available Health-care administration; nursing administration; nursing education. *Nurse practitioner programs in:* family health.
Site Options Modesto, CA; Lathrop, CA; Fairfield, CA.
Study Options Full-time and part-time.
Program Entrance Requirements Clinical experience, computer literacy, minimum overall college GPA of 2.5, transcript of college record. *Application deadline:* Applications are processed on a rolling basis. *Application fee:* $110.
Advanced Placement Credit given for nursing courses completed elsewhere dependent upon specific evaluations.
Degree Requirements 39 total credit hours, thesis or project.

POST-MASTER'S PROGRAM
Areas of Study *Nurse practitioner programs in:* family health.

University of Phoenix–San Diego Campus
College of Health and Human Services
San Diego, California

Founded in 1988
DEGREES • BSN • MSN

Nursing Program Faculty 85 (28% with doctorates).
Baccalaureate Enrollment 115
Women 84.35% **Men** 15.65% **Minority** 26.09%
Graduate Enrollment 55
Women 78.18% **Men** 21.82% **Minority** 27.27%
Nursing Student Activities Sigma Theta Tau.
Nursing Student Resources Academic advising; academic or career counseling; assistance for students with disabilities; bookstore; computer lab; Internet.
Library Facilities 444 volumes; 666 periodical subscriptions.

BACCALAUREATE PROGRAMS
Degree BSN

Available Programs Accelerated Baccalaureate.
Site Options Palm Desert, CA; Chula Vista, CA; Imperial, CA.
Study Options Full-time.
Program Entrance Requirements Transcript of college record, 1 letter of recommendation, RN licensure. Transfer students are accepted.
Standardized tests *Required:* TOEFL for international students. **Application** *Deadline:* rolling (freshmen), rolling (transfer). *Application fee:* $110.
Advanced Placement Credit by examination available. Credit given for nursing courses completed elsewhere dependent upon specific evaluations.
Expenses (2006–07) *Tuition:* full-time $12,425. *International tuition:* $12,425 full-time. *Required fees:* full-time $750.
Contact Campus College Chair, Nursing, College of Health and Human Services, University of Phoenix–San Diego Campus, 3870 Murphy Canyon Road, #100, San Diego, CA 92123-4403. *Telephone:* 888-867-4636.

GRADUATE PROGRAMS
Expenses (2006–07) *Tuition:* full-time $11,880. *International tuition:* $11,880 full-time. *Required fees:* full-time $760.
Contact Campus College Chair, Nursing, College of Health and Human Services, University of Phoenix–San Diego Campus, 3870 Murphy Canyon Road, #100, San Diego, CA 92123-4403. *Telephone:* 888-867-4636.

MASTER'S DEGREE PROGRAM
Degree MSN
Available Programs Master's.
Concentrations Available Health-care administration; nursing administration; nursing education.
Site Options Palm Desert, CA; Chula Vista, CA; Imperial, CA.
Study Options Full-time.
Program Entrance Requirements Clinical experience, computer literacy, minimum overall college GPA of 2.5, transcript of college record. *Application deadline:* Applications are processed on a rolling basis. *Application fee:* $110.
Advanced Placement Credit given for nursing courses completed elsewhere dependent upon specific evaluations.
Degree Requirements 39 total credit hours, thesis or project.

University of Phoenix–Southern California Campus
College of Health and Human Services
Costa Mesa, California

Founded in 1980

University of Phoenix–Southern California Campus (continued)
DEGREES • BSN • MSN • MSN/MBA

Nursing Program Faculty 239 (41% with doctorates).

Baccalaureate Enrollment 560
Women 91.43% **Men** 8.57% **Minority** 19.64%

Graduate Enrollment 409
Women 83.13% **Men** 16.87% **Minority** 27.14%

Nursing Student Activities Sigma Theta Tau.

Nursing Student Resources Academic advising; academic or career counseling; assistance for students with disabilities; bookstore; computer lab; library services.

Library Facilities 444 volumes; 666 periodical subscriptions.

BACCALAUREATE PROGRAMS

Degree BSN

Available Programs Accelerated Baccalaureate.

Site Options La Marada, CA; Diamond Bar, CA; Lancaster, CA.

Study Options Full-time.

Program Entrance Requirements Transcript of college record, 1 letter of recommendation, RN licensure. Transfer students are accepted. **Standardized tests** *Required:* TOEFL for international students. **Application** *Deadline:* rolling (freshmen), rolling (transfer). *Application fee:* $110.

Advanced Placement Credit by examination available. Credit given for nursing courses completed elsewhere dependent upon specific evaluations.

Expenses (2006–07) *Tuition:* full-time $13,710. *International tuition:* $13,710 full-time. *Required fees:* full-time $750.

Contact Campus College Chair, Nursing, College of Health and Human Services, University of Phoenix–Southern California Campus, 10540 Talbert Avenue, West Tower, Suite 120, Fountain Valley, CA 92708-6027. *Telephone:* 800-697-8223.

GRADUATE PROGRAMS

Expenses (2006–07) *Tuition:* full-time $14,112. *International tuition:* $14,112 full-time. *Required fees:* full-time $760.

Contact Campus College Chair, Nursing, College of Health and Human Services, University of Phoenix–Southern California Campus, 10540 Talbert Avenue, West Tower, Suite 120, Fountain Valley, CA 92708-6027. *Telephone:* 800-697-8223.

MASTER'S DEGREE PROGRAM

Degrees MSN; MSN/MBA

Available Programs Master's.

Concentrations Available Health-care administration; nursing administration; nursing education. *Nurse practitioner programs in:* family health.

Site Options La Marada, CA; Diamond Bar, CA; Lancaster, CA.

Study Options Full-time.

Program Entrance Requirements Clinical experience, computer literacy, minimum overall college GPA of 2.5, transcript of college record, 1 letter of recommendation. *Application deadline:* Applications are processed on a rolling basis. *Application fee:* $110.

Advanced Placement Credit given for nursing courses completed elsewhere dependent upon specific evaluations.

Degree Requirements 39 total credit hours, thesis or project.

POST-MASTER'S PROGRAM

Areas of Study *Nurse practitioner programs in:* family health.

University of San Diego
Hahn School of Nursing and Health Sciences
San Diego, California

http://www.sandiego.edu
Founded in 1949

DEGREES • BSN • MSN • MSN/MBA • PHD

Nursing Program Faculty 40 (65% with doctorates).

Baccalaureate Enrollment 9
Women 89% **Men** 11% **Minority** 90% **Part-time** 33%

Graduate Enrollment 245
Women 90% **Men** 10% **Minority** 25% **International** 3% **Part-time** 48%

Nursing Student Activities Nursing Honor Society, Sigma Theta Tau, Student Nurses' Association.

Nursing Student Resources Academic advising; academic or career counseling; assistance for students with disabilities; bookstore; campus computer network; career placement assistance; computer lab; computer-assisted instruction; daycare for children of students; e-mail services; employment services for current students; externships; interactive nursing skills videos; Internet; learning resource lab; library services; nursing audiovisuals; resume preparation assistance; skills, simulation, or other laboratory; tutoring.

Library Facilities 714,082 volumes (41,573 in health, 22,465 in nursing); 10,451 periodical subscriptions (1,764 health-care related).

BACCALAUREATE PROGRAMS

Degree BSN

Available Programs ADN to Baccalaureate; RN Baccalaureate.

Study Options Full-time and part-time.

Program Entrance Requirements Minimum overall college GPA of 3.0, transcript of college record, CPR certification, written essay, health exam, health insurance, high school transcript, immunizations, interview, 3 letters of recommendation, professional liability insurance/malpractice insurance, prerequisite course work, RN licensure. Transfer students are accepted. **Standardized tests** *Required:* TOEFL for international students. **Application** *Deadline:* 3/1 (fall), 11/1 (spring). *Application fee:* $55.

Advanced Placement Credit by examination available. Credit given for nursing courses completed elsewhere dependent upon specific evaluations.

Expenses (2006–07) *Tuition:* full-time $30,480; part-time $1050 per unit. *International tuition:* $30,480 full-time. *Required fees:* full-time $450; part-time $225 per term.

Financial Aid 100% of baccalaureate students in nursing programs received some form of financial aid in 2005–06.

Contact Ms. Cathleen Mumper, Director of Student Services and Admissions Officer, Hahn School of Nursing and Health Sciences, University of San Diego, 5998 Alcala Park, San Diego, CA 92110-2492. *Telephone:* 619-260-4548. *Fax:* 619-260-6814. *E-mail:* cmm@sandiego.edu.

GRADUATE PROGRAMS

Expenses (2006–07) *Tuition:* full-time $21,000; part-time $1050 per unit. *International tuition:* $21,000 full-time. *Required fees:* full-time $550; part-time $225 per term.

Financial Aid 80% of graduate students in nursing programs received some form of financial aid in 2005–06. 27 fellowships with partial tuition reimbursements available (averaging $4,831 per year) were awarded; institutionally sponsored loans, scholarships, traineeships, tuition waivers (partial), and graduate work program also available. Aid available to part-time students. *Financial aid application deadline:* 5/1.

Contact Ms. Cathleen Mumper, Director of Student Services and Admissions Officer, Hahn School of Nursing and Health Sciences, University of San Diego, 5998 Alcala Park, San Diego, CA 92110-2492. *Telephone:* 619-260-4548. *Fax:* 619-260-6814. *E-mail:* cmm@sandiego.edu.

MASTER'S DEGREE PROGRAM

Degrees MSN; MSN/MBA

Available Programs Accelerated AD/RN to Master's; Accelerated RN to Master's; Master's; Master's for Non-Nursing College Graduates; Master's for Nurses with Non-Nursing Degrees.

Concentrations Available Nursing administration; nursing education. *Clinical nurse specialist programs in:* acute care, adult health, medical-surgical. *Nurse practitioner programs in:* adult health, family health, gerontology, pediatric.

Study Options Full-time and part-time.

Program Entrance Requirements Computer literacy, minimum overall college GPA of 3.0, transcript of college record, CPR certification, written essay, immunizations, interview, 3 letters of recommendation, professional liability insurance/malpractice insurance, prerequisite course work, resume, statistics course, GRE General Test. *Application deadline:* For fall admission, 5/1 (priority date); for spring admission, 11/1 (priority date). Applications are processed on a rolling basis. *Application fee:* $45.

Advanced Placement Credit by examination available. Credit given for nursing courses completed elsewhere dependent upon specific evaluations.

POST-MASTER'S PROGRAM

Areas of Study Nursing administration. *Clinical nurse specialist programs in:* acute care, adult health, medical-surgical. *Nurse practitioner programs in:* adult health, family health, gerontology, pediatric.

DOCTORAL DEGREE PROGRAM

Degree PhD

Available Programs Doctorate.

Areas of Study Advanced practice nursing, aging, clinical practice, community health, ethics, faculty preparation, family health, health policy, health promotion/disease prevention, health-care systems, human health and illness, illness and transition, individualized study, maternity-newborn, nursing administration, nursing education, nursing research, nursing science, oncology, women's health.

Program Entrance Requirements Clinical experience, minimum overall college GPA of 3.5, interview by faculty committee, interview, 3 letters of recommendation, MSN or equivalent, scholarly papers, statistics course, vita, writing sample, GRE General Test. *Application deadline:* For fall admission, 5/1 (priority date); for spring admission, 11/1 (priority date). Applications are processed on a rolling basis. *Application fee:* $45.

Degree Requirements 48 total credit hours, dissertation, oral exam, residency.

See full description on page 558.

University of San Francisco
School of Nursing
San Francisco, California

http://www.usfca.edu/nursing/

Founded in 1855

DEGREES • BSN • MSN • MSN/MS

Nursing Program Faculty 83 (79% with doctorates).

Baccalaureate Enrollment 650
Women 76% **Men** 24% **Minority** 51% **International** 9% **Part-time** 7%

Graduate Enrollment 175
Women 80% **Men** 20% **Minority** 47% **International** 5% **Part-time** 11%

Nursing Student Activities Nursing Honor Society, Sigma Theta Tau, Student Nurses' Association, nursing club.

Nursing Student Resources Academic advising; academic or career counseling; assistance for students with disabilities; bookstore; campus computer network; career placement assistance; computer lab; computer-assisted instruction; e-mail services; employment services for current students; housing assistance; interactive nursing skills videos; Internet; learning resource lab; library services; nursing audiovisuals; placement services for program completers; remedial services; resume preparation assistance; skills, simulation, or other laboratory; tutoring.

Library Facilities 1.1 million volumes; 5,560 periodical subscriptions.

BACCALAUREATE PROGRAMS

Degree BSN

Available Programs Baccalaureate for Second Degree; Generic Baccalaureate.

Study Options Full-time and part-time.

Program Entrance Requirements Minimum overall college GPA of 3.0, transcript of college record, CPR certification, written essay, health exam, health insurance, high school biology, high school chemistry, 3 years high school math, 2 years high school science, high school transcript, immunizations, 2 letters of recommendation, minimum high school GPA of 3.0, professional liability insurance/malpractice insurance, prerequisite course work. Transfer students are accepted. **Standardized tests**

Required: SAT or ACT, TOEFL for international students. **Application** *Deadline:* 2/1 (freshmen), rolling (transfer). *Early decision:* 11/15. *Notification:* continuous until 8/15 (freshmen), 1/16 (early action). *Application fee:* $55.

Advanced Placement Credit given for nursing courses completed elsewhere dependent upon specific evaluations.

Expenses (2006–07) *Tuition:* full-time $28,420; part-time $1015 per unit. *Room and board:* $11,840; room only: $6490 per academic year. *Required fees:* full-time $340.

Financial Aid 91% of baccalaureate students in nursing programs received some form of financial aid in 2005–06.

Contact Mr. Robert J. Reed, Assistant Dean, School of Nursing, University of San Francisco, 2130 Fulton Street, Cowell Hall 102, San Francisco, CA 94117-1080. *Telephone:* 415-422-6681. *Fax:* 415-422-6877. *E-mail:* reedr@usfca.edu.

GRADUATE PROGRAMS

Expenses (2006–07) *Tuition:* part-time $860 per unit. *Room and board:* $11,840; room only: $6490 per academic year.

Financial Aid 87% of graduate students in nursing programs received some form of financial aid in 2005–06. Institutionally sponsored loans available. *Financial aid application deadline:* 3/2.

Contact Mr. Robert J. Reed, Assistant Dean, School of Nursing, University of San Francisco, 2130 Fulton Street, Cowell Hall 102, San Francisco, CA 94117-1080. *Telephone:* 415-422-6681. *Fax:* 415-422-6877. *E-mail:* reedr@usfca.edu.

MASTER'S DEGREE PROGRAM

Degrees MSN; MSN/MS

Available Programs Accelerated Master's; Accelerated Master's for Non-Nursing College Graduates; Accelerated Master's for Nurses with Non-Nursing Degrees; Master's; Master's for Non-Nursing College Graduates; Master's for Nurses with Non-Nursing Degrees.

Concentrations Available Health-care administration; nurse case management; nursing informatics. *Clinical nurse specialist programs in:* family health. *Nurse practitioner programs in:* family health.

Study Options Full-time and part-time.

Program Entrance Requirements Clinical experience, minimum overall college GPA of 3.25, transcript of college record, written essay, immunizations, 2 letters of recommendation, nursing research course, prerequisite course work, resume, statistics course. *Application deadline:* Applications are processed on a rolling basis. *Application fee:* $40.

Advanced Placement Credit given for nursing courses completed elsewhere dependent upon specific evaluations.

Degree Requirements 53 total credit hours, comprehensive exam.

CONTINUING EDUCATION PROGRAM

Contact Mr. Robert J. Reed, Assistant Dean, School of Nursing, University of San Francisco, 2130 Fulton Street, Cowell Hall 102, San Francisco, CA 94117-1080. *Telephone:* 415-422-6681. *Fax:* 415-422-6877. *E-mail:* reedr@usfca.edu.

Western University of Health Sciences
College of Graduate Nursing
Pomona, California

http://www.westernu.edu/cogn.html

Founded in 1975

DEGREE • MSN

Nursing Program Faculty 13 (62% with doctorates).

Graduate Enrollment 156
Women 87% **Men** 13% **Minority** 53% **International** 1% **Part-time** 4%

Nursing Student Resources Academic advising; assistance for students with disabilities; bookstore; campus computer network; computer-assisted instruction; e-mail services; Internet; library services; tutoring.

Library Facilities 23,463 volumes in health, 563 volumes in nursing; 7,671 periodical subscriptions health-care related.

Western University of Health Sciences (continued)
GRADUATE PROGRAMS
Expenses (2006–07) *Tuition:* full-time $15,660; part-time $580 per unit. *International tuition:* $15,660 full-time. *Required fees:* full-time $165.

Financial Aid 80% of graduate students in nursing programs received some form of financial aid in 2005–06. Institutionally sponsored loans, scholarships, and Veterans Educational Benefits available. *Financial aid application deadline:* 3/2.

Contact Mitzi McKay, Director of Student Services, College of Graduate Nursing, Western University of Health Sciences, 309 East Second Street, College Plaza, Pomona, CA 91766. *Telephone:* 909-469-5255. *Fax:* 909-469-5521. *E-mail:* mmckay@westernu.edu.

MASTER'S DEGREE PROGRAM
Degree MSN

Available Programs Accelerated Master's; Master's for Nurses with Non-Nursing Degrees.

Concentrations Available Nursing administration. *Nurse practitioner programs in:* family health.

Study Options Full-time and part-time.

Program Entrance Requirements Computer literacy, minimum overall college GPA of 3.0, transcript of college record, CPR certification, written essay, immunizations, interview, 3 letters of recommendation, prerequisite course work, statistics course, GRE General Test. *Application deadline:* For fall admission, 3/1 (priority date). Applications are processed on a rolling basis. *Application fee:* $60.

Advanced Placement Credit given for nursing courses completed elsewhere dependent upon specific evaluations.

Degree Requirements 27 total credit hours, thesis or project.

POST-MASTER'S PROGRAM
Areas of Study *Nurse practitioner programs in:* family health.

COLORADO

Colorado State University-Pueblo
Department of Nursing
Pueblo, Colorado

Founded in 1933
DEGREES • BSN • MS

Nursing Program Faculty 30 (10% with doctorates).
Baccalaureate Enrollment 190
Women 84% **Men** 16% **Minority** 27% **International** 1%
Graduate Enrollment 25
Women 76% **Men** 24% **Minority** 16%
Nursing Student Activities Sigma Theta Tau, Student Nurses' Association.

Nursing Student Resources Academic advising; academic or career counseling; assistance for students with disabilities; bookstore; campus computer network; computer lab; computer-assisted instruction; daycare for children of students; e-mail services; employment services for current students; housing assistance; Internet; learning resource lab; library services; nursing audiovisuals; remedial services; resume preparation assistance; skills, simulation, or other laboratory; tutoring.

Library Facilities 270,761 volumes (2,891 in health, 1,168 in nursing); 1,327 periodical subscriptions (101 health-care related).

BACCALAUREATE PROGRAMS
Degree BSN

Available Programs ADN to Baccalaureate; Accelerated Baccalaureate for Second Degree; Accelerated RN Baccalaureate; Baccalaureate for Second Degree; Generic Baccalaureate; LPN to Baccalaureate; LPN to RN Baccalaureate; RN Baccalaureate.

Study Options Full-time.

Program Entrance Requirements Minimum overall college GPA of 2.75, transcript of college record, CPR certification, health exam, immunizations, minimum GPA in nursing prerequisites of 2.75, professional liability insurance/malpractice insurance, prerequisite course work. Transfer students are accepted. **Standardized tests** *Required:* SAT or ACT, TOEFL for international students. *Placement:* Required: SAT or ACT. **Application** *Deadline:* 8/1 (freshmen), 8/1 (transfer). *Notification:* continuous until 8/1 (freshmen). *Application fee:* $25.

Advanced Placement Credit by examination available. Credit given for nursing courses completed elsewhere dependent upon specific evaluations.

Expenses (2006–07) *Tuition, state resident:* full-time $4640; part-time $179 per credit hour. *Tuition, nonresident:* full-time $15,206; part-time $620 per credit hour. *International tuition:* $15,206 full-time. *Room and board:* $5810 per academic year. *Required fees:* full-time $340.

Financial Aid 80% of baccalaureate students in nursing programs received some form of financial aid in 2005–06. *Gift aid (need-based):* Federal Pell, FSEOG, state, private, college/university gift aid from institutional funds. *Loans:* FFEL (Subsidized and Unsubsidized Stafford PLUS), Perkins. *Work-Study:* Federal Work-Study, part-time campus jobs. *Application deadline (priority):* 3/1.

Contact Ruth DePalma, RN, Nursing Undergraduate Coordinator, MSN, Department of Nursing, Colorado State University-Pueblo, 2200 Bonforte Boulevard, Pueblo, CO 81001. *Telephone:* 719-549-2422. *Fax:* 719-549-2113. *E-mail:* ruth.depalma@colostate-pueblo.edu.

GRADUATE PROGRAMS
Expenses (2006–07) *Tuition, state resident:* full-time $5090; part-time $194 per credit hour. *Tuition, nonresident:* full-time $15,656; part-time $635 per credit hour.

Financial Aid 50% of graduate students in nursing programs received some form of financial aid in 2005–06.

Contact Dr. Barbara Sabo, Nursing Graduate Coordinator, Department of Nursing, Colorado State University-Pueblo, 2200 Bonforte Boulevard, Pueblo, CO 81001. *Telephone:* 719-549-2477. *Fax:* 719-549-2113. *E-mail:* barbara.sabo@colostate-pueblo.edu.

MASTER'S DEGREE PROGRAM
Degree MS

Available Programs Master's.

Concentrations Available Nursing education. *Clinical nurse specialist programs in:* acute care, psychiatric/mental health. *Nurse practitioner programs in:* acute care, family health, pediatric.

Study Options Full-time and part-time.

Program Entrance Requirements Clinical experience, computer literacy, minimum overall college GPA of 3.0, transcript of college record, CPR certification, written essay, immunizations, 3 letters of recommendation, nursing research course, professional liability insurance/malpractice insurance, prerequisite course work, resume, statistics course.

Advanced Placement Credit given for nursing courses completed elsewhere dependent upon specific evaluations.

Degree Requirements 46 total credit hours, thesis or project, comprehensive exam.

POST-MASTER'S PROGRAM
Areas of Study Nursing education. *Clinical nurse specialist programs in:* acute care, psychiatric/mental health. *Nurse practitioner programs in:* acute care, family health, pediatric.

Mesa State College
Department of Nursing and Radiologic Sciences
Grand Junction, Colorado

http://www.mesastate.edu/schools/sbps/nars/nursing.htm
Founded in 1925
DEGREE • BSN

Nursing Program Faculty 37 (5% with doctorates).

Baccalaureate Enrollment 170

Women 88% **Men** 12% **Minority** 11% **International** 4% **Part-time** 8%

Nursing Student Activities Sigma Theta Tau, Student Nurses' Association.

Nursing Student Resources Academic advising; academic or career counseling; assistance for students with disabilities; bookstore; campus computer network; career placement assistance; computer lab; computer-assisted instruction; daycare for children of students; e-mail services; employment services for current students; housing assistance; interactive nursing skills videos; Internet; learning resource lab; library services; nursing audiovisuals; placement services for program completers; resume preparation assistance; skills, simulation, or other laboratory; tutoring; unpaid internships.

Library Facilities 260,784 volumes (200 in health, 150 in nursing); 31,992 periodical subscriptions (25 health-care related).

BACCALAUREATE PROGRAMS

Degree BSN

Available Programs ADN to Baccalaureate; Generic Baccalaureate; LPN to Baccalaureate; LPN to RN Baccalaureate; RN Baccalaureate.

Site Options *Distance Learning:* Montrose, CO; Craig, CO; Cortez, CO.

Study Options Full-time and part-time.

Program Entrance Requirements Minimum overall college GPA of 2.0, transcript of college record, CPR certification, written essay, health exam, immunizations, minimum GPA in nursing prerequisites of 2.0, professional liability insurance/malpractice insurance, prerequisite course work. Transfer students are accepted. **Standardized tests** *Required:* SAT or ACT. *Recommended:* TOEFL for international students. **Application** *Deadline:* rolling (freshmen), rolling (transfer). *Notification:* continuous (freshmen). *Application fee:* $30.

Advanced Placement Credit by examination available. Credit given for nursing courses completed elsewhere dependent upon specific evaluations.

Expenses (2005–06) *Tuition, state resident:* full-time $2359; part-time $140 per credit hour. *Tuition, nonresident:* full-time $9546; part-time $398 per credit hour. *Room and board:* $6702; room only: $3364 per academic year. *Required fees:* full-time $721; part-time $41 per credit.

Financial Aid 90% of baccalaureate students in nursing programs received some form of financial aid in 2004–05. *Gift aid (need-based):* Federal Pell, FSEOG, state, private, college/university gift aid from institutional funds. *Loans:* FFEL (Subsidized and Unsubsidized Stafford PLUS), Perkins. *Work-Study:* Federal Work-Study, part-time campus jobs. *Application deadline (priority):* 3/1.

Contact Judy Goodhart, Program Director, Department of Nursing and Radiologic Sciences, Mesa State College, 1100 North Avenue, Grand Junction, CO 81501. *Telephone:* 970-248-1774. *Fax:* 970-248-1133. *E-mail:* goodhart@mesastate.edu.

Metropolitan State College of Denver

Department of Health Professions
Denver, Colorado

http://www.mscd.edu/~nursing

Founded in 1963

DEGREE • BS

Nursing Program Faculty 6 (35% with doctorates).

Baccalaureate Enrollment 74

Women 88% **Men** 12% **Minority** 23% **Part-time** 72%

Nursing Student Activities Nursing club.

Nursing Student Resources Academic advising; academic or career counseling; assistance for students with disabilities; bookstore; campus computer network; computer lab; computer-assisted instruction; daycare for children of students; e-mail services; Internet; library services; nursing audiovisuals; remedial services; resume preparation assistance.

Library Facilities 607,971 volumes (21,503 in health); 2,380 periodical subscriptions (204 health-care related).

BACCALAUREATE PROGRAMS

Degree BS

Available Programs ADN to Baccalaureate; RN Baccalaureate.

Study Options Full-time and part-time.

Program Entrance Requirements Transcript of college record, CPR certification, immunizations, professional liability insurance/malpractice insurance, prerequisite course work, RN licensure. Transfer students are accepted. **Standardized tests** *Required:* TOEFL for international students. *Required for some:* SAT or ACT. **Application** *Deadline:* 8/7 (freshmen), rolling (transfer). *Notification:* continuous (freshmen). *Application fee:* $25.

Advanced Placement Credit given for nursing courses completed elsewhere dependent upon specific evaluations.

Contact *Telephone:* 303-556-8415. *Fax:* 303-556-3439.

Regis University

Department of Nursing
Denver, Colorado

Founded in 1877

DEGREES • BSN • MS

Nursing Program Faculty 18 (55% with doctorates).

Nursing Student Activities Nursing Honor Society, Sigma Theta Tau, Student Nurses' Association.

Nursing Student Resources Academic advising; academic or career counseling; assistance for students with disabilities; bookstore; campus computer network; computer lab; computer-assisted instruction; e-mail services; interactive nursing skills videos; Internet; learning resource lab; library services; nursing audiovisuals; resume preparation assistance; skills, simulation, or other laboratory; tutoring; unpaid internships.

Library Facilities 350,000 volumes; 20,800 periodical subscriptions.

BACCALAUREATE PROGRAMS

Degree BSN

Available Programs Accelerated Baccalaureate; Generic Baccalaureate; RN Baccalaureate.

Study Options Full-time.

Program Entrance Requirements Minimum overall college GPA of 2.5, transcript of college record, written essay, 2 letters of recommendation, prerequisite course work. Transfer students are accepted. **Standardized tests** *Required:* SAT or ACT, TOEFL for international students. *Recommended:* SAT Subject Tests. **Application** *Deadline:* rolling (freshmen), rolling (out-of-state freshmen), rolling (transfer). *Notification:* continuous (freshmen). *Application fee:* $40.

Advanced Placement Credit by examination available.

Contact *Telephone:* 303-458-4958. *Fax:* 303-964-5533.

GRADUATE PROGRAMS

Contact *Telephone:* 303-458-4938. *Fax:* 303-964-5533.

MASTER'S DEGREE PROGRAM

Degree MS

Available Programs Master's.

Concentrations Available Health-care administration; nursing administration; nursing education. *Nurse practitioner programs in:* family health, neonatal health.

Study Options Full-time and part-time.

Program Entrance Requirements Minimum overall college GPA of 2.75, transcript of college record, written essay, 3 letters of recommendation, prerequisite course work, statistics course.

Advanced Placement Credit by examination available.

Degree Requirements 42 total credit hours, thesis or project.

University of Colorado at Colorado Springs

Beth-El College of Nursing and Health Sciences
Colorado Springs, Colorado

http://www.uccs.edu

Founded in 1965

DEGREES • BSN • DNP • MSN

Nursing Program Faculty 47 (32% with doctorates).

Baccalaureate Enrollment 627
Women 92% **Men** 8% **Minority** 6.5% **Part-time** 5%

Graduate Enrollment 138
Women 94% **Men** 6% **Minority** 8% **Part-time** 31%

Nursing Student Activities Nursing Honor Society, Sigma Theta Tau, Student Nurses' Association, nursing club.

Nursing Student Resources Academic advising; academic or career counseling; assistance for students with disabilities; bookstore; campus computer network; career placement assistance; computer lab; computer-assisted instruction; daycare for children of students; e-mail services; employment services for current students; externships; housing assistance; interactive nursing skills videos; Internet; learning resource lab; library services; nursing audiovisuals; resume preparation assistance; skills, simulation, or other laboratory.

Library Facilities 391,638 volumes (10,416 in health, 1,031 in nursing); 2,201 periodical subscriptions (331 health-care related).

BACCALAUREATE PROGRAMS

Degree BSN

Available Programs Accelerated Baccalaureate for Second Degree; Generic Baccalaureate; RN Baccalaureate.
Study Options Full-time.
Program Entrance Requirements Minimum overall college GPA of 3.0, transcript of college record, CPR certification, high school biology, high school chemistry, high school foreign language, 3 years high school math, 1 year of high school science, high school transcript, immunizations, minimum high school GPA of 3.0, minimum high school rank 30%, minimum GPA in nursing prerequisites of 3.0. Transfer students are accepted. **Standardized tests** *Required:* SAT or ACT, TOEFL for international students. **Application** *Deadline:* 7/1 (freshmen), 7/1 (transfer). *Notification:* continuous (freshmen). *Application fee:* $50.
Advanced Placement Credit given for nursing courses completed elsewhere dependent upon specific evaluations.
Expenses (2006–07) *Tuition, state resident:* full-time $8160; part-time $340 per credit. *Tuition, nonresident:* full-time $18,360; part-time $765 per credit. *Room and board:* $6438; room only: $5600 per academic year. *Required fees:* full-time $540; part-time $30 per credit; part-time $93 per term.
Financial Aid 68% of baccalaureate students in nursing programs received some form of financial aid in 2005–06. *Gift aid (need-based):* Federal Pell, FSEOG, state, private, college/university gift aid from institutional funds. *Loans:* FFEL (Subsidized and Unsubsidized Stafford PLUS), Perkins, college/university. *Work-Study:* Federal Work-Study, part-time campus jobs. *Application deadline (priority):* 4/1.
Contact Mr. Robert King, Advisor, Baccalaureate Nursing and Health Sciences, Beth-El College of Nursing and Health Sciences, University of Colorado at Colorado Springs, 1460 Austin Bluffs Parkway, PO Box 7150, Colorado Springs, CO 80933. *Telephone:* 719-262-3473. *Fax:* 719-262-3316. *E-mail:* rking@uccs.edu.

GRADUATE PROGRAMS

Expenses (2006–07) *Tuition, state resident:* full-time $5654; part-time $371 per credit. *Tuition, nonresident:* full-time $11,700; part-time $900 per credit. *Required fees:* full-time $940; part-time $30 per credit; part-time $52 per term.
Financial Aid 34% of graduate students in nursing programs received some form of financial aid in 2005–06.

Contact Dr. Kathy LaSala, Chair, Department of Graduate Studies, Beth-El College of Nursing and Health Sciences, University of Colorado at Colorado Springs, 1420 Austin Bluffs Parkway, PO Box 7150, Colorado Springs, CO 80933-7150. *Telephone:* 719-262-4411. *Fax:* 719-262-4416. *E-mail:* klasala@uccs.edu.

MASTER'S DEGREE PROGRAM

Degree MSN
Available Programs Master's.
Concentrations Available Nursing administration. *Clinical nurse specialist programs in:* adult health, community health. *Nurse practitioner programs in:* adult health, family health, gerontology.
Study Options Full-time and part-time.
Program Entrance Requirements Clinical experience, computer literacy, minimum overall college GPA of 3.0, transcript of college record, CPR certification, immunizations, 4 letters of recommendation, nursing research course, physical assessment course, professional liability insurance/malpractice insurance, prerequisite course work, resume, statistics course.
Advanced Placement Credit by examination available. Credit given for nursing courses completed elsewhere dependent upon specific evaluations.
Degree Requirements 45 total credit hours, thesis or project, comprehensive exam.

POST-MASTER'S PROGRAM

Areas of Study *Clinical nurse specialist programs in:* adult health. *Nurse practitioner programs in:* adult health, family health, gerontology.

DOCTORAL DEGREE PROGRAM

Degree DNP
Available Programs Doctorate.
Areas of Study Forensic nursing, gerontology, nursing education.
Program Entrance Requirements Clinical experience, minimum overall college GPA of 3.3, interview, 4 letters of recommendation, MSN or equivalent, statistics course, vita.
Degree Requirements 36 total credit hours, written exam, residency.

CONTINUING EDUCATION PROGRAM

Contact Dr. William Crouch, Director, Extended Studies, Beth-El College of Nursing and Health Sciences, University of Colorado at Colorado Springs, 1460 Austin Bluffs Parkway, Mail Stop UH-1, Colorado Springs, CO 80917. *Telephone:* 719-262-4651. *Fax:* 719-262-4416. *E-mail:* wcrouch@uccs.edu.

University of Colorado at Denver and Health Sciences Center

School of Nursing
Denver, Colorado

http://www.uchsc.edu/nursing

Founded in 1883

DEGREES • BS • MS • MSN/MBA • PHD

Nursing Program Faculty 75 (66% with doctorates).

Baccalaureate Enrollment 267
Women 92% **Men** 8% **Minority** 12% **Part-time** 7%

Graduate Enrollment 262
Women 95% **Men** 5% **Minority** 7% **International** 1% **Part-time** 18%

Nursing Student Activities Sigma Theta Tau, Student Nurses' Association, nursing club.

Nursing Student Resources Academic advising; academic or career counseling; assistance for students with disabilities; bookstore; campus computer network; computer lab; computer-assisted instruction; e-mail services; externships; interactive nursing skills videos; Internet; learning resource lab; library services; nursing audiovisuals; paid internships; remedial services; skills, simulation, or other laboratory; tutoring; unpaid internships.

Library Facilities 250,000 volumes (1,000 in health, 40 in nursing); 1,650 periodical subscriptions (200 health-care related).

BACCALAUREATE PROGRAMS

Degree BS

Available Programs Generic Baccalaureate; RN Baccalaureate.

Site Options *Distance Learning:* Denver, CO.

Study Options Full-time and part-time.

Program Entrance Requirements Minimum overall college GPA of 2.75, transcript of college record, written essay, health exam, health insurance, immunizations, minimum GPA in nursing prerequisites of 2.0, prerequisite course work. Transfer students are accepted. **Standardized tests** *Required:* TOEFL for international students. **Application** *Deadline:* 10/1 (transfer). *Application fee:* $50.

Advanced Placement Credit given for nursing courses completed elsewhere dependent upon specific evaluations.

Contact *Telephone:* 303-315-5592. *Fax:* 303-315-8920.

GRADUATE PROGRAMS

Contact *Telephone:* 303-315-5592. *Fax:* 303-315-5648.

MASTER'S DEGREE PROGRAM

Degrees MS; MSN/MBA

Available Programs Master's; RN to Master's.

Concentrations Available Health-care administration; nurse-midwifery; nursing administration; nursing informatics. *Clinical nurse specialist programs in:* adult health, community health, psychiatric/mental health, public health. *Nurse practitioner programs in:* adult health, family health, gerontology, pediatric, psychiatric/mental health, women's health.

Site Options *Distance Learning:* Denver, CO.

Study Options Full-time and part-time.

Program Entrance Requirements Computer literacy, minimum overall college GPA of 3.0, transcript of college record, written essay, immunizations, 4 letters of recommendation, nursing research course, resume, statistics course. *Application deadline:* For fall admission, 5/1 (priority date); for spring admission, 10/1. *Application fee:* $65.

Advanced Placement Credit given for nursing courses completed elsewhere dependent upon specific evaluations.

Degree Requirements 35 total credit hours, comprehensive exam.

POST-MASTER'S PROGRAM

Areas of Study Health-care administration; nurse-midwifery; nursing administration; nursing informatics. *Clinical nurse specialist programs in:* adult health, community health, psychiatric/mental health, public health. *Nurse practitioner programs in:* adult health, family health, gerontology, pediatric, psychiatric/mental health, women's health.

DOCTORAL DEGREE PROGRAM

Degree PhD

Available Programs Doctorate; Post-Baccalaureate Doctorate.

Areas of Study Community health, health-care systems, human health and illness, illness and transition, individualized study, nursing research, nursing science.

Site Options *Distance Learning:* Denver, CO.

Program Entrance Requirements Minimum overall college GPA of 3.0, interview by faculty committee, interview, 4 letters of recommendation, MSN or equivalent, statistics course, vita, writing sample. *Application deadline:* For fall admission, 5/1 (priority date); for spring admission, 10/1. *Application fee:* $65.

Degree Requirements 75 total credit hours, dissertation, oral exam, written exam.

POSTDOCTORAL PROGRAM

Areas of Study Adolescent health, cancer care, community health, gerontology, individualized study, information systems, nursing informatics, nursing interventions, nursing research, nursing science, outcomes, vulnerable population.

Postdoctoral Program Contact *Telephone:* 303-315-5592. *Fax:* 303-315-5648.

CONTINUING EDUCATION PROGRAM

Contact *Telephone:* 303-315-8691. *Fax:* 303-315-0907.

University of Northern Colorado
School of Nursing
Greeley, Colorado

http://www.unco.edu/HHS/son/son.htm

Founded in 1890

DEGREES • BS • MS • PHD

Nursing Program Faculty 31 (65% with doctorates).

Baccalaureate Enrollment 162
Women 94% **Men** 6% **Minority** 18%

Graduate Enrollment 42
Women 98% **Men** 2% **Minority** 11% **Part-time** 59%

Nursing Student Activities Sigma Theta Tau, Student Nurses' Association.

Nursing Student Resources Academic advising; academic or career counseling; assistance for students with disabilities; bookstore; campus computer network; career placement assistance; computer lab; computer-assisted instruction; e-mail services; employment services for current students; housing assistance; Internet; learning resource lab; library services; nursing audiovisuals; paid internships; placement services for program completers; resume preparation assistance; skills, simulation, or other laboratory; tutoring.

Library Facilities 1 million volumes (43,602 in health, 25,700 in nursing); 3,417 periodical subscriptions (140 health-care related).

BACCALAUREATE PROGRAMS

Degree BS

Available Programs Accelerated Baccalaureate; Generic Baccalaureate; RN Baccalaureate.

Site Options *Distance Learning:* Greeley, CO.

Study Options Full-time.

Program Entrance Requirements Minimum overall college GPA of 2.5, transcript of college record, CPR certification, written essay, health exam, immunizations, 1 letter of recommendation, minimum GPA in nursing prerequisites of 2.5, professional liability insurance/malpractice insurance, prerequisite course work. Transfer students are accepted. **Standardized tests** *Required:* SAT or ACT. **Application** *Deadline:* 8/1 (freshmen), rolling (transfer). *Notification:* continuous (freshmen). *Application fee:* $40.

Advanced Placement Credit given for nursing courses completed elsewhere dependent upon specific evaluations.

Contact *Telephone:* 970-351-1692. *Fax:* 970-351-1707.

GRADUATE PROGRAMS

Contact *Telephone:* 970-351-2662. *Fax:* 970-351-1707.

MASTER'S DEGREE PROGRAM

Degree MS

Concentrations Available Nursing education. *Nurse practitioner programs in:* family health.

Site Options *Distance Learning:* Greeley, CO.

Study Options Full-time and part-time.

Program Entrance Requirements Clinical experience, minimum overall college GPA of 3.0, transcript of college record, CPR certification, immunizations, 2 letters of recommendation, nursing research course, physical assessment course, GRE General Test. *Application deadline:* Applications are processed on a rolling basis. *Application fee:* $50 ($60 for international students).

Advanced Placement Credit given for nursing courses completed elsewhere dependent upon specific evaluations.

Degree Requirements 45 total credit hours, thesis or project, comprehensive exam.

POST-MASTER'S PROGRAM

Areas of Study *Nurse practitioner programs in:* family health.

DOCTORAL DEGREE PROGRAM

Degree PhD

Available Programs Doctorate.

University of Northern Colorado (continued)

Areas of Study Nursing education.

Program Entrance Requirements Clinical experience, minimum overall college GPA of 3.0, interview, GRE General Test. *Application deadline:* Applications are processed on a rolling basis. *Application fee:* $50 ($60 for international students).

Degree Requirements 30 total credit hours, dissertation.

University of Phoenix–Denver Campus

College of Health and Human Services
Lone Tree, Colorado

DEGREES • BSN • MSN

Nursing Program Faculty 32 (22% with doctorates).

Baccalaureate Enrollment 72
Women 88.24% **Men** 11.76% **Minority** 11.76%

Graduate Enrollment 11
Women 90.91% **Men** 9.09% **Minority** 9.09%

Nursing Student Activities Sigma Theta Tau.

Nursing Student Resources Academic advising; academic or career counseling; assistance for students with disabilities; bookstore; computer lab; library services.

Library Facilities 444 volumes; 666 periodical subscriptions.

BACCALAUREATE PROGRAMS

Degree BSN

Available Programs Accelerated Baccalaureate.

Site Options Aurora, CO; Ft. Collins, CO; Westminister, CO.

Study Options Full-time.

Program Entrance Requirements Transcript of college record, 1 letter of recommendation, RN licensure. Transfer students are accepted. **Standardized tests** *Required:* TOEFL for international students. **Application** *Deadline:* rolling (freshmen), rolling (transfer). *Application fee:* $110.

Advanced Placement Credit by examination available. Credit given for nursing courses completed elsewhere dependent upon specific evaluations.

Expenses (2006–07) *Tuition:* full-time $9750. *International tuition:* $9750 full-time. *Required fees:* full-time $750.

Contact Campus College Chair, Nursing, College of Health and Human Services, University of Phoenix–Denver Campus, 10004 Park Meadow Drive, Lone Tree, CO 80124-5453. *Telephone:* 303-694-9093.

GRADUATE PROGRAMS

Expenses (2006–07) *Tuition:* full-time $10,680. *International tuition:* $10,680 full-time. *Required fees:* full-time $760.

Contact Campus College Chair, Nursing, College of Health and Human Services, University of Phoenix–Denver Campus, 10004 Park Meadow Drive, Lone Tree, CO 80124-5453. *Telephone:* 303-694-9003.

MASTER'S DEGREE PROGRAM

Degree MSN

Available Programs Master's; Master's for Non-Nursing College Graduates.

Concentrations Available Nursing administration; nursing education.

Site Options Aurora, CO; Westminister, CO.

Study Options Full-time.

Program Entrance Requirements Clinical experience, computer literacy, minimum overall college GPA of 2.5, transcript of college record. *Application deadline:* Applications are processed on a rolling basis. *Application fee:* $110.

Advanced Placement Credit given for nursing courses completed elsewhere dependent upon specific evaluations.

Degree Requirements 39 total credit hours, thesis or project.

University of Phoenix–Southern Colorado Campus

College of Health and Human Services
Colorado Springs, Colorado

Founded in 1999

DEGREES • BSN • MSN

Nursing Program Faculty 57 (12% with doctorates).

Baccalaureate Enrollment 2
Women 100%

Nursing Student Activities Sigma Theta Tau.

Nursing Student Resources Academic advising; academic or career counseling; assistance for students with disabilities; bookstore; computer lab; library services.

Library Facilities 444 volumes; 666 periodical subscriptions.

BACCALAUREATE PROGRAMS

Degree BSN

Available Programs Accelerated Baccalaureate; LPN to Baccalaureate.

Study Options Full-time.

Program Entrance Requirements Transcript of college record, 1 letter of recommendation, RN licensure. Transfer students are accepted. **Standardized tests** *Required:* TOEFL for international students. **Application** *Deadline:* rolling (freshmen), rolling (transfer). *Application fee:* $110.

Advanced Placement Credit by examination available. Credit given for nursing courses completed elsewhere dependent upon specific evaluations.

Expenses (2006–07) *Tuition:* full-time $9750. *International tuition:* $9750 full-time. *Required fees:* full-time $750.

Contact Campus College Chair, Nursing, College of Health and Human Services, University of Phoenix–Southern Colorado Campus, 5475 Tech Center Drive, #130, Colorado Springs, CO 80919-2335. *Telephone:* 719-599-5282.

GRADUATE PROGRAMS

Expenses (2006–07) *Tuition:* full-time $10,680. *International tuition:* $10,680 full-time. *Required fees:* full-time $760.

Contact Campus College Chair, Nursing, College of Health and Human Services, University of Phoenix–Southern Colorado Campus, 5475 Tech Center Drive, #130, Colorado Springs, CO 80919-2335. *Telephone:* 719-599-5282.

MASTER'S DEGREE PROGRAM

Degree MSN

Available Programs Master's.

Concentrations Available Health-care administration; nursing administration; nursing education.

Study Options Full-time.

Program Entrance Requirements Clinical experience, computer literacy, minimum overall college GPA of 2.5, transcript of college record. *Application deadline:* Applications are processed on a rolling basis. *Application fee:* $110.

Advanced Placement Credit given for nursing courses completed elsewhere dependent upon specific evaluations.

Degree Requirements 39 total credit hours, thesis or project.

CONNECTICUT

Central Connecticut State University
Department of Counseling and Family Therapy
New Britain, Connecticut

http://www.ccsu.edu/nursing/
Founded in 1849
DEGREE • BSN

Nursing Program Faculty 5 (80% with doctorates).
Nursing Student Activities Nursing Honor Society.
Library Facilities 688,604 volumes; 2,705 periodical subscriptions.

BACCALAUREATE PROGRAMS
Degree BSN
Available Programs RN Baccalaureate.
Site Options New London, CT.
Program Entrance Requirements Minimum overall college GPA of 2.7, transcript of college record, CPR certification, health exam, immunizations, minimum GPA in nursing prerequisites of 2.7, professional liability insurance/malpractice insurance, prerequisite course work, RN licensure. Transfer students are accepted. **Standardized tests** *Required:* SAT, TOEFL for international students. **Application** *Deadline:* 6/1 (freshmen), 6/1 (transfer). *Notification:* continuous until 7/1 (freshmen). *Application fee:* $50.
Advanced Placement Credit by examination available. Credit given for nursing courses completed elsewhere dependent upon specific evaluations.
Contact *Telephone:* 860-832-0032. *Fax:* 860-832-2188.

Fairfield University
School of Nursing
Fairfield, Connecticut

http://www.fairfield.edu/academic/nursing/
Founded in 1942
DEGREES • BS • MSN

Nursing Program Faculty 19 (69% with doctorates).
Baccalaureate Enrollment 318
Women 95% **Men** 5% **Minority** 9% **Part-time** 26%
Graduate Enrollment 42
Women 98% **Men** 2% **Minority** 17% **Part-time** 93%
Nursing Student Activities Nursing Honor Society, Sigma Theta Tau, Student Nurses' Association.
Nursing Student Resources Academic advising; academic or career counseling; bookstore; career placement assistance; computer lab; e-mail services; Internet; library services; skills, simulation, or other laboratory.
Library Facilities 347,244 volumes (9,580 in health); 1,614 periodical subscriptions (129 health-care related).

BACCALAUREATE PROGRAMS
Degree BS
Available Programs Accelerated Baccalaureate for Second Degree; Baccalaureate for Second Degree; Generic Baccalaureate; RN Baccalaureate.
Study Options Full-time.
Program Entrance Requirements Written essay, health exam, high school biology, high school chemistry, high school foreign language, 3 years high school math, 3 years high school science, high school transcript, letters of recommendation, minimum high school GPA of 3.0, minimum

high school rank 40%. Transfer students are accepted. **Standardized tests** *Required:* SAT or ACT, TOEFL for international students. **Application** *Deadline:* 1/15 (freshmen), 5/1 (transfer). *Notification:* 4/1 (freshmen), continuous (early decision). *Application fee:* $55.
Advanced Placement Credit given for nursing courses completed elsewhere dependent upon specific evaluations.
Expenses (2006–07) *Tuition:* full-time $31,450; part-time $545 per credit hour. *Room and board:* $9980 per academic year. *Required fees:* full-time $505; part-time $115 per credit; part-time $115 per term.
Financial Aid 63% of baccalaureate students in nursing programs received some form of financial aid in 2005–06. *Gift aid (need-based):* Federal Pell, FSEOG, state, private, college/university gift aid from institutional funds, United Negro College Fund. *Loans:* Federal Nursing Student Loans, FFEL (Subsidized and Unsubsidized Stafford PLUS), Perkins, alternative loans. *Work-Study:* Federal Work-Study. *Application deadline:* 2/15 (priority: 2/15).
Contact Ms. Karen Pellegrino, Director of Admission, School of Nursing, Fairfield University, 1073 North Benson Road, Fairfield, CT 06824-5195. *Telephone:* 203-254-4100. *Fax:* 203-254-4199. *E-mail:* admis@mail.fairfield.edu.

GRADUATE PROGRAMS
Expenses (2006–07) *Tuition:* part-time $475 per credit hour. *Required fees:* part-time $25 per credit; part-time $25 per term.
Financial Aid 7% of graduate students in nursing programs received some form of financial aid in 2005–06. Traineeships available.
Contact Ms. Marianne Gumpper, Director of Graduate and Continuing Studies Admission, School of Nursing, Fairfield University, 1073 North Benson Road, KEL 122, Fairfield, CT 06824-5195. *Telephone:* 203-254-4000 Ext. 2908. *Fax:* 203-254-4073. *E-mail:* gradadmis@mail.fairfield.edu.

MASTER'S DEGREE PROGRAM
Degree MSN
Available Programs Master's.
Concentrations Available Health-care administration; nurse anesthesia. *Nurse practitioner programs in:* family health, psychiatric/mental health.
Study Options Full-time and part-time.
Program Entrance Requirements Computer literacy, minimum overall college GPA of 3.0, transcript of college record, written essay, immunizations, interview, 2 letters of recommendation, physical assessment course, prerequisite course work, resume, statistics course, MAT or GRE. *Application deadline:* For fall admission, 4/1 (priority date); for spring admission, 11/1 (priority date). Applications are processed on a rolling basis. *Application fee:* $55.
Degree Requirements 39 total credit hours, thesis or project.

POST-MASTER'S PROGRAM
Areas of Study Health-care administration. *Nurse practitioner programs in:* family health, psychiatric/mental health.

Quinnipiac University
Department of Nursing
Hamden, Connecticut

Founded in 1929
DEGREES • BSN • MSN

Nursing Program Faculty 50 (90% with doctorates).
Baccalaureate Enrollment 385
Women 98% **Men** 2% **Minority** 7% **International** 2%
Graduate Enrollment 92
Women 98% **Men** 2% **Minority** 6% **International** 1% **Part-time** 60%
Nursing Student Activities Sigma Theta Tau, Student Nurses' Association.
Nursing Student Resources Academic advising; academic or career counseling; bookstore; campus computer network; career placement assistance; computer lab; computer-assisted instruction; e-mail services; employment services for current students; externships; housing assistance; interactive nursing skills videos; Internet; learning resource lab; library

Quinnipiac University (continued)

services; nursing audiovisuals; paid internships; placement services for program completers; remedial services; resume preparation assistance; skills, simulation, or other laboratory; tutoring; unpaid internships.

Library Facilities 285,000 volumes (1,500 in nursing); 5,500 periodical subscriptions.

BACCALAUREATE PROGRAMS

Degree BSN

Available Programs Accelerated Baccalaureate for Second Degree; Generic Baccalaureate.

Study Options Full-time.

Program Entrance Requirements Minimum overall college GPA of 3.0, transcript of college record, CPR certification, written essay, health exam, high school biology, high school chemistry, 4 years high school math, 3 years high school science, high school transcript, immunizations, 1 letter of recommendation, minimum high school GPA of 3.0, minimum high school rank 50%, minimum GPA in nursing prerequisites of 3.0. Transfer students are accepted. **Standardized tests** *Required:* SAT or ACT, TOEFL for international students. **Application** *Deadline:* 2/1 (freshmen), 2/1 (out-of-state freshmen), 4/1 (transfer). *Notification:* 3/1 (freshmen), 3/1 (out-of-state freshmen). *Application fee:* $45.

Advanced Placement Credit given for nursing courses completed elsewhere dependent upon specific evaluations.

Expenses (2006–07) *Tuition:* full-time $25,240; part-time $610 per credit. *International tuition:* $25,240 full-time. *Room and board:* $10,700 per academic year. *Required fees:* full-time $1040; part-time $30 per credit.

Financial Aid 70% of baccalaureate students in nursing programs received some form of financial aid in 2005–06. *Gift aid (need-based):* Federal Pell, FSEOG, state, private, college/university gift aid from institutional funds. *Loans:* Federal Nursing Student Loans, FFEL (Subsidized and Unsubsidized Stafford PLUS), Perkins. *Work-Study:* Federal Work-Study, part-time campus jobs. *Application deadline (priority):* 3/1.

Contact Ms. Carla Knowlton, Director of Undergraduate Admissions, Department of Nursing, Quinnipiac University, 275 Mount Carmel Avenue, Hamden, CT 06518. *Telephone:* 203-582-8600. *Fax:* 203-582-8906. *E-mail:* admissions@quinnipiac.edu.

GRADUATE PROGRAMS

Expenses (2006–07) *Tuition:* part-time $625 per credit. *Required fees:* part-time $30 per credit.

Financial Aid 30% of graduate students in nursing programs received some form of financial aid in 2005–06.

Contact Scott Farber, Director of Graduate Admissions, Department of Nursing, Quinnipiac University, 275 Mount Carmel Avenue, Hamden, CT 06518. *Telephone:* 203-582-8672. *Fax:* 203-582-3443. *E-mail:* graduate@quinnipiac.edu.

MASTER'S DEGREE PROGRAM

Degree MSN

Available Programs Master's.

Concentrations Available Health-care administration. *Clinical nurse specialist programs in:* forensic nursing. *Nurse practitioner programs in:* adult health, family health.

Study Options Full-time and part-time.

Program Entrance Requirements Clinical experience, minimum overall college GPA of 3.0, transcript of college record, CPR certification, written essay, immunizations, interview, 3 letters of recommendation, prerequisite course work, resume.

Advanced Placement Credit given for nursing courses completed elsewhere dependent upon specific evaluations.

Degree Requirements 47 total credit hours, thesis or project.

POST-MASTER'S PROGRAM

Areas of Study *Clinical nurse specialist programs in:* forensic nursing. *Nurse practitioner programs in:* adult health, family health.

CONTINUING EDUCATION PROGRAM

Contact Ms. Mary Wargo, Director of Transfer and Part-Time Admissions, Department of Nursing, Quinnipiac University, 275 Mount Carmel Avenue, Hamden, CT 06518. *Telephone:* 203-582-8612. *Fax:* 203-582-8906. *E-mail:* mary.wargo@quinnipiac.edu.

See full description on page 524.

Sacred Heart University
Program in Nursing
Fairfield, Connecticut

http://nursing.sacredheart.edu/
Founded in 1963

DEGREES • BS • MSN • MSN/MBA

Nursing Program Faculty 26 (30% with doctorates).

Baccalaureate Enrollment 254
Women 93% **Men** 7% **Minority** 22% **Part-time** 51%

Graduate Enrollment 59
Women 91% **Men** 9% **Minority** 14% **Part-time** 94%

Nursing Student Activities Nursing Honor Society, Sigma Theta Tau, Student Nurses' Association, nursing club.

Nursing Student Resources Academic advising; academic or career counseling; assistance for students with disabilities; bookstore; campus computer network; career placement assistance; computer lab; computer-assisted instruction; e-mail services; employment services for current students; interactive nursing skills videos; Internet; learning resource lab; library services; nursing audiovisuals; paid internships; placement services for program completers; remedial services; resume preparation assistance; skills, simulation, or other laboratory; tutoring; unpaid internships.

Library Facilities 134,348 volumes (3,829 in health, 1,920 in nursing); 860 periodical subscriptions (145 health-care related).

BACCALAUREATE PROGRAMS

Degree BS

Available Programs ADN to Baccalaureate; Generic Baccalaureate; RN Baccalaureate.

Site Options *Distance Learning:* Fairfield, CT.

Study Options Full-time and part-time.

Program Entrance Requirements Minimum overall college GPA of 2.5, transcript of college record, CPR certification, written essay, health exam, health insurance, high school biology, 3 years high school math, 3 years high school science, high school transcript, immunizations, interview, 2 letters of recommendation, minimum high school GPA of 3.0, minimum high school rank 50%, minimum GPA in nursing prerequisites of 2.5, prerequisite course work. Transfer students are accepted. **Standardized tests** *Required:* SAT or ACT, TOEFL for international students. **Application** *Early decision:* 11/15. *Notification:* continuous (freshmen), 12/15 (out-of-state freshmen), 12/15 (early decision). *Application fee:* $50.

Advanced Placement Credit given for nursing courses completed elsewhere dependent upon specific evaluations.

Expenses (2005–06) *Tuition:* full-time $23,750; part-time $390 per credit. *Room and board:* $9820; room only: $7160 per academic year. *Required fees:* full-time $1450.

Financial Aid 72% of baccalaureate students in nursing programs received some form of financial aid in 2004–05. *Gift aid (need-based):* Federal Pell, FSEOG, state, private, college/university gift aid from institutional funds, Federal Nursing. *Loans:* FFEL (Subsidized and Unsubsidized Stafford PLUS), Perkins, state. *Work-Study:* Federal Work-Study. *Application deadline (priority):* 2/15.

Contact Ms. Alma C. Haluch, Departmental Assistant, Program in Nursing, Sacred Heart University, 5151 Park Avenue, Fairfield, CT 06825-1000. *Telephone:* 203-371-7715. *Fax:* 203-365-7662. *E-mail:* halucha@sacredheart.edu.

GRADUATE PROGRAMS

Expenses (2005–06) *Tuition:* part-time $445 per credit. *Required fees:* part-time $145 per term.

Contact Dr. Dori Taylor Sullivan, Chair and Director, Program in Nursing, Sacred Heart University, 5151 Park Avenue, Fairfield, CT 06825-1000. *Telephone:* 203-371-7715. *Fax:* 203-365-7662. *E-mail:* sullivand@sacredheart.edu.

MASTER'S DEGREE PROGRAM

Degrees MSN; MSN/MBA

Available Programs Accelerated AD/RN to Master's; Accelerated Master's for Nurses with Non-Nursing Degrees; Accelerated RN to Master's; Master's; Master's for Nurses with Non-Nursing Degrees; RN to Master's.

Concentrations Available Nursing administration. *Nurse practitioner programs in:* family health.

Site Options *Distance Learning:* Fairfield, CT.

Study Options Full-time and part-time.

Program Entrance Requirements Clinical experience, minimum overall college GPA of 3.0, transcript of college record, written essay, interview, 2 letters of recommendation, physical assessment course, professional liability insurance/malpractice insurance, prerequisite course work, resume, statistics course.

Advanced Placement Credit given for nursing courses completed elsewhere dependent upon specific evaluations.

Degree Requirements 36 total credit hours, thesis or project.

POST-MASTER'S PROGRAM

Areas of Study Nursing administration. *Nurse practitioner programs in:* family health.

CONTINUING EDUCATION PROGRAM

Contact Department of Nursing, Program in Nursing, Sacred Heart University, 5151 Park Avenue, Fairfield, CT 06825-1000. *Telephone:* 203-371-7715. *Fax:* 203-365-7662. *E-mail:* halucha@sacredheart.edu.

Saint Joseph College
Department of Nursing
West Hartford, Connecticut

Founded in 1932

DEGREES • BS • MS

Nursing Program Faculty 23 (44% with doctorates).

Baccalaureate Enrollment 176
Women 98% **Men** 2% **Minority** 22% **International** 2% **Part-time** 40%

Graduate Enrollment 60
Women 90% **Men** 10% **Minority** 10% **International** 1% **Part-time** 95%

Nursing Student Activities Sigma Theta Tau, Student Nurses' Association, nursing club.

Nursing Student Resources Academic advising; academic or career counseling; assistance for students with disabilities; bookstore; campus computer network; career placement assistance; computer lab; computer-assisted instruction; daycare for children of students; e-mail services; employment services for current students; externships; housing assistance; interactive nursing skills videos; Internet; learning resource lab; library services; nursing audiovisuals; paid internships; remedial services; resume preparation assistance; skills, simulation, or other laboratory; tutoring; unpaid internships.

Library Facilities 7,058 volumes in health, 1,949 volumes in nursing; 1,495 periodical subscriptions health-care related.

BACCALAUREATE PROGRAMS

Degree BS

Available Programs Accelerated Baccalaureate; Accelerated Baccalaureate for Second Degree; Baccalaureate for Second Degree; Generic Baccalaureate; RN Baccalaureate.

Site Options *Distance Learning:* Middletown, CT.

Study Options Full-time and part-time.

Program Entrance Requirements Minimum overall college GPA of 2.8, transcript of college record, CPR certification, written essay, health exam, health insurance, high school biology, high school chemistry, 3 years high school math, high school transcript, immunizations, minimum high school GPA, minimum GPA in nursing prerequisites of 2.8. Transfer

students are accepted. **Standardized tests** *Required:* SAT or ACT, TOEFL for international students. *Recommended:* SAT. **Application** *Deadline:* rolling (freshmen), rolling (out-of-state freshmen), rolling (transfer). *Notification:* continuous (freshmen), continuous (out-of-state freshmen). *Application fee:* $35.

Advanced Placement Credit given for nursing courses completed elsewhere dependent upon specific evaluations.

Expenses (2006–07) *Tuition:* full-time $23,960; part-time $530 per credit. *International tuition:* $23,960 full-time. *Room and board:* $11,680; room only: $6140 per academic year. *Required fees:* full-time $1100; part-time $250 per term.

Financial Aid 85% of baccalaureate students in nursing programs received some form of financial aid in 2005–06. *Gift aid (need-based):* Federal Pell, FSEOG, state, private, college/university gift aid from institutional funds. *Loans:* FFEL (Subsidized and Unsubsidized Stafford PLUS), Perkins, state, Connecticut Family Education Loan Program. *Work-Study:* Federal Work-Study, part-time campus jobs. *Application deadline (priority):* 3/15.

Contact Dr. Terry Lee Bosworth, Chairperson, Department of Nursing, Saint Joseph College, 1678 Asylum Avenue, West Hartford, CT 06117. *Telephone:* 860-231-5304. *E-mail:* tbosworth@sjc.edu.

GRADUATE PROGRAMS

Expenses (2006–07) *Tuition:* part-time $540 per credit. *Required fees:* part-time $25 per credit.

Financial Aid 85% of graduate students in nursing programs received some form of financial aid in 2005–06.

Contact Dr. Marylouise Welch, Director, Department of Nursing, Saint Joseph College, 1678 Asylum Avenue, West Hartford, CT 06117-2700. *Telephone:* 860-231-5211. *Fax:* 860-231-8396. *E-mail:* mwelch@sjc.edu.

MASTER'S DEGREE PROGRAM

Degree MS

Available Programs Accelerated AD/RN to Master's; Accelerated RN to Master's; Master's; Master's for Nurses with Non-Nursing Degrees; RN to Master's.

Concentrations Available *Clinical nurse specialist programs in:* family health, psychiatric/mental health. *Nurse practitioner programs in:* family health.

Site Options *Distance Learning:* Middletown, CT.

Study Options Full-time and part-time.

Program Entrance Requirements Clinical experience, minimum overall college GPA of 3.0, transcript of college record, CPR certification, written essay, immunizations, interview, 2 letters of recommendation, nursing research course, physical assessment course, professional liability insurance/malpractice insurance, statistics course.

Advanced Placement Credit given for nursing courses completed elsewhere dependent upon specific evaluations.

Degree Requirements 36 total credit hours, thesis or project.

POST-MASTER'S PROGRAM

Areas of Study *Clinical nurse specialist programs in:* family health, psychiatric/mental health. *Nurse practitioner programs in:* family health.

Southern Connecticut State University
Department of Nursing
New Haven, Connecticut

http://www.southernct.edu/departments/nursing

Founded in 1893

DEGREES • BSN • MSN

Nursing Program Faculty 13 (55% with doctorates).

Nursing Student Activities Nursing Honor Society, Sigma Theta Tau, Student Nurses' Association.

Library Facilities 495,660 volumes (35,540 in health, 2,279 in nursing); 3,549 periodical subscriptions (318 health-care related).

Southern Connecticut State University (continued)

BACCALAUREATE PROGRAMS

Degree BSN

Available Programs ADN to Baccalaureate; Generic Baccalaureate; RN Baccalaureate.

Study Options Full-time and part-time.

Program Entrance Requirements Minimum overall college GPA of 2.4, transcript of college record, high school math, high school transcript, prerequisite course work. Transfer students are accepted. **Standardized tests** *Required:* SAT or ACT, TOEFL for international students. **Application** *Deadline:* 7/1 (freshmen), 8/1 (transfer). *Notification:* continuous (freshmen). *Application fee:* $50.

Advanced Placement Credit given for nursing courses completed elsewhere dependent upon specific evaluations.

Contact *Telephone:* 203-392-6483. *Fax:* 203-392-6493.

GRADUATE PROGRAMS

Contact *Telephone:* 203-392-6486. *Fax:* 203-392-6493.

MASTER'S DEGREE PROGRAM

Degree MSN

Concentrations Available Nursing administration; nursing education. *Nurse practitioner programs in:* family health.

Study Options Full-time and part-time.

Program Entrance Requirements Clinical experience, minimum overall college GPA of 2.8, transcript of college record, interview, 2 letters of recommendation, nursing research course, professional liability insurance/malpractice insurance, prerequisite course work, resume, statistics course, GRE, MAT. *Application deadline:* For fall admission, 7/15 (priority date). Applications are processed on a rolling basis. *Application fee:* $50.

Advanced Placement Credit given for nursing courses completed elsewhere dependent upon specific evaluations.

Degree Requirements 42 total credit hours, thesis or project.

POST-MASTER'S PROGRAM

Areas of Study *Nurse practitioner programs in:* family health.

University of Connecticut
School of Nursing
Storrs, Connecticut

http://www.nursing.uconn.edu

Founded in 1881

DEGREES • BS • MS • MSN/MBA • MSN/MPH • PHD

Nursing Program Faculty 77 (26% with doctorates).

Baccalaureate Enrollment 554
Women 90% **Men** 10% **Minority** 25% **Part-time** 5%

Graduate Enrollment 140
Women 91% **Men** 9% **Minority** 15% **International** 1% **Part-time** 61%

Nursing Student Activities Sigma Theta Tau, Student Nurses' Association.

Nursing Student Resources Academic advising; academic or career counseling; assistance for students with disabilities; bookstore; campus computer network; career placement assistance; computer lab; daycare for children of students; e-mail services; externships; housing assistance; interactive nursing skills videos; Internet; learning resource lab; library services; nursing audiovisuals; paid internships; placement services for program completers; resume preparation assistance; skills, simulation, or other laboratory; tutoring.

Library Facilities 3 million volumes (46,250 in health, 1,170 in nursing); 17,378 periodical subscriptions (4,553 health-care related).

BACCALAUREATE PROGRAMS

Degree BS

Available Programs RN Baccalaureate.

Site Options *Distance Learning:* Waterbury, Stamford, CT; Torrington, Avery Point, CT; West Hartford, CT.

Study Options Full-time and part-time.

Program Entrance Requirements Minimum overall college GPA of 2.5, transcript of college record, written essay, health exam, health insurance, high school chemistry, high school foreign language, 3 years high school math, high school physics, 2 years high school science, high school transcript, immunizations, minimum high school GPA of 3.0, minimum GPA in nursing prerequisites of 2.0, prerequisite course work. Transfer students are accepted. **Standardized tests** *Required:* SAT or ACT, TOEFL for international students. **Application** *Deadline:* 2/1 (freshmen), 4/1 (transfer). *Early decision:* 12/1. *Notification:* continuous until 1/1 (freshmen), 1/1 (early action). *Application fee:* $70.

Advanced Placement Credit by examination available. Credit given for nursing courses completed elsewhere dependent upon specific evaluations.

Expenses (2006–07) *Tuition, state resident:* full-time $6456. *Tuition, nonresident:* full-time $19,656. *International tuition:* $19,656 full-time. *Room and board:* $8266; room only: $4350 per academic year. *Required fees:* full-time $1906; part-time $650 per term.

Financial Aid 77% of baccalaureate students in nursing programs received some form of financial aid in 2005–06. *Gift aid (need-based):* Federal Pell, FSEOG, state, private, college/university gift aid from institutional funds. *Loans:* FFEL (Subsidized and Unsubsidized Stafford PLUS), Perkins, state. *Work-Study:* Federal Work-Study, part-time campus jobs. *Application deadline (priority):* 3/1.

Contact Mr. John James McNulty, RN, Instructor/Academic Advisor, School of Nursing, University of Connecticut, 231 Glenbrook Road, Unit 2026, Storrs, CT 06269-2026. *Telephone:* 860-486-1968. *Fax:* 860-486-0906. *E-mail:* John.McNulty@UConn.edu.

GRADUATE PROGRAMS

Expenses (2006–07) *Tuition, state resident:* full-time $3996; part-time $444 per credit. *Tuition, nonresident:* full-time $10,386; part-time $1154 per credit. *International tuition:* $10,386 full-time. *Room and board:* $8864; room only: $4948 per academic year. *Required fees:* full-time $759; part-time $509 per term.

Financial Aid 24% of graduate students in nursing programs received some form of financial aid in 2005–06. 4 research assistantships with full tuition reimbursements available, 13 teaching assistantships with full tuition reimbursements available were awarded; fellowships, Federal Work-Study, scholarships, and unspecified assistantships also available. *Financial aid application deadline:* 2/1.

Contact Ms. Lisa Santor, Office of Academic Advising Services, School of Nursing, University of Connecticut, 231 Glenbrook Road, Unit 2026, Storrs, CT 06269-2026. *Telephone:* 860-486-1968. *Fax:* 860-486-0906. *E-mail:* Lisa.Santor@UConn.edu.

MASTER'S DEGREE PROGRAM

Degrees MS; MSN/MBA; MSN/MPH

Available Programs Master's; RN to Master's.

Concentrations Available Nursing administration. *Clinical nurse specialist programs in:* adult health, community health. *Nurse practitioner programs in:* acute care, adult health, neonatal health, primary care.

Site Options *Distance Learning:* Waterbury, Stamford, CT; West Hartford, CT.

Study Options Full-time and part-time.

Program Entrance Requirements Clinical experience, computer literacy, minimum overall college GPA of 3.0, transcript of college record, CPR certification, written essay, immunizations, interview, 3 letters of recommendation, nursing research course, physical assessment course, professional liability insurance/malpractice insurance, resume, statistics course. *Application deadline:* For fall admission, 2/1 (priority date); for spring admission, 11/1. Applications are processed on a rolling basis. *Application fee:* $55.

Advanced Placement Credit given for nursing courses completed elsewhere dependent upon specific evaluations.

Degree Requirements 24 total credit hours, comprehensive exam.

POST-MASTER'S PROGRAM

Areas of Study Nursing administration. *Clinical nurse specialist programs in:* adult health, community health. *Nurse practitioner programs in:* acute care, adult health, neonatal health, primary care, psychiatric/mental health.

DOCTORAL DEGREE PROGRAM

Degree PhD

Available Programs Doctorate.

Areas of Study Nursing research, nursing science.

Program Entrance Requirements Minimum overall college GPA of 3.25, interview by faculty committee, interview, 3 letters of recommendation, MSN or equivalent, statistics course, vita, writing sample. *Application deadline:* For fall admission, 2/1 (priority date); for spring admission, 11/1. Applications are processed on a rolling basis. *Application fee:* $55.

Degree Requirements 48 total credit hours, dissertation, oral exam, written exam, residency.

CONTINUING EDUCATION PROGRAM

Contact Center for Academic Advising Services, School of Nursing, University of Connecticut, 231 Glenbrook Road, Unit 2026, Storrs, CT 06269-2026. *Telephone:* 860-486-1968. *Fax:* 860-486-0906. *E-mail:* nuradm11@uconnvm.uconn.edu.

University of Hartford
College of Education, Nursing, and Health Professions
West Hartford, Connecticut

http://www.hartford.edu/enhp

Founded in 1877

DEGREES • BSN • MSN • MSN/MSOB

Nursing Program Faculty 8 (70% with doctorates).

Baccalaureate Enrollment 92
Women 98% **Men** 2% **Minority** 30% **Part-time** 100%

Graduate Enrollment 148
Women 96% **Men** 4% **Minority** 8% **Part-time** 100%

Nursing Student Activities Sigma Theta Tau.

Library Facilities 473,115 volumes; 2,425 periodical subscriptions.

BACCALAUREATE PROGRAMS

Degree BSN

Available Programs ADN to Baccalaureate; RN Baccalaureate.

Study Options Part-time.

Program Entrance Requirements Transcript of college record, RN licensure. Transfer students are accepted. **Standardized tests** *Required:* SAT or ACT, TOEFL for international students. **Application** *Deadline:* rolling (freshmen), rolling (transfer). *Notification:* continuous (freshmen). *Application fee:* $35.

Advanced Placement Credit by examination available. Credit given for nursing courses completed elsewhere dependent upon specific evaluations.

Financial Aid 60% of baccalaureate students in nursing programs received some form of financial aid in 2005–06.

Contact Dr. Mary Jane Williams, RN, Interim Chair, Department of Nursing, College of Education, Nursing, and Health Professions, University of Hartford, 200 Bloomfield Avenue, West Hartford, CT 06117-1599. *Telephone:* 860-768-4213. *Fax:* 860-768-5346. *E-mail:* mjwilliam@hartford.edu.

GRADUATE PROGRAMS

Expenses (2006–07) *Tuition:* part-time $345 per credit hour. *Required fees:* part-time $100 per term.

Financial Aid 60% of graduate students in nursing programs received some form of financial aid in 2005–06. 2 teaching assistantships (averaging $6,000 per year) were awarded; institutionally sponsored loans and unspecified assistantships also available. *Financial aid application deadline:* 6/1.

Contact Dr. Mary Jane Williams, RN, Interim Chair, Department of Nursing, College of Education, Nursing, and Health Professions, University of Hartford, 200 Bloomfield Avenue, West Hartford, CT 06117-1599. *Telephone:* 860-768-4213. *Fax:* 860-768-5346. *E-mail:* mjwilliam@hartford.edu.

MASTER'S DEGREE PROGRAM

Degrees MSN; MSN/MSOB

Available Programs Master's; Master's for Nurses with Non-Nursing Degrees.

Concentrations Available Nursing administration; nursing education.

Study Options Part-time.

Program Entrance Requirements Clinical experience, minimum overall college GPA of 3.0, transcript of college record, written essay, 2 letters of recommendation, professional liability insurance/malpractice insurance, resume. *Application deadline:* Applications are processed on a rolling basis. *Application fee:* $40 ($55 for international students).

Advanced Placement Credit given for nursing courses completed elsewhere dependent upon specific evaluations.

Degree Requirements 34 total credit hours, thesis or project.

POST-MASTER'S PROGRAM

Areas of Study Nursing education.

DOCTORAL DEGREE PROGRAM

Program Entrance Requirements MAT. *Application deadline:* Applications are processed on a rolling basis. *Application fee:* $40 ($55 for international students).

CONTINUING EDUCATION PROGRAM

Contact Dr. Mary Jane Williams, RN, Interim Chair, Department of Nursing, College of Education, Nursing, and Health Professions, University of Hartford, 200 Bloomfield Avenue, West Hartford, CT 06117-1599. *Telephone:* 860-768-4213. *Fax:* 860-768-5346. *E-mail:* mjwilliam@hartford.edu.

Western Connecticut State University
Department of Nursing
Danbury, Connecticut

Founded in 1903

DEGREES • BS • MS

Nursing Program Faculty 18 (56% with doctorates).

Baccalaureate Enrollment 247
Women 95% **Men** 5% **Minority** 20% **Part-time** 30%

Graduate Enrollment 30
Women 100% **Minority** 2% **Part-time** 100%

Nursing Student Activities Sigma Theta Tau, Student Nurses' Association.

Nursing Student Resources Academic advising; academic or career counseling; assistance for students with disabilities; bookstore; campus computer network; career placement assistance; computer lab; computer-assisted instruction; daycare for children of students; e-mail services; employment services for current students; externships; interactive nursing skills videos; Internet; learning resource lab; library services; nursing audiovisuals; remedial services; resume preparation assistance; skills, simulation, or other laboratory; tutoring.

Library Facilities 182,915 volumes; 1,273 periodical subscriptions.

BACCALAUREATE PROGRAMS

Degree BS

Available Programs Generic Baccalaureate; RN Baccalaureate.

Site Options Waterbury, CT.

Study Options Full-time.

Program Entrance Requirements Transcript of college record, CPR certification, health exam, high school biology, high school chemistry, high school foreign language, 3 years high school math, 2 years high school science, high school transcript, immunizations, minimum GPA in nursing prerequisites of 2.25, prerequisite course work. Transfer students are accepted. **Standardized tests** *Required:* SAT or ACT, TOEFL for international students. **Application** *Deadline:* 5/1 (freshmen), 7/1 (transfer). *Notification:* continuous (freshmen). *Application fee:* $50.

Western Connecticut State University (continued)

Advanced Placement Credit by examination available. Credit given for nursing courses completed elsewhere dependent upon specific evaluations.

Contact Barbara Piscopo, EdD, Chair, Department of Nursing, Western Connecticut State University, 181 White Street, Danbury, CT 06810. *Telephone:* 203-837-8556. *Fax:* 203-837-8550. *E-mail:* piscopob@wcsu.edu.

GRADUATE PROGRAMS

Expenses (2005–06) *Tuition, area resident:* full-time $1890; part-time $330 per credit hour. *Tuition, nonresident:* full-time $5265; part-time $330 per credit hour. *Required fees:* part-time $60 per term.

Contact Patricia Z. Lund, EdD, Graduate Program Coordinator, Department of Nursing, Western Connecticut State University, 181 White Street, Danbury, CT 06810. *Telephone:* 203-837-8567. *Fax:* 203-837-8550. *E-mail:* lundp@wcsu.edu.

MASTER'S DEGREE PROGRAM

Degree MS

Available Programs Master's.

Concentrations Available *Clinical nurse specialist programs in:* adult health. *Nurse practitioner programs in:* adult health.

Study Options Full-time and part-time.

Program Entrance Requirements Clinical experience, computer literacy, minimum overall college GPA of 3.3, transcript of college record, CPR certification, immunizations, interview, 2 letters of recommendation, nursing research course, professional liability insurance/malpractice insurance, resume, statistics course.

Advanced Placement Credit given for nursing courses completed elsewhere dependent upon specific evaluations.

Degree Requirements 36 total credit hours, thesis or project.

POST-MASTER'S PROGRAM

Areas of Study *Clinical nurse specialist programs in:* adult health. *Nurse practitioner programs in:* adult health.

Yale University
School of Nursing
New Haven, Connecticut

http://www.nursing.yale.edu

Founded in 1701

DEGREES • MSN • MSN/MDIV • MSN/MPH • PHD

Nursing Program Faculty 75 (50% with doctorates).

Graduate Enrollment 285
Women 92% **Men** 8% **Minority** 15% **International** 5% **Part-time** 17%

Nursing Student Activities Sigma Theta Tau.

Nursing Student Resources Academic advising; academic or career counseling; assistance for students with disabilities; bookstore; campus computer network; career placement assistance; computer lab; computer-assisted instruction; e-mail services; employment services for current students; housing assistance; interactive nursing skills videos; Internet; learning resource lab; library services; nursing audiovisuals; placement services for program completers; resume preparation assistance; skills, simulation, or other laboratory; tutoring.

Library Facilities 11.1 million volumes (400,000 in health); 61,649 periodical subscriptions (2,900 health-care related).

GRADUATE PROGRAMS

Financial Aid 82% of graduate students in nursing programs received some form of financial aid in 2005–06. 63 fellowships (averaging $2,004 per year), 11 research assistantships with tuition reimbursements available (averaging $29,895 per year) were awarded; Federal Work-Study, institutionally sponsored loans, scholarships, and traineeships also available. Aid available to part-time students.

Contact Mr. Frank A. Grosso, Assistant Dean for Student Affairs, School of Nursing, Yale University, PO Box 9740, New Haven, CT 06536-0740. *Telephone:* 203-737-2257. *Fax:* 203-737-5409. *E-mail:* frank.grosso@yale.edu.

MASTER'S DEGREE PROGRAM

Degrees MSN; MSN/MDIV; MSN/MPH

Available Programs Master's; Master's for Non-Nursing College Graduates; RN to Master's.

Concentrations Available Nurse case management; nurse-midwifery; nursing administration. *Clinical nurse specialist programs in:* acute care, cardiovascular, critical care, oncology, psychiatric/mental health. *Nurse practitioner programs in:* acute care, adult health, family health, gerontology, oncology, pediatric, psychiatric/mental health, women's health.

Study Options Full-time.

Program Entrance Requirements Transcript of college record, CPR certification, written essay, immunizations, interview, 3 letters of recommendation, GRE General Test. *Application deadline:* For fall admission, 11/15 (priority date); for spring admission, 1/15 (priority date). Applications are processed on a rolling basis. *Application fee:* $50.

Degree Requirements 40 total credit hours, thesis or project.

POST-MASTER'S PROGRAM

Areas of Study *Clinical nurse specialist programs in:* psychiatric/mental health. *Nurse practitioner programs in:* acute care, adult health, gerontology, oncology, pediatric.

DOCTORAL DEGREE PROGRAM

Degree PhD

Available Programs Doctorate.

Areas of Study Aging, critical care, family health, gerontology, health policy, health promotion/disease prevention, health-care systems, human health and illness, maternity-newborn, neuro-behavior, nursing policy, nursing research, oncology.

Program Entrance Requirements Minimum overall college GPA of 3.2, interview by faculty committee, interview, 3 letters of recommendation, MSN or equivalent, statistics course, writing sample, GRE General Test. *Application deadline:* For fall admission, 11/15 (priority date); for spring admission, 1/15 (priority date). Applications are processed on a rolling basis. *Application fee:* $50.

Degree Requirements 60 total credit hours, dissertation, oral exam, written exam.

POSTDOCTORAL PROGRAM

Areas of Study Adolescent health, chronic illness.

Postdoctoral Program Contact Ms. Sarah Zaino, Assistant Director, Research Activities, School of Nursing, Yale University, PO Box 9740, New Haven, CT 06536-0740. *Telephone:* 203-737-2420. *Fax:* 203-737-4480. *E-mail:* sarah.zaino@yale.edu.

DELAWARE

Delaware State University
Department of Nursing
Dover, Delaware

http://www.dsc.edu/schools/professional_studies/nursing

Founded in 1891

DEGREE • BSN

Nursing Program Faculty 11.

Nursing Student Activities Sigma Theta Tau, Student Nurses' Association.

Library Facilities 360,616 volumes.

BACCALAUREATE PROGRAMS

Degree BSN

Available Programs Generic Baccalaureate; LPN to Baccalaureate.

Study Options Full-time and part-time.

Program Entrance Requirements High school biology, high school chemistry, high school transcript, minimum high school GPA of 2.0, prerequisite course work. Transfer students are accepted. **Standardized tests** *Required:* SAT or ACT. *Recommended:* TOEFL for international students. **Application** *Deadline:* 4/1 (freshmen), 4/1 (out-of-state freshmen), 4/1 (transfer). *Application fee:* $25.

Advanced Placement Credit by examination available. Credit given for nursing courses completed elsewhere dependent upon specific evaluations.

Contact *Telephone:* 302-857-6750. *Fax:* 302-857-6755.

University of Delaware
School of Nursing
Newark, Delaware

http://www.udel.edu/nursing/udnursing.html

Founded in 1743

DEGREES • BSN • MSN

Nursing Program Faculty 56 (54% with doctorates).

Baccalaureate Enrollment 666
Women 92% **Men** 8% **Minority** 15% **International** 1% **Part-time** 21%

Graduate Enrollment 132
Women 92% **Men** 8% **Minority** 14.8% **Part-time** 79%

Nursing Student Activities Sigma Theta Tau, Student Nurses' Association.

Nursing Student Resources Academic advising; academic or career counseling; assistance for students with disabilities; bookstore; campus computer network; career placement assistance; computer lab; computer-assisted instruction; e-mail services; employment services for current students; housing assistance; interactive nursing skills videos; Internet; learning resource lab; library services; nursing audiovisuals; resume preparation assistance; skills, simulation, or other laboratory; tutoring.

Library Facilities 2.7 million volumes (2.7 million in health, 40,000 in nursing); 12,532 periodical subscriptions (240 health-care related).

BACCALAUREATE PROGRAMS
Degree BSN

Available Programs Accelerated Baccalaureate for Second Degree; Generic Baccalaureate; RN Baccalaureate.

Study Options Full-time.

Program Entrance Requirements Written essay, high school biology, high school chemistry, high school foreign language, 3 years high school math, 4 years high school science, high school transcript, 1 letter of recommendation, minimum high school GPA of 3.0. Transfer students are accepted. **Standardized tests** *Required:* SAT or ACT, TOEFL for international students. *Recommended:* SAT Subject Tests. **Application** *Deadline:* 1/15 (freshmen), 5/1 (transfer). *Notification:* 3/15 (freshmen), continuous (early decision). *Application fee:* $60.

Advanced Placement Credit given for nursing courses completed elsewhere dependent upon specific evaluations.

Expenses (2006–07) *Tuition, state resident:* full-time $6980; part-time $291 per credit hour. *Tuition, nonresident:* full-time $17,690; part-time $737 per credit hour. *International tuition:* $17,690 full-time. *Room and board:* $3683; room only: $1515 per academic year. *Required fees:* full-time $650; part-time $25 per credit.

Financial Aid *Gift aid (need-based):* Federal Pell, FSEOG, state, private, college/university gift aid from institutional funds. *Loans:* Federal Nursing Student Loans, Federal Direct (Subsidized and Unsubsidized Stafford PLUS), Perkins. *Work-Study:* Federal Work-Study, part-time campus jobs. *Application deadline:* 3/15 (priority: 2/1).

Contact Ms. Patricia G. Grim, Assistant to the Director, School of Nursing, University of Delaware, 385 McDowell Hall, Newark, DE 19716. *Telephone:* 302-831-1117. *Fax:* 302-831-2382. *E-mail:* spring@udel.edu.

GRADUATE PROGRAMS
Expenses (2006–07) *Tuition, state resident:* full-time $3490; part-time $388 per credit hour. *Tuition, nonresident:* full-time $8845; part-time $983 per credit hour. *International tuition:* $8845 full-time. *Required fees:* full-time $735; part-time $25 per term.

Financial Aid 11% of graduate students in nursing programs received some form of financial aid in 2005–06. 5 fellowships with tuition reimbursements available were awarded; institutionally sponsored loans, scholarships, traineeships, tuition waivers (full), and unspecified assistantships also available. Aid available to part-time students. *Financial aid application deadline:* 7/1.

Contact Ms. Joanne Marra, Senior Secretary, School of Nursing, University of Delaware, 349 McDowell Hall, Newark, DE 19716. *Telephone:* 302-831-8386. *Fax:* 302-831-2382. *E-mail:* ud-gradnursing@udel.edu.

MASTER'S DEGREE PROGRAM
Degree MSN

Available Programs Master's; Master's for Nurses with Non-Nursing Degrees; RN to Master's.

Concentrations Available Health-care administration. *Clinical nurse specialist programs in:* adult health, pediatric, psychiatric/mental health, school health. *Nurse practitioner programs in:* adult health, family health.

Study Options Full-time and part-time.

Program Entrance Requirements Clinical experience, minimum overall college GPA of 3.0, transcript of college record, CPR certification, written essay, immunizations, interview, 3 letters of recommendation, professional liability insurance/malpractice insurance, resume. *Application deadline:* For fall admission, 7/1; for spring admission, 12/1. Applications are processed on a rolling basis. *Application fee:* $60.

Advanced Placement Credit given for nursing courses completed elsewhere dependent upon specific evaluations.

Degree Requirements 34 total credit hours.

POST-MASTER'S PROGRAM
Areas of Study Health-care administration. *Clinical nurse specialist programs in:* adult health, pediatric, psychiatric/mental health. *Nurse practitioner programs in:* adult health, family health.

See full description on page 542.

Wesley College
Nursing Program
Dover, Delaware

http://www.wesley.edu

Founded in 1873

DEGREES • BSN • MSN

Nursing Program Faculty 8 (70% with doctorates).

Baccalaureate Enrollment 210
Women 85% **Men** 15% **Minority** 35% **Part-time** 2%

Graduate Enrollment 63
Women 90% **Men** 10% **Minority** 25% **Part-time** 15%

Nursing Student Activities Sigma Theta Tau, Student Nurses' Association.

Nursing Student Resources Academic advising; academic or career counseling; assistance for students with disabilities; bookstore; campus computer network; career placement assistance; computer lab; computer-assisted instruction; e-mail services; employment services for current students; externships; housing assistance; interactive nursing skills videos; Internet; learning resource lab; library services; nursing audiovisuals; placement services for program completers; remedial services; resume preparation assistance; skills, simulation, or other laboratory; tutoring; unpaid internships.

Library Facilities 102,528 volumes (15,000 in health, 1,500 in nursing); 270 periodical subscriptions (40 health-care related).

BACCALAUREATE PROGRAMS
Degree BSN

Available Programs Generic Baccalaureate; LPN to Baccalaureate.

Study Options Full-time and part-time.

Program Entrance Requirements CPR certification, written essay, health exam, high school biology, high school chemistry, 2 years high school math, 2 years high school science, high school transcript, immunizations, minimum high school GPA of 2.5, minimum GPA in nursing

Wesley College (continued)

prerequisites of 3.0, professional liability insurance/malpractice insurance. Transfer students are accepted. **Standardized tests** *Required:* TOEFL for international students. **Application** *Deadline:* rolling (freshmen), rolling (transfer). *Early decision:* 11/15. *Notification:* 12/1 (out-of-state freshmen), 12/1 (early decision). *Application fee:* $25.

Advanced Placement Credit by examination available. Credit given for nursing courses completed elsewhere dependent upon specific evaluations.

Expenses (2006–07) *Tuition:* full-time $15,000; part-time $610 per credit. *Room and board:* $3725; room only: $3700 per academic year. *Required fees:* full-time $400; part-time $100 per term.

Financial Aid 90% of baccalaureate students in nursing programs received some form of financial aid in 2005–06.

Contact Dr. Nancy D. Rubino, Program Director, Nursing Program, Wesley College, 120 North State Street, Dulany Hall, Dover, DE 19901. *Telephone:* 302-736-2550. *Fax:* 302-736-2548. *E-mail:* rubinona@wesley. edu.

GRADUATE PROGRAMS

Expenses (2006–07) *Tuition:* part-time $325 per credit. *Required fees:* full-time $125; part-time $65 per term.

Financial Aid 100% of graduate students in nursing programs received some form of financial aid in 2005–06. 4 teaching assistantships with full tuition reimbursements available were awarded; traineeships also available.

Contact Dr. Lucille C. Gambardella, Chairperson, Nursing Program, Wesley College, 120 North State Street, Dover, DE 19901. *Telephone:* 302-736-2512. *Fax:* 302-736-2548. *E-mail:* gambarlu@wesley.edu.

MASTER'S DEGREE PROGRAM

Degree MSN

Available Programs Accelerated AD/RN to Master's; Accelerated RN to Master's; Master's.

Concentrations Available *Clinical nurse specialist programs in:* community health.

Site Options New Castle, DE.

Study Options Full-time and part-time.

Program Entrance Requirements Clinical experience, computer literacy, minimum overall college GPA of 3.0, transcript of college record, written essay, interview, 3 letters of recommendation, professional liability insurance/malpractice insurance, resume, statistics course, GRE or MAT. *Application deadline:* Applications are processed on a rolling basis. *Application fee:* $25.

Advanced Placement Credit by examination available. Credit given for nursing courses completed elsewhere dependent upon specific evaluations.

Degree Requirements 36 total credit hours, thesis or project.

POST-MASTER'S PROGRAM

Areas of Study Nursing education.

CONTINUING EDUCATION PROGRAM

Contact Dr. Lucille C. Gambardella, Chairperson, Nursing Program, Wesley College, 120 North State Street, Dover, DE 19901. *Telephone:* 302-736-2512. *Fax:* 302-736-2548. *E-mail:* gambarlu@wesley.edu.

Wilmington College
Division of Nursing
New Castle, Delaware

Founded in 1967

DEGREES • BSN • MSN • MSN/MBA • MSN/MS

Nursing Program Faculty 10 (50% with doctorates).

Baccalaureate Enrollment 150
Women 96% **Men** 4% **Minority** 8% **Part-time** 90%

Graduate Enrollment 170
Women 92% **Men** 8% **Minority** 17% **International** 5% **Part-time** 50%

Nursing Student Activities Sigma Theta Tau.

Nursing Student Resources Academic advising; academic or career counseling; assistance for students with disabilities; bookstore; career placement assistance; computer lab; computer-assisted instruction; employment services for current students; housing assistance; interactive nursing skills videos; learning resource lab; library services; nursing audiovisuals; remedial services; resume preparation assistance; tutoring.

Library Facilities 98,713 volumes (6,000 in health, 3,500 in nursing); 425 periodical subscriptions (60 health-care related).

BACCALAUREATE PROGRAMS

Degree BSN

Available Programs Accelerated RN Baccalaureate; International Nurse to Baccalaureate; RN Baccalaureate.

Site Options Dover, DE; Georgetown, DE.

Study Options Full-time and part-time.

Program Entrance Requirements Transcript of college record, CPR certification, health exam, immunizations, prerequisite course work, RN licensure. Transfer students are accepted. **Standardized tests** *Required:* TOEFL for international students. **Application** *Deadline:* rolling (freshmen), rolling (transfer). *Notification:* continuous (freshmen). *Application fee:* $25.

Advanced Placement Credit by examination available. Credit given for nursing courses completed elsewhere dependent upon specific evaluations.

Financial Aid 60% of baccalaureate students in nursing programs received some form of financial aid in 2004–05.

Contact Ms. Sheila Sharbaugh, BSN Program Coordinator, Division of Nursing, Wilmington College, 320 DuPont Highway, New Castle, DE 19720. *Telephone:* 302-328-9401 Ext. 296. *Fax:* 302-322-7081. *E-mail:* Sheila.M. Sharbaugh@wilmcoll.edu.

GRADUATE PROGRAMS

Expenses (2005–06) *Tuition:* part-time $312 per credit. *Required fees:* full-time $250.

Financial Aid 65% of graduate students in nursing programs received some form of financial aid in 2004–05. 28 fellowships with tuition reimbursements available (averaging $2,200 per year) were awarded; traineeships also available.

Contact Ms. Kim Christensen, Admissions Associate, Division of Nursing, Wilmington College, Wilson Graduate Center, 31 Read's Way, New Castle, DE 19720. *Telephone:* 302-295-1120. *E-mail:* kimberly.a.christensen@ wilmcoll.edu.

MASTER'S DEGREE PROGRAM

Degrees MSN; MSN/MBA; MSN/MS

Available Programs Master's.

Concentrations Available Nursing administration; nursing education. *Nurse practitioner programs in:* adult health, family health, gerontology, women's health.

Site Options Georgetown, DE; New Castle—Graduate Center, DE.

Study Options Full-time and part-time.

Program Entrance Requirements Clinical experience, computer literacy, minimum overall college GPA of 3.0, transcript of college record, CPR certification, written essay, immunizations, interview, 2 letters of recommendation, nursing research course, physical assessment course, professional liability insurance/malpractice insurance, prerequisite course work, resume, statistics course. *Application deadline:* For fall admission, 3/31 (priority date). Applications are processed on a rolling basis. *Application fee:* $25.

Advanced Placement Credit given for nursing courses completed elsewhere dependent upon specific evaluations.

Degree Requirements 42 total credit hours, thesis or project.

POST-MASTER'S PROGRAM

Areas of Study Nursing administration; nursing education. *Nurse practitioner programs in:* adult health, family health, gerontology.

DISTRICT OF COLUMBIA

The Catholic University of America

School of Nursing
Washington, District of Columbia

http://www.nursing.cua.edu

Founded in 1887

DEGREES • BSN • DN SC • MA/MSM • MSN

Nursing Program Faculty 27 (74% with doctorates).

Baccalaureate Enrollment 177
Women 91% **Men** 9% **Minority** 18% **International** 2% **Part-time** 3%

Graduate Enrollment 110
Women 98% **Men** 2% **Minority** 22% **International** 9% **Part-time** 69%

Nursing Student Activities Nursing Honor Society, Sigma Theta Tau, Student Nurses' Association.

Nursing Student Resources Academic advising; academic or career counseling; assistance for students with disabilities; bookstore; computer lab; computer-assisted instruction; e-mail services; interactive nursing skills videos; Internet; learning resource lab; library services; nursing audiovisuals.

Library Facilities 1.6 million volumes (39,000 in health, 17,500 in nursing); 10,448 periodical subscriptions (250 health-care related).

BACCALAUREATE PROGRAMS

Degree BSN

Available Programs Accelerated Baccalaureate for Second Degree; Baccalaureate for Second Degree; Generic Baccalaureate.

Study Options Full-time and part-time.

Program Entrance Requirements Transcript of college record, written essay, health exam, health insurance, high school biology, high school chemistry, 3 years high school math, 2 years high school science, high school transcript, immunizations, 1 letter of recommendation, minimum high school GPA of 3.0, minimum GPA in nursing prerequisites of 2.75, professional liability insurance/malpractice insurance. Transfer students are accepted. **Standardized tests** *Required:* SAT or ACT. *Recommended:* SAT Subject Tests. **Application** *Deadline:* 2/15 (freshmen), 7/15 (transfer). *Notification:* continuous until 3/15 (freshmen), continuous (early decision). *Application fee:* $55.

Advanced Placement Credit given for nursing courses completed elsewhere dependent upon specific evaluations.

Expenses (2005–06) *Tuition:* full-time $24,800; part-time $940 per credit hour. *International tuition:* $24,800 full-time. *Room and board:* $12,000; room only: $8000 per academic year. *Required fees:* full-time $1200; part-time $300 per term.

Financial Aid 50% of baccalaureate students in nursing programs received some form of financial aid in 2004–05. *Gift aid (need-based):* Federal Pell, FSEOG, state, private, college/university gift aid from institutional funds, Federal Nursing. *Loans:* Federal Nursing Student Loans, FFEL (Subsidized and Unsubsidized Stafford PLUS), Perkins, college/university, Commercial Loans. *Work-Study:* Federal Work-Study. *Application deadline:* 4/15 (priority: 2/1).

Contact Mr. Jacques Grooms, Program Contact, School of Nursing, The Catholic University of America, 124 Gowan Hall, Washington, DC 20064. *Telephone:* 202-319-6457. *Fax:* 202-319-6485. *E-mail:* grooms@cua.edu.

GRADUATE PROGRAMS

Expenses (2005–06) *Tuition:* full-time $24,800; part-time $940 per credit hour. *International tuition:* $24,800 full-time. *Room and board:* $12,000; room only: $8000 per academic year. *Required fees:* full-time $1200; part-time $300 per term.

Financial Aid 60% of graduate students in nursing programs received some form of financial aid in 2004–05. Research assistantships, teaching assistantships, career-related internships or fieldwork, Federal Work-Study, scholarships, tuition waivers (full and partial), and unspecified assistantships available. Aid available to part-time students. *Financial aid application deadline:* 2/1.

Contact Rita Rooney, Academic Affairs Liaison, School of Nursing, The Catholic University of America, 122 Gowan Hall, Washington, DC 20064. *Telephone:* 202-319-6290. *Fax:* 202-319-6485. *E-mail:* rooneyr@cua.edu.

MASTER'S DEGREE PROGRAM

Degrees MA/MSM; MSN

Available Programs Master's.

Concentrations Available Nursing education. *Clinical nurse specialist programs in:* adult health, community health, pediatric, psychiatric/mental health. *Nurse practitioner programs in:* family health, gerontology, pediatric, school health.

Site Options Silver Spring, MD.

Study Options Full-time and part-time.

Program Entrance Requirements Clinical experience, minimum overall college GPA of 3.0, transcript of college record, written essay, immunizations, 3 letters of recommendation, professional liability insurance/malpractice insurance, prerequisite course work, statistics course, GRE General Test or MAT. *Application deadline:* For fall admission, 2/1 (priority date); for spring admission, 11/15 (priority date). Applications are processed on a rolling basis. *Application fee:* $55.

Advanced Placement Credit given for nursing courses completed elsewhere dependent upon specific evaluations.

Degree Requirements 44 total credit hours, comprehensive exam.

POST-MASTER'S PROGRAM

Areas of Study Nursing education. *Clinical nurse specialist programs in:* adult health, community health, pediatric, psychiatric/mental health. *Nurse practitioner programs in:* gerontology, pediatric, school health.

DOCTORAL DEGREE PROGRAM

Degree DN Sc

Available Programs Doctorate.

Areas of Study Clinical practice, nursing research, nursing science.

Program Entrance Requirements Clinical experience, minimum overall college GPA of 3.5, interview by faculty committee, interview, 3 letters of recommendation, MSN or equivalent, scholarly papers, statistics course, writing sample, GRE General Test. *Application deadline:* For fall admission, 2/1 (priority date); for spring admission, 11/15 (priority date). Applications are processed on a rolling basis. *Application fee:* $55.

Degree Requirements 66 total credit hours, dissertation, oral exam, written exam, residency.

Georgetown University

School of Nursing and Health Studies
Washington, District of Columbia

http://snhs.georgetown.edu

Founded in 1789

DEGREES • BSN • MS

Nursing Program Faculty 72 (50% with doctorates).

Baccalaureate Enrollment 480
Women 85% **Men** 15% **Minority** 26% **International** 1% **Part-time** 2%

Graduate Enrollment 235
Women 73% **Men** 27% **Minority** 24% **International** 1% **Part-time** 20%

Nursing Student Activities Sigma Theta Tau, Student Nurses' Association.

Nursing Student Resources Academic advising; academic or career counseling; assistance for students with disabilities; bookstore; campus computer network; career placement assistance; computer lab; computer-assisted instruction; e-mail services; housing assistance; interactive nursing skills videos; Internet; learning resource lab; library services; nursing audiovisuals; resume preparation assistance; skills, simulation, or other laboratory; tutoring; unpaid internships.

Library Facilities 2.5 million volumes (36,000 in health, 20,000 in nursing); 31,099 periodical subscriptions (92 health-care related).

BACCALAUREATE PROGRAMS

Degree BSN

Georgetown University (continued)

Available Programs Accelerated Baccalaureate for Second Degree; Generic Baccalaureate; RN Baccalaureate.

Study Options Full-time.

Program Entrance Requirements Minimum overall college GPA of 3.0, transcript of college record, CPR certification, written essay, health exam, health insurance, high school biology, high school chemistry, high school math, 4 years high school science, high school transcript, immunizations, interview, 2 letters of recommendation. Transfer students are accepted. **Standardized tests** *Required:* SAT or ACT, TOEFL for international students. *Recommended:* SAT Subject Tests. **Application** *Deadline:* 1/10 (freshmen), 3/1 (transfer). *Early decision:* 11/1. *Notification:* 4/1 (freshmen), 12/15 (early action). *Application fee:* $65.

Advanced Placement Credit by examination available.

Financial Aid *Gift aid (need-based):* Federal Pell, FSEOG, state, private, college/university gift aid from institutional funds. *Loans:* Federal Nursing Student Loans, FFEL (Subsidized and Unsubsidized Stafford PLUS), Perkins. *Work-Study:* Federal Work-Study. *Application deadline:* 2/1.

Contact Office of Undergraduate Admissions, School of Nursing and Health Studies, Georgetown University, 37th and O Street NW, Washington, DC 20057. *Telephone:* 202-687-3600.

GRADUATE PROGRAMS

Financial Aid 95% of graduate students in nursing programs received some form of financial aid in 2005–06. Scholarships and traineeships available.

Contact Office of Graduate Admissions, School of Nursing and Health Studies, Georgetown University, 37th and O Street NW, Washington, DC 20057. *Telephone:* 202-687-5568.

MASTER'S DEGREE PROGRAM

Degree MS

Available Programs Master's; Master's for Non-Nursing College Graduates; RN to Master's.

Concentrations Available Health-care administration; nurse anesthesia; nurse-midwifery; nursing education. *Clinical nurse specialist programs in:* critical care. *Nurse practitioner programs in:* acute care, family health, women's health.

Study Options Full-time and part-time.

Program Entrance Requirements Clinical experience, minimum overall college GPA of 3.0, transcript of college record, written essay, interview, 3 letters of recommendation, resume, statistics course, GRE General Test or MAT. *Application fee:* $50 ($55 for international students).

Advanced Placement Credit given for nursing courses completed elsewhere dependent upon specific evaluations.

Degree Requirements 40 total credit hours, thesis or project.

POST-MASTER'S PROGRAM

Areas of Study Nurse-midwifery; nursing education. *Clinical nurse specialist programs in:* critical care. *Nurse practitioner programs in:* acute care, family health, women's health.

CONTINUING EDUCATION PROGRAM

Contact Ms. Marianne Lyons, Director of Continuing Education, School of Nursing and Health Studies, Georgetown University, 3700 Reservoir Road NW, Washington, DC 20007. *Telephone:* 202-687-1561. *Fax:* 202-687-3703. *E-mail:* lyonsm@georgetown.edu.

See full description on page 486.

Howard University
Division of Nursing
Washington, District of Columbia

http://www.howard.edu

Founded in 1867

DEGREES • BSN • MSN

Nursing Program Faculty 32 (25% with doctorates).

Baccalaureate Enrollment 476
Women 88% **Men** 12% **Minority** 88% **International** 12% **Part-time** 20%
Graduate Enrollment 20
Women 90% **Men** 10% **Minority** 55% **International** 45% **Part-time** 75%

Nursing Student Activities Sigma Theta Tau, Student Nurses' Association.

Nursing Student Resources Academic advising; academic or career counseling; assistance for students with disabilities; bookstore; campus computer network; career placement assistance; computer lab; computer-assisted instruction; e-mail services; externships; housing assistance; interactive nursing skills videos; Internet; learning resource lab; library services; nursing audiovisuals; paid internships; placement services for program completers; remedial services; resume preparation assistance; skills, simulation, or other laboratory.

Library Facilities 2.5 million volumes (219,448 in health, 4,500 in nursing); 12,795 periodical subscriptions (5,247 health-care related).

BACCALAUREATE PROGRAMS

Degree BSN

Available Programs ADN to Baccalaureate; Accelerated Baccalaureate for Second Degree; Accelerated RN Baccalaureate; Baccalaureate for Second Degree; Generic Baccalaureate; LPN to Baccalaureate; LPN to RN Baccalaureate; RN Baccalaureate.

Study Options Full-time and part-time.

Program Entrance Requirements Minimum overall college GPA of 2.8, transcript of college record, CPR certification, written essay, health exam, high school biology, high school chemistry, 2 years high school math, 2 years high school science, high school transcript, immunizations, 2 letters of recommendation, minimum high school GPA of 2.5, minimum high school rank 50%, minimum GPA in nursing prerequisites of 2.5. Transfer students are accepted. **Standardized tests** *Required:* SAT or ACT, TOEFL for international students. **Application** *Deadline:* 2/15 (freshmen), 4/1 (transfer). *Early decision:* 11/1. *Notification:* continuous (freshmen), 12/24 (early action). *Application fee:* $45.

Advanced Placement Credit by examination available. Credit given for nursing courses completed elsewhere dependent upon specific evaluations.

Expenses (2006–07) *Tuition:* full-time $6090; part-time $508 per credit. *International tuition:* $6090 full-time. *Room and board:* $6110; room only: $5474 per academic year. *Required fees:* full-time $12,985; part-time $508 per credit; part-time $6493 per term.

Financial Aid 92% of baccalaureate students in nursing programs received some form of financial aid in 2005–06.

Contact Mrs. Charmaine McKie, Director of Student Affairs, Division of Nursing, Howard University, 501 Bryant Street NW, Room 119, Washington, DC 20059. *Telephone:* 202-806-6509. *Fax:* 202-806-5958. *E-mail:* cmcKie@howard.edu.

GRADUATE PROGRAMS

Expenses (2006–07) *Tuition:* full-time $14,910; part-time $828 per credit. *International tuition:* $14,910 full-time. *Room and board:* $16,200; room only: $10,200 per academic year. *Required fees:* full-time $387; part-time $387 per term.

Financial Aid 52% of graduate students in nursing programs received some form of financial aid in 2005–06. Teaching assistantships, career-related internships or fieldwork, institutionally sponsored loans, and scholarships available. *Financial aid application deadline:* 4/1.

Contact Dean Mamie Clark Montague, PhD, Interim Associate Dean for Nursing, Division of Nursing, Howard University, 501 Bryant Street NW, Washington, DC 20059. *Telephone:* 202-806-7460. *Fax:* 202-806-5978. *E-mail:* mmontague@howard.edu.

MASTER'S DEGREE PROGRAM

Degree MSN

Available Programs Master's.

Concentrations Available *Nurse practitioner programs in:* family health.

Study Options Full-time and part-time.

Program Entrance Requirements Minimum overall college GPA of 3.0, transcript of college record, CPR certification, written essay, immunizations, interview, 3 letters of recommendation, physical assessment course, professional liability insurance/malpractice insurance, statistics course. *Application deadline:* For fall admission, 4/1 (priority date); for spring admission, 11/1. Applications are processed on a rolling basis. *Application fee:* $45.

Advanced Placement Credit given for nursing courses completed elsewhere dependent upon specific evaluations.

Degree Requirements 46 total credit hours, comprehensive exam.

POST-MASTER'S PROGRAM

Areas of Study *Nurse practitioner programs in:* family health.

University of the District of Columbia
Nursing Education Program
Washington, District of Columbia

Founded in 1976

DEGREE • BSN

Nursing Program Faculty 11 (1% with doctorates).

Nursing Student Activities Student Nurses' Association.

Nursing Student Resources Learning resource lab; library services; skills, simulation, or other laboratory.

Library Facilities 544,412 volumes (100 in health, 20 in nursing); 594 periodical subscriptions (35 health-care related).

BACCALAUREATE PROGRAMS

Degree BSN

Available Programs ADN to Baccalaureate.

Site Options Washington, DC.

Program Entrance Requirements CPR certification, professional liability insurance/malpractice insurance, prerequisite course work. Transfer students are accepted. **Standardized tests** *Required:* TOEFL for international students. *Recommended:* SAT. **Application** *Deadline:* 8/1 (freshmen), 8/1 (transfer). *Notification:* continuous until 8/15 (freshmen). *Application fee:* $20.

Contact *Telephone:* 202-274-5899. *Fax:* 202-274-5952.

FLORIDA

Barry University
School of Nursing
Miami Shores, Florida

http://www.barry.edu/nursing

Founded in 1940

DEGREES • BSN • MSN • MSN/MBA • PHD

Nursing Program Faculty 30 (46% with doctorates).

Baccalaureate Enrollment 250

Women 90% **Men** 10% **Minority** 51% **International** 3% **Part-time** 49%

Graduate Enrollment 150

Nursing Student Activities Sigma Theta Tau, Student Nurses' Association.

Nursing Student Resources Academic advising; academic or career counseling; assistance for students with disabilities; bookstore; campus computer network; career placement assistance; computer lab; computer-assisted instruction; e-mail services; employment services for current students; housing assistance; interactive nursing skills videos; Internet;

learning resource lab; library services; nursing audiovisuals; paid internships; remedial services; resume preparation assistance; skills, simulation, or other laboratory; tutoring.

Library Facilities 233,938 volumes (15,000 in health, 8,500 in nursing); 2,880 periodical subscriptions (400 health-care related).

BACCALAUREATE PROGRAMS

Degree BSN

Available Programs ADN to Baccalaureate; Accelerated Baccalaureate; Accelerated Baccalaureate for Second Degree; Baccalaureate for Second Degree; Generic Baccalaureate; LPN to Baccalaureate; LPN to RN Baccalaureate; RN Baccalaureate.

Study Options Full-time and part-time.

Program Entrance Requirements Minimum overall college GPA of 2.7, transcript of college record, CPR certification, health exam, health insurance, high school biology, high school chemistry, high school math, high school science, high school transcript, immunizations, 2 letters of recommendation, minimum high school GPA of 2.7, minimum GPA in nursing prerequisites of 2.7, professional liability insurance/malpractice insurance. Transfer students are accepted. **Standardized tests** *Required:* SAT or ACT. **Application** *Deadline:* rolling (freshmen), rolling (transfer). *Notification:* continuous (freshmen). *Application fee:* $30.

Advanced Placement Credit given for nursing courses completed elsewhere dependent upon specific evaluations.

Expenses (2006–07) *Tuition:* full-time $24,000; part-time $705 per credit. *Room and board:* $16,755; room only: $13,155 per academic year. *Required fees:* full-time $24,000; part-time $705 per credit.

Financial Aid 90% of baccalaureate students in nursing programs received some form of financial aid in 2005–06.

Contact Ms. Jennifer Morejon, Administrative Assistant, School of Nursing, Barry University, 11300 NE Second Avenue, Miami Shores, FL 33161-6695. *Telephone:* 305-899-3837. *Fax:* 305-899-3831. *E-mail:* jmorejon@mail.barry.edu.

GRADUATE PROGRAMS

Expenses (2006–07) *Tuition:* full-time $12,600; part-time $725 per credit. *Room and board:* $18,075; room only: $14,675 per academic year.

Financial Aid 100% of graduate students in nursing programs received some form of financial aid in 2005–06. 3 research assistantships (averaging $5,000 per year), 3 teaching assistantships (averaging $5,000 per year) were awarded; scholarships and tuition waivers (full) also available. *Financial aid application deadline:* 5/1.

Contact Dr. Claudette Spalding, Associate Dean, School of Nursing, Barry University, 11300 NE Second Avenue, Miami Shores, FL 33161-6695. *Telephone:* 305-899-3849. *Fax:* 305-899-3831. *E-mail:* cspalding@mail.barry.edu.

MASTER'S DEGREE PROGRAM

Degrees MSN; MSN/MBA

Available Programs Master's.

Concentrations Available Nursing administration; nursing education. *Nurse practitioner programs in:* acute care, family health.

Study Options Part-time.

Program Entrance Requirements Clinical experience, computer literacy, minimum overall college GPA of 3.0, transcript of college record, written essay, 2 letters of recommendation, nursing research course, professional liability insurance/malpractice insurance, statistics course, GRE General Test or MAT. *Application deadline:* For fall admission, 5/1 (priority date). Applications are processed on a rolling basis. *Application fee:* $30.

Advanced Placement Credit given for nursing courses completed elsewhere dependent upon specific evaluations.

Degree Requirements 45 total credit hours.

POST-MASTER'S PROGRAM

Areas of Study Nursing administration; nursing education. *Nurse practitioner programs in:* acute care, family health.

DOCTORAL DEGREE PROGRAM

Degree PhD

Available Programs Doctorate.

Areas of Study Nursing research, nursing science.

Barry University (continued)

Program Entrance Requirements Clinical experience, minimum overall college GPA of 3.0, interview, 2 letters of recommendation, MSN or equivalent, statistics course, writing sample, GRE General Test or MAT. *Application deadline:* For fall admission, 5/1 (priority date). Applications are processed on a rolling basis. *Application fee:* $30.

Degree Requirements 45 total credit hours, dissertation, written exam, residency.

Bethune-Cookman College
School of Nursing
Daytona Beach, Florida

http://www.cookman.edu/Nursing

Founded in 1904

DEGREE • BSN

Nursing Program Faculty 11 (2% with doctorates).

Baccalaureate Enrollment 137
Women 93% **Men** 7% **Minority** 95% **International** 2%

Nursing Student Activities Nursing Honor Society, Student Nurses' Association.

Nursing Student Resources Academic advising; bookstore; campus computer network; computer lab; computer-assisted instruction; e-mail services; interactive nursing skills videos; Internet; learning resource lab; library services; nursing audiovisuals; resume preparation assistance; skills, simulation, or other laboratory; tutoring; unpaid internships.

Library Facilities 187,908 volumes; 800 periodical subscriptions.

BACCALAUREATE PROGRAMS

Degree BSN

Available Programs Generic Baccalaureate; RN Baccalaureate.
Study Options Full-time.
Program Entrance Requirements Minimum overall college GPA of 2.8, transcript of college record, CPR certification, written essay, health exam, high school transcript, immunizations, interview, 2 letters of recommendation, minimum GPA in nursing prerequisites of 2.8, prerequisite course work. Transfer students are accepted. **Standardized tests** *Required:* SAT or ACT, TOEFL for international students. **Application** *Deadline:* 6/30 (freshmen), 6/30 (transfer). *Notification:* continuous (freshmen). *Application fee:* $25.
Advanced Placement Credit by examination available. Credit given for nursing courses completed elsewhere dependent upon specific evaluations.
Expenses (2005–06) *Tuition:* full-time $11,230; part-time $5615 per semester. *International tuition:* $11,230 full-time. *Room and board:* $6692 per academic year. *Required fees:* full-time $330.
Financial Aid 99% of baccalaureate students in nursing programs received some form of financial aid in 2004–05.
Contact Dr. Alma Dixon, RN, Chair and Associate Professor, School of Nursing, Bethune-Cookman College, 640 Dr. Mary McLeod Bethune Boulevard, Daytona Beach, FL 32114-3099. *Telephone:* 386-481-2000. *E-mail:* dixonal@cookman.edu.

Florida Agricultural and Mechanical University
School of Nursing
Tallahassee, Florida

http://www.famu.edu/acad/colleges/son

Founded in 1887

DEGREES • BSN • MSN • PHD

Nursing Program Faculty 28 (18% with doctorates).

Baccalaureate Enrollment 161
Women 90% **Men** 10% **Minority** 98%

Graduate Enrollment 17
Women 83% **Men** 17% **Minority** 76% **Part-time** 12%

Nursing Student Activities Sigma Theta Tau, Student Nurses' Association.

Nursing Student Resources Academic advising; academic or career counseling; bookstore; campus computer network; career placement assistance; computer lab; computer-assisted instruction; daycare for children of students; e-mail services; employment services for current students; externships; interactive nursing skills videos; Internet; library services; nursing audiovisuals; placement services for program completers; remedial services; resume preparation assistance; skills, simulation, or other laboratory; tutoring.

Library Facilities 484,801 volumes (5,000 in health, 4,091 in nursing); 7,672 periodical subscriptions (385 health-care related).

BACCALAUREATE PROGRAMS

Degree BSN

Available Programs Generic Baccalaureate.
Study Options Part-time.
Program Entrance Requirements CPR certification, health exam, immunizations, 3 letters of recommendation, minimum high school GPA of 2.5, prerequisite course work. Transfer students are accepted. **Standardized tests** *Required:* SAT or ACT, TOEFL for international students. **Application** *Deadline:* 5/9 (freshmen), 5/1 (transfer). *Notification:* continuous until 8/1 (freshmen). *Application fee:* $20.
Contact *Telephone:* 850-599-3458. *Fax:* 850-599-3508.

GRADUATE PROGRAMS

Contact *Telephone:* 850-599-3017. *Fax:* 850-599-3508.

MASTER'S DEGREE PROGRAM

Degree MSN

Available Programs Master's.
Concentrations Available *Nurse practitioner programs in:* adult health, gerontology, women's health.
Study Options Full-time and part-time.
Program Entrance Requirements Clinical experience, minimum overall college GPA of 3.0, CPR certification, immunizations, interview, nursing research course, physical assessment course, professional liability insurance/malpractice insurance, statistics course.
Degree Requirements 42 total credit hours, thesis or project.

POST-MASTER'S PROGRAM

Areas of Study *Nurse practitioner programs in:* adult health, gerontology, women's health.

DOCTORAL DEGREE PROGRAM

Degree PhD

Program Entrance Requirements Minimum overall college GPA of 3.5, 3 letters of recommendation, MSN or equivalent.
Degree Requirements 90 total credit hours, dissertation, oral exam, written exam.

CONTINUING EDUCATION PROGRAM

Contact *Telephone:* 850-599-3017. *Fax:* 850-599-3508.

Florida Atlantic University
College of Nursing
Boca Raton, Florida

http://www.fau.edu/nursing

Founded in 1961

DEGREES • BSN • MS • MS/MBA • PHD

Nursing Program Faculty 73 (49% with doctorates).

Baccalaureate Enrollment 600
Women 85% **Men** 15% **Minority** 30% **International** 10% **Part-time** 30%

Graduate Enrollment 209
Women 89% **Men** 11% **Minority** 39% **Part-time** 85%
Nursing Student Activities Sigma Theta Tau, Student Nurses' Association.

Nursing Student Resources Academic advising; assistance for students with disabilities; bookstore; campus computer network; computer lab; computer-assisted instruction; e-mail services; housing assistance; Internet; learning resource lab; library services; nursing audiovisuals; skills, simulation, or other laboratory; tutoring.

Library Facilities 1.3 million volumes (18,735 in health, 4,713 in nursing); 12,811 periodical subscriptions (333 health-care related).

BACCALAUREATE PROGRAMS

Degree BSN

Available Programs ADN to Baccalaureate; Accelerated Baccalaureate for Second Degree; Generic Baccalaureate; RN Baccalaureate.
Site Options *Distance Learning:* Port St. Lucie, FL; Davie, FL.
Study Options Full-time.
Program Entrance Requirements Minimum overall college GPA of 3.0, transcript of college record, CPR certification, written essay, health exam, health insurance, high school transcript, immunizations, minimum GPA in nursing prerequisites of 2.0, professional liability insurance/malpractice insurance, prerequisite course work. Transfer students are accepted. **Standardized tests** *Required:* SAT or ACT, TOEFL for international students. **Application** *Deadline:* 6/1 (freshmen), 6/1 (transfer). *Notification:* continuous (freshmen). *Application fee:* $30.
Advanced Placement Credit by examination available. Credit given for nursing courses completed elsewhere dependent upon specific evaluations.
Financial Aid 75% of baccalaureate students in nursing programs received some form of financial aid in 2005–06. *Gift aid (need-based):* Federal Pell, FSEOG, state, private, college/university gift aid from institutional funds, Federal Nursing. *Loans:* FFEL (Subsidized and Unsubsidized Stafford PLUS), Perkins, college/university. *Work-Study:* Federal Work-Study, part-time campus jobs. *Application deadline (priority):* 3/1.
Contact Dr. Debera Thomas, Assistant Dean for Undergraduate Programs, College of Nursing, Florida Atlantic University, 777 Glades Road, Boca Raton, FL 33431. *Telephone:* 561-297-2535. *Fax:* 561-297-3652. *E-mail:* dthomas@fau.edu.

GRADUATE PROGRAMS

Financial Aid 11 research assistantships, 6 teaching assistantships were awarded; career-related internships or fieldwork, Federal Work-Study, institutionally sponsored loans, scholarships, and traineeships also available.
Contact Dr. Susan Chase, Assistant Dean for Graduate Programs, College of Nursing, Florida Atlantic University, 777 Glades Road, Boca Raton, FL 33431. *Telephone:* 561-297-3389. *Fax:* 561-297-3652. *E-mail:* schase@fau.edu.

MASTER'S DEGREE PROGRAM

Degrees MS; MS/MBA

Available Programs Master's; Master's for Nurses with Non-Nursing Degrees; RN to Master's.
Concentrations Available Nursing administration; nursing education. *Clinical nurse specialist programs in:* gerontology. *Nurse practitioner programs in:* adult health, family health, gerontology.
Site Options *Distance Learning:* Port St. Lucie, FL; Davie, FL.
Study Options Full-time and part-time.
Program Entrance Requirements Minimum overall college GPA of 3.0, transcript of college record, CPR certification, written essay, immunizations, 2 letters of recommendation, nursing research course, physical assessment course, professional liability insurance/malpractice insurance, prerequisite course work, resume, statistics course, GRE General Test. *Application deadline:* For fall admission, 6/2; for spring admission, 10/20. Applications are processed on a rolling basis. *Application fee:* $30.

POST-MASTER'S PROGRAM

Areas of Study Nursing administration; nursing education. *Clinical nurse specialist programs in:* gerontology. *Nurse practitioner programs in:* adult health, family health, gerontology.

DOCTORAL DEGREE PROGRAM

Degree PhD

Available Programs Doctorate.
Areas of Study Advanced practice nursing, aging, clinical practice, community health, faculty preparation, family health, gerontology, health policy, health promotion/disease prevention, individualized study, nursing administration, nursing education, nursing policy, nursing research, nursing science.
Program Entrance Requirements Minimum overall college GPA of 3.5, interview by faculty committee, 3 letters of recommendation, MSN or equivalent, statistics course, vita, writing sample, GRE General Test. *Application deadline:* For fall admission, 6/2; for spring admission, 10/20. Applications are processed on a rolling basis. *Application fee:* $30.
Degree Requirements 62 total credit hours, dissertation, written exam, residency.

CONTINUING EDUCATION PROGRAM

Contact Dr. Beth King, Director, College of Nursing, Florida Atlantic University, 777 Glades Road, Boca Raton, FL 33431. *Telephone:* 561-297-3887. *Fax:* 561-297-3652. *E-mail:* bking@fau.edu.

Florida Gulf Coast University
School of Nursing
Fort Myers, Florida

Founded in 1991
DEGREES • BSN • MSN

Nursing Program Faculty 21 (52% with doctorates).
Baccalaureate Enrollment 192
Women 89% **Men** 11% **Minority** 11% **International** 15% **Part-time** 3%
Graduate Enrollment 140
Women 54% **Men** 46% **Minority** 20% **Part-time** 15%
Nursing Student Activities Sigma Theta Tau, Student Nurses' Association.

Nursing Student Resources Academic advising; academic or career counseling; assistance for students with disabilities; bookstore; campus computer network; career placement assistance; computer lab; computer-assisted instruction; daycare for children of students; e-mail services; employment services for current students; housing assistance; Internet; library services; nursing audiovisuals; remedial services; skills, simulation, or other laboratory; tutoring.

Library Facilities 312,132 volumes (13,943 in health, 6,742 in nursing); 7,119 periodical subscriptions (471 health-care related).

BACCALAUREATE PROGRAMS

Degree BSN

Available Programs ADN to Baccalaureate; Accelerated Baccalaureate for Second Degree; Accelerated RN Baccalaureate; Generic Baccalaureate.
Site Options *Distance Learning:* Port Charlotte, FL.
Study Options Full-time.
Program Entrance Requirements Minimum overall college GPA of 3.0, transcript of college record, CPR certification, health insurance, high school foreign language, immunizations, minimum GPA in nursing prerequisites of 3.0, professional liability insurance/malpractice insurance, prerequisite course work. Transfer students are accepted. **Standardized tests** *Required:* SAT or ACT, TOEFL for international students. **Application** *Deadline:* 8/1 (freshmen), 8/1 (transfer). *Notification:* continuous (freshmen). *Application fee:* $30.
Advanced Placement Credit by examination available. Credit given for nursing courses completed elsewhere dependent upon specific evaluations.
Expenses (2006–07) *Tuition, state resident:* part-time $117 per credit. *Tuition, nonresident:* part-time $514 per credit. *Room and board:* room only: $4440 per academic year.
Contact Mrs. Peggy Raynor, Advisor, School of Nursing, Florida Gulf Coast University, 10501 FGCU Boulevard South, Fort Myers, FL 33965-6565. *Telephone:* 239-590-7455. *Fax:* 239-590-7474. *E-mail:* praynor@fgcu.edu.

Florida Gulf Coast University (continued)
GRADUATE PROGRAMS
Expenses (2006–07) *Tuition, state resident:* part-time $229 per credit. *Tuition, nonresident:* part-time $850 per credit. *Room and board:* room only: $4400 per academic year.

Contact Dr. Marydelle Polk, Program Director, School of Nursing, Florida Gulf Coast University, 10501 FGCU Boulevard South, Fort Myers, FL 33965-6565. *Telephone:* 239-590-7518. *Fax:* 239-590-7474. *E-mail:* mpolk@fgcu.edu.

MASTER'S DEGREE PROGRAM
Degree MSN

Available Programs Accelerated AD/RN to Master's; Accelerated RN to Master's; Master's.

Concentrations Available Nurse anesthesia; nursing education. *Nurse practitioner programs in:* family health.

Study Options Full-time and part-time.

Program Entrance Requirements Clinical experience, minimum overall college GPA of 3.0, transcript of college record, CPR certification, written essay, immunizations, interview, 1 letter of recommendation, nursing research course, physical assessment course, professional liability insurance/malpractice insurance, prerequisite course work, resume, statistics course.

Advanced Placement Credit given for nursing courses completed elsewhere dependent upon specific evaluations.

Degree Requirements 40 total credit hours.

POST-MASTER'S PROGRAM
Areas of Study *Nurse practitioner programs in:* family health.

CONTINUING EDUCATION PROGRAM
Contact Dr. Anne Nolan, Associate Professor, School of Nursing, Florida Gulf Coast University, 10501 FGCU Boulevard South, Fort Myers, FL 33931. *Telephone:* 239-590-7513. *Fax:* 239-590-7474. *E-mail:* anolan@fgcu.edu.

Florida Hospital College of Health Sciences
Department of Nursing
Orlando, Florida

http://www.fhchs.edu/
Founded in 1913
DEGREE • BS

Nursing Program Faculty 12 (16% with doctorates).

Nursing Student Resources Campus computer network; computer lab; computer-assisted instruction; Internet; learning resource lab; library services; nursing audiovisuals; skills, simulation, or other laboratory.

Library Facilities 74,581 volumes; 158 periodical subscriptions.

BACCALAUREATE PROGRAMS
Degree BS

Available Programs Generic Baccalaureate; RN Baccalaureate.

Study Options Full-time and part-time.

Program Entrance Requirements Minimum overall college GPA of 2.5, transcript of college record, health exam, 1 letter of recommendation, prerequisite course work, RN licensure. Transfer students are accepted. **Standardized tests** *Required for some:* SAT or ACT. **Application** *Deadline:* 7/18 (freshmen), 7/18 (out-of-state freshmen), 7/18 (transfer). *Notification:* continuous until 8/30 (freshmen), continuous until 8/30 (out-of-state freshmen). *Application fee:* $20.

Advanced Placement Credit by examination available. Credit given for nursing courses completed elsewhere dependent upon specific evaluations.

Contact *Telephone:* 407-303-9798. *Fax:* 407-303-9408.

Florida International University
College of Nursing and Health Sciences
Miami, Florida

http://www.fiu.edu
Founded in 1965
DEGREES • BSN • MSN • PHD

Nursing Program Faculty 72 (38% with doctorates).

Baccalaureate Enrollment 495
Women 78% **Men** 22% **Minority** 88% **International** 1% **Part-time** 69%

Graduate Enrollment 276
Women 73% **Men** 27% **Minority** 71% **International** 1% **Part-time** 55%

Nursing Student Activities Sigma Theta Tau, Student Nurses' Association.

Nursing Student Resources Academic advising; academic or career counseling; assistance for students with disabilities; bookstore; campus computer network; career placement assistance; computer lab; computer-assisted instruction; daycare for children of students; e-mail services; externships; housing assistance; interactive nursing skills videos; Internet; learning resource lab; library services; nursing audiovisuals; paid internships; remedial services; resume preparation assistance; skills, simulation, or other laboratory; tutoring.

Library Facilities 1.8 million volumes (201,000 in health, 10,000 in nursing); 16,920 periodical subscriptions (1,500 health-care related).

BACCALAUREATE PROGRAMS
Degree BSN

Available Programs Accelerated Baccalaureate; Accelerated Baccalaureate for Second Degree; Generic Baccalaureate; RN Baccalaureate.

Site Options *Distance Learning:* North Miami, FL.

Study Options Full-time.

Program Entrance Requirements Minimum overall college GPA of 3.0, transcript of college record, CPR certification, written essay, health exam, health insurance, high school foreign language, high school transcript, immunizations, minimum GPA in nursing prerequisites of 3.0, prerequisite course work. Transfer students are accepted. **Standardized tests** *Required:* SAT or ACT, TOEFL for international students. **Application** *Deadline:* rolling (freshmen), rolling (transfer). *Notification:* continuous until 8/1 (freshmen). *Application fee:* $25.

Advanced Placement Credit by examination available. Credit given for nursing courses completed elsewhere dependent upon specific evaluations.

Expenses (2006–07) *Tuition, state resident:* full-time $3339; part-time $104 per credit. *Tuition, nonresident:* full-time $16,563; part-time $517 per credit. *International tuition:* $16,563 full-time. *Room and board:* $14,610; room only: $9780 per academic year. *Required fees:* full-time $1578; part-time $49 per credit; part-time $526 per term.

Financial Aid 75% of baccalaureate students in nursing programs received some form of financial aid in 2005–06.

Contact Dr. Suzanne Phillips, EdD, Director of Administration, College of Nursing and Health Sciences, Florida International University, University Park Campus, HLS 2, 11200 SW 8th Street, Miami, FL 33199. *Telephone:* 305-348-7743. *Fax:* 305-348-7764. *E-mail:* phillips@fiu.edu.

GRADUATE PROGRAMS
Expenses (2006–07) *Tuition, state resident:* full-time $7020; part-time $260 per credit. *Tuition, nonresident:* full-time $20,628; part-time $764 per credit. *International tuition:* $20,628 full-time. *Room and board:* $14,610; room only: $9780 per academic year. *Required fees:* full-time $1554; part-time $58 per credit; part-time $518 per term.

Financial Aid 60% of graduate students in nursing programs received some form of financial aid in 2005–06.

Contact Dr. Suzanne Phillips, EdD, Director of Administration, College of Nursing and Health Sciences, Florida International University, University Park Campus, HLS 2, 11200 SW 8th Street, Miami, FL 33199. *Telephone:* 305-348-7743. *Fax:* 305-348-7764. *E-mail:* phillips@fiu.edu.

MASTER'S DEGREE PROGRAM
Degree MSN

Available Programs Master's; Master's for Nurses with Non-Nursing Degrees.

Concentrations Available Nurse anesthesia; nursing administration. *Clinical nurse specialist programs in:* adult health, family health, pediatric, psychiatric/mental health. *Nurse practitioner programs in:* adult health, family health, pediatric, psychiatric/mental health.

Study Options Full-time and part-time.

Program Entrance Requirements Clinical experience, computer literacy, minimum overall college GPA of 3.0, transcript of college record, CPR certification, written essay, immunizations, interview, 3 letters of recommendation, nursing research course, physical assessment course, professional liability insurance/malpractice insurance, prerequisite course work, statistics course, GRE General Test. *Application deadline:* For fall admission, 4/1 (priority date); for spring admission, 10/1. Applications are processed on a rolling basis. *Application fee:* $25.

Advanced Placement Credit given for nursing courses completed elsewhere dependent upon specific evaluations.

Degree Requirements 43 total credit hours.

POST-MASTER'S PROGRAM

Areas of Study Nursing administration. *Clinical nurse specialist programs in:* adult health, family health, pediatric, psychiatric/mental health. *Nurse practitioner programs in:* adult health, family health, pediatric, psychiatric/mental health.

DOCTORAL DEGREE PROGRAM

Degree PhD

Available Programs Doctorate.

Areas of Study Faculty preparation, health policy, health-care systems, individualized study, information systems, nursing administration, nursing education, nursing policy, nursing research, nursing science.

Program Entrance Requirements Clinical experience, minimum overall college GPA of 3.0, interview by faculty committee, 3 letters of recommendation, MSN or equivalent, statistics course. *Application deadline:* For fall admission, 4/1 (priority date); for spring admission, 10/1. Applications are processed on a rolling basis. *Application fee:* $25.

Degree Requirements 84 total credit hours, dissertation, oral exam, written exam.

Florida Southern College
Department of Nursing
Lakeland, Florida

http://www.flsouthern.edu/nursing/

Founded in 1885

DEGREES • BSN • MS

Nursing Program Faculty 6 (83% with doctorates).

Baccalaureate Enrollment 75
Women 93% **Men** 7% **Minority** 24% **International** 2% **Part-time** 70%

Graduate Enrollment 38
Women 100% **Minority** 35% **Part-time** 90%

Nursing Student Activities Nursing Honor Society.

Nursing Student Resources Academic advising; academic or career counseling; assistance for students with disabilities; bookstore; campus computer network; career placement assistance; computer lab; computer-assisted instruction; e-mail services; externships; interactive nursing skills videos; Internet; learning resource lab; library services; nursing audiovisuals; paid internships; remedial services; resume preparation assistance; skills, simulation, or other laboratory; tutoring.

Library Facilities 182,765 volumes (4,000 in health, 3,500 in nursing); 939 periodical subscriptions (12 health-care related).

BACCALAUREATE PROGRAMS

Degree BSN

Available Programs ADN to Baccalaureate; Baccalaureate for Second Degree; Generic Baccalaureate.

Site Options Orlando, FL.

Study Options Full-time.

Program Entrance Requirements Minimum overall college GPA of 3.2, transcript of college record, CPR certification, health exam, immunizations, minimum high school GPA of 3.2, minimum GPA in nursing prerequisites of 3.0, prerequisite course work, RN licensure. Transfer students are accepted. **Standardized tests** *Required:* SAT or ACT, TOEFL for international students. **Application** *Deadline:* 3/1 (freshmen), rolling (transfer). *Early decision:* 12/1. *Notification:* continuous (freshmen), 12/15 (out-of-state freshmen), 12/15 (early decision). *Application fee:* $30.

Advanced Placement Credit given for nursing courses completed elsewhere dependent upon specific evaluations.

Expenses (2006–07) *Tuition:* full-time $9850. *Room and board:* $3070; room only: $1970 per academic year. *Required fees:* full-time $276; part-time $138 per term.

Financial Aid 50% of baccalaureate students in nursing programs received some form of financial aid in 2005–06. *Gift aid (need-based):* Federal Pell, FSEOG, state, private, college/university gift aid from institutional funds. *Loans:* FFEL (Subsidized and Unsubsidized Stafford PLUS), Perkins. *Work-Study:* Federal Work-Study, part-time campus jobs. *Application deadline:* 8/1 (priority: 4/1).

Contact Dr. Mavra E. Kear, Department Chair, Department of Nursing, Florida Southern College, 111 Lake Hollingsworth Drive, Lakeland, FL 33801. *Telephone:* 863-680-4310. *Fax:* 863-680-3860. *E-mail:* mkear@flsouthern.edu.

GRADUATE PROGRAMS

Expenses (2006–07) *Tuition:* part-time $330 per credit hour. *Required fees:* part-time $10 per term.

Financial Aid 10% of graduate students in nursing programs received some form of financial aid in 2005–06.

Contact Dr. Mavra E. Kear, Department Chair, Department of Nursing, Florida Southern College, 111 Lake Hollingsworth Drive, Lakeland, FL 33801. *Telephone:* 863-680-4310. *Fax:* 863-680-3860. *E-mail:* mkear@flsouthern.edu.

MASTER'S DEGREE PROGRAM

Degree MS

Available Programs Accelerated AD/RN to Master's; Master's; Master's for Nurses with Non-Nursing Degrees.

Concentrations Available Nursing education. *Clinical nurse specialist programs in:* medical-surgical.

Study Options Full-time and part-time.

Program Entrance Requirements Computer literacy, minimum overall college GPA of 3.0, transcript of college record, written essay, immunizations, 3 letters of recommendation, nursing research course, physical assessment course, resume, statistics course.

Advanced Placement Credit given for nursing courses completed elsewhere dependent upon specific evaluations.

Degree Requirements 39 total credit hours, thesis or project.

POST-MASTER'S PROGRAM

Areas of Study Nursing education. *Clinical nurse specialist programs in:* medical-surgical.

CONTINUING EDUCATION PROGRAM

Contact Deborah Stanley, Assistant Director, Evening Program, Department of Nursing, Florida Southern College, 111 Lake Hollingsworth Drive, Lakeland, FL 33801. *Telephone:* 863-680-4205. *Fax:* 863-680-3872. *E-mail:* dstanley@flsouthern.edu.

Florida State University
School of Nursing
Tallahassee, Florida

Founded in 1851

DEGREES • BSN • MSN

Nursing Program Faculty 49 (43% with doctorates).

Baccalaureate Enrollment 389
Women 89% **Men** 11% **Minority** 21% **Part-time** 31%

Florida State University (continued)
Graduate Enrollment 80
Women 94% **Men** 6% **Minority** 20% **International** 1% **Part-time** 75%
Nursing Student Activities Nursing Honor Society, Sigma Theta Tau, Student Nurses' Association, nursing club.
Nursing Student Resources Academic advising; academic or career counseling; assistance for students with disabilities; bookstore; campus computer network; career placement assistance; computer lab; computer-assisted instruction; e-mail services; externships; housing assistance; interactive nursing skills videos; Internet; learning resource lab; library services; nursing audiovisuals; resume preparation assistance; skills, simulation, or other laboratory; unpaid internships.
Library Facilities 2.9 million volumes (220,248 in nursing); 58,093 periodical subscriptions.

BACCALAUREATE PROGRAMS

Degree BSN

Available Programs ADN to Baccalaureate; Baccalaureate for Second Degree; Generic Baccalaureate; RN Baccalaureate.
Site Options Panama City, FL. *Distance Learning:* Pensacola, FL; Marianna, FL.
Study Options Full-time.
Program Entrance Requirements Minimum overall college GPA of 3.0, transcript of college record, CPR certification, health exam, health insurance, high school foreign language, immunizations, minimum GPA in nursing prerequisites of 3.0, professional liability insurance/malpractice insurance, prerequisite course work. Transfer students are accepted. **Standardized tests** *Required:* SAT or ACT, TOEFL for international students. **Application** *Deadline:* 2/14 (freshmen), 7/1 (transfer). *Notification:* 3/28 (freshmen). *Application fee:* $30.
Advanced Placement Credit given for nursing courses completed elsewhere dependent upon specific evaluations.
Expenses (2006–07) *Tuition, state resident:* full-time $3335; part-time $104 per credit hour. *Tuition, nonresident:* full-time $17,342; part-time $542 per credit hour. *International tuition:* $17,342 full-time. *Room and board:* $7800; room only: $4500 per academic year. *Required fees:* full-time $192; part-time $6 per credit; part-time $84 per term.
Financial Aid 92% of baccalaureate students in nursing programs received some form of financial aid in 2005–06. *Gift aid (need-based):* Federal Pell, FSEOG, state, private, college/university gift aid from institutional funds. *Loans:* FFEL (Subsidized and Unsubsidized Stafford PLUS), Perkins, college/university. *Work-Study:* Federal Work-Study, part-time campus jobs. *Application deadline (priority):* 2/15.
Contact Ms. Brenda Arosemena, Academic Coordinator, School of Nursing, Florida State University, 104H Vivian M. Duxbury Hall, Tallahassee, FL 32306-4310. *Telephone:* 850-644-5107. *Fax:* 850-644-7660. *E-mail:* barosemena@nursing.fsu.edu.

GRADUATE PROGRAMS

Expenses (2006–07) *Tuition, state resident:* full-time $10,300; part-time $312 per credit hour. *Tuition, nonresident:* full-time $31,350; part-time $950 per credit hour.
Financial Aid 50% of graduate students in nursing programs received some form of financial aid in 2005–06. 1 fellowship with partial tuition reimbursement available (averaging $6,300 per year), 3 research assistantships with partial tuition reimbursements available (averaging $3,000 per year), 13 teaching assistantships with partial tuition reimbursements available (averaging $3,000 per year) were awarded; career-related internships or fieldwork, Federal Work-Study, institutionally sponsored loans, traineeships, and tuition waivers (partial) also available. *Financial aid application deadline:* 4/15.
Contact Mr. Eddie Page, Graduate Program Advisor, School of Nursing, Florida State University, 461C Vivian M. Duxbury Hall, Tallahassee, FL 32306-4310. *Telephone:* 850-644-5638. *Fax:* 850-645-7321. *E-mail:* epage@nursing.fsu.edu.

MASTER'S DEGREE PROGRAM

Degree MSN

Available Programs Master's; RN to Master's.
Concentrations Available Nurse case management; nursing education. *Nurse practitioner programs in:* family health, pediatric.
Site Options *Distance Learning:* Pensacola, FL; Marianna, FL.
Study Options Full-time and part-time.

Program Entrance Requirements Computer literacy, minimum overall college GPA of 3.0, transcript of college record, CPR certification, written essay, immunizations, 2 letters of recommendation, professional liability insurance/malpractice insurance, prerequisite course work, GRE General Test. *Application deadline:* For fall admission, 7/1 (priority date); for spring admission, 10/15 (priority date). Applications are processed on a rolling basis. *Application fee:* $30.
Advanced Placement Credit given for nursing courses completed elsewhere dependent upon specific evaluations.
Degree Requirements 51 total credit hours, thesis or project.

POST-MASTER'S PROGRAM

Areas of Study Nursing education. *Nurse practitioner programs in:* family health, pediatric.

CONTINUING EDUCATION PROGRAM

Contact Dr. Katherine P. Mason, Dean and Professor, School of Nursing, Florida State University, 102 Vivian M. Duxbury Hall, Tallahassee, FL 32306-4310. *Telephone:* 850-644-3299. *Fax:* 850-644-7660. *E-mail:* kmason@nursing.fsu.edu.

Jacksonville University
School of Nursing
Jacksonville, Florida

http://www.jacksonville.edu
Founded in 1934
DEGREES • BSN • MSN • MSN/MBA

Nursing Program Faculty 28 (32% with doctorates).
Graduate Enrollment 60
Nursing Student Activities Nursing Honor Society, Sigma Theta Tau, Student Nurses' Association, nursing club.
Nursing Student Resources Academic advising; academic or career counseling; assistance for students with disabilities; bookstore; campus computer network; career placement assistance; computer lab; computer-assisted instruction; e-mail services; employment services for current students; externships; interactive nursing skills videos; Internet; learning resource lab; library services; nursing audiovisuals; placement services for program completers; remedial services; resume preparation assistance; skills, simulation, or other laboratory; tutoring; unpaid internships.
Library Facilities 385,016 volumes; 686 periodical subscriptions.

BACCALAUREATE PROGRAMS

Degree BSN

Available Programs ADN to Baccalaureate; Accelerated Baccalaureate; Accelerated Baccalaureate for Second Degree; Accelerated RN Baccalaureate; Baccalaureate for Second Degree; Generic Baccalaureate; RN Baccalaureate.
Site Options *Distance Learning:* Not limited.
Study Options Full-time and part-time.
Program Entrance Requirements Minimum overall college GPA of 2.5, transcript of college record, CPR certification, written essay, health exam, 3 years high school math, 2 years high school science, high school transcript, immunizations, interview, 3 letters of recommendation, minimum high school GPA of 2.5, minimum GPA in nursing prerequisites of 2.5, prerequisite course work. Transfer students are accepted. **Standardized tests** *Required:* SAT or ACT, TOEFL for international students. **Application** *Deadline:* rolling (freshmen), rolling (transfer). *Application fee:* $30.
Advanced Placement Credit given for nursing courses completed elsewhere dependent upon specific evaluations.
Financial Aid 92% of baccalaureate students in nursing programs received some form of financial aid in 2004–05. *Gift aid (need-based):* Federal Pell, FSEOG, state, private, college/university gift aid from institutional funds. *Loans:* FFEL (Subsidized and Unsubsidized Stafford PLUS), Perkins, college/university, Navy ROTC. *Work-Study:* Federal Work-Study. *Application deadline:* 3/15 (priority: 2/1).

Contact Becky Cromwell, Coordinator of Nursing, School of Nursing, Jacksonville University, 2800 University Boulevard North, Jacksonville, FL 32211. *Telephone:* 904-256-7286. *Fax:* 904-256-7287. *E-mail:* bcromwe@ju.edu.

GRADUATE PROGRAMS

Contact Ms. Laura Winn, Coordinator, RN-BSN Program and MSN Program, School of Nursing, Jacksonville University, 2800 University Boulevard North, Jacksonville, FL 32211. *Telephone:* 904-256-7034. *Fax:* 904-256-7287. *E-mail:* lwinn@ju.edu.

MASTER'S DEGREE PROGRAM

Degrees MSN; MSN/MBA

Available Programs Accelerated RN to Master's; Master's; RN to Master's.

Concentrations Available Nursing administration; nursing education.

Site Options JAcksonville, FL.

Study Options Full-time and part-time.

Program Entrance Requirements Clinical experience, minimum overall college GPA of 3.0, transcript of college record, CPR certification, written essay, immunizations, interview, 2 letters of recommendation, prerequisite course work, resume.

Advanced Placement Credit given for nursing courses completed elsewhere dependent upon specific evaluations.

Degree Requirements 36 total credit hours, thesis or project.

Nova Southeastern University
College of Allied Health and Nursing
Fort Lauderdale, Florida

Founded in 1964

DEGREES • BSN • MSN • MSN/MBA

Library Facilities 725,000 volumes; 22,295 periodical subscriptions.

BACCALAUREATE PROGRAMS

Degree BSN

Available Programs Generic Baccalaureate; RN Baccalaureate.

Study Options Full-time.

Program Entrance Requirements Minimum overall college GPA of 2.75, transcript of college record, written essay, health exam, immunizations, 2 letters of recommendation, prerequisite course work. **Standardized tests** *Required:* SAT or ACT, TOEFL for international students. **Application** *Deadline:* rolling (freshmen), rolling (out-of-state freshmen), rolling (transfer). *Notification:* continuous (freshmen), continuous (out-of-state freshmen). *Application fee:* $50.

Financial Aid *Gift aid (need-based):* Federal Pell, FSEOG, state, private, college/university gift aid from institutional funds. *Loans:* FFEL (Subsidized and Unsubsidized Stafford PLUS), Perkins, college/university. *Work-Study:* Federal Work-Study, part-time campus jobs. *Application deadline (priority):* 4/15.

Contact Dr. Gale Woolley, Nursing Department, College of Allied Health and Nursing, Nova Southeastern University, Health Professions Division/Nursing, 3200 South University Drive, Fort Lauderdale, FL 33328. *Telephone:* 800-356-0026 Ext. 1983. *Fax:* 954-262-1036. *E-mail:* nursinginfo@nsu.nova.edu.

GRADUATE PROGRAMS

Expenses (2005–06) *Tuition:* part-time $445 per credit hour. *Required fees:* full-time $850.

Financial Aid 100% of graduate students in nursing programs received some form of financial aid in 2004–05. Teaching assistantships, institutionally sponsored loans and unspecified assistantships available.

Contact Dr. Jean Davis, Program Director, College of Allied Health and Nursing, Nova Southeastern University, Health Professions Division/Nursing, 3200 South University Drive, Fort Lauderdale, FL 33328-2018. *Telephone:* 954-262-1956. *Fax:* 954-262-1036. *E-mail:* djean@nsu.nova.edu.

MASTER'S DEGREE PROGRAM

Degrees MSN; MSN/MBA

Available Programs Master's.

Concentrations Available Nursing administration; nursing education.

Study Options Full-time and part-time.

Program Entrance Requirements Minimum overall college GPA of 3.0, transcript of college record, 3 letters of recommendation, GRE General Test. *Application deadline:* Applications are processed on a rolling basis. *Application fee:* $50.

Degree Requirements 42 total credit hours, thesis or project.

DOCTORAL DEGREE PROGRAM

Program Entrance Requirements GRE General Test. *Application deadline:* Applications are processed on a rolling basis. *Application fee:* $50.

St. Petersburg College
Department of Nursing
St. Petersburg, Florida

http://www.spcollege.edu

Founded in 1927

DEGREE • BSN

Nursing Program Faculty 70 (10% with doctorates).

Baccalaureate Enrollment 234
Women 91% **Men** 9% **Minority** 20%

Nursing Student Activities Nursing Honor Society, Student Nurses' Association, nursing club.

Nursing Student Resources Academic advising; academic or career counseling; assistance for students with disabilities; bookstore; campus computer network; career placement assistance; computer lab; computer-assisted instruction; e-mail services; employment services for current students; interactive nursing skills videos; Internet; learning resource lab; library services; nursing audiovisuals; paid internships; placement services for program completers; remedial services; skills, simulation, or other laboratory; unpaid internships.

Library Facilities 222,990 volumes (1,000 in health, 1,000 in nursing); 1,393 periodical subscriptions (50 health-care related).

BACCALAUREATE PROGRAMS

Degree BSN

Available Programs ADN to Baccalaureate; RN Baccalaureate.

Site Options *Distance Learning:* Bayonet Point, FL; Pinellas Park, FL.

Program Entrance Requirements Minimum overall college GPA of 2.0, RN licensure. Transfer students are accepted. **Standardized tests** *Required:* TOEFL for international students. **Application** *Deadline:* rolling (freshmen). *Notification:* continuous (freshmen). *Application fee:* $35.

Advanced Placement Credit given for nursing courses completed elsewhere dependent upon specific evaluations.

Expenses (2006–07) *Tuition, state resident:* full-time $1631; part-time $78 per credit hour. *Tuition, nonresident:* full-time $6113; part-time $291 per credit hour. *Required fees:* full-time $95; part-time $95 per credit.

Financial Aid 80% of baccalaureate students in nursing programs received some form of financial aid in 2005–06. *Gift aid (need-based):* Federal Pell, FSEOG, state, private, college/university gift aid from institutional funds. *Loans:* FFEL (Subsidized and Unsubsidized Stafford PLUS), college/university. *Work-Study:* Federal Work-Study. *Application deadline (priority):* 4/15.

Contact Dr. Jean M. Wortock, Dean, Department of Nursing, St. Petersburg College, PO Box 13489, St. Petersburg, FL 33733. *Telephone:* 727-341-3640. *Fax:* 727-341-3546. *E-mail:* Wortock.Jean@spcollege.edu.

CONTINUING EDUCATION PROGRAM

Contact Denise Kerwin, Program Director, Department of Nursing, St. Petersburg College, PO Box 13489, St. Petersburg, FL 33733. *Telephone:* 727-341-4549. *Fax:* 727-341-3494. *E-mail:* kerwin.denise@spcollege.edu.

South University
Nursing Program
West Palm Beach, Florida

Founded in 1899

DEGREE • BSN

Library Facilities 8,400 volumes; 67 periodical subscriptions.

BACCALAUREATE PROGRAMS

Degree BSN

Available Programs Generic Baccalaureate.

Program Entrance Requirements Standardized tests *Required:* TOEFL for international students. *Recommended:* SAT or ACT. **Application** *Deadline:* rolling (freshmen), rolling (transfer). *Notification:* continuous (freshmen). *Application fee:* $25.

Contact West Palm Beach Campus, Nursing Program, South University, 1760 North Congress Avenue, West Palm Beach, FL 33409-5178. *Telephone:* 561-697-9200. *Fax:* 561-697-9944. *E-mail:* wpbfdesk@southuniversity.edu.

University of Central Florida
School of Nursing
Orlando, Florida

http://www.cohpa.ucf.edu/nursing

Founded in 1963

DEGREES • BSN • MSN • PHD

Nursing Program Faculty 56 (43% with doctorates).

Baccalaureate Enrollment 379
Women 91% **Men** 9% **Minority** 25% **Part-time** 32%

Graduate Enrollment 136
Women 87% **Men** 13% **Minority** 10% **Part-time** 75%

Nursing Student Activities Sigma Theta Tau, Student Nurses' Association.

Nursing Student Resources Academic advising; academic or career counseling; assistance for students with disabilities; bookstore; campus computer network; computer lab; computer-assisted instruction; daycare for children of students; e-mail services; employment services for current students; externships; housing assistance; interactive nursing skills videos; Internet; learning resource lab; library services; nursing audiovisuals; skills, simulation, or other laboratory; tutoring.

Library Facilities 1.4 million volumes (38,944 in health, 2,848 in nursing); 16,368 periodical subscriptions (360 health-care related).

BACCALAUREATE PROGRAMS

Degree BSN

Available Programs Accelerated Baccalaureate for Second Degree; Generic Baccalaureate; RN Baccalaureate.

Site Options *Distance Learning:* Cocoa Beach, FL; Daytona Beach, FL; Leesburg, FL.

Study Options Full-time and part-time.

Program Entrance Requirements Minimum overall college GPA of 2.5, transcript of college record, CPR certification, health exam, health insurance, high school foreign language, high school math, high school transcript, immunizations, minimum high school GPA of 2.5, prerequisite course work. Transfer students are accepted. **Standardized tests** *Required:* SAT or ACT, TOEFL for international students. **Application** *Deadline:* 3/1 (freshmen), 5/1 (transfer). *Notification:* continuous (freshmen). *Application fee:* $30.

Advanced Placement Credit given for nursing courses completed elsewhere dependent upon specific evaluations.

Contact *Telephone:* 407-823-2744. *Fax:* 407-823-5675.

GRADUATE PROGRAMS

Contact *Telephone:* 407-823-2744. *Fax:* 407-823-5675.

MASTER'S DEGREE PROGRAM

Degree MSN

Available Programs Master's; RN to Master's.

Concentrations Available Nurse case management; nursing administration; nursing education. *Clinical nurse specialist programs in:* acute care, critical care. *Nurse practitioner programs in:* adult health, family health, pediatric.

Study Options Full-time and part-time.

Program Entrance Requirements Clinical experience, minimum overall college GPA of 3.0, transcript of college record, CPR certification, written essay, immunizations, 3 letters of recommendation, physical assessment course, resume, statistics course.

Advanced Placement Credit given for nursing courses completed elsewhere dependent upon specific evaluations.

Degree Requirements 47 total credit hours, thesis or project.

POST-MASTER'S PROGRAM

Areas of Study *Nurse practitioner programs in:* adult health, family health, pediatric.

DOCTORAL DEGREE PROGRAM

Degree PhD

Available Programs Doctorate.

Areas of Study Health policy, health-care systems, individualized study, information systems, nursing research.

Program Entrance Requirements Minimum overall college GPA of 3.5, interview by faculty committee, 3 letters of recommendation, MSN or equivalent, statistics course, vita.

Degree Requirements 57 total credit hours, dissertation.

University of Florida
College of Nursing
Gainesville, Florida

http://www.nursing.ufl.edu

Founded in 1853

DEGREES • BSN • MSN • MSN/PHD

Nursing Program Faculty 63 (54% with doctorates).

Baccalaureate Enrollment 323
Women 95% **Men** 5% **Minority** 24%

Graduate Enrollment 270
Women 87% **Men** 13% **Minority** 19% **Part-time** 63%

Nursing Student Activities Sigma Theta Tau, Student Nurses' Association.

Nursing Student Resources Academic advising; academic or career counseling; assistance for students with disabilities; bookstore; campus computer network; career placement assistance; computer lab; computer-assisted instruction; daycare for children of students; e-mail services; employment services for current students; housing assistance; interactive nursing skills videos; Internet; learning resource lab; library services; nursing audiovisuals; placement services for program completers; remedial services; resume preparation assistance; skills, simulation, or other laboratory; tutoring.

Library Facilities 5.3 million volumes (260,000 in health, 3,000 in nursing); 25,342 periodical subscriptions (200 health-care related).

BACCALAUREATE PROGRAMS

Degree BSN

Available Programs Accelerated Baccalaureate for Second Degree; Generic Baccalaureate; RN Baccalaureate.

Site Options Jacksonville, FL.

Study Options Full-time.

Program Entrance Requirements Minimum GPA in nursing prerequisites of 2.8, prerequisite course work. Transfer students are accepted. **Standardized tests** *Required:* SAT or ACT, TOEFL for international students. **Application** *Deadline:* 1/17 (freshmen). *Early decision:* 10/1. *Notification:* continuous (freshmen), 12/1 (out-of-state freshmen), 12/1 (early decision). *Application fee:* $30.

Advanced Placement   Credit by examination available.

Expenses (2006–07) *Tuition, state resident:* part-time $107 per credit hour. *Tuition, nonresident:* part-time $571 per credit hour.

Financial Aid   90% of baccalaureate students in nursing programs received some form of financial aid in 2005–06.

Contact   Mr. Kenneth H. Foote, Program Assistant, College of Nursing, University of Florida, PO Box 100197, Health Professions, Nursing and Pharmacy Complex, Gainesville, FL 32610-0197. *Telephone:* 352-273-6383. *Fax:* 352-273-6440. *E-mail:* kfoote@ufl.edu.

GRADUATE PROGRAMS

Expenses (2006–07) *Tuition, state resident:* part-time $284 per credit hour. *Tuition, nonresident:* part-time $915 per credit hour.

Financial Aid   Fellowships, research assistantships, teaching assistantships, career-related internships or fieldwork and Federal Work-Study available.

Contact   Ms. Cecile Kiley, Coordinator, Academic Support Services, College of Nursing, University of Florida, PO Box 100197, HPNP Building, Gainesville, FL 32610-0197. *Telephone:* 352-273-6331. *Fax:* 352-273-6440. *E-mail:* ckiley@ufl.edu.

MASTER'S DEGREE PROGRAM

Degrees   MSN; MSN/PhD

Available Programs   Master's.

Concentrations Available   Nurse-midwifery. *Clinical nurse specialist programs in:* medical-surgical, psychiatric/mental health, public health. *Nurse practitioner programs in:* acute care, adult health, family health, neonatal health, pediatric, psychiatric/mental health.

Site Options   Jacksonville, FL.

Study Options   Full-time and part-time.

Program Entrance Requirements   Minimum overall college GPA of 3.0, transcript of college record, written essay, 2 letters of recommendation, resume, GRE General Test. *Application deadline:* For fall admission, 3/1 (priority date). Applications are processed on a rolling basis. *Application fee:* $30.

Advanced Placement   Credit given for nursing courses completed elsewhere dependent upon specific evaluations.

Degree Requirements   46 total credit hours, comprehensive exam.

POST-MASTER'S PROGRAM

Areas of Study   Nurse-midwifery. *Clinical nurse specialist programs in:* medical-surgical, psychiatric/mental health, public health. *Nurse practitioner programs in:* acute care, adult health, family health, neonatal health, oncology, pediatric, psychiatric/mental health.

DOCTORAL DEGREE PROGRAM

Degree   PhD

Available Programs   Doctorate.

Areas of Study   Aging, bio-behavioral research, health policy, nursing policy, nursing science, oncology, women's health.

Site Options   Jacksonville, FL.

Program Entrance Requirements   Minimum overall college GPA of 3.5, 3 letters of recommendation, MSN or equivalent, vita, writing sample, GRE General Test. *Application deadline:* For fall admission, 3/1 (priority date). Applications are processed on a rolling basis. *Application fee:* $30.

Degree Requirements   92 total credit hours, dissertation.

University of Miami

School of Nursing and Health Studies
Coral Gables, Florida

http://www.miami.edu/nur

Founded in 1925

DEGREES • BSN • MSN • PHD

Nursing Program Faculty 60 (32% with doctorates).

Baccalaureate Enrollment 592

Women 85% **Men** 15% **Minority** 65% **International** 1% **Part-time** 25%

Graduate Enrollment 51

Women 97% **Men** 3% **Minority** 55% **International** 1% **Part-time** 50%

Nursing Student Activities Sigma Theta Tau, Student Nurses' Association.

Nursing Student Resources Academic advising; academic or career counseling; assistance for students with disabilities; bookstore; campus computer network; career placement assistance; computer lab; computer-assisted instruction; daycare for children of students; e-mail services; employment services for current students; externships; housing assistance; interactive nursing skills videos; Internet; learning resource lab; library services; nursing audiovisuals; placement services for program completers; remedial services; resume preparation assistance; skills, simulation, or other laboratory; tutoring; unpaid internships.

Library Facilities 3 million volumes (2,000 in nursing); 45,953 periodical subscriptions (89 health-care related).

BACCALAUREATE PROGRAMS

Degree BSN

Available Programs   Accelerated Baccalaureate; Accelerated Baccalaureate for Second Degree; Baccalaureate for Second Degree; Generic Baccalaureate; RN Baccalaureate.

Study Options   Full-time and part-time.

Program Entrance Requirements   Transcript of college record, written essay, 1 letter of recommendation, minimum high school GPA of 2.8, prerequisite course work. Transfer students are accepted. **Standardized tests** *Required:* SAT or ACT, TOEFL for international students. *Required for some:* SAT and SAT Subject Tests or ACT, SAT Subject Tests. **Application** *Deadline:* 2/1 (freshmen), 3/1 (transfer). *Early decision:* 11/1, 11/1. *Notification:* 4/15 (freshmen), 12/15 (out-of-state freshmen), 12/15 (early decision), 2/1 (early action). *Application fee:* $65.

Advanced Placement   Credit given for nursing courses completed elsewhere dependent upon specific evaluations.

Expenses (2005–06) *Tuition:* full-time $30,732; part-time $1280 per credit. *Room and board:* $10,714; room only: $7032 per academic year. *Required fees:* full-time $173; part-time $13 per credit.

Financial Aid   85% of baccalaureate students in nursing programs received some form of financial aid in 2004–05. *Gift aid (need-based):* Federal Pell, FSEOG, state, private, college/university gift aid from institutional funds, Federal Nursing. *Loans:* Federal Nursing Student Loans, FFEL (Subsidized and Unsubsidized Stafford PLUS), Perkins, Private Alternative Education Loans. *Work-Study:* Federal Work-Study, part-time campus jobs. *Application deadline (priority):* 2/1.

Contact   Dr. Denise M. Korniewicz, RN, Interim Associate Dean for Student Services, School of Nursing and Health Studies, University of Miami, 5801 Red Road, Coral Gables, FL 33143. *Telephone:* 305-284-4325. *Fax:* 305-284-4827. *E-mail:* dkorniewicz@miami.edu.

GRADUATE PROGRAMS

Expenses (2005–06) *Tuition:* full-time $23,040; part-time $1208 per credit.

Financial Aid   95% of graduate students in nursing programs received some form of financial aid in 2004–05. 3 research assistantships with tuition reimbursements available (averaging $9,000 per year), 5 teaching assistantships with tuition reimbursements available (averaging $9,000 per year) were awarded; fellowships, Federal Work-Study, institutionally sponsored loans, scholarships, and unspecified assistantships also available. Aid available to part-time students. *Financial aid application deadline:* 3/1.

Contact   Dr. Denise M. Korniewicz, RN, Interim Associate Dean for Student Services, School of Nursing and Health Studies, University of Miami, 5801 Red Road, Coral Gables, FL 33143-2343. *Telephone:* 305-284-4325. *Fax:* 305-284-4827. *E-mail:* dkorniewicz@miami.edu.

MASTER'S DEGREE PROGRAM

Degree MSN

Available Programs   Accelerated Master's; Master's.

Concentrations Available   Nurse anesthesia; nurse-midwifery. *Clinical nurse specialist programs in:* acute care, adult health, community health, family health, psychiatric/mental health, women's health. *Nurse practitioner programs in:* acute care, adult health, community health, family health, primary care, psychiatric/mental health, women's health.

Study Options   Full-time and part-time.

University of Miami (continued)

Program Entrance Requirements Clinical experience, minimum overall college GPA of 3.0, transcript of college record, written essay, interview, 3 letters of recommendation, resume, statistics course, GRE General Test. *Application deadline:* For fall admission, 3/1 (priority date); for spring admission, 10/1 (priority date). Applications are processed on a rolling basis. *Application fee:* $50.

Degree Requirements 39 total credit hours.

POST-MASTER'S PROGRAM

Areas of Study Nursing administration; nursing education. *Clinical nurse specialist programs in:* adult health, family health, psychiatric/mental health, women's health. *Nurse practitioner programs in:* adult health, family health, psychiatric/mental health, women's health.

DOCTORAL DEGREE PROGRAM

Degree PhD

Available Programs Doctorate.

Areas of Study Faculty preparation, nursing education, nursing research, nursing science.

Program Entrance Requirements Minimum overall college GPA of 3.0, interview by faculty committee, interview, 3 letters of recommendation, MSN or equivalent, vita, writing sample, GRE General Test. *Application deadline:* For fall admission, 3/1 (priority date); for spring admission, 10/1 (priority date). Applications are processed on a rolling basis. *Application fee:* $50.

Degree Requirements 60 total credit hours, dissertation, written exam.

CONTINUING EDUCATION PROGRAM

Contact Dr. Denise M. Korniewicz, RN, Interim Associate Dean for Student Services, School of Nursing and Health Studies, University of Miami, 5801 Red Road, Coral Gables, FL 33124. *Telephone:* 305-284-4325. *Fax:* 305-284-4827. *E-mail:* dkorniewicz@miami.edu.

University of North Florida
School of Nursing
Jacksonville, Florida

http://www.unf.edu/coh/cohnursi.htm

Founded in 1965

DEGREES • BSN • MSN

Nursing Program Faculty 19 (50% with doctorates).

Baccalaureate Enrollment 279
Women 85% **Men** 15% **Minority** 20% **International** 1% **Part-time** 27%

Graduate Enrollment 35
Women 86% **Men** 14% **Minority** 6% **Part-time** 70%

Nursing Student Activities Sigma Theta Tau, Student Nurses' Association.

Nursing Student Resources Academic advising; academic or career counseling; assistance for students with disabilities; bookstore; campus computer network; career placement assistance; computer lab; computer-assisted instruction; e-mail services; interactive nursing skills videos; Internet; learning resource lab; library services; nursing audiovisuals; resume preparation assistance; skills, simulation, or other laboratory.

Library Facilities 798,321 volumes (30,466 in health, 3,000 in nursing); 3,101 periodical subscriptions (200 health-care related).

BACCALAUREATE PROGRAMS

Degree BSN

Available Programs Accelerated Baccalaureate for Second Degree; Generic Baccalaureate; RN Baccalaureate.

Study Options Full-time.

Program Entrance Requirements Minimum overall college GPA of 2.7, CPR certification, written essay, health exam, immunizations, interview, minimum high school GPA, minimum GPA in nursing prerequisites of 3.0, professional liability insurance/malpractice insurance, prerequisite course

work. Transfer students are accepted. **Standardized tests** *Required:* SAT or ACT. **Application** *Deadline:* 7/2 (freshmen), 7/2 (transfer). *Early decision:* 11/15. *Notification:* continuous (freshmen), 12/2 (early action). *Application fee:* $30.

Advanced Placement Credit given for nursing courses completed elsewhere dependent upon specific evaluations.

Contact *Telephone:* 904-620-2418.

GRADUATE PROGRAMS

Contact *Telephone:* 904-620-2684. *Fax:* 904-620-2848.

MASTER'S DEGREE PROGRAM

Degree MSN

Available Programs Master's; RN to Master's.

Concentrations Available *Clinical nurse specialist programs in:* adult health, cardiovascular, community health, critical care, gerontology, maternity-newborn, medical-surgical, pediatric, psychiatric/mental health, women's health. *Nurse practitioner programs in:* family health, primary care.

Study Options Full-time and part-time.

Program Entrance Requirements Clinical experience, computer literacy, minimum overall college GPA of 3.0, transcript of college record, CPR certification, written essay, immunizations, 2 letters of recommendation, nursing research course, physical assessment course, professional liability insurance/malpractice insurance, resume, statistics course.

Advanced Placement Credit given for nursing courses completed elsewhere dependent upon specific evaluations.

Degree Requirements 43 total credit hours, thesis or project.

POST-MASTER'S PROGRAM

Areas of Study *Nurse practitioner programs in:* family health, primary care.

University of Phoenix–Central Florida Campus
College of Health and Human Services
Maitland, Florida

Founded in 1996

DEGREES • BSN • MSN • MSN/MBA • MSN/MHA

Nursing Program Faculty 67 (55% with doctorates).

Baccalaureate Enrollment 77
Women 96.1% **Men** 3.9% **Minority** 11.69%

Graduate Enrollment 49
Women 93.88% **Men** 6.12% **Minority** 20.41%

Nursing Student Activities Sigma Theta Tau.

Nursing Student Resources Academic advising; academic or career counseling; assistance for students with disabilities; bookstore; computer lab; library services.

Library Facilities 444 volumes; 666 periodical subscriptions.

BACCALAUREATE PROGRAMS

Degree BSN

Available Programs Accelerated Baccalaureate.

Site Options Orlando, FL.

Study Options Full-time.

Program Entrance Requirements Transcript of college record, 1 letter of recommendation, RN licensure. Transfer students are accepted. **Standardized tests** *Required:* TOEFL for international students. **Application** *Deadline:* rolling (freshmen), rolling (transfer). *Application fee:* $110.

Advanced Placement Credit by examination available. Credit given for nursing courses completed elsewhere dependent upon specific evaluations.

Expenses (2006–07) *Tuition:* full-time $10,260. *International tuition:* $10,260 full-time. *Required fees:* full-time $750.

Contact Campus College Chair, Nursing, College of Health and Human Services, University of Phoenix–Central Florida Campus, 2290 Lucien Way, Suite 400, Maitland, FL 32751-7057. *Telephone:* 407-667-0555.

GRADUATE PROGRAMS

Expenses (2006–07) *Tuition:* full-time $9576. *International tuition:* $9576 full-time. *Required fees:* full-time $760.

Contact Campus College Chair, Nursing, College of Health and Human Services, University of Phoenix–Central Florida Campus, 2290 Lucien Way, Suite 400, Maitland, FL 32751-7057. *Telephone:* 407-667-0555.

MASTER'S DEGREE PROGRAM

Degrees MSN; MSN/MBA; MSN/MHA

Available Programs Master's.

Concentrations Available Health-care administration; nursing administration; nursing education.

Site Options Orlando, FL.

Study Options Full-time.

Program Entrance Requirements Clinical experience, computer literacy, minimum overall college GPA of 2.5, transcript of college record. *Application deadline:* Applications are processed on a rolling basis. *Application fee:* $110.

Advanced Placement Credit given for nursing courses completed elsewhere dependent upon specific evaluations.

Degree Requirements 39 total credit hours, thesis or project.

University of Phoenix–North Florida Campus
College of Health and Human Services
Jacksonville, Florida

Founded in 1976

DEGREES • BSN • MSN

Nursing Program Faculty 75 (44% with doctorates).

Baccalaureate Enrollment 69
Women 86.96% **Men** 13.04% **Minority** 28.99%

Graduate Enrollment 69
Women 75.36% **Men** 24.64% **Minority** 44.93%

Nursing Student Activities Sigma Theta Tau.

Nursing Student Resources Academic advising; academic or career counseling; assistance for students with disabilities; bookstore; computer lab; library services.

Library Facilities 444 volumes; 666 periodical subscriptions.

BACCALAUREATE PROGRAMS

Degree BSN

Available Programs Accelerated Baccalaureate.

Site Options Orange Park, FL.

Study Options Full-time.

Program Entrance Requirements Transcript of college record, 1 letter of recommendation, RN licensure. Transfer students are accepted. **Standardized tests** *Required:* TOEFL for international students. **Application** *Deadline:* rolling (freshmen), rolling (transfer). *Application fee:* $110.

Advanced Placement Credit by examination available. Credit given for nursing courses completed elsewhere dependent upon specific evaluations.

Expenses (2006–07) *Tuition:* full-time $10,260. *International tuition:* $10,260 full-time. *Required fees:* full-time $750.

Contact Campus College Chair, Nursing, College of Health and Human Services, University of Phoenix–North Florida Campus, 4500 Salisbury Road, Suite 200, Jacksonville, FL 32216-0959. *Telephone:* 904-636-6645.

GRADUATE PROGRAMS

Expenses (2006–07) *Tuition:* full-time $9576. *International tuition:* $9576 full-time. *Required fees:* full-time $760.

Contact Campus College Chair, Nursing, College of Health and Human Services, University of Phoenix–North Florida Campus, 4500 Salisbury Road, Suite 200, Jacksonville, FL 32216-0959. *Telephone:* 904-636-6645.

MASTER'S DEGREE PROGRAM

Degree MSN

Available Programs Master's.

Concentrations Available Health-care administration; nursing administration; nursing education.

Site Options Orange Park, FL.

Study Options Full-time.

Program Entrance Requirements Clinical experience, computer literacy, minimum overall college GPA of 2.5, transcript of college record. *Application deadline:* Applications are processed on a rolling basis. *Application fee:* $110.

Advanced Placement Credit given for nursing courses completed elsewhere dependent upon specific evaluations.

Degree Requirements 39 total credit hours, thesis or project.

University of Phoenix–South Florida Campus
College of Health and Human Services
Fort Lauderdale, Florida

DEGREES • BSN • MSN • MSN/MBA • MSN/MHA

Nursing Program Faculty 76 (37% with doctorates).

Baccalaureate Enrollment 211
Women 90.52% **Men** 9.48% **Minority** 34.12%

Graduate Enrollment 197
Women 87.82% **Men** 12.18% **Minority** 31.47%

Nursing Student Activities Sigma Theta Tau.

Nursing Student Resources Academic advising; academic or career counseling; assistance for students with disabilities; bookstore; computer lab; library services.

BACCALAUREATE PROGRAMS

Degree BSN

Available Programs RN Baccalaureate.

Site Options Palm Beach Gardens, FL; Ft. Lauderdale, FL; Miramar, FL.

Study Options Full-time.

Program Entrance Requirements Transcript of college record, 1 letter of recommendation, RN licensure. Transfer students are accepted. **Standardized tests** *Required:* TOEFL for international students. **Application** *Deadline:* rolling (freshmen), rolling (transfer). *Application fee:* $110.

Advanced Placement Credit by examination available. Credit given for nursing courses completed elsewhere dependent upon specific evaluations.

Expenses (2006–07) *Tuition:* full-time $10,260. *International tuition:* $10,260 full-time. *Required fees:* full-time $750.

Contact Campus College Chair, Nursing, College of Health and Human Services, University of Phoenix–South Florida Campus, 600 North Pine Island Road, Suite #500, Plantation, FL 33324-1393. *Telephone:* 954-382-5303.

GRADUATE PROGRAMS

Expenses (2006–07) *Tuition:* full-time $9576. *International tuition:* $9576 full-time. *Required fees:* full-time $760.

Contact Campus College Chair, Nursing, College of Health and Human Services, University of Phoenix–South Florida Campus, 600 North Pine Island Road, Suite #500, Plantation, FL 33324-1393. *Telephone:* 954-382-5303.

MASTER'S DEGREE PROGRAM

Degrees MSN; MSN/MBA; MSN/MHA

Available Programs Master's.

University of Phoenix–South Florida Campus (continued)

Concentrations Available Health-care administration; nursing administration; nursing education.

Site Options Palm Beach Gardens, FL; Ft. Lauderdale, FL; Miramar, FL.

Study Options Full-time.

Program Entrance Requirements Clinical experience, computer literacy, minimum overall college GPA of 2.5, transcript of college record. *Application deadline:* Applications are processed on a rolling basis. *Application fee:* $110.

Advanced Placement Credit given for nursing courses completed elsewhere dependent upon specific evaluations.

Degree Requirements 39 total credit hours, thesis or project.

University of Phoenix–West Florida Campus
College of Health and Human Services
Temple Terrace, Florida

DEGREES • BSN • MSN • MSN/MBA • MSN/MHA

Nursing Program Faculty 62 (22% with doctorates).

Baccalaureate Enrollment 47
Women 91.49% **Men** 8.51% **Minority** 12.77%

Graduate Enrollment 87
Women 90.8% **Men** 9.2% **Minority** 14.94%

Nursing Student Activities Sigma Theta Tau.

Nursing Student Resources Academic advising; academic or career counseling; assistance for students with disabilities; bookstore; computer lab; library services.

Library Facilities 444 volumes; 666 periodical subscriptions.

BACCALAUREATE PROGRAMS

Degree BSN

Available Programs Accelerated Baccalaureate.

Site Options Clearwater, FL; Sarasota, FL; Tampa, FL.

Study Options Full-time.

Program Entrance Requirements Transcript of college record, 1 letter of recommendation, RN licensure. Transfer students are accepted. **Standardized tests** *Required:* TOEFL for international students. **Application** *Deadline:* rolling (freshmen), rolling (transfer). *Application fee:* $110.

Advanced Placement Credit by examination available. Credit given for nursing courses completed elsewhere dependent upon specific evaluations.

Expenses (2006–07) *Tuition:* full-time $10,260. *International tuition:* $10,260 full-time. *Required fees:* full-time $750.

Contact Campus College Chair, Nursing, College of Health and Human Services, University of Phoenix–West Florida Campus, 100 Tampa Oaks Boulevard, Suite #200, Temple Terrace, FL 33637-1920. *Telephone:* 813-626-7911.

GRADUATE PROGRAMS

Expenses (2006–07) *Tuition:* full-time $9576. *International tuition:* $9576 full-time. *Required fees:* full-time $760.

Contact Campus College Chair, Nursing, College of Health and Human Services, University of Phoenix–West Florida Campus, 100 Tampa Oaks Boulevard, Suite #200, Temple Terrace, FL 33637-1920. *Telephone:* 813-626-7911.

MASTER'S DEGREE PROGRAM

Degrees MSN; MSN/MBA; MSN/MHA

Available Programs Master's.

Concentrations Available Health-care administration; nursing administration; nursing education.

Site Options Clearwater, FL; Sarasota, FL; Tampa, FL.

Study Options Full-time.

Program Entrance Requirements Clinical experience, computer literacy, minimum overall college GPA of 2.5, transcript of college record. *Application deadline:* Applications are processed on a rolling basis. *Application fee:* $110.

Advanced Placement Credit given for nursing courses completed elsewhere dependent upon specific evaluations.

Degree Requirements 39 total credit hours, thesis or project.

University of South Florida
College of Nursing
Tampa, Florida

http://hsc.usf.edu/nursing

Founded in 1956

DEGREES • BS • MS • MSN/MPH • PHD

Nursing Program Faculty 51 (49% with doctorates).

Baccalaureate Enrollment 554
Women 86% **Men** 14% **Minority** 49% **International** 2% **Part-time** 46%

Graduate Enrollment 323
Women 91% **Men** 9% **Minority** 19% **International** .6% **Part-time** 62%

Nursing Student Activities Nursing Honor Society, Sigma Theta Tau, Student Nurses' Association.

Nursing Student Resources Academic advising; academic or career counseling; assistance for students with disabilities; bookstore; campus computer network; career placement assistance; computer lab; computer-assisted instruction; daycare for children of students; e-mail services; employment services for current students; housing assistance; Internet; learning resource lab; library services; nursing audiovisuals; remedial services; resume preparation assistance; skills, simulation, or other laboratory; tutoring.

Library Facilities 2.1 million volumes (106,028 in health, 3,898 in nursing); 20,440 periodical subscriptions (1,581 health-care related).

BACCALAUREATE PROGRAMS

Degree BS

Available Programs ADN to Baccalaureate; Accelerated Baccalaureate; Accelerated Baccalaureate for Second Degree; Baccalaureate for Second Degree; Generic Baccalaureate; RN Baccalaureate.

Site Options Winterhaven, FL; Sarasota/Bradenton, FL.

Study Options Full-time.

Program Entrance Requirements Minimum overall college GPA of 3.0, transcript of college record, CPR certification, health insurance, high school foreign language, immunizations, prerequisite course work. Transfer students are accepted. **Standardized tests** *Required:* SAT or ACT, TOEFL for international students. **Application** *Deadline:* 4/15 (freshmen), 4/15 (transfer). *Notification:* continuous (freshmen). *Application fee:* $30.

Advanced Placement Credit given for nursing courses completed elsewhere dependent upon specific evaluations.

Expenses (2006–07) *Tuition, state resident:* part-time $111 per credit hour. *Tuition, nonresident:* part-time $535 per credit hour. *Room and board:* $6900 per academic year.

Financial Aid 40% of baccalaureate students in nursing programs received some form of financial aid in 2005–06.

Contact Ms. Victoria Wise-Neely, Director of Student Affairs, College of Nursing, University of South Florida, 12901 Bruce B. Downs Boulevard, MDC Box 22, Tampa, FL 33612-4766. *Telephone:* 813-974-2191. *Fax:* 813-974-3118. *E-mail:* vwisenee@health.usf.edu.

GRADUATE PROGRAMS

Expenses (2006–07) *Tuition, state resident:* part-time $252 per credit hour. *Tuition, nonresident:* part-time $897 per credit hour. *Room and board:* $7840 per academic year.

Financial Aid 40% of graduate students in nursing programs received some form of financial aid in 2005–06. 3 fellowships with partial tuition reimbursements available (averaging $7,500 per year), 6 research assistantships with partial tuition reimbursements available (averaging $20,500 per year), 9 teaching assistantships with partial tuition reimbursements available (averaging $16,000 per year) were awarded; Federal Work-Study, institutionally sponsored loans, scholarships, traineeships, tuition waivers (partial), and unspecified assistantships also available. *Financial aid application deadline:* 2/1.

Contact Ms. Victoria Wise-Neely, Director of Student Affairs, College of Nursing, University of South Florida, 12901 Bruce B. Downs Boulevard, MDC Box 22, Tampa, FL 33612-4766. *Telephone:* 813-974-2191. *Fax:* 813-974-3118. *E-mail:* vwisenee@health.usf.edu.

MASTER'S DEGREE PROGRAM

Degrees MS; MSN/MPH

Available Programs Master's; Master's for Nurses with Non-Nursing Degrees; RN to Master's.

Concentrations Available Nurse anesthesia; nursing education. *Clinical nurse specialist programs in:* gerontology, oncology, psychiatric/mental health. *Nurse practitioner programs in:* acute care, adult health, family health, gerontology, occupational health, oncology, pediatric, psychiatric/mental health.

Site Options Sarasota/Bradenton, FL.

Study Options Full-time and part-time.

Program Entrance Requirements Computer literacy, minimum overall college GPA of 3.0, transcript of college record, CPR certification, written essay, immunizations, interview, 3 letters of recommendation, nursing research course, physical assessment course, prerequisite course work, resume, statistics course, GRE General Test. *Application deadline:* For fall admission, 6/1 (priority date); for spring admission, 10/15 (priority date). Applications are processed on a rolling basis. *Application fee:* $30.

Advanced Placement Credit given for nursing courses completed elsewhere dependent upon specific evaluations.

Degree Requirements 44 total credit hours, thesis or project, comprehensive exam.

POST-MASTER'S PROGRAM

Areas of Study Nursing education; nursing informatics. *Nurse practitioner programs in:* adult health, family health, gerontology, oncology, pediatric, psychiatric/mental health.

DOCTORAL DEGREE PROGRAM

Degree PhD

Available Programs Doctorate; Post-Baccalaureate Doctorate.

Areas of Study Addiction/substance abuse, advanced practice nursing, aging, faculty preparation, family health, gerontology, health policy, health promotion/disease prevention, health-care systems, human health and illness, information systems, nurse case management, nursing administration, nursing education, nursing policy, nursing research, oncology.

Program Entrance Requirements Minimum overall college GPA of 3.5, interview by faculty committee, interview, 3 letters of recommendation, MSN or equivalent, scholarly papers, vita, writing sample, GRE General Test. *Application deadline:* For fall admission, 6/1 (priority date); for spring admission, 10/15 (priority date). Applications are processed on a rolling basis. *Application fee:* $30.

Degree Requirements 94 total credit hours, dissertation.

CONTINUING EDUCATION PROGRAM

Contact Dr. Patricia Gorzka, Coordinator of Continuing Medical Education, College of Nursing, University of South Florida, 12901 Bruce B. Downs Boulevard, MDC Box 22, Tampa, FL 33612-4766. *Telephone:* 813-974-4392. *Fax:* 813-974-5418. *E-mail:* pgorzka@hsc.usf.edu.

The University of Tampa
Department of Nursing
Tampa, Florida

http://www.utampa.edu/academics/liberalarts/departments/nursingbsn.html

Founded in 1931

DEGREES • BSN • MSN

Nursing Program Faculty 38.

Baccalaureate Enrollment 156

Graduate Enrollment 84

Nursing Student Activities Nursing Honor Society, Sigma Theta Tau, Student Nurses' Association.

Nursing Student Resources Academic advising; academic or career counseling; assistance for students with disabilities; bookstore; campus computer network; career placement assistance; computer lab; computer-assisted instruction; e-mail services; employment services for current students; externships; housing assistance; interactive nursing skills videos; Internet; learning resource lab; library services; nursing audiovisuals; paid internships; placement services for program completers; remedial services; resume preparation assistance; skills, simulation, or other laboratory; tutoring; unpaid internships.

Library Facilities 288,857 volumes (252,147 in health); 24,122 periodical subscriptions (10,854 health-care related).

BACCALAUREATE PROGRAMS

Degree BSN

Available Programs ADN to Baccalaureate; Generic Baccalaureate; RN Baccalaureate.

Study Options Full-time.

Program Entrance Requirements Minimum overall college GPA of 3.25, transcript of college record, CPR certification, written essay, health exam, high school transcript, immunizations, 1 letter of recommendation, professional liability insurance/malpractice insurance, prerequisite course work. Transfer students are accepted. **Standardized tests** *Required:* SAT or ACT, TOEFL for international students. **Application** *Deadline:* rolling (freshmen), rolling (transfer). *Application fee:* $35.

Advanced Placement Credit by examination available. Credit given for nursing courses completed elsewhere dependent upon specific evaluations.

Expenses (2006–07) *Tuition:* full-time $18,666; part-time $398 per credit hour. *Room and board:* $7254; room only: $3900 per academic year. *Required fees:* full-time $962.

Contact Admissions Office, Department of Nursing, The University of Tampa, 401 West Kennedy Boulevard, Tampa, FL 33606. *Telephone:* 813-253-6273. *Fax:* 813-258-7398. *E-mail:* nursing@ut.edu.

GRADUATE PROGRAMS

Expenses (2006–07) *Tuition:* part-time $426 per credit hour.

Contact Graduate Studies Office, Department of Nursing, The University of Tampa, 401 West Kennedy Boulevard, Tampa, FL 33606. *Telephone:* 813-258-7409. *E-mail:* utgrad@ut.edu.

MASTER'S DEGREE PROGRAM

Degree MSN

Available Programs Accelerated RN to Master's; Master's.

Concentrations Available Nursing education. *Nurse practitioner programs in:* adult health, family health.

Study Options Full-time and part-time.

Program Entrance Requirements Computer literacy, minimum overall college GPA of 3.0, transcript of college record, CPR certification, written essay, immunizations, interview, 2 letters of recommendation, physical assessment course, professional liability insurance/malpractice insurance, resume, statistics course.

Advanced Placement Credit by examination available.

Degree Requirements 48 total credit hours, comprehensive exam.

POST-MASTER'S PROGRAM

Areas of Study Nursing education. *Nurse practitioner programs in:* adult health, family health.

See full description on page 562.

University of West Florida
Department of Nursing
Pensacola, Florida

http://uwf.edu/nursing

Founded in 1963

University of West Florida (continued)
DEGREE • BSN

Nursing Program Faculty 10 (10% with doctorates).

Baccalaureate Enrollment 95

Women 98% **Men** 2% **Minority** 20% **International** 5% **Part-time** 25%

Nursing Student Activities Nursing Honor Society, Student Nurses' Association.

Nursing Student Resources Academic advising; academic or career counseling; assistance for students with disabilities; campus computer network; computer lab; e-mail services; interactive nursing skills videos; Internet; learning resource lab; nursing audiovisuals; skills, simulation, or other laboratory.

Library Facilities 792,733 volumes (3,500 in health, 1,950 in nursing); 5,122 periodical subscriptions (54 health-care related).

BACCALAUREATE PROGRAMS

Degree BSN

Available Programs ADN to Baccalaureate; Baccalaureate for Second Degree; Generic Baccalaureate; RN Baccalaureate.

Site Options Niceville, FL.

Study Options Full-time.

Program Entrance Requirements Minimum overall college GPA of 2.75, transcript of college record, CPR certification, health exam, health insurance, immunizations, minimum GPA in nursing prerequisites of 2.75, professional liability insurance/malpractice insurance, prerequisite course work. Transfer students are accepted. **Standardized tests** *Required:* SAT or ACT, TOEFL for international students. **Application** *Deadline:* 6/30 (freshmen), 6/30 (transfer). *Notification:* continuous (freshmen). *Application fee:* $30.

Advanced Placement Credit given for nursing courses completed elsewhere dependent upon specific evaluations.

Expenses (2006–07) *Tuition, area resident:* full-time $9982. *Tuition, state resident:* full-time $13,232. *Tuition, nonresident:* full-time $24,620. *International tuition:* $24,620 full-time. *Room and board:* $3000 per academic year. *Required fees:* full-time $450.

Financial Aid 70% of baccalaureate students in nursing programs received some form of financial aid in 2005–06.

Contact Nursing Contact, Department of Nursing, University of West Florida, 11000 University Parkway, Pensacola, FL 32514. *Telephone:* 850-494-3802. *E-mail:* nursing@uwf.edu.

GEORGIA

Albany State University
College of Health Professions
Albany, Georgia

http://asuweb.asurams.edu
Founded in 1903
DEGREES • BSN • MSN

Nursing Program Faculty 15 (27% with doctorates).

Baccalaureate Enrollment 349

Women 92% **Men** 8% **Minority** 1% **International** 1% **Part-time** 11%

Graduate Enrollment 55

Women 87% **Men** 13% **Minority** 31% **International** 1% **Part-time** 49%

Nursing Student Activities Nursing Honor Society, Student Nurses' Association, nursing club.

Nursing Student Resources Academic advising; academic or career counseling; assistance for students with disabilities; bookstore; campus computer network; career placement assistance; computer lab; computer-assisted instruction; e-mail services; interactive nursing skills videos; Internet; learning resource lab; library services; nursing audiovisuals; paid internships; placement services for program completers; remedial services; resume preparation assistance; skills, simulation, or other laboratory; tutoring; unpaid internships.

Library Facilities 191,117 volumes (10,000 in health, 7,000 in nursing); 323 periodical subscriptions (75 health-care related).

BACCALAUREATE PROGRAMS

Degree BSN

Available Programs ADN to Baccalaureate; Accelerated RN Baccalaureate; Baccalaureate for Second Degree; Generic Baccalaureate; RN Baccalaureate.

Site Options Bainbridge, GA.

Study Options Full-time.

Program Entrance Requirements Minimum overall college GPA of 2.75, transcript of college record, CPR certification, written essay, health exam, health insurance, high school biology, high school foreign language, 4 years high school math, 3 years high school science, high school transcript, immunizations, interview, minimum GPA in nursing prerequisites of 2.75, professional liability insurance/malpractice insurance, prerequisite course work. Transfer students are accepted. **Standardized tests** *Required:* SAT or ACT, TOEFL for international students. **Application** *Deadline:* 7/1 (freshmen), 7/1 (transfer). *Application fee:* $20.

Advanced Placement Credit given for nursing courses completed elsewhere dependent upon specific evaluations.

Expenses (2006–07) *Tuition, state resident:* full-time $3154; part-time $107 per credit hour. *Tuition, nonresident:* full-time $10,738; part-time $427 per credit hour. *International tuition:* $10,738 full-time. *Room and board:* $5464; room only: $3300 per academic year. *Required fees:* full-time $664.

Financial Aid 84% of baccalaureate students in nursing programs received some form of financial aid in 2005–06.

Contact Dr. Linda P. Grimsley, RN, Chair, College of Health Professions, Albany State University, 504 College Drive, Albany, GA 31705. *Telephone:* 229-430-4724. *Fax:* 229-430-3937. *E-mail:* linda.grimsley@asurams.edu.

GRADUATE PROGRAMS

Expenses (2006–07) *Tuition, state resident:* full-time $3638; part-time $127 per credit hour. *Tuition, nonresident:* full-time $12,172; part-time $508 per credit hour. *International tuition:* $12,172 full-time. *Room and board:* $5464; room only: $3300 per academic year. *Required fees:* full-time $597.

Financial Aid 70% of graduate students in nursing programs received some form of financial aid in 2005–06. Scholarships and traineeships available.

Contact Dr. Linda P. Grimsley, RN, Chair, College of Health Professions, Albany State University, 504 College Drive, Albany, GA 31705. *Telephone:* 229-430-4727. *Fax:* 229-430-3937. *E-mail:* linda.grimsley@asurams.edu.

MASTER'S DEGREE PROGRAM

Degree MSN

Available Programs Accelerated Master's; Master's; RN to Master's.

Concentrations Available Nursing education. *Nurse practitioner programs in:* family health.

Study Options Full-time and part-time.

Program Entrance Requirements Clinical experience, computer literacy, minimum overall college GPA of 3.0, transcript of college record, CPR certification, immunizations, interview, 2 letters of recommendation, nursing research course, physical assessment course, professional liability insurance/malpractice insurance, prerequisite course work, resume, statistics course, GRE General Test or MAT. *Application deadline:* For fall admission, 4/15; for spring admission, 11/15. Applications are processed on a rolling basis. *Application fee:* $20.

Advanced Placement Credit given for nursing courses completed elsewhere dependent upon specific evaluations.

Degree Requirements 36 total credit hours, thesis or project, comprehensive exam.

POST-MASTER'S PROGRAM

Areas of Study Nursing education. *Nurse practitioner programs in:* family health.

Armstrong Atlantic State University
Program in Nursing
Savannah, Georgia

http://www.don.armstrong.edu/

Founded in 1935

DEGREES • BSN • MS/MHSA • MSN

Nursing Program Faculty 35 (31% with doctorates).

Baccalaureate Enrollment 222
Women 85% **Men** 15% **Minority** 30% **Part-time** 10%

Graduate Enrollment 45
Women 93% **Men** 7% **Minority** 38% **Part-time** 70%

Nursing Student Activities Nursing Honor Society, Sigma Theta Tau, Student Nurses' Association.

Nursing Student Resources Academic advising; assistance for students with disabilities; bookstore; campus computer network; career placement assistance; computer lab; computer-assisted instruction; e-mail services; employment services for current students; housing assistance; interactive nursing skills videos; Internet; learning resource lab; library services; nursing audiovisuals; placement services for program completers; remedial services; resume preparation assistance; skills, simulation, or other laboratory; tutoring.

Library Facilities 227,439 volumes (8,200 in nursing); 990 periodical subscriptions (171 health-care related).

BACCALAUREATE PROGRAMS

Degree BSN

Available Programs ADN to Baccalaureate; Baccalaureate for Second Degree; Generic Baccalaureate; LPN to Baccalaureate; RN Baccalaureate.

Site Options *Distance Learning:* Brunswick, GA.

Study Options Full-time and part-time.

Program Entrance Requirements Transcript of college record, CPR certification, health exam, health insurance, immunizations, minimum GPA in nursing prerequisites of 2.7, professional liability insurance/malpractice insurance, prerequisite course work. Transfer students are accepted. **Standardized tests** *Required:* SAT or ACT, TOEFL for international students. *Required for some:* SAT Subject Tests. **Application** *Deadline:* 6/30 (freshmen), 6/30 (transfer). *Notification:* continuous (freshmen). *Application fee:* $20.

Advanced Placement Credit by examination available.

Expenses (2006–07) *Tuition, state resident:* full-time $1462. *Tuition, nonresident:* full-time $5120.

Financial Aid 90% of baccalaureate students in nursing programs received some form of financial aid in 2005–06.

Contact Dr. Helen Taggart, Undergraduate Coordinator, Program in Nursing, Armstrong Atlantic State University, 11935 Abercorn Street, Savannah, GA 31419-1997. *Telephone:* 912-927-5302. *Fax:* 912-920-6579. *E-mail:* taggarhe@mail.armstrong.edu.

GRADUATE PROGRAMS

Expenses (2006–07) *Tuition, state resident:* full-time $1341. *Tuition, nonresident:* full-time $4635.

Financial Aid 85% of graduate students in nursing programs received some form of financial aid in 2005–06. Research assistantships with partial tuition reimbursements available (averaging $2,500 per year); Federal Work-Study, scholarships, and unspecified assistantships also available. Aid available to part-time students.

Contact Dr. Anita Nivens, Graduate Program Coordinator, Program in Nursing, Armstrong Atlantic State University, 11935 Abercorn Street, Savannah, GA 31419-1997. *Telephone:* 912-927-5311. *Fax:* 912-920-6579. *E-mail:* nivensan@mail.armstrong.edu.

MASTER'S DEGREE PROGRAM

Degrees MS/MHSA; MSN

Available Programs Master's; RN to Master's.

Concentrations Available Nursing administration. *Clinical nurse specialist programs in:* adult health. *Nurse practitioner programs in:* adult health.

Study Options Full-time and part-time.

Program Entrance Requirements Clinical experience, minimum overall college GPA of 3.0, transcript of college record, CPR certification, written essay, immunizations, interview, 3 letters of recommendation, nursing research course, physical assessment course, professional liability insurance/malpractice insurance, prerequisite course work, statistics course, GRE General Test or MAT. *Application deadline:* For fall admission, 7/1 (priority date); for spring admission, 11/15 (priority date). Applications are processed on a rolling basis. *Application fee:* $25.

Advanced Placement Credit by examination available.

Degree Requirements 36 total credit hours, thesis or project.

POST-MASTER'S PROGRAM

Areas of Study Nursing administration. *Clinical nurse specialist programs in:* adult health. *Nurse practitioner programs in:* adult health.

Brenau University
School of Health and Science
Gainesville, Georgia

Founded in 1878

DEGREES • BSN • MSN

Nursing Program Faculty 14 (65% with doctorates).

Baccalaureate Enrollment 130
Women 95% **Men** 5% **Minority** 40% **International** 10% **Part-time** 30%

Graduate Enrollment 20
Women 100% **Minority** 10% **Part-time** 100%

Nursing Student Activities Sigma Theta Tau, Student Nurses' Association.

Nursing Student Resources Academic advising; academic or career counseling; assistance for students with disabilities; bookstore; campus computer network; computer lab; computer-assisted instruction; e-mail services; employment services for current students; housing assistance; interactive nursing skills videos; Internet; learning resource lab; library services; nursing audiovisuals; remedial services; resume preparation assistance; skills, simulation, or other laboratory; tutoring.

Library Facilities 6,000 volumes in health, 5,000 volumes in nursing; 75 periodical subscriptions health-care related.

BACCALAUREATE PROGRAMS

Degree BSN

Available Programs ADN to Baccalaureate; Generic Baccalaureate; RN Baccalaureate.

Study Options Full-time and part-time.

Program Entrance Requirements Minimum overall college GPA of 2.5, transcript of college record, health exam, high school chemistry, high school foreign language, 2 years high school math, 1 year of high school science, high school transcript, immunizations, minimum high school GPA of 2.5, minimum GPA in nursing prerequisites of 2.5, professional liability insurance/malpractice insurance, prerequisite course work. Transfer students are accepted. **Standardized tests** *Required:* SAT or ACT, TOEFL for international students. **Application** *Deadline:* rolling (freshmen), rolling (transfer). *Notification:* continuous (freshmen). *Application fee:* $35.

Expenses (2006–07) *Tuition:* part-time $425 per credit hour.

Financial Aid 75% of baccalaureate students in nursing programs received some form of financial aid in 2005–06. *Gift aid (need-based):* Federal Pell, FSEOG, state, private, college/university gift aid from institutional funds. *Loans:* FFEL (Subsidized and Unsubsidized Stafford PLUS), Perkins, state. *Work-Study:* Federal Work-Study, part-time campus jobs. *Application deadline (priority):* 4/1.

Contact Ms. Teresa Chastain, Undergraduate Admissions Coordinator for Women's College, School of Health and Science, Brenau University, One Centennial Circle, Gainesville, GA 30501. *Telephone:* 770-534-6100. *Fax:* 770-538-4306. *E-mail:* tchastain@lib.brenau.edu.

GRADUATE PROGRAMS

Financial Aid 70% of graduate students in nursing programs received some form of financial aid in 2005–06. Scholarships available. Aid available to part-time students. *Financial aid application deadline:* 7/15.

Brenau University (continued)

Contact Ms. Michelle Leavell, Graduate Admissions Coordinator, School of Health and Science, Brenau University, One Centennial Circle, Gainesville, GA 30501. *Telephone:* 770-534-6162. *E-mail:* lminish@lib.brenau.edu.

MASTER'S DEGREE PROGRAM

Degree MSN

Available Programs Master's.

Concentrations Available Nursing education. *Nurse practitioner programs in:* family health.

Site Options Atlanta, GA.

Study Options Part-time.

Program Entrance Requirements Clinical experience, minimum overall college GPA of 3.0, transcript of college record, written essay, 3 letters of recommendation, nursing research course, physical assessment course, statistics course, GRE General Test or MAT. *Application deadline:* Applications are processed on a rolling basis. *Application fee:* $30.

Degree Requirements 42 total credit hours.

POST-MASTER'S PROGRAM

Areas of Study *Nurse practitioner programs in:* family health.

CONTINUING EDUCATION PROGRAM

Contact Dr. Keeta Wilborn, Chair, Department of Nursing, School of Health and Science, Brenau University, 500 Washington Street, Gainesville, GA 30501. *Telephone:* 770-534-6206. *Fax:* 770-538-4666. *E-mail:* kwilborn@brenau.edu.

Clayton State University
Department of Nursing
Morrow, Georgia

http://www.healthsci.clayton.edu

Founded in 1969

DEGREE • BSN

Nursing Program Faculty 30 (45% with doctorates).

Baccalaureate Enrollment 135

Women 88% **Men** 12% **Minority** 50% **International** 10%

Nursing Student Activities Sigma Theta Tau, Student Nurses' Association.

Nursing Student Resources Academic advising; academic or career counseling; assistance for students with disabilities; bookstore; campus computer network; career placement assistance; computer lab; computer-assisted instruction; e-mail services; employment services for current students; externships; housing assistance; interactive nursing skills videos; Internet; learning resource lab; library services; nursing audiovisuals; paid internships; placement services for program completers; remedial services; resume preparation assistance; skills, simulation, or other laboratory; tutoring.

Library Facilities 77,043 volumes (3,450 in health, 1,800 in nursing); 4,250 periodical subscriptions (151 health-care related).

BACCALAUREATE PROGRAMS

Degree BSN

Available Programs Generic Baccalaureate; RN Baccalaureate.

Study Options Full-time.

Program Entrance Requirements Minimum overall college GPA of 2.5, transcript of college record, CPR certification, health exam, health insurance, immunizations, interview, minimum GPA in nursing prerequisites of 2.5, professional liability insurance/malpractice insurance, prerequisite course work. Transfer students are accepted. **Standardized tests** *Required:* SAT or ACT, TOEFL for international students. *Required for some:* SAT Subject Tests. **Application** *Deadline:* 7/17 (freshmen). *Notification:* continuous (freshmen). *Application fee:* $40.

Advanced Placement Credit by examination available.

Expenses (2006–07) *Tuition, state resident:* full-time $1280; part-time $107 per contact hour. *Tuition, nonresident:* full-time $5121; part-time $427 per credit. *International tuition:* $5121 full-time. *Required fees:* full-time $282; part-time $282 per term.

Financial Aid 25% of baccalaureate students in nursing programs received some form of financial aid in 2005–06.

Contact Dr. Sue E. Odom, Acting Chair, Department of Nursing, Clayton State University, 2000 Clayton State Boulevard, Business and Health Sciences Building, Morrow, GA 30260. *Telephone:* 770-961-3484. *Fax:* 770-961-3639. *E-mail:* sueodom@clayton.edu.

Columbus State University
Nursing Program
Columbus, Georgia

http://nursing.colstate.edu

Founded in 1958

DEGREE • BSN

Nursing Program Faculty 29 (13% with doctorates).

Baccalaureate Enrollment 144

Women 85% **Men** 15% **Minority** 37% **International** 1%

Nursing Student Activities Sigma Theta Tau, Student Nurses' Association.

Nursing Student Resources Academic advising; academic or career counseling; assistance for students with disabilities; bookstore; campus computer network; career placement assistance; computer lab; computer-assisted instruction; e-mail services; housing assistance; interactive nursing skills videos; Internet; learning resource lab; library services; nursing audiovisuals; remedial services; resume preparation assistance; skills, simulation, or other laboratory; tutoring.

Library Facilities 387,026 volumes (13,300 in health, 3,125 in nursing); 1,400 periodical subscriptions (475 health-care related).

BACCALAUREATE PROGRAMS

Degree BSN

Available Programs Accelerated RN Baccalaureate; Generic Baccalaureate.

Study Options Full-time.

Program Entrance Requirements Minimum overall college GPA of 2.75, transcript of college record, CPR certification, health exam, immunizations, 3 letters of recommendation, minimum GPA in nursing prerequisites of 2.75, professional liability insurance/malpractice insurance, prerequisite course work. Transfer students are accepted. **Standardized tests** *Required:* SAT or ACT, TOEFL for international students. **Application** *Deadline:* 7/1 (freshmen), 7/1 (transfer). *Notification:* continuous (freshmen). *Application fee:* $25.

Advanced Placement Credit given for nursing courses completed elsewhere dependent upon specific evaluations.

Expenses (2006–07) *Tuition, state resident:* full-time $2536; part-time $106 per credit hour. *Tuition, nonresident:* full-time $10,144; part-time $423 per credit hour. *International tuition:* $10,144 full-time. *Room and board:* $9110; room only: $4320 per academic year. *Required fees:* full-time $640; part-time $260 per credit; part-time $520 per term.

Financial Aid 95% of baccalaureate students in nursing programs received some form of financial aid in 2005–06. *Gift aid (need-based):* Federal Pell, FSEOG, state, private, college/university gift aid from institutional funds. *Loans:* Federal Direct (Subsidized and Unsubsidized Stafford PLUS), Perkins, state, college/university. *Work-Study:* Federal Work-Study. *Application deadline (priority):* 5/1.

Contact Dr. June S. Goyne, Department Chair and Director of BSN Program, Nursing Program, Columbus State University, 4225 University Avenue, Columbus, GA 31907. *Telephone:* 706-565-3649. *Fax:* 706-569-3101. *E-mail:* goyne_june@colstate.edu.

Emory University
Nell Hodgson Woodruff School of Nursing
Atlanta, Georgia

http://www.nursing.emory.edu

Founded in 1836

DEGREES • BSN • MSN • MSN/MPH • PHD

Nursing Program Faculty 70 (35% with doctorates).

Baccalaureate Enrollment 213
Women 91% **Men** 9% **Minority** 36% **International** 1%

Graduate Enrollment 177
Women 95% **Men** 5% **Minority** 32% **International** 1% **Part-time** 40%

Nursing Student Activities Sigma Theta Tau, Student Nurses' Association.

Nursing Student Resources Academic advising; academic or career counseling; assistance for students with disabilities; bookstore; campus computer network; career placement assistance; computer lab; computer-assisted instruction; daycare for children of students; e-mail services; housing assistance; interactive nursing skills videos; Internet; learning resource lab; library services; nursing audiovisuals; other; skills, simulation, or other laboratory; tutoring; unpaid internships.

Library Facilities 3.2 million volumes (250,000 in health); 51,500 periodical subscriptions (1,800 health-care related).

BACCALAUREATE PROGRAMS

Degree BSN

Available Programs Baccalaureate for Second Degree; Generic Baccalaureate.

Study Options Full-time.

Program Entrance Requirements Minimum overall college GPA of 3.0, transcript of college record, CPR certification, written essay, health exam, health insurance, immunizations, 3 letters of recommendation, minimum GPA in nursing prerequisites of 3.0, prerequisite course work. Transfer students are accepted. **Standardized tests** *Recommended:* TOEFL for international students. **Application** *Deadline:* 1/15. *Application fee:* $50.

Advanced Placement Credit given for nursing courses completed elsewhere dependent upon specific evaluations.

Expenses (2006–07) *Tuition:* full-time $28,800; part-time $1200 per hour. *International tuition:* $28,800 full-time. *Room and board:* room only: $13,176 per academic year. *Required fees:* full-time $394.

Financial Aid 95% of baccalaureate students in nursing programs received some form of financial aid in 2005–06. *Gift aid (need-based):* Federal Pell, FSEOG, state, private, college/university gift aid from institutional funds. *Loans:* Federal Nursing Student Loans, FFEL (Subsidized and Unsubsidized Stafford PLUS), Perkins, state, college/university. *Work-Study:* Federal Work-Study, part-time campus jobs. *Application deadline:* 4/1 (priority: 3/1).

Contact Mr. Robert N. Hoover, Assistant Dean for Admission and Student Services, Nell Hodgson Woodruff School of Nursing, Emory University, 1520 Clifton Road NE, Atlanta, GA 30322. *Telephone:* 404-727-7980. *Fax:* 404-727-8509. *E-mail:* admit@nursing.emory.edu.

GRADUATE PROGRAMS

Expenses (2006–07) *Tuition:* full-time $28,800; part-time $1200 per hour. *International tuition:* $28,800 full-time. *Room and board:* room only: $13,176 per academic year. *Required fees:* full-time $334; part-time $167 per term.

Financial Aid 96% of graduate students in nursing programs received some form of financial aid in 2005–06. Fellowships, career-related internships or fieldwork, Federal Work-Study, institutionally sponsored loans, scholarships, traineeships, and tuition waivers (full and partial) available. Aid available to part-time students. *Financial aid application deadline:* 3/15.

Contact Mr. Robert N. Hoover, Assistant Dean for Admission and Student Services, Nell Hodgson Woodruff School of Nursing, Emory University, 1520 Clifton Road NE, Atlanta, GA 30322. *Telephone:* 404-727-7980. *Fax:* 404-727-8509. *E-mail:* admit@nursing.emory.edu.

MASTER'S DEGREE PROGRAM

Degrees MSN; MSN/MPH

Available Programs Master's; RN to Master's.

Concentrations Available Health-care administration; nurse-midwifery; nursing administration. *Clinical nurse specialist programs in:* public health. *Nurse practitioner programs in:* acute care, adult health, family health, gerontology, oncology, pediatric, women's health.

Study Options Full-time and part-time.

Program Entrance Requirements Clinical experience, minimum overall college GPA of 3.0, transcript of college record, CPR certification, written essay, immunizations, interview, 3 letters of recommendation, physical assessment course, prerequisite course work, resume, statistics course, GRE General Test or MAT. *Application deadline:* For fall admission, 1/15 (priority date); for spring admission, 10/1 (priority date). Applications are processed on a rolling basis. *Application fee:* $50.

Advanced Placement Credit given for nursing courses completed elsewhere dependent upon specific evaluations.

Degree Requirements 36 total credit hours.

POST-MASTER'S PROGRAM

Areas of Study Health-care administration; nurse-midwifery; nursing administration; nursing education. *Clinical nurse specialist programs in:* public health. *Nurse practitioner programs in:* acute care, adult health, family health, gerontology, oncology, pediatric, women's health.

DOCTORAL DEGREE PROGRAM

Degree PhD

Available Programs Doctorate; Post-Baccalaureate Doctorate.

Areas of Study Biology of health and illness, ethics, faculty preparation, gerontology, health policy, human health and illness, illness and transition, individualized study, neuro-behavior, nursing policy, nursing research, nursing science, women's health.

Program Entrance Requirements Minimum overall college GPA of 3.0, interview by faculty committee, interview, 3 letters of recommendation, MSN or equivalent, statistics course, vita, writing sample. *Application deadline:* For fall admission, 2/15 (priority date); for spring admission, 10/1 (priority date). Applications are processed on a rolling basis. *Application fee:* $50.

Degree Requirements 50 total credit hours, dissertation, oral exam, written exam, residency.

POSTDOCTORAL PROGRAM

Postdoctoral Program Contact Ms. Teresa Fosque, Senior Business Manager, Nell Hodgson Woodruff School of Nursing, Emory University, 1520 Clifton Road NE, Atlanta, GA 30322. *E-mail:* tfosque@emory.edu.

See full description on page 478.

Georgia Baptist College of Nursing of Mercer University
Department of Nursing
Atlanta, Georgia

http://nursing.mercer.edu

Founded in 1988

DEGREES • BSN • MSN

Nursing Program Faculty 34 (29% with doctorates).

Baccalaureate Enrollment 402
Women 95% **Men** 5% **Minority** 38% **Part-time** 12%

Graduate Enrollment 13
Women 100% **Minority** 38% **Part-time** 15%

Nursing Student Activities Nursing Honor Society, Sigma Theta Tau, Student Nurses' Association, nursing club.

Nursing Student Resources Academic advising; academic or career counseling; assistance for students with disabilities; bookstore; campus computer network; computer lab; computer-assisted instruction; e-mail services; employment services for current students; housing assistance; interactive nursing skills videos; Internet; learning resource lab; library services; nursing audiovisuals; skills, simulation, or other laboratory; tutoring.

Library Facilities 12,836 volumes (10,912 in health, 2,897 in nursing); 182 periodical subscriptions (218 health-care related).

BACCALAUREATE PROGRAMS

Degree BSN

Georgia Baptist College of Nursing of Mercer University (continued)
Available Programs Generic Baccalaureate; RN Baccalaureate.
Study Options Full-time.

Program Entrance Requirements Transcript of college record, written essay, health exam, health insurance, high school biology, high school foreign language, 3 years high school math, 3 years high school science, high school transcript, immunizations, prerequisite course work. Transfer students are accepted. **Standardized tests** *Required:* SAT or ACT, TOEFL for international students. **Application** *Deadline:* 5/15 (freshmen), 5/15 (transfer). *Notification:* continuous until 6/1 (freshmen). *Application fee:* $35.

Advanced Placement Credit by examination available. Credit given for nursing courses completed elsewhere dependent upon specific evaluations.

Expenses (2006–07) *Tuition:* full-time $16,416; part-time $684 per contact hour. *International tuition:* $16,416 full-time. *Room and board:* room only: $6330 per academic year. *Required fees:* full-time $500.

Financial Aid 79% of baccalaureate students in nursing programs received some form of financial aid in 2005–06.

Contact Ms. Lynn Vines, Director of Admissions, Department of Nursing, Georgia Baptist College of Nursing of Mercer University, 3001 Mercer University Drive, Atlanta, GA 30341. *Telephone:* 678-547-6700. *Fax:* 678-547-6794. *E-mail:* vines_ml@mercer.edu.

GRADUATE PROGRAMS

Expenses (2006–07) *Tuition:* full-time $14,468; part-time $809 per contact hour. *International tuition:* $14,468 full-time. *Room and board:* room only: $6330 per academic year. *Required fees:* full-time $300.

Financial Aid 69% of graduate students in nursing programs received some form of financial aid in 2005–06.

Contact Dr. Linda Streit, Associate Dean for the Graduate Program, Department of Nursing, Georgia Baptist College of Nursing of Mercer University, 3001 Mercer University Drive, Atlanta, GA 30341. *Telephone:* 678-547-6774. *Fax:* 678-547-6777. *E-mail:* streit_la@mercer.edu.

MASTER'S DEGREE PROGRAM

Degree MSN

Available Programs Master's.

Concentrations Available Nursing education. *Clinical nurse specialist programs in:* acute care.

Study Options Full-time and part-time.

Program Entrance Requirements Clinical experience, computer literacy, minimum overall college GPA of 3.0, transcript of college record, CPR certification, immunizations, interview, letters of recommendation, nursing research course, physical assessment course, statistics course.

Advanced Placement Credit given for nursing courses completed elsewhere dependent upon specific evaluations.

Degree Requirements 42 total credit hours, thesis or project.

POST-MASTER'S PROGRAM

Areas of Study Nursing education.

CONTINUING EDUCATION PROGRAM

Contact Dr. Susan S. Gunby, Dean, Department of Nursing, Georgia Baptist College of Nursing of Mercer University, 3001 Mercer University Drive, Atlanta, GA 30341. *Telephone:* 678-547-6798. *Fax:* 678-547-6796. *E-mail:* gunby_ss@mercer.edu.

Georgia College & State University
School of Health Sciences
Milledgeville, Georgia

http://www.gcsu.edu/acad_affairs/ school_healthsci/healthsci

Founded in 1889

DEGREES • BSN • MSN • MSN/MBA

Nursing Program Faculty 36 (25% with doctorates).

Baccalaureate Enrollment 267
Women 85% **Men** 15% **Minority** 12% **International** 1% **Part-time** 30%
Graduate Enrollment 70
Women 80% **Men** 20% **Minority** 16% **International** 1% **Part-time** 100%
Nursing Student Activities Sigma Theta Tau, Student Nurses' Association.

Nursing Student Resources Academic advising; academic or career counseling; assistance for students with disabilities; bookstore; campus computer network; career placement assistance; computer lab; computer-assisted instruction; e-mail services; employment services for current students; housing assistance; interactive nursing skills videos; Internet; learning resource lab; library services; nursing audiovisuals; remedial services; resume preparation assistance; skills, simulation, or other laboratory; tutoring; unpaid internships.

Library Facilities 175,299 volumes (3,095 in health, 1,465 in nursing); 22,955 periodical subscriptions (315 health-care related).

BACCALAUREATE PROGRAMS

Degree BSN

Available Programs Generic Baccalaureate; RN Baccalaureate.
Site Options Macon, GA.
Study Options Full-time and part-time.

Program Entrance Requirements Minimum overall college GPA of 2.5, transcript of college record, CPR certification, health exam, health insurance, high school biology, high school foreign language, 4 years high school math, 3 years high school science, high school transcript, immunizations, minimum GPA in nursing prerequisites of 2.5, professional liability insurance/malpractice insurance, prerequisite course work. Transfer students are accepted. **Standardized tests** *Required:* SAT or ACT, TOEFL for international students. *Required for some:* SAT Subject Tests. **Application** *Deadline:* 4/1 (freshmen), 7/1 (transfer). *Early decision:* 11/1. *Notification:* continuous (freshmen), 12/1 (early action). *Application fee:* $25.

Advanced Placement Credit by examination available. Credit given for nursing courses completed elsewhere dependent upon specific evaluations.

Financial Aid 87% of baccalaureate students in nursing programs received some form of financial aid in 2005–06.

Contact Dr. Cheryl Pope Kish, Interim Dean, School of Health Sciences, Georgia College & State University, Campus Box 064, Milledgeville, GA 31061. *Telephone:* 478-445-4004. *Fax:* 478-445-1913. *E-mail:* cheryl.kish@gcsu.edu.

GRADUATE PROGRAMS

Financial Aid 51% of graduate students in nursing programs received some form of financial aid in 2005–06. 14 research assistantships with tuition reimbursements available (averaging $3,800 per year) were awarded; career-related internships or fieldwork, Federal Work-Study, and unspecified assistantships also available. Aid available to part-time students. *Financial aid application deadline:* 3/1.

Contact Dr. Karen Frith, Graduate Coordinator, School of Health Sciences, Georgia College & State University, CBX 64, 231 West Hancock Street, Milledgeville, GA 31061. *Telephone:* 478-445-1795. *Fax:* 478-445-1913. *E-mail:* karen.frith@gcsu.edu.

MASTER'S DEGREE PROGRAM

Degrees MSN; MSN/MBA

Available Programs Master's; RN to Master's.

Concentrations Available Nursing administration; nursing education; nursing informatics. *Clinical nurse specialist programs in:* adult health. *Nurse practitioner programs in:* family health.

Site Options Macon, GA.

Study Options Part-time.

Program Entrance Requirements Clinical experience, computer literacy, minimum overall college GPA of 2.75, transcript of college record, CPR certification, immunizations, interview, nursing research course, professional liability insurance/malpractice insurance, resume, statistics course, GRE, GMAT or MAT. *Application deadline:* For fall admission, 7/1 (priority date). Applications are processed on a rolling basis. *Application fee:* $25.

Advanced Placement Credit given for nursing courses completed elsewhere dependent upon specific evaluations.

Degree Requirements 36 total credit hours, thesis or project, comprehensive exam.

POST-MASTER'S PROGRAM

Areas of Study Nursing education; nursing informatics. *Nurse practitioner programs in:* family health.

Georgia Southern University
School of Nursing
Statesboro, Georgia

http://www.georgiasouthern.edu

Founded in 1906

DEGREES • BSN • MSN

Nursing Program Faculty 27 (59% with doctorates).

Baccalaureate Enrollment 285
Women 89% **Men** 11% **Minority** 23% **International** 1% **Part-time** 35%

Graduate Enrollment 45
Women 96% **Men** 4% **Minority** 13% **Part-time** 3%

Nursing Student Activities Sigma Theta Tau, Student Nurses' Association.

Nursing Student Resources Academic advising; academic or career counseling; assistance for students with disabilities; bookstore; campus computer network; career placement assistance; computer lab; computer-assisted instruction; daycare for children of students; e-mail services; housing assistance; interactive nursing skills videos; Internet; learning resource lab; library services; nursing audiovisuals; placement services for program completers; resume preparation assistance; skills, simulation, or other laboratory; tutoring.

Library Facilities 588,997 volumes (25,000 in health, 12,000 in nursing); 2,690 periodical subscriptions (20,000 health-care related).

BACCALAUREATE PROGRAMS

Degree BSN

Available Programs ADN to Baccalaureate; Generic Baccalaureate; LPN to RN Baccalaureate.

Study Options Full-time.

Program Entrance Requirements Minimum overall college GPA of 3.0, transcript of college record, CPR certification, written essay, health exam, health insurance, high school biology, high school chemistry, high school foreign language, 2 years high school math, 4 years high school science, high school transcript, immunizations, minimum GPA in nursing prerequisites of 3.0, professional liability insurance/malpractice insurance, prerequisite course work. Transfer students are accepted. **Standardized tests** *Required:* SAT or ACT, TOEFL for international students. **Application** *Deadline:* 5/1 (freshmen), 5/1 (out-of-state freshmen), 8/1 (transfer). *Notification:* continuous (freshmen), continuous (out-of-state freshmen). *Application fee:* $30.

Advanced Placement Credit by examination available. Credit given for nursing courses completed elsewhere dependent upon specific evaluations.

Expenses (2006–07) *Tuition, state resident:* full-time $2536; part-time $106 per hour. *Tuition, nonresident:* full-time $10,144; part-time $423 per hour. *International tuition:* $10,144 full-time. *Room and board:* $7484; room only: $5036 per academic year. *Required fees:* full-time $1052; part-time $57 per term.

Financial Aid 86% of baccalaureate students in nursing programs received some form of financial aid in 2005–06.

Contact Dr. Danette Wood, BSN Program Director, School of Nursing, Georgia Southern University, PO Box 8158, Statesboro, GA 30460-8158. *Telephone:* 912-681-5454. *Fax:* 912-681-0536. *E-mail:* danette_wood@ georgiasouthern.edu.

GRADUATE PROGRAMS

Expenses (2006–07) *Tuition, state resident:* full-time $3044; part-time $127 per hour. *Tuition, nonresident:* full-time $12,172; part-time $508 per hour. *International tuition:* $12,172 full-time. *Room and board:* $7484; room only: $5036 per academic year. *Required fees:* full-time $1052; part-time $57 per term.

Financial Aid 35% of graduate students in nursing programs received some form of financial aid in 2005–06. Research assistantships with partial tuition reimbursements available (averaging $5,500 per year), teaching assistantships with partial tuition reimbursements available (averaging $5,500 per year) were awarded; career-related internships or fieldwork, Federal Work-Study, scholarships, traineeships, and unspecified assistantships also available. Aid available to part-time students. *Financial aid application deadline:* 4/15.

Contact Dr. Donna Hodnicki, Director, Graduate Program, School of Nursing, Georgia Southern University, PO Box 8158, Statesboro, GA 30460-8158. *Telephone:* 912-681-5056. *Fax:* 912-681-0536. *E-mail:* dhodnick@georgiasouthern.edu.

MASTER'S DEGREE PROGRAM

Degree MSN

Available Programs Master's; RN to Master's.

Concentrations Available *Clinical nurse specialist programs in:* community health. *Nurse practitioner programs in:* family health, women's health.

Study Options Full-time and part-time.

Program Entrance Requirements Clinical experience, computer literacy, minimum overall college GPA of 3.0, transcript of college record, CPR certification, immunizations, interview, 3 letters of recommendation, professional liability insurance/malpractice insurance, prerequisite course work, statistics course, GRE General Test or MAT. *Application deadline:* For fall admission, 3/1 (priority date); for spring admission, 10/1 (priority date). Applications are processed on a rolling basis. *Application fee:* $50.

Advanced Placement Credit given for nursing courses completed elsewhere dependent upon specific evaluations.

Degree Requirements 48 total credit hours, thesis or project, comprehensive exam.

POST-MASTER'S PROGRAM

Areas of Study *Clinical nurse specialist programs in:* community health. *Nurse practitioner programs in:* family health, women's health.

Georgia Southwestern State University
School of Nursing
Americus, Georgia

http://www.gsw.edu

Founded in 1906

DEGREE • BSN

Nursing Program Faculty 8 (50% with doctorates).

Baccalaureate Enrollment 73
Women 90% **Men** 10% **Minority** 24% **Part-time** 20%

Nursing Student Activities Sigma Theta Tau, Student Nurses' Association.

Nursing Student Resources Academic advising; academic or career counseling; assistance for students with disabilities; bookstore; campus computer network; career placement assistance; computer lab; computer-assisted instruction; e-mail services; employment services for current students; interactive nursing skills videos; Internet; learning resource lab; library services; nursing audiovisuals; placement services for program completers; remedial services; resume preparation assistance; skills, simulation, or other laboratory; tutoring.

Library Facilities 428,197 volumes (627 in health, 528 in nursing); 516 periodical subscriptions (141 health-care related).

BACCALAUREATE PROGRAMS

Degree BSN

Available Programs Baccalaureate for Second Degree; Generic Baccalaureate; RN Baccalaureate.

Study Options Full-time and part-time.

Georgia Southwestern State University (continued)

Program Entrance Requirements Minimum overall college GPA of 2.7, transcript of college record, CPR certification, written essay, health exam, health insurance, high school foreign language, 4 years high school math, 4 years high school science, high school transcript, immunizations, 2 letters of recommendation, minimum GPA in nursing prerequisites of 2.7, professional liability insurance/malpractice insurance, prerequisite course work. Transfer students are accepted. **Standardized tests** *Required:* SAT or ACT, TOEFL for international students. **Application** *Deadline:* 7/21 (freshmen), 7/21 (transfer). *Early decision:* 12/15. *Notification:* continuous (freshmen), 1/15 (out-of-state freshmen), 1/15 (early decision). *Application fee:* $25.

Advanced Placement Credit given for nursing courses completed elsewhere dependent upon specific evaluations.

Expenses (2006–07) *Tuition, state resident:* full-time $2536; part-time $106 per credit hour. *Tuition, nonresident:* full-time $10,144; part-time $423 per credit hour. *International tuition:* $10,144 full-time. *Room and board:* $2700 per academic year. *Required fees:* full-time $800; part-time $106 per credit; part-time $273 per term.

Financial Aid 91% of baccalaureate students in nursing programs received some form of financial aid in 2005–06. *Gift aid (need-based):* Federal Pell, FSEOG, state, private, college/university gift aid from institutional funds. *Loans:* FFEL (Subsidized and Unsubsidized Stafford PLUS), Perkins, state, college/university. *Work-Study:* Federal Work-Study, part-time campus jobs. *Application deadline (priority):* 4/1.

Contact Dr. Maria R. Warda, Dean, School of Nursing, Georgia Southwestern State University, Americus, GA 31709. *Telephone:* 229-931-2289. *Fax:* 229-931-2288. *E-mail:* mwarda@canes.gsw.edu.

CONTINUING EDUCATION PROGRAM

Contact Dr. Judith M. Malachowski, Assistant Professor, School of Nursing, Georgia Southwestern State University, 800 Georgia Southwestern State University Drive, Americus, GA 31709. *Telephone:* 229-931-2662. *Fax:* 229-931-2288. *E-mail:* jmm@canes.gsw.edu.

Georgia State University
School of Nursing
Atlanta, Georgia

http://chhs.gsu.edu/nursing/

Founded in 1913

DEGREES • BS • MS • PHD

Nursing Program Faculty 52 (32% with doctorates).

Baccalaureate Enrollment 250

Graduate Enrollment 195

Nursing Student Activities Sigma Theta Tau, Student Nurses' Association.

Nursing Student Resources Academic advising; academic or career counseling; assistance for students with disabilities; bookstore; campus computer network; career placement assistance; computer lab; computer-assisted instruction; daycare for children of students; e-mail services; externships; interactive nursing skills videos; Internet; learning resource lab; library services; nursing audiovisuals; skills, simulation, or other laboratory.

Library Facilities 1.5 million volumes (52,835 in health, 20,856 in nursing); 7,788 periodical subscriptions (725 health-care related).

BACCALAUREATE PROGRAMS

Degree BS

Available Programs Accelerated Baccalaureate; Accelerated RN Baccalaureate; Generic Baccalaureate; RN Baccalaureate.

Study Options Full-time and part-time.

Program Entrance Requirements Minimum overall college GPA of 2.5, transcript of college record, CPR certification, written essay, health exam, immunizations, interview, 2 letters of recommendation, minimum GPA in nursing prerequisites of 2.5, professional liability insurance/malpractice insurance, prerequisite course work. Transfer students are accepted. **Standardized tests** *Required:* SAT or ACT, TOEFL for international students. *Required for some:* SAT Subject Tests. **Application** *Deadline:* 3/1 (freshmen), 6/1 (transfer). *Notification:* continuous until 10/1 (freshmen). *Application fee:* $50.

Advanced Placement Credit given for nursing courses completed elsewhere dependent upon specific evaluations.

Contact Office of Academic Assistance, School of Nursing, Georgia State University, College of Health and Human Sciences, Atlanta, GA 30303-3083. *Telephone:* 404-651-3083. *Fax:* 404-651-4871. *E-mail:* schoolofnursing@gsu.edu.

GRADUATE PROGRAMS

Financial Aid 80 fellowships, 34 research assistantships (averaging $1,500 per year) were awarded; teaching assistantships, Federal Work-Study, institutionally sponsored loans, scholarships, traineeships, and tuition waivers (partial) also available.

Contact Office of Academic Assistance, School of Nursing, Georgia State University, College of Health and Human Sciences, Atlanta, GA 30303-3083. *Telephone:* 404-651-3064. *Fax:* 404-651-4871. *E-mail:* schoolofnursing@gsu.edu.

MASTER'S DEGREE PROGRAM

Degree MS

Available Programs Master's; RN to Master's.

Concentrations Available *Clinical nurse specialist programs in:* adult health, pediatric, perinatal, psychiatric/mental health. *Nurse practitioner programs in:* family health, pediatric, women's health.

Study Options Full-time and part-time.

Program Entrance Requirements Clinical experience, minimum overall college GPA of 2.75, transcript of college record, CPR certification, interview, 2 letters of recommendation, professional liability insurance/malpractice insurance, GRE or MAT. *Application deadline:* For fall admission, 3/1 (priority date); for spring admission, 10/1 (priority date). Applications are processed on a rolling basis. *Application fee:* $50.

Advanced Placement Credit given for nursing courses completed elsewhere dependent upon specific evaluations.

Degree Requirements 48 total credit hours, thesis or project.

POST-MASTER'S PROGRAM

Areas of Study *Clinical nurse specialist programs in:* adult health, pediatric, perinatal, psychiatric/mental health. *Nurse practitioner programs in:* family health, pediatric, women's health.

DOCTORAL DEGREE PROGRAM

Degree PhD

Available Programs Doctorate.

Areas of Study Faculty preparation, family health, health promotion/disease prevention, individualized study, nursing research, nursing science.

Program Entrance Requirements Minimum overall college GPA of 3.0, interview by faculty committee, interview, 3 letters of recommendation, MSN or equivalent, scholarly papers, vita, GRE General Test. *Application deadline:* For fall admission, 3/1 (priority date); for spring admission, 10/1 (priority date). Applications are processed on a rolling basis. *Application fee:* $50.

Degree Requirements 60 total credit hours, dissertation, written exam, residency.

Kennesaw State University
School of Nursing
Kennesaw, Georgia

http://www.kennesaw.edu/chhs/schoolofnursing

Founded in 1963

DEGREES • BSN • MSN

Nursing Program Faculty 63 (41% with doctorates).

Baccalaureate Enrollment 372
Women 89% **Men** 11% **Minority** 13% **International** 7% **Part-time** 37%

Graduate Enrollment 80
Women 92% **Men** 8% **Minority** 13% **International** 6% **Part-time** 4%

Nursing Student Activities Sigma Theta Tau, Student Nurses' Association.

Nursing Student Resources Academic advising; academic or career counseling; assistance for students with disabilities; bookstore; campus computer network; career placement assistance; computer lab; computer-assisted instruction; e-mail services; employment services for current students; externships; housing assistance; interactive nursing skills videos; Internet; learning resource lab; library services; nursing audiovisuals; paid internships; placement services for program completers; resume preparation assistance; skills, simulation, or other laboratory.

Library Facilities 630,614 volumes (20,000 in health, 10,000 in nursing); 4,410 periodical subscriptions (503 health-care related).

BACCALAUREATE PROGRAMS

Degree BSN

Available Programs ADN to Baccalaureate; Accelerated Baccalaureate; Accelerated Baccalaureate for Second Degree; Baccalaureate for Second Degree; Generic Baccalaureate; RN Baccalaureate.

Site Options *Distance Learning:* Rome, GA.

Study Options Full-time and part-time.

Program Entrance Requirements Minimum overall college GPA of 2.7, transcript of college record, CPR certification, health exam, health insurance, 2 years high school math, 2 years high school science, high school transcript, immunizations, interview, 1 letter of recommendation, minimum high school GPA of 2.5, minimum GPA in nursing prerequisites of 2.7, professional liability insurance/malpractice insurance, prerequisite course work. Transfer students are accepted. **Standardized tests** *Required:* SAT or ACT, TOEFL for international students. **Application** *Deadline:* 5/18 (freshmen), 6/30 (transfer). *Notification:* continuous (freshmen). *Application fee:* $40.

Advanced Placement Credit by examination available. Credit given for nursing courses completed elsewhere dependent upon specific evaluations.

Expenses (2006–07) *Tuition, state resident:* full-time $2536; part-time $107 per credit hour. *Tuition, nonresident:* full-time $10,144; part-time $423 per credit hour. *Room and board:* room only: $5700 per academic year. *Required fees:* full-time $489.

Financial Aid 60% of baccalaureate students in nursing programs received some form of financial aid in 2005–06. *Gift aid (need-based):* Federal Pell, FSEOG, state, private, college/university gift aid from institutional funds. *Loans:* Federal Nursing Student Loans, FFEL (Subsidized and Unsubsidized Stafford PLUS), Perkins, state. *Work-Study:* Federal Work-Study. *Application deadline (priority):* 4/1.

Contact Fran Herzig, Admissions Coordinator, School of Nursing, Kennesaw State University, 1000 Chastain Road, Kennesaw, GA 30144. *Telephone:* 770-499-3211. *Fax:* 770-423-6627. *E-mail:* fpaul@kennesaw.edu.

GRADUATE PROGRAMS

Financial Aid 50% of graduate students in nursing programs received some form of financial aid in 2005–06.

Contact Dr. Regina Dorman, Coordinator, School of Nursing, Kennesaw State University, 1000 Chastain Road, Kennesaw, GA 30144. *Telephone:* 770-423-6061. *Fax:* 770-423-6627. *E-mail:* gdorman@ksumail.kennesaw.edu.

MASTER'S DEGREE PROGRAM

Degree MSN

Available Programs Master's.

Concentrations Available *Clinical nurse specialist programs in:* adult health. *Nurse practitioner programs in:* adult health, family health, primary care.

Study Options Full-time.

Program Entrance Requirements Clinical experience, minimum overall college GPA of 3.0, transcript of college record, CPR certification, written essay, immunizations, 2 letters of recommendation, nursing research course, physical assessment course, professional liability insurance/malpractice insurance, prerequisite course work, resume.

Advanced Placement Credit given for nursing courses completed elsewhere dependent upon specific evaluations.

Degree Requirements 40 total credit hours, thesis or project.

Contact Dr. Vanice Wise Roberts, Associate Dean, School of Nursing, Kennesaw State University, 1000 Chastain Road, #1601, Kennesaw, GA 30144. *Telephone:* 770-423-6064. *Fax:* 770-423-6627. *E-mail:* vroberts@kennesaw.edu.

See full description on page 500.

LaGrange College
Department of Nursing
LaGrange, Georgia

http://www.lagrange.edu

Founded in 1831

DEGREE • BSN

Nursing Program Faculty 6 (20% with doctorates).

Baccalaureate Enrollment 65
Women 90% **Men** 10% **Minority** 20%

Nursing Student Activities Nursing Honor Society, Student Nurses' Association.

Nursing Student Resources Academic advising; academic or career counseling; assistance for students with disabilities; bookstore; campus computer network; career placement assistance; computer lab; computer-assisted instruction; e-mail services; employment services for current students; externships; interactive nursing skills videos; Internet; learning resource lab; library services; nursing audiovisuals; paid internships; placement services for program completers; remedial services; resume preparation assistance; skills, simulation, or other laboratory; tutoring; unpaid internships.

Library Facilities 108,389 volumes (19,000 in health, 10,000 in nursing); 512 periodical subscriptions (100 health-care related).

BACCALAUREATE PROGRAMS

Degree BSN

Available Programs Generic Baccalaureate; RN Baccalaureate.

Study Options Full-time.

Program Entrance Requirements Minimum overall college GPA of 2.5, transcript of college record, CPR certification, written essay, health exam, health insurance, immunizations, interview, 2 letters of recommendation, minimum GPA in nursing prerequisites of 2.5, professional liability insurance/malpractice insurance, prerequisite course work. Transfer students are accepted. **Standardized tests** *Required:* SAT or ACT, TOEFL for international students. **Application** *Deadline:* 8/30 (freshmen), 8/15 (transfer). *Notification:* continuous (freshmen). *Application fee:* $20.

Advanced Placement Credit given for nursing courses completed elsewhere dependent upon specific evaluations.

Expenses (2006–07) *Tuition:* full-time $8626. *Room and board:* $7100 per academic year. *Required fees:* full-time $1050.

Financial Aid 95% of baccalaureate students in nursing programs received some form of financial aid in 2005–06.

Contact Dr. Celia G. Hay, RN, Chair, Department of Nursing, LaGrange College, 601 Broad Street, LaGrange, GA 30240-2999. *Telephone:* 706-880-8220. *Fax:* 706-880-8029. *E-mail:* chay@lagrange.edu.

Macon State College
Division of Nursing and Health Sciences
Macon, Georgia

Founded in 1968

DEGREE • BSN

Nursing Program Faculty 24 (16% with doctorates).

Baccalaureate Enrollment 28

Nursing Student Activities Sigma Theta Tau, Student Nurses' Association.

Macon State College (continued)

Nursing Student Resources Academic advising; academic or career counseling; assistance for students with disabilities; bookstore; campus computer network; career placement assistance; computer lab; computer-assisted instruction; e-mail services; externships; interactive nursing skills videos; Internet; learning resource lab; library services; nursing audiovisuals; resume preparation assistance; skills, simulation, or other laboratory; tutoring.

Library Facilities 80,000 volumes; 513 periodical subscriptions.

BACCALAUREATE PROGRAMS

Degree BSN

Available Programs ADN to Baccalaureate.

Site Options *Distance Learning:* Warner Robins, GA.

Program Entrance Requirements Standardized tests *Required:* SAT or ACT, TOEFL for international students. *Required for some:* SAT Subject Tests. **Application** *Deadline:* rolling (freshmen), rolling (transfer). *Notification:* continuous (freshmen). *Application fee:* $20.

Expenses (2006–07) *Tuition, state resident:* full-time $1280; part-time $107 per credit hour. *Tuition, nonresident:* full-time $5121; part-time $427 per credit hour. *Required fees:* full-time $1000; part-time $1000 per credit.

Financial Aid 50% of baccalaureate students in nursing programs received some form of financial aid in 2005–06.

Contact Dr. Rebecca Corvey, Division Chair, Nursing and Health Sciences, Division of Nursing and Health Sciences, Macon State College, 100 College Station Drive, Macon, GA 31206-5145. *Telephone:* 478-471-2734. *Fax:* 478-471-2787. *E-mail:* rcorvey@mail.maconstate.edu.

Medical College of Georgia
School of Nursing
Augusta, Georgia

http://www.mcg.edu/son

Founded in 1828

DEGREES • BSN • MSN • PHD

Nursing Program Faculty 77 (49% with doctorates).

Baccalaureate Enrollment 339
Women 92% **Men** 8% **Minority** 14%

Graduate Enrollment 136
Women 77% **Men** 23% **Minority** 14% **Part-time** 40%

Nursing Student Activities Sigma Theta Tau, Student Nurses' Association, nursing club.

Nursing Student Resources Academic advising; academic or career counseling; assistance for students with disabilities; bookstore; campus computer network; career placement assistance; computer lab; computer-assisted instruction; daycare for children of students; e-mail services; employment services for current students; externships; housing assistance; interactive nursing skills videos; Internet; learning resource lab; library services; nursing audiovisuals; paid internships; remedial services; skills, simulation, or other laboratory; tutoring.

Library Facilities 164,138 volumes (178,650 in health, 14,650 in nursing); 2,429 periodical subscriptions (1,307 health-care related).

BACCALAUREATE PROGRAMS

Degree BSN

Available Programs ADN to Baccalaureate; Generic Baccalaureate; RN Baccalaureate.

Site Options *Distance Learning:* Athens, GA; Barnesville, GA; Columbus, GA.

Study Options Full-time.

Program Entrance Requirements Minimum overall college GPA of 2.8, transcript of college record, CPR certification, written essay, immunizations, 2 letters of recommendation, prerequisite course work. Transfer students are accepted. **Standardized tests** *Required:* TOEFL for international students. **Application** *Application fee:* $30.

Expenses (2006–07) *Tuition, state resident:* full-time $1910; part-time $160 per credit hour. *Tuition, nonresident:* full-time $7640; part-time $637 per credit hour. *Room and board:* room only: $1500 per academic year. *Required fees:* full-time $532.

Contact Office of Academic Admissions, School of Nursing, Medical College of Georgia, AA-170 Kelly Building, Augusta, GA 30912. *Telephone:* 706-721-2725. *Fax:* 706-721-0186. *E-mail:* underadm@mail.mcg.edu.

GRADUATE PROGRAMS

Expenses (2006–07) *Tuition, state resident:* full-time $2293; part-time $192 per credit hour. *Tuition, nonresident:* full-time $9169; part-time $765 per credit hour. *Required fees:* full-time $1000.

Contact Director, Academic Admissions, School of Nursing, Medical College of Georgia, AA-170 Kelly Building, Augusta, GA 30912. *Telephone:* 706-721-2725. *Fax:* 706-721-0186. *E-mail:* gradadm@mail.mcg.edu.

MASTER'S DEGREE PROGRAM

Degree MSN

Available Programs Accelerated Master's for Non-Nursing College Graduates; Master's; RN to Master's.

Concentrations Available Nurse anesthesia. *Clinical nurse specialist programs in:* acute care, adult health, critical care. *Nurse practitioner programs in:* family health, pediatric.

Site Options *Distance Learning:* Athens, GA; Columbus, GA.

Study Options Full-time and part-time.

Program Entrance Requirements Clinical experience, minimum overall college GPA of 3.0, transcript of college record, written essay, interview, 3 letters of recommendation, physical assessment course, professional liability insurance/malpractice insurance, statistics course.

Degree Requirements 36 total credit hours.

POST-MASTER'S PROGRAM

Areas of Study Nurse anesthesia. *Nurse practitioner programs in:* family health.

DOCTORAL DEGREE PROGRAM

Degree PhD

Available Programs Doctorate; Post-Baccalaureate Doctorate.

Areas of Study Bio-behavioral research, nursing research.

Program Entrance Requirements Clinical experience, minimum overall college GPA of 3.2, interview by faculty committee, interview, 3 letters of recommendation, MSN or equivalent, scholarly papers, statistics course, vita, writing sample.

Degree Requirements 60 total credit hours, dissertation, oral exam, written exam.

See full description on page 512.

North Georgia College & State University
Department of Nursing
Dahlonega, Georgia

Founded in 1873

DEGREES • BSN • MS

Nursing Program Faculty 42 (19% with doctorates).

Baccalaureate Enrollment 59
Women 93% **Men** 7% **Minority** 24% **Part-time** 46%

Graduate Enrollment 58
Women 90% **Men** 10% **Minority** 9% **Part-time** 3%

Nursing Student Activities Nursing Honor Society, Student Nurses' Association.

Nursing Student Resources Academic advising; academic or career counseling; assistance for students with disabilities; bookstore; campus computer network; career placement assistance; computer lab; computer-assisted instruction; e-mail services; interactive nursing skills videos; Internet; learning resource lab; library services; nursing audiovisuals; remedial services; resume preparation assistance; skills, simulation, or other laboratory; tutoring.

Library Facilities 146,888 volumes (6,665 in health, 619 in nursing); 2,548 periodical subscriptions (2,377 health-care related).

BACCALAUREATE PROGRAMS

Degree BSN

Available Programs RN Baccalaureate.

Study Options Full-time and part-time.

Program Entrance Requirements Minimum overall college GPA of 2.5, transcript of college record, CPR certification, health exam, health insurance, high school biology, high school chemistry, high school foreign language, 3 years high school math, 2 years high school science, high school transcript, immunizations, 2 letters of recommendation, professional liability insurance/malpractice insurance, prerequisite course work, RN licensure. Transfer students are accepted. **Standardized tests** *Required:* SAT or ACT, TOEFL for international students. **Application** *Deadline:* 7/1 (freshmen), rolling (transfer). *Notification:* continuous (freshmen). *Application fee:* $25.

Expenses (2006–07) *Tuition, state resident:* full-time $2560; part-time $107 per credit hour. *Tuition, nonresident:* full-time $10,242; part-time $427 per credit hour. *International tuition:* $10,242 full-time. *Room and board:* $2390; room only: $1192 per academic year. *Required fees:* full-time $892; part-time $446 per term.

Financial Aid 90% of baccalaureate students in nursing programs received some form of financial aid in 2005–06.

Contact Mrs. Nancy Stahl, RN, Coordinator, BSN Program, Department of Nursing, North Georgia College & State University, 82 College Circle, Dahlonega, GA 30597. *Telephone:* 706-864-1937. *Fax:* 706-864-1845. *E-mail:* nstahl@ngcsu.edu.

GRADUATE PROGRAMS

Expenses (2006–07) *Tuition, state resident:* full-time $3044; part-time $127 per credit hour. *Tuition, nonresident:* full-time $12,172; part-time $508 per credit hour. *International tuition:* $12,172 full-time. *Room and board:* $2390; room only: $1192 per academic year. *Required fees:* full-time $892; part-time $446 per term.

Financial Aid 100% of graduate students in nursing programs received some form of financial aid in 2005–06.

Contact Dr. Grace Newsome, Coordinator, MS Program, Department of Nursing, North Georgia College & State University, 82 College Circle, Dahlonega, GA 30597. *Telephone:* 706-864-1489. *Fax:* 706-864-1845. *E-mail:* gnewsome@ngsu.edu.

MASTER'S DEGREE PROGRAM

Degree MS

Available Programs Master's.

Concentrations Available Nursing education. *Nurse practitioner programs in:* family health.

Study Options Full-time and part-time.

Program Entrance Requirements Clinical experience, computer literacy, minimum overall college GPA of 2.75, transcript of college record, CPR certification, written essay, immunizations, interview, 3 letters of recommendation, nursing research course, physical assessment course, professional liability insurance/malpractice insurance, prerequisite course work.

Degree Requirements 46 total credit hours, thesis or project, comprehensive exam.

POST-MASTER'S PROGRAM

Areas of Study Nursing education. *Nurse practitioner programs in:* family health.

Piedmont College

School of Nursing
Demorest, Georgia

http://www.piedmont.edu/schools/index.html#nursing

Founded in 1897

DEGREE • BSN

Nursing Program Faculty 7 (12% with doctorates).

Baccalaureate Enrollment 50
Women 98% **Men** 2% **Minority** 10% **International** 1% **Part-time** 20%

Nursing Student Activities Nursing Honor Society, Student Nurses' Association.

Nursing Student Resources Academic advising; academic or career counseling; assistance for students with disabilities; bookstore; campus computer network; career placement assistance; computer lab; computer-assisted instruction; e-mail services; externships; housing assistance; interactive nursing skills videos; Internet; learning resource lab; library services; nursing audiovisuals; other; paid internships; resume preparation assistance; skills, simulation, or other laboratory; tutoring.

Library Facilities 115,400 volumes (3,000 in health, 500 in nursing); 365 periodical subscriptions (75 health-care related).

BACCALAUREATE PROGRAMS

Degree BSN

Available Programs Generic Baccalaureate; RN Baccalaureate.

Study Options Full-time.

Program Entrance Requirements Transcript of college record, CPR certification, health exam, health insurance, high school foreign language, 2 years high school math, 3 years high school science, high school transcript, immunizations, minimum GPA in nursing prerequisites of 3.0, professional liability insurance/malpractice insurance, prerequisite course work. Transfer students are accepted. **Standardized tests** *Required:* SAT or ACT, TOEFL for international students. **Application** *Deadline:* 7/1 (freshmen), 7/1 (transfer).

Advanced Placement Credit given for nursing courses completed elsewhere dependent upon specific evaluations.

Expenses (2006–07) *Tuition:* full-time $15,500; part-time $646 per credit hour. *International tuition:* $15,500 full-time. *Room and board:* $5000; room only: $5000 per academic year. *Required fees:* part-time $646 per credit; part-time $7750 per term.

Financial Aid 90% of baccalaureate students in nursing programs received some form of financial aid in 2005–06. *Gift aid (need-based):* Federal Pell, FSEOG, state, private, college/university gift aid from institutional funds. *Loans:* Federal Direct (Subsidized and Unsubsidized Stafford PLUS), state. *Work-Study:* Federal Work-Study, part-time campus jobs. *Application deadline (priority):* 5/1.

Contact Dr. Linda Scott, Dean, School of Nursing, Piedmont College, 165 Central Avenue, Demorest, GA 30535. *Telephone:* 706-776-0116. *Fax:* 706-778-0701. *E-mail:* lscott@piedmont.edu.

Thomas University

Division of Nursing
Thomasville, Georgia

http://www.thomasu.edu/nursing.htm

Founded in 1950

DEGREES • BSN • MSN

Nursing Program Faculty 5 (40% with doctorates).

Baccalaureate Enrollment 28
Women 80% **Men** 20% **Minority** 30%

Graduate Enrollment 12

Nursing Student Activities Nursing club.

Nursing Student Resources Academic advising; academic or career counseling; assistance for students with disabilities; bookstore; campus computer network; career placement assistance; computer lab; computer-assisted instruction; e-mail services; housing assistance; interactive nursing skills videos; Internet; library services; nursing audiovisuals; resume preparation assistance; skills, simulation, or other laboratory; tutoring.

Library Facilities 61,096 volumes (600 in health, 200 in nursing); 408 periodical subscriptions (30 health-care related).

BACCALAUREATE PROGRAMS

Degree BSN

Available Programs ADN to Baccalaureate; RN Baccalaureate.

Site Options Tallahassee, FL.

Study Options Full-time.

Thomas University (continued)

Program Entrance Requirements Minimum overall college GPA of 2.5, transcript of college record, CPR certification, health exam, health insurance, immunizations, professional liability insurance/malpractice insurance, prerequisite course work, RN licensure. Transfer students are accepted. **Standardized tests** *Required:* TOEFL for international students. **Application** *Deadline:* rolling (freshmen), rolling (transfer). *Notification:* continuous (freshmen). *Application fee:* $25.

Advanced Placement Credit given for nursing courses completed elsewhere dependent upon specific evaluations.

Financial Aid *Gift aid (need-based):* Federal Pell, FSEOG, state, private, college/university gift aid from institutional funds. *Loans:* FFEL (Subsidized and Unsubsidized Stafford PLUS), state, alternative loans. *Work-Study:* Federal Work-Study. *Application deadline:* Continuous.

Contact Kerri Knight, Assistant Director of Admissions, Division of Nursing, Thomas University, 1501 Millpond Road, Thomasville, GA 31792-7490. *Telephone:* 229-226-1621 Ext. 174. *Fax:* 229-226-1653. *E-mail:* kknight@thomasu.edu.

GRADUATE PROGRAMS

Contact Adrienne Diggs, Assistant Director of Admissions, Division of Nursing, Thomas University, 1501 Millpond Road, Thomasville, GA 31792. *Telephone:* 229-226-1621 Ext. 127. *E-mail:* adiggs@thomasu.edu.

MASTER'S DEGREE PROGRAM

Degree MSN

Available Programs Master's; Master's for Nurses with Non-Nursing Degrees.

Concentrations Available Nursing administration; nursing education.

Study Options Full-time and part-time.

Program Entrance Requirements Computer literacy, minimum overall college GPA of 2.8, transcript of college record, CPR certification, written essay, immunizations, 3 letters of recommendation, professional liability insurance/malpractice insurance, resume, statistics course.

Degree Requirements 36 total credit hours, thesis or project.

POST-MASTER'S PROGRAM

Areas of Study Nursing administration; nursing education.

University of Phoenix–Atlanta Campus
College of Health and Human Services
Atlanta, Georgia

DEGREES • BSN • MSN

Nursing Program Faculty 38 (18% with doctorates).

Baccalaureate Enrollment 12
Women 100% **Minority** 41.67%

Nursing Student Resources Academic advising; academic or career counseling; assistance for students with disabilities; bookstore; library services.

Library Facilities 444 volumes; 666 periodical subscriptions.

BACCALAUREATE PROGRAMS

Degree BSN

Available Programs Accelerated Baccalaureate.

Site Options Duluth, GA; Marietta, GA; Alpharetta, GA.

Study Options Full-time.

Program Entrance Requirements Transcript of college record, 1 letter of recommendation, RN licensure. Transfer students are accepted. **Standardized tests** *Required:* TOEFL for international students. **Application** *Deadline:* rolling (freshmen), rolling (transfer). *Application fee:* $110.

Advanced Placement Credit by examination available. Credit given for nursing courses completed elsewhere dependent upon specific evaluations.

Expenses (2006–07) *Tuition:* full-time $11,010. *International tuition:* $11,010 full-time. *Required fees:* full-time $750.

Contact Campus College Chair, Nursing. *Telephone:* 678-731-0555. *Fax:* 678-731-9666.

GRADUATE PROGRAMS

Expenses (2006–07) *Tuition:* full-time $10,560. *International tuition:* $10,560 full-time. *Required fees:* full-time $760.

Contact Campus College Chair, Nursing. *Telephone:* 678-731-0555. *Fax:* 678-731-9666.

MASTER'S DEGREE PROGRAM

Degree MSN

Available Programs Accelerated Master's.

Site Options Duluth, GA; Marietta, GA; Alpharetta, GA.

Study Options Full-time.

Program Entrance Requirements Clinical experience, transcript of college record. *Application deadline:* Applications are processed on a rolling basis. *Application fee:* $100.

Advanced Placement Credit given for nursing courses completed elsewhere dependent upon specific evaluations.

Degree Requirements 39 total credit hours, thesis or project.

University of West Georgia
Department of Nursing
Carrollton, Georgia

http://www.westga.edu/~nurs/
Founded in 1933

DEGREES • BSN • MSN

Nursing Program Faculty 28 (39% with doctorates).

Baccalaureate Enrollment 205
Women 87% **Men** 13% **Minority** 20% **International** .01% **Part-time** 59%
Graduate Enrollment 26
Women 100% **Minority** 12% **Part-time** 24%

Nursing Student Activities Sigma Theta Tau, Student Nurses' Association.

Nursing Student Resources Academic advising; academic or career counseling; assistance for students with disabilities; bookstore; campus computer network; career placement assistance; computer lab; computer-assisted instruction; e-mail services; employment services for current students; externships; housing assistance; interactive nursing skills videos; Internet; learning resource lab; library services; nursing audiovisuals; placement services for program completers; remedial services; resume preparation assistance; skills, simulation, or other laboratory; tutoring.

Library Facilities 563,677 volumes (9,029 in health, 651 in nursing); 14,884 periodical subscriptions (92 health-care related).

BACCALAUREATE PROGRAMS

Degree BSN

Available Programs Generic Baccalaureate; RN Baccalaureate.

Site Options Newnan, GA. *Distance Learning:* Rome, GA; Dalton, GA.

Study Options Full-time and part-time.

Program Entrance Requirements Minimum overall college GPA of 2.75, transcript of college record, CPR certification, health exam, health insurance, immunizations, minimum GPA in nursing prerequisites of 2.75, professional liability insurance/malpractice insurance, prerequisite course work. Transfer students are accepted. **Standardized tests** *Required:* SAT or ACT, TOEFL for international students. **Application** *Deadline:* 7/1 (freshmen), 7/1 (transfer). *Notification:* continuous until 9/1 (freshmen). *Application fee:* $20.

Advanced Placement Credit given for nursing courses completed elsewhere dependent upon specific evaluations.

Expenses (2006–07) *Tuition, state resident:* full-time $2881; part-time $963 per semester. *Tuition, nonresident:* full-time $11,523; part-time $2562 per semester. *International tuition:* $11,523 full-time. *Room and board:* $5922; room only: $3110 per academic year. *Required fees:* full-time $1200; part-time $27 per credit; part-time $240 per term.

Financial Aid 74% of baccalaureate students in nursing programs received some form of financial aid in 2005–06. *Gift aid (need-based):* Federal Pell, FSEOG, state, private, college/university gift aid from institutional funds. *Loans:* Federal Direct (Subsidized and Unsubsidized Stafford PLUS), Perkins, state, college/university. *Work-Study:* Federal Work-Study, part-time campus jobs. *Application deadline (priority):* 4/1.

Contact Dr. Kathryn Mary Grams, RN, Chair and Professor, Department of Nursing, University of West Georgia, 1601 Maple Street, Carrollton, GA 30118. *Telephone:* 678-839-5624. *Fax:* 678-839-6553. *E-mail:* kgrams@westga.edu.

GRADUATE PROGRAMS

Expenses (2006–07) *Tuition, state resident:* full-time $3044; part-time $127 per credit hour. *Tuition, nonresident:* full-time $12,172; part-time $508 per credit hour. *International tuition:* $12,172 full-time. *Room and board:* $6632; room only: $4070 per academic year. *Required fees:* full-time $1100; part-time $27 per credit; part-time $209 per term.

Financial Aid 19% of graduate students in nursing programs received some form of financial aid in 2005–06.

Contact Dr. Laurie Taylor, RN, Coordinator of Graduate Program and Professor, Department of Nursing, University of West Georgia, 1601 Maple Street, Carrollton, GA 30118. *Telephone:* 678-839-5631. *Fax:* 678-839-6553. *E-mail:* ltaylor@westga.edu.

MASTER'S DEGREE PROGRAM

Degree MSN

Available Programs Master's.

Concentrations Available Nursing administration; nursing education.

Study Options Full-time and part-time.

Program Entrance Requirements Clinical experience, computer literacy, minimum overall college GPA of 3.0, transcript of college record, CPR certification, immunizations, 3 letters of recommendation, nursing research course, professional liability insurance/malpractice insurance, prerequisite course work, resume, statistics course.

Degree Requirements 36 total credit hours, thesis or project, comprehensive exam.

POST-MASTER'S PROGRAM

Areas of Study Nursing administration; nursing education.

Valdosta State University
College of Nursing
Valdosta, Georgia

http://www.valdosta.edu/nursing/

Founded in 1906

DEGREES • BSN • MSN

Nursing Program Faculty 23 (52% with doctorates).

Baccalaureate Enrollment 183
Women 87% **Men** 13% **Minority** 21% **International** 1% **Part-time** 7%

Graduate Enrollment 25
Women 99% **Men** 1% **Minority** 15% **International** 1% **Part-time** 49%

Nursing Student Activities Sigma Theta Tau, Student Nurses' Association.

Nursing Student Resources Academic advising; academic or career counseling; assistance for students with disabilities; bookstore; campus computer network; career placement assistance; computer lab; computer-assisted instruction; e-mail services; employment services for current students; externships; housing assistance; Internet; learning resource lab; library services; nursing audiovisuals; placement services for program completers; resume preparation assistance; skills, simulation, or other laboratory; tutoring; unpaid internships.

Library Facilities 467,560 volumes (21,688 in health); 2,815 periodical subscriptions (75 health-care related).

BACCALAUREATE PROGRAMS

Degree BSN

Available Programs Generic Baccalaureate; RN Baccalaureate.

Site Options *Distance Learning:* Kings Bay, GA; Tifton, GA; Waycross, GA.

Study Options Full-time.

Program Entrance Requirements Minimum overall college GPA of 2.8, transcript of college record, CPR certification, health exam, health insurance, immunizations, minimum GPA in nursing prerequisites of 2.8, professional liability insurance/malpractice insurance, prerequisite course work. Transfer students are accepted. **Standardized tests** *Required:* SAT or ACT, TOEFL for international students. *Required for some:* SAT and SAT Subject Tests or ACT, SAT Subject Tests. **Application** *Deadline:* 7/1 (freshmen), 8/1 (transfer). *Notification:* continuous (freshmen). *Application fee:* $20.

Advanced Placement Credit given for nursing courses completed elsewhere dependent upon specific evaluations.

Contact *Telephone:* 229-333-5959. *Fax:* 229-333-7300.

GRADUATE PROGRAMS

Contact *Telephone:* 229-333-5959. *Fax:* 229-333-7300.

MASTER'S DEGREE PROGRAM

Degree MSN

Available Programs Master's; RN to Master's.

Concentrations Available Nurse case management; nursing administration; nursing education. *Clinical nurse specialist programs in:* adult health, family health, psychiatric/mental health.

Site Options *Distance Learning:* Kings Bay, GA; Tifton, GA; Waycross, GA.

Study Options Full-time and part-time.

Program Entrance Requirements Minimum overall college GPA of 2.8, transcript of college record, CPR certification, immunizations, 3 letters of recommendation, physical assessment course, professional liability insurance/malpractice insurance, statistics course, GRE General Test. *Application deadline:* For fall admission, 7/1; for spring admission, 11/15. Applications are processed on a rolling basis. *Application fee:* $20.

Advanced Placement Credit given for nursing courses completed elsewhere dependent upon specific evaluations.

Degree Requirements 36 total credit hours, thesis or project, comprehensive exam.

CONTINUING EDUCATION PROGRAM

Contact *Telephone:* 229-333-5960.

GUAM

University of Guam
College of Nursing and Health Sciences
Mangilao, Guam

http://www.uog.edu/cnhs/index.html

Founded in 1952

DEGREE • BSN

Nursing Program Faculty 10 (30% with doctorates).

Baccalaureate Enrollment 175
Women 97% **Men** 3% **International** 2%

Nursing Student Activities Student Nurses' Association.

Nursing Student Resources Academic advising; academic or career counseling; assistance for students with disabilities; bookstore; campus computer network; career placement assistance; computer lab; daycare for children of students; e-mail services; employment services for current students; interactive nursing skills videos; Internet; learning resource lab; library services; nursing audiovisuals; remedial services; skills, simulation, or other laboratory; tutoring.

Library Facilities 386,539 volumes (5,246 in health, 982 in nursing); 2,276 periodical subscriptions (53 health-care related).

University of Guam (continued)
BACCALAUREATE PROGRAMS
Degree BSN

Available Programs ADN to Baccalaureate; Generic Baccalaureate; RN Baccalaureate.

Study Options Full-time and part-time.

Program Entrance Requirements Transcript of college record, CPR certification, written essay, health exam, high school biology, high school chemistry, 1 year of high school math, 1 year of high school science, high school transcript, immunizations, interview, minimum high school GPA of 2.5, minimum GPA in nursing prerequisites of 2.7, prerequisite course work. Transfer students are accepted. **Application** *Deadline:* 6/1 (freshmen), 6/1 (transfer). *Notification:* continuous (freshmen). *Application fee:* $49.

Advanced Placement Credit by examination available. Credit given for nursing courses completed elsewhere dependent upon specific evaluations.

Contact *Telephone:* 671-735-2210. *Fax:* 671-734-4245.

HAWAII

Hawai'i Pacific University
School of Nursing
Honolulu, Hawaii

http://www.hpu.edu
Founded in 1965

DEGREES • BSN • MSN • MSN/MBA

Nursing Program Faculty 93 (13% with doctorates).

Baccalaureate Enrollment 1,521
Women 86% **Men** 14% **Minority** 74% **International** 4% **Part-time** 32%

Graduate Enrollment 37
Women 92% **Men** 8% **Minority** 49% **Part-time** 27%

Nursing Student Activities Nursing Honor Society, Sigma Theta Tau, Student Nurses' Association.

Nursing Student Resources Academic advising; academic or career counseling; assistance for students with disabilities; bookstore; campus computer network; career placement assistance; computer lab; computer-assisted instruction; e-mail services; employment services for current students; externships; housing assistance; Internet; learning resource lab; library services; paid internships; placement services for program compl-eters; resume preparation assistance; tutoring.

Library Facilities 162,000 volumes (5,587 in health, 1,950 in nursing); 12,000 periodical subscriptions (1,033 health-care related).

■ Hawai'i Pacific University's B.S.N. program offers hands-on experiences in both classroom and clinical settings in which multicultural nursing is an everyday opportunity. Students are accepted directly into the nursing major when they apply to the University but must achieve a minimum 2.75 GPA in courses required for the major before progressing into nursing courses. In the sophomore year, HPU students begin their clinical experiences. Small clinical laboratories (8–10 students) utilize health-care facilities all over the island of Oahu for clinical experiences. The M.S.N. is available to registered nurses and offers three concentrations: community clinical nurse specialist (CNS) studies, community clinical nurse specialist educator option (CNS), and family nurse practitioner (FNP) studies. Hawai'i Pacific's B.S.N. and M.S.N. programs are accredited by the National League for Nursing Accrediting Commission and approved by the State of Hawai'i Board of Nursing.

BACCALAUREATE PROGRAMS
Degree BSN

Available Programs Accelerated Baccalaureate; Generic Baccalaureate; International Nurse to Baccalaureate; LPN to Baccalaureate; RN Baccalaureate.

Site Options Kailua, Kaneohe, Honolulu, Aiea, Kahuku, Wahiawa, HI.

Study Options Full-time and part-time.

Program Entrance Requirements Minimum overall college GPA of 2.75, transcript of college record, 2 years high school math, 2 years high school science, high school transcript, minimum high school GPA of 2.75. Transfer students are accepted. **Standardized tests** *Required:* SAT or ACT. *Recommended:* TOEFL for international students. **Application** *Deadline:* rolling (freshmen), rolling (transfer). *Application fee:* $50.

Advanced Placement Credit given for nursing courses completed elsewhere dependent upon specific evaluations.

Expenses (2006–07) *Tuition:* full-time $17,400; part-time $725 per credit hour. *International tuition:* $17,400 full-time. *Room and board:* $9840 per academic year.

Financial Aid 60% of baccalaureate students in nursing programs received some form of financial aid in 2005–06. *Gift aid (need-based):* Federal Pell, FSEOG, state, private, college/university gift aid from institutional funds. *Loans:* Federal Nursing Student Loans, FFEL (Subsidized and Unsubsidized Stafford PLUS), Perkins. *Work-Study:* Federal Work-Study. *Application deadline (priority):* 3/1.

Contact Miss Sara Sato, Director of Admissions, School of Nursing, Hawai'i Pacific University, 1164 Bishop Street, Honolulu, HI 96813. *Telephone:* 808-544-0238. *Fax:* 808-544-1136. *E-mail:* ssato@hpu.edu.

GRADUATE PROGRAMS
Expenses (2006–07) *Tuition:* full-time $9360; part-time $520 per credit. *International tuition:* $9360 full-time. *Room and board:* $9840 per academic year.

Financial Aid 50% of graduate students in nursing programs received some form of financial aid in 2005–06. Career-related internships or fieldwork, Federal Work-Study, scholarships, and traineeships available. Aid available to part-time students. *Financial aid application deadline:* 3/1.

Contact Dr. Dale Allison, Coordinator for Nursing Graduate Program, School of Nursing, Hawai'i Pacific University, 45-045 Kamehameha Highway, Kaneohe, HI 96744-5297. *Telephone:* 808-236-5852. *Fax:* 808-236-5818. *E-mail:* dallison@hpu.edu.

MASTER'S DEGREE PROGRAM
Degrees MSN; MSN/MBA

Available Programs Master's.

Concentrations Available *Clinical nurse specialist programs in:* community health. *Nurse practitioner programs in:* community health, family health.

Study Options Full-time and part-time.

Program Entrance Requirements Clinical experience, minimum overall college GPA of 3.0, transcript of college record, CPR certification, written essay, immunizations, 2 letters of recommendation, nursing research course, physical assessment course, professional liability insurance/malpractice insurance, resume, statistics course. *Application deadline:* Applications are processed on a rolling basis. *Application fee:* $50.

Advanced Placement Credit given for nursing courses completed elsewhere dependent upon specific evaluations.

Degree Requirements 48 total credit hours, thesis or project.

POST-MASTER'S PROGRAM
Areas of Study Nursing education. *Clinical nurse specialist programs in:* family health.

See full description on page 492.

University of Hawaii at Hilo
Department in Nursing
Hilo, Hawaii

http://www.uhh.hawaii.edu
Founded in 1970

DEGREE • BSN

Nursing Program Faculty 11 (27% with doctorates).

Baccalaureate Enrollment 53

Women 97% **Men** 3% **Minority** 75% **International** 2% **Part-time** 6%

Nursing Student Activities Sigma Theta Tau, Student Nurses' Association, nursing club.

Nursing Student Resources Academic advising; academic or career counseling; assistance for students with disabilities; bookstore; campus computer network; career placement assistance; computer lab; computer-assisted instruction; daycare for children of students; e-mail services; employment services for current students; externships; housing assistance; Internet; learning resource lab; library services; nursing audiovisuals; remedial services; resume preparation assistance; skills, simulation, or other laboratory; tutoring; unpaid internships.

Library Facilities 250,000 volumes; 2,500 periodical subscriptions (15,000 health-care related).

BACCALAUREATE PROGRAMS

Degree BSN

Available Programs ADN to Baccalaureate; Generic Baccalaureate; RN Baccalaureate.

Site Options *Distance Learning:* Lihue, HI; Kahalui, HI; Kona, HI.

Study Options Full-time.

Program Entrance Requirements Minimum overall college GPA of 2.7, transcript of college record, CPR certification, written essay, health exam, health insurance, 4 years high school math, 3 years high school science, high school transcript, immunizations, 2 letters of recommendation, minimum high school GPA of 3.0, minimum GPA in nursing prerequisites of 3.0, professional liability insurance/malpractice insurance, prerequisite course work. **Standardized tests** *Required:* SAT or ACT. *Recommended:* TOEFL for international students. **Application** *Deadline:* 7/1 (freshmen), 7/1 (transfer). *Notification:* 7/31 (freshmen). *Application fee:* $50.

Expenses (2006–07) *Required fees:* full-time $1000; part-time $500 per term.

Financial Aid 65% of baccalaureate students in nursing programs received some form of financial aid in 2005–06. *Gift aid (need-based):* Federal Pell, FSEOG, state, private, college/university gift aid from institutional funds. *Loans:* FFEL (Subsidized and Unsubsidized Stafford PLUS), Perkins, state. *Work-Study:* Federal Work-Study, part-time campus jobs. *Application deadline (priority):* 3/1.

Contact Dr. Katharyn Daub, Chair, Department in Nursing, University of Hawaii at Hilo, 200 West Kawili Street, UCB 239, Hilo, HI 96720. *Telephone:* 808-974-7760. *Fax:* 808-974-7665. *E-mail:* katharyn@hawaii.edu.

University of Hawaii at Manoa
School of Nursing and Dental Hygiene
Honolulu, Hawaii

http://www.nursing.hawaii.edu

Founded in 1907

DEGREES • BS • MS • PHD

Nursing Student Activities Nursing Honor Society, Sigma Theta Tau, Student Nurses' Association, nursing club.

Nursing Student Resources Academic advising; academic or career counseling; assistance for students with disabilities; bookstore; computer lab; computer-assisted instruction; e-mail services; employment services for current students; housing assistance; Internet; learning resource lab; library services; nursing audiovisuals; resume preparation assistance; skills, simulation, or other laboratory.

Library Facilities 3.2 million volumes; 27,328 periodical subscriptions.

BACCALAUREATE PROGRAMS

Degree BS

Available Programs ADN to Baccalaureate; Generic Baccalaureate; RN Baccalaureate.

Site Options *Distance Learning:* Lihue, HI; Kailua Kona, HI; Kahului, HI.

Study Options Full-time and part-time.

Program Entrance Requirements Minimum overall college GPA of 2.5, transcript of college record, CPR certification, health exam, health insurance, immunizations, minimum GPA in nursing prerequisites of 2.5, professional liability insurance/malpractice insurance, prerequisite course work. Transfer students are accepted. **Standardized tests** *Required:* SAT or ACT, TOEFL for international students. **Application** *Deadline:* 5/1 (freshmen), 5/1 (transfer). *Notification:* continuous (freshmen). *Application fee:* $50.

Advanced Placement Credit by examination available. Credit given for nursing courses completed elsewhere dependent upon specific evaluations.

Contact Katherine Thompson, Academic Advisor, School of Nursing and Dental Hygiene, University of Hawaii at Manoa, 2528 McCarthy Mall, Honolulu, HI 96822. *Telephone:* 808-956-8939. *Fax:* 808-956-5977. *E-mail:* nursing@hawaii.edu.

GRADUATE PROGRAMS

Financial Aid 1 research assistantship (averaging $16,284 per year) was awarded.

Contact Dr. Jillian Inouye, Graduate Chair, School of Nursing and Dental Hygiene, University of Hawaii at Manoa, 2528 McCarthy Mall, Honolulu, HI 96822. *Telephone:* 808-956-5326. *Fax:* 808-956-5296. *E-mail:* jinouye@hawaii.edu.

MASTER'S DEGREE PROGRAM

Degree MS

Available Programs Master's.

Concentrations Available Health-care administration; nursing education. *Clinical nurse specialist programs in:* psychiatric/mental health. *Nurse practitioner programs in:* adult health, family health, gerontology, primary care.

Site Options *Distance Learning:* Kailua Kona, HI; Kahului, HI.

Study Options Full-time and part-time.

Program Entrance Requirements Minimum overall college GPA of 3.0, transcript of college record, CPR certification, written essay, immunizations, interview, 2 letters of recommendation, nursing research course, professional liability insurance/malpractice insurance, resume, statistics course. *Application deadline:* For fall admission, 3/1; for spring admission, 10/1. *Application fee:* $50.

Advanced Placement Credit given for nursing courses completed elsewhere dependent upon specific evaluations.

Degree Requirements 52 total credit hours.

POST-MASTER'S PROGRAM

Areas of Study Health-care administration. *Clinical nurse specialist programs in:* psychiatric/mental health. *Nurse practitioner programs in:* adult health, family health, gerontology, pediatric, women's health.

DOCTORAL DEGREE PROGRAM

Degree PhD

Available Programs Doctorate.

Areas of Study Faculty preparation, nursing education, nursing research, nursing science.

Program Entrance Requirements Clinical experience, minimum overall college GPA of 3.0, interview by faculty committee, interview, 3 letters of recommendation, MSN or equivalent, scholarly papers, statistics course, vita, writing sample. *Application deadline:* For fall admission, 3/1; for spring admission, 10/1. *Application fee:* $50.

Degree Requirements 46 total credit hours, dissertation, oral exam, residency.

University of Phoenix–Hawaii Campus
College of Health and Human Services
Honolulu, Hawaii

DEGREES • BSN • MSN

Nursing Program Faculty 51 (18% with doctorates).

University of Phoenix–Hawaii Campus (continued)
Baccalaureate Enrollment 21
Women 85.71% **Men** 14.29% **Minority** 23.81%
Graduate Enrollment 33
Women 78.79% **Men** 21.21% **Minority** 30.3%
Nursing Student Activities Sigma Theta Tau.

Nursing Student Resources Academic advising; academic or career counseling; assistance for students with disabilities; bookstore; computer lab; library services.

BACCALAUREATE PROGRAMS

Degree BSN

Available Programs Accelerated Baccalaureate; LPN to Baccalaureate.
Site Options Maui, HI; Mililani, HI; Kapolei, HI.
Study Options Full-time.
Program Entrance Requirements Transcript of college record, 1 letter of recommendation, RN licensure. Transfer students are accepted.
Standardized tests *Required:* TOEFL for international students. **Application** *Deadline:* rolling (freshmen), rolling (transfer). *Application fee:* $110.
Advanced Placement Credit by examination available. Credit given for nursing courses completed elsewhere dependent upon specific evaluations.
Expenses (2006–07) *Tuition:* full-time $11,700. *International tuition:* $11,700 full-time. *Required fees:* full-time $750.
Contact Campus College Chair, Nursing, College of Health and Human Services, University of Phoenix–Hawaii Campus, 827 Fort Street, Hololulu, HI 96813-4317. *Telephone:* 808-536-2686.

GRADUATE PROGRAMS

Expenses (2006–07) *Tuition:* full-time $11,520. *International tuition:* $11,520 full-time. *Required fees:* full-time $760.
Contact Campus College Chair, Nursing, College of Health and Human Services, University of Phoenix–Hawaii Campus, 827 Fort Street, Hololulu, HI 96813-4317. *Telephone:* 808-536-2686.

MASTER'S DEGREE PROGRAM

Degree MSN

Available Programs Master's.
Concentrations Available Health-care administration; nursing administration; nursing education. *Nurse practitioner programs in:* family health.
Site Options Maui, HI; Mililani, HI; Kapolei, HI.
Study Options Full-time.
Program Entrance Requirements Clinical experience, computer literacy, minimum overall college GPA of 2.5, transcript of college record. *Application deadline:* Applications are processed on a rolling basis. *Application fee:* $110.
Advanced Placement Credit given for nursing courses completed elsewhere dependent upon specific evaluations.
Degree Requirements 39 total credit hours, thesis or project.

POST-MASTER'S PROGRAM

Areas of Study *Nurse practitioner programs in:* family health.

IDAHO

Boise State University
Department of Nursing
Boise, Idaho

http://nursing.boisestate.edu
Founded in 1932
DEGREES • BS • MS • MSN/MS
Nursing Program Faculty 40 (20% with doctorates).

Baccalaureate Enrollment 475
Women 90% **Men** 10% **International** 1%
Nursing Student Activities Nursing Honor Society, Sigma Theta Tau, Student Nurses' Association.

Nursing Student Resources Academic advising; academic or career counseling; assistance for students with disabilities; bookstore; campus computer network; career placement assistance; computer lab; computer-assisted instruction; daycare for children of students; e-mail services; employment services for current students; housing assistance; interactive nursing skills videos; Internet; learning resource lab; library services; nursing audiovisuals; placement services for program completers; remedial services; resume preparation assistance; skills, simulation, or other laboratory; tutoring.

Library Facilities 675,000 volumes; 5,000 periodical subscriptions.

BACCALAUREATE PROGRAMS

Degree BS

Available Programs Generic Baccalaureate; LPN to Baccalaureate; RN Baccalaureate.
Site Options *Distance Learning:* Nampa, ID.
Study Options Full-time.
Program Entrance Requirements Transcript of college record, CPR certification, health exam, health insurance, immunizations, minimum GPA in nursing prerequisites, professional liability insurance/malpractice insurance, RN licensure. Transfer students are accepted. **Standardized tests** *Required:* TOEFL for international students. *Required for some:* SAT or ACT.
Application *Deadline:* 7/12 (freshmen), 7/12 (transfer). *Notification:* continuous (freshmen). *Application fee:* $30.
Advanced Placement Credit by examination available. Credit given for nursing courses completed elsewhere dependent upon specific evaluations.
Contact Pat Taylor, Associate Chair of Student Affairs, Department of Nursing, Boise State University, 1910 University Drive, Boise, ID 83725-0399. *Telephone:* 208-426-3783. *Fax:* 208-426-1370. *E-mail:* ptaylor@boisestate.edu.

GRADUATE PROGRAMS

Contact Dr. Ingrid Brudenell, Associate Chair of Graduate Studies, Department of Nursing, Boise State University, 1910 University Drive, Boise, ID 83725. *Telephone:* 208-426-3789. *E-mail:* ibruden@boisestate.edu.

MASTER'S DEGREE PROGRAM

Degrees MS; MSN/MS
Available Programs Master's.
Study Options Part-time.
Program Entrance Requirements Transcript of college record, CPR certification, written essay, letters of recommendation, nursing research course, professional liability insurance/malpractice insurance, prerequisite course work, resume, statistics course.
Degree Requirements 39 total credit hours, thesis or project.

Idaho State University
Department of Nursing
Pocatello, Idaho

Founded in 1901
DEGREES • BSN • MS
Nursing Program Faculty 25 (60% with doctorates).
Baccalaureate Enrollment 230
Women 89% **Men** 11% **Minority** 5%
Graduate Enrollment 70
Women 90% **Men** 10% **Minority** 2% **Part-time** 40%
Nursing Student Activities Sigma Theta Tau, Student Nurses' Association.

Nursing Student Resources Academic advising; assistance for students with disabilities; bookstore; campus computer network; computer lab; computer-assisted instruction; daycare for children of students; e-mail services; employment services for current students; interactive nursing skills videos; Internet; learning resource lab; library services; nursing audiovisuals; skills, simulation, or other laboratory; tutoring.

Library Facilities 1.2 million volumes (500 in health, 35 in nursing); 444 periodical subscriptions (3,391 health-care related).

BACCALAUREATE PROGRAMS

Degree BSN

Available Programs ADN to Baccalaureate; Accelerated Baccalaureate for Second Degree; Generic Baccalaureate; LPN to Baccalaureate.

Site Options *Distance Learning:* Boise, ID; Twin Falls, ID.

Study Options Full-time.

Program Entrance Requirements Transcript of college record, CPR certification, health exam, health insurance, high school transcript, immunizations, minimum high school GPA of 2.0, minimum GPA in nursing prerequisites of 3.0, prerequisite course work. Transfer students are accepted. **Standardized tests** *Required:* SAT or ACT, TOEFL for international students. *Recommended:* ACT. **Application** *Deadline:* 8/1 (freshmen), 8/1 (transfer). *Notification:* 3/1 (freshmen). *Application fee:* $40.

Advanced Placement Credit given for nursing courses completed elsewhere dependent upon specific evaluations.

Expenses (2006–07) *Tuition, area resident:* full-time $2095; part-time $214 per credit hour. *Tuition, nonresident:* full-time $6230; part-time $332 per credit hour. *International tuition:* $12,460 full-time. *Required fees:* full-time $930.

Financial Aid 75% of baccalaureate students in nursing programs received some form of financial aid in 2005–06. *Gift aid (need-based):* Federal Pell, FSEOG, state, private. *Loans:* Federal Direct (Subsidized and Unsubsidized Stafford PLUS), Perkins. *Work-Study:* Federal Work-Study, part-time campus jobs. *Application deadline:* Continuous.

Contact Dr. Diana McLaughlin, RN, Associate Chair, Undergraduate Studies, Department of Nursing, Idaho State University, Campus Box 8101, Pocatello, ID 83209. *Telephone:* 208-236-2152. *Fax:* 208-236-4476. *E-mail:* mcladian@isu.edu.

GRADUATE PROGRAMS

Expenses (2006–07) *Tuition, state resident:* full-time $5860; part-time $251 per credit hour. *Tuition, nonresident:* full-time $14,130; part-time $369 per credit hour. *International tuition:* $14,130 full-time. *Required fees:* full-time $930.

Financial Aid 35% of graduate students in nursing programs received some form of financial aid in 2005–06. 2 teaching assistantships with full and partial tuition reimbursements available (averaging $8,276 per year) were awarded; research assistantships, career-related internships or fieldwork, Federal Work-Study, scholarships, traineeships, and unspecified assistantships also available. Aid available to part-time students. *Financial aid application deadline:* 1/1.

Contact Dr. Susan Steiner, Associate Chair, Graduate Studies, Department of Nursing, Idaho State University, 921 South 8th Avenue, Stop 8101, Pocatello, ID 83209-8101. *Telephone:* 208-282-5278. *Fax:* 208-282-4476. *E-mail:* steisus2@isu.edu.

MASTER'S DEGREE PROGRAM

Degree MS

Available Programs Accelerated AD/RN to Master's; Master's.

Concentrations Available Nursing administration; nursing education. *Clinical nurse specialist programs in:* adult health. *Nurse practitioner programs in:* family health.

Study Options Full-time and part-time.

Program Entrance Requirements Minimum overall college GPA of 3.0, transcript of college record, interview, 3 letters of recommendation, nursing research course, physical assessment course, professional liability insurance/malpractice insurance, prerequisite course work, statistics course, GRE General Test. *Application deadline:* For fall admission, 7/1 (priority date); for spring admission, 12/1 (priority date). Applications are processed on a rolling basis. *Application fee:* $35.

Advanced Placement Credit given for nursing courses completed elsewhere dependent upon specific evaluations.

Degree Requirements 44 total credit hours, comprehensive exam.

POST-MASTER'S PROGRAM

Areas of Study Nursing administration; nursing education. *Clinical nurse specialist programs in:* adult health. *Nurse practitioner programs in:* family health.

Lewis-Clark State College
Division of Nursing and Health Sciences
Lewiston, Idaho

http://www.lcsc.edu/Nurdiv/

Founded in 1893

DEGREE • BSN

Nursing Program Faculty 22 (36% with doctorates).

Baccalaureate Enrollment 203
Women 86% **Men** 14% **Minority** 3% **International** .4% **Part-time** 41%

Nursing Student Activities Student Nurses' Association, nursing club.

Nursing Student Resources Academic advising; academic or career counseling; assistance for students with disabilities; bookstore; campus computer network; career placement assistance; computer lab; computer-assisted instruction; daycare for children of students; e-mail services; employment services for current students; housing assistance; interactive nursing skills videos; Internet; learning resource lab; library services; nursing audiovisuals; remedial services; resume preparation assistance; skills, simulation, or other laboratory; tutoring; unpaid internships.

Library Facilities 139,499 volumes (19,920 in health, 5,101 in nursing); 1,612 periodical subscriptions (12,058 health-care related).

BACCALAUREATE PROGRAMS

Degree BSN

Available Programs ADN to Baccalaureate; Generic Baccalaureate; LPN to Baccalaureate; RN Baccalaureate.

Site Options *Distance Learning:* Coeur d'Alene, ID.

Study Options Full-time.

Program Entrance Requirements Minimum overall college GPA of 2.5, transcript of college record, CPR certification, health exam, health insurance, high school biology, high school chemistry, high school transcript, immunizations, 2 letters of recommendation, minimum high school GPA of 2.0, minimum GPA in nursing prerequisites of 2.0, professional liability insurance/malpractice insurance, prerequisite course work. Transfer students are accepted. **Standardized tests** *Required:* TOEFL for international students. *Required for some:* SAT or ACT, ACT COMPASS. **Application** *Deadline:* rolling (freshmen), rolling (transfer). *Notification:* continuous (freshmen). *Application fee:* $35.

Advanced Placement Credit by examination available. Credit given for nursing courses completed elsewhere dependent upon specific evaluations.

Contact *Telephone:* 208-792-2250. *Fax:* 208-792-2062.

CONTINUING EDUCATION PROGRAM

Contact *Telephone:* 208-792-2250. *Fax:* 208-792-2062.

Northwest Nazarene University
School of Health and Science
Nampa, Idaho

Founded in 1913

DEGREE • BSN

Nursing Program Faculty 7 (40% with doctorates).

Baccalaureate Enrollment 77
Women 95% **Men** 5% **Minority** 5%

Nursing Student Activities Student Nurses' Association, nursing club.

Nursing Student Resources Academic advising; academic or career counseling; assistance for students with disabilities; bookstore; campus computer network; computer lab; computer-assisted instruction; e-mail services; housing assistance; interactive nursing skills videos; Internet; learning resource lab; library services; nursing audiovisuals; remedial services; resume preparation assistance; skills, simulation, or other laboratory; tutoring; unpaid internships.

Library Facilities 100,966 volumes; 821 periodical subscriptions.

Northwest Nazarene University (continued)

BACCALAUREATE PROGRAMS

Degree BSN

Available Programs Generic Baccalaureate.

Study Options Full-time.

Program Entrance Requirements Minimum overall college GPA of 2.75, minimum GPA in nursing prerequisites of 2.75, prerequisite course work. Transfer students are accepted. **Standardized tests** *Required:* SAT or ACT, TOEFL for international students. **Application** *Deadline:* 8/8 (freshmen). *Early decision:* 12/15. *Notification:* continuous (freshmen), 1/15 (early action). *Application fee:* $25.

Advanced Placement Credit given for nursing courses completed elsewhere dependent upon specific evaluations.

Expenses (2006–07) *Tuition:* full-time $18,430; part-time $798 per credit. *Room and board:* $4860; room only: $3060 per academic year. *Required fees:* full-time $340; part-time $35 per credit.

Financial Aid 90% of baccalaureate students in nursing programs received some form of financial aid in 2005–06. *Gift aid (need-based):* Federal Pell, FSEOG, state, private, college/university gift aid from institutional funds. *Loans:* FFEL (Subsidized and Unsubsidized Stafford PLUS), Perkins, college/university. *Work-Study:* Federal Work-Study. *Application deadline (priority):* 3/1.

Contact Dr. Patricia D. Kissell, Chair, School of Health and Science, Northwest Nazarene University, 623 Holly Street, Nampa, ID 83686. *Telephone:* 208-467-8650. *Fax:* 208-467-8651. *E-mail:* nursing@nnu.edu.

ILLINOIS

Aurora University
School of Nursing
Aurora, Illinois

http://www.aurora.edu

Founded in 1893

DEGREE • BSN

Nursing Program Faculty 8 (25% with doctorates).

Baccalaureate Enrollment 104
Women 94% **Men** 6% **Minority** 35% **Part-time** 6%

Nursing Student Activities Sigma Theta Tau, Student Nurses' Association, nursing club.

Nursing Student Resources Academic advising; academic or career counseling; assistance for students with disabilities; bookstore; campus computer network; career placement assistance; computer lab; computer-assisted instruction; e-mail services; externships; interactive nursing skills videos; Internet; learning resource lab; library services; nursing audiovisuals; remedial services; resume preparation assistance; skills, simulation, or other laboratory; tutoring.

Library Facilities 115,642 volumes (5,285 in health, 86 in nursing); 748 periodical subscriptions (698 health-care related).

BACCALAUREATE PROGRAMS

Degree BSN

Available Programs Generic Baccalaureate; RN Baccalaureate.

Site Options Aurora, IL.

Study Options Full-time and part-time.

Program Entrance Requirements Minimum overall college GPA of 2.75, transcript of college record, CPR certification, written essay, health exam, health insurance, 3 years high school math, 3 years high school science, high school transcript, immunizations, interview, minimum high school GPA of 2.75, minimum high school rank 50%, minimum GPA in nursing prerequisites of 2.75, prerequisite course work. Transfer students are accepted. **Standardized tests** *Required:* TOEFL for international students. **Application** *Deadline:* rolling (freshmen), rolling (transfer). *Notification:* continuous (freshmen). *Application fee:* $25.

Advanced Placement Credit given for nursing courses completed elsewhere dependent upon specific evaluations.

Expenses (2005–06) *Tuition:* full-time $14,750. *Room and board:* $1823; room only: $1529 per academic year. *Required fees:* full-time $480; part-time $240 per credit.

Financial Aid 85% of baccalaureate students in nursing programs received some form of financial aid in 2004–05. *Gift aid (need-based):* Federal Pell, FSEOG, state, private, college/university gift aid from institutional funds. *Loans:* FFEL (Subsidized and Unsubsidized Stafford PLUS), Perkins, college/university. *Work-Study:* Federal Work-Study. *Application deadline (priority):* 4/15.

Contact Dr. Maryanne Phyllis Locklin, Director and Associate Professor, School of Nursing, Aurora University, 347 South Gladstone Avenue, Aurora, IL 60506-4892. *Telephone:* 630-844-5130. *Fax:* 630-844-7822. *E-mail:* mlocklin@aurora.edu.

Benedictine University
Department of Nursing
Lisle, Illinois

Founded in 1887

DEGREE • BSN

Nursing Program Faculty 5 (40% with doctorates).

Baccalaureate Enrollment 30
Women 90% **Men** 10% **Minority** 25% **Part-time** 100%

Nursing Student Activities Nursing Honor Society, Sigma Theta Tau.

Nursing Student Resources Academic advising; academic or career counseling; assistance for students with disabilities; bookstore; campus computer network; computer lab; computer-assisted instruction; e-mail services; interactive nursing skills videos; Internet; learning resource lab; library services; nursing audiovisuals; resume preparation assistance; skills, simulation, or other laboratory.

Library Facilities 201,190 volumes (1,350 in health, 850 in nursing); 14,177 periodical subscriptions (291 health-care related).

BACCALAUREATE PROGRAMS

Degree BSN

Available Programs Accelerated RN Baccalaureate.

Site Options College of DuPage, Glen Ellyn, IL.

Study Options Full-time and part-time.

Program Entrance Requirements Transcript of college record, RN licensure. Transfer students are accepted. **Standardized tests** *Required:* ACT, TOEFL for international students. **Application** *Deadline:* rolling (freshmen), rolling (transfer). *Notification:* continuous (freshmen). *Application fee:* $40.

Advanced Placement Credit given for nursing courses completed elsewhere dependent upon specific evaluations.

Expenses (2006–07) *Tuition:* part-time $215 per credit.

Financial Aid *Gift aid (need-based):* Federal Pell, FSEOG, state, private, college/university gift aid from institutional funds. *Loans:* FFEL (Subsidized and Unsubsidized Stafford PLUS), Perkins, alternative loans. *Work-Study:* Federal Work-Study. *Application deadline:* Continuous.

Contact Dr. Ethel C. Ragland, Department Chair, Department of Nursing, Benedictine University, 5700 College Road, Lisle, IL 60532-0900. *Telephone:* 630-829-6583. *Fax:* 630-829-6551. *E-mail:* eragland@ben.edu.

Blessing–Rieman College of Nursing
Blessing–Rieman College of Nursing
Quincy, Illinois

DEGREE • BSN

Nursing Program Faculty 18 (25% with doctorates).

Baccalaureate Enrollment 275
Women 95% **Men** 5% **Minority** 5% **Part-time** 8%
Nursing Student Activities Sigma Theta Tau, Student Nurses' Association.

Nursing Student Resources Academic advising; academic or career counseling; bookstore; campus computer network; computer lab; computer-assisted instruction; daycare for children of students; e-mail services; employment services for current students; externships; interactive nursing skills videos; Internet; learning resource lab; library services; nursing audiovisuals; paid internships; resume preparation assistance; skills, simulation, or other laboratory; tutoring.

Library Facilities 3,767 volumes in health, 3,767 volumes in nursing; 125 periodical subscriptions health-care related.

BACCALAUREATE PROGRAMS

Degree BSN

Available Programs Accelerated Baccalaureate for Second Degree; Generic Baccalaureate; LPN to Baccalaureate; RN Baccalaureate.
Study Options Full-time and part-time.
Program Entrance Requirements Minimum overall college GPA of 2.5, transcript of college record, CPR certification, health insurance, high school biology, high school chemistry, 2 years high school math, 2 years high school science, high school transcript, immunizations, minimum high school GPA of 3.0, minimum high school rank 50%, minimum GPA in nursing prerequisites of 2.5, prerequisite course work. Transfer students are accepted.
Advanced Placement Credit by examination available. Credit given for nursing courses completed elsewhere dependent upon specific evaluations.
Expenses (2006–07) *Tuition:* full-time $16,800; part-time $319 per credit hour. *International tuition:* $16,800 full-time. *Room and board:* $6550; room only: $3500 per academic year. *Required fees:* full-time $500; part-time $500 per term.
Financial Aid 99% of baccalaureate students in nursing programs received some form of financial aid in 2005–06.
Contact Ms. Kate Boster, Admission Counselor, Blessing–Rieman College of Nursing, Broadway at 11th Street, PO Box 7005, Quincy, IL 62305-7005. *Telephone:* 217-228-5520 Ext. 6949. *Fax:* 217-223-4661. *E-mail:* admissions@brcn.edu.

See full description on page 458.

Bradley University
Department of Nursing
Peoria, Illinois

http://www.bradley.edu/academics/ebs/nur/nur_index.html
Founded in 1897

DEGREES • BSN • BSC PN • MSN

Nursing Program Faculty 36 (25% with doctorates).
Baccalaureate Enrollment 325
Women 91.1% **Men** 8.9% **Minority** 13.2% **Part-time** 3%
Graduate Enrollment 50
Women 58% **Men** 42% **Minority** 14% **Part-time** 94%
Nursing Student Activities Sigma Theta Tau, Student Nurses' Association.

Nursing Student Resources Academic advising; bookstore; campus computer network; career placement assistance; computer lab; computer-assisted instruction; e-mail services; housing assistance; Internet; learning resource lab; library services; nursing audiovisuals; placement services for program completers; resume preparation assistance; skills, simulation, or other laboratory; tutoring.

Library Facilities 518,000 volumes (11,159 in health, 2,214 in nursing); 3,529 periodical subscriptions (210 health-care related).

BACCALAUREATE PROGRAMS

Degrees BSN; BSc PN

Available Programs Generic Baccalaureate; LPN to Baccalaureate; RN Baccalaureate.
Study Options Full-time and part-time.
Program Entrance Requirements Minimum overall college GPA of 2.5, transcript of college record, health exam, high school biology, high school chemistry, 3 years high school math, 3 years high school science, high school transcript, immunizations, minimum high school GPA of 2.5, minimum GPA in nursing prerequisites of 2.0. Transfer students are accepted. **Standardized tests** *Required:* SAT or ACT, TOEFL for international students. **Application** *Deadline:* rolling (freshmen). *Notification:* continuous (freshmen). *Application fee:* $35.
Advanced Placement Credit by examination available. Credit given for nursing courses completed elsewhere dependent upon specific evaluations.
Expenses (2006–07) *Tuition:* full-time $19,900; part-time $550 per credit hour. *Room and board:* $6750 per academic year.
Financial Aid 93% of baccalaureate students in nursing programs received some form of financial aid in 2005–06.
Contact Ms. Marilyn Miller, Student Records Coordinator, Department of Nursing, Bradley University, 1501 West Bradley Avenue, Peoria, IL 61625. *Telephone:* 309-677-2530. *Fax:* 309-677-2566. *E-mail:* mmiller@bradley.edu.

GRADUATE PROGRAMS

Expenses (2006–07) *Tuition:* part-time $565 per credit hour. *Room and board:* $6750 per academic year.
Financial Aid 93% of graduate students in nursing programs received some form of financial aid in 2005–06. 3 research assistantships with full and partial tuition reimbursements available (averaging $5,060 per year) were awarded; scholarships, tuition waivers (partial), and unspecified assistantships also available. *Financial aid application deadline:* 4/1.
Contact Ms. Marilyn Miller, Student Records Coordinator, Department of Nursing, Bradley University, 1501 West Bradley Avenue, Peoria, IL 61625. *Telephone:* 309-677-2530. *Fax:* 309-677-2527. *E-mail:* mmiller@bradley.edu.

MASTER'S DEGREE PROGRAM

Degree MSN

Available Programs Accelerated Master's for Nurses with Non-Nursing Degrees; Master's.
Concentrations Available Nurse anesthesia; nursing administration.
Site Options Decatur, IL.
Study Options Full-time and part-time.
Program Entrance Requirements Clinical experience, minimum overall college GPA of 3.0, transcript of college record, interview, 3 letters of recommendation, nursing research course, physical assessment course, prerequisite course work, resume, statistics course, GRE General Test or MAT. *Application deadline:* For fall admission, 5/15 (priority date); for spring admission, 10/15 (priority date). Applications are processed on a rolling basis. *Application fee:* $40 ($50 for international students).
Advanced Placement Credit given for nursing courses completed elsewhere dependent upon specific evaluations.
Degree Requirements Thesis or project, comprehensive exam.

Chicago State University
College of Nursing and Allied Health Professions
Chicago, Illinois

http://www.csu.edu
Founded in 1867

DEGREE • BSN

Nursing Program Faculty 23 (60% with doctorates).
Baccalaureate Enrollment 372
Women 90% **Men** 10% **Minority** 97% **International** 15% **Part-time** 24%
Nursing Student Activities Nursing Honor Society, Student Nurses' Association.

Chicago State University (continued)

Nursing Student Resources Academic advising; academic or career counseling; assistance for students with disabilities; bookstore; campus computer network; computer lab; computer-assisted instruction; daycare for children of students; e-mail services; employment services for current students; externships; interactive nursing skills videos; Internet; learning resource lab; library services; nursing audiovisuals; remedial services; resume preparation assistance; skills, simulation, or other laboratory; tutoring; unpaid internships.

Library Facilities 320,000 volumes; 1,539 periodical subscriptions.

BACCALAUREATE PROGRAMS

Degree BSN

Available Programs Generic Baccalaureate; LPN to Baccalaureate; RN Baccalaureate.

Site Options *Distance Learning:* Chicago, IL.

Study Options Full-time.

Program Entrance Requirements Minimum overall college GPA of 2.5, transcript of college record, written essay, health exam, health insurance, 3 years high school math, 3 years high school science, high school transcript, immunizations, interview, 3 letters of recommendation, minimum GPA in nursing prerequisites of 2.5, professional liability insurance/malpractice insurance, prerequisite course work. Transfer students are accepted. **Standardized tests** *Required:* TOEFL for international students. *Recommended:* SAT or ACT. **Application** *Notification:* continuous (freshmen). *Application fee:* $25.

Advanced Placement Credit by examination available.

Contact *Telephone:* 773-995-3992. *Fax:* 773-821-2438.

DePaul University
Department of Nursing
Chicago, Illinois

http://www.depaul.edu/~nursing

Founded in 1898

DEGREES • BS • MS

Nursing Program Faculty 19 (89% with doctorates).

Baccalaureate Enrollment 5

Graduate Enrollment 131

Women 87% **Men** 13% **Minority** 23% **Part-time** 35%

Nursing Student Activities Sigma Theta Tau, Student Nurses' Association.

Nursing Student Resources Academic advising; academic or career counseling; assistance for students with disabilities; bookstore; campus computer network; computer lab; computer-assisted instruction; e-mail services; employment services for current students; externships; housing assistance; interactive nursing skills videos; Internet; learning resource lab; library services; nursing audiovisuals; resume preparation assistance; skills, simulation, or other laboratory; tutoring.

Library Facilities 897,564 volumes; 28,514 periodical subscriptions (193 health-care related).

BACCALAUREATE PROGRAMS

Degree BS

Available Programs Accelerated RN Baccalaureate.

Study Options Full-time and part-time.

Program Entrance Requirements Minimum overall college GPA of 2.5, transcript of college record, CPR certification, health exam, immunizations, professional liability insurance/malpractice insurance, RN licensure. Transfer students are accepted. **Standardized tests** *Required:* SAT or ACT, TOEFL for international students. **Application** *Deadline:* rolling (freshmen), rolling (transfer). *Early decision:* 11/15. *Notification:* 10/15 (freshmen), 1/1 (early action). *Application fee:* $40.

Advanced Placement Credit given for nursing courses completed elsewhere dependent upon specific evaluations.

Contact *Telephone:* 773-325-7280. *Fax:* 773-325-7282.

GRADUATE PROGRAMS

Contact *Telephone:* 773-325-7280. *Fax:* 773-325-7282.

MASTER'S DEGREE PROGRAM

Degree MS

Available Programs Master's; Master's for Non-Nursing College Graduates; Master's for Nurses with Non-Nursing Degrees; RN to Master's.

Concentrations Available Nurse anesthesia; nurse case management; nursing administration; nursing education. *Clinical nurse specialist programs in:* community health, medical-surgical. *Nurse practitioner programs in:* adult health, community health, family health, pediatric, women's health.

Study Options Full-time and part-time.

Program Entrance Requirements Computer literacy, minimum overall college GPA of 2.75, transcript of college record, CPR certification, physical assessment course, professional liability insurance/malpractice insurance, prerequisite course work, statistics course, GRE. *Application fee:* $25.

Advanced Placement Credit given for nursing courses completed elsewhere dependent upon specific evaluations.

Degree Requirements 52 total credit hours, thesis or project.

POST-MASTER'S PROGRAM

Areas of Study Nurse anesthesia. *Nurse practitioner programs in:* adult health, community health, family health, pediatric, women's health.

Elmhurst College
Deicke Center for Nursing Education
Elmhurst, Illinois

Founded in 1871

DEGREE • BSN

Nursing Program Faculty 8 (50% with doctorates).

Library Facilities 222,441 volumes (6,000 in health); 2,010 periodical subscriptions (80 health-care related).

BACCALAUREATE PROGRAMS

Degree BSN

Available Programs Generic Baccalaureate; RN Baccalaureate.

Study Options Full-time.

Program Entrance Requirements Minimum overall college GPA of 2.75, transcript of college record, CPR certification, immunizations, minimum GPA in nursing prerequisites of 2.0, prerequisite course work. Transfer students are accepted. **Standardized tests** *Required:* SAT or ACT, TOEFL for international students. **Application** *Deadline:* 7/15 (freshmen). *Notification:* continuous (freshmen). *Application fee:* $25.

Advanced Placement Credit given for nursing courses completed elsewhere dependent upon specific evaluations.

Contact *Telephone:* 630-617-3344. *Fax:* 630-617-3237.

Governors State University
Division of Nursing, Communication Disorders, Occupational Therapy, and Physical Therapy
University Park, Illinois

http://www.govst.edu/nursing/index.html

Founded in 1969

DEGREES • BS • MS

Nursing Program Faculty 7 (85% with doctorates).

Baccalaureate Enrollment 31

Women 98% **Men** 2% **Minority** 92% **International** 1% **Part-time** 100%

Graduate Enrollment 72

Women 97% **Men** 3% **Minority** 89% **International** 6% **Part-time** 4%

Nursing Student Activities Sigma Theta Tau.

Nursing Student Resources Academic advising; assistance for students with disabilities; bookstore; campus computer network; computer lab; daycare for children of students; e-mail services; Internet; learning resource lab; library services; nursing audiovisuals; tutoring.

Library Facilities 260,000 volumes; 2,200 periodical subscriptions.

BACCALAUREATE PROGRAMS

Degree BS

Available Programs RN Baccalaureate.

Study Options Part-time.

Program Entrance Requirements Transcript of college record, CPR certification, health exam, health insurance, immunizations, minimum GPA in nursing prerequisites of 2.0, professional liability insurance/malpractice insurance, prerequisite course work, RN licensure. Transfer students are accepted. **Standardized tests** *Required:* TOEFL for international students. **Application** *Deadline:* 7/15 (transfer).

Expenses (2005–06) *Tuition, state resident:* part-time $149 per credit hour. *Tuition, nonresident:* part-time $408 per credit hour.

Financial Aid *Gift aid (need-based):* Federal Pell, FSEOG, state, private, college/university gift aid from institutional funds. *Loans:* Federal Direct (Subsidized and Unsubsidized Stafford), Perkins. *Work-Study:* Federal Work-Study, part-time campus jobs. *Application deadline (priority):* 5/1.

Contact Linda McCann, Program Advisor, Division of Nursing, Communication Disorders, Occupational Therapy, and Physical Therapy, Governors State University, University Park, IL 60466-0975. *Telephone:* 708-534-4053. *Fax:* 708-534-2197. *E-mail:* l-mccann@govst.edu.

GRADUATE PROGRAMS

Expenses (2005–06) *Tuition, state resident:* part-time $157 per credit hour. *Tuition, nonresident:* part-time $471 per credit hour.

Financial Aid Research assistantships, career-related internships or fieldwork, Federal Work-Study, institutionally sponsored loans, scholarships, and tuition waivers (full and partial) available.

Contact Linda McCann, Program Advisor, Division of Nursing, Communication Disorders, Occupational Therapy, and Physical Therapy, Governors State University, University Park, IL 60466-0975. *Telephone:* 708-534-4053. *Fax:* 708-534-2197. *E-mail:* l-mccann@govst.edu.

MASTER'S DEGREE PROGRAM

Degree MS

Available Programs Master's.

Concentrations Available *Clinical nurse specialist programs in:* adult health.

Study Options Full-time and part-time.

Program Entrance Requirements Clinical experience, computer literacy, minimum overall college GPA of 3.0, transcript of college record, CPR certification, written essay, immunizations, nursing research course, physical assessment course, professional liability insurance/malpractice insurance, prerequisite course work, statistics course. *Application deadline:* Applications are processed on a rolling basis.

Degree Requirements 42 total credit hours, comprehensive exam.

POST-MASTER'S PROGRAM

Areas of Study Nursing education.

Illinois State University
Mennonite College of Nursing
Normal, Illinois

http://www.mcn.ilstu.edu

Founded in 1857

DEGREES • BSN • MSN

Nursing Program Faculty 35 (37% with doctorates).

Baccalaureate Enrollment 239

Graduate Enrollment 42

Nursing Student Activities Nursing Honor Society, Sigma Theta Tau, Student Nurses' Association.

Nursing Student Resources Academic advising; academic or career counseling; assistance for students with disabilities; bookstore; campus computer network; career placement assistance; computer lab; computer-assisted instruction; daycare for children of students; e-mail services; employment services for current students; externships; interactive nursing skills videos; Internet; learning resource lab; library services; nursing audiovisuals; placement services for program completers; resume preparation assistance; skills, simulation, or other laboratory; tutoring.

Library Facilities 1.6 million volumes (18,000 in health, 4,000 in nursing); 14,166 periodical subscriptions (700 health-care related).

BACCALAUREATE PROGRAMS

Degree BSN

Available Programs ADN to Baccalaureate; Accelerated Baccalaureate for Second Degree; Generic Baccalaureate; RN Baccalaureate.

Study Options Full-time.

Program Entrance Requirements Minimum overall college GPA of 2.7, transcript of college record, CPR certification, health exam, health insurance, immunizations, minimum GPA in nursing prerequisites of 2.0, prerequisite course work. Transfer students are accepted. **Standardized tests** *Required:* SAT or ACT, TOEFL for international students. **Application** *Deadline:* 3/1 (freshmen), rolling (transfer). *Notification:* continuous (freshmen). *Application fee:* $30.

Advanced Placement Credit given for nursing courses completed elsewhere dependent upon specific evaluations.

Expenses (2006–07) *Tuition, area resident:* full-time $4920; part-time $205 per credit hour. *Tuition, nonresident:* full-time $10,272; part-time $428 per credit hour. *Room and board:* room only: $1600 per academic year. *Required fees:* full-time $1258; part-time $52 per credit.

Financial Aid 70% of baccalaureate students in nursing programs received some form of financial aid in 2005–06. *Gift aid (need-based):* Federal Pell, FSEOG, state, private, college/university gift aid from institutional funds, Federal Nursing. *Loans:* Federal Nursing Student Loans, Federal Direct (Subsidized and Unsubsidized Stafford PLUS), Perkins, alternative loans. *Work-Study:* Federal Work-Study, part-time campus jobs. *Application deadline (priority):* 3/1.

Contact Mrs. Tenna Webb, Academic Advising Secretary, Mennonite College of Nursing, Illinois State University, 5810 Edwards Hall, Normal, IL 61790-5810. *Telephone:* 309-438-2252. *Fax:* 309-438-2620. *E-mail:* tlwebb@ilstu.edu.

GRADUATE PROGRAMS

Expenses (2006–07) *Tuition, state resident:* full-time $3330; part-time $185 per credit hour. *Tuition, nonresident:* full-time $6948; part-time $386 per credit hour. *Required fees:* full-time $944; part-time $52 per credit.

Financial Aid 56% of graduate students in nursing programs received some form of financial aid in 2005–06. 3 research assistantships (averaging $6,375 per year) were awarded; teaching assistantships.

Contact Dr. Brenda R. Jeffers, Director of Graduate Program and Research, Mennonite College of Nursing, Illinois State University, 5810 Edwards Hall, Normal, IL 61790-5810. *Telephone:* 309-438-2349. *Fax:* 309-438-2280. *E-mail:* brjeffe@ilstu.edu.

MASTER'S DEGREE PROGRAM

Degree MSN

Available Programs Master's.

Concentrations Available Nursing administration. *Nurse practitioner programs in:* family health.

Study Options Full-time and part-time.

Program Entrance Requirements Minimum overall college GPA of 3.0, transcript of college record, CPR certification, written essay, immunizations, 3 letters of recommendation, prerequisite course work, resume, statistics course. *Application fee:* $30.

Advanced Placement Credit given for nursing courses completed elsewhere dependent upon specific evaluations.

Degree Requirements 44 total credit hours.

POST-MASTER'S PROGRAM

Areas of Study Nursing education. *Nurse practitioner programs in:* family health.

See full description on page 494.

Illinois Wesleyan University
School of Nursing
Bloomington, Illinois

http://titan.iwu.edu/~nursing

Founded in 1850

DEGREE • BSN

Nursing Program Faculty 23 (44% with doctorates).

Baccalaureate Enrollment 111
Women 94% **Men** 6% **Minority** 10% **International** .01%

Nursing Student Activities Nursing Honor Society, Sigma Theta Tau, Student Nurses' Association, nursing club.

Nursing Student Resources Academic advising; academic or career counseling; assistance for students with disabilities; bookstore; campus computer network; career placement assistance; computer lab; computer-assisted instruction; e-mail services; employment services for current students; externships; housing assistance; interactive nursing skills videos; Internet; learning resource lab; library services; nursing audiovisuals; paid internships; placement services for program completers; resume preparation assistance; skills, simulation, or other laboratory; tutoring; unpaid internships.

Library Facilities 313,495 volumes (4,459 in health, 3,373 in nursing); 12,238 periodical subscriptions (266 health-care related).

BACCALAUREATE PROGRAMS

Degree BSN

Available Programs Generic Baccalaureate; RN Baccalaureate.

Study Options Full-time and part-time.

Program Entrance Requirements Minimum overall college GPA of 3.0, transcript of college record, written essay, health exam, health insurance, high school biology, high school chemistry, 2 years high school math, 2 years high school science, high school transcript, immunizations, interview, minimum high school GPA of 3.0, minimum high school rank 25%. Transfer students are accepted. **Standardized tests** *Required:* SAT or ACT, TOEFL for international students. **Application** *Notification:* continuous (freshmen), continuous (out-of-state freshmen).

Expenses (2006–07) *Tuition:* full-time $28,986. *International tuition:* $28,986 full-time. *Room and board:* $6714; room only: $4104 per academic year.

Financial Aid 89% of baccalaureate students in nursing programs received some form of financial aid in 2005–06. *Gift aid (need-based):* Federal Pell, FSEOG, state, private, college/university gift aid from institutional funds. *Loans:* Federal Nursing Student Loans, FFEL (Subsidized and Unsubsidized Stafford PLUS), Perkins, college/university. *Work-Study:* Federal Work-Study, part-time campus jobs. *Application deadline:* 3/1 (priority: 3/1).

Contact Dr. Donna L. Hartweg, Director, Caroline F. Rupert Professor of Nursing, School of Nursing, Illinois Wesleyan University, PO Box 2900, Bloomington, IL 61701-2900. *Telephone:* 309-556-3051. *Fax:* 309-556-3043. *E-mail:* dhartweg@iwu.edu.

Lakeview College of Nursing
Lakeview College of Nursing
Danville, Illinois

http://www.lakeviewcol.edu

Founded in 1987

DEGREE • BSN

Nursing Program Faculty 13.

Baccalaureate Enrollment 233
Women 87% **Men** 13% **Minority** 20% **Part-time** 8%

Nursing Student Activities Nursing Honor Society, Sigma Theta Tau, Student Nurses' Association.

Nursing Student Resources Academic advising; academic or career counseling; assistance for students with disabilities; bookstore; campus computer network; career placement assistance; computer lab; Internet; library services; nursing audiovisuals; resume preparation assistance; skills, simulation, or other laboratory; tutoring.

Library Facilities 1,500 volumes; 60 periodical subscriptions.

BACCALAUREATE PROGRAMS

Degree BSN

Available Programs Accelerated RN Baccalaureate; Generic Baccalaureate; RN Baccalaureate.

Site Options *Distance Learning:* Charleston, IL.

Study Options Full-time and part-time.

Program Entrance Requirements Minimum overall college GPA of 2.5, transcript of college record, CPR certification, written essay, health exam, immunizations, 2 letters of recommendation, prerequisite course work. Transfer students are accepted. **Application** *Deadline:* rolling (transfer). *Application fee:* $50.

Advanced Placement Credit given for nursing courses completed elsewhere dependent upon specific evaluations.

Expenses (2006–07) *Tuition:* full-time $310. *Required fees:* full-time $1870.

Financial Aid 42% of baccalaureate students in nursing programs received some form of financial aid in 2005–06.

Contact Mrs. Connie Young, Coordinator of Admissions and Records/Registrar, Lakeview College of Nursing, 903 North Logan Avenue, Danville, IL 61832. *Telephone:* 217-554-6899. *Fax:* 217-442-2279. *E-mail:* cyoung@lakeviewcol.edu.

Lewis University
Program in Nursing
Romeoville, Illinois

http://www.lewisu.edu/academics/nursing/index.htm

Founded in 1932

DEGREES • BSN • MSN • MSN/MBA

Nursing Program Faculty 25 (29% with doctorates).

Baccalaureate Enrollment 632
Women 95% **Men** 5% **Minority** 31% **International** 8% **Part-time** 69%

Graduate Enrollment 185
Women 90% **Men** 10% **Minority** 16% **International** 2%

Nursing Student Activities Sigma Theta Tau, Student Nurses' Association.

Nursing Student Resources Academic advising; academic or career counseling; assistance for students with disabilities; bookstore; campus computer network; career placement assistance; computer lab; computer-assisted instruction; e-mail services; employment services for current students; Internet; learning resource lab; library services; nursing audiovisuals; remedial services; resume preparation assistance; skills, simulation, or other laboratory; tutoring.

Library Facilities 149,870 volumes (3,100 in health, 2,038 in nursing); 1,990 periodical subscriptions (85 health-care related).

BACCALAUREATE PROGRAMS

Degree BSN

Available Programs Accelerated Baccalaureate for Second Degree; Accelerated RN Baccalaureate; Generic Baccalaureate.

Site Options Hickory Hills, IL; Oak Brook, IL; Tinley Park, IL.

Study Options Full-time.

Program Entrance Requirements Minimum overall college GPA of 2.5, transcript of college record, CPR certification, health exam, health insurance, high school transcript, immunizations, minimum high school GPA of 2.5, minimum GPA in nursing prerequisites of 2.0, prerequisite course work. Transfer students are accepted. **Standardized tests** *Required:* SAT or ACT, TOEFL for international students. **Application** *Deadline:* 8/1 (freshmen), rolling (transfer). *Application fee:* $40.

Advanced Placement Credit given for nursing courses completed elsewhere dependent upon specific evaluations.

Contact *Telephone:* 815-836-5245. *Fax:* 815-838-8306.

GRADUATE PROGRAMS

Contact *Telephone:* 815-836-5355 Ext. 5363. *Fax:* 815-838-8306.

MASTER'S DEGREE PROGRAM

Degrees MSN; MSN/MBA

Available Programs Accelerated Master's; RN to Master's.

Concentrations Available Health-care administration; nurse case management; nursing administration; nursing education. *Clinical nurse specialist programs in:* community health.

Site Options Hickory Hills, IL; Oak Brook, IL.

Study Options Full-time and part-time.

Program Entrance Requirements Clinical experience, minimum overall college GPA of 2.75, transcript of college record, CPR certification, immunizations, 3 letters of recommendation, nursing research course, professional liability insurance/malpractice insurance, prerequisite course work, resume, statistics course, GRE General Test, GRE Subject Test. *Application deadline:* Applications are processed on a rolling basis. *Application fee:* $40.

Degree Requirements 45 total credit hours, thesis or project.

POST-MASTER'S PROGRAM

Areas of Study *Clinical nurse specialist programs in:* community health.

CONTINUING EDUCATION PROGRAM

Contact *Telephone:* 815-836-5798. *Fax:* 815-838-8306.

Loyola University Chicago
Marcella Niehoff School of Nursing
Chicago, Illinois

http://www.luc.edu/schools/nursing/

Founded in 1870

DEGREES • BSN • MSN • MSN/MBA • MSN/MDIV • PHD

Nursing Program Faculty 40 (90% with doctorates).

Nursing Student Activities Nursing Honor Society, Sigma Theta Tau, Student Nurses' Association.

Library Facilities 1.4 million volumes (51,674 in health, 4,966 in nursing); 136,663 periodical subscriptions (2,630 health-care related).

BACCALAUREATE PROGRAMS

Degree BSN

Available Programs Accelerated Baccalaureate; Generic Baccalaureate; RN Baccalaureate.

Site Options Maywood, IL; Chicago, IL.

Study Options Full-time and part-time.

Program Entrance Requirements Transcript of college record, CPR certification, written essay, health exam, health insurance, high school biology, high school chemistry, 2 years high school math, high school transcript, immunizations, 2 letters of recommendation, minimum high school GPA of 3.0, minimum high school rank 25%, prerequisite course work. Transfer students are accepted. **Standardized tests** *Required:* SAT or ACT, TOEFL for international students. **Application** *Deadline:* 4/1 (freshmen), 7/1 (transfer). *Notification:* continuous (freshmen). *Application fee:* $25.

Advanced Placement Credit given for nursing courses completed elsewhere dependent upon specific evaluations.

Contact *Telephone:* 773-508-3249. *Fax:* 773-508-3241.

GRADUATE PROGRAMS

Contact *Telephone:* 773-508-3249. *Fax:* 773-508-3241.

MASTER'S DEGREE PROGRAM

Degrees MSN; MSN/MBA; MSN/MDIV

Available Programs Master's; RN to Master's.

Concentrations Available Nurse-midwifery; nursing administration. *Clinical nurse specialist programs in:* acute care, cardiovascular, oncology. *Nurse practitioner programs in:* acute care, adult health, family health, pediatric, women's health.

Site Options Maywood, IL; Chicago, IL.

Study Options Full-time and part-time.

Program Entrance Requirements Clinical experience, minimum overall college GPA of 3.0, transcript of college record, CPR certification, written essay, immunizations, interview, 3 letters of recommendation, physical assessment course, professional liability insurance/malpractice insurance, statistics course. *Application deadline:* For fall admission, 8/1 (priority date); for spring admission, 12/1 (priority date). Applications are processed on a rolling basis. *Application fee:* $40.

Advanced Placement Credit given for nursing courses completed elsewhere dependent upon specific evaluations.

Degree Requirements 48 total credit hours, comprehensive exam.

DOCTORAL DEGREE PROGRAM

Degree PhD

Available Programs Post-Baccalaureate Doctorate.

Areas of Study Ethics, nursing education, nursing research, nursing science.

Site Options Maywood, IL; Chicago, IL.

Program Entrance Requirements interview by faculty committee, interview, 3 letters of recommendation, scholarly papers, statistics course, vita, writing sample, GRE General Test. *Application deadline:* For fall admission, 8/1 (priority date); for spring admission, 12/1 (priority date). Applications are processed on a rolling basis. *Application fee:* $40.

Degree Requirements 64 total credit hours, dissertation, oral exam, written exam.

MacMurray College
Department of Nursing
Jacksonville, Illinois

http://www.mac.edu/academics/nursing.html

Founded in 1846

DEGREE • BSN

Nursing Program Faculty 7 (30% with doctorates).

Baccalaureate Enrollment 110
Women 95% **Men** 5% **Minority** 5% **Part-time** 12%

Nursing Student Activities Nursing club.

Nursing Student Resources Academic advising; academic or career counseling; assistance for students with disabilities; bookstore; campus computer network; career placement assistance; computer lab; computer-assisted instruction; e-mail services; employment services for current students; externships; interactive nursing skills videos; Internet; learning resource lab; library services; nursing audiovisuals; placement services for program completers; resume preparation assistance; skills, simulation, or other laboratory; tutoring.

Library Facilities 1.8 million volumes (1,800 in health, 1,000 in nursing); 185 periodical subscriptions (40 health-care related).

BACCALAUREATE PROGRAMS

Degree BSN

Available Programs ADN to Baccalaureate; Baccalaureate for Second Degree; Generic Baccalaureate; RN Baccalaureate.

Study Options Full-time and part-time.

Program Entrance Requirements Minimum overall college GPA of 2.5, transcript of college record, CPR certification, health exam, high school transcript, immunizations, interview, minimum high school GPA of 2.5, minimum GPA in nursing prerequisites of 2.5. Transfer students are accepted. **Standardized tests** *Required:* SAT or ACT, TOEFL for international students. **Application** *Deadline:* rolling (freshmen), rolling (transfer). *Notification:* continuous (freshmen).

Advanced Placement Credit given for nursing courses completed elsewhere dependent upon specific evaluations.

MacMurray College (continued)

Expenses (2006–07) *Tuition:* full-time $15,500. *Room and board:* $5732; room only: $2732 per academic year. *Required fees:* full-time $530.

Financial Aid 98% of baccalaureate students in nursing programs received some form of financial aid in 2005–06. *Gift aid (need-based):* Federal Pell, FSEOG, state, private, college/university gift aid from institutional funds. *Loans:* FFEL (Subsidized and Unsubsidized Stafford PLUS), Perkins. *Work-Study:* Federal Work-Study, part-time campus jobs. *Application deadline (priority):* 5/31.

Contact Devonna L. Dugan, Administrative Assistant, Department of Nursing, MacMurray College, 447 East College Avenue, Jacksonville, IL 62650. *Telephone:* 217-479-7083. *Fax:* 217-479-7078. *E-mail:* nursing.dept@mac.edu.

McKendree College
Department of Nursing
Lebanon, Illinois

Founded in 1828

DEGREES • BSN • MSN

Nursing Program Faculty 31 (60% with doctorates).

Baccalaureate Enrollment 344
Women 93% **Men** 7% **Minority** 12% **International** 1% **Part-time** 90%

Graduate Enrollment 88
Women 95.5% **Men** 4.5% **Minority** 9%

Nursing Student Activities Nursing Honor Society.

Nursing Student Resources Academic advising; academic or career counseling; assistance for students with disabilities; bookstore; campus computer network; career placement assistance; computer lab; computer-assisted instruction; e-mail services; interactive nursing skills videos; Internet; learning resource lab; library services; nursing audiovisuals; resume preparation assistance; tutoring.

Library Facilities 109,000 volumes (1,929 in health, 760 in nursing); 450 periodical subscriptions (100 health-care related).

BACCALAUREATE PROGRAMS

Degree BSN

Available Programs ADN to Baccalaureate.

Site Options Marion, IL; Belleville, IL; Louisville, KY.

Program Entrance Requirements Minimum overall college GPA of 2.0, transcript of college record, CPR certification, health exam, high school transcript, immunizations, prerequisite course work, RN licensure. Transfer students are accepted. **Standardized tests** *Required:* SAT or ACT, TOEFL for international students. **Application** *Deadline:* rolling (freshmen), rolling (transfer). *Notification:* continuous (freshmen). *Application fee:* $40.

Advanced Placement Credit given for nursing courses completed elsewhere dependent upon specific evaluations.

Expenses (2006–07) *Tuition:* part-time $245 per credit hour.

Financial Aid 90% of baccalaureate students in nursing programs received some form of financial aid in 2005–06. *Gift aid (need-based):* Federal Pell, FSEOG, state, private, college/university gift aid from institutional funds. *Loans:* FFEL (Subsidized and Unsubsidized Stafford PLUS), Perkins. *Work-Study:* Federal Work-Study, part-time campus jobs. *Application deadline (priority):* 5/31.

Contact Kim Eichelberger, Director of Nursing Admissions, Department of Nursing, McKendree College, 701 College Road, Lebanon, IL 62254. *Telephone:* 800-232-7228 Ext. 6411. *Fax:* 618-537-6259. *E-mail:* kaeichelberger@mckendree.edu.

GRADUATE PROGRAMS

Financial Aid 90% of graduate students in nursing programs received some form of financial aid in 2005–06.

Contact Kim Eichelberger, Director of Nursing Admissions, Department of Nursing, McKendree College, 701 College Road, Lebanon, IL 62254. *Telephone:* 618-537-6411. *Fax:* 618-537-6410. *E-mail:* kaeichelberger@mckendree.edu.

MASTER'S DEGREE PROGRAM

Degree MSN

Available Programs Master's; RN to Master's.

Concentrations Available Nursing administration; nursing education.

Site Options Marion, IL; Belleville, IL; Louisville, KY.

Study Options Full-time and part-time.

Program Entrance Requirements Minimum overall college GPA of 2.75, transcript of college record, CPR certification, immunizations, 3 letters of recommendation.

Advanced Placement Credit given for nursing courses completed elsewhere dependent upon specific evaluations.

Degree Requirements 33 total credit hours, thesis or project.

Millikin University
School of Nursing
Decatur, Illinois

Founded in 1901

DEGREE • BSN

Nursing Program Faculty 10 (60% with doctorates).

Baccalaureate Enrollment 210
Women 86% **Men** 14% **Minority** 19% **Part-time** 4%

Nursing Student Activities Nursing Honor Society, Student Nurses' Association.

Nursing Student Resources Academic advising; academic or career counseling; assistance for students with disabilities; bookstore; campus computer network; career placement assistance; computer lab; computer-assisted instruction; e-mail services; employment services for current students; housing assistance; interactive nursing skills videos; Internet; learning resource lab; library services; nursing audiovisuals; other; remedial services; resume preparation assistance; skills, simulation, or other laboratory; tutoring; unpaid internships.

Library Facilities 199,660 volumes (10,000 in health, 6,000 in nursing); 927 periodical subscriptions (64 health-care related).

BACCALAUREATE PROGRAMS

Degree BSN

Available Programs Accelerated RN Baccalaureate; Generic Baccalaureate.

Site Options Decatur, IL; Springfield, IL.

Study Options Full-time and part-time.

Program Entrance Requirements Minimum overall college GPA of 2.3, transcript of college record, CPR certification, written essay, health exam, high school biology, high school chemistry, 2 years high school math, 2 years high school science, high school transcript, immunizations, minimum high school GPA of 3.0, minimum high school rank 75%, minimum GPA in nursing prerequisites of 2.3. Transfer students are accepted. **Standardized tests** *Required:* SAT or ACT, TOEFL for international students. **Application** *Deadline:* rolling (freshmen). *Notification:* continuous (freshmen).

Advanced Placement Credit given for nursing courses completed elsewhere dependent upon specific evaluations.

Expenses (2005–06) *Tuition:* full-time $20,696; part-time $609 per credit hour. *Room and board:* $6613; room only: $3763 per academic year. *Required fees:* full-time $595.

Financial Aid 97% of baccalaureate students in nursing programs received some form of financial aid in 2004–05.

Contact Dr. Kathy J. Booker, RN, Dean, School of Nursing, Millikin University, 1184 West Main Street, Decatur, IL 62522. *Telephone:* 217-424-6393. *Fax:* 217-420-6731. *E-mail:* kbooker@mail.millikin.edu.

Northern Illinois University
School of Nursing
De Kalb, Illinois

http://www.nursing.niu.edu

Founded in 1895

DEGREES • BS • MS • MSN/MPH

Nursing Program Faculty 40 (52% with doctorates).

Baccalaureate Enrollment 364
Women 96% **Men** 4% **Minority** 25% **Part-time** 31%

Graduate Enrollment 122
Women 97% **Men** 3% **Minority** 21% **Part-time** 86%

Nursing Student Activities Nursing Honor Society, Sigma Theta Tau, Student Nurses' Association, nursing club.

Nursing Student Resources Academic advising; academic or career counseling; assistance for students with disabilities; bookstore; campus computer network; career placement assistance; computer lab; computer-assisted instruction; daycare for children of students; e-mail services; employment services for current students; externships; housing assistance; interactive nursing skills videos; Internet; learning resource lab; library services; nursing audiovisuals; paid internships; placement services for program completers; remedial services; resume preparation assistance; skills, simulation, or other laboratory; tutoring; unpaid internships.

Library Facilities 3.1 million volumes (39,869 in health, 7,600 in nursing); 24,696 periodical subscriptions (676 health-care related).

BACCALAUREATE PROGRAMS

Degree BS

Available Programs Generic Baccalaureate; RN Baccalaureate.

Site Options *Distance Learning:* Highland, IL; Rockford, IL; Hoffman Estates, IL.

Study Options Full-time and part-time.

Program Entrance Requirements Transcript of college record, CPR certification, health exam, health insurance, high school transcript, immunizations, minimum high school rank 50%, professional liability insurance/malpractice insurance. Transfer students are accepted. **Standardized tests** *Required:* SAT or ACT, TOEFL for international students. **Application** *Deadline:* 8/1 (freshmen), 8/1 (transfer). *Notification:* continuous (freshmen).

Advanced Placement Credit given for nursing courses completed elsewhere dependent upon specific evaluations.

Contact *Telephone:* 815-753-6557. *Fax:* 815-753-0814.

GRADUATE PROGRAMS

Contact *Telephone:* 815-753-6557. *Fax:* 815-753-0814.

MASTER'S DEGREE PROGRAM

Degrees MS; MSN/MPH

Available Programs Master's.

Concentrations Available *Clinical nurse specialist programs in:* adult health, community health. *Nurse practitioner programs in:* adult health, family health.

Site Options *Distance Learning:* Rockford, IL; Hoffman Estates, IL.

Study Options Full-time and part-time.

Program Entrance Requirements Minimum overall college GPA of 3.0, transcript of college record, CPR certification, written essay, immunizations, 2 letters of recommendation, nursing research course, physical assessment course, professional liability insurance/malpractice insurance, statistics course. *Application deadline:* For fall admission, 6/1; for spring admission, 11/1. Applications are processed on a rolling basis. *Application fee:* $30.

Degree Requirements 48 total credit hours.

POST-MASTER'S PROGRAM

Areas of Study *Nurse practitioner programs in:* family health.

North Park University
School of Nursing
Chicago, Illinois

http://www.northpark.edu
Founded in 1891

DEGREES • BS • MS • MSN/MA • MSN/MBA • MSN/MM

Nursing Program Faculty 35 (63% with doctorates).

Baccalaureate Enrollment 192
Women 90% **Men** 10% **Minority** 47% **International** 3% **Part-time** 27%

Graduate Enrollment 140
Women 93% **Men** 7% **Minority** 36% **International** .5% **Part-time** 73%

Nursing Student Activities Sigma Theta Tau, Student Nurses' Association.

Nursing Student Resources Academic advising; academic or career counseling; assistance for students with disabilities; bookstore; campus computer network; career placement assistance; computer lab; computer-assisted instruction; e-mail services; employment services for current students; interactive nursing skills videos; Internet; learning resource lab; library services; nursing audiovisuals; remedial services; skills, simulation, or other laboratory; tutoring.

Library Facilities 260,685 volumes (3,959 in health, 1,791 in nursing); 1,178 periodical subscriptions (239 health-care related).

BACCALAUREATE PROGRAMS

Degree BS

Available Programs Generic Baccalaureate; RN Baccalaureate.

Site Options Evanston, IL; Arlington Heights, IL; Grayslake, IL.

Study Options Full-time.

Program Entrance Requirements Minimum overall college GPA of 2.75, transcript of college record, CPR certification, health exam, health insurance, immunizations, 1 letter of recommendation, minimum GPA in nursing prerequisites of 2.75, prerequisite course work. Transfer students are accepted. **Standardized tests** *Required:* SAT or ACT, TOEFL for international students. **Application** *Deadline:* rolling (freshmen), rolling (transfer). *Notification:* continuous (freshmen). *Application fee:* $20.

Expenses (2006–07) *Tuition:* full-time $14,900; part-time $650 per credit hour. *Room and board:* $7050; room only: $3950 per academic year. *Required fees:* full-time $1500.

Financial Aid 92% of baccalaureate students in nursing programs received some form of financial aid in 2005–06.

Contact Mr. Robert Berki, Admissions Counselor, School of Nursing, North Park University, 3225 West Foster Avenue, Chicago, IL 60625. *Telephone:* 773-244-5516. *E-mail:* rberki@northpark.edu.

GRADUATE PROGRAMS

Expenses (2006–07) *Tuition:* part-time $565 per credit hour. *Required fees:* full-time $90.

Financial Aid 95% of graduate students in nursing programs received some form of financial aid in 2005–06.

Contact Ms. Jennifer Hulting, Assistant Director of Admissions, School of Nursing, North Park University, 3225 West Foster Avenue, Chicago, IL 60625. *Telephone:* 773-244-5508. *Fax:* 773-279-7082. *E-mail:* jhulting@northpark.edu.

MASTER'S DEGREE PROGRAM

Degrees MS; MSN/MA; MSN/MBA; MSN/MM

Available Programs Master's.

Concentrations Available Nursing administration. *Clinical nurse specialist programs in:* community health. *Nurse practitioner programs in:* adult health, family health.

Site Options Arlington Heights, IL; Grayslake, IL.

Study Options Full-time and part-time.

Program Entrance Requirements Clinical experience, minimum overall college GPA of 3.0, transcript of college record, CPR certification, immunizations, 2 letters of recommendation, nursing research course, physical assessment course, professional liability insurance/malpractice insurance, prerequisite course work, resume, statistics course.

Degree Requirements 37 total credit hours, thesis or project.

POST-MASTER'S PROGRAM

Areas of Study *Nurse practitioner programs in:* adult health, family health.

Olivet Nazarene University
Division of Nursing
Bourbonnais, Illinois

http://www.olivet.edu/academics/divisions/nursing

Founded in 1907

DEGREES • BSN • MSN

Nursing Program Faculty 10 (33% with doctorates).

Baccalaureate Enrollment 377
Women 93% **Men** 7% **Minority** 17% **International** 10%

Graduate Enrollment 8
Women 100% **Minority** 13%

Nursing Student Activities Sigma Theta Tau, nursing club.

Nursing Student Resources Academic advising; academic or career counseling; assistance for students with disabilities; bookstore; campus computer network; career placement assistance; computer lab; computer-assisted instruction; e-mail services; employment services for current students; externships; housing assistance; interactive nursing skills videos; Internet; learning resource lab; library services; nursing audiovisuals; placement services for program completers; remedial services; resume preparation assistance; skills, simulation, or other laboratory; tutoring.

Library Facilities 160,039 volumes (8,847 in health, 5,489 in nursing); 925 periodical subscriptions (722 health-care related).

BACCALAUREATE PROGRAMS
Degree BSN

Available Programs Accelerated RN Baccalaureate; Generic Baccalaureate.

Site Options Chicago, IL.

Study Options Full-time.

Program Entrance Requirements Minimum overall college GPA of 2.75, transcript of college record, CPR certification, health exam, health insurance, high school biology, high school chemistry, 2 years high school science, high school transcript, immunizations, minimum GPA in nursing prerequisites of 2.75. Transfer students are accepted. **Standardized tests** *Required:* ACT, TOEFL for international students. **Application** *Deadline:* rolling (freshmen), rolling (transfer). *Notification:* continuous (freshmen).

Expenses (2006–07) *Tuition:* full-time $16,750; part-time $698 per credit hour. *Room and board:* $6400; room only: $3200 per academic year. *Required fees:* full-time $840.

Financial Aid 98% of baccalaureate students in nursing programs received some form of financial aid in 2005–06. *Gift aid (need-based):* Federal Pell, FSEOG, state, private, college/university gift aid from institutional funds. *Loans:* FFEL (Subsidized and Unsubsidized Stafford PLUS), Perkins, alternative loans. *Work-Study:* Federal Work-Study, part-time campus jobs. *Application deadline (priority):* 3/1.

Contact Mr. Brian Parker, Director of Admissions, Division of Nursing, Olivet Nazarene University, One University Avenue, Bourbonnais, IL 60914-2345. *Telephone:* 815-939-5203. *Fax:* 815-939-5203. *E-mail:* bparker@olivet.edu.

GRADUATE PROGRAMS
Expenses (2006–07) *Tuition:* part-time $574 per credit hour. *Required fees:* full-time $650.

Financial Aid 84% of graduate students in nursing programs received some form of financial aid in 2005–06.

Contact Linda Westerberg, Division of Nursing, Olivet Nazarene University, One University Avenue, Bourbonnais, IL 60914-2345. *Telephone:* 815-939-5186. *Fax:* 815-935-4991. *E-mail:* lwester@olivet.edu.

MASTER'S DEGREE PROGRAM
Degree MSN

Available Programs Master's.

Study Options Full-time.

Program Entrance Requirements Computer literacy, minimum overall college GPA of 2.5, transcript of college record, CPR certification, immunizations, nursing research course, professional liability insurance/malpractice insurance, statistics course.

Degree Requirements 36 total credit hours, thesis or project.

Quincy University
Blessing–Rieman College of Nursing
Quincy, Illinois

http://www.quincy.edu/

See description of programs under
Blessing–Rieman College of Nursing (Quincy, Illinois).

Rockford College
Department of Nursing
Rockford, Illinois

http://www.rockford.edu

Founded in 1847

DEGREE • BSN

Nursing Program Faculty 5 (20% with doctorates).

Baccalaureate Enrollment 82
Women 91% **Men** 9% **Minority** 16% **Part-time** 14%

Nursing Student Activities Student Nurses' Association.

Nursing Student Resources Academic advising; academic or career counseling; assistance for students with disabilities; bookstore; campus computer network; career placement assistance; computer lab; computer-assisted instruction; e-mail services; employment services for current students; externships; housing assistance; interactive nursing skills videos; Internet; learning resource lab; library services; nursing audiovisuals; paid internships; placement services for program completers; remedial services; resume preparation assistance; skills, simulation, or other laboratory; tutoring.

Library Facilities 140,000 volumes (655 in health, 600 in nursing); 831 periodical subscriptions (55 health-care related).

BACCALAUREATE PROGRAMS
Degree BSN

Available Programs ADN to Baccalaureate; Generic Baccalaureate; RN Baccalaureate.

Site Options Rockford, IL.

Study Options Full-time and part-time.

Program Entrance Requirements Minimum overall college GPA of 2.75, transcript of college record, CPR certification, written essay, health exam, health insurance, high school biology, high school chemistry, 2 years high school math, 2 years high school science, high school transcript, immunizations, minimum high school GPA of 3.00, minimum high school rank 50%, minimum GPA in nursing prerequisites of 2.75, prerequisite course work. Transfer students are accepted. **Standardized tests** *Required:* SAT or ACT, TOEFL for international students. **Application** *Deadline:* 8/1 (freshmen), 8/1 (transfer). *Application fee:* $35.

Advanced Placement Credit given for nursing courses completed elsewhere dependent upon specific evaluations.

Expenses (2006–07) *Tuition:* full-time $22,950; part-time $610 per credit hour. *International tuition:* $22,950 full-time. *Room and board:* $6630; room only: $3850 per academic year. *Required fees:* part-time $30 per term.

Financial Aid 90% of baccalaureate students in nursing programs received some form of financial aid in 2005–06.

Contact Ms. Jennifer Nordstrom, Director of Admissions, Department of Nursing, Rockford College, 5050 East State Street, Rockford, IL 61108-2393. *Telephone:* 815-226-4050. *E-mail:* jnordstrom@rockford.edu.

Rush University
College of Nursing
Chicago, Illinois

http://www.rushu.rush.edu/nursing

Founded in 1969

DEGREES • BSN • MSN • PHD

Nursing Program Faculty 90 (75% with doctorates).

Baccalaureate Enrollment 194
Women 89% **Men** 11% **Minority** 27% **Part-time** 3.6%

Graduate Enrollment 363
Women 91% **Men** 9% **Minority** 15% **Part-time** 81%

Nursing Student Activities Nursing Honor Society, Sigma Theta Tau, Student Nurses' Association.

Nursing Student Resources Academic advising; academic or career counseling; assistance for students with disabilities; bookstore; campus computer network; computer lab; computer-assisted instruction; daycare for children of students; e-mail services; employment services for current students; housing assistance; interactive nursing skills videos; Internet; learning resource lab; library services; nursing audiovisuals; other; resume preparation assistance; skills, simulation, or other laboratory; tutoring.

Library Facilities 120,042 volumes; 1,100 periodical subscriptions.

BACCALAUREATE PROGRAMS

Degree BSN

Available Programs ADN to Baccalaureate; Accelerated Baccalaureate for Second Degree; Generic Baccalaureate; RN Baccalaureate.

Study Options Full-time.

Program Entrance Requirements Minimum overall college GPA of 2.75, transcript of college record, written essay, health exam, immunizations, 3 letters of recommendation, minimum GPA in nursing prerequisites of 2.75, prerequisite course work. **Standardized tests** *Required:* TOEFL for international students. **Application** *Deadline:* rolling (transfer). *Application fee:* $40.

Expenses (2006–07) *Tuition:* full-time $22,288; part-time $551 per credit hour. *Room and board:* room only: $9216 per academic year.

Financial Aid 82% of baccalaureate students in nursing programs received some form of financial aid in 2005–06.

Contact Ms. Hicela Castruita-Woods, Director of Admissions, College of Nursing, Rush University, 600 South Paulina Street, Armour Academic Center, Room 440, Chicago, IL 60612. *Telephone:* 312-942-7100. *Fax:* 312-942-2219. *E-mail:* Rush_Admissions@rush.edu.

GRADUATE PROGRAMS

Expenses (2006–07) *Tuition:* full-time $26,772; part-time $588 per credit hour. *Room and board:* room only: $9216 per academic year.

Financial Aid 60% of graduate students in nursing programs received some form of financial aid in 2005–06. 6 teaching assistantships with partial tuition reimbursements available (averaging $22,000 per year) were awarded; fellowships, research assistantships, Federal Work-Study, institutionally sponsored loans, scholarships, and traineeships also available. Aid available to part-time students. *Financial aid application deadline:* 4/15.

Contact Ms. Hicela Castruita-Woods, Director of Admissions, College of Nursing, Rush University, 600 South Paulina Street, Armour Academic Center, Room 440, Chicago, IL 60612. *Telephone:* 312-942-7100. *Fax:* 312-942-2219. *E-mail:* Rush_Admissions@rush.edu.

MASTER'S DEGREE PROGRAM

Degree MSN

Available Programs Accelerated AD/RN to Master's; Master's; Master's for Nurses with Non-Nursing Degrees; RN to Master's.

Concentrations Available Nurse anesthesia. *Clinical nurse specialist programs in:* community health, critical care, gerontology, medical-surgical, pediatric, psychiatric/mental health, public health. *Nurse practitioner programs in:* acute care, adult health, family health, gerontology, neonatal health, pediatric, psychiatric/mental health.

Study Options Full-time and part-time.

Program Entrance Requirements Minimum overall college GPA of 3.0, transcript of college record, CPR certification, written essay, immunizations, interview, 3 letters of recommendation, resume, GRE General Test (waived if nursing GPA is greater than 3.0 or cumulative GPA is greater than 3.25. *Application deadline:* For fall admission, 7/1; for winter admission, 11/1; for spring admission, 1/15. Applications are processed on a rolling basis. *Application fee:* $40.

Advanced Placement Credit given for nursing courses completed elsewhere dependent upon specific evaluations.

Degree Requirements 55 total credit hours, thesis or project.

POST-MASTER'S PROGRAM

Areas of Study Nurse anesthesia. *Clinical nurse specialist programs in:* community health, critical care, gerontology, medical-surgical, pediatric, psychiatric/mental health, public health. *Nurse practitioner programs in:* acute care, adult health, family health, gerontology, neonatal health, pediatric, psychiatric/mental health.

DOCTORAL DEGREE PROGRAM

Degree PhD

Available Programs Doctorate; Post-Baccalaureate Doctorate.

Areas of Study Addiction/substance abuse, advanced practice nursing, aging, bio-behavioral research, biology of health and illness, clinical practice, community health, critical care, ethics, family health, gerontology, health policy, health promotion/disease prevention, health-care systems, human health and illness, illness and transition, individualized study, maternity-newborn, neuro-behavior, nursing policy, nursing research, oncology, urban health, women's health.

Program Entrance Requirements Minimum overall college GPA of 3.25, interview, 3 letters of recommendation, MSN or equivalent, statistics course, vita, writing sample, GRE General Test. *Application deadline:* For fall admission, 7/1; for winter admission, 11/1; for spring admission, 1/15. Applications are processed on a rolling basis. *Application fee:* $40.

Degree Requirements 72 total credit hours, dissertation, oral exam.

POSTDOCTORAL PROGRAM

Areas of Study Aging, cancer care, chronic illness, community health, family health, gerontology, health promotion/disease prevention, individualized study, neuro-behavior, nursing interventions, nursing research, outcomes, vulnerable population, women's health.

Postdoctoral Program Contact Dr. Carol Farran, PhD Program Director, College of Nursing, Rush University, 600 South Paulina Street, 1064 AR, Chicago, IL 60612. *Telephone:* 312-942-6955. *Fax:* 312-942-3043. *E-mail:* Carol_J_Farran@rush.edu.

CONTINUING EDUCATION PROGRAM

Contact Dr. Ruth Kleinpell, College of Nursing, Rush University, 600 South Paulina Street, Suite 1080 AR, Chicago, IL 60612-3832. *Telephone:* 312-942-7117. *Fax:* 312-942-3043. *E-mail:* Ruth_Kleinpell@rush.edu.

Saint Anthony College of Nursing
Saint Anthony College of Nursing
Rockford, Illinois

http://www.sacn.edu

Founded in 1915

DEGREES • BSN • MSN

Nursing Program Faculty 21 (15% with doctorates).

Baccalaureate Enrollment 146
Women 90% **Men** 10% **Minority** 8% **Part-time** 12%

Graduate Enrollment 15

Nursing Student Activities Student Nurses' Association.

Nursing Student Resources Academic advising; academic or career counseling; campus computer network; computer lab; computer-assisted instruction; e-mail services; interactive nursing skills videos; Internet; learning resource lab; library services; paid internships; skills, simulation, or other laboratory; tutoring.

Library Facilities 1,394 volumes (48 in health, 47 in nursing); 3,136 periodical subscriptions (12 health-care related).

Saint Anthony College of Nursing (continued)

BACCALAUREATE PROGRAMS

Degree BSN

Available Programs Baccalaureate for Second Degree; Generic Baccalaureate; RN Baccalaureate.

Site Options Woodstock, IL.

Study Options Full-time and part-time.

Program Entrance Requirements Minimum overall college GPA of 2.5, transcript of college record, CPR certification, written essay, health exam, health insurance, immunizations, interview, 3 letters of recommendation, minimum GPA in nursing prerequisites of 2.7, prerequisite course work. Transfer students are accepted. **Application** *Deadline:* 8/15 (transfer). *Application fee:* $50.

Advanced Placement Credit by examination available. Credit given for nursing courses completed elsewhere dependent upon specific evaluations.

Expenses (2006–07) *Tuition:* full-time $8085; part-time $506 per credit hour. *Required fees:* full-time $285; part-time $129 per term.

Financial Aid 85% of baccalaureate students in nursing programs received some form of financial aid in 2005–06.

Contact Ms. Cheryl Delgado, Admissions Representative, Saint Anthony College of Nursing, 5658 East State Street, Rockford, IL 61108-2468. *Telephone:* 815-227-2141. *Fax:* 815-227-2730. *E-mail:* cheryldelgado@sacn.edu.

GRADUATE PROGRAMS

Expenses (2006–07) *Tuition:* part-time $600 per credit hour. *Required fees:* part-time $50 per term.

Contact Ms. Deetra S. Sallis, Graduate Affairs Representative, Saint Anthony College of Nursing, 5658 East State Street, Rockford, IL 61108-2468. *Telephone:* 815-395-5476. *Fax:* 815-227-2730. *E-mail:* deetrasallis@sacn.edu.

MASTER'S DEGREE PROGRAM

Degree MSN

Available Programs Master's.

Concentrations Available Nursing education. *Clinical nurse specialist programs in:* adult health.

Study Options Part-time.

Program Entrance Requirements Minimum overall college GPA of 2.7, transcript of college record, CPR certification, written essay, immunizations, interview, 3 letters of recommendation, professional liability insurance/malpractice insurance, prerequisite course work, resume, statistics course.

Advanced Placement Credit given for nursing courses completed elsewhere dependent upon specific evaluations.

Degree Requirements 39 total credit hours, thesis or project.

POST-MASTER'S PROGRAM

Areas of Study Nursing education.

See full description on page 528.

Saint Francis Medical Center College of Nursing
Baccalaureate Nursing Program
Peoria, Illinois

http://www.sfmccon.edu

Founded in 1986

DEGREES • BSN • MSN

Nursing Program Faculty 28 (18% with doctorates).

Baccalaureate Enrollment 270

Women 87% **Men** 13% **Minority** 7% **Part-time** 33%

Graduate Enrollment 77

Women 94% **Men** 6% **Minority** 8% **Part-time** 97%

Nursing Student Activities Nursing Honor Society, Student Nurses' Association.

Nursing Student Resources Academic advising; academic or career counseling; campus computer network; computer lab; computer-assisted instruction; e-mail services; externships; housing assistance; interactive nursing skills videos; Internet; learning resource lab; library services; nursing audiovisuals; skills, simulation, or other laboratory; tutoring.

Library Facilities 6,215 volumes (4,000 in nursing); 125 periodical subscriptions (117 health-care related).

BACCALAUREATE PROGRAMS

Degree BSN

Available Programs Generic Baccalaureate; RN Baccalaureate.

Study Options Full-time and part-time.

Program Entrance Requirements Transcript of college record, CPR certification, written essay, health exam, high school transcript, immunizations, minimum GPA in nursing prerequisites of 2.5, professional liability insurance/malpractice insurance, prerequisite course work. Transfer students are accepted. **Application** *Application fee:* $50.

Advanced Placement Credit given for nursing courses completed elsewhere dependent upon specific evaluations.

Expenses (2006–07) *Tuition:* full-time $13,200; part-time $440 per credit hour. *Room and board:* room only: $1880 per academic year. *Required fees:* full-time $220; part-time $110 per term.

Financial Aid 90% of baccalaureate students in nursing programs received some form of financial aid in 2005–06. *Gift aid (need-based):* Federal Pell, state, private, college/university gift aid from institutional funds. *Loans:* FFEL (Subsidized and Unsubsidized Stafford PLUS), college/university. *Application deadline (priority):* 3/1.

Contact Ms. Janice E. Farquharson, Director of Admissions/Registrar, Baccalaureate Nursing Program, Saint Francis Medical Center College of Nursing, 511 NE Greenleaf Street, Peoria, IL 61603-3783. *Telephone:* 309-624-8980. *Fax:* 309-624-8973. *E-mail:* janice.farquharson@osfhealthcare.org.

GRADUATE PROGRAMS

Expenses (2006–07) *Tuition:* full-time $5280; part-time $440 per credit hour. *Room and board:* room only: $1880 per academic year. *Required fees:* full-time $220; part-time $110 per term.

Financial Aid 87% of graduate students in nursing programs received some form of financial aid in 2005–06.

Contact Dr. Janice F. Boundy, Associate Dean of Graduate Program, Baccalaureate Nursing Program, Saint Francis Medical Center College of Nursing, 511 NE Greenleaf Street, Peoria, IL 61603. *Telephone:* 309-655-2230. *Fax:* 309-655-3648. *E-mail:* jan.f.boundy@osfhealthcare.org.

MASTER'S DEGREE PROGRAM

Degree MSN

Available Programs Master's; Master's for Nurses with Non-Nursing Degrees; RN to Master's.

Concentrations Available Nursing education. *Clinical nurse specialist programs in:* medical-surgical, parent-child.

Study Options Full-time and part-time.

Program Entrance Requirements Clinical experience, computer literacy, minimum overall college GPA of 2.8, transcript of college record, CPR certification, written essay, immunizations, interview, 3 letters of recommendation, nursing research course, physical assessment course, professional liability insurance/malpractice insurance, prerequisite course work, statistics course.

Advanced Placement Credit given for nursing courses completed elsewhere dependent upon specific evaluations.

Degree Requirements 45 total credit hours, thesis or project.

St. John's College
Department of Nursing
Springfield, Illinois

http://www.st-johns.org/collegeofnursing

Founded in 1886

DEGREE • BSN

Nursing Program Faculty 15 (13% with doctorates).

Baccalaureate Enrollment 81
Women 93% **Men** 7% **Minority** 4% **International** 1% **Part-time** 5%

Nursing Student Activities Student Nurses' Association.

Nursing Student Resources Academic advising; computer lab; daycare for children of students; interactive nursing skills videos; Internet; library services; resume preparation assistance; skills, simulation, or other laboratory.

Library Facilities 7,715 volumes; 349 periodical subscriptions.

BACCALAUREATE PROGRAMS

Degree BSN

Available Programs Generic Baccalaureate.

Study Options Full-time and part-time.

Program Entrance Requirements Transcript of college record, CPR certification, health exam, high school transcript, immunizations, 2 letters of recommendation, minimum GPA in nursing prerequisites of 2.4, professional liability insurance/malpractice insurance, prerequisite course work. Transfer students are accepted. **Application** *Application fee:* $35.

Advanced Placement Credit given for nursing courses completed elsewhere dependent upon specific evaluations.

Contact *Telephone:* 217-525-5628. *Fax:* 217-757-6870.

Saint Xavier University
School of Nursing
Chicago, Illinois

http://www.sxu.edu/son
Founded in 1847

DEGREES • BSN • MSN • MSN/MBA

Nursing Program Faculty 38 (53% with doctorates).

Baccalaureate Enrollment 655
Women 93% **Men** 7% **Minority** 44% **International** 1% **Part-time** 25%

Graduate Enrollment 96
Women 95% **Men** 5% **Minority** 38% **Part-time** 42%

Nursing Student Activities Nursing Honor Society, Sigma Theta Tau, Student Nurses' Association.

Nursing Student Resources Academic advising; academic or career counseling; assistance for students with disabilities; bookstore; campus computer network; career placement assistance; computer lab; computer-assisted instruction; daycare for children of students; e-mail services; employment services for current students; externships; interactive nursing skills videos; Internet; learning resource lab; library services; nursing audiovisuals; other; placement services for program completers; remedial services; resume preparation assistance; skills, simulation, or other laboratory; tutoring; unpaid internships.

Library Facilities 170,753 volumes (6,545 in health, 5,680 in nursing); 717 periodical subscriptions (2,045 health-care related).

BACCALAUREATE PROGRAMS

Degree BSN

Available Programs Generic Baccalaureate; LPN to RN Baccalaureate; RN Baccalaureate.

Site Options Orland Park, IL; Chicago, IL; Elk Grove Village, IL.

Study Options Full-time and part-time.

Program Entrance Requirements Minimum overall college GPA of 2.75, transcript of college record, CPR certification, written essay, health exam, health insurance, high school biology, high school chemistry, high school foreign language, 3 years high school math, 4 years high school science, high school transcript, immunizations, minimum high school GPA of 2.75, minimum GPA in nursing prerequisites of 2.75, prerequisite course work. Transfer students are accepted. **Standardized tests** *Required:* SAT or ACT, TOEFL for international students. **Application** *Deadline:* rolling (freshmen), rolling (transfer). *Notification:* continuous (freshmen). *Application fee:* $25.

Advanced Placement Credit by examination available. Credit given for nursing courses completed elsewhere dependent upon specific evaluations.

Expenses (2006–07) *Tuition:* full-time $19,640; part-time $658 per credit hour. *International tuition:* $19,640 full-time. *Room and board:* $7414 per academic year. *Required fees:* full-time $490; part-time $200 per term.

Financial Aid 94% of baccalaureate students in nursing programs received some form of financial aid in 2005–06. *Gift aid (need-based):* Federal Pell, FSEOG, state, private, college/university gift aid from institutional funds, United Negro College Fund, Federal Nursing. *Loans:* FFEL (Subsidized and Unsubsidized Stafford PLUS), Perkins. *Work-Study:* Federal Work-Study, part-time campus jobs. *Application deadline (priority):* 3/1.

Contact Dr. Phyllis Baker, Associate Dean, Undergraduate Nursing Program, School of Nursing, Saint Xavier University, 3700 West 103rd Street, Chicago, IL 60655. *Telephone:* 773-298-3707. *Fax:* 773-298-3704. *E-mail:* baker@sxu.edu.

GRADUATE PROGRAMS

Expenses (2006–07) *Tuition:* part-time $625 per credit hour. *Room and board:* $7442 per academic year. *Required fees:* full-time $370; part-time $140 per term.

Financial Aid 23% of graduate students in nursing programs received some form of financial aid in 2005–06. Available to part-time students.

Contact Dr. Kay Thurn, Associate Dean, Graduate Program, School of Nursing, Saint Xavier University, 3700 West 103rd Street, Chicago, IL 60655. *Telephone:* 773-298-3708. *Fax:* 773-298-3704. *E-mail:* thurn@sxu.edu.

MASTER'S DEGREE PROGRAM

Degrees MSN; MSN/MBA

Available Programs Master's; Master's for Nurses with Non-Nursing Degrees.

Concentrations Available Nursing administration. *Clinical nurse specialist programs in:* adult health. *Nurse practitioner programs in:* family health.

Site Options Orland Park, IL; Chicago, IL; Elk Grove Village, IL.

Study Options Full-time and part-time.

Program Entrance Requirements Minimum overall college GPA of 3.0, transcript of college record, written essay, interview, 2 letters of recommendation, prerequisite course work, GRE General Test or MAT. *Application deadline:* For fall admission, 2/15; for spring admission, 9/15. Applications are processed on a rolling basis. *Application fee:* $35.

Advanced Placement Credit given for nursing courses completed elsewhere dependent upon specific evaluations.

Degree Requirements 36 total credit hours.

POST-MASTER'S PROGRAM

Areas of Study Nursing education. *Nurse practitioner programs in:* family health.

CONTINUING EDUCATION PROGRAM

Contact Darlene O'Callaghan, RN, Assistant Dean, Special Projects, School of Nursing, Saint Xavier University, 3700 West 103rd Street, Chicago, IL 60655. *Telephone:* 773-298-3742. *Fax:* 773-298-3704. *E-mail:* ocallaghan@sxu.edu.

Southern Illinois University Edwardsville
School of Nursing
Edwardsville, Illinois

http://www.siue.edu/NURSING
Founded in 1957

DEGREES • BS • MS

Nursing Program Faculty 67 (83% with doctorates).

Baccalaureate Enrollment 381
Women 88% **Men** 12% **Minority** 12% **International** 3% **Part-time** 4%

Southern Illinois University Edwardsville (continued)
Graduate Enrollment 243
Women 90% **Men** 10% **Minority** 9% **Part-time** 73%
Nursing Student Activities Nursing Honor Society, Sigma Theta Tau, Student Nurses' Association, nursing club.

Nursing Student Resources Academic advising; academic or career counseling; assistance for students with disabilities; bookstore; campus computer network; career placement assistance; computer lab; computer-assisted instruction; daycare for children of students; e-mail services; employment services for current students; housing assistance; interactive nursing skills videos; Internet; learning resource lab; library services; nursing audiovisuals; placement services for program completers; remedial services; skills, simulation, or other laboratory; tutoring.

Library Facilities 788,003 volumes; 14,371 periodical subscriptions.

BACCALAUREATE PROGRAMS

Degree BS

Available Programs Accelerated Baccalaureate; Generic Baccalaureate; RN Baccalaureate.

Site Options *Distance Learning:* Springfield, IL.

Study Options Full-time.

Program Entrance Requirements Minimum overall college GPA of 2.5, transcript of college record, CPR certification, written essay, health exam, health insurance, high school transcript, immunizations, minimum high school GPA of 2.5, minimum GPA in nursing prerequisites of 2.7, prerequisite course work. Transfer students are accepted. **Standardized tests** *Required:* SAT or ACT, TOEFL for international students. **Application Deadline:** 5/1 (freshmen), 7/21 (transfer). *Notification:* continuous (freshmen). *Application fee:* $50.

Expenses (2006–07) *Tuition, area resident:* full-time $6000; part-time $159 per credit hour. *Tuition, nonresident:* full-time $12,000; part-time $397 per credit hour. *Room and board:* $6000 per academic year. *Required fees:* full-time $1000.

Financial Aid 77% of baccalaureate students in nursing programs received some form of financial aid in 2005–06.

Contact Mr. Stephen Wayne Held, Director of Admission, School of Nursing, Southern Illinois University Edwardsville, Box 1066, Edwardsville, IL 62026-1066. *Telephone:* 618-650-5612. *Fax:* 618-650-3854. *E-mail:* sheld@siue.edu.

GRADUATE PROGRAMS

Expenses (2006–07) *Tuition, state resident:* full-time $6400; part-time $225 per credit hour. *Tuition, nonresident:* full-time $14,300; part-time $563 per credit hour. *Required fees:* full-time $1500.

Financial Aid 73% of graduate students in nursing programs received some form of financial aid in 2005–06. Fellowships with full tuition reimbursements available, research assistantships, teaching assistantships, career-related internships or fieldwork, Federal Work-Study, institutionally sponsored loans, scholarships, traineeships, and unspecified assistantships available. Aid available to part-time students. *Financial aid application deadline:* 3/1.

Contact Ms. Angela White, Academic Advisor, School of Nursing, Southern Illinois University Edwardsville, Alumni Hall, Room 2107, Edwardsville, IL 62026-1066. *Telephone:* 618-650-3956. *Fax:* 618-650-2522. *E-mail:* angewhi@siue.edu.

MASTER'S DEGREE PROGRAM

Degree MS

Available Programs Master's.

Concentrations Available Health-care administration; nurse anesthesia; nursing education. *Nurse practitioner programs in:* family health.

Site Options *Distance Learning:* Springfield, IL.

Study Options Full-time and part-time.

Program Entrance Requirements Clinical experience, minimum overall college GPA of 3.0, transcript of college record, CPR certification, written essay, immunizations, interview, 3 letters of recommendation, nursing research course, physical assessment course, prerequisite course work, statistics course. *Application deadline:* For fall admission, 1/1. *Application fee:* $30.

Advanced Placement Credit by examination available. Credit given for nursing courses completed elsewhere dependent upon specific evaluations.

Degree Requirements 33 total credit hours, thesis or project, comprehensive exam.

POST-MASTER'S PROGRAM

Areas of Study Health-care administration; nurse anesthesia; nursing education. *Nurse practitioner programs in:* family health.

CONTINUING EDUCATION PROGRAM

Contact Dr. Karen Kelly, School of Nursing, Southern Illinois University Edwardsville, Box 1066, Edwardsville, IL 62026-1066. *Telephone:* 618-650-3908. *Fax:* 618-650-3854. *E-mail:* kkelly@siue.edu.

Trinity Christian College
Department of Nursing
Palos Heights, Illinois

http://www.trnty/depts/nursing/
Founded in 1959

DEGREE • BSN

Nursing Program Faculty 8 (37% with doctorates).
Baccalaureate Enrollment 145
Women 94.5% **Men** 5.5% **Minority** 14% **International** 3%
Nursing Student Activities Student Nurses' Association.

Nursing Student Resources Academic advising; academic or career counseling; assistance for students with disabilities; bookstore; campus computer network; career placement assistance; computer lab; computer-assisted instruction; e-mail services; interactive nursing skills videos; Internet; learning resource lab; library services; nursing audiovisuals; resume preparation assistance; skills, simulation, or other laboratory; tutoring; unpaid internships.

Library Facilities 81,714 volumes (2,500 in health, 500 in nursing); 435 periodical subscriptions (100 health-care related).

BACCALAUREATE PROGRAMS

Degree BSN

Available Programs Generic Baccalaureate; RN Baccalaureate.

Study Options Full-time.

Program Entrance Requirements Minimum overall college GPA of 2.5, transcript of college record, CPR certification, health exam, health insurance, high school biology, 3 years high school math, 2 years high school science, high school transcript, immunizations, minimum high school GPA of 2.0, minimum GPA in nursing prerequisites of 2.5, prerequisite course work. Transfer students are accepted. **Standardized tests** *Required:* SAT or ACT, TOEFL for international students. *Recommended:* ACT. **Application** *Deadline:* rolling (freshmen). *Notification:* continuous (freshmen). *Application fee:* $20.

Advanced Placement Credit given for nursing courses completed elsewhere dependent upon specific evaluations.

Expenses (2005–06) *Tuition:* full-time $16,986; part-time $570 per credit hour. *International tuition:* $16,986 full-time. *Room and board:* $6600; room only: $3400 per academic year. *Required fees:* full-time $200.

Financial Aid 90% of baccalaureate students in nursing programs received some form of financial aid in 2004–05.

Contact Admissions Office, Department of Nursing, Trinity Christian College, 6601 West College Drive, Palos Heights, IL 60463. *Telephone:* 866-874-6463. *Fax:* 708-385-5665. *E-mail:* admissions@trnty.edu.

Trinity College of Nursing and Health Sciences
Trinity College of Nursing and Health Sciences
Rock Island, Illinois

http://www.trinityqc.com/college/default.htm
Founded in 1994

DEGREE • BSN

Nursing Program Faculty 9 (33% with doctorates).

Baccalaureate Enrollment 78
Women 100% **Minority** 2% **Part-time** 80%

Nursing Student Activities Nursing Honor Society, Student Nurses' Association.

Nursing Student Resources Academic advising; assistance for students with disabilities; computer lab; computer-assisted instruction; daycare for children of students; e-mail services; interactive nursing skills videos; Internet; library services; nursing audiovisuals; remedial services; skills, simulation, or other laboratory; tutoring.

Library Facilities 6,000 volumes in health, 3,400 volumes in nursing; 794 periodical subscriptions health-care related.

BACCALAUREATE PROGRAMS

Degree BSN

Available Programs ADN to Baccalaureate; RN Baccalaureate.
Study Options Full-time and part-time.

Program Entrance Requirements Transcript of college record, CPR certification, health exam, RN licensure. Transfer students are accepted. **Standardized tests** *Required:* SAT or ACT, TOEFL for international students. **Application** *Deadline:* 6/1 (freshmen), 6/1 (transfer). *Application fee:* $50.

Expenses (2006–07) *Tuition:* part-time $380 per credit hour. *Required fees:* full-time $340.

Financial Aid 95% of baccalaureate students in nursing programs received some form of financial aid in 2005–06. *Gift aid (need-based):* Federal Pell, FSEOG, state, college/university gift aid from institutional funds. *Loans:* Federal Nursing Student Loans, FFEL (Subsidized and Unsubsidized Stafford PLUS). *Work-Study:* Federal Work-Study. *Application deadline:* Continuous.

Contact Tracy Poelvoorde, Director, Nursing Programs, Trinity College of Nursing and Health Sciences, 2122 25th Avenue, Rock Island, IL 61201. *Telephone:* 309-779-7708. *Fax:* 309-779-7798. *E-mail:* poelvoordet@trinityqc.com.

University of Illinois at Chicago
College of Nursing
Chicago, Illinois

http://www.uic.edu/nursing
Founded in 1946
DEGREES • BSN • MS • MS/MBA • MS/MPH • PHD

Nursing Program Faculty 150 (68% with doctorates).

Baccalaureate Enrollment 330
Women 90% **Men** 10% **Minority** 23% **International** 3% **Part-time** 20%

Graduate Enrollment 600
Women 95% **Men** 5% **Minority** 10% **International** 6%

Nursing Student Activities Sigma Theta Tau, Student Nurses' Association.

Nursing Student Resources Academic advising; academic or career counseling; assistance for students with disabilities; bookstore; campus computer network; computer lab; computer-assisted instruction; daycare for children of students; e-mail services; externships; Internet; learning resource lab; library services; resume preparation assistance; skills, simulation, or other laboratory; tutoring.

Library Facilities 3 million volumes (500,000 in health); 38,392 periodical subscriptions (5,100 health-care related).

■ The University of Illinois at Chicago College of Nursing, consistently rated among the top ten colleges of nursing in the United States, continues at the forefront of nursing education and research. In 2004, the College was third in the nation in total NIH research and research training dollars. Graduates guide the nursing practice of tomorrow, create and maintain high-quality health-care delivery sys-

tems, and ensure that excellent nursing services are available to the public. Diversity is a characteristic of both the specializations available for study and the students, whose backgrounds and clinical experiences enrich the broad range of topics that are the focus of study and investigation.

BACCALAUREATE PROGRAMS

Degree BSN

Available Programs Generic Baccalaureate; RN Baccalaureate.
Site Options *Distance Learning:* Urbana, IL.
Study Options Full-time and part-time.

Program Entrance Requirements Minimum overall college GPA of 2.5, transcript of college record, written essay, 2 letters of recommendation, minimum GPA in nursing prerequisites of 2.5, prerequisite course work. Transfer students are accepted. **Standardized tests** *Required:* SAT or ACT, TOEFL for international students. **Application** *Deadline:* 1/15 (freshmen), 3/1 (transfer). *Notification:* continuous (freshmen). *Application fee:* $40.

Expenses (2006–07) *Tuition, state resident:* full-time $5671. *Tuition, nonresident:* full-time $11,866. *International tuition:* $11,866 full-time.

Financial Aid 80% of baccalaureate students in nursing programs received some form of financial aid in 2005–06.

Contact Ms. Andrea Schmoyer, Undergraduate Program Coordinator, College of Nursing, University of Illinois at Chicago, 845 South Damen Avenue, Chicago, IL 60612-7350. *Telephone:* 312-996-5786. *Fax:* 312-996-8066. *E-mail:* schmoyer@uic.edu.

GRADUATE PROGRAMS

Expenses (2006–07) *Tuition, state resident:* full-time $8038. *Tuition, nonresident:* full-time $14,037. *International tuition:* $14,037 full-time.

Financial Aid 75% of graduate students in nursing programs received some form of financial aid in 2005–06. 3 fellowships with full tuition reimbursements available were awarded; research assistantships with full tuition reimbursements available, teaching assistantships with full tuition reimbursements available, career-related internships or fieldwork, Federal Work-Study, institutionally sponsored loans, scholarships, traineeships, tuition waivers (full and partial), and unspecified assistantships also available. Aid available to part-time students. *Financial aid application deadline:* 3/1.

Contact Ms. Kate DiAna, Graduate Program Coordinator, College of Nursing, University of Illinois at Chicago, 845 South Damen Avenue, MC 802, Chicago, IL 60612-7350. *Telephone:* 312-996-2184. *Fax:* 312-996-8066. *E-mail:* kdiana@uic.edu.

MASTER'S DEGREE PROGRAM

Degrees MS; MS/MBA; MS/MPH

Available Programs Master's; Master's for Non-Nursing College Graduates; Master's for Nurses with Non-Nursing Degrees.

Concentrations Available Health-care administration; nurse-midwifery; nursing administration; nursing informatics. *Clinical nurse specialist programs in:* acute care, adult health, cardiovascular, community health, family health, gerontology, maternity-newborn, medical-surgical, occupational health, pediatric, perinatal, psychiatric/mental health, public health, school health, women's health. *Nurse practitioner programs in:* acute care, adult health, family health, gerontology, occupational health, pediatric, psychiatric/mental health, school health, women's health.

Site Options *Distance Learning:* Rockford, IL; Urbana, IL; Peoria, IL.
Study Options Full-time and part-time.

Program Entrance Requirements Clinical experience, computer literacy, minimum overall college GPA of 3.0, transcript of college record, CPR certification, written essay, immunizations, interview, 3 letters of recommendation, nursing research course, physical assessment course, prerequisite course work, resume, statistics course, GRE General Test. *Application deadline:* For fall admission, 5/15; for spring admission, 10/15. Applications are processed on a rolling basis. *Application fee:* $40 ($50 for international students).

Advanced Placement Credit given for nursing courses completed elsewhere dependent upon specific evaluations.

Degree Requirements Thesis or project.

University of Illinois at Chicago (continued)
POST-MASTER'S PROGRAM

Areas of Study Health-care administration; nurse-midwifery; nursing administration; nursing education; nursing informatics. *Clinical nurse specialist programs in:* acute care, adult health, cardiovascular, family health, gerontology, medical-surgical, occupational health, pediatric, psychiatric/mental health, public health, school health, women's health. *Nurse practitioner programs in:* acute care, adult health, family health, gerontology, occupational health, pediatric, psychiatric/mental health, school health, women's health.

DOCTORAL DEGREE PROGRAM

Degree PhD

Available Programs Doctorate; Post-Baccalaureate Doctorate.

Areas of Study Bio-behavioral research, clinical practice, community health, faculty preparation, family health, gerontology, health policy, health-care systems, individualized study, maternity-newborn, nursing administration, nursing policy, nursing research, nursing science, women's health.

Program Entrance Requirements Minimum overall college GPA of 3.0, interview by faculty committee, interview, 3 letters of recommendation, MSN or equivalent, statistics course, vita, writing sample, GRE General Test. *Application deadline:* For fall admission, 5/15; for spring admission, 10/15. Applications are processed on a rolling basis. *Application fee:* $40 ($50 for international students).

Degree Requirements 96 total credit hours, dissertation.

POSTDOCTORAL PROGRAM

Areas of Study Individualized study, nursing interventions, nursing research, nursing science.

Postdoctoral Program Contact Jan Larson, Department Head, Medical-Surgical Nursing, College of Nursing, University of Illinois at Chicago, 845 South Damen Avenue, Chicago, IL 60612-7350. *Telephone:* 312-996-7900. *E-mail:* jllarson@uic.edu.

CONTINUING EDUCATION PROGRAM

Contact Dr. Judith Storfjell, Associate Dean for Academic Practice, College of Nursing, University of Illinois at Chicago, 845 South Damen Avenue, Chicago, IL 60612-7350. *Telephone:* 312-996-4299. *E-mail:* jstorfjl@uic.edu.

See full description on page 544.

University of St. Francis
College of Nursing and Allied Health
Joliet, Illinois

http://www.stfrancis.edu/conah/

Founded in 1920

DEGREES • BSN • MSN

Nursing Program Faculty 33 (24% with doctorates).

Baccalaureate Enrollment 460

Women 91% **Men** 9% **Minority** 29% **International** 1% **Part-time** 21%

Graduate Enrollment 65

Women 95% **Men** 5% **Minority** 26% **Part-time** 91%

Nursing Student Activities Nursing Honor Society, Student Nurses' Association.

Nursing Student Resources Academic advising; academic or career counseling; assistance for students with disabilities; bookstore; campus computer network; career placement assistance; computer lab; computer-assisted instruction; e-mail services; employment services for current students; externships; housing assistance; interactive nursing skills videos; Internet; learning resource lab; library services; nursing audiovisuals; remedial services; skills, simulation, or other laboratory; tutoring.

Library Facilities 111,546 volumes (2,768 in health, 902 in nursing); 24,985 periodical subscriptions (149 health-care related).

BACCALAUREATE PROGRAMS

Degree BSN

Available Programs Accelerated RN Baccalaureate; Generic Baccalaureate.

Study Options Full-time and part-time.

Program Entrance Requirements Minimum overall college GPA of 2.75, transcript of college record, CPR certification, health exam, 2 years high school math, 2 years high school science, high school transcript, immunizations, minimum high school GPA of 2.0, minimum high school rank 50%, minimum GPA in nursing prerequisites of 2.0, prerequisite course work. Transfer students are accepted. **Standardized tests** *Required:* SAT or ACT, TOEFL for international students. **Application** *Deadline:* 8/1 (freshmen). *Notification:* continuous (freshmen). *Application fee:* $30.

Advanced Placement Credit by examination available. Credit given for nursing courses completed elsewhere dependent upon specific evaluations.

Expenses (2006–07) *Tuition:* full-time $19,150; part-time $625 per credit hour. *International tuition:* $19,150 full-time. *Room and board:* $7280 per academic year. *Required fees:* full-time $390.

Financial Aid 78% of baccalaureate students in nursing programs received some form of financial aid in 2005–06. *Gift aid (need-based):* Federal Pell, FSEOG, state, private, college/university gift aid from institutional funds. *Loans:* Federal Direct (Subsidized and Unsubsidized Stafford PLUS), Perkins, alternative loans. *Work-Study:* Federal Work-Study, part-time campus jobs. *Application deadline (priority):* 4/1.

Contact Ms. Meghan Connolly, Director, Undergraduate Admissions, College of Nursing and Allied Health, University of St. Francis, 500 Wilcox Street, Joliet, IL 60435. *Telephone:* 800-735-7500. *Fax:* 815-740-5032. *E-mail:* mconnolly1@stfrancis.edu.

GRADUATE PROGRAMS

Expenses (2006–07) *Tuition:* part-time $495 per credit hour.

Financial Aid 46% of graduate students in nursing programs received some form of financial aid in 2005–06.

Contact Ms. Sandee Sloka, Director, Graduate Off-Campus Admissions, College of Nursing and Allied Health, University of St. Francis, 500 Wilcox Street, Joliet, IL 60435. *Telephone:* 815-740-5026. *Fax:* 815-740-3431. *E-mail:* ssloka@stfrancis.edu.

MASTER'S DEGREE PROGRAM

Degree MSN

Available Programs Master's for Nurses with Non-Nursing Degrees; RN to Master's.

Concentrations Available Nursing education. *Clinical nurse specialist programs in:* adult health. *Nurse practitioner programs in:* adult health, family health.

Site Options Albuquerque, NM.

Study Options Part-time.

Program Entrance Requirements Clinical experience, computer literacy, minimum overall college GPA of 3.0, transcript of college record, CPR certification, written essay, immunizations, interview, 3 letters of recommendation, nursing research course, physical assessment course, professional liability insurance/malpractice insurance, prerequisite course work, resume, statistics course.

Advanced Placement Credit given for nursing courses completed elsewhere dependent upon specific evaluations.

Degree Requirements 44 total credit hours, thesis or project.

See full description on page 556.

West Suburban College of Nursing
West Suburban College of Nursing
Oak Park, Illinois

Founded in 1982

DEGREES • BSN • MSN

Nursing Program Faculty 16 (30% with doctorates).

Baccalaureate Enrollment 175

Women 92% **Men** 8% **Minority** 50% **Part-time** 15%

Nursing Student Activities Student Nurses' Association.

Nursing Student Resources Academic advising; academic or career counseling; bookstore; campus computer network; career placement assistance; computer lab; computer-assisted instruction; e-mail services; employment services for current students; externships; Internet; learning resource lab; library services; nursing audiovisuals; skills, simulation, or other laboratory; tutoring.

Library Facilities 2,400 volumes in health, 1,100 volumes in nursing; 300 periodical subscriptions health-care related.

BACCALAUREATE PROGRAMS

Degree BSN

Available Programs ADN to Baccalaureate; Accelerated Baccalaureate for Second Degree; Baccalaureate for Second Degree; Generic Baccalaureate; RN Baccalaureate.

Study Options Full-time and part-time.

Program Entrance Requirements Minimum overall college GPA of 2.75, transcript of college record, CPR certification, written essay, health exam, health insurance, immunizations, 1 letter of recommendation, minimum GPA in nursing prerequisites of 2.75, prerequisite course work. Transfer students are accepted. **Standardized tests** *Required:* TOEFL for international students. **Application** *Deadline:* rolling (freshmen), rolling (transfer). *Notification:* continuous until 8/21 (freshmen).

Advanced Placement Credit by examination available. Credit given for nursing courses completed elsewhere dependent upon specific evaluations.

Expenses (2006–07) *Tuition:* full-time $19,204; part-time $649 per credit hour. *Required fees:* full-time $400; part-time $200 per term.

Financial Aid 95% of baccalaureate students in nursing programs received some form of financial aid in 2005–06.

Contact Mr. Sujith Zachariah, Admissions Counselor, West Suburban College of Nursing, 3 Erie Court, Oak Park, IL 60302. *Telephone:* 708-763-6532. *Fax:* 708-763-1531. *E-mail:* admissions@wscn.edu.

GRADUATE PROGRAMS

Expenses (2006–07) *Tuition:* part-time $677 per credit hour. *Required fees:* part-time $125 per term.

Contact Mr. Sujith Zachariah, Admissions Counselor, West Suburban College of Nursing, 3 Erie Court, Oak Park, IL 60302. *Telephone:* 708-763-6532. *Fax:* 708-763-1531. *E-mail:* zachariahs@wscn.edu.

MASTER'S DEGREE PROGRAM

Degree MSN

Available Programs Accelerated AD/RN to Master's; Accelerated RN to Master's; Master's; Master's for Nurses with Non-Nursing Degrees; RN to Master's.

Concentrations Available Nursing administration; nursing education. *Clinical nurse specialist programs in:* adult health.

Study Options Part-time.

Program Entrance Requirements Computer literacy, minimum overall college GPA of 3.0, transcript of college record, CPR certification, written essay, immunizations, 3 letters of recommendation, resume.

Advanced Placement Credit given for nursing courses completed elsewhere dependent upon specific evaluations.

Degree Requirements 32 total credit hours, thesis or project.

POST-MASTER'S PROGRAM

Areas of Study Nursing administration; nursing education. *Clinical nurse specialist programs in:* adult health.

INDIANA

Ball State University
School of Nursing
Muncie, Indiana

http://www.bsu.edu/nursing
Founded in 1918

DEGREES • BS • MS

Nursing Program Faculty 42 (33% with doctorates).

Baccalaureate Enrollment 338
Women 92% **Men** 8% **Minority** 7% **International** 1%

Graduate Enrollment 300
Women 95% **Men** 5% **Minority** 10% **Part-time** 100%

Nursing Student Activities Nursing Honor Society, Sigma Theta Tau, Student Nurses' Association, nursing club.

Nursing Student Resources Academic advising; academic or career counseling; assistance for students with disabilities; bookstore; campus computer network; career placement assistance; computer lab; computer-assisted instruction; e-mail services; employment services for current students; housing assistance; interactive nursing skills videos; Internet; learning resource lab; library services; nursing audiovisuals; remedial services; resume preparation assistance; skills, simulation, or other laboratory; tutoring.

Library Facilities 1.1 million volumes; 2,937 periodical subscriptions.

BACCALAUREATE PROGRAMS

Degree BS

Available Programs Accelerated Baccalaureate for Second Degree; Generic Baccalaureate; LPN to Baccalaureate; RN Baccalaureate.

Study Options Full-time and part-time.

Program Entrance Requirements Minimum overall college GPA of 3.00, transcript of college record, CPR certification, health exam, immunizations, prerequisite course work. Transfer students are accepted. **Standardized tests** *Required:* SAT or ACT, TOEFL for international students. **Application** *Deadline:* rolling (freshmen), rolling (transfer). *Notification:* continuous (freshmen). *Application fee:* $25.

Expenses (2006–07) *Tuition, area resident:* full-time $3180. *Tuition, nonresident:* full-time $8368. *Room and board:* $7886 per academic year. *Required fees:* full-time $597; part-time $302 per credit; part-time $302 per term.

Financial Aid 90% of baccalaureate students in nursing programs received some form of financial aid in 2005–06. *Gift aid (need-based):* Federal Pell, FSEOG, state, private, college/university gift aid from institutional funds. *Loans:* Federal Direct (Subsidized and Unsubsidized Stafford PLUS), Perkins. *Work-Study:* Federal Work-Study, part-time campus jobs. *Application deadline (priority):* 3/1.

Contact Dr. Nancy Dillard, RN, Associate Director, Baccalaureate Nursing, School of Nursing, Ball State University, CN 418, Muncie, IN 47306. *Telephone:* 765-285-5589. *Fax:* 765-285-2169. *E-mail:* ndillard@bsu.edu.

GRADUATE PROGRAMS

Expenses (2006–07) *Tuition, state resident:* part-time $212 per credit hour. *Tuition, nonresident:* part-time $364 per credit hour.

Financial Aid 2 teaching assistantships (averaging $9,307 per year) were awarded; research assistantships, career-related internships or fieldwork also available.

Contact Dr. Marilyn Ryan, RN, Associate Director, Graduate Program, School of Nursing, Ball State University, Muncie, IN 47306. *Telephone:* 765-285-5764. *Fax:* 765-285-2169. *E-mail:* mryan@bsu.edu.

MASTER'S DEGREE PROGRAM

Degree MS

Available Programs Master's; RN to Master's.

Concentrations Available Nursing administration; nursing education. *Clinical nurse specialist programs in:* adult health. *Nurse practitioner programs in:* adult health, family health.

Study Options Part-time.

Program Entrance Requirements Clinical experience, computer literacy, minimum overall college GPA of 2.8, transcript of college record, CPR certification, written essay, interview, 1 letter of recommendation, nursing research course, physical assessment course. *Application fee:* $25 ($35 for international students).

Advanced Placement Credit given for nursing courses completed elsewhere dependent upon specific evaluations.

POST-MASTER'S PROGRAM

Areas of Study Nursing education. *Nurse practitioner programs in:* adult health, family health.

Bethel College
Department of Nursing
Mishawaka, Indiana

http://www.bethelcollege.edu

Founded in 1947

DEGREES • BSN • MSN

Nursing Program Faculty 25 (8% with doctorates).

Baccalaureate Enrollment 125
Women 90% **Men** 10% **Minority** 5% **Part-time** 40%

Graduate Enrollment 15

Nursing Student Activities Sigma Theta Tau, Student Nurses' Association.

Nursing Student Resources Academic advising; academic or career counseling; assistance for students with disabilities; campus computer network; career placement assistance; computer lab; computer-assisted instruction; e-mail services; employment services for current students; housing assistance; Internet; learning resource lab; library services; nursing audiovisuals; placement services for program completers; remedial services; resume preparation assistance; skills, simulation, or other laboratory; tutoring.

Library Facilities 106,584 volumes (3,000 in health, 2,000 in nursing); 450 periodical subscriptions (150 health-care related).

BACCALAUREATE PROGRAMS

Degree BSN

Available Programs ADN to Baccalaureate; Generic Baccalaureate; LPN to Baccalaureate; RN Baccalaureate.

Site Options Mishawaka, IN; Winona Lake, IN; St. Joseph, MI.

Study Options Full-time and part-time.

Program Entrance Requirements Minimum overall college GPA of 2.5, transcript of college record, CPR certification, written essay, health exam, high school chemistry, high school transcript, immunizations, 1 letter of recommendation, minimum high school GPA of 2.5, minimum high school rank 35%, minimum GPA in nursing prerequisites of 2.5. Transfer students are accepted. **Standardized tests** *Required:* SAT or ACT, TOEFL for international students. **Application** *Deadline:* 8/6 (freshmen), 8/6 (transfer). *Notification:* continuous (freshmen). *Application fee:* $25.

Advanced Placement Credit by examination available. Credit given for nursing courses completed elsewhere dependent upon specific evaluations.

Expenses (2006–07) *Tuition:* full-time $17,400; part-time $350 per credit hour. *International tuition:* $17,400 full-time. *Room and board:* $5000; room only: $2800 per academic year. *Required fees:* full-time $600; part-time $70 per term.

Financial Aid 90% of baccalaureate students in nursing programs received some form of financial aid in 2005–06.

Contact Dr. Ruth Davidhizar, Dean of Nursing, Department of Nursing, Bethel College, 1001 West McKinley Avenue, Mishawaka, IN 46545. *Telephone:* 574-257-2594. *Fax:* 574-257-2683. *E-mail:* davidhr@bethelcollege.edu.

GRADUATE PROGRAMS

Expenses (2006–07) *Tuition:* part-time $330 per credit hour. *Room and board:* $5000; room only: $2800 per academic year.

Financial Aid 100% of graduate students in nursing programs received some form of financial aid in 2005–06.

Contact Dr. Karon Schwartz, Graduate Nursing Program Director, Department of Nursing, Bethel College, 1001 West McKinley Avenue, Mishawaka, IN 46545. *Telephone:* 574-257-3382. *Fax:* 574-257-7616. *E-mail:* schwark@bethelcollege.edu.

MASTER'S DEGREE PROGRAM

Degree MSN

Available Programs Master's.

Concentrations Available Nursing administration; nursing education.

Site Options Mishawaka, IN.

Study Options Full-time and part-time.

Program Entrance Requirements Clinical experience, minimum overall college GPA of 3.0, transcript of college record, CPR certification, immunizations, 3 letters of recommendation, nursing research course, physical assessment course, statistics course.

Advanced Placement Credit given for nursing courses completed elsewhere dependent upon specific evaluations.

Degree Requirements 36 total credit hours, thesis or project.

POST-MASTER'S PROGRAM

Areas of Study Nursing administration; nursing education.

Goshen College
Department of Nursing
Goshen, Indiana

http://www.goshen.edu

Founded in 1894

DEGREE • BSN

Nursing Program Faculty 9 (22% with doctorates).

Baccalaureate Enrollment 150
Women 91% **Men** 9% **Minority** 11% **International** 9%

Nursing Student Activities Sigma Theta Tau, Student Nurses' Association.

Nursing Student Resources Academic advising; academic or career counseling; bookstore; campus computer network; career placement assistance; computer lab; e-mail services; employment services for current students; externships; library services; nursing audiovisuals; placement services for program completers; resume preparation assistance.

Library Facilities 136,550 volumes (80 in health, 80 in nursing); 496 periodical subscriptions (68 health-care related).

BACCALAUREATE PROGRAMS

Degree BSN

Available Programs Generic Baccalaureate; RN Baccalaureate.

Site Options Elkhart, IN.

Study Options Full-time and part-time.

Program Entrance Requirements Minimum overall college GPA of 2.5, transcript of college record, CPR certification, health exam, high school chemistry, high school foreign language, 2 years high school math, high school science, high school transcript, immunizations, 2 letters of recommendation, minimum high school GPA of 2.5, minimum high school rank 50%. Transfer students are accepted. **Standardized tests** *Required:* SAT or ACT, TOEFL for international students. **Application** *Deadline:* 8/15 (freshmen), 8/15 (transfer). *Early decision:* 12/1. *Notification:* continuous (freshmen), 12/15 (early action). *Application fee:* $25.

Advanced Placement Credit by examination available. Credit given for nursing courses completed elsewhere dependent upon specific evaluations.

Expenses (2006–07) *Tuition:* full-time $20,300. *International tuition:* $20,300 full-time. *Room and board:* $6700; room only: $3600 per academic year. *Required fees:* full-time $500.

Financial Aid 98% of baccalaureate students in nursing programs received some form of financial aid in 2005–06. *Gift aid (need-based):* Federal Pell, FSEOG, state, private, college/university gift aid from institutional funds. *Loans:* Federal Nursing Student Loans, Federal Direct (Subsidized and Unsubsidized Stafford PLUS), Perkins, college/university. *Work-Study:* Federal Work-Study, part-time campus jobs. *Application deadline (priority):* 2/15.

Contact Admissions, Department of Nursing, Goshen College, 1700 South Main Street, Goshen, IN 46526. *Telephone:* 219-535-7535. *Fax:* 219-535-7609. *E-mail:* admissions@goshen.edu.

See full description on page 488.

Indiana State University
College of Nursing
Terre Haute, Indiana

http://www.indstate.edu/nurs/

Founded in 1865

DEGREES • BS • MS

Nursing Program Faculty 34 (29% with doctorates).

Baccalaureate Enrollment 357
Women 89% **Men** 11% **Minority** 12% **International** 1% **Part-time** 34%

Graduate Enrollment 160
Women 91% **Men** 9% **Minority** 18% **International** 1% **Part-time** 77%

Nursing Student Activities Sigma Theta Tau, Student Nurses' Association.

Nursing Student Resources Academic advising; academic or career counseling; assistance for students with disabilities; bookstore; campus computer network; career placement assistance; computer lab; computer-assisted instruction; daycare for children of students; e-mail services; employment services for current students; externships; housing assistance; interactive nursing skills videos; Internet; learning resource lab; library services; nursing audiovisuals; paid internships; placement services for program completers; remedial services; resume preparation assistance; skills, simulation, or other laboratory; tutoring; unpaid internships.

Library Facilities 1.3 million volumes (54,890 in health, 33,560 in nursing); 43,464 periodical subscriptions (104 health-care related).

BACCALAUREATE PROGRAMS

Degree BS

Available Programs Generic Baccalaureate; LPN to RN Baccalaureate; RN Baccalaureate.

Site Options *Distance Learning:* Terre Haute, IN.

Study Options Full-time and part-time.

Program Entrance Requirements Minimum overall college GPA of 2.25, transcript of college record, CPR certification, health exam, high school chemistry, high school foreign language, 3 years high school math, 3 years high school science, high school transcript, immunizations, minimum high school GPA of 2.5, minimum high school rank 40%, minimum GPA in nursing prerequisites of 2.5, prerequisite course work. Transfer students are accepted. **Standardized tests** *Required:* SAT or ACT, TOEFL for international students. **Application** *Deadline:* 8/15 (freshmen). *Notification:* continuous (freshmen). *Application fee:* $25.

Advanced Placement Credit by examination available. Credit given for nursing courses completed elsewhere dependent upon specific evaluations.

Expenses (2006–07) *Tuition, state resident:* full-time $6102; part-time $220 per credit hour. *Tuition, nonresident:* full-time $13,518; part-time $476 per credit hour. *International tuition:* $13,518 full-time. *Room and board:* $6770; room only: $6413 per academic year.

Financial Aid 7.5% of baccalaureate students in nursing programs received some form of financial aid in 2005–06.

Contact Ms. Lynn C. Foster, Director of Student Affairs, College of Nursing, Indiana State University, 749 Chestnut Street, Terre Haute, IN 47809. *Telephone:* 812-237-2316. *Fax:* 812-237-8022. *E-mail:* lfoster@isugw.indstate.edu.

GRADUATE PROGRAMS

Expenses (2006–07) *Tuition, state resident:* full-time $5004; part-time $278 per credit hour. *Tuition, nonresident:* full-time $9936; part-time $552 per credit hour. *International tuition:* $9936 full-time.

Financial Aid 7.5% of graduate students in nursing programs received some form of financial aid in 2005–06. 3 research assistantships with partial tuition reimbursements available (averaging $5,510 per year) were awarded; teaching assistantships with partial tuition reimbursements available, career-related internships or fieldwork and Federal Work-Study also available. Aid available to part-time students. *Financial aid application deadline:* 3/1.

Contact Ms. Lynn C. Foster, Director of Student Affairs, College of Nursing, Indiana State University, 749 Chestnut Street, Terre Haute, IN 47809. *Telephone:* 812-237-2316. *Fax:* 812-237-8022. *E-mail:* lfoster@isugw.indstate.edu.

MASTER'S DEGREE PROGRAM

Degree MS

Available Programs Master's.

Concentrations Available Nursing administration. *Nurse practitioner programs in:* family health.

Site Options *Distance Learning:* Terre Haute, IN.

Study Options Full-time and part-time.

Program Entrance Requirements Clinical experience, minimum overall college GPA of 3.0, transcript of college record, CPR certification, written essay, immunizations, 3 letters of recommendation, nursing research course, prerequisite course work, statistics course. *Application deadline:* For fall admission, 7/1 (priority date); for spring admission, 11/1 (priority date). Applications are processed on a rolling basis. *Application fee:* $35.

Advanced Placement Credit given for nursing courses completed elsewhere dependent upon specific evaluations.

Degree Requirements 36 total credit hours, thesis or project.

POST-MASTER'S PROGRAM

Areas of Study *Nurse practitioner programs in:* family health.

CONTINUING EDUCATION PROGRAM

Contact Ms. Michelle Pantle, RN, Director of Continuing Education, College of Nursing, Indiana State University, Landsbaum Center, LCHE 111, 1433 North 61/2 Street, Terre Haute, IN 47807. *Telephone:* 812-237-3696. *Fax:* 812-237-8248. *E-mail:* nupantle@isugw.indstate.edu.

Indiana University Bloomington
Department of Nursing–Bloomington Division
Bloomington, Indiana

Founded in 1820

DEGREE • BSN

Nursing Program Faculty 19 (1.5% with doctorates).

Baccalaureate Enrollment 144
Women 98% **Men** 2% **Minority** 1%

Nursing Student Activities Nursing Honor Society, Sigma Theta Tau, Student Nurses' Association, nursing club.

Nursing Student Resources Academic advising; academic or career counseling; campus computer network; computer lab; computer-assisted instruction; e-mail services; employment services for current students; interactive nursing skills videos; Internet; learning resource lab; library services; nursing audiovisuals; remedial services; resume preparation assistance; skills, simulation, or other laboratory; tutoring.

Library Facilities 6.5 million volumes (8,500 in nursing); 60,019 periodical subscriptions (1,000 health-care related).

BACCALAUREATE PROGRAMS

Degree BSN

Available Programs Generic Baccalaureate; RN Baccalaureate.

Site Options Bloomington, IN.

Study Options Full-time.

Program Entrance Requirements Minimum overall college GPA of 2.5, CPR certification, written essay, health exam, health insurance, 3 years high school math, high school transcript, immunizations, interview, minimum GPA in nursing prerequisites of 2.7, prerequisite course work. Transfer students are accepted. **Standardized tests** *Required:* SAT or ACT. *Recommended:* SAT Subject Tests, TOEFL for international students. **Application** *Deadline:* rolling (freshmen), rolling (transfer). *Notification:* continuous (freshmen). *Application fee:* $50.

Advanced Placement Credit given for nursing courses completed elsewhere dependent upon specific evaluations.

Expenses (2006–07) *Tuition, state resident:* full-time $5507; part-time $172 per credit hour. *Tuition, nonresident:* full-time $18,498; part-time $578 per credit hour. *Room and board:* $5684 per academic year. *Required fees:* full-time $803; part-time $338 per credit; part-time $676 per term.

Indiana University Bloomington (continued)

Financial Aid 50% of baccalaureate students in nursing programs received some form of financial aid in 2005–06. *Gift aid (need-based):* Federal Pell, FSEOG, state, private, college/university gift aid from institutional funds. *Loans:* Federal Nursing Student Loans, Federal Direct (Subsidized and Unsubsidized Stafford PLUS), Perkins, college/university. *Work-Study:* Federal Work-Study. *Application deadline:* Continuous.

Contact Mrs. Deborah Hrisomalos, Academic Advisor, Department of Nursing–Bloomington Division, Indiana University Bloomington, Sycamore Hall, Room 401, Bloomington, IN 47405. *Telephone:* 812-855-2592. *Fax:* 812-855-6986. *E-mail:* dhrisoma@indiana.edu.

Indiana University East
Division of Nursing
Richmond, Indiana

http://www.indiana.edu/nursing

Founded in 1971

DEGREE • BSN

Nursing Program Faculty 15 (7% with doctorates).

Baccalaureate Enrollment 125
Women 94% **Men** 6% **Minority** 4%

Nursing Student Activities Sigma Theta Tau, Student Nurses' Association.

Nursing Student Resources Academic advising; academic or career counseling; assistance for students with disabilities; bookstore; campus computer network; career placement assistance; computer lab; computer-assisted instruction; daycare for children of students; e-mail services; externships; interactive nursing skills videos; Internet; learning resource lab; library services; nursing audiovisuals; placement services for program completers; remedial services; resume preparation assistance; skills, simulation, or other laboratory; tutoring; unpaid internships.

Library Facilities 67,036 volumes (5,039 in health, 3,418 in nursing); 435 periodical subscriptions (70 health-care related).

BACCALAUREATE PROGRAMS

Degree BSN

Available Programs ADN to Baccalaureate; Generic Baccalaureate; RN Baccalaureate.

Study Options Full-time.

Program Entrance Requirements Minimum overall college GPA of 2.7, transcript of college record, CPR certification, high school biology, high school chemistry, 3 years high school math, 3 years high school science, high school transcript, immunizations, minimum high school GPA of 2.0, minimum high school rank 50%, minimum GPA in nursing prerequisites of 2.0, prerequisite course work. Transfer students are accepted. **Standardized tests** *Recommended:* SAT or ACT. **Application** *Deadline:* rolling (freshmen), rolling (transfer). *Notification:* continuous (freshmen). *Application fee:* $25.

Advanced Placement Credit by examination available. Credit given for nursing courses completed elsewhere dependent upon specific evaluations.

Expenses (2006–07) *Tuition, state resident:* full-time $1879; part-time $157 per credit hour. *Tuition, nonresident:* full-time $4662; part-time $389 per credit hour. *Required fees:* full-time $950; part-time $475 per term.

Financial Aid 75% of baccalaureate students in nursing programs received some form of financial aid in 2005–06. *Gift aid (need-based):* Federal Pell, FSEOG, state, private, college/university gift aid from institutional funds. *Loans:* Federal Nursing Student Loans, FFEL (Subsidized and Unsubsidized Stafford PLUS), Perkins, college/university. *Work-Study:* Federal Work-Study. *Application deadline (priority):* 3/1.

Contact Miss Josephine Robinson, Pre-nursing Advisor, Division of Nursing, Indiana University East, 2325 Chester Boulevard, Richmond, IN 47374-1289. *Telephone:* 765-973-8235. *Fax:* 765-973-8220. *E-mail:* jr47@indiana.edu.

Indiana University Kokomo
Indiana University School of Nursing
Kokomo, Indiana

Founded in 1945

DEGREE • BSN

Nursing Program Faculty 14 (43% with doctorates).

Baccalaureate Enrollment 198
Women 95% **Men** 5% **Minority** 1% **International** 1% **Part-time** 32%

Nursing Student Activities Student Nurses' Association.

Nursing Student Resources Academic advising; academic or career counseling; assistance for students with disabilities; bookstore; campus computer network; career placement assistance; computer lab; computer-assisted instruction; daycare for children of students; e-mail services; employment services for current students; externships; interactive nursing skills videos; Internet; learning resource lab; library services; nursing audiovisuals; paid internships; remedial services; resume preparation assistance; skills, simulation, or other laboratory; tutoring.

Library Facilities 132,424 volumes (2,881 in health, 1,513 in nursing); 1,513 periodical subscriptions (75 health-care related).

BACCALAUREATE PROGRAMS

Degree BSN

Available Programs Accelerated RN Baccalaureate; Generic Baccalaureate.

Site Options Marion, IN; Peru, IN; Logansport, IN.

Study Options Full-time.

Program Entrance Requirements Minimum overall college GPA of 2.5, transcript of college record, CPR certification, high school biology, high school chemistry, 4 years high school math, high school transcript, immunizations, minimum high school GPA of 2.0, minimum high school rank 50%, minimum GPA in nursing prerequisites of 2.7, prerequisite course work. Transfer students are accepted. **Standardized tests** *Required:* SAT or ACT. **Application** *Deadline:* rolling (freshmen). *Notification:* continuous (freshmen). *Application fee:* $30.

Financial Aid 75% of baccalaureate students in nursing programs received some form of financial aid in 2005–06. *Gift aid (need-based):* Federal Pell, FSEOG, state, private, college/university gift aid from institutional funds. *Loans:* Federal Nursing Student Loans, FFEL (Subsidized and Unsubsidized Stafford PLUS), Perkins, college/university. *Work-Study:* Federal Work-Study. *Application deadline (priority):* 3/1.

Contact Mr. Morris S. Starkey, Coordinator, Indiana University School of Nursing, Indiana University Kokomo, 2300 South Washington Street, PO Box 9003, Kokomo, IN 46904-9003. *Telephone:* 765-455-9384. *Fax:* 765-455-9421. *E-mail:* mstarke@iuk.edu.

CONTINUING EDUCATION PROGRAM

Contact Mr. Morris S. Starkey, Coordinator, Indiana University School of Nursing, Indiana University Kokomo, 2300 South Washington Street, PO Box 9003, Kokomo, IN 46904-9003. *Telephone:* 765-455-9384. *Fax:* 765-455-9421. *E-mail:* mstarke@iuk.edu.

Indiana University Northwest
School of Nursing and Health Professions
Gary, Indiana

http://www.iun.edu/~nurse

Founded in 1959

DEGREE • BSN

Nursing Program Faculty 14 (15% with doctorates).

Baccalaureate Enrollment 155
Women 95% **Men** 5% **Minority** 25%

Nursing Student Activities Sigma Theta Tau, Student Nurses' Association.

Nursing Student Resources Academic advising; academic or career counseling; assistance for students with disabilities; bookstore; campus computer network; career placement assistance; computer lab; computer-assisted instruction; daycare for children of students; e-mail services; externships; interactive nursing skills videos; Internet; learning resource lab; library services; nursing audiovisuals; placement services for program completers; skills, simulation, or other laboratory; tutoring.

Library Facilities 251,508 volumes (42,000 in health, 15,000 in nursing); 1,541 periodical subscriptions (200 health-care related).

BACCALAUREATE PROGRAMS

Degree BSN

Available Programs Baccalaureate for Second Degree; Generic Baccalaureate; RN Baccalaureate.

Study Options Full-time.

Program Entrance Requirements Minimum overall college GPA of 2.5, transcript of college record, CPR certification, health exam, health insurance, high school biology, high school chemistry, high school foreign language, 4 years high school science, high school transcript, immunizations, minimum high school rank 25%, minimum GPA in nursing prerequisites, prerequisite course work. Transfer students are accepted. **Standardized tests** *Required:* SAT or ACT. *Recommended:* TOEFL for international students. **Application** *Deadline:* rolling (freshmen), rolling (transfer). *Notification:* continuous (freshmen). *Application fee:* $25.

Advanced Placement Credit given for nursing courses completed elsewhere dependent upon specific evaluations.

Expenses (2006–07) *Tuition, state resident:* part-time $138 per credit hour. *Tuition, nonresident:* part-time $369 per credit hour. *Required fees:* full-time $830.

Financial Aid 54% of baccalaureate students in nursing programs received some form of financial aid in 2005–06. *Gift aid (need-based):* Federal Pell, FSEOG, state, private, college/university gift aid from institutional funds, Federal Nursing. *Loans:* FFEL (Subsidized and Unsubsidized Stafford PLUS), Perkins, college/university. *Work-Study:* Federal Work-Study. *Application deadline (priority):* 3/1.

Contact Ms. Anne Mitchell, Nursing Student Services Coordinator, School of Nursing and Health Professions, Indiana University Northwest, 3400 Broadway, Gary, IN 46408. *Telephone:* 219-980-6611. *Fax:* 219-980-6578. *E-mail:* amitchel@iun.edu.

Indiana University–Purdue University Fort Wayne
Department of Nursing
Fort Wayne, Indiana

http://www.ipfw.edu/nursing

Founded in 1917

DEGREES • BS • MS

Nursing Program Faculty 40 (17% with doctorates).

Baccalaureate Enrollment 55
Women 85% **Men** 15% **Minority** 11% **Part-time** 71%

Graduate Enrollment 7
Women 100% **Part-time** 100%

Nursing Student Activities Sigma Theta Tau, nursing club.

Nursing Student Resources Academic advising; academic or career counseling; assistance for students with disabilities; bookstore; campus computer network; career placement assistance; computer lab; computer-assisted instruction; daycare for children of students; e-mail services; employment services for current students; housing assistance; interactive nursing skills videos; Internet; learning resource lab; library services; nursing audiovisuals; placement services for program completers; remedial services; resume preparation assistance; skills, simulation, or other laboratory; tutoring.

Library Facilities 478,091 volumes (1,100 in health, 500 in nursing); 24,872 periodical subscriptions (120 health-care related).

BACCALAUREATE PROGRAMS

Degree BS

Available Programs RN Baccalaureate.

Study Options Full-time and part-time.

Program Entrance Requirements Minimum overall college GPA, transcript of college record, CPR certification, health exam, high school transcript, immunizations, professional liability insurance/malpractice insurance, prerequisite course work, RN licensure. Transfer students are accepted. **Standardized tests** *Required:* SAT or ACT, TOEFL for international students. **Application** *Deadline:* 8/1 (freshmen). *Notification:* continuous (freshmen). *Application fee:* $30.

Advanced Placement Credit by examination available. Credit given for nursing courses completed elsewhere dependent upon specific evaluations.

Expenses (2005–06) *Tuition, state resident:* full-time $5025; part-time $1256 per semester. *Tuition, nonresident:* full-time $12,380; part-time $3095 per semester. *International tuition:* $12,984 full-time. *Room and board:* room only: $4256 per academic year. *Required fees:* full-time $780; part-time $390 per credit.

Financial Aid 50% of baccalaureate students in nursing programs received some form of financial aid in 2004–05.

Contact Dr. Linda H. Meyer, Director of Undergraduate Programs/Associate Professor in Nursing, Department of Nursing, Indiana University–Purdue University Fort Wayne, 2101 East Coliseum Boulevard, Fort Wayne, IN 46805. *Telephone:* 260-481-6276. *Fax:* 260-481-5767. *E-mail:* meyer@ipfw.edu.

GRADUATE PROGRAMS

Expenses (2005–06) *Tuition, state resident:* full-time $3812; part-time $953 per semester. *Tuition, nonresident:* full-time $8699; part-time $2175 per semester. *International tuition:* $8699 full-time. *Room and board:* room only: $4256 per academic year. *Required fees:* full-time $780; part-time $520 per credit.

Financial Aid 5% of graduate students in nursing programs received some form of financial aid in 2004–05.

Contact Dr. Katherine Willock, Director of Graduate Programs and Associate Professor, Department of Nursing, Indiana University–Purdue University Fort Wayne, 2101 East Coliseum Boulevard, Fort Wayne, IN 46805-1499. *Telephone:* 260-481-6284. *Fax:* 260-481-5767. *E-mail:* willockk@ipfw.edu.

MASTER'S DEGREE PROGRAM

Degree MS

Available Programs Master's.

Concentrations Available Nursing administration.

Study Options Full-time and part-time.

Program Entrance Requirements Clinical experience, minimum overall college GPA of 3.0, transcript of college record, interview, prerequisite course work, statistics course.

Advanced Placement Credit by examination available. Credit given for nursing courses completed elsewhere dependent upon specific evaluations.

Degree Requirements 40 total credit hours, thesis or project.

CONTINUING EDUCATION PROGRAM

Contact Roberta Barnes, Registrar, Continuing Studies, Department of Nursing, Indiana University–Purdue University Fort Wayne, 2101 East Coliseum Boulevard, Fort Wayne, IN 46805. *Telephone:* 260-481-6626. *E-mail:* barnes@ipfw.edu.

Indiana University–Purdue University Indianapolis
School of Nursing
Indianapolis, Indiana

http://www.nursing.iupui.edu

Founded in 1969

DEGREES • BSN • MSN • MSN/MPH • PHD

Nursing Program Faculty 182 (37% with doctorates).

Indiana University–Purdue University Indianapolis (continued)

Baccalaureate Enrollment 771
Women 92% **Men** 8% **Minority** 13% **International** 1% **Part-time** 21%
Graduate Enrollment 411
Women 96% **Men** 4% **Minority** 8% **International** .5% **Part-time** 85%
Nursing Student Activities Sigma Theta Tau, Student Nurses' Association.

Nursing Student Resources Academic advising; academic or career counseling; assistance for students with disabilities; bookstore; campus computer network; career placement assistance; computer lab; computer-assisted instruction; e-mail services; employment services for current students; externships; housing assistance; interactive nursing skills videos; Internet; learning resource lab; library services; nursing audiovisuals; other; paid internships; remedial services; resume preparation assistance; skills, simulation, or other laboratory; tutoring; unpaid internships.

Library Facilities 1.5 million volumes (318,211 in health, 8,258 in nursing); 14,673 periodical subscriptions (1,951 health-care related).

BACCALAUREATE PROGRAMS

Degree BSN

Available Programs ADN to Baccalaureate; Accelerated Baccalaureate for Second Degree; Generic Baccalaureate; RN Baccalaureate.
Site Options Columbus, IN.
Study Options Full-time and part-time.
Program Entrance Requirements Minimum overall college GPA of 2.5, transcript of college record, CPR certification, health insurance, 2 years high school math, 1 year of high school science, high school transcript, immunizations, interview, minimum GPA in nursing prerequisites of 2.7, prerequisite course work. Transfer students are accepted. **Standardized tests** *Required:* SAT or ACT, TOEFL for international students. **Application Deadline:** 6/1 (freshmen), rolling (transfer). *Notification:* continuous (freshmen). *Application fee:* $50.
Advanced Placement Credit by examination available. Credit given for nursing courses completed elsewhere dependent upon specific evaluations.
Expenses (2006–07) *Tuition, state resident:* part-time $197 per credit hour. *Tuition, nonresident:* part-time $559 per credit hour. *Room and board:* $4834; room only: $2434 per academic year. *Required fees:* full-time $600; part-time $300 per term.
Financial Aid 52% of baccalaureate students in nursing programs received some form of financial aid in 2005–06. *Gift aid (need-based):* Federal Pell, FSEOG, state, private, college/university gift aid from institutional funds. *Loans:* Federal Nursing Student Loans, FFEL (Subsidized and Unsubsidized Stafford PLUS), Perkins, college/university. *Work-Study:* Federal Work-Study. *Application deadline (priority):* 3/1.
Contact Dr. Pamela R. Jeffries, Associate Dean for Undergraduate Programs, School of Nursing, Indiana University–Purdue University Indianapolis, 1111 Middle Drive, NU 140, Indianapolis, IN 46202-5107. *Telephone:* 317-274-8010. *Fax:* 317-274-2996. *E-mail:* prjeffri@iupui.edu.

GRADUATE PROGRAMS

Expenses (2006–07) *Tuition, state resident:* part-time $273 per credit hour. *Tuition, nonresident:* part-time $825 per credit hour. *Room and board:* $8705 per academic year. *Required fees:* full-time $660; part-time $204 per term.
Financial Aid 29% of graduate students in nursing programs received some form of financial aid in 2005–06. Fellowships with full tuition reimbursements available, research assistantships with full tuition reimbursements available, teaching assistantships with full tuition reimbursements available, Federal Work-Study, institutionally sponsored loans, scholarships, and tuition waivers (full) available. Aid available to part-time students. *Financial aid application deadline:* 5/1.
Contact Dr. Daniel J. Pesut, Associate Dean for Graduate Programs, School of Nursing, Indiana University–Purdue University Indianapolis, 1111 Middle Drive, NU 136, Indianapolis, IN 46202-5107. *Telephone:* 317-274-3115. *Fax:* 317-274-2996. *E-mail:* dpesut@iupui.edu.

MASTER'S DEGREE PROGRAM

Degrees MSN; MSN/MPH
Available Programs Master's; RN to Master's.

Concentrations Available Nursing administration. *Clinical nurse specialist programs in:* acute care, adult health, community health, critical care, oncology, pediatric, psychiatric/mental health. *Nurse practitioner programs in:* acute care, adult health, family health, neonatal health, pediatric, women's health.
Study Options Full-time and part-time.
Program Entrance Requirements Clinical experience, computer literacy, minimum overall college GPA of 3.0, transcript of college record, written essay, immunizations, 3 letters of recommendation, physical assessment course, resume, statistics course, GRE General Test. *Application deadline:* For fall admission, 2/15; for spring admission, 9/15. *Application fee:* $50 ($60 for international students).
Advanced Placement Credit given for nursing courses completed elsewhere dependent upon specific evaluations.
Degree Requirements 42 total credit hours, thesis or project.

POST-MASTER'S PROGRAM

Areas of Study Nursing administration. *Clinical nurse specialist programs in:* adult health, community health, pediatric, psychiatric/mental health. *Nurse practitioner programs in:* acute care, adult health, family health, neonatal health, pediatric, women's health.

DOCTORAL DEGREE PROGRAM

Degree PhD

Available Programs Doctorate; Post-Baccalaureate Doctorate.
Areas of Study Aging, bio-behavioral research, faculty preparation, family health, health policy, health promotion/disease prevention, health-care systems, human health and illness, information systems, nursing administration, nursing education, nursing policy, nursing research, nursing science, oncology.
Program Entrance Requirements Minimum overall college GPA of 3.0, interview by faculty committee, 3 letters of recommendation, scholarly papers, statistics course, vita, GRE General Test. *Application deadline:* For fall admission, 2/15; for spring admission, 9/15. *Application fee:* $50 ($60 for international students).
Degree Requirements 90 total credit hours, dissertation, oral exam, written exam, residency.

POSTDOCTORAL PROGRAM

Areas of Study Adolescent health, cancer care, chronic illness, family health, health promotion/disease prevention, individualized study, nursing informatics, nursing research, nursing science.
Postdoctoral Program Contact Dr. Joan K. Austin, Distinguished Professor, School of Nursing, Indiana University–Purdue University Indianapolis, 1111 Middle Drive, Indianapolis, IN 46202-5107. *Telephone:* 317-274-8254. *Fax:* 317-278-1811. *E-mail:* joausti@iupui.edu.

CONTINUING EDUCATION PROGRAM

Contact Janice Ward, Director, Lifelong Learning, School of Nursing, Indiana University–Purdue University Indianapolis, 1111 Middle Drive, NU 347, Indianapolis, IN 46202-5107. *Telephone:* 317-274-7779. *Fax:* 317-274-0012. *E-mail:* jaward@iupui.edu.

See full description on page 496.

Indiana University South Bend
Division of Nursing and Health Professions
South Bend, Indiana

http://www.iusb.edu/~health/
Founded in 1922
DEGREE • BSN

Nursing Program Faculty 24 (25% with doctorates).
Baccalaureate Enrollment 170
Women 94% **Men** 6% **Minority** 11% **International** 1% **Part-time** 36%
Nursing Student Activities Sigma Theta Tau, Student Nurses' Association.

Nursing Student Resources Academic advising; academic or career counseling; assistance for students with disabilities; bookstore; campus computer network; career placement assistance; computer lab; computer-assisted instruction; daycare for children of students; e-mail services; employment services for current students; externships; interactive nursing skills videos; Internet; learning resource lab; library services; nursing audiovisuals; placement services for program completers; resume preparation assistance; skills, simulation, or other laboratory; tutoring.

Library Facilities 300,202 volumes (4,300 in health, 2,300 in nursing); 1,937 periodical subscriptions (145 health-care related).

BACCALAUREATE PROGRAMS

Degree BSN

Available Programs Accelerated Baccalaureate for Second Degree; Generic Baccalaureate; RN Baccalaureate.

Study Options Full-time and part-time.

Program Entrance Requirements Minimum overall college GPA of 2.3, transcript of college record, CPR certification, written essay, health exam, health insurance, high school biology, high school chemistry, high school transcript, immunizations, minimum high school GPA of 2.0, minimum high school rank 50%, minimum GPA in nursing prerequisites of 2.5, prerequisite course work. Transfer students are accepted. **Standardized tests** *Required:* SAT or ACT. *Recommended:* TOEFL for international students. **Application** *Deadline:* rolling (freshmen), rolling (transfer). *Notification:* continuous (freshmen). *Application fee:* $45.

Advanced Placement Credit given for nursing courses completed elsewhere dependent upon specific evaluations.

Expenses (2006–07) *Tuition, area resident:* part-time $161 per credit hour. *Tuition, nonresident:* part-time $420 per credit hour. *Required fees:* full-time $1500.

Financial Aid 65% of baccalaureate students in nursing programs received some form of financial aid in 2005–06. *Gift aid (need-based):* Federal Pell, FSEOG, state, private, college/university gift aid from institutional funds. *Loans:* Federal Nursing Student Loans, Federal Direct (Subsidized and Unsubsidized Stafford PLUS), Perkins, college/university. *Work-Study:* Federal Work-Study. *Application deadline (priority):* 3/1.

Contact Office of Student Services, Division of Nursing and Health Professions, Indiana University South Bend, 1700 Mishawaka Avenue, PO Box 7111, South Bend, IN 46634-7111. *Telephone:* 574-520-4571. *Fax:* 574-520-4461. *E-mail:* nursing@iusb.edu.

Indiana University Southeast
Division of Nursing
New Albany, Indiana

http://www.ius.edu/Nursing/homepage1.htm

Founded in 1941

DEGREE • BSN

Nursing Program Faculty 10 (35% with doctorates).

Baccalaureate Enrollment 154
Women 96% **Men** 4% **Minority** 1% **International** 2%

Nursing Student Activities Sigma Theta Tau, Student Nurses' Association.

Nursing Student Resources Academic advising; academic or career counseling; assistance for students with disabilities; bookstore; career placement assistance; computer lab; computer-assisted instruction; daycare for children of students; e-mail services; externships; Internet; learning resource lab; library services; skills, simulation, or other laboratory; tutoring.

Library Facilities 215,429 volumes; 962 periodical subscriptions.

BACCALAUREATE PROGRAMS

Degree BSN

Available Programs Generic Baccalaureate; RN Baccalaureate.
Study Options Full-time.

Program Entrance Requirements Transcript of college record, CPR certification, immunizations, minimum GPA in nursing prerequisites of 3.6, prerequisite course work. Transfer students are accepted. **Standardized tests** *Required:* SAT or ACT, TOEFL for international students. **Application** *Deadline:* rolling (freshmen), rolling (transfer). *Notification:* continuous (freshmen). *Application fee:* $30.

Advanced Placement Credit given for nursing courses completed elsewhere dependent upon specific evaluations.

Expenses (2006–07) *Tuition, state resident:* full-time $6200; part-time $175 per credit hour. *Tuition, nonresident:* full-time $13,599; part-time $389 per credit hour. *Required fees:* full-time $576.

Financial Aid 90% of baccalaureate students in nursing programs received some form of financial aid in 2005–06. *Gift aid (need-based):* Federal Pell, FSEOG, state, private, college/university gift aid from institutional funds. *Loans:* Federal Nursing Student Loans, FFEL (Subsidized and Unsubsidized Stafford PLUS), Perkins, college/university. *Work-Study:* Federal Work-Study. *Application deadline (priority):* 3/1.

Contact Ms. Brenda Hackett, Nursing Advisor, Division of Nursing, Indiana University Southeast, 4201 Grant Line Road, Life Sciences Building, Room 276, New Albany, IN 47150-6405. *Telephone:* 812-941-2283. *Fax:* 812-941-2687. *E-mail:* bhackett@ius.edu.

Indiana Wesleyan University
Division of Nursing
Marion, Indiana

http://www.indwes.edu/academics/Nursing

Founded in 1920

DEGREES • BS • MS

Nursing Program Faculty 264 (21% with doctorates).

Baccalaureate Enrollment 1,160
Women 93% **Men** 7% **Minority** 14% **Part-time** 4%

Graduate Enrollment 314
Women 95% **Men** 5% **Minority** 16% **Part-time** 1%

Nursing Student Activities Nursing Honor Society, Sigma Theta Tau, Student Nurses' Association, nursing club.

Nursing Student Resources Academic advising; academic or career counseling; assistance for students with disabilities; bookstore; campus computer network; career placement assistance; computer lab; computer-assisted instruction; e-mail services; housing assistance; Internet; learning resource lab; library services; nursing audiovisuals; remedial services; resume preparation assistance; skills, simulation, or other laboratory; tutoring.

Library Facilities 141,236 volumes (6,821 in health, 5,292 in nursing); 76,011 periodical subscriptions (155 health-care related).

BACCALAUREATE PROGRAMS

Degree BS

Available Programs ADN to Baccalaureate; Accelerated Baccalaureate for Second Degree; Generic Baccalaureate; RN Baccalaureate.
Site Options Indianapolis, IN; Fort Wayne, IN; Terre Haute, IN.
Study Options Full-time and part-time.

Program Entrance Requirements Minimum overall college GPA of 2.75, transcript of college record, CPR certification, written essay, health exam, high school biology, high school chemistry, high school foreign language, 3 years high school math, 3 years high school science, high school transcript, immunizations, minimum high school GPA of 2.8, minimum GPA in nursing prerequisites of 2.75, prerequisite course work. Transfer students are accepted. **Standardized tests** *Required:* SAT or ACT, TOEFL for international students. **Application** *Deadline:* rolling (freshmen), rolling (transfer). *Notification:* continuous (freshmen). *Application fee:* $25.

Advanced Placement Credit given for nursing courses completed elsewhere dependent upon specific evaluations.

Expenses (2006–07) *Tuition:* full-time $17,164; part-time $365 per credit hour. *International tuition:* $17,164 full-time. *Room and board:* $6124; room only: $2940 per academic year. *Required fees:* full-time $135; part-time $15 per credit.

Indiana Wesleyan University (continued)

Financial Aid 82% of baccalaureate students in nursing programs received some form of financial aid in 2005–06. *Gift aid (need-based):* Federal Pell, FSEOG, state, private, college/university gift aid from institutional funds. *Loans:* FFEL (Subsidized and Unsubsidized Stafford PLUS), Perkins, college/university. *Work-Study:* Federal Work-Study, part-time campus jobs. *Application deadline (priority):* 3/1.

Contact Sandy Mindach, Divisional Secretary, Division of Nursing, Indiana Wesleyan University, 4201 South Washington Street, Marion, IN 46953. *Telephone:* 765-677-2269. *Fax:* 765-677-2284. *E-mail:* sandy. mindach@indwes.edu.

GRADUATE PROGRAMS

Expenses (2006–07) *Tuition:* full-time $8300; part-time $415 per credit hour. *International tuition:* $8300 full-time. *Required fees:* full-time $80.

Financial Aid 62% of graduate students in nursing programs received some form of financial aid in 2005–06. 15 fellowships were awarded; career-related internships or fieldwork, scholarships, and traineeships also available. Aid available to part-time students. *Financial aid application deadline:* 3/15.

Contact Mrs. Pam Giles, Chair, Department of Graduate Nursing Studies, Division of Nursing, Indiana Wesleyan University, 4201 South Washington Street, Marion, IN 46953. *Telephone:* 765-677-1716 Ext. 2357. *Fax:* 765-677-2380. *E-mail:* pam.giles@indwes.edu.

MASTER'S DEGREE PROGRAM

Degree MS

Available Programs Master's.

Concentrations Available Nursing administration; nursing education. *Nurse practitioner programs in:* family health, gerontology.

Site Options Indianapolis, IN; Fort Wayne, IN; Terre Haute, IN.

Study Options Full-time and part-time.

Program Entrance Requirements Clinical experience, minimum overall college GPA of 3.0, transcript of college record, immunizations, interview, 3 letters of recommendation, nursing research course, physical assessment course, resume, statistics course, GRE. *Application deadline:* For fall admission, 7/31 (priority date); for winter admission, 11/15 (priority date); for spring admission, 4/15 (priority date).

Advanced Placement Credit given for nursing courses completed elsewhere dependent upon specific evaluations.

Degree Requirements 43 total credit hours, thesis or project.

POST-MASTER'S PROGRAM

Areas of Study Nursing administration; nursing education. *Nurse practitioner programs in:* family health, gerontology.

Marian College
Department of Nursing and Nutritional Science
Indianapolis, Indiana

http://www.sonak.marian.edu/academ/nursing/ index.html

Founded in 1851

DEGREE • BSN

Nursing Program Faculty 16 (1% with doctorates).

Nursing Student Activities Nursing Honor Society, Sigma Theta Tau, Student Nurses' Association.

Nursing Student Resources Academic advising; academic or career counseling; assistance for students with disabilities; bookstore; campus computer network; career placement assistance; computer lab; computer-assisted instruction; e-mail services; employment services for current students; interactive nursing skills videos; Internet; learning resource lab; library services; nursing audiovisuals; resume preparation assistance; skills, simulation, or other laboratory; tutoring.

Library Facilities 132,000 volumes (3,250 in health, 2,000 in nursing); 300 periodical subscriptions (116 health-care related).

BACCALAUREATE PROGRAMS

Degree BSN

Available Programs Accelerated Baccalaureate for Second Degree; Generic Baccalaureate; LPN to Baccalaureate; RN Baccalaureate.

Study Options Full-time and part-time.

Program Entrance Requirements Minimum overall college GPA of 2.5, transcript of college record, CPR certification, high school biology, high school chemistry, high school transcript, immunizations, minimum high school GPA of 2.7, minimum GPA in nursing prerequisites of 2.67, prerequisite course work. Transfer students are accepted. **Standardized tests** *Required:* SAT or ACT, TOEFL for international students. **Application** *Deadline:* 8/15 (freshmen), 8/1 (transfer). *Notification:* continuous until 8/24 (freshmen). *Application fee:* $20.

Advanced Placement Credit by examination available. Credit given for nursing courses completed elsewhere dependent upon specific evaluations.

Contact *Telephone:* 317-955-6157. *Fax:* 317-955-6135.

Purdue University
School of Nursing
West Lafayette, Indiana

http://www.nursing.purdue.edu

Founded in 1869

DEGREES • BS • DNP • MS

Nursing Program Faculty 60 (15% with doctorates).

Baccalaureate Enrollment 552
Women 95% **Men** 5% **Minority** 2% **International** .5% **Part-time** .06%

Graduate Enrollment 48
Women 99% **Men** 1% **Part-time** .25%

Nursing Student Activities Sigma Theta Tau, Student Nurses' Association.

Nursing Student Resources Academic advising; academic or career counseling; assistance for students with disabilities; bookstore; campus computer network; career placement assistance; computer lab; computer-assisted instruction; e-mail services; interactive nursing skills videos; Internet; learning resource lab; library services; nursing audiovisuals; remedial services; resume preparation assistance; skills, simulation, or other laboratory; tutoring.

Library Facilities 2.5 million volumes (200,000 in health, 10,000 in nursing); 20,829 periodical subscriptions (1,000 health-care related).

BACCALAUREATE PROGRAMS

Degree BS

Available Programs ADN to Baccalaureate; Baccalaureate for Second Degree; Generic Baccalaureate; RN Baccalaureate.

Site Options Indianapolis, IN.

Study Options Full-time and part-time.

Program Entrance Requirements Transcript of college record, CPR certification, health exam, health insurance, high school biology, high school chemistry, high school foreign language, 3 years high school math, 3 years high school science, high school transcript, immunizations, letters of recommendation, minimum high school GPA of 3.0. Transfer students are accepted. **Standardized tests** *Required:* SAT or ACT, TOEFL for international students. **Application** *Deadline:* 3/1 (freshmen), rolling (transfer). *Notification:* continuous (freshmen). *Application fee:* $30.

Advanced Placement Credit by examination available. Credit given for nursing courses completed elsewhere dependent upon specific evaluations.

Expenses (2006–07) *Tuition, state resident:* full-time $7096; part-time $254 per credit hour. *Tuition, nonresident:* full-time $21,266; part-time $706 per credit hour. *International tuition:* $21,316 full-time. *Room and board:* $7076 per academic year. *Required fees:* full-time $300; part-time $150 per term.

Financial Aid 75% of baccalaureate students in nursing programs received some form of financial aid in 2005–06. *Gift aid (need-based):* Federal Pell, FSEOG, state, private, college/university gift aid from institutional funds. *Loans:* FFEL (Subsidized and Unsubsidized Stafford PLUS), Perkins, college/university. *Work-Study:* Federal Work-Study. *Application deadline (priority):* 3/1.

Contact Office of Admissions, School of Nursing, Purdue University, Schleman Hall of Student Services, West Lafayette, IN 47907-2069. *Telephone:* 765-494-1776. *Fax:* 765-494-0544. *E-mail:* admissions@purdue.edu.

GRADUATE PROGRAMS

Expenses (2006–07) *Tuition, state resident:* full-time $7096; part-time $254 per credit hour. *Tuition, nonresident:* full-time $21,266; part-time $706 per credit hour. *International tuition:* $21,316 full-time. *Room and board:* $7076 per academic year. *Required fees:* full-time $300; part-time $150 per term.

Financial Aid 100% of graduate students in nursing programs received some form of financial aid in 2005–06.

Contact Dr. Nancy Edwards, Interim Program Director, School of Nursing, Purdue University, 502 North University Street, West Lafayette, IN 47907-2069. *Telephone:* 765-494-4015. *Fax:* 765-496-1800. *E-mail:* edwardsn@purdue.edu.

MASTER'S DEGREE PROGRAM

Degree MS

Available Programs Master's.

Concentrations Available *Nurse practitioner programs in:* adult health, pediatric.

Study Options Full-time and part-time.

Program Entrance Requirements Clinical experience, computer literacy, minimum overall college GPA of 3.0, transcript of college record, CPR certification, written essay, interview, 3 letters of recommendation, professional liability insurance/malpractice insurance, prerequisite course work, resume, statistics course.

Advanced Placement Credit given for nursing courses completed elsewhere dependent upon specific evaluations.

Degree Requirements 46 total credit hours, thesis or project.

POST-MASTER'S PROGRAM

Areas of Study *Nurse practitioner programs in:* adult health, pediatric.

DOCTORAL DEGREE PROGRAM

Degree DNP

Available Programs Doctorate; Doctorate for Nurses with Non-Nursing Degrees.

Areas of Study Advanced practice nursing, aging, biology of health and illness, clinical practice, critical care, ethics, gerontology, health policy, health promotion/disease prevention, health-care systems, illness and transition, individualized study, information systems, nursing administration, nursing education, nursing policy, nursing research, nursing science, oncology, urban health, women's health.

Program Entrance Requirements Clinical experience, minimum overall college GPA of 3.0, interview by faculty committee, MSN or equivalent, vita, writing sample.

Degree Requirements 40 total credit hours, oral exam, residency.

CONTINUING EDUCATION PROGRAM

Contact Dr. Patricia G. Coyle-Rogers, Director of Lifelong Learning, School of Nursing, Purdue University, 502 North University Street, West Lafayette, IN 47907-2069. *Telephone:* 765-494-4030. *Fax:* 765-494-6339. *E-mail:* pcrogers@purdue.edu.

Purdue University Calumet

School of Nursing
Hammond, Indiana

Founded in 1951

DEGREES • BS • MS

Nursing Program Faculty 30 (45% with doctorates).

Baccalaureate Enrollment 408
Women 96% **Men** 4% **Minority** 39% **Part-time** 30%

Graduate Enrollment 100
Women 95% **Men** 5% **Minority** 19% **Part-time** 86%

Nursing Student Activities Sigma Theta Tau, Student Nurses' Association, nursing club.

Nursing Student Resources Academic advising; academic or career counseling; assistance for students with disabilities; bookstore; campus computer network; career placement assistance; computer lab; computer-assisted instruction; daycare for children of students; e-mail services; employment services for current students; externships; housing assistance; interactive nursing skills videos; Internet; learning resource lab; library services; nursing audiovisuals; paid internships; placement services for program completers; remedial services; resume preparation assistance; skills, simulation, or other laboratory; tutoring; unpaid internships.

Library Facilities 269,648 volumes (400 in health, 300 in nursing); 1,228 periodical subscriptions (110 health-care related).

BACCALAUREATE PROGRAMS

Degree BS

Available Programs Baccalaureate for Second Degree; Generic Baccalaureate; RN Baccalaureate.

Study Options Full-time and part-time.

Program Entrance Requirements Minimum overall college GPA of 2.5, transcript of college record, CPR certification, health exam, high school biology, high school chemistry, 2 years high school math, 3 years high school science, high school transcript, immunizations, minimum high school rank 65%, minimum GPA in nursing prerequisites of 2.0, prerequisite course work. Transfer students are accepted. **Standardized tests** *Required for some:* SAT or ACT. **Application** *Deadline:* rolling (freshmen), rolling (transfer).

Advanced Placement Credit by examination available. Credit given for nursing courses completed elsewhere dependent upon specific evaluations.

Expenses (2006–07) *Tuition, area resident:* full-time $5733; part-time $146 per credit hour. *Tuition, nonresident:* full-time $12,856; part-time $369 per credit hour. *Room and board:* room only: $4000 per academic year. *Required fees:* full-time $293; part-time $16 per credit.

Financial Aid 35% of baccalaureate students in nursing programs received some form of financial aid in 2005–06.

Contact Kathleen Nix, Undergraduate Program Coordinator, School of Nursing, Purdue University Calumet, 2200 169th Street, Hammond, IN 46323-2094. *Telephone:* 219-989-2814. *Fax:* 219-989-2848. *E-mail:* nix@calumet.purdue.edu.

GRADUATE PROGRAMS

Expenses (2006–07) *Tuition, state resident:* full-time $4781; part-time $213 per credit hour. *Tuition, nonresident:* full-time $10,257; part-time $456 per credit hour. *Required fees:* full-time $298; part-time $11 per credit.

Financial Aid 30% of graduate students in nursing programs received some form of financial aid in 2005–06.

Contact Dr. Jane Walker, Graduate Program Coordinator, School of Nursing, Purdue University Calumet, 2200 169th Street, Hammond, IN 46323-2094. *Telephone:* 219-989-2815. *Fax:* 219-989-2848. *E-mail:* walkerj@calumet.purdue.edu.

MASTER'S DEGREE PROGRAM

Degree MS

Available Programs Accelerated RN to Master's; Master's.

Concentrations Available Nursing administration. *Clinical nurse specialist programs in:* adult health, critical care. *Nurse practitioner programs in:* family health.

Site Options Crown Point, IN. *Distance Learning:* Fort Wayne, IN; West Lafayette, IN.

Study Options Full-time and part-time.

Program Entrance Requirements Clinical experience, minimum overall college GPA of 3.0, transcript of college record, written essay, interview, 3 letters of recommendation, physical assessment course, resume, statistics course.

Advanced Placement Credit given for nursing courses completed elsewhere dependent upon specific evaluations.

Degree Requirements 45 total credit hours.

Purdue University Calumet (continued)
POST-MASTER'S PROGRAM
Areas of Study Nursing education. *Nurse practitioner programs in:* family health.

Purdue University North Central
Department of Nursing
Westville, Indiana

Founded in 1967

DEGREE • BS

Library Facilities 87,675 volumes; 403 periodical subscriptions.

BACCALAUREATE PROGRAMS
Degree BS

Available Programs RN Baccalaureate.

Program Entrance Requirements Standardized tests *Required:* TOEFL for international students. *Recommended:* SAT, ACT. *Required for some:* SAT or ACT. **Application** *Deadline:* 8/6 (freshmen), 8/1 (transfer). *Notification:* continuous (freshmen).

Contact Nursing Contact, Department of Nursing, Purdue University North Central, 1404 South U.S. 421, Westville, IN 46391. *Telephone:* 219-785-5200. *E-mail:* nursing@pnc.edu.

Saint Mary's College
Department of Nursing
Notre Dame, Indiana

http://www.saintmarys.edu

Founded in 1844

DEGREE • BS

Nursing Program Faculty 14 (13% with doctorates).

Baccalaureate Enrollment 157
Women 100% **Minority** 4%

Nursing Student Activities Nursing Honor Society, Sigma Theta Tau, Student Nurses' Association.

Nursing Student Resources Academic advising; academic or career counseling; assistance for students with disabilities; bookstore; campus computer network; career placement assistance; computer lab; computer-assisted instruction; daycare for children of students; e-mail services; employment services for current students; externships; interactive nursing skills videos; Internet; learning resource lab; library services; nursing audiovisuals; paid internships; placement services for program completers; remedial services; resume preparation assistance; skills, simulation, or other laboratory; tutoring; unpaid internships.

Library Facilities 215,616 volumes (9,787 in health, 5,149 in nursing); 759 periodical subscriptions (70 health-care related).

BACCALAUREATE PROGRAMS
Degree BS

Available Programs Accelerated Baccalaureate; Generic Baccalaureate.
Site Options Goshen, IN; South Bend, IN.
Study Options Full-time.
Program Entrance Requirements Minimum overall college GPA of 3.0, transcript of college record, CPR certification, written essay, health exam, high school foreign language, 3 years high school math, 2 years high school science, high school transcript, immunizations, interview, 2 letters of recommendation, minimum GPA in nursing prerequisites of 2.5. Transfer students are accepted. **Standardized tests** *Required:* SAT or ACT, TOEFL for international students. **Application** *Deadline:* 3/1 (freshmen), rolling (transfer). *Early decision:* 11/15. *Notification:* continuous (freshmen), 12/15 (out-of-state freshmen), 12/15 (early decision). *Application fee:* $30.
Advanced Placement Credit given for nursing courses completed elsewhere dependent upon specific evaluations.

Expenses (2006–07) *Tuition:* full-time $23,838; part-time $942 per credit hour. *Room and board:* $9430 per academic year. *Required fees:* full-time $500.
Financial Aid 75% of baccalaureate students in nursing programs received some form of financial aid in 2005–06. *Gift aid (need-based):* Federal Pell, FSEOG, state, private, college/university gift aid from institutional funds. *Loans:* FFEL (Subsidized and Unsubsidized Stafford PLUS), Perkins, college/university. *Work-Study:* Federal Work-Study, part-time campus jobs. *Application deadline (priority):* 3/1.
Contact Mr. Daniel L. Meyer, Vice President for Enrollment Management, Department of Nursing, Saint Mary's College, 124 LeMans, Notre Dame, IN 46556. *Telephone:* 574-284-4587. *Fax:* 574-284-4716. *E-mail:* dmeyer@ saintmarys.edu.

University of Evansville
Department of Nursing
Evansville, Indiana

http://nursing.evansville.edu

Founded in 1854

DEGREE • BSN

Nursing Program Faculty 8 (12% with doctorates).

Baccalaureate Enrollment 67
Women 99% **Men** 1% **Minority** 2%

Nursing Student Activities Sigma Theta Tau, Student Nurses' Association.

Nursing Student Resources Academic advising; academic or career counseling; assistance for students with disabilities; bookstore; campus computer network; career placement assistance; computer lab; computer-assisted instruction; e-mail services; employment services for current students; externships; housing assistance; Internet; learning resource lab; library services; nursing audiovisuals; paid internships; placement services for program completers; remedial services; resume preparation assistance; skills, simulation, or other laboratory; tutoring; unpaid internships.

Library Facilities 289,593 volumes (11,000 in nursing); 970 periodical subscriptions (155 health-care related).

BACCALAUREATE PROGRAMS
Degree BSN

Available Programs Generic Baccalaureate.
Study Options Full-time.
Program Entrance Requirements Health exam, health insurance, high school biology, high school chemistry, 4 years high school math, 4 years high school science, high school transcript, immunizations, minimum high school rank 67%, professional liability insurance/malpractice insurance. Transfer students are accepted. **Standardized tests** *Required:* SAT or ACT, TOEFL for international students. **Application** *Deadline:* 2/1 (freshmen), 2/1 (out-of-state freshmen), rolling (transfer). *Early decision:* 12/1. *Notification:* continuous until 3/1 (freshmen), continuous until 3/1 (out-of-state freshmen), 12/15 (early action). *Application fee:* $35.
Contact *Telephone:* 812-479-2584. *Fax:* 812-479-2717.

University of Indianapolis
School of Nursing
Indianapolis, Indiana

http://www.uindy.edu

Founded in 1902

DEGREES • BSN • MSN • MSN/MBA

Nursing Program Faculty 46 (45% with doctorates).

Baccalaureate Enrollment 241
Women 92% **Men** 8% **Minority** 10% **International** 2% **Part-time** 2%
Graduate Enrollment 121
Women 98% **Men** 2% **Minority** 2% **International** 1% **Part-time** 90%

Nursing Student Activities Nursing Honor Society, Sigma Theta Tau, Student Nurses' Association.

Nursing Student Resources Academic advising; academic or career counseling; assistance for students with disabilities; bookstore; campus computer network; career placement assistance; computer lab; computer-assisted instruction; e-mail services; employment services for current students; housing assistance; interactive nursing skills videos; Internet; learning resource lab; library services; nursing audiovisuals; remedial services; resume preparation assistance; skills, simulation, or other laboratory; tutoring.

Library Facilities 173,363 volumes (15,350 in health, 960 in nursing); 1,015 periodical subscriptions (202 health-care related).

BACCALAUREATE PROGRAMS

Degree BSN

Available Programs Accelerated RN Baccalaureate; Generic Baccalaureate.

Site Options Indianapolis, IN.

Study Options Full-time and part-time.

Program Entrance Requirements Minimum overall college GPA of 2.82, transcript of college record, CPR certification, health exam, health insurance, high school biology, high school chemistry, high school foreign language, 2 years high school math, 2 years high school science, high school transcript, immunizations, minimum high school GPA of 2.82, minimum GPA in nursing prerequisites of 2.82, prerequisite course work. Transfer students are accepted. **Standardized tests** *Required:* SAT or ACT. **Application** *Deadline:* rolling (freshmen), rolling (transfer). *Notification:* continuous (freshmen). *Application fee:* $20.

Advanced Placement Credit by examination available. Credit given for nursing courses completed elsewhere dependent upon specific evaluations.

Expenses (2006–07) *Tuition:* full-time $18,700; part-time $780 per credit hour. *International tuition:* $18,700 full-time. *Room and board:* $5090; room only: $3450 per academic year. *Required fees:* full-time $200; part-time $200 per credit; part-time $200 per term.

Financial Aid 88% of baccalaureate students in nursing programs received some form of financial aid in 2005–06.

Contact Erna Karla Backer, BSN Program Coordinator, School of Nursing, University of Indianapolis, 1400 East Hanna Avenue, Indianapolis, IN 46227-3697. *Telephone:* 317-788-3324. *Fax:* 317-788-3542. *E-mail:* backer@uindy.edu.

GRADUATE PROGRAMS

Expenses (2006–07) *Tuition:* full-time $4680; part-time $520 per credit hour. *International tuition:* $4680 full-time. *Required fees:* full-time $150; part-time $150 per credit; part-time $150 per term.

Financial Aid 90% of graduate students in nursing programs received some form of financial aid in 2005–06.

Contact Anita Siccardi, MSN Program Coordinator, School of Nursing, University of Indianapolis, 1400 East Hanna Avenue, Indianapolis, IN 46227-3697. *Telephone:* 317-788-3471. *Fax:* 317-788-3542. *E-mail:* siccardi@uindy.edu.

MASTER'S DEGREE PROGRAM

Degrees MSN; MSN/MBA

Available Programs Master's.

Concentrations Available Nurse-midwifery; nursing administration; nursing education. *Nurse practitioner programs in:* family health, gerontology.

Site Options Indianapolis, IN.

Study Options Full-time and part-time.

Program Entrance Requirements Clinical experience, minimum overall college GPA of 3.0, transcript of college record, CPR certification, written essay, immunizations, interview, 3 letters of recommendation.

Advanced Placement Credit given for nursing courses completed elsewhere dependent upon specific evaluations.

Degree Requirements 46 total credit hours, thesis or project.

POST-MASTER'S PROGRAM

Areas of Study Nurse-midwifery; nursing administration; nursing education. *Nurse practitioner programs in:* family health, gerontology.

University of Saint Francis
Department of Nursing
Fort Wayne, Indiana

http://www.sf.edu

Founded in 1890

DEGREES • BSN • MSN

Nursing Program Faculty 69 (9% with doctorates).

Baccalaureate Enrollment 291
Women 95% **Men** 5% **Minority** 4% **Part-time** 8%

Graduate Enrollment 34
Women 94% **Men** 6% **Minority** 3% **International** 3% **Part-time** 88%

Nursing Student Activities Sigma Theta Tau, Student Nurses' Association.

Nursing Student Resources Academic advising; academic or career counseling; assistance for students with disabilities; bookstore; campus computer network; career placement assistance; computer lab; computer-assisted instruction; e-mail services; employment services for current students; externships; housing assistance; interactive nursing skills videos; Internet; learning resource lab; library services; nursing audiovisuals; paid internships; remedial services; resume preparation assistance; skills, simulation, or other laboratory; tutoring; unpaid internships.

Library Facilities 50,186 volumes (7,826 in health, 1,746 in nursing); 549 periodical subscriptions (142 health-care related).

BACCALAUREATE PROGRAMS

Degree BSN

Available Programs ADN to Baccalaureate; Generic Baccalaureate; RN Baccalaureate.

Site Options *Distance Learning:* Fort Wayne, IN.

Study Options Full-time and part-time.

Program Entrance Requirements Minimum overall college GPA of 2.7, transcript of college record, CPR certification, health exam, high school biology, high school chemistry, 1 year of high school math, high school transcript, immunizations, minimum high school GPA of 2.7, minimum GPA in nursing prerequisites of 2.7, prerequisite course work. Transfer students are accepted. **Standardized tests** *Required:* SAT or ACT, TOEFL for international students. **Application** *Deadline:* rolling (freshmen), rolling (transfer). *Notification:* continuous until 8/15 (freshmen). *Application fee:* $20.

Advanced Placement Credit given for nursing courses completed elsewhere dependent upon specific evaluations.

Expenses (2006–07) *Tuition:* full-time $17,760; part-time $560 per credit. *International tuition:* $17,760 full-time. *Room and board:* $5834 per academic year. *Required fees:* full-time $798; part-time $17 per credit; part-time $155 per term.

Financial Aid 97% of baccalaureate students in nursing programs received some form of financial aid in 2005–06.

Contact Amy Knepp, BSN/MSN Program Director, Department of Nursing, University of Saint Francis, 2701 Spring Street, Fort Wayne, IN 46808. *Telephone:* 260-434-7447. *Fax:* 260-434-7404. *E-mail:* aknepp@sf.edu.

GRADUATE PROGRAMS

Expenses (2006–07) *Tuition:* part-time $590 per credit. *Room and board:* $5834 per academic year. *Required fees:* full-time $768; part-time $17 per credit; part-time $155 per term.

Financial Aid 90% of graduate students in nursing programs received some form of financial aid in 2005–06. Federal Work-Study and unspecified assistantships available.

Contact Amy Knepp, BSN/MSN Program Director, Department of Nursing, University of Saint Francis, 2701 Spring Street, Fort Wayne, IN 46808. *Telephone:* 260-434-3239. *Fax:* 260-434-7404. *E-mail:* aknepp@sf.edu.

MASTER'S DEGREE PROGRAM

Degree MSN

Available Programs Accelerated RN to Master's; Master's; Master's for Nurses with Non-Nursing Degrees.

University of Saint Francis (continued)

Concentrations Available *Nurse practitioner programs in:* family health.

Study Options Full-time and part-time.

Program Entrance Requirements Computer literacy, minimum overall college GPA of 3.2, transcript of college record, CPR certification, written essay, immunizations, interview, 3 letters of recommendation, nursing research course, physical assessment course, resume, statistics course, GRE. *Application deadline:* For fall admission, 7/1 (priority date); for spring admission, 11/1 (priority date). Applications are processed on a rolling basis. *Application fee:* $20.

Advanced Placement Credit given for nursing courses completed elsewhere dependent upon specific evaluations.

Degree Requirements 48 total credit hours.

POST-MASTER'S PROGRAM

Areas of Study *Nurse practitioner programs in:* family health.

University of Southern Indiana
College of Nursing and Health Professions
Evansville, Indiana

http://health.usi.edu

Founded in 1965

DEGREES • BSN • MSN

Nursing Program Faculty 25 (42% with doctorates).

Baccalaureate Enrollment 179
Women 95% **Men** 5% **Minority** 1% **Part-time** 30%

Graduate Enrollment 196
Women 94% **Men** 6% **Minority** 5% **Part-time** 62%

Nursing Student Activities Sigma Theta Tau, Student Nurses' Association.

Nursing Student Resources Academic advising; academic or career counseling; assistance for students with disabilities; bookstore; campus computer network; career placement assistance; computer lab; computer-assisted instruction; daycare for children of students; e-mail services; employment services for current students; housing assistance; interactive nursing skills videos; Internet; learning resource lab; library services; nursing audiovisuals; placement services for program completers; remedial services; resume preparation assistance; skills, simulation, or other laboratory; tutoring; unpaid internships.

Library Facilities 328,734 volumes (9,200 in health, 1,345 in nursing); 15,153 periodical subscriptions (1,470 health-care related).

BACCALAUREATE PROGRAMS

Degree BSN

Available Programs Generic Baccalaureate; RN Baccalaureate.

Study Options Full-time.

Program Entrance Requirements Minimum overall college GPA of 3.0, transcript of college record, CPR certification, written essay, health exam, high school transcript, immunizations, minimum high school GPA of 3.0, minimum GPA in nursing prerequisites of 3.0, professional liability insurance/malpractice insurance, prerequisite course work. Transfer students are accepted. **Standardized tests** *Required:* SAT or ACT, TOEFL for international students. **Application** *Deadline:* 8/15 (freshmen). *Notification:* continuous until 8/27 (freshmen). *Application fee:* $25.

Advanced Placement Credit given for nursing courses completed elsewhere dependent upon specific evaluations.

Expenses (2006–07) *Tuition, state resident:* full-time $4460; part-time $149 per credit hour. *Tuition, nonresident:* full-time $10,630; part-time $354 per credit hour. *International tuition:* $10,630 full-time. *Room and board:* $7165; room only: $3900 per academic year. *Required fees:* full-time $330; part-time $165 per term.

Financial Aid 70% of baccalaureate students in nursing programs received some form of financial aid in 2005–06. *Gift aid (need-based):* Federal Pell, FSEOG, state, private, college/university gift aid from institutional funds. *Loans:* FFEL (Subsidized and Unsubsidized Stafford PLUS), Perkins. *Work-Study:* Federal Work-Study. *Application deadline:* 3/1.

Contact Dr. Ann H. White, Assistant Dean for Nursing, College of Nursing and Health Professions, University of Southern Indiana, 8600 University Boulevard, Evansville, IN 47712. *Telephone:* 812-465-1173. *Fax:* 812-465-7092. *E-mail:* awhite@usi.edu.

GRADUATE PROGRAMS

Expenses (2006–07) *Tuition, state resident:* full-time $5180; part-time $216 per credit hour. *Tuition, nonresident:* full-time $5180; part-time $216 per credit hour. *International tuition:* $5180 full-time. *Room and board:* $7164; room only: $3900 per academic year. *Required fees:* full-time $670; part-time $335 per term.

Financial Aid 35% of graduate students in nursing programs received some form of financial aid in 2005–06. Federal Work-Study, scholarships, tuition waivers (full and partial), and unspecified assistantships available. *Financial aid application deadline:* 3/1.

Contact Dr. Ann H. White, Assistant Dean for Nursing, College of Nursing and Health Professions, University of Southern Indiana, 8600 University Boulevard, Evansville, IN 47712. *Telephone:* 812-465-1173. *Fax:* 812-465-7092. *E-mail:* awhite@usi.edu.

MASTER'S DEGREE PROGRAM

Degree MSN

Available Programs Master's; RN to Master's.

Concentrations Available Nursing administration; nursing education. *Nurse practitioner programs in:* acute care, family health.

Study Options Full-time and part-time.

Program Entrance Requirements Clinical experience, computer literacy, minimum overall college GPA of 3.0, transcript of college record, CPR certification, written essay, immunizations, 2 letters of recommendation, professional liability insurance/malpractice insurance, resume, statistics course. *Application deadline:* Applications are processed on a rolling basis. *Application fee:* $25.

Advanced Placement Credit given for nursing courses completed elsewhere dependent upon specific evaluations.

Degree Requirements 42 total credit hours, thesis or project.

POST-MASTER'S PROGRAM

Areas of Study Nursing administration; nursing education. *Nurse practitioner programs in:* acute care, family health.

CONTINUING EDUCATION PROGRAM

Contact Peggy Graul, Coordinator of Continuing Education for Nursing and Health Professions, College of Nursing and Health Professions, University of Southern Indiana, 8600 University Boulevard, Evansville, IN 47712. *Telephone:* 812-465-1161. *Fax:* 812-465-7092. *E-mail:* pgraul@usi.edu.

See full description on page 560.

Valparaiso University
College of Nursing
Valparaiso, Indiana

http://www.valpo.edu/nursing

Founded in 1859

DEGREES • BSN • MSN • MSN/MBA

Nursing Program Faculty 12 (33% with doctorates).

Baccalaureate Enrollment 268
Women 93% **Men** 7% **Minority** 12% **International** 1% **Part-time** 7%

Graduate Enrollment 39
Women 95% **Men** 5% **Minority** 26% **Part-time** 59%

Nursing Student Activities Sigma Theta Tau, Student Nurses' Association.

Nursing Student Resources Academic advising; academic or career counseling; assistance for students with disabilities; bookstore; campus computer network; career placement assistance; computer lab; computer-assisted instruction; e-mail services; employment services for current students; externships; housing assistance; interactive nursing skills videos; Internet; learning resource lab; library services; nursing audiovisuals;

placement services for program completers; remedial services; resume preparation assistance; skills, simulation, or other laboratory; tutoring; unpaid internships.

Library Facilities 471,645 volumes (9,500 in health, 995 in nursing); 41,649 periodical subscriptions (1,000 health-care related).

BACCALAUREATE PROGRAMS

Degree BSN

Available Programs Accelerated Baccalaureate; Generic Baccalaureate; RN Baccalaureate.

Study Options Full-time and part-time.

Program Entrance Requirements Minimum overall college GPA of 3.0, transcript of college record, written essay, high school biology, high school chemistry, 2 years high school math, 4 years high school science, high school transcript, immunizations, minimum high school GPA of 2.0, minimum GPA in nursing prerequisites of 2.5. Transfer students are accepted. **Standardized tests** *Required:* SAT or ACT, TOEFL for international students. **Application** *Deadline:* 8/15 (freshmen). *Early decision:* 11/1. *Notification:* 12/1 (early action). *Application fee:* $30.

Advanced Placement Credit by examination available. Credit given for nursing courses completed elsewhere dependent upon specific evaluations.

Expenses (2006–07) *Tuition:* full-time $23,200; part-time $1100 per credit hour. *International tuition:* $23,200 full-time. *Room and board:* $6640; room only: $4140 per academic year. *Required fees:* full-time $1324; part-time $20 per credit.

Financial Aid 75% of baccalaureate students in nursing programs received some form of financial aid in 2005–06. *Gift aid (need-based):* Federal Pell, FSEOG, state, private, college/university gift aid from institutional funds. *Loans:* Federal Direct (Subsidized and Unsubsidized Stafford PLUS), Perkins, college/university. *Work-Study:* Federal Work-Study, part-time campus jobs. *Application deadline (priority):* 3/1.

Contact Admissions Counselor, College of Nursing, Valparaiso University, Office of Admission, Kretzmann Hall, Valparaiso, IN 46383. *Telephone:* 219-464-5011. *Fax:* 219-464-6888. *E-mail:* admitinfo@valpo.edu.

GRADUATE PROGRAMS

Expenses (2006–07) *Tuition:* full-time $11,160; part-time $465 per credit hour. *International tuition:* $11,160 full-time. *Required fees:* full-time $264; part-time $60 per term.

Financial Aid 79% of graduate students in nursing programs received some form of financial aid in 2005–06. Scholarships available. Aid available to part-time students.

Contact Dr. Janet M. Brown, Dean, College of Nursing, Valparaiso University, 836 LaPorte Avenue, Valparaiso, IN 46383-6493. *Telephone:* 219-464-5289. *Fax:* 219-464-5425. *E-mail:* janet.brown@valpo.edu.

MASTER'S DEGREE PROGRAM

Degrees MSN; MSN/MBA

Available Programs Master's; RN to Master's.

Concentrations Available *Clinical nurse specialist programs in:* adult health, gerontology, women's health.

Study Options Full-time and part-time.

Program Entrance Requirements Minimum overall college GPA of 3.0, transcript of college record, CPR certification, written essay, immunizations, 2 letters of recommendation, nursing research course, physical assessment course, statistics course. *Application deadline:* Applications are processed on a rolling basis. *Application fee:* $30 ($50 for international students).

Advanced Placement Credit given for nursing courses completed elsewhere dependent upon specific evaluations.

Degree Requirements 36 total credit hours, thesis or project.

POST-MASTER'S PROGRAM

Areas of Study *Nurse practitioner programs in:* family health.

CONTINUING EDUCATION PROGRAM

Contact Mrs. Julie Koch, Assistant Professor, College of Nursing, Valparaiso University, 836 LaPorte Avenue, Valparaiso, IN 46383. *Telephone:* 219-464-5291. *Fax:* 219-464-5425. *E-mail:* julie.koch@valpo.edu.

IOWA

Allen College
Program in Nursing
Waterloo, Iowa

http://www.allencollege.edu
Founded in 1989
DEGREES • BSN • MSN

Nursing Program Faculty 28 (14% with doctorates).

Baccalaureate Enrollment 324
Women 94% **Men** 6% **Minority** 3% **Part-time** 14%

Graduate Enrollment 67
Women 93% **Men** 7% **Part-time** 70%

Nursing Student Activities Sigma Theta Tau, Student Nurses' Association, nursing club.

Nursing Student Resources Academic advising; academic or career counseling; campus computer network; career placement assistance; computer lab; computer-assisted instruction; daycare for children of students; employment services for current students; housing assistance; Internet; library services; nursing audiovisuals; other; placement services for program completers; resume preparation assistance; tutoring.

Library Facilities 2,797 volumes (3,100 in health, 2,975 in nursing); 199 periodical subscriptions (202 health-care related).

BACCALAUREATE PROGRAMS

Degree BSN

Available Programs ADN to Baccalaureate; Accelerated Baccalaureate; Accelerated Baccalaureate for Second Degree; Accelerated RN Baccalaureate; Baccalaureate for Second Degree; Generic Baccalaureate; LPN to Baccalaureate; RN Baccalaureate.

Study Options Full-time and part-time.

Program Entrance Requirements Minimum overall college GPA of 2.7, transcript of college record, CPR certification, health exam, high school biology, high school chemistry, 3 years high school math, 3 years high school science, high school transcript, immunizations, 1 letter of recommendation, minimum high school GPA of 3.0, minimum high school rank 50%. Transfer students are accepted. **Standardized tests** *Required:* ACT, TOEFL for international students. **Application** *Deadline:* 7/1 (freshmen), 7/1 (transfer). *Early decision:* 3/1. *Notification:* continuous until 8/20 (freshmen), 3/15 (out-of-state freshmen), 3/15 (early decision). *Application fee:* $50.

Advanced Placement Credit given for nursing courses completed elsewhere dependent upon specific evaluations.

Expenses (2006–07) *Tuition:* full-time $12,306; part-time $415 per credit. *Room and board:* $5712; room only: $2856 per academic year. *Required fees:* full-time $1513; part-time $37 per credit; part-time $170 per term.

Financial Aid 86% of baccalaureate students in nursing programs received some form of financial aid in 2005–06.

Contact Diane DeGroote, Student Services Assistant, Program in Nursing, Allen College, 1825 Logan Avenue, Waterloo, IA 50703. *Telephone:* 319-226-2000. *Fax:* 319-226-2051. *E-mail:* AllenCollegeAdmissions@ihs.org.

GRADUATE PROGRAMS

Expenses (2006–07) *Tuition:* full-time $9827; part-time $562 per credit. *Room and board:* $5712; room only: $2856 per academic year. *Required fees:* full-time $481; part-time $37 per credit; part-time $170 per term.

Financial Aid 70% of graduate students in nursing programs received some form of financial aid in 2005–06. Institutionally sponsored loans, scholarships, and traineeships available. Aid available to part-time students. *Financial aid application deadline:* 8/15.

Contact Diane DeGroote, Student Services Assistant, Program in Nursing, Allen College, 1825 Logan Avenue, Waterloo, IA 50703. *Telephone:* 319-226-2000. *Fax:* 319-226-2051. *E-mail:* AllenCollegeAdmissions@ihs.org.

Allen College (continued)

MASTER'S DEGREE PROGRAM

Degree MSN

Available Programs Master's; Master's for Nurses with Non-Nursing Degrees; RN to Master's.

Concentrations Available Nursing administration; nursing education. *Nurse practitioner programs in:* family health.

Study Options Full-time and part-time.

Program Entrance Requirements Clinical experience, computer literacy, minimum overall college GPA of 3.0, transcript of college record, CPR certification, written essay, immunizations, interview, 3 letters of recommendation, nursing research course, professional liability insurance/ malpractice insurance, prerequisite course work, resume, statistics course. *Application deadline:* For fall admission, 7/15 (priority date); for spring admission, 12/1 (priority date). Applications are processed on a rolling basis. *Application fee:* $50.

Advanced Placement Credit given for nursing courses completed elsewhere dependent upon specific evaluations.

Degree Requirements 40 total credit hours, thesis or project.

POST-MASTER'S PROGRAM

Areas of Study Nursing administration; nursing education. *Nurse practitioner programs in:* family health.

POSTDOCTORAL PROGRAM

Postdoctoral Program Contact Dr. Diane Young, Department Chair, MSN Program, Program in Nursing, Allen College, 1825 Logan Avenue, Waterloo, IA 50703. *Telephone:* 319-226-2047. *Fax:* 319-226-2070. *E-mail:* YoungDM@ihs.org.

CONTINUING EDUCATION PROGRAM

Contact Mrs. Mary Kay Frost, Continuing Education Coordinator, Program in Nursing, Allen College, 1825 Logan Avenue, Waterloo, IA 50703. *Telephone:* 319-226-2028. *Fax:* 319-226-2051. *E-mail:* FrostMK@ihs.org.

Briar Cliff University
Department of Nursing
Sioux City, Iowa

http://www.briarcliff.edu/nursing

Founded in 1930

DEGREES • BSN • MSN

Nursing Program Faculty 9 (11% with doctorates).

Baccalaureate Enrollment 200
Women 90% **Men** 10% **Minority** 5% **Part-time** 50%

Graduate Enrollment 25
Women 95% **Men** 5% **Minority** 5% **Part-time** 50%

Nursing Student Activities Sigma Theta Tau, Student Nurses' Association.

Nursing Student Resources Academic advising; academic or career counseling; assistance for students with disabilities; bookstore; campus computer network; career placement assistance; computer lab; computer-assisted instruction; e-mail services; employment services for current students; externships; interactive nursing skills videos; Internet; learning resource lab; library services; nursing audiovisuals; placement services for program completers; remedial services; resume preparation assistance; skills, simulation, or other laboratory; tutoring.

Library Facilities 84,540 volumes; 10,409 periodical subscriptions.

BACCALAUREATE PROGRAMS

Degree BSN

Available Programs ADN to Baccalaureate; Generic Baccalaureate; LPN to Baccalaureate; RN Baccalaureate.

Study Options Full-time and part-time.

Program Entrance Requirements Minimum overall college GPA of 2.5, transcript of college record, CPR certification, written essay, health exam, high school transcript, immunizations, minimum GPA in nursing prerequisites of 2.5, prerequisite course work. Transfer students are accepted. **Standardized tests** *Required:* SAT or ACT. *Recommended:* TOEFL for international students. **Application** *Deadline:* rolling (freshmen), rolling (out-of-state freshmen), rolling (transfer). *Application fee:* $20.

Advanced Placement Credit by examination available. Credit given for nursing courses completed elsewhere dependent upon specific evaluations.

Expenses (2006–07) *Tuition:* full-time $18,714; part-time $624 per credit. *Room and board:* $5034; room only: $2835 per academic year. *Required fees:* full-time $400; part-time $18 per credit.

Financial Aid 90% of baccalaureate students in nursing programs received some form of financial aid in 2005–06.

Contact Dr. Richard A. Petersen, EdD, Department Chair and Associate Professor, Department of Nursing, Briar Cliff University, 3303 Rebecca Street, Sioux City, IA 51104. *Telephone:* 712-279-1662. *E-mail:* rick. petersen@briarcliff.edu.

GRADUATE PROGRAMS

Expenses (2006–07) *Tuition:* part-time $395 per credit. *Room and board:* $6034; room only: $2835 per academic year.

Financial Aid 60% of graduate students in nursing programs received some form of financial aid in 2005–06.

Contact Dr. Richard A. Petersen, EdD, Department Chair and Associate Professor, Department of Nursing, Briar Cliff University, 3303 Rebecca Street, Sioux City, IA 51104. *Telephone:* 712-279-1662. *E-mail:* rick. petersen@briarcliff.edu.

MASTER'S DEGREE PROGRAM

Degree MSN

Available Programs Master's.

Concentrations Available Nursing education. *Nurse practitioner programs in:* family health.

Study Options Full-time and part-time.

Program Entrance Requirements Clinical experience, computer literacy, minimum overall college GPA of 3.0, transcript of college record, CPR certification, written essay, immunizations, 2 letters of recommendation, nursing research course, physical assessment course, resume, statistics course.

Advanced Placement Credit given for nursing courses completed elsewhere dependent upon specific evaluations.

Degree Requirements 40 total credit hours, thesis or project.

CONTINUING EDUCATION PROGRAM

Contact Judith Scherer Connealy, Director of Continuing Education, Department of Nursing, Briar Cliff University, 3303 Rebecca Street, Sioux City, IA 51104. *Telephone:* 712-279-1774. *Fax:* 712-279-5497. *E-mail:* schererj@briarcliff.edu.

Clarke College
Department of Nursing and Health
Dubuque, Iowa

Founded in 1843

DEGREES • BS • MSN

Nursing Program Faculty 21.

Baccalaureate Enrollment 146
Women 95% **Men** 5% **Minority** 1% **Part-time** 1%

Graduate Enrollment 30
Men 4% **Part-time** 50%

Nursing Student Activities Nursing Honor Society, Sigma Theta Tau, Student Nurses' Association.

Nursing Student Resources Academic advising; academic or career counseling; assistance for students with disabilities; bookstore; campus computer network; career placement assistance; computer lab; computer-assisted instruction; e-mail services; employment services for current students; externships; housing assistance; interactive nursing skills videos; Internet; learning resource lab; library services; nursing audiovisuals; paid internships; placement services for program completers; remedial services; resume preparation assistance; skills, simulation, or other laboratory; tutoring; unpaid internships.

Library Facilities 182,649 volumes (7,000 in health, 2,856 in nursing); 508 periodical subscriptions (124 health-care related).

BACCALAUREATE PROGRAMS

Degree BS

Available Programs Baccalaureate for Second Degree; Generic Baccalaureate; RN Baccalaureate.

Study Options Full-time and part-time.

Program Entrance Requirements Minimum overall college GPA of 2.75, transcript of college record, CPR certification, written essay, health exam, health insurance, high school chemistry, high school foreign language, high school math, high school transcript, immunizations, interview, 2 letters of recommendation, minimum high school GPA of 2.0, minimum high school rank 50%, professional liability insurance/malpractice insurance, prerequisite course work. Transfer students are accepted. **Standardized tests** *Required:* SAT or ACT, TOEFL for international students. **Application** *Deadline:* rolling (freshmen), rolling (transfer). *Notification:* continuous until 7/15 (freshmen). *Application fee:* $25.

Advanced Placement Credit given for nursing courses completed elsewhere dependent upon specific evaluations.

Expenses (2006–07) *Tuition:* full-time $19,682; part-time $498 per credit. *Room and board:* $6576; room only: $3198 per academic year. *Required fees:* full-time $308; part-time $21 per credit.

Financial Aid 98% of baccalaureate students in nursing programs received some form of financial aid in 2005–06. *Gift aid (need-based):* Federal Pell, FSEOG, state, private, college/university gift aid from institutional funds. *Loans:* Federal Nursing Student Loans, FFEL (Subsidized and Unsubsidized Stafford PLUS), Perkins, state, college/university, alternative loans. *Work-Study:* Federal Work-Study, part-time campus jobs. *Application deadline (priority):* 4/15.

Contact Dr. Katherine Helen Frommelt, Chair, Department of Nursing and Health, Clarke College, 1550 Clarke Drive, Dubuque, IA 52001. *Telephone:* 563-588-6361. *Fax:* 563-588-8684. *E-mail:* kay.frommelt@clarke.edu.

GRADUATE PROGRAMS

Expenses (2006–07) *Tuition:* full-time $19,682; part-time $520 per credit hour. *Room and board:* $6574; room only: $3198 per academic year. *Required fees:* full-time $615; part-time $21 per credit.

Financial Aid 30% of graduate students in nursing programs received some form of financial aid in 2005–06. Career-related internships or fieldwork available. Aid available to part-time students.

Contact Dr. Katherine Helen Frommelt, Chair, Department of Nursing and Health, Clarke College, 1550 Clarke Drive, Dubuque, IA 52001. *Telephone:* 563-588-6361. *Fax:* 563-588-8684. *E-mail:* kay.frommelt@clarke.edu.

MASTER'S DEGREE PROGRAM

Degree MSN

Available Programs Master's.

Concentrations Available Nursing administration; nursing education. *Nurse practitioner programs in:* family health.

Study Options Full-time and part-time.

Program Entrance Requirements Computer literacy, minimum overall college GPA of 3.0, transcript of college record, CPR certification, written essay, immunizations, interview, 3 letters of recommendation, nursing research course, physical assessment course, prerequisite course work, resume, statistics course, GRE General Test or MAT. *Application deadline:* For fall admission, 2/15 (priority date); for spring admission, 12/15 (priority date). Applications are processed on a rolling basis. *Application fee:* $25.

Advanced Placement Credit given for nursing courses completed elsewhere dependent upon specific evaluations.

Degree Requirements 37 total credit hours, thesis or project.

POST-MASTER'S PROGRAM

Areas of Study *Nurse practitioner programs in:* family health.

CONTINUING EDUCATION PROGRAM

Contact Scott Schneider, Director of Adult Education and Timesaver Programs, Department of Nursing and Health, Clarke College, 1550 Clarke Drive, Dubuque, IA 52001. *Telephone:* 563-588-6378. *Fax:* 563-588-8684. *E-mail:* scott.schneider@clarke.edu.

Coe College
Department of Nursing
Cedar Rapids, Iowa

Founded in 1851

DEGREE • BSN

Nursing Program Faculty 6 (33% with doctorates).

Baccalaureate Enrollment 44
Women 95% **Men** 5%

Nursing Student Activities Student Nurses' Association.

Nursing Student Resources Academic advising; academic or career counseling; assistance for students with disabilities; bookstore; campus computer network; career placement assistance; computer lab; e-mail services; employment services for current students; housing assistance; Internet; learning resource lab; library services; nursing audiovisuals; remedial services; resume preparation assistance; skills, simulation, or other laboratory; tutoring; unpaid internships.

Library Facilities 218,881 volumes (2,929 in health, 492 in nursing); 1,576 periodical subscriptions (34 health-care related).

BACCALAUREATE PROGRAMS

Degree BSN

Available Programs Generic Baccalaureate; RN Baccalaureate.

Study Options Full-time and part-time.

Program Entrance Requirements Minimum overall college GPA of 2.7, transcript of college record, CPR certification, written essay, health exam, health insurance, high school chemistry, high school transcript, immunizations, minimum high school GPA of 2.0, minimum GPA in nursing prerequisites of 2.7, prerequisite course work. Transfer students are accepted. **Standardized tests** *Required:* SAT or ACT, TOEFL for international students. **Application** *Deadline:* 3/1 (freshmen), rolling (transfer). *Early decision:* 12/10. *Notification:* 3/15 (freshmen), 1/20 (early action). *Application fee:* $30.

Advanced Placement Credit given for nursing courses completed elsewhere dependent upon specific evaluations.

Expenses (2005–06) *Tuition:* full-time $23,570; part-time $1120 per course. *Room and board:* $6260; room only: $2880 per academic year.

Financial Aid *Gift aid (need-based):* Federal Pell, FSEOG, state, private, college/university gift aid from institutional funds, ROTC. *Loans:* Federal Direct (Subsidized and Unsubsidized Stafford PLUS), Perkins, college/university. *Work-Study:* Federal Work-Study, part-time campus jobs. *Application deadline (priority):* 3/1.

Contact Dr. H. Jule Ohrt, Chair, Department of Nursing, Coe College, 1220 First Avenue, NE, Cedar Rapids, IA 52402. *Telephone:* 319-369-8120. *Fax:* 319-369-8121. *E-mail:* johrt@coe.edu.

Grand View College
Division of Nursing
Des Moines, Iowa

http://www.gvc.edu/academics/nursing/

Founded in 1896

DEGREE • BSN

Nursing Program Faculty 16 (25% with doctorates).

Nursing Student Activities Student Nurses' Association.

Library Facilities 106,432 volumes (3,868 in health); 13,068 periodical subscriptions (91 health-care related).

Grand View College (continued)

BACCALAUREATE PROGRAMS

Degree BSN

Available Programs Generic Baccalaureate; RN Baccalaureate.

Study Options Full-time and part-time.

Program Entrance Requirements Minimum overall college GPA of 2.2, transcript of college record, CPR certification, health exam, high school chemistry, high school transcript, immunizations, 3 letters of recommendation, minimum GPA in nursing prerequisites of 2.2, prerequisite course work. Transfer students are accepted. **Standardized tests** *Required:* SAT or ACT, TOEFL for international students. **Application** *Deadline:* 8/15 (freshmen), 8/15 (transfer). *Notification:* continuous until 9/15 (freshmen). *Application fee:* $35.

Advanced Placement Credit by examination available. Credit given for nursing courses completed elsewhere dependent upon specific evaluations.

Contact *Telephone:* 515-263-2866. *Fax:* 515-263-6077.

CONTINUING EDUCATION PROGRAM

Contact *Telephone:* 515-263-2912. *Fax:* 515-263-6190.

Iowa Wesleyan College
Division of Health and Natural Sciences
Mount Pleasant, Iowa

http://www.iwc.edu

Founded in 1842

DEGREE • BSN

Nursing Program Faculty 8 (12% with doctorates).

Baccalaureate Enrollment 70
Women 89% **Men** 11% **Minority** 14% **Part-time** 11%

Nursing Student Activities Student Nurses' Association.

Nursing Student Resources Academic advising; academic or career counseling; assistance for students with disabilities; bookstore; campus computer network; career placement assistance; computer lab; computer-assisted instruction; e-mail services; Internet; learning resource lab; library services; nursing audiovisuals; remedial services; resume preparation assistance; skills, simulation, or other laboratory; tutoring; unpaid internships.

Library Facilities 107,227 volumes (500 in health, 300 in nursing); 431 periodical subscriptions (40 health-care related).

BACCALAUREATE PROGRAMS

Degree BSN

Available Programs ADN to Baccalaureate; LPN to RN Baccalaureate; RN Baccalaureate.

Study Options Full-time and part-time.

Program Entrance Requirements Minimum overall college GPA of 2.0, transcript of college record, CPR certification, health exam, high school transcript, immunizations, minimum high school GPA of 2.0, minimum high school rank 50%, minimum GPA in nursing prerequisites of 2.0, professional liability insurance/malpractice insurance, prerequisite course work. Transfer students are accepted. **Standardized tests** *Required:* SAT or ACT, TOEFL for international students. **Placement:** *Required:* SAT or ACT. **Application** *Deadline:* 8/15 (freshmen), 8/15 (transfer).

Advanced Placement Credit given for nursing courses completed elsewhere dependent upon specific evaluations.

Financial Aid 98% of baccalaureate students in nursing programs received some form of financial aid in 2005–06. *Gift aid (need-based):* Federal Pell, FSEOG, state, private, college/university gift aid from institutional funds. *Loans:* FFEL (Subsidized and Unsubsidized Stafford PLUS), Perkins, state, alternative loans. *Work-Study:* Federal Work-Study, part-time campus jobs. *Application deadline (priority):* 4/1.

Contact Mr. Mark Petty, Director, Enrollment Management, Division of Health and Natural Sciences, Iowa Wesleyan College, 601 North Main Street, Mount Pleasant, IA 52641. *Telephone:* 800-582-2383 Ext. 6231. *Fax:* 319-385-6296. *E-mail:* mpetty@iwc.edu.

CONTINUING EDUCATION PROGRAM

Contact David File, Dean of Extended Learning, Division of Health and Natural Sciences, Iowa Wesleyan College, 601 North Main Street, Mount Pleasant, IA 52641. *Telephone:* 800-582-2383 Ext. 6245. *Fax:* 319-385-6296. *E-mail:* dfile@iwc.edu.

Luther College
Department of Nursing
Decorah, Iowa

http://nursing.luther.edu/

Founded in 1861

DEGREE • BA

Nursing Program Faculty 16 (31% with doctorates).

Baccalaureate Enrollment 130
Women 96% **Men** 4% **Minority** 3% **International** 2% **Part-time** 1%

Nursing Student Activities Sigma Theta Tau, nursing club.

Nursing Student Resources Academic advising; academic or career counseling; assistance for students with disabilities; bookstore; campus computer network; career placement assistance; computer lab; e-mail services; Internet; learning resource lab; library services; nursing audiovisuals; placement services for program completers; remedial services; resume preparation assistance; skills, simulation, or other laboratory; tutoring; unpaid internships.

Library Facilities 334,814 volumes (4,324 in health, 3,337 in nursing); 831 periodical subscriptions (35 health-care related).

BACCALAUREATE PROGRAMS

Degree BA

Available Programs ADN to Baccalaureate; Generic Baccalaureate.

Site Options Rochester, MN.

Study Options Full-time and part-time.

Program Entrance Requirements Minimum overall college GPA of 2.5, transcript of college record, written essay, health exam, high school foreign language, 3 years high school math, 2 years high school science, high school transcript, immunizations, 1 letter of recommendation, minimum high school rank 50%, minimum GPA in nursing prerequisites of 2.0. Transfer students are accepted. **Standardized tests** *Required:* SAT or ACT, TOEFL for international students. **Application** *Notification:* continuous (freshmen), continuous (out-of-state freshmen). *Application fee:* $25.

Advanced Placement Credit given for nursing courses completed elsewhere dependent upon specific evaluations.

Expenses (2006–07) *Tuition:* full-time $26,380; part-time $942 per credit hour. *Room and board:* $4290; room only: $2100 per academic year.

Financial Aid 98% of baccalaureate students in nursing programs received some form of financial aid in 2005–06. *Gift aid (need-based):* Federal Pell, FSEOG, state, private, college/university gift aid from institutional funds. *Loans:* Federal Direct (Subsidized and Unsubsidized Stafford PLUS), Perkins, college/university. *Work-Study:* Federal Work-Study, part-time campus jobs. *Application deadline (priority):* 3/1.

Contact Ms. Ruth Green, Administrative Assistant, Department of Nursing, Luther College, 700 College Drive, Decorah, IA 52101. *Telephone:* 563-387-1057. *Fax:* 563-387-2149. *E-mail:* greenru@luther.edu.

CONTINUING EDUCATION PROGRAM

Contact Ms. Ruth Green, Administrative Assistant, Department of Nursing, Luther College, 700 College Drive, Decorah, IA 52101. *Telephone:* 563-387-1057. *Fax:* 563-387-2149. *E-mail:* greenru@luther.edu.

See full description on page 508.

Mercy College of Health Sciences
Division of Nursing
Des Moines, Iowa

http://www.mchs.edu/divnurs.html

Founded in 1995

DEGREE • BSN

Nursing Program Faculty 22 (2% with doctorates).

Baccalaureate Enrollment 71
Women 98% **Men** 2% **Part-time** 98%

Nursing Student Activities Sigma Theta Tau, Student Nurses' Association.

Nursing Student Resources Academic advising; academic or career counseling; assistance for students with disabilities; campus computer network; career placement assistance; computer lab; computer-assisted instruction; daycare for children of students; e-mail services; employment services for current students; interactive nursing skills videos; Internet; learning resource lab; library services; nursing audiovisuals; placement services for program completers; skills, simulation, or other laboratory.

BACCALAUREATE PROGRAMS

Degree BSN

Available Programs ADN to Baccalaureate; Accelerated Baccalaureate; Accelerated Baccalaureate for Second Degree; RN Baccalaureate.

Study Options Full-time and part-time.

Program Entrance Requirements Minimum overall college GPA of 2.7, transcript of college record, prerequisite course work. Transfer students are accepted. **Standardized tests** *Required:* ACT, TOEFL for international students. **Application** *Deadline:* rolling (freshmen). *Notification:* continuous (freshmen). *Application fee:* $25.

Contact *Telephone:* 515-643-3180. *Fax:* 515-643-6698.

Morningside College
Department of Nursing Education
Sioux City, Iowa

http://www.morningside.edu/
academicdepartments/nursing.htm
Founded in 1894

DEGREE • BSN

Nursing Program Faculty 9 (11% with doctorates).

Baccalaureate Enrollment 57
Women 96% **Men** 4% **Minority** 7% **International** 4% **Part-time** 5%

Nursing Student Activities Student Nurses' Association, nursing club.

Nursing Student Resources Academic advising; academic or career counseling; assistance for students with disabilities; bookstore; campus computer network; computer lab; computer-assisted instruction; e-mail services; employment services for current students; externships; housing assistance; interactive nursing skills videos; Internet; learning resource lab; library services; nursing audiovisuals; resume preparation assistance; skills, simulation, or other laboratory; tutoring; unpaid internships.

Library Facilities 113,169 volumes (2,464 in health, 2,464 in nursing); 528 periodical subscriptions (43 health-care related).

BACCALAUREATE PROGRAMS

Degree BSN

Available Programs Baccalaureate for Second Degree; Generic Baccalaureate; International Nurse to Baccalaureate; LPN to Baccalaureate; RN Baccalaureate.

Study Options Full-time and part-time.

Program Entrance Requirements Minimum overall college GPA of 2.5, transcript of college record, CPR certification, high school transcript, immunizations, interview, minimum GPA in nursing prerequisites of 2.5, professional liability insurance/malpractice insurance, prerequisite course work. Transfer students are accepted. **Standardized tests** *Required:* SAT or ACT, TOEFL for international students. **Application** *Deadline:* rolling (freshmen), rolling (transfer). *Notification:* continuous (freshmen). *Application fee:* $25.

Advanced Placement Credit given for nursing courses completed elsewhere dependent upon specific evaluations.

Expenses (2005–06) *Tuition:* full-time $17,170; part-time $330 per credit hour. *Room and board:* $5624 per academic year. *Required fees:* full-time $230.

Financial Aid 99% of baccalaureate students in nursing programs received some form of financial aid in 2004–05. *Gift aid (need-based):* Federal Pell, FSEOG, state, private, college/university gift aid from institutional funds. *Loans:* FFEL (Subsidized and Unsubsidized Stafford PLUS), Perkins, state, college/university, private loans. *Work-Study:* Federal Work-Study, part-time campus jobs. *Application deadline (priority):* 3/1.

Contact Mary Kovarna, RN, Chair, Associate Professor, Department of Nursing Education, Morningside College, 1501 Morningside Avenue, Sioux City, IA 51106-1751. *Telephone:* 712-274-5154. *Fax:* 712-274-5101. *E-mail:* kovarna@morningside.edu.

Mount Mercy College
Department of Nursing
Cedar Rapids, Iowa

http://www.mtmercy.edu
Founded in 1928

DEGREE • BSN

Nursing Program Faculty 36 (15% with doctorates).

Baccalaureate Enrollment 207
Women 97% **Men** 3% **Minority** 1% **Part-time** 30%

Nursing Student Activities Sigma Theta Tau, Student Nurses' Association, nursing club.

Nursing Student Resources Academic advising; academic or career counseling; assistance for students with disabilities; bookstore; campus computer network; career placement assistance; computer lab; computer-assisted instruction; e-mail services; employment services for current students; externships; housing assistance; interactive nursing skills videos; Internet; learning resource lab; library services; nursing audiovisuals; paid internships; placement services for program completers; remedial services; resume preparation assistance; skills, simulation, or other laboratory; tutoring; unpaid internships.

Library Facilities 125,000 volumes (4,775 in health, 1,450 in nursing); 10,900 periodical subscriptions (130 health-care related).

BACCALAUREATE PROGRAMS

Degree BSN

Available Programs Accelerated RN Baccalaureate; Generic Baccalaureate.

Study Options Full-time and part-time.

Program Entrance Requirements Minimum overall college GPA of 2.5, transcript of college record, CPR certification, health exam, health insurance, high school chemistry, 2 years high school math, 2 years high school science, high school transcript, immunizations, minimum high school rank 75%, minimum GPA in nursing prerequisites of 2.5, prerequisite course work. Transfer students are accepted. **Standardized tests** *Required:* SAT or ACT, TOEFL for international students. **Application** *Deadline:* 8/15 (freshmen), 8/15 (transfer). *Notification:* continuous (freshmen). *Application fee:* $20.

Advanced Placement Credit by examination available. Credit given for nursing courses completed elsewhere dependent upon specific evaluations.

Expenses (2006–07) *Tuition:* full-time $18,930; part-time $525 per credit hour. *International tuition:* $18,930 full-time. *Room and board:* $2985; room only: $1150 per academic year. *Required fees:* full-time $200.

Financial Aid 90% of baccalaureate students in nursing programs received some form of financial aid in 2005–06. *Gift aid (need-based):* Federal Pell, FSEOG, state, college/university gift aid from institutional funds. *Loans:* Federal Direct (Subsidized and Unsubsidized Stafford PLUS), Perkins, state, college/university. *Work-Study:* Federal Work-Study, part-time campus jobs. *Application deadline (priority):* 3/1.

Contact Dr. Mary P. Tarbox, Professor and Chair, Department of Nursing, Mount Mercy College, 1330 Elmhurst Drive NE, Cedar Rapids, IA 52402. *Telephone:* 800-248-4504 Ext. 6460. *Fax:* 319-368-6479. *E-mail:* mtarbox@mtmercy.edu.

Mount Mercy College (continued)
CONTINUING EDUCATION PROGRAM
Contact Dr. Mary P. Tarbox, Professor and Chair, Department of Nursing, Mount Mercy College, 1330 Elmhurst Drive NE, Cedar Rapids, IA 52402. *Telephone:* 319-368-6471. *Fax:* 319-368-6479. *E-mail:* mtarbox@mtmercy.edu.

St. Ambrose University
Program in Nursing (BSN)
Davenport, Iowa

Founded in 1882

DEGREE • BSN

Library Facilities 143,634 volumes; 739 periodical subscriptions.

BACCALAUREATE PROGRAMS
Degree BSN

Available Programs Generic Baccalaureate; RN Baccalaureate.

Program Entrance Requirements Standardized tests *Required:* SAT or ACT, TOEFL for international students. *Recommended:* ACT. **Application** *Deadline:* rolling (freshmen), rolling (transfer). *Notification:* 10/1 (freshmen). *Application fee:* $25.

Contact *Telephone:* 563-333-6076.

The University of Iowa
College of Nursing
Iowa City, Iowa

http://www.nursing.uiowa.edu

Founded in 1847

DEGREES • BSN • MSN • MSN/MBA • MSN/MPH • PHD

Nursing Program Faculty 67 (63% with doctorates).

Baccalaureate Enrollment 618
Women 93% **Men** 7% **Minority** 6% **Part-time** 25%

Graduate Enrollment 258
Women 89% **Men** 11% **Minority** 4% **International** 7% **Part-time** 50%

Nursing Student Activities Sigma Theta Tau, Student Nurses' Association.

Nursing Student Resources Academic advising; academic or career counseling; assistance for students with disabilities; campus computer network; career placement assistance; computer lab; computer-assisted instruction; e-mail services; employment services for current students; Internet; learning resource lab; nursing audiovisuals; placement services for program completers; resume preparation assistance; skills, simulation, or other laboratory; tutoring.

Library Facilities 4 million volumes (273,469 in health); 44,644 periodical subscriptions (2,500 health-care related).

BACCALAUREATE PROGRAMS
Degree BSN

Available Programs Generic Baccalaureate; RN Baccalaureate.

Site Options *Distance Learning:* Mason City & Calmar, IA; Spencer & Orange City, IA; Fort Dodge & Ottumwa, IA.

Study Options Full-time and part-time.

Program Entrance Requirements Minimum overall college GPA of 2.7, transcript of college record, CPR certification, written essay, health exam, health insurance, high school biology, high school chemistry, high school foreign language, 3 years high school math, 3 years high school science, high school transcript, immunizations, minimum GPA in nursing prerequisites of 2.7, professional liability insurance/malpractice insurance, prerequisite course work. Transfer students are accepted. **Standardized tests** *Required:* SAT or ACT, TOEFL for international students. **Application** *Deadline:* 4/1 (freshmen), 4/1 (transfer). *Notification:* continuous (freshmen). *Application fee:* $40.

Advanced Placement Credit given for nursing courses completed elsewhere dependent upon specific evaluations.

Expenses (2006–07) *Tuition, area resident:* full-time $5935. *Tuition, nonresident:* full-time $18,159. *Room and board:* $6912 per academic year.

Financial Aid 64% of baccalaureate students in nursing programs received some form of financial aid in 2005–06. *Gift aid (need-based):* Federal Pell, FSEOG, state, private, college/university gift aid from institutional funds. *Loans:* Federal Nursing Student Loans, Federal Direct (Subsidized and Unsubsidized Stafford PLUS), Perkins, college/university. *Work-Study:* Federal Work-Study, part-time campus jobs. *Application deadline:* Continuous.

Contact Linda Myers, College of Nursing, The University of Iowa, 37 Nursing Building, Iowa City, IA 52242. *Telephone:* 319-335-7016. *Fax:* 319-384-4423. *E-mail:* linda-myers@uiowa.edu.

GRADUATE PROGRAMS
Expenses (2006–07) *Required fees:* full-time $777.

Financial Aid 8 fellowships, 19 research assistantships, 23 teaching assistantships were awarded.

Contact Program Associate, Nursing Graduate Program, College of Nursing, The University of Iowa, 444 Nursing Building, Iowa City, IA 52242. *Telephone:* 319-335-7021. *Fax:* 319-335-9990. *E-mail:* nursing-graduateprogram@uiowa.edu.

MASTER'S DEGREE PROGRAM
Degrees MSN; MSN/MBA; MSN/MPH

Available Programs Accelerated RN to Master's; Master's; Master's for Nurses with Non-Nursing Degrees.

Concentrations Available Nurse anesthesia; nursing administration; nursing education; nursing informatics. *Clinical nurse specialist programs in:* adult health, community health, gerontology, occupational health, psychiatric/mental health. *Nurse practitioner programs in:* adult health, family health, gerontology, neonatal health, pediatric, psychiatric/mental health.

Site Options *Distance Learning:* Mason City & Calmar, IA; Spencer & Orange City, IA; Fort Dodge & Ottumwa, IA.

Study Options Full-time and part-time.

Program Entrance Requirements Computer literacy, minimum overall college GPA of 3.0, transcript of college record, written essay, immunizations, 3 letters of recommendation, nursing research course, physical assessment course, professional liability insurance/malpractice insurance, prerequisite course work, resume, statistics course, GRE General Test. *Application fee:* $60 ($85 for international students).

Advanced Placement Credit given for nursing courses completed elsewhere dependent upon specific evaluations.

Degree Requirements 33 total credit hours, thesis or project.

POST-MASTER'S PROGRAM
Areas of Study Nursing informatics. *Clinical nurse specialist programs in:* adult health, psychiatric/mental health. *Nurse practitioner programs in:* adult health, family health, gerontology, pediatric, psychiatric/mental health.

DOCTORAL DEGREE PROGRAM
Degree PhD

Available Programs Doctorate; Post-Baccalaureate Doctorate.

Areas of Study Aging, family health, gerontology, individualized study, information systems, nursing administration.

Program Entrance Requirements Minimum overall college GPA of 3.0, interview, 3 letters of recommendation, statistics course, vita, GRE General Test. *Application fee:* $60 ($85 for international students).

Degree Requirements 60 total credit hours, dissertation, oral exam, written exam, residency.

POSTDOCTORAL PROGRAM
Areas of Study Family health, nursing informatics, nursing interventions, outcomes.

Postdoctoral Program Contact Jennifer Clougherty, Program Associate, College of Nursing, The University of Iowa, 101NB, Iowa City, IA 52242. *Telephone:* 319-335-7021. *Fax:* 319-335-9990. *E-mail:* jennifer-clougherty@uiowa.edu.

CONTINUING EDUCATION PROGRAM

Contact Ms. Nancy Lathrop, College of Nursing, The University of Iowa, 342 Nursing Building, Iowa City, IA 52242. *Telephone:* 319-335-7075. *Fax:* 319-335-9990. *E-mail:* nancy-lathrop@uiowa.edu.

KANSAS

Baker University
School of Nursing
Topeka, Kansas

http://www.bakeru.edu

Founded in 1858

DEGREE • BSN

Nursing Program Faculty 15 (13% with doctorates).

Baccalaureate Enrollment 142
Women 89% **Men** 11% **Minority** 6% **Part-time** 3%

Nursing Student Activities Sigma Theta Tau, Student Nurses' Association.

Nursing Student Resources Academic advising; campus computer network; computer lab; e-mail services; Internet; learning resource lab; library services; nursing audiovisuals; resume preparation assistance; skills, simulation, or other laboratory; tutoring.

Library Facilities 132,325 volumes (5,000 in health, 2,716 in nursing); 678 periodical subscriptions (414 health-care related).

BACCALAUREATE PROGRAMS

Degree BSN

Available Programs Generic Baccalaureate; RN Baccalaureate.

Study Options Full-time and part-time.

Program Entrance Requirements Transcript of college record, CPR certification, written essay, health exam, health insurance, high school transcript, immunizations, interview, 1 letter of recommendation, minimum GPA in nursing prerequisites of 2.7, prerequisite course work. Transfer students are accepted. **Standardized tests** *Required:* SAT or ACT, TOEFL for international students. **Application** *Deadline:* rolling (freshmen), rolling (transfer).

Advanced Placement Credit given for nursing courses completed elsewhere dependent upon specific evaluations.

Expenses (2006–07) *Tuition:* full-time $11,400; part-time $380 per credit hour. *Required fees:* full-time $466; part-time $247 per term.

Financial Aid 89% of baccalaureate students in nursing programs received some form of financial aid in 2005–06.

Contact Ms. Janet Creager, Student Affairs Specialist, School of Nursing, Baker University, 1500 Southwest 10th Avenue, Topeka, KS 66604-1353. *Telephone:* 785-354-5850. *Fax:* 785-354-5832. *E-mail:* janet.creager@bakeru.edu.

See full description on page 456.

Bethel College
Department of Nursing
North Newton, Kansas

http://www.bethelks.edu

Founded in 1887

DEGREE • BSN

Nursing Program Faculty 9.

Baccalaureate Enrollment 100
Women 75% **Men** 25% **Minority** 30% **International** 25% **Part-time** 1%

Nursing Student Activities Nursing Honor Society, Sigma Theta Tau, Student Nurses' Association.

Nursing Student Resources Academic advising; academic or career counseling; assistance for students with disabilities; bookstore; computer lab; e-mail services; employment services for current students; housing assistance; Internet; learning resource lab; library services; nursing audio-visuals; resume preparation assistance; skills, simulation, or other laboratory; tutoring.

Library Facilities 162,327 volumes (5,690 in health, 3,150 in nursing); 38,356 periodical subscriptions (445 health-care related).

BACCALAUREATE PROGRAMS

Degree BSN

Available Programs Generic Baccalaureate; LPN to Baccalaureate; RN Baccalaureate.

Study Options Full-time and part-time.

Program Entrance Requirements Minimum overall college GPA of 3.0, transcript of college record, CPR certification, written essay, health exam, health insurance, high school transcript, immunizations, interview, 2 letters of recommendation, minimum high school GPA of 3.0, minimum GPA in nursing prerequisites of 2.0, prerequisite course work. Transfer students are accepted. **Standardized tests** *Required:* SAT or ACT, TOEFL for international students. **Application** *Deadline:* rolling (freshmen), rolling (transfer). *Notification:* continuous (freshmen). *Application fee:* $20.

Advanced Placement Credit given for nursing courses completed elsewhere dependent upon specific evaluations.

Expenses (2006–07) *Tuition:* full-time $16,700; part-time $325 per credit. *International tuition:* $16,700 full-time. *Room and board:* $2500; room only: $1450 per academic year. *Required fees:* full-time $550.

Financial Aid 99% of baccalaureate students in nursing programs received some form of financial aid in 2005–06.

Contact Mr. Gregg Schroeder, Director, Department of Nursing, Bethel College, 300 East 27th Street, North Newton, KS 67117. *Telephone:* 316-283-2500 Ext. 377. *Fax:* 316-284-5286. *E-mail:* gls58@bethelks.edu.

Emporia State University
Newman Division of Nursing
Emporia, Kansas

http://www.emporia.edu/ndn

Founded in 1863

DEGREE • BSN

Nursing Program Faculty 11 (36% with doctorates).

Baccalaureate Enrollment 111
Women 93% **Men** 7% **International** 7% **Part-time** 4%

Nursing Student Activities Student Nurses' Association.

Nursing Student Resources Academic advising; academic or career counseling; assistance for students with disabilities; bookstore; campus computer network; career placement assistance; computer lab; computer-assisted instruction; daycare for children of students; e-mail services; employment services for current students; housing assistance; interactive nursing skills videos; Internet; learning resource lab; library services; nursing audiovisuals; placement services for program completers; remedial services; resume preparation assistance; skills, simulation, or other laboratory; tutoring.

Library Facilities 2.4 million volumes (51,624 in health, 2,545 in nursing); 15,645 periodical subscriptions (244 health-care related).

BACCALAUREATE PROGRAMS

Degree BSN

Available Programs ADN to Baccalaureate; Generic Baccalaureate; LPN to Baccalaureate; RN Baccalaureate.

Study Options Full-time and part-time.

Program Entrance Requirements Transcript of college record, written essay, minimum GPA in nursing prerequisites of 2.5, prerequisite course work. Transfer students are accepted. **Standardized tests** *Required:* SAT or ACT, TOEFL for international students. **Application** *Deadline:* rolling (freshmen), rolling (transfer). *Application fee:* $30.

Emporia State University (continued)

Advanced Placement Credit given for nursing courses completed elsewhere dependent upon specific evaluations.

Expenses (2006–07) *Tuition, area resident:* full-time $2862; part-time $95 per credit hour. *Tuition, state resident:* full-time $4296; part-time $143 per credit hour. *Tuition, nonresident:* full-time $10,214; part-time $340 per credit hour. *International tuition:* $10,214 full-time. *Room and board:* $5200; room only: $4266 per academic year. *Required fees:* full-time $724; part-time $44 per credit.

Financial Aid 89% of baccalaureate students in nursing programs received some form of financial aid in 2005–06.

Contact Dr. Judith E. Calhoun, RN, Division Chair, Newman Division of Nursing, Emporia State University, 1127 Chestnut Street, Emporia, KS 66801. *Telephone:* 620-343-6800 Ext. 5641. *Fax:* 620-341-7871. *E-mail:* jcalhoun@emporia.edu.

Fort Hays State University
Department of Nursing
Hays, Kansas

http://www.fhsu.edu/nursing/

Founded in 1902

DEGREES • BSN • MSN

Nursing Program Faculty 21 (24% with doctorates).

Baccalaureate Enrollment 117
Women 92% **Men** 8% **Minority** 4% **International** 2% **Part-time** 32%

Graduate Enrollment 62
Women 95% **Men** 5% **Minority** 3% **Part-time** 100%

Nursing Student Activities Sigma Theta Tau, Student Nurses' Association, nursing club.

Nursing Student Resources Academic advising; academic or career counseling; assistance for students with disabilities; bookstore; campus computer network; career placement assistance; computer lab; computer-assisted instruction; daycare for children of students; e-mail services; employment services for current students; housing assistance; interactive nursing skills videos; Internet; learning resource lab; library services; nursing audiovisuals; paid internships; placement services for program completers; remedial services; resume preparation assistance; skills, simulation, or other laboratory; tutoring.

Library Facilities 624,637 volumes (9,950 in health, 1,550 in nursing); 1,689 periodical subscriptions (187 health-care related).

BACCALAUREATE PROGRAMS

Degree BSN

Available Programs Generic Baccalaureate; RN Baccalaureate.
Site Options *Distance Learning:* Pratt, Liberal, Salina, Garden City, Dodge City, KS; Colby, KS.
Study Options Full-time and part-time.
Program Entrance Requirements Minimum overall college GPA of 2.5, transcript of college record, CPR certification, written essay, health exam, health insurance, high school transcript, immunizations, 2 letters of recommendation, minimum GPA in nursing prerequisites of 2.0, professional liability insurance/malpractice insurance, prerequisite course work. Transfer students are accepted. **Standardized tests** *Required:* ACT, SAT or ACT, TOEFL for international students. **Application** *Deadline:* rolling (freshmen), rolling (transfer). *Notification:* continuous (freshmen). *Application fee:* $30.
Advanced Placement Credit by examination available. Credit given for nursing courses completed elsewhere dependent upon specific evaluations.
Expenses (2006–07) *Tuition, area resident:* full-time $2554; part-time $106 per credit hour. *Tuition, state resident:* full-time $3544; part-time $148 per credit hour. *Tuition, nonresident:* full-time $8030; part-time $335 per credit hour. *International tuition:* $8030 full-time. *Room and board:* $5500; room only: $2823 per academic year.
Financial Aid 92% of baccalaureate students in nursing programs received some form of financial aid in 2005–06.

Contact Mrs. Sally Dineen Schmidt, Coordinator of Quality and Advising, Department of Nursing, Fort Hays State University, 600 Park Street, Stroup Hall, 122D, Hays, KS 67601-4099. *Telephone:* 785-628-5559. *Fax:* 785-628-4080. *E-mail:* sschmidt@fhsu.edu.

GRADUATE PROGRAMS

Expenses (2006–07) *Tuition, area resident:* full-time $3500; part-time $147 per credit hour. *Tuition, state resident:* full-time $4593; part-time $209 per credit hour. *Tuition, nonresident:* full-time $9338; part-time $389 per credit hour. *International tuition:* $9338 full-time.

Financial Aid 90% of graduate students in nursing programs received some form of financial aid in 2005–06. 1 teaching assistantship (averaging $5,000 per year) was awarded; research assistantships.

Contact Dr. Liane Connelly, Chair, Department of Nursing, Fort Hays State University, 600 Park Street, Stroup Hall, 127, Hays, KS 67601-4099. *Telephone:* 785-628-4511. *Fax:* 785-628-4080. *E-mail:* lconnell@fhsu.edu.

MASTER'S DEGREE PROGRAM

Degree MSN

Available Programs Master's.
Concentrations Available Nursing administration; nursing education. *Nurse practitioner programs in:* family health.
Site Options *Distance Learning:* Pratt, Liberal, Salina, Garden City, Dodge City, KS; Colby, KS.
Study Options Full-time and part-time.
Program Entrance Requirements Clinical experience, computer literacy, minimum overall college GPA of 3.0, transcript of college record, CPR certification, written essay, immunizations, 2 letters of recommendation, physical assessment course, professional liability insurance/malpractice insurance, prerequisite course work, statistics course, GRE General Test or MAT. *Application deadline:* For fall admission, 7/1 (priority date). Applications are processed on a rolling basis. *Application fee:* $30 ($35 for international students).
Advanced Placement Credit given for nursing courses completed elsewhere dependent upon specific evaluations.
Degree Requirements 34 total credit hours, thesis or project, comprehensive exam.

POST-MASTER'S PROGRAM

Areas of Study Nursing administration; nursing education. *Nurse practitioner programs in:* family health.

Kansas Wesleyan University
Department of Nursing Education
Salina, Kansas

http://www.kwu.edu/nursing

Founded in 1886

DEGREE • BSN

Nursing Program Faculty 7 (29% with doctorates).

Baccalaureate Enrollment 49
Women 92% **Men** 8% **Minority** 8% **Part-time** 26%

Nursing Student Activities Nursing club.

Nursing Student Resources Academic advising; academic or career counseling; assistance for students with disabilities; bookstore; campus computer network; career placement assistance; computer lab; computer-assisted instruction; e-mail services; employment services for current students; housing assistance; Internet; learning resource lab; library services; nursing audiovisuals; resume preparation assistance; skills, simulation, or other laboratory; tutoring.

Library Facilities 2,914 volumes in health, 1,861 volumes in nursing; 370 periodical subscriptions (1,959 health-care related).

BACCALAUREATE PROGRAMS

Degree BSN

Available Programs ADN to Baccalaureate; Generic Baccalaureate; RN Baccalaureate.
Study Options Full-time.

Program Entrance Requirements Minimum overall college GPA of 2.6, transcript of college record, high school transcript, minimum GPA in nursing prerequisites of 2.6, prerequisite course work. Transfer students are accepted. **Standardized tests** *Required:* SAT or ACT, TOEFL for international students. *Recommended:* SAT, ACT. **Application** *Deadline:* rolling (freshmen), rolling (transfer). *Notification:* continuous (freshmen). *Application fee:* $20.

Advanced Placement Credit by examination available. Credit given for nursing courses completed elsewhere dependent upon specific evaluations.

Expenses (2006–07) *Tuition:* full-time $16,600; part-time $200 per credit hour. *International tuition:* $16,600 full-time. *Room and board:* $5800 per academic year. *Required fees:* part-time $50 per credit.

Financial Aid 100% of baccalaureate students in nursing programs received some form of financial aid in 2005–06.

Contact Dr. Patricia L. Brown, RN, Professor and Director, Department of Nursing Education, Kansas Wesleyan University, 100 East Claflin Avenue, Campus Box 39, Salina, KS 67401-6196. *Telephone:* 785-827-5541 Ext. 2311. *Fax:* 785-827-0927. *E-mail:* pbrown@kwu.edu.

MidAmerica Nazarene University
Division of Nursing
Olathe, Kansas

http://www.mnu.edu

Founded in 1966

DEGREE • BSN

Nursing Program Faculty 14 (36% with doctorates).

Baccalaureate Enrollment 63
Women 81% **Men** 19% **Minority** 16% **International** 17%

Nursing Student Activities Student Nurses' Association, nursing club.

Nursing Student Resources Academic advising; academic or career counseling; assistance for students with disabilities; bookstore; campus computer network; career placement assistance; computer lab; computer-assisted instruction; e-mail services; employment services for current students; housing assistance; Internet; learning resource lab; library services; nursing audiovisuals; resume preparation assistance; skills, simulation, or other laboratory; tutoring; unpaid internships.

Library Facilities 132,991 volumes (1,903 in health, 547 in nursing); 1,250 periodical subscriptions (115 health-care related).

BACCALAUREATE PROGRAMS

Degree BSN

Available Programs ADN to Baccalaureate; Accelerated Baccalaureate; Accelerated Baccalaureate for Second Degree; Accelerated LPN to Baccalaureate; Accelerated RN Baccalaureate; Generic Baccalaureate; RN Baccalaureate.

Study Options Full-time.

Program Entrance Requirements Minimum overall college GPA of 2.6, transcript of college record, CPR certification, written essay, health exam, health insurance, high school transcript, immunizations, 2 letters of recommendation, minimum GPA in nursing prerequisites of 2.6, prerequisite course work. Transfer students are accepted. **Standardized tests** *Required:* SAT or ACT, TOEFL for international students. **Application** *Deadline:* 8/1 (freshmen), 8/1 (transfer). *Notification:* continuous (freshmen). *Application fee:* $25.

Advanced Placement Credit by examination available. Credit given for nursing courses completed elsewhere dependent upon specific evaluations.

Expenses (2006–07) *Tuition:* full-time $14,968; part-time $500 per credit hour. *International tuition:* $14,968 full-time. *Room and board:* $6112; room only: $5830 per academic year. *Required fees:* full-time $1750; part-time $1480 per term.

Financial Aid 80% of baccalaureate students in nursing programs received some form of financial aid in 2005–06. *Gift aid (need-based):* Federal Pell, FSEOG, state, private, college/university gift aid from institutional funds. *Loans:* Federal Nursing Student Loans, FFEL (Subsidized and Unsubsidized Stafford PLUS), Perkins. *Work-Study:* Federal Work-Study. *Application deadline (priority):* 3/1.

Contact Dr. Palma L. Smith, Chair and Professor, Division of Nursing, MidAmerica Nazarene University, 2030 East College Way, Olathe, KS 66062-1899. *Telephone:* 913-971-3698. *Fax:* 913-971-3408. *E-mail:* psmith@mnu.edu.

CONTINUING EDUCATION PROGRAM

Contact Dr. Joyce A. Lasseter, Continuing Education Coordinator, Division of Nursing, MidAmerica Nazarene University, 2030 East College Way, Olathe, KS 66062-1899. *Telephone:* 913-971-3696. *Fax:* 913-971-3408. *E-mail:* jalasseter@mnu.edu.

Newman University
Division of Nursing
Wichita, Kansas

http://www.newmanu.edu

Founded in 1933

DEGREE • BSN

Nursing Program Faculty 16 (25% with doctorates).

Baccalaureate Enrollment 122
Women 88% **Men** 12% **Minority** 26% **International** 11% **Part-time** 3%

Graduate Enrollment 24
Women 54% **Men** 46% **Minority** 8%

Nursing Student Activities Sigma Theta Tau, nursing club.

Nursing Student Resources Academic advising; academic or career counseling; assistance for students with disabilities; bookstore; campus computer network; career placement assistance; computer lab; computer-assisted instruction; e-mail services; employment services for current students; housing assistance; Internet; learning resource lab; library services; nursing audiovisuals; placement services for program completers; remedial services; resume preparation assistance; skills, simulation, or other laboratory; tutoring.

Library Facilities 108,735 volumes (7,377 in health, 5,441 in nursing); 267 periodical subscriptions (147 health-care related).

BACCALAUREATE PROGRAMS

Degree BSN

Available Programs Generic Baccalaureate; LPN to Baccalaureate; RN Baccalaureate.

Study Options Full-time and part-time.

Program Entrance Requirements Minimum overall college GPA of 2.75, transcript of college record, CPR certification, written essay, health exam, health insurance, immunizations, interview, 2 letters of recommendation, minimum GPA in nursing prerequisites, professional liability insurance/malpractice insurance, prerequisite course work. Transfer students are accepted. **Standardized tests** *Required:* SAT or ACT, TOEFL for international students. **Application** *Deadline:* rolling (freshmen), rolling (transfer). *Notification:* continuous (freshmen). *Application fee:* $20.

Advanced Placement Credit given for nursing courses completed elsewhere dependent upon specific evaluations.

Expenses (2006–07) *Tuition:* full-time $17,008; part-time $567 per credit hour. *Room and board:* $6662 per academic year. *Required fees:* full-time $870; part-time $10 per credit.

Financial Aid 97% of baccalaureate students in nursing programs received some form of financial aid in 2005–06.

Contact Dr. Joan Felts, RN, Dean, School of Science, Nursing, and Allied Health, Division of Nursing, Newman University, 3100 McCormick Avenue, Wichita, KS 67213. *Telephone:* 316-942-4291 Ext. 2244. *Fax:* 316-942-4483. *E-mail:* feltsj@newmanu.edu.

GRADUATE PROGRAMS

Expenses (2006–07) *Tuition:* full-time $16,500; part-time $623 per credit hour. *Required fees:* full-time $300.

Financial Aid 100% of graduate students in nursing programs received some form of financial aid in 2005–06. *Application deadline:* 8/15.

Contact Ms. Sharon Niemann, Director, Master of Science in Nurse Anesthesia Program, Division of Nursing, Newman University, 3100 McCormick Avenue, Wichita, KS 67213. *Telephone:* 316-942-4291 Ext. 2272. *Fax:* 316-942-4483. *E-mail:* niemanns@newmanu.edu.

Newman University (continued)
MASTER'S DEGREE PROGRAM
Program Entrance Requirements MAT. *Application deadline:* For fall admission, 8/15. Applications are processed on a rolling basis. *Application fee:* $25.

Pittsburg State University
Department of Nursing
Pittsburg, Kansas

http://www.pittstate.edu/nurs
Founded in 1903
DEGREES • BSN • MSN

Nursing Program Faculty 29 (34% with doctorates).
Baccalaureate Enrollment 130
Graduate Enrollment 15
Nursing Student Activities Nursing Honor Society, Sigma Theta Tau, Student Nurses' Association.
Nursing Student Resources Academic advising; academic or career counseling; assistance for students with disabilities; bookstore; career placement assistance; computer lab; computer-assisted instruction; e-mail services; employment services for current students; externships; housing assistance; interactive nursing skills videos; Internet; learning resource lab; library services; nursing audiovisuals; placement services for program completers; resume preparation assistance; skills, simulation, or other laboratory; tutoring; unpaid internships.
Library Facilities 705,267 volumes (2,717 in nursing); 9,436 periodical subscriptions.

BACCALAUREATE PROGRAMS
Degree BSN
Available Programs Generic Baccalaureate; RN Baccalaureate.
Study Options Full-time and part-time.
Program Entrance Requirements Minimum overall college GPA of 2.5, transcript of college record, CPR certification, health exam, immunizations, 3 letters of recommendation, professional liability insurance/malpractice insurance, prerequisite course work. Transfer students are accepted. **Standardized tests** *Required:* ACT, TOEFL for international students. **Application** *Deadline:* rolling (freshmen), rolling (transfer). *Application fee:* $30.
Advanced Placement Credit by examination available. Credit given for nursing courses completed elsewhere dependent upon specific evaluations.
Contact *Telephone:* 620-235-4437. *Fax:* 620-235-4449.

GRADUATE PROGRAMS
Contact *Telephone:* 316-235-4435. *Fax:* 316-235-4449.

MASTER'S DEGREE PROGRAM
Degree MSN
Available Programs RN to Master's.
Concentrations Available *Clinical nurse specialist programs in:* family health, gerontology. *Nurse practitioner programs in:* family health.
Study Options Full-time and part-time.
Program Entrance Requirements Clinical experience, minimum overall college GPA of 3.0, transcript of college record, CPR certification, written essay, immunizations, 3 letters of recommendation, nursing research course, physical assessment course, professional liability insurance/malpractice insurance, statistics course, GRE General Test. *Application fee:* $30 ($60 for international students).
Advanced Placement Credit given for nursing courses completed elsewhere dependent upon specific evaluations.
Degree Requirements 45 total credit hours, thesis or project, comprehensive exam.

POST-MASTER'S PROGRAM
Areas of Study *Nurse practitioner programs in:* family health.

CONTINUING EDUCATION PROGRAM
Contact *Telephone:* 620-235-4440. *Fax:* 620-235-4449.

Southwestern College
Nursing Program
Winfield, Kansas

Founded in 1885
DEGREE • BSN

Nursing Program Faculty 6 (33% with doctorates).
Baccalaureate Enrollment 79
Nursing Student Activities Nursing Honor Society, Sigma Theta Tau, Student Nurses' Association, nursing club.
Nursing Student Resources Academic advising; academic or career counseling; assistance for students with disabilities; bookstore; campus computer network; career placement assistance; computer lab; computer-assisted instruction; e-mail services; externships; housing assistance; interactive nursing skills videos; Internet; learning resource lab; library services; nursing audiovisuals; paid internships; placement services for program completers; remedial services; resume preparation assistance; skills, simulation, or other laboratory; tutoring; unpaid internships.
Library Facilities 50,720 volumes; 19,999 periodical subscriptions.

BACCALAUREATE PROGRAMS
Degree BSN
Available Programs Generic Baccalaureate; RN Baccalaureate.
Site Options Wichita, KS.
Study Options Full-time and part-time.
Program Entrance Requirements Transcript of college record, minimum high school GPA of 2.5. Transfer students are accepted. **Standardized tests** *Required:* SAT or ACT, TOEFL for international students. **Application** *Deadline:* 8/25 (freshmen), 8/25 (transfer). *Notification:* continuous (freshmen). *Application fee:* $20.
Advanced Placement Credit given for nursing courses completed elsewhere dependent upon specific evaluations.
Contact *Telephone:* 620-229-6306.

Tabor College
Department of Nursing
Hillsboro, Kansas

http://www.tabor.edu/
Founded in 1908
DEGREE • BSN

Nursing Program Faculty 8.
Baccalaureate Enrollment 45
Women 90% **Men** 10% **Minority** 10% **Part-time** 100%
Nursing Student Activities Nursing Honor Society.
Nursing Student Resources Academic advising; bookstore; campus computer network; computer lab; e-mail services; Internet; library services; nursing audiovisuals; remedial services; resume preparation assistance; skills, simulation, or other laboratory; tutoring.
Library Facilities 80,099 volumes (240 in health, 140 in nursing); 265 periodical subscriptions.

BACCALAUREATE PROGRAMS
Degree BSN
Available Programs Accelerated RN Baccalaureate.
Site Options Wichita, KS.
Study Options Full-time and part-time.

Program Entrance Requirements Minimum overall college GPA of 2.5, transcript of college record, CPR certification, written essay, health exam, health insurance, immunizations, interview, professional liability insurance/malpractice insurance, prerequisite course work, RN licensure. Transfer students are accepted. **Standardized tests** *Required:* SAT or ACT, TOEFL for international students. **Application** *Deadline:* 8/1 (freshmen), 8/1 (transfer). *Early decision:* 1/1. *Notification:* continuous (freshmen). *Application fee:* $30.

Advanced Placement Credit by examination available. Credit given for nursing courses completed elsewhere dependent upon specific evaluations.

Expenses (2006–07) *Tuition:* part-time $310 per credit hour.

Financial Aid 90% of baccalaureate students in nursing programs received some form of financial aid in 2005–06. *Gift aid (need-based):* Federal Pell, FSEOG, state, private, college/university gift aid from institutional funds. *Loans:* FFEL (Subsidized and Unsubsidized Stafford PLUS), Perkins. *Work-Study:* Federal Work-Study, part-time campus jobs. *Application deadline:* 8/15 (priority: 3/1).

Contact Ms. Tona L. Leiker, Chairperson, Department of Nursing, Tabor College, 7348 West 21st Street, Suite 117, Wichita, KS 67205. *Telephone:* 316-729-6333 Ext. 207. *Fax:* 316-773-5436. *E-mail:* tleiker@tabor.edu.

University of Kansas
School of Nursing
Kansas City, Kansas

http://www2.kumc.edu/son

Founded in 1866

DEGREES • BSN • MS • PHD

Nursing Program Faculty 65 (63% with doctorates).

Baccalaureate Enrollment 613
Women 95% **Men** 5% **Minority** 9% **International** 2% **Part-time** 20%

Graduate Enrollment 249
Women 96% **Men** 4% **Minority** 15% **International** 2% **Part-time** 87%

Nursing Student Activities Nursing Honor Society, Sigma Theta Tau, Student Nurses' Association, nursing club.

Nursing Student Resources Academic advising; academic or career counseling; assistance for students with disabilities; bookstore; campus computer network; computer lab; computer-assisted instruction; e-mail services; employment services for current students; interactive nursing skills videos; Internet; learning resource lab; library services; nursing audiovisuals; remedial services; resume preparation assistance; skills, simulation, or other laboratory.

Library Facilities 4.9 million volumes (51,563 in health, 1,554 in nursing); 50,992 periodical subscriptions (1,491 health-care related).

BACCALAUREATE PROGRAMS

Degree BSN

Available Programs ADN to Baccalaureate; Generic Baccalaureate; RN Baccalaureate.

Study Options Full-time and part-time.

Program Entrance Requirements Minimum overall college GPA of 2.5, transcript of college record, CPR certification, written essay, health exam, health insurance, immunizations, 3 letters of recommendation, minimum GPA in nursing prerequisites of 2.5, prerequisite course work. Transfer students are accepted. **Standardized tests** *Required:* SAT or ACT. *Recommended:* TOEFL for international students. **Application** *Deadline:* 4/1 (freshmen), 5/1 (transfer). *Notification:* continuous (freshmen). *Application fee:* $30.

Advanced Placement Credit given for nursing courses completed elsewhere dependent upon specific evaluations.

Expenses (2006–07) *Tuition, state resident:* full-time $5512; part-time $184 per credit hour. *Tuition, nonresident:* full-time $14,482; part-time $483 per credit hour. *International tuition:* $14,482 full-time. *Required fees:* full-time $318.

Financial Aid 71% of baccalaureate students in nursing programs received some form of financial aid in 2005–06.

Contact Office of Student Affairs, School of Nursing, University of Kansas, 3901 Rainbow Boulevard, Mail Stop 2029, Kansas City, KS 66160. *Telephone:* 913-588-1619. *Fax:* 913-588-1615. *E-mail:* soninfo@kumc.edu.

GRADUATE PROGRAMS

Expenses (2006–07) *Tuition, state resident:* full-time $5904; part-time $227 per credit hour. *Tuition, nonresident:* full-time $14,104; part-time $543 per credit hour. *International tuition:* $14,104 full-time. *Required fees:* full-time $378; part-time $166 per term.

Financial Aid 26% of graduate students in nursing programs received some form of financial aid in 2005–06. Research assistantships, teaching assistantships with full and partial tuition reimbursements available, traineeships available.

Contact Dr. Rita Clifford, RN, Associate Dean, Student Affairs, School of Nursing, University of Kansas, 3901 Rainbow Boulevard, Mail Stop 2029, Kansas City, KS 66160. *Telephone:* 913-588-1619. *Fax:* 913-588-1615. *E-mail:* soninfo@kumc.edu.

MASTER'S DEGREE PROGRAM

Degree MS

Available Programs Accelerated AD/RN to Master's; Master's; RN to Master's.

Concentrations Available Health-care administration; nurse-midwifery; nursing administration; nursing education; nursing informatics. *Clinical nurse specialist programs in:* adult health, gerontology. *Nurse practitioner programs in:* adult health, family health, gerontology, psychiatric/mental health.

Site Options *Distance Learning:* Garden City, KS.

Study Options Full-time and part-time.

Program Entrance Requirements Clinical experience, minimum overall college GPA of 3.0, transcript of college record, interview, 3 letters of recommendation, physical assessment course, resume, statistics course, GRE General Test. *Application deadline:* For fall admission, 4/1; for winter admission, 7/1; for spring admission, 9/1. *Application fee:* $35.

Advanced Placement Credit given for nursing courses completed elsewhere dependent upon specific evaluations.

Degree Requirements 47 total credit hours, thesis or project, comprehensive exam.

POST-MASTER'S PROGRAM

Areas of Study Health-care administration; nurse-midwifery; nursing administration; nursing education; nursing informatics. *Clinical nurse specialist programs in:* adult health, gerontology. *Nurse practitioner programs in:* adult health, family health, gerontology, psychiatric/mental health.

DOCTORAL DEGREE PROGRAM

Degree PhD

Available Programs Doctorate; Post-Baccalaureate Doctorate.

Areas of Study Nursing research.

Program Entrance Requirements Minimum overall college GPA of 3.5, interview by faculty committee, interview, 3 letters of recommendation, statistics course, vita, writing sample, GRE General Test. *Application deadline:* For fall admission, 4/1; for winter admission, 7/1; for spring admission, 9/1. *Application fee:* $35.

Degree Requirements 65 total credit hours, dissertation, oral exam, written exam, residency.

CONTINUING EDUCATION PROGRAM

Contact Mary Kinnaman, PhD, Director, School of Nursing, University of Kansas, 3901 Rainbow Boulevard, Mail Stop 4001, Kansas City, KS 66160. *Telephone:* 913-588-4488. *Fax:* 913-588-4486. *E-mail:* ceinfo@kumc.edu.

Washburn University
School of Nursing
Topeka, Kansas

http://www.washburn.edu/sonu/index.html

Founded in 1865

Washburn University (continued)
DEGREES • BSN • MSN

Nursing Program Faculty 29 (24% with doctorates).

Baccalaureate Enrollment 201
Women 89% **Men** 11% **Minority** 10% **International** 1% **Part-time** 1%

Nursing Student Activities Sigma Theta Tau, Student Nurses' Association, nursing club.

Nursing Student Resources Academic advising; academic or career counseling; assistance for students with disabilities; bookstore; campus computer network; career placement assistance; computer lab; computer-assisted instruction; e-mail services; employment services for current students; interactive nursing skills videos; Internet; learning resource lab; library services; nursing audiovisuals; remedial services; resume preparation assistance; skills, simulation, or other laboratory; tutoring; unpaid internships.

Library Facilities 345,642 volumes (12,880 in health, 1,612 in nursing); 1,672 periodical subscriptions (84 health-care related).

BACCALAUREATE PROGRAMS

Degree BSN

Available Programs ADN to Baccalaureate; Baccalaureate for Second Degree; Generic Baccalaureate; LPN to Baccalaureate; RN Baccalaureate.
Study Options Full-time.

Program Entrance Requirements Minimum overall college GPA of 2.7, transcript of college record, CPR certification, written essay, health exam, health insurance, immunizations, interview, 2 letters of recommendation, minimum GPA in nursing prerequisites of 2.0, professional liability insurance/malpractice insurance, prerequisite course work. Transfer students are accepted. **Standardized tests** *Required:* ACT, TOEFL for international students. **Application** *Deadline:* 8/1 (freshmen), 8/1 (transfer). *Notification:* continuous (freshmen). *Application fee:* $20.

Advanced Placement Credit by examination available. Credit given for nursing courses completed elsewhere dependent upon specific evaluations.

Contact *Telephone:* 785-231-1032 Ext. 1525. *Fax:* 785-231-1032.

GRADUATE PROGRAMS

Contact *Telephone:* 785-231-1010 Ext. 1533. *Fax:* 785-213-1032.

MASTER'S DEGREE PROGRAM

Degree MSN

Available Programs Master's.

Concentrations Available Nursing administration. *Clinical nurse specialist programs in:* gerontology. *Nurse practitioner programs in:* adult health, community health.

Study Options Full-time and part-time.

Program Entrance Requirements Computer literacy, transcript of college record, CPR certification, written essay, immunizations, 2 letters of recommendation, nursing research course, physical assessment course, professional liability insurance/malpractice insurance, prerequisite course work, resume, statistics course.

Degree Requirements 42 total credit hours, thesis or project.

POST-MASTER'S PROGRAM

Areas of Study Nursing education.

CONTINUING EDUCATION PROGRAM

Contact *Telephone:* 785-231-1010 Ext. 1526. *Fax:* 785-231-1032.

Wichita State University
School of Nursing
Wichita, Kansas

http://www.wichita.edu/nurs
Founded in 1895

DEGREES • BSN • DNP • MSN • MSN/MBA

Nursing Program Faculty 38 (35% with doctorates).

Baccalaureate Enrollment 240
Women 88% **Men** 12% **Minority** 13% **International** 1% **Part-time** 1%
Graduate Enrollment 163
Women 94% **Men** 6% **Minority** 6% **International** 1% **Part-time** 60%

Nursing Student Activities Sigma Theta Tau, Student Nurses' Association.

Nursing Student Resources Academic advising; academic or career counseling; assistance for students with disabilities; bookstore; campus computer network; computer lab; computer-assisted instruction; daycare for children of students; e-mail services; employment services for current students; housing assistance; interactive nursing skills videos; Internet; learning resource lab; library services; nursing audiovisuals; skills, simulation, or other laboratory.

Library Facilities 1.6 million volumes (31,320 in health, 2,746 in nursing); 15,169 periodical subscriptions (406 health-care related).

■ Wichita State University School of Nursing, located in the major medical referral center for south-central Kansas, provides high-quality and diverse clinical learning experiences in urban and rural agencies throughout the state. Progression to the baccalaureate degree is facilitated for traditional and nontraditional students through both fall and spring admissions and includes an LPN to RN option. Internet courses provide RN to B.S.N., RN to M.S.N., and continuing education students with convenience and flexibility in scheduling. The graduate program prepares advanced practice nurses as clinical nurse specialists, nurse practitioners, nurse midwives, administrators, and educators. An M.S.N./M.B.A. dual degree and graduate (post-master's) certificate options are offered.

BACCALAUREATE PROGRAMS

Degree BSN

Available Programs ADN to Baccalaureate; Generic Baccalaureate; LPN to RN Baccalaureate; RN Baccalaureate.
Study Options Full-time.

Program Entrance Requirements Minimum overall college GPA of 2.75, transcript of college record, CPR certification, health exam, health insurance, immunizations, interview, minimum GPA in nursing prerequisites of 2.0, professional liability insurance/malpractice insurance, prerequisite course work. Transfer students are accepted. **Standardized tests** *Required:* TOEFL for international students. *Required for some:* SAT and SAT Subject Tests or ACT. **Application** *Deadline:* rolling (freshmen), rolling (transfer). *Notification:* continuous (freshmen). *Application fee:* $30.

Advanced Placement Credit given for nursing courses completed elsewhere dependent upon specific evaluations.

Expenses (2006–07) *Tuition, state resident:* full-time $2092; part-time $146 per credit hour. *Tuition, nonresident:* full-time $5520; part-time $391 per credit hour. *International tuition:* $5520 full-time. *Room and board:* $5276 per academic year. *Required fees:* full-time $250; part-time $96 per term.

Financial Aid 80% of baccalaureate students in nursing programs received some form of financial aid in 2005–06.

Contact Mrs. Alice Henry, RN, Senior Academic Advisor, School of Nursing, Wichita State University, 1845 Fairmount Street, Wichita, KS 67260-0041. *Telephone:* 316-978-5732. *Fax:* 316-978-3094. *E-mail:* alice.henry@wichita.edu.

GRADUATE PROGRAMS

Expenses (2006–07) *Tuition, state resident:* part-time $198 per credit hour. *Tuition, nonresident:* part-time $548 per credit hour. *International tuition:* $9864 full-time. *Room and board:* $5276 per academic year. *Required fees:* part-time $33 per credit.

Financial Aid 60% of graduate students in nursing programs received some form of financial aid in 2005–06. 3 teaching assistantships with full tuition reimbursements available (averaging $8,243 per year) were awarded; fellowships, research assistantships, Federal Work-Study, institutionally sponsored loans, scholarships, traineeships, and unspecified assistantships also available. Aid available to part-time students. *Financial aid application deadline:* 4/1.

Contact Dr. Alicia Huckstadt, Director, Graduate Program, School of Nursing, Wichita State University, 1845 Fairmount Street, Wichita, KS 67260-0041. *Telephone:* 316-978-3610. *Fax:* 316-978-3094. *E-mail:* alicia. huckstadt@wichita.edu.

MASTER'S DEGREE PROGRAM

Degrees MSN; MSN/MBA

Available Programs Master's; Master's for Nurses with Non-Nursing Degrees; RN to Master's.

Concentrations Available Nursing administration. *Clinical nurse specialist programs in:* acute care, pediatric. *Nurse practitioner programs in:* acute care, family health, pediatric, psychiatric/mental health.

Study Options Full-time and part-time.

Program Entrance Requirements Clinical experience, computer literacy, minimum overall college GPA of 3.0, transcript of college record, CPR certification, immunizations, professional liability insurance/ malpractice insurance, resume, statistics course, GRE. *Application deadline:* For fall admission, 6/30 (priority date); for spring admission, 1/1. Applications are processed on a rolling basis. *Application fee:* $35 ($50 for international students).

Advanced Placement Credit given for nursing courses completed elsewhere dependent upon specific evaluations.

Degree Requirements 42 total credit hours, comprehensive exam.

POST-MASTER'S PROGRAM

Areas of Study *Clinical nurse specialist programs in:* acute care, pediatric. *Nurse practitioner programs in:* acute care, family health, pediatric, psychiatric/mental health.

DOCTORAL DEGREE PROGRAM

Degree DNP

Available Programs Post-Baccalaureate Doctorate.

Areas of Study Nursing administration, nursing science.

Program Entrance Requirements Clinical experience, minimum overall college GPA of 3.0, interview, statistics course. *Application deadline:* For fall admission, 6/30 (priority date); for spring admission, 1/1. Applications are processed on a rolling basis. *Application fee:* $35 ($50 for international students).

Degree Requirements 74 total credit hours, oral exam, residency.

KENTUCKY

Bellarmine University
Donna and Allan Lansing School of Nursing and Health Sciences
Louisville, Kentucky

http://www.bellarmine.edu

Founded in 1950

DEGREES • BSN • MSN • MSN/MBA

Nursing Program Faculty 76 (8% with doctorates).

Baccalaureate Enrollment 210
Women 90% **Men** 10% **Part-time** 100%

Graduate Enrollment 79
Women 95% **Men** 5% **Part-time** 100%

Nursing Student Activities Sigma Theta Tau, Student Nurses' Association.

Nursing Student Resources Academic advising; academic or career counseling; assistance for students with disabilities; bookstore; campus computer network; career placement assistance; computer lab; computer-assisted instruction; e-mail services; employment services for current students; externships; housing assistance; interactive nursing skills videos; Internet; learning resource lab; library services; nursing audiovisuals; paid internships; placement services for program completers; remedial services; resume preparation assistance; skills, simulation, or other laboratory; tutoring; unpaid internships.

Library Facilities 118,707 volumes (1,795 in health, 1,395 in nursing); 19,687 periodical subscriptions (93 health-care related).

BACCALAUREATE PROGRAMS

Degree BSN

Available Programs ADN to Baccalaureate; Accelerated Baccalaureate for Second Degree; Generic Baccalaureate; RN Baccalaureate.

Study Options Full-time and part-time.

Program Entrance Requirements Minimum overall college GPA of 2.5, transcript of college record, CPR certification, health exam, health insurance, high school transcript, immunizations, minimum GPA in nursing prerequisites of 2.5, prerequisite course work. Transfer students are accepted. **Standardized tests** *Required:* SAT or ACT, TOEFL for international students. **Application** *Deadline:* 2/1 (freshmen), 8/15 (transfer). *Early decision:* 11/1. *Notification:* 12/1 (early action). *Application fee:* $25.

Advanced Placement Credit by examination available. Credit given for nursing courses completed elsewhere dependent upon specific evaluations.

Expenses (2006–07) *Tuition:* full-time $11,650; part-time $550 per credit hour. *Room and board:* $3600; room only: $2200 per academic year.

Financial Aid 90% of baccalaureate students in nursing programs received some form of financial aid in 2005–06.

Contact Ms. Julie Armstrong-Binnix, Lansing School Marketing/ Recruiter, Donna and Allan Lansing School of Nursing and Health Sciences, Bellarmine University, Miles Hall, #201, 2001 Newburg Road, Louisville, KY 40205-0671. *Telephone:* 502-452-8364. *Fax:* 502-452-8058. *E-mail:* julieab@ bellarmine.edu.

GRADUATE PROGRAMS

Expenses (2006–07) *Tuition:* full-time $23,300; part-time $550 per contact hour. *Room and board:* $3600; room only: $2400 per academic year.

Financial Aid 90% of graduate students in nursing programs received some form of financial aid in 2005–06. Career-related internships or fieldwork and scholarships available.

Contact Mrs. Julie Armstrong-Binnix, Lansing School Marketing/ Recruiter, Donna and Allan Lansing School of Nursing and Health Sciences, Bellarmine University, Miles Hall, #201, 2001 Newburg Road, Louisville, KY 40205-0671. *Telephone:* 502-452-8364. *Fax:* 502-452-8058. *E-mail:* julieab@ bellarmine.edu.

MASTER'S DEGREE PROGRAM

Degrees MSN; MSN/MBA

Available Programs Master's; Master's for Nurses with Non-Nursing Degrees; RN to Master's.

Concentrations Available Nursing administration; nursing education.

Study Options Part-time.

Program Entrance Requirements Minimum overall college GPA of 2.75, transcript of college record, professional liability insurance/ malpractice insurance, GRE General Test. *Application deadline:* For fall admission, 8/1 (priority date). Applications are processed on a rolling basis. *Application fee:* $25.

Advanced Placement Credit given for nursing courses completed elsewhere dependent upon specific evaluations.

Degree Requirements 38 total credit hours, thesis or project.

CONTINUING EDUCATION PROGRAM

Contact Ms. Linda Bailey, Director, Continuing Education, Donna and Allan Lansing School of Nursing and Health Sciences, Bellarmine University, Continuing Education Office, 2001 Newburg Road, Louisville, KY 40205-0671. *Telephone:* 502-452-8161. *Fax:* 502-452-8203. *E-mail:* lbailey@ bellarmine.edu.

Berea College
Department of Nursing
Berea, Kentucky

http://www.berea.edu

Founded in 1855

Berea College (continued)
DEGREE • BS

Nursing Program Faculty 8 (25% with doctorates).

Baccalaureate Enrollment 66
Women 90% **Men** 10% **Minority** 20% **International** 10%

Nursing Student Activities Student Nurses' Association.

Nursing Student Resources Academic advising; academic or career counseling; assistance for students with disabilities; bookstore; campus computer network; career placement assistance; computer lab; computer-assisted instruction; daycare for children of students; e-mail services; employment services for current students; externships; housing assistance; interactive nursing skills videos; Internet; learning resource lab; library services; nursing audiovisuals; paid internships; placement services for program completers; remedial services; resume preparation assistance; skills, simulation, or other laboratory; tutoring; unpaid internships.

Library Facilities 366,926 volumes (5,760 in health, 4,871 in nursing); 1,067 periodical subscriptions (95 health-care related).

BACCALAUREATE PROGRAMS

Degree BS

Available Programs Generic Baccalaureate.

Study Options Full-time.

Program Entrance Requirements Transcript of college record, written essay, high school transcript, immunizations, 3 letters of recommendation, minimum high school rank 20%. Transfer students are accepted. **Standardized tests** *Required:* SAT or ACT, TOEFL for international students. **Application** *Deadline:* 4/30 (freshmen), rolling (transfer). *Notification:* continuous (freshmen).

Advanced Placement Credit given for nursing courses completed elsewhere dependent upon specific evaluations.

Contact *Telephone:* 859-985-3384. *Fax:* 859-985-3917.

CONTINUING EDUCATION PROGRAM

Contact *Telephone:* 859-985-3384. *Fax:* 859-985-3917.

Eastern Kentucky University
Department of Baccalaureate and Graduate Nursing
Richmond, Kentucky

http://www.bsn-gn.eku.edu

Founded in 1906

DEGREES • BSN • MSN

Nursing Program Faculty 22.

Nursing Student Activities Sigma Theta Tau.

Library Facilities 799,496 volumes; 2,901 periodical subscriptions.

BACCALAUREATE PROGRAMS

Degree BSN

Available Programs Generic Baccalaureate; RN Baccalaureate.

Site Options *Distance Learning:* Corbin, KY; Hazard, KY; Somerset, KY.

Study Options Full-time and part-time.

Program Entrance Requirements Minimum high school GPA of 2.5, prerequisite course work. Transfer students are accepted. **Standardized tests** *Required:* SAT or ACT, TOEFL for international students. **Application** *Deadline:* 8/1 (freshmen), rolling (transfer). *Notification:* continuous (freshmen). *Application fee:* $30.

Advanced Placement Credit by examination available. Credit given for nursing courses completed elsewhere dependent upon specific evaluations.

Contact *Telephone:* 859-622-1956. *Fax:* 859-622-1972.

GRADUATE PROGRAMS

Contact *Telephone:* 859-622-1827. *Fax:* 859-622-1972.

MASTER'S DEGREE PROGRAM

Degree MSN

Available Programs Master's.

Concentrations Available *Nurse practitioner programs in:* community health, family health.

Site Options *Distance Learning:* Corbin, KY.

Study Options Full-time and part-time.

Program Entrance Requirements Minimum overall college GPA of 2.75, transcript of college record, written essay, 3 letters of recommendation, physical assessment course, prerequisite course work.

Kentucky Christian University
School of Nursing
Grayson, Kentucky

Founded in 1919

DEGREE • BSN

Nursing Program Faculty 6 (20% with doctorates).

Baccalaureate Enrollment 63
Women 90% **Men** 10% **Minority** 1% **International** 1%

Nursing Student Activities Student Nurses' Association.

Nursing Student Resources Academic advising; assistance for students with disabilities; bookstore; campus computer network; computer lab; e-mail services; housing assistance; interactive nursing skills videos; Internet; learning resource lab; library services; nursing audiovisuals; other; remedial services; skills, simulation, or other laboratory.

Library Facilities 103,323 volumes (400 in health, 300 in nursing); 395 periodical subscriptions (200 health-care related).

BACCALAUREATE PROGRAMS

Degree BSN

Available Programs Generic Baccalaureate.

Study Options Full-time.

Program Entrance Requirements Transcript of college record, written essay, health exam, health insurance, high school transcript, immunizations, minimum GPA in nursing prerequisites of 2.5, prerequisite course work. Transfer students are accepted. **Standardized tests** *Required:* TOEFL for international students. *Recommended:* SAT or ACT. **Application** *Deadline:* rolling (freshmen), rolling (transfer). *Notification:* continuous (freshmen). *Application fee:* $30.

Expenses (2006–07) *Tuition:* full-time $13,000. *Room and board:* $1000 per academic year. *Required fees:* full-time $500.

Financial Aid 90% of baccalaureate students in nursing programs received some form of financial aid in 2005–06. *Gift aid (need-based):* Federal Pell, FSEOG, state, private, college/university gift aid from institutional funds. *Loans:* FFEL (Subsidized and Unsubsidized Stafford PLUS), Perkins. *Work-Study:* Federal Work-Study, part-time campus jobs. *Application deadline (priority):* 4/1.

Contact Nursing Department, School of Nursing, Kentucky Christian University, 100 Academic Parkway, Grayson, KY 41143-2205. *Telephone:* 606-474-3255. *Fax:* 606-474-3342. *E-mail:* nursing@kcu.edu.

CONTINUING EDUCATION PROGRAM

Contact Gail Elaine Wise, EdD, Dean, School of Nursing, Kentucky Christian University, 100 Academic Parkway, Grayson, KY 41143-2205. *Telephone:* 606-474-3271. *Fax:* 606-474-3342. *E-mail:* gailwise@kcu.edu.

Kentucky State University
School of Nursing
Frankfort, Kentucky

Founded in 1886

DEGREE • BSN

Nursing Program Faculty 18 (11% with doctorates).

Baccalaureate Enrollment 25

Nursing Student Activities Student Nurses' Association.

Nursing Student Resources Academic advising; academic or career counseling; assistance for students with disabilities; bookstore; campus computer network; career placement assistance; computer lab; computer-assisted instruction; e-mail services; externships; housing assistance; inter-active nursing skills videos; Internet; learning resource lab; library services; nursing audiovisuals; other; placement services for program completers; remedial services; resume preparation assistance; skills, simulation, or other laboratory; tutoring.

Library Facilities 457,728 volumes; 809 periodical subscriptions.

BACCALAUREATE PROGRAMS

Degree BSN

Available Programs ADN to Baccalaureate.

Program Entrance Requirements Transfer students are accepted. **Standardized tests** *Required:* SAT or ACT, TOEFL for international students. *Recommended:* ACT. **Application** *Deadline:* rolling (freshmen), rolling (transfer). *Application fee:* $30.

Contact Mrs. Catherine Cooke, Associate Professor, School of Nursing, Kentucky State University, 400 East Main Street, Frankfort, KY 40601. *Telephone:* 502-597-6963. *Fax:* 502-597-5818. *E-mail:* catherine.cooke@ kysu.edu.

Midway College

Program in Nursing (Baccalaureate)
Midway, Kentucky

http://www.midway.edu/degreeprograms/nursing. html

Founded in 1847

DEGREE • BSN

Nursing Program Faculty 3.

Baccalaureate Enrollment 17
Women 100% **Minority** 5% **Part-time** 100%

Nursing Student Activities Nursing club.

Nursing Student Resources Academic advising; academic or career counseling; assistance for students with disabilities; campus computer network; computer lab; computer-assisted instruction; e-mail services; interactive nursing skills videos; Internet; learning resource lab; library services; nursing audiovisuals; remedial services; resume preparation assistance; skills, simulation, or other laboratory; tutoring.

Library Facilities 96,236 volumes (1,200 in health, 800 in nursing); 250 periodical subscriptions (102 health-care related).

BACCALAUREATE PROGRAMS

Degree BSN

Available Programs ADN to Baccalaureate; Accelerated RN Baccalaureate; RN Baccalaureate.
Site Options Somerset, KY; Frankfort, KY.
Study Options Full-time and part-time.
Program Entrance Requirements Minimum overall college GPA of 2.3, transcript of college record, CPR certification, high school transcript, immunizations, interview, 1 letter of recommendation, minimum GPA in nursing prerequisites of 2.0, prerequisite course work, RN licensure. Transfer students are accepted. **Standardized tests** *Required:* SAT or ACT, TOEFL for international students. **Application** *Deadline:* rolling (freshmen), rolling (transfer). *Notification:* continuous (freshmen). *Application fee:* $25.
Advanced Placement Credit given for nursing courses completed elsewhere dependent upon specific evaluations.
Expenses (2006–07) *Tuition:* part-time $654 per credit hour. *Room and board:* $6000 per academic year. *Required fees:* part-time $654 per credit.
Financial Aid 95% of baccalaureate students in nursing programs received some form of financial aid in 2005–06.

Contact Dr. Barbara R. Kitchen, RN, Chair, Nursing and Science Programs, Program in Nursing (Baccalaureate), Midway College, 512 East Stephens Street, Midway, KY 40347. *Telephone:* 859-846-5335. *Fax:* 859-846-5876. *E-mail:* bkitchen@midway.edu.

CONTINUING EDUCATION PROGRAM

Contact Dr. Barbara R. Kitchen, RN, Chair, Nursing and Science Programs, Program in Nursing (Baccalaureate), Midway College, 512 East Stephens Street, Midway, KY 40347. *Telephone:* 859-846-5335. *Fax:* 859-846-5876. *E-mail:* bkitchen@midway.edu.

Morehead State University

Department of Nursing
Morehead, Kentucky

http://www.moreheadstate.edu/colleges/science/ nahs/

Founded in 1922

DEGREE • BSN

Nursing Program Faculty 17 (18% with doctorates).

Baccalaureate Enrollment 94
Women 88% **Men** 12% **Minority** 4% **Part-time** 8%

Nursing Student Activities Student Nurses' Association.

Nursing Student Resources Academic advising; academic or career counseling; assistance for students with disabilities; bookstore; campus computer network; career placement assistance; computer lab; computer-assisted instruction; daycare for children of students; e-mail services; interactive nursing skills videos; Internet; learning resource lab; library services; nursing audiovisuals; remedial services; resume preparation assistance; skills, simulation, or other laboratory; tutoring.

Library Facilities 523,767 volumes (2,000 in health, 850 in nursing); 26,817 periodical subscriptions (45 health-care related).

BACCALAUREATE PROGRAMS

Degree BSN

Available Programs Generic Baccalaureate; RN Baccalaureate.
Site Options *Distance Learning:* Maysville, KY; Ashland, KY; Prestonsburg, KY.
Study Options Full-time.
Program Entrance Requirements Minimum overall college GPA of 2.0, transcript of college record, CPR certification, health exam, immunizations, minimum GPA in nursing prerequisites of 2.7, prerequisite course work. Transfer students are accepted. **Standardized tests** *Required:* SAT or ACT, TOEFL for international students. *Recommended:* ACT. **Application** *Deadline:* rolling (freshmen), rolling (transfer). *Notification:* continuous (freshmen).
Advanced Placement Credit by examination available. Credit given for nursing courses completed elsewhere dependent upon specific evaluations.
Expenses (2006–07) *Tuition, area resident:* full-time $2435; part-time $205 per credit hour. *Tuition, state resident:* full-time $3045; part-time $255 per credit hour. *Tuition, nonresident:* full-time $6475; part-time $540 per credit hour. *Room and board:* $1310 per academic year.
Financial Aid 75% of baccalaureate students in nursing programs received some form of financial aid in 2005–06. *Gift aid (need-based):* Federal Pell, FSEOG, state, private, college/university gift aid from institutional funds. *Loans:* Federal Direct (Subsidized and Unsubsidized Stafford PLUS), FFEL (Subsidized and Unsubsidized Stafford PLUS), Perkins, college/university. *Work-Study:* Federal Work-Study, part-time campus jobs. *Application deadline (priority):* 3/15.
Contact Misty Lilley, Academic Counseling Coordinator, Department of Nursing, Morehead State University, Reed Hall 234, Morehead, KY 40351. *Telephone:* 606-783-2639. *Fax:* 606-783-9104. *E-mail:* m.lilley@ moreheadstate.edu.

Murray State University
Program in Nursing
Murray, Kentucky

http://www.murraystate.edu/

Founded in 1922

DEGREES • BSN • M SC N

Nursing Program Faculty 17 (47% with doctorates).

Baccalaureate Enrollment 254
Women 94% **Men** 6% **Minority** 3%

Graduate Enrollment 50
Women 85% **Men** 15%

Nursing Student Activities Sigma Theta Tau, Student Nurses' Association.

Nursing Student Resources Academic advising; academic or career counseling; assistance for students with disabilities; bookstore; campus computer network; career placement assistance; computer lab; computer-assisted instruction; daycare for children of students; e-mail services; employment services for current students; externships; housing assistance; interactive nursing skills videos; Internet; learning resource lab; library services; nursing audiovisuals; placement services for program completers; remedial services; resume preparation assistance; skills, simulation, or other laboratory; tutoring; unpaid internships.

Library Facilities 518,450 volumes (4,060 in health, 2,160 in nursing); 1,381 periodical subscriptions (124 health-care related).

BACCALAUREATE PROGRAMS

Degree BSN

Available Programs Generic Baccalaureate; RN Baccalaureate.
Site Options *Distance Learning:* Madisonville, KY; Paducah, KY; Hopkinsville, KY.
Study Options Full-time.
Program Entrance Requirements Transcript of college record, CPR certification, immunizations, minimum GPA in nursing prerequisites of 2.5, professional liability insurance/malpractice insurance, prerequisite course work. Transfer students are accepted. **Standardized tests** *Required:* ACT, TOEFL for international students. **Application** *Notification:* continuous until 8/1 (freshmen), continuous until 1/8 (out-of-state freshmen). *Application fee:* $30.
Advanced Placement Credit by examination available. Credit given for nursing courses completed elsewhere dependent upon specific evaluations.
Expenses (2006–07) *Tuition, state resident:* full-time $4998; part-time $208 per credit hour. *Tuition, nonresident:* full-time $13,566; part-time $565 per credit hour. *International tuition:* $13,566 full-time. *Room and board:* $5398; room only: $2698 per academic year.
Financial Aid 70% of baccalaureate students in nursing programs received some form of financial aid in 2005–06. *Gift aid (need-based):* Federal Pell, FSEOG, state, private, college/university gift aid from institutional funds. *Loans:* Federal Nursing Student Loans, FFEL (Subsidized and Unsubsidized Stafford PLUS), Perkins, state, college/university. *Work-Study:* Federal Work-Study, part-time campus jobs. *Application deadline (priority):* 4/1.
Contact Dr. Marcia B. Hobbs, Chair, Program in Nursing, Murray State University, 120 Mason Hall, Murray, KY 42071-0009. *Telephone:* 270-809-2193. *Fax:* 270-809-6662. *E-mail:* marcia.hobbs@murraystate.edu.

GRADUATE PROGRAMS

Expenses (2006–07) *Tuition, state resident:* full-time $5679; part-time $316 per credit hour. *Tuition, nonresident:* full-time $15,966; part-time $887 per credit hour. *International tuition:* $15,966 full-time. *Room and board:* $5398; room only: $2698 per academic year.
Financial Aid 70% of graduate students in nursing programs received some form of financial aid in 2005–06. Traineeships available. *Financial aid application deadline:* 4/1.
Contact Dr. Nancey E.M. France, RN, Graduate Coordinator, Program in Nursing, Murray State University, 120 Mason Hall, Murray, KY 42071-0009. *Telephone:* 270-809-6671. *Fax:* 270-809-6662. *E-mail:* nancey.france@murraystate.edu.

MASTER'S DEGREE PROGRAM

Degree M Sc N

Available Programs Master's.
Concentrations Available Nurse anesthesia. *Clinical nurse specialist programs in:* adult health, critical care, medical-surgical. *Nurse practitioner programs in:* family health.
Site Options *Distance Learning:* Madisonville, KY; Paducah, KY; Hopkinsville, KY.
Study Options Full-time and part-time.
Program Entrance Requirements Clinical experience, minimum overall college GPA of 3.0, transcript of college record, CPR certification, immunizations, interview, 3 letters of recommendation, nursing research course, physical assessment course, professional liability insurance/malpractice insurance, prerequisite course work, statistics course, GRE General Test. *Application deadline:* For fall admission, 4/15. *Application fee:* $30.
Advanced Placement Credit given for nursing courses completed elsewhere dependent upon specific evaluations.
Degree Requirements 46 total credit hours.

POST-MASTER'S PROGRAM

Areas of Study Nurse anesthesia. *Clinical nurse specialist programs in:* adult health, critical care, medical-surgical. *Nurse practitioner programs in:* family health.

CONTINUING EDUCATION PROGRAM

Contact Sandy Minor, Program in Nursing, Murray State University, 120 Mason Hall, Murray, KY 42071-0009. *Telephone:* 270-809-6674. *Fax:* 270-809-6662. *E-mail:* ann.minor@murraystate.edu.

Northern Kentucky University
Department of Nursing
Highland Heights, Kentucky

Founded in 1968

DEGREES • BSN • MSN

Nursing Program Faculty 42 (50% with doctorates).

Baccalaureate Enrollment 1,000
Women 95% **Men** 5% **Minority** 2% **International** 1% **Part-time** 50%

Graduate Enrollment 150
Women 95% **Men** 5% **Minority** 1%

Nursing Student Activities Sigma Theta Tau, Student Nurses' Association.

Nursing Student Resources Academic advising; academic or career counseling; assistance for students with disabilities; bookstore; campus computer network; career placement assistance; computer lab; computer-assisted instruction; daycare for children of students; e-mail services; interactive nursing skills videos; Internet; learning resource lab; library services; nursing audiovisuals; resume preparation assistance; skills, simulation, or other laboratory; tutoring.

Library Facilities 667,064 volumes (6,380 in health, 3,500 in nursing); 1,731 periodical subscriptions (100 health-care related).

BACCALAUREATE PROGRAMS

Degree BSN

Available Programs Accelerated Baccalaureate for Second Degree; Generic Baccalaureate; RN Baccalaureate.
Study Options Full-time and part-time.
Program Entrance Requirements Minimum overall college GPA of 2.5, transcript of college record, CPR certification, health exam, health insurance, high school biology, high school chemistry, 1 year of high school math, high school transcript, immunizations, prerequisite course work. Transfer students are accepted. **Standardized tests** *Required:* SAT or ACT, TOEFL for international students. *Recommended:* ACT. **Application** *Deadline:* 8/1 (freshmen), 8/1 (transfer). *Notification:* continuous (freshmen). *Application fee:* $40.

Advanced Placement Credit by examination available. Credit given for nursing courses completed elsewhere dependent upon specific evaluations.

Expenses (2006–07) *Tuition, area resident:* full-time $2724; part-time $227 per credit hour. *Tuition, nonresident:* full-time $5100; part-time $425 per credit hour. *Room and board:* $1875; room only: $1725 per academic year. *Required fees:* full-time $176; part-time $176 per term.

Financial Aid 10% of baccalaureate students in nursing programs received some form of financial aid in 2005–06.

Contact Dr. Louise Niemer, Director, BSN Program, Department of Nursing, Northern Kentucky University, Nunn Drive, AHC 303, Highland Heights, KY 41099. *Telephone:* 859-572-5248. *Fax:* 859-572-6098. *E-mail:* niemer@nku.edu.

GRADUATE PROGRAMS

Expenses (2006–07) *Room and board:* $1875; room only: $1725 per academic year. *Required fees:* full-time $146.

Financial Aid 15% of graduate students in nursing programs received some form of financial aid in 2005–06.

Contact Dr. Denise Robinson, Director of Graduate Nursing Program, Department of Nursing, Northern Kentucky University, Highland Heights, KY 41099. *Telephone:* 859-572-5178. *Fax:* 859-572-6098. *E-mail:* robinson@nku.edu.

MASTER'S DEGREE PROGRAM

Degree MSN

Available Programs Master's.

Concentrations Available Nursing administration; nursing education. *Nurse practitioner programs in:* adult health, family health, gerontology, pediatric, psychiatric/mental health.

Study Options Full-time and part-time.

Program Entrance Requirements Clinical experience, minimum overall college GPA of 3.0, transcript of college record, CPR certification, immunizations, nursing research course, physical assessment course, professional liability insurance/malpractice insurance, statistics course.

Advanced Placement Credit by examination available. Credit given for nursing courses completed elsewhere dependent upon specific evaluations.

Degree Requirements 44 total credit hours, thesis or project.

POST-MASTER'S PROGRAM

Areas of Study Nursing administration; nursing education. *Nurse practitioner programs in:* adult health, family health, gerontology, pediatric, psychiatric/mental health.

Spalding University
School of Nursing
Louisville, Kentucky

http://www.spalding.edu/nursing
Founded in 1814
DEGREES • BSN • MSN

Nursing Program Faculty 33 (18% with doctorates).

Baccalaureate Enrollment 159
Women 94% **Men** 6% **Minority** 24%

Graduate Enrollment 41
Women 100% **Minority** 2% **Part-time** 50%

Nursing Student Activities Sigma Theta Tau, Student Nurses' Association.

Nursing Student Resources Academic advising; academic or career counseling; assistance for students with disabilities; bookstore; campus computer network; career placement assistance; computer lab; computer-assisted instruction; e-mail services; employment services for current students; externships; interactive nursing skills videos; Internet; learning resource lab; library services; nursing audiovisuals; remedial services; resume preparation assistance; skills, simulation, or other laboratory; tutoring; unpaid internships.

Library Facilities 160,954 volumes (2,875 in health, 1,125 in nursing); 655 periodical subscriptions (367 health-care related).

BACCALAUREATE PROGRAMS

Degree BSN

Available Programs Accelerated Baccalaureate for Second Degree; Accelerated RN Baccalaureate; Generic Baccalaureate.

Study Options Full-time and part-time.

Program Entrance Requirements Minimum overall college GPA of 2.5, transcript of college record, CPR certification, health exam, health insurance, high school transcript, immunizations, interview, minimum GPA in nursing prerequisites of 2.5, professional liability insurance/malpractice insurance, prerequisite course work. Transfer students are accepted.

Standardized tests *Required:* SAT or ACT, TOEFL for international students. **Application** *Deadline:* rolling (freshmen), rolling (transfer). *Notification:* continuous (freshmen). *Application fee:* $20.

Advanced Placement Credit given for nursing courses completed elsewhere dependent upon specific evaluations.

Contact *Telephone:* 502-585-7125. *Fax:* 502-588-7175.

GRADUATE PROGRAMS

Contact *Telephone:* 502-585-7125. *Fax:* 502-588-7175.

MASTER'S DEGREE PROGRAM

Degree MSN

Available Programs Accelerated Master's for Non-Nursing College Graduates; Accelerated RN to Master's; Master's.

Concentrations Available Nursing administration; nursing education. *Nurse practitioner programs in:* adult health, family health, pediatric.

Site Options Louisville, KY.

Study Options Full-time and part-time.

Program Entrance Requirements Minimum overall college GPA of 2.7, transcript of college record, CPR certification, written essay, immunizations, interview, 2 letters of recommendation, physical assessment course, professional liability insurance/malpractice insurance, prerequisite course work, resume, statistics course, GRE General Test. *Application deadline:* For fall admission, 8/15 (priority date); for spring admission, 12/15 (priority date). Applications are processed on a rolling basis. *Application fee:* $30.

Advanced Placement Credit by examination available. Credit given for nursing courses completed elsewhere dependent upon specific evaluations.

Degree Requirements 40 total credit hours, thesis or project.

POST-MASTER'S PROGRAM

Areas of Study Nursing administration; nursing education. *Nurse practitioner programs in:* adult health, family health, pediatric.

CONTINUING EDUCATION PROGRAM

Contact *Telephone:* 502-585-7125. *Fax:* 502-588-7175.

Thomas More College
Program in Nursing
Crestview Hills, Kentucky

http://www.thomasmore.edu
Founded in 1921
DEGREE • BSN

Nursing Program Faculty 6 (33% with doctorates).

Baccalaureate Enrollment 70
Women 98% **Men** 2% **Minority** 1% **International** 1% **Part-time** 5%

Nursing Student Activities Student Nurses' Association, nursing club.

Nursing Student Resources Academic advising; academic or career counseling; assistance for students with disabilities; bookstore; campus computer network; career placement assistance; computer lab; computer-assisted instruction; e-mail services; employment services for current students; externships; interactive nursing skills videos; Internet; learning resource lab; library services; nursing audiovisuals; other; placement

Thomas More College (continued)

services for program completers; remedial services; resume preparation assistance; skills, simulation, or other laboratory; tutoring.

Library Facilities 115,345 volumes (350 in health, 200 in nursing); 498 periodical subscriptions (50 health-care related).

BACCALAUREATE PROGRAMS

Degree BSN

Available Programs Generic Baccalaureate.

Study Options Full-time.

Program Entrance Requirements CPR certification, health exam, health insurance, 1 year of high school math, immunizations, minimum GPA in nursing prerequisites of 2.5, professional liability insurance/malpractice insurance, prerequisite course work. Transfer students are accepted. **Standardized tests** *Required:* SAT or ACT, TOEFL for international students. **Application** *Deadline:* 8/15 (freshmen), 8/15 (transfer). *Notification:* continuous (freshmen). *Application fee:* $25.

Advanced Placement Credit given for nursing courses completed elsewhere dependent upon specific evaluations.

Contact *Telephone:* 859-344-3413. *Fax:* 859-344-3537.

University of Kentucky
Graduate School Programs in the College of Nursing
Lexington, Kentucky

http://www.mc.uky.edu/nursing

Founded in 1865

DEGREES • BSN • MSN • PHD

Nursing Program Faculty 65 (54% with doctorates).

Baccalaureate Enrollment 260
Women 97% **Men** 3% **Minority** 6% **Part-time** 14%

Graduate Enrollment 221
Women 92% **Men** 8% **Minority** 9% **International** 5% **Part-time** 35%

Nursing Student Activities Sigma Theta Tau, Student Nurses' Association.

Nursing Student Resources Academic advising; academic or career counseling; assistance for students with disabilities; bookstore; campus computer network; career placement assistance; computer lab; computer-assisted instruction; e-mail services; interactive nursing skills videos; Internet; learning resource lab; library services; nursing audiovisuals; skills, simulation, or other laboratory.

Library Facilities 3.1 million volumes (105,793 in health); 29,633 periodical subscriptions (3,347 health-care related).

BACCALAUREATE PROGRAMS

Degree BSN

Available Programs Baccalaureate for Second Degree; Generic Baccalaureate; RN Baccalaureate.

Study Options Full-time and part-time.

Program Entrance Requirements Minimum overall college GPA of 2.5, transcript of college record, CPR certification, written essay, high school transcript, immunizations, minimum GPA in nursing prerequisites of 2.5, prerequisite course work. Transfer students are accepted. **Standardized tests** *Required:* SAT or ACT, TOEFL for international students. **Application** *Deadline:* 2/15 (freshmen), 8/1 (transfer). *Notification:* continuous (freshmen). *Application fee:* $40.

Advanced Placement Credit by examination available. Credit given for nursing courses completed elsewhere dependent upon specific evaluations.

Expenses (2006–07) *Tuition, state resident:* full-time $3255; part-time $258 per credit hour. *Tuition, nonresident:* full-time $6985; part-time $569 per credit hour. *International tuition:* $6985 full-time. *Required fees:* full-time $165.

Financial Aid 60% of baccalaureate students in nursing programs received some form of financial aid in 2005–06. *Gift aid (need-based):* Federal Pell, FSEOG, state, private, college/university gift aid from institutional funds. *Loans:* Federal Nursing Student Loans, Federal Direct

(Subsidized and Unsubsidized Stafford PLUS), FFEL (Subsidized and Unsubsidized Stafford PLUS), Perkins, college/university. *Work-Study:* Federal Work-Study, part-time campus jobs. *Application deadline (priority):* 2/15.

Contact Office of Student Services, Graduate School Programs in the College of Nursing, University of Kentucky, Room 309, College of Nursing Building, Lexington, KY 40536-0232. *Telephone:* 859-323-5108. *Fax:* 859-323-1057. *E-mail:* conss@uky.edu.

GRADUATE PROGRAMS

Expenses (2006–07) *Tuition, state resident:* full-time $3518; part-time $368 per credit hour. *Tuition, nonresident:* full-time $7577; part-time $819 per credit hour. *International tuition:* $7577 full-time. *Required fees:* full-time $180.

Financial Aid 40% of graduate students in nursing programs received some form of financial aid in 2005–06. 4 fellowships with full tuition reimbursements available (averaging $25,000 per year), 12 research assistantships with full tuition reimbursements available (averaging $10,000 per year), 6 teaching assistantships with full tuition reimbursements available (averaging $8,160 per year) were awarded; Federal Work-Study, institutionally sponsored loans, scholarships, traineeships, tuition waivers (partial), and unspecified assistantships also available. Aid available to part-time students. *Financial aid application deadline:* 3/15.

Contact Office of Student Services, Graduate School Programs in the College of Nursing, University of Kentucky, Room 309, College of Nursing Building, Lexington, KY 40536-0232. *Telephone:* 859-323-5108. *Fax:* 859-323-1057. *E-mail:* conss@uky.edu.

MASTER'S DEGREE PROGRAM

Degree MSN

Available Programs Master's; RN to Master's.

Concentrations Available Nurse case management; nursing administration. *Clinical nurse specialist programs in:* acute care, adult health, community health, critical care, gerontology, medical-surgical, oncology, parent-child, pediatric, perinatal, psychiatric/mental health, public health, women's health. *Nurse practitioner programs in:* acute care, adult health, family health, gerontology, pediatric, psychiatric/mental health.

Site Options Morehead, KY.

Study Options Full-time and part-time.

Program Entrance Requirements Clinical experience, minimum overall college GPA of 2.75, transcript of college record, written essay, interview, 3 letters of recommendation, physical assessment course, statistics course, GRE General Test. *Application deadline:* For fall admission, 7/17 (priority date); for spring admission, 12/13 (priority date). Applications are processed on a rolling basis. *Application fee:* $40 ($55 for international students).

Advanced Placement Credit given for nursing courses completed elsewhere dependent upon specific evaluations.

Degree Requirements 40 total credit hours, comprehensive exam.

POST-MASTER'S PROGRAM

Areas of Study Nurse case management. *Nurse practitioner programs in:* acute care, adult health, family health, gerontology, pediatric, psychiatric/mental health.

DOCTORAL DEGREE PROGRAM

Degree PhD

Available Programs Doctorate.

Areas of Study Nursing research.

Program Entrance Requirements Minimum overall college GPA of 3.3, interview, 3 letters of recommendation, MSN or equivalent, statistics course, writing sample, GRE General Test. *Application deadline:* For fall admission, 7/17 (priority date); for spring admission, 12/13 (priority date). Applications are processed on a rolling basis. *Application fee:* $40 ($55 for international students).

Degree Requirements 63 total credit hours, dissertation, oral exam, written exam, residency.

CONTINUING EDUCATION PROGRAM

Contact Hazel Chappell, Assistant Director, Graduate School Programs in the College of Nursing, University of Kentucky, Room 315, College of Nursing Building, Lexington, KY 40536-0232. *Telephone:* 859-323-3851. *Fax:* 859-323-1057. *E-mail:* hwchap1@uky.edu.

University of Louisville
School of Nursing
Louisville, Kentucky

http://www.louisville.edu/nursing

Founded in 1798

DEGREES • BSN • MSN • PHD

Nursing Program Faculty 51 (39% with doctorates).

Baccalaureate Enrollment 287
Women 89.5% **Men** 10.5% **Minority** 18% **Part-time** 1%

Graduate Enrollment 81
Women 91% **Men** 9% **Minority** 12% **Part-time** 65%

Nursing Student Activities Sigma Theta Tau, Student Nurses' Association.

Nursing Student Resources Academic advising; academic or career counseling; assistance for students with disabilities; bookstore; campus computer network; career placement assistance; computer lab; computer-assisted instruction; e-mail services; employment services for current students; housing assistance; interactive nursing skills videos; Internet; learning resource lab; library services; nursing audiovisuals; skills, simulation, or other laboratory; tutoring.

Library Facilities 2.1 million volumes (253,595 in health, 2,806 in nursing); 37,931 periodical subscriptions (4,329 health-care related).

BACCALAUREATE PROGRAMS

Degree BSN

Available Programs Accelerated Baccalaureate for Second Degree; Accelerated RN Baccalaureate; Generic Baccalaureate.

Study Options Full-time.

Program Entrance Requirements Minimum overall college GPA of 2.5, transcript of college record, CPR certification, written essay, health insurance, high school foreign language, 3 years high school math, 3 years high school science, high school transcript, immunizations, minimum high school GPA of 2.5, minimum GPA in nursing prerequisites of 2.5, professional liability insurance/malpractice insurance, prerequisite course work. Transfer students are accepted. **Standardized tests** *Required:* SAT or ACT, TOEFL for international students. **Application** *Deadline:* rolling (freshmen). *Notification:* continuous (freshmen). *Application fee:* $30.

Advanced Placement Credit by examination available. Credit given for nursing courses completed elsewhere dependent upon specific evaluations.

Expenses (2006–07) *Tuition, area resident:* full-time $6252; part-time $261 per credit hour. *Tuition, state resident:* full-time $6752; part-time $282 per credit hour. *Tuition, nonresident:* full-time $16,072; part-time $670 per credit hour. *Room and board:* $5432; room only: $3732 per academic year. *Required fees:* full-time $325; part-time $163 per term.

Financial Aid *Gift aid (need-based):* Federal Pell, FSEOG, state, private, college/university gift aid from institutional funds. *Loans:* Federal Nursing Student Loans, FFEL (Subsidized and Unsubsidized Stafford PLUS), Perkins, college/university. *Work-Study:* Federal Work-Study. *Application deadline (priority):* 3/15.

Contact Trish Hart, Director of Student Services, School of Nursing, University of Louisville, 555 South Floyd Street, Louisville, KY 40202. *Telephone:* 502-852-8298. *Fax:* 502-852-8783. *E-mail:* ddfost01@louisville.edu.

GRADUATE PROGRAMS

Expenses (2006–07) *Tuition, area resident:* full-time $6787; part-time $377 per credit hour. *Tuition, state resident:* full-time $7286; part-time $405 per credit hour. *Tuition, nonresident:* full-time $17,348; part-time $964 per credit hour. *Required fees:* full-time $325; part-time $163 per term.

Financial Aid 1 research assistantship (averaging $10,800 per year) was awarded; institutionally sponsored loans, scholarships, and traineeships also available.

Contact Dr. Cynthia McCurren, Interim Dean, School of Nursing, University of Louisville, 555 South Floyd Street, Louisville, KY 40202. *Telephone:* 502-852-8300. *Fax:* 502-852-8783. *E-mail:* camccu01@louisville.edu.

MASTER'S DEGREE PROGRAM

Degree MSN

Available Programs Master's.

Concentrations Available *Clinical nurse specialist programs in:* adult health, oncology, psychiatric/mental health. *Nurse practitioner programs in:* adult health, family health, neonatal health, psychiatric/mental health, women's health.

Study Options Full-time and part-time.

Program Entrance Requirements Clinical experience, minimum overall college GPA of 3.0, transcript of college record, CPR certification, written essay, immunizations, 2 letters of recommendation, physical assessment course, professional liability insurance/malpractice insurance, statistics course, GRE General Test. *Application deadline:* For fall admission, 5/1 (priority date); for spring admission, 10/1 (priority date). Applications are processed on a rolling basis. *Application fee:* $50.

Advanced Placement Credit given for nursing courses completed elsewhere dependent upon specific evaluations.

Degree Requirements 45 total credit hours, thesis or project.

POST-MASTER'S PROGRAM

Areas of Study *Clinical nurse specialist programs in:* adult health, oncology, psychiatric/mental health. *Nurse practitioner programs in:* adult health, family health, gerontology, neonatal health, psychiatric/mental health, women's health.

DOCTORAL DEGREE PROGRAM

Degree PhD

Available Programs Doctorate; Post-Baccalaureate Doctorate.

Areas of Study Faculty preparation, health policy, individualized study, nursing research, nursing science.

Program Entrance Requirements Minimum overall college GPA of 3.0, interview by faculty committee, 3 letters of recommendation, statistics course, vita, writing sample. *Application deadline:* For fall admission, 5/1 (priority date); for spring admission, 10/1 (priority date). Applications are processed on a rolling basis. *Application fee:* $50.

Degree Requirements 54 total credit hours, dissertation, written exam.

Western Kentucky University
Department of Nursing
Bowling Green, Kentucky

http://www.wku.edu

Founded in 1906

DEGREES • BSN • MSN

Nursing Program Faculty 18 (58% with doctorates).

Baccalaureate Enrollment 163
Women 89% **Men** 11% **Minority** 3% **Part-time** 40%

Graduate Enrollment 34
Women 89% **Men** 11% **Minority** 2%

Nursing Student Activities Nursing Honor Society, Sigma Theta Tau, Student Nurses' Association.

Nursing Student Resources Academic advising; academic or career counseling; assistance for students with disabilities; bookstore; campus computer network; career placement assistance; computer lab; computer-assisted instruction; e-mail services; employment services for current students; externships; housing assistance; interactive nursing skills videos; Internet; learning resource lab; library services; nursing audiovisuals; paid internships; placement services for program completers; remedial services; resume preparation assistance; skills, simulation, or other laboratory; tutoring; unpaid internships.

Library Facilities 1.2 million volumes (17,880 in health, 1,697 in nursing); 4,080 periodical subscriptions (217 health-care related).

BACCALAUREATE PROGRAMS

Degree BSN

Site Options *Distance Learning:* Elizabethtown, KY; Glasgow, KY; Owensboro, KY.

Study Options Full-time.

Western Kentucky University (continued)

Program Entrance Requirements Minimum overall college GPA of 2.75, transcript of college record, CPR certification, health exam, health insurance, high school transcript, immunizations, professional liability insurance/malpractice insurance. Transfer students are accepted. **Standardized tests** *Required:* SAT or ACT, TOEFL for international students. **Application** *Deadline:* 8/1 (freshmen), 8/1 (out-of-state freshmen), 8/1 (transfer). *Notification:* continuous (freshmen), continuous (out-of-state freshmen). *Application fee:* $35.

Advanced Placement Credit given for nursing courses completed elsewhere dependent upon specific evaluations.

Contact *Telephone:* 270-745-3391. *Fax:* 270-745-3392.

GRADUATE PROGRAMS

Contact *Telephone:* 270-745-3490. *Fax:* 270-745-3392.

MASTER'S DEGREE PROGRAM

Degree MSN

Concentrations Available Nursing administration; nursing education. *Nurse practitioner programs in:* primary care.

Site Options *Distance Learning:* Elizabethtown, KY; Glasgow, KY; Owensboro, KY.

Study Options Full-time and part-time.

Program Entrance Requirements Computer literacy, minimum overall college GPA of 2.75, transcript of college record, CPR certification, written essay, immunizations, interview, 3 letters of recommendation, nursing research course, physical assessment course, professional liability insurance/malpractice insurance, statistics course, GRE General Test. *Application deadline:* For fall admission, 8/1 (priority date); for spring admission, 4/14. Applications are processed on a rolling basis. *Application fee:* $35.

Advanced Placement Credit given for nursing courses completed elsewhere dependent upon specific evaluations.

Degree Requirements 45 total credit hours, thesis or project, comprehensive exam.

POST-MASTER'S PROGRAM

Areas of Study *Nurse practitioner programs in:* primary care.

CONTINUING EDUCATION PROGRAM

Contact *Telephone:* 270-745-3762. *Fax:* 270-745-3392.

LOUISIANA

Dillard University
Division of Nursing
New Orleans, Louisiana

http://www.dillard.edu/academic/nursing

Founded in 1869

DEGREE • BSN

Nursing Program Faculty 14 (14% with doctorates).

Baccalaureate Enrollment 58
Women 99% **Men** 1% **Minority** 100%

Nursing Student Activities Student Nurses' Association.

Nursing Student Resources Academic advising; academic or career counseling; bookstore; campus computer network; career placement assistance; computer lab; computer-assisted instruction; e-mail services; externships; interactive nursing skills videos; Internet; learning resource lab; library services; nursing audiovisuals; paid internships; placement services for program completers; remedial services; resume preparation assistance; skills, simulation, or other laboratory; tutoring.

BACCALAUREATE PROGRAMS

Degree BSN

Available Programs Generic Baccalaureate; RN Baccalaureate.

Study Options Full-time.

Program Entrance Requirements Minimum overall college GPA of 2.5, transcript of college record, CPR certification, health exam, health insurance, high school transcript, immunizations, letters of recommendation, prerequisite course work. Transfer students are accepted. **Standardized tests** *Required:* SAT or ACT, TOEFL for international students. **Application** *Deadline:* 7/1 (freshmen), 7/1 (transfer). *Notification:* continuous until 8/1 (freshmen). *Application fee:* $20.

Contact *Telephone:* 504-816-4717. *Fax:* 504-816-4861.

Grambling State University
School of Nursing
Grambling, Louisiana

Founded in 1901

DEGREES • BSN • MSN

Nursing Program Faculty 18 (17% with doctorates).

Baccalaureate Enrollment 350
Women 88% **Men** 12% **Minority** 94% **International** 5% **Part-time** 6%
Graduate Enrollment 35
Women 86% **Men** 14% **Minority** 17% **Part-time** 9%

Nursing Student Activities Student Nurses' Association.

Nursing Student Resources Academic advising; academic or career counseling; assistance for students with disabilities; bookstore; campus computer network; career placement assistance; computer lab; computer-assisted instruction; e-mail services; Internet; learning resource lab; library services; nursing audiovisuals; skills, simulation, or other laboratory.

Library Facilities 275,048 volumes (10,000 in health, 5,000 in nursing); 1,600 periodical subscriptions (65 health-care related).

BACCALAUREATE PROGRAMS

Degree BSN

Available Programs Generic Baccalaureate; LPN to Baccalaureate; RN Baccalaureate.

Study Options Full-time.

Program Entrance Requirements Transcript of college record, CPR certification, health exam, immunizations, minimum GPA in nursing prerequisites of 2.75, professional liability insurance/malpractice insurance, prerequisite course work. Transfer students are accepted. **Standardized tests** *Required:* TOEFL for international students. **Application** *Deadline:* 6/30 (freshmen), 6/30 (transfer). *Early decision:* 4/15. *Notification:* continuous until 8/1 (freshmen), 4/20 (out-of-state freshmen), 4/20 (early decision). *Application fee:* $20.

Advanced Placement Credit given for nursing courses completed elsewhere dependent upon specific evaluations.

Contact *Telephone:* 318-274-2672. *Fax:* 318-274-3491.

GRADUATE PROGRAMS

Contact *Telephone:* 318-274-2897. *Fax:* 318-274-3491.

MASTER'S DEGREE PROGRAM

Degree MSN

Available Programs Master's.

Concentrations Available Nursing education. *Nurse practitioner programs in:* family health.

Study Options Full-time and part-time.

Program Entrance Requirements Clinical experience, minimum overall college GPA of 3.0, transcript of college record, CPR certification, immunizations, interview, 3 letters of recommendation, physical assessment course, professional liability insurance/malpractice insurance, prerequisite course work, statistics course, GRE. *Application deadline:* For fall admission, 7/1; for spring admission, 12/1. Applications are processed on a rolling basis. *Application fee:* $20 ($30 for international students).

Advanced Placement Credit given for nursing courses completed elsewhere dependent upon specific evaluations.

Degree Requirements 49 total credit hours, thesis or project, comprehensive exam.

POST-MASTER'S PROGRAM

Areas of Study *Nurse practitioner programs in:* family health.

Louisiana College
Department of Nursing
Pineville, Louisiana

http://www.lacollege.edu

Founded in 1906

DEGREE • BSN

Nursing Program Faculty 6 (17% with doctorates).

Baccalaureate Enrollment 100

Nursing Student Activities Sigma Theta Tau, Student Nurses' Association.

Nursing Student Resources Academic advising; academic or career counseling; assistance for students with disabilities; bookstore; campus computer network; career placement assistance; computer lab; computer-assisted instruction; e-mail services; employment services for current students; externships; Internet; learning resource lab; library services; nursing audiovisuals; skills, simulation, or other laboratory; tutoring; unpaid internships.

Library Facilities 135,566 volumes (3,426 in health, 500 in nursing); 380 periodical subscriptions (142 health-care related).

BACCALAUREATE PROGRAMS

Degree BSN

Available Programs Generic Baccalaureate.

Study Options Full-time.

Program Entrance Requirements Minimum overall college GPA of 2.6, transcript of college record, CPR certification, health exam, health insurance, immunizations, interview, minimum high school GPA of 2.0, minimum high school rank 50%, minimum GPA in nursing prerequisites of 2.6, professional liability insurance/malpractice insurance, prerequisite course work. Transfer students are accepted. **Standardized tests** *Required:* SAT or ACT, TOEFL for international students. **Application** *Deadline:* 8/15 (freshmen). *Notification:* continuous (freshmen). *Application fee:* $25.

Advanced Placement Credit given for nursing courses completed elsewhere dependent upon specific evaluations.

Contact *Telephone:* 318-487-7127. *Fax:* 318-487-7488.

Louisiana State University Health Sciences Center
School of Nursing
New Orleans, Louisiana

http://nursing.lsuhsc.edu

Founded in 1931

DEGREES • BSN • DNS • MN

Nursing Program Faculty 77 (33% with doctorates).

Nursing Student Activities Nursing Honor Society, Sigma Theta Tau, Student Nurses' Association.

Nursing Student Resources Academic advising; academic or career counseling; bookstore; computer lab; computer-assisted instruction; e-mail services; housing assistance; interactive nursing skills videos; Internet; learning resource lab; library services; nursing audiovisuals; skills, simulation, or other laboratory.

Library Facilities 232,617 volumes (181,235 in health); 2,359 periodical subscriptions (1,964 health-care related).

BACCALAUREATE PROGRAMS

Degree BSN

Available Programs Generic Baccalaureate; RN Baccalaureate.

Study Options Full-time and part-time.

Program Entrance Requirements Minimum overall college GPA of 2.8, transcript of college record, interview, prerequisite course work. Transfer students are accepted. **Application** *Deadline:* 3/1 (transfer). *Application fee:* $50.

Contact *Telephone:* 504-568-4197.

GRADUATE PROGRAMS

Contact *Telephone:* 504-568-4213.

MASTER'S DEGREE PROGRAM

Degree MN

Available Programs Master's.

Concentrations Available Health-care administration; nurse anesthesia; nursing administration; nursing education. *Clinical nurse specialist programs in:* adult health, community health, parent-child, psychiatric/mental health. *Nurse practitioner programs in:* neonatal health, primary care.

Study Options Full-time and part-time.

Program Entrance Requirements Clinical experience, minimum overall college GPA of 3.0, transcript of college record, CPR certification, interview, 3 letters of recommendation, statistics course, GRE General Test, MAT. *Application deadline:* For spring admission, 6/1. *Application fee:* $50.

Degree Requirements 38 total credit hours.

DOCTORAL DEGREE PROGRAM

Degree DNS

Available Programs Doctorate.

Areas of Study Clinical practice, nursing education.

Program Entrance Requirements Clinical experience, minimum overall college GPA of 3.5, 3 letters of recommendation, MSN or equivalent, scholarly papers, writing sample, GRE General Test. *Application deadline:* For spring admission, 6/1. *Application fee:* $50.

Degree Requirements 54 total credit hours, dissertation, oral exam.

POSTDOCTORAL PROGRAM

Postdoctoral Program Contact *Telephone:* 504-568-4107. *Fax:* 504-568-5853.

CONTINUING EDUCATION PROGRAM

Contact *Telephone:* 504-568-4202. *Fax:* 504-568-5859.

Loyola University New Orleans
Program in Nursing
New Orleans, Louisiana

http://www.loyno.edu/~nursing

Founded in 1912

DEGREES • BSN • MSN

Nursing Program Faculty 10 (70% with doctorates).

Baccalaureate Enrollment 107
Women 90% **Men** 10% **Minority** 32% **Part-time** 100%

Graduate Enrollment 226
Women 95% **Men** 5% **Minority** 26% **Part-time** 96%

Nursing Student Activities Sigma Theta Tau.

Nursing Student Resources Academic advising; academic or career counseling; assistance for students with disabilities; bookstore; campus computer network; career placement assistance; computer lab; computer-assisted instruction; e-mail services; Internet; library services; tutoring.

Library Facilities 409,782 volumes; 37,520 periodical subscriptions.

BACCALAUREATE PROGRAMS

Degree BSN

Available Programs RN Baccalaureate.

Site Options Baton Rouge, LA.

Study Options Part-time.

Loyola University New Orleans (continued)

Program Entrance Requirements Minimum overall college GPA of 2.5, transcript of college record, written essay, immunizations, minimum GPA in nursing prerequisites of 2.0, professional liability insurance/malpractice insurance, RN licensure. Transfer students are accepted. **Standardized tests** *Required:* TOEFL for international students. *Required for some:* SAT or ACT, PAA. **Application** *Deadline:* 1/15 (freshmen), rolling (transfer). *Notification:* continuous (freshmen). *Application fee:* $20.

Advanced Placement Credit by examination available. Credit given for nursing courses completed elsewhere dependent upon specific evaluations.

Expenses (2006–07) *Tuition:* part-time $289 per credit hour. *Required fees:* part-time $183 per term.

Financial Aid 98% of baccalaureate students in nursing programs received some form of financial aid in 2005–06.

Contact Dr. Gail Tumulty, RN, Associate Professor, Program in Nursing, Loyola University New Orleans, 6363 St. Charles Avenue, Campus Box 42, New Orleans, LA 70118. *Telephone:* 504-865-3142. *Fax:* 504-865-3254. *E-mail:* nursing@loyno.edu.

GRADUATE PROGRAMS

Expenses (2006–07) *Tuition:* part-time $365 per credit hour. *Required fees:* part-time $183 per term.

Financial Aid 100% of graduate students in nursing programs received some form of financial aid in 2005–06. Scholarships available. Aid available to part-time students. *Financial aid application deadline:* 5/1.

Contact Dr. Gail Tumulty, RN, Associate Professor, Program in Nursing, Loyola University New Orleans, 6363 St. Charles Avenue, Campus Box 42, New Orleans, LA 70118. *Telephone:* 504-865-3142. *Fax:* 504-865-3254. *E-mail:* nursing@loyno.edu.

MASTER'S DEGREE PROGRAM

Degree MSN

Available Programs Master's; Master's for Nurses with Non-Nursing Degrees; RN to Master's.

Concentrations Available Health-care administration; nurse case management. *Nurse practitioner programs in:* adult health, family health.

Study Options Full-time and part-time.

Program Entrance Requirements Clinical experience, minimum overall college GPA of 2.8, transcript of college record, written essay, interview, 3 letters of recommendation, nursing research course, professional liability insurance/malpractice insurance, prerequisite course work, statistics course, GRE. *Application deadline:* For fall admission, 3/1 (priority date). *Application fee:* $20.

Advanced Placement Credit given for nursing courses completed elsewhere dependent upon specific evaluations.

Degree Requirements 39 total credit hours, comprehensive exam.

POST-MASTER'S PROGRAM

Areas of Study *Nurse practitioner programs in:* adult health, family health.

McNeese State University

College of Nursing
Lake Charles, Louisiana

http://www.mcneese.edu
Founded in 1939
DEGREES • BSN • MSN

Nursing Program Faculty 43 (12% with doctorates).

Baccalaureate Enrollment 850
Women 68% **Men** 32% **Minority** 25% **International** 2% **Part-time** 16%

Graduate Enrollment 69
Women 86% **Men** 14% **Minority** 14% **Part-time** 78%

Nursing Student Activities Sigma Theta Tau, Student Nurses' Association.

Nursing Student Resources Academic advising; academic or career counseling; assistance for students with disabilities; bookstore; campus computer network; career placement assistance; computer lab; computer-assisted instruction; daycare for children of students; e-mail services; employment services for current students; housing assistance; interactive nursing skills videos; Internet; learning resource lab; library services; nursing audiovisuals; placement services for program completers; resume preparation assistance; skills, simulation, or other laboratory; tutoring.

Library Facilities 351,708 volumes (40,956 in health, 27,504 in nursing); 1,679 periodical subscriptions (113 health-care related).

BACCALAUREATE PROGRAMS

Degree BSN

Available Programs ADN to Baccalaureate; Accelerated LPN to Baccalaureate; Generic Baccalaureate; LPN to Baccalaureate; LPN to RN Baccalaureate.

Study Options Full-time and part-time.

Program Entrance Requirements Minimum overall college GPA of 2.7, transcript of college record, CPR certification, health exam, health insurance, high school transcript, immunizations, minimum high school GPA of 2.5, minimum GPA in nursing prerequisites of 2.7, prerequisite course work. Transfer students are accepted. **Standardized tests** *Required:* SAT or ACT, TOEFL for international students. **Application** *Deadline:* rolling (freshmen), rolling (transfer). *Notification:* continuous (freshmen). *Application fee:* $20.

Advanced Placement Credit by examination available. Credit given for nursing courses completed elsewhere dependent upon specific evaluations.

Expenses (2006–07) *Tuition, state resident:* full-time $2792; part-time $1396 per semester. *Tuition, nonresident:* full-time $8858; part-time $4429 per semester. *International tuition:* $8858 full-time. *Room and board:* $4380; room only: $3580 per academic year. *Required fees:* full-time $1080; part-time $150 per credit.

Financial Aid 70% of baccalaureate students in nursing programs received some form of financial aid in 2005–06.

Contact Dr. Peggy L. Wolfe, Dean and Professor, College of Nursing, McNeese State University, PO Box 90415, Lake Charles, LA 70609-0415. *Telephone:* 337-475-5820. *Fax:* 337-475-5924. *E-mail:* pwolfe@mail.mcneese.edu.

GRADUATE PROGRAMS

Expenses (2006–07) *Tuition, state resident:* full-time $3132; part-time $1566 per semester. *Tuition, nonresident:* full-time $8858; part-time $4429 per semester. *International tuition:* $8858 full-time. *Room and board:* $4380; room only: $3580 per academic year. *Required fees:* full-time $80; part-time $40 per term.

Financial Aid 15% of graduate students in nursing programs received some form of financial aid in 2005–06. *Application deadline:* 5/1.

Contact Dr. Ruth Brewer, MSN Co-Coordinator, College of Nursing, McNeese State University, PO Box 90415, Lake Charles, LA 70609-0415. *Telephone:* 337-475-5753. *Fax:* 337-475-5702. *E-mail:* rbrewer@acc.mcneese.edu.

MASTER'S DEGREE PROGRAM

Degree MSN

Available Programs Master's.

Concentrations Available Nursing education. *Clinical nurse specialist programs in:* adult health, psychiatric/mental health. *Nurse practitioner programs in:* adult health, psychiatric/mental health.

Site Options *Distance Learning:* Lake Charles, LA; Lafayette, LA; Baton Rouge, LA.

Study Options Full-time and part-time.

Program Entrance Requirements Minimum overall college GPA of 2.7, transcript of college record, physical assessment course, statistics course, GRE. *Application deadline:* For fall admission, 7/15 (priority date). Applications are processed on a rolling basis. *Application fee:* $20 ($30 for international students).

Advanced Placement Credit given for nursing courses completed elsewhere dependent upon specific evaluations.

Degree Requirements 43 total credit hours, thesis or project.

CONTINUING EDUCATION PROGRAM

Contact Mrs. Patsy Trahan, Continuing Education Coordinator, College of Nursing, McNeese State University, PO Box 90415, Lake Charles, LA 70609-0415. *Telephone:* 337-475-5832. *Fax:* 337-475-5924. *E-mail:* ptrahan@acc.mcneese.edu.

Nicholls State University
Department of Nursing
Thibodaux, Louisiana

http://www.nicholls.edu/nursing/
Founded in 1948
DEGREE • BSN

Nursing Program Faculty 19 (21% with doctorates).

BACCALAUREATE PROGRAMS

Degree BSN

Available Programs Generic Baccalaureate; LPN to Baccalaureate; RN Baccalaureate.

Program Entrance Requirements Minimum overall college GPA of 2.75, transcript of college record, minimum GPA in nursing prerequisites of 2.0, prerequisite course work. Transfer students are accepted. **Standardized tests** *Required:* SAT or ACT. **Application** *Deadline:* rolling (freshmen), rolling (transfer). *Notification:* 9/1 (freshmen). *Application fee:* $20.
Contact *Telephone:* 985-448-4696. *Fax:* 985-448-4932.

CONTINUING EDUCATION PROGRAM

Contact *Telephone:* 985-448-4696. *Fax:* 985-448-4932.

Northwestern State University of Louisiana
College of Nursing
Shreveport, Louisiana

http://www.nsula.edu
Founded in 1884
DEGREES • BSN • MSN

Nursing Program Faculty 56 (16% with doctorates).
Baccalaureate Enrollment 1,256
Women 87% **Men** 13% **Minority** 34% **Part-time** 33%
Graduate Enrollment 136
Women 92% **Men** 8% **Minority** 14% **Part-time** 80%
Nursing Student Activities Sigma Theta Tau, Student Nurses' Association.
Nursing Student Resources Academic advising; academic or career counseling; assistance for students with disabilities; bookstore; campus computer network; computer lab; computer-assisted instruction; e-mail services; employment services for current students; interactive nursing skills videos; Internet; learning resource lab; library services; nursing audiovisuals; remedial services; skills, simulation, or other laboratory; tutoring.
Library Facilities 861,048 volumes (4,328 in health, 3,030 in nursing); 1,403 periodical subscriptions (1,298 health-care related).

BACCALAUREATE PROGRAMS

Degree BSN

Available Programs ADN to Baccalaureate; Generic Baccalaureate; LPN to Baccalaureate; RN Baccalaureate.
Site Options *Distance Learning:* Alexandria, LA; Ferriday, LA.
Study Options Full-time and part-time.

Program Entrance Requirements Minimum overall college GPA of 2.0, transcript of college record, CPR certification, health exam, immunizations, minimum GPA in nursing prerequisites of 2.7, prerequisite course work. Transfer students are accepted. **Standardized tests** *Required:* SAT or ACT, TOEFL for international students. **Application** *Deadline:* 7/6 (freshmen), 7/6 (transfer). *Notification:* continuous (freshmen). *Application fee:* $20.
Advanced Placement Credit by examination available. Credit given for nursing courses completed elsewhere dependent upon specific evaluations.
Expenses (2006–07) *Tuition, state resident:* full-time $6231; part-time $1095 per semester. *Tuition, nonresident:* full-time $10,392; part-time $1986 per semester. *Required fees:* full-time $1275; part-time $213 per term.
Financial Aid 75% of baccalaureate students in nursing programs received some form of financial aid in 2005–06.
Contact Mrs. Shirley Cashio, Director, Undergraduate Studies in Nursing, College of Nursing, Northwestern State University of Louisiana, 1800 Line Avenue, Shreveport, LA 71101. *Telephone:* 318-677-3100. *Fax:* 318-677-3127. *E-mail:* cashios@nsula.edu.

GRADUATE PROGRAMS

Expenses (2006–07) *Tuition, state resident:* full-time $5991; part-time $987 per semester. *Tuition, nonresident:* full-time $10,392; part-time $1480 per semester. *Required fees:* full-time $1275; part-time $213 per term.
Financial Aid 15% of graduate students in nursing programs received some form of financial aid in 2005–06. Career-related internships or fieldwork and Federal Work-Study available. Aid available to part-time students. *Financial aid application deadline:* 7/15.
Contact Dr. Sally Cook, Director, Graduate Studies and Research in Nursing, College of Nursing, Northwestern State University of Louisiana, 1800 Line Avenue, Shreveport, LA 71101. *Telephone:* 318-677-3100. *Fax:* 318-677-3127. *E-mail:* cooks@nsula.edu.

MASTER'S DEGREE PROGRAM

Degree MSN

Available Programs Master's.
Concentrations Available Nursing administration; nursing education. *Clinical nurse specialist programs in:* adult health, critical care, psychiatric/mental health. *Nurse practitioner programs in:* acute care, family health, neonatal health, pediatric, women's health.
Site Options *Distance Learning:* Alexandria, LA; Ferriday, LA.
Study Options Full-time and part-time.
Program Entrance Requirements Clinical experience, minimum overall college GPA of 3.0, transcript of college record, written essay, immunizations, 2 letters of recommendation, nursing research course, physical assessment course, professional liability insurance/malpractice insurance, statistics course, GRE General Test. *Application deadline:* For fall admission, 8/1 (priority date); for spring admission, 1/10. Applications are processed on a rolling basis. *Application fee:* $20 ($30 for international students).
Degree Requirements 42 total credit hours, thesis or project, comprehensive exam.

POST-MASTER'S PROGRAM

Areas of Study *Nurse practitioner programs in:* acute care, family health, neonatal health, pediatric, women's health.

CONTINUING EDUCATION PROGRAM

Contact Ms. Diane Graham Webb, Director, Non-Traditional Studies in Nursing, College of Nursing, Northwestern State University of Louisiana, 1800 Line Avenue, Shreveport, LA 71101. *Telephone:* 318-677-3100. *Fax:* 318-677-3127. *E-mail:* grahamd@nsula.edu.

Our Lady of Holy Cross College
Division of Nursing
New Orleans, Louisiana

http://www.olhcc.edu
Founded in 1916

Our Lady of Holy Cross College (continued)
DEGREE • BSN

Nursing Program Faculty 16 (32% with doctorates).

Baccalaureate Enrollment 168
Women 90% **Men** 10% **Minority** 15% **Part-time** 11%

Nursing Student Activities Sigma Theta Tau, Student Nurses' Association, nursing club.

Nursing Student Resources Academic advising; academic or career counseling; assistance for students with disabilities; bookstore; campus computer network; career placement assistance; computer lab; computer-assisted instruction; e-mail services; interactive nursing skills videos; Internet; learning resource lab; library services; nursing audiovisuals; remedial services; resume preparation assistance; skills, simulation, or other laboratory; tutoring.

Library Facilities 83,631 volumes (5,000 in health, 3,100 in nursing); 1,002 periodical subscriptions (103 health-care related).

BACCALAUREATE PROGRAMS

Degree BSN

Available Programs Generic Baccalaureate.

Study Options Full-time.

Program Entrance Requirements Minimum overall college GPA of 2.5, transcript of college record, CPR certification, written essay, health exam, health insurance, high school transcript, immunizations, 3 letters of recommendation, minimum high school GPA of 2.0, minimum GPA in nursing prerequisites of 2.5, professional liability insurance/malpractice insurance, prerequisite course work. Transfer students are accepted. **Standardized tests** *Required:* TOEFL for international students. **Placement:** *Required:* SAT or ACT. *Recommended:* ACT. **Application** *Deadline:* 7/20 (freshmen), rolling (transfer). *Notification:* continuous (freshmen). *Application fee:* $15.

Advanced Placement Credit by examination available. Credit given for nursing courses completed elsewhere dependent upon specific evaluations.

Expenses (2006–07) *Tuition:* full-time $6000. *Required fees:* full-time $300.

Financial Aid 80% of baccalaureate students in nursing programs received some form of financial aid in 2005–06. *Gift aid (need-based):* Federal Pell, FSEOG, state, private, college/university gift aid from institutional funds, Federal Nursing. *Loans:* FFEL (Subsidized and Unsubsidized Stafford PLUS). *Work-Study:* Federal Work-Study. *Application deadline (priority):* 4/15.

Contact Miss Tami Valadie, Administrative Assistant for Nursing, Division of Nursing, Our Lady of Holy Cross College, 4123 Woodland Drive, New Orleans, LA 70131. *Telephone:* 504-398-2215. *Fax:* 504-391-2421. *E-mail:* tvaladie@olhcc.edu.

Our Lady of the Lake College
Division of Nursing
Baton Rouge, Louisiana

http://www.ololcollege.edu
Founded in 1990
DEGREES • BSN • MSN

Nursing Program Faculty 23 (4% with doctorates).

Baccalaureate Enrollment 110
Women 90% **Men** 10% **Minority** 5% **Part-time** 45%

Graduate Enrollment 67
Women 55% **Men** 45% **Minority** 3%

Nursing Student Activities Student Nurses' Association.

Nursing Student Resources Academic advising; academic or career counseling; assistance for students with disabilities; bookstore; campus computer network; career placement assistance; computer lab; computer-assisted instruction; e-mail services; employment services for current students; interactive nursing skills videos; Internet; learning resource lab; library services; nursing audiovisuals; paid internships; remedial services; resume preparation assistance; skills, simulation, or other laboratory; tutoring.

Library Facilities 12,409 volumes (10,000 in health, 1,000 in nursing); 328 periodical subscriptions (200 health-care related).

BACCALAUREATE PROGRAMS

Degree BSN

Available Programs RN Baccalaureate.

Study Options Full-time and part-time.

Program Entrance Requirements Minimum overall college GPA of 2.0, CPR certification, written essay, health exam, immunizations, minimum high school GPA of 2.0, professional liability insurance/malpractice insurance, RN licensure. Transfer students are accepted. **Standardized tests** *Required:* ACT, ACT ASSET. **Application** *Deadline:* rolling (freshmen), rolling (transfer). *Notification:* 8/1 (freshmen). *Application fee:* $35.

Advanced Placement Credit by examination available.

Expenses (2006–07) *Tuition:* full-time $5500; part-time $226 per credit hour. *Required fees:* full-time $410.

Financial Aid 83% of baccalaureate students in nursing programs received some form of financial aid in 2005–06.

Contact Ms. Cathy Groeger, RN-BSN Program Director, Division of Nursing, Our Lady of the Lake College, 7434 Perkins Road, Baton Rouge, LA 70808. *Telephone:* 225-768-1788. *Fax:* 225-768-1760. *E-mail:* cgroeger@ololcollege.edu.

GRADUATE PROGRAMS

Expenses (2006–07) *Tuition:* full-time $4500; part-time $500 per credit hour. *Required fees:* full-time $610.

Financial Aid 95% of graduate students in nursing programs received some form of financial aid in 2005–06.

Contact Dr. Joan Ellis, Dean, Graduate Programs in Nursing, Division of Nursing, Our Lady of the Lake College, 7500 Hennessy Boulevard, Baton Rouge, LA 70808. *Telephone:* 225-768-1715. *Fax:* 225-768-1760. *E-mail:* jellis@ololcollege.edu.

MASTER'S DEGREE PROGRAM

Degree MSN

Available Programs Master's.

Concentrations Available Nurse anesthesia; nursing administration; nursing education.

Study Options Full-time and part-time.

Program Entrance Requirements Clinical experience, minimum overall college GPA of 3.3, transcript of college record, interview, letters of recommendation, nursing research course, physical assessment course, statistics course.

Advanced Placement Credit given for nursing courses completed elsewhere dependent upon specific evaluations.

Degree Requirements 42 total credit hours, thesis or project.

CONTINUING EDUCATION PROGRAM

Contact Mrs. Marie Kelley, Vice President, HCI, Division of Nursing, Our Lady of the Lake College, 7434 Perkins Road, Baton Rouge, LA 70808. *Telephone:* 225-768-1789. *Fax:* 225-214-1940. *E-mail:* mkelley@ololcollege.edu.

Southeastern Louisiana University
School of Nursing
Hammond, Louisiana

Founded in 1925
DEGREES • BS • MSN

Nursing Program Faculty 58 (26% with doctorates).

Baccalaureate Enrollment 1,814
Women 84.5% **Men** 15.5% **Minority** 21.3% **International** .6% **Part-time** 18%

Graduate Enrollment 73
Women 84.9% **Men** 15.1% **Minority** 9.6% **International** 2.7% **Part-time** 82.2%

Nursing Student Activities Nursing Honor Society, Sigma Theta Tau, Student Nurses' Association.

Nursing Student Resources Academic advising; academic or career counseling; assistance for students with disabilities; bookstore; campus computer network; career placement assistance; computer lab; computer-assisted instruction; e-mail services; employment services for current students; housing assistance; interactive nursing skills videos; Internet; learning resource lab; library services; nursing audiovisuals; other; paid internships; placement services for program completers; remedial services; resume preparation assistance; skills, simulation, or other laboratory; tutoring; unpaid internships.

Library Facilities 623,746 volumes (11,403 in health, 5,910 in nursing); 2,707 periodical subscriptions (324 health-care related).

BACCALAUREATE PROGRAMS

Degree BS

Available Programs Accelerated Baccalaureate; Accelerated RN Baccalaureate; Generic Baccalaureate; LPN to RN Baccalaureate; RN Baccalaureate.

Site Options *Distance Learning:* Baton Rouge, LA.

Study Options Full-time and part-time.

Program Entrance Requirements Health exam, immunizations, minimum GPA in nursing prerequisites of 2.7. Transfer students are accepted. **Standardized tests** *Required:* SAT or ACT, TOEFL for international students. *Recommended:* SAT Subject Tests. **Application** *Deadline:* 8/15 (freshmen), 8/15 (out-of-state freshmen), 8/15 (transfer). *Notification:* continuous (freshmen), continuous (out-of-state freshmen). *Application fee:* $20.

Advanced Placement Credit by examination available. Credit given for nursing courses completed elsewhere dependent upon specific evaluations.

Expenses (2006–07) *Tuition, state resident:* full-time $2216; part-time $92 per credit hour. *Tuition, nonresident:* full-time $7544; part-time $314 per credit hour. *International tuition:* $7544 full-time. *Room and board:* $5750; room only: $3600 per academic year. *Required fees:* full-time $1407; part-time $50 per credit.

Financial Aid 83% of baccalaureate students in nursing programs received some form of financial aid in 2005–06.

Contact Dr. Barbara Moffett, Director, School of Nursing, Southeastern Louisiana University, SLU 10835, Hammond, LA 70402. *Telephone:* 985-549-2156. *Fax:* 985-549-2869. *E-mail:* nursing@selu.edu.

GRADUATE PROGRAMS

Expenses (2006–07) *Tuition, state resident:* full-time $2216; part-time $123 per credit hour. *Tuition, nonresident:* full-time $6212; part-time $345 per credit hour. *International tuition:* $6212 full-time. *Room and board:* $5750; room only: $3600 per academic year. *Required fees:* full-time $1066; part-time $55 per credit.

Financial Aid 29% of graduate students in nursing programs received some form of financial aid in 2005–06. 1 fellowship with full tuition reimbursement available (averaging $2,450 per year) was awarded; career-related internships or fieldwork, Federal Work-Study, institutionally sponsored loans, unspecified assistantships, and administrative assistantship also available. Aid available to part-time students. *Financial aid application deadline:* 5/1.

Contact Dr. Anne Carruth, Graduate Nursing Program Coordinator, School of Nursing, Southeastern Louisiana University, SLU 10835, Hammond, LA 70402. *Telephone:* 985-549-5045. *Fax:* 985-549-2869. *E-mail:* acarruth@selu.edu.

MASTER'S DEGREE PROGRAM

Degree MSN

Available Programs Master's.

Concentrations Available Nursing administration; nursing education. *Clinical nurse specialist programs in:* adult health, community health, family health. *Nurse practitioner programs in:* adult health.

Site Options *Distance Learning:* Lafayette, LA; Lake Charles, LA.

Study Options Full-time and part-time.

Program Entrance Requirements Clinical experience, minimum overall college GPA of 2.7, transcript of college record, immunizations, physical assessment course, statistics course, GRE General Test. *Application deadline:* For fall admission, 7/15 (priority date); for spring admission, 12/1 (priority date). Applications are processed on a rolling basis. *Application fee:* $20 ($30 for international students).

Degree Requirements 36 total credit hours, thesis or project, comprehensive exam.

DOCTORAL DEGREE PROGRAM

Site Options *Distance Learning:* Baton Rouge, LA.

Southern University and Agricultural and Mechanical College
School of Nursing
Baton Rouge, Louisiana

http://www.subr.edu/suson

Founded in 1880

DEGREES • BSN • MSN • PHD

Nursing Program Faculty 36 (3% with doctorates).

Baccalaureate Enrollment 1,020
Women 91% **Men** 9% **Minority** 96% **International** 1% **Part-time** 12%

Nursing Student Activities Nursing Honor Society, Student Nurses' Association, nursing club.

Nursing Student Resources Academic advising; academic or career counseling; assistance for students with disabilities; bookstore; campus computer network; computer lab; computer-assisted instruction; e-mail services; interactive nursing skills videos; Internet; learning resource lab; library services; nursing audiovisuals; resume preparation assistance; skills, simulation, or other laboratory; tutoring.

Library Facilities 835,325 volumes (4,220 in health, 716 in nursing); 2,921 periodical subscriptions (114 health-care related).

BACCALAUREATE PROGRAMS

Degree BSN

Available Programs Generic Baccalaureate.

Study Options Full-time and part-time.

Program Entrance Requirements Minimum overall college GPA of 2.6, CPR certification, health exam, immunizations, minimum GPA in nursing prerequisites, prerequisite course work. Transfer students are accepted. **Standardized tests** *Required:* SAT or ACT, TOEFL for international students. *Recommended:* SAT, ACT. **Placement:** *Required:* SAT or ACT. **Application** *Deadline:* 7/1 (freshmen), 7/1 (transfer). *Notification:* continuous (freshmen). *Application fee:* $20.

Contact *Telephone:* 225-771-3416. *Fax:* 225-771-2651.

GRADUATE PROGRAMS

Contact *Telephone:* 225-771-2663. *Fax:* 225-771-3547.

MASTER'S DEGREE PROGRAM

Degree MSN

Available Programs Master's.

Concentrations Available Health-care administration; nursing education. *Clinical nurse specialist programs in:* family health. *Nurse practitioner programs in:* family health.

Study Options Full-time and part-time.

Program Entrance Requirements Minimum overall college GPA of 3.0, transcript of college record, 3 letters of recommendation, physical assessment course, statistics course, GRE General Test. *Application deadline:* For fall admission, 4/15 (priority date); for spring admission, 11/1. Applications are processed on a rolling basis. *Application fee:* $25.

Degree Requirements 46 total credit hours, thesis or project, comprehensive exam.

POST-MASTER'S PROGRAM

Areas of Study *Nurse practitioner programs in:* family health.

DOCTORAL DEGREE PROGRAM

Degree PhD

Areas of Study Advanced practice nursing, nursing education, nursing research, women's health.

Southern University and Agricultural and Mechanical College (continued)

Program Entrance Requirements Clinical experience, minimum overall college GPA of 3.2, interview by faculty committee, 3 letters of recommendation, MSN or equivalent, scholarly papers, statistics course, vita, writing sample, GRE General Test. *Application deadline:* For fall admission, 4/15 (priority date); for spring admission, 11/1. Applications are processed on a rolling basis. *Application fee:* $25.

Degree Requirements 60 total credit hours, dissertation, written exam.

University of Louisiana at Lafayette
College of Nursing
Lafayette, Louisiana

http://www.nursing.louisiana.edu

Founded in 1898

DEGREES • BSN • MSN

Nursing Program Faculty 47 (23% with doctorates).

Baccalaureate Enrollment 1,577
Women 83% **Men** 17% **Minority** 30% **Part-time** 11.6%

Nursing Student Activities Nursing Honor Society, Sigma Theta Tau, Student Nurses' Association.

Nursing Student Resources Academic advising; academic or career counseling; assistance for students with disabilities; bookstore; campus computer network; career placement assistance; computer lab; computer-assisted instruction; daycare for children of students; e-mail services; employment services for current students; externships; housing assistance; interactive nursing skills videos; Internet; learning resource lab; library services; nursing audiovisuals; other; paid internships; placement services for program completers; remedial services; resume preparation assistance; skills, simulation, or other laboratory; tutoring; unpaid internships.

Library Facilities 999,913 volumes (6,883 in health, 4,593 in nursing); 2,851 periodical subscriptions (184 health-care related).

BACCALAUREATE PROGRAMS

Degree BSN

Available Programs ADN to Baccalaureate; Accelerated Baccalaureate for Second Degree; Generic Baccalaureate; LPN to RN Baccalaureate; RN Baccalaureate.

Study Options Full-time and part-time.

Program Entrance Requirements Minimum overall college GPA of 2.5, transcript of college record, CPR certification, health exam, health insurance, high school biology, high school chemistry, high school foreign language, 2 years high school math, 3 years high school science, high school transcript, immunizations, minimum high school GPA of 2.0, minimum high school rank 25%, prerequisite course work. Transfer students are accepted. **Standardized tests** *Required:* SAT or ACT, TOEFL for international students. **Application** *Deadline:* rolling (freshmen), rolling (transfer). *Application fee:* $25.

Advanced Placement Credit by examination available. Credit given for nursing courses completed elsewhere dependent upon specific evaluations.

Expenses (2006–07) *Tuition, state resident:* full-time $3422; part-time $430 per credit hour. *Tuition, nonresident:* full-time $9602; part-time $430 per credit hour. *International tuition:* $9738 full-time. *Room and board:* $3770; room only: $3770 per academic year. *Required fees:* part-time $202 per credit; part-time $1215 per term.

Financial Aid 80% of baccalaureate students in nursing programs received some form of financial aid in 2005–06.

Contact Ms. Jan Byrd, Administrative Assistant II, College of Nursing, University of Louisiana at Lafayette, PO Box 43810, Lafayette, LA 70504-3810. *Telephone:* 337-482-5604. *Fax:* 337-482-5700. *E-mail:* jmb6110@louisiana.edu.

GRADUATE PROGRAMS

Expenses (2006–07) *Tuition, state resident:* full-time $3256. *Tuition, nonresident:* full-time $9436. *International tuition:* $9572 full-time. *Room and board:* $4000 per academic year. *Required fees:* full-time $200.

Financial Aid 20% of graduate students in nursing programs received some form of financial aid in 2005–06. Fellowships with full tuition reimbursements available available.

Contact Dr. Paula Broussard, Graduate Coordinator, College of Nursing, University of Louisiana at Lafayette, PO Box 43810, Lafayette, LA 70504-3810. *Telephone:* 337-482-5617. *Fax:* 337-482-5650. *E-mail:* pcbroussard@louisiana.edu.

MASTER'S DEGREE PROGRAM

Degree MSN

Available Programs Master's.

Concentrations Available Nursing education. *Clinical nurse specialist programs in:* adult health, psychiatric/mental health. *Nurse practitioner programs in:* adult health, psychiatric/mental health.

Site Options *Distance Learning:* Hammond, LA; Baton Rouge, LA; Lake Charles, LA.

Study Options Full-time and part-time.

Program Entrance Requirements Minimum overall college GPA of 2.75, transcript of college record, immunizations, 3 letters of recommendation, physical assessment course, statistics course, GRE General Test. *Application deadline:* For fall admission, 5/15; for spring admission, 10/1. Applications are processed on a rolling basis. *Application fee:* $20 ($30 for international students).

Advanced Placement Credit given for nursing courses completed elsewhere dependent upon specific evaluations.

Degree Requirements 38 total credit hours, thesis or project.

POST-MASTER'S PROGRAM

Areas of Study *Clinical nurse specialist programs in:* adult health, psychiatric/mental health. *Nurse practitioner programs in:* adult health, psychiatric/mental health.

CONTINUING EDUCATION PROGRAM

Contact Patricia Miller, Director of Continuing Education, College of Nursing, University of Louisiana at Lafayette, PO Box 43810, Lafayette, LA 70504-3810. *Telephone:* 337-482-5648. *Fax:* 337-482-5053.

University of Louisiana at Monroe
Nursing
Monroe, Louisiana

http://www.ulm.edu/nursing

Founded in 1931

DEGREE • BS

Nursing Program Faculty 32 (1% with doctorates).

Baccalaureate Enrollment 220
Women 88% **Men** 12% **Minority** 20% **International** 1% **Part-time** 100%

Nursing Student Activities Sigma Theta Tau, Student Nurses' Association.

Nursing Student Resources Academic advising; academic or career counseling; assistance for students with disabilities; bookstore; campus computer network; computer lab; computer-assisted instruction; daycare for children of students; e-mail services; employment services for current students; interactive nursing skills videos; Internet; learning resource lab; library services; nursing audiovisuals; placement services for program completers; remedial services; resume preparation assistance; skills, simulation, or other laboratory; tutoring.

Library Facilities 645,612 volumes (20,924 in health, 3,000 in nursing); 425 periodical subscriptions health-care related.

BACCALAUREATE PROGRAMS

Degree BS

Available Programs ADN to Baccalaureate; Accelerated Baccalaureate; Generic Baccalaureate; LPN to Baccalaureate; RN Baccalaureate.

Study Options Full-time and part-time.

Program Entrance Requirements Transcript of college record, CPR certification, health exam, high school transcript, immunizations, minimum high school GPA of 2.0, minimum high school rank 50%, minimum GPA in nursing prerequisites of 2.8, professional liability insurance/malpractice insurance, prerequisite course work. Transfer students are accepted. **Standardized tests** *Required:* SAT or ACT, TOEFL for international students. **Application** *Deadline:* rolling (freshmen), rolling (transfer). *Notification:* continuous (freshmen). *Application fee:* $20.

Advanced Placement Credit given for nursing courses completed elsewhere dependent upon specific evaluations.

Financial Aid 82% of baccalaureate students in nursing programs received some form of financial aid in 2005–06. *Gift aid (need-based):* Federal Pell, FSEOG, state, private, college/university gift aid from institutional funds, Leveraging Educational Assistance Partnership Program (LEAPP). *Loans:* FFEL (Subsidized and Unsubsidized Stafford PLUS), Perkins, college/university, Federal Health Professions Student Loans. *Work-Study:* Federal Work-Study, part-time campus jobs. *Application deadline (priority):* 4/1.

Contact Dr. Florencetta H. Gibson, Director, Nursing, University of Louisiana at Monroe, 700 University Avenue, Monroe, LA 71209-0460. *Telephone:* 318-342-1640. *Fax:* 318-342-1567. *E-mail:* fgibson@ulm.edu.

CONTINUING EDUCATION PROGRAM

Contact Mrs. Celia Laird, Coordinator of Continuing Education, Nursing, University of Louisiana at Monroe, 700 University Avenue, Monroe, LA 71209-0460. *Telephone:* 318-342-1679. *Fax:* 318-342-1567. *E-mail:* laird@ulm.edu.

University of Phoenix–Louisiana Campus
College of Health and Human Services
Metairie, Louisiana

Founded in 1976
DEGREES • BSN • MSN • MSN/MBA • MSN/MHA

Nursing Program Faculty 35 (23% with doctorates).

Baccalaureate Enrollment 34
Women 91.18% **Men** 8.82% **Minority** 20.59%

Graduate Enrollment 29
Women 79.31% **Men** 20.69% **Minority** 66.67%

Nursing Student Activities Sigma Theta Tau.

Nursing Student Resources Academic advising; academic or career counseling; assistance for students with disabilities; bookstore; computer lab; library services.

Library Facilities 444 volumes; 666 periodical subscriptions.

BACCALAUREATE PROGRAMS

Degree BSN

Available Programs Accelerated Baccalaureate.

Site Options Baton Rouge, LA; Lafayette, LA.

Study Options Full-time.

Program Entrance Requirements Transcript of college record, 1 letter of recommendation, RN licensure. Transfer students are accepted. **Standardized tests** *Required:* TOEFL for international students. **Application** *Deadline:* rolling (freshmen), rolling (transfer). *Application fee:* $110.

Advanced Placement Credit by examination available. Credit given for nursing courses completed elsewhere dependent upon specific evaluations.

Expenses (2006–07) *Tuition:* full-time $9090. *International tuition:* $9090 full-time. *Required fees:* full-time $750.

Contact Campus College Chair, Nursing, College of Health and Human Services, University of Phoenix–Louisiana Campus, One Galleria Boulevard, Suite 725, Metairie, LA 70001-2082. *Telephone:* 504-461-8852.

GRADUATE PROGRAMS

Expenses (2006–07) *Tuition:* full-time $8760. *International tuition:* $8760 full-time. *Required fees:* full-time $760.

Contact Campus College Chair, Nursing, College of Health and Human Services, University of Phoenix–Louisiana Campus, One Galleria Boulevard, Suite 725, Metairie, LA 70001-2082. *Telephone:* 504-461-8852.

MASTER'S DEGREE PROGRAM

Degrees MSN; MSN/MBA; MSN/MHA

Available Programs Master's.

Concentrations Available Health-care administration; nursing administration; nursing education.

Site Options Baton Rouge, LA; Lafayette, LA.

Study Options Full-time.

Program Entrance Requirements Clinical experience, computer literacy, minimum overall college GPA of 2.5, transcript of college record. *Application deadline:* Applications are processed on a rolling basis. *Application fee:* $110.

Advanced Placement Credit given for nursing courses completed elsewhere dependent upon specific evaluations.

Degree Requirements 39 total credit hours, thesis or project.

MAINE

Husson College
School of Nursing
Bangor, Maine

http://www.husson.edu
Founded in 1898
DEGREES • BSN • MSN

Nursing Program Faculty 15 (33% with doctorates).

Baccalaureate Enrollment 237
Women 94% **Men** 6% **Minority** 6% **International** 3% **Part-time** 6%

Graduate Enrollment 54
Women 89% **Men** 11% **Minority** 2% **International** 2% **Part-time** 24%

Nursing Student Activities Sigma Theta Tau, Student Nurses' Association, nursing club.

Nursing Student Resources Academic advising; academic or career counseling; assistance for students with disabilities; bookstore; campus computer network; career placement assistance; computer lab; computer-assisted instruction; e-mail services; employment services for current students; externships; interactive nursing skills videos; Internet; learning resource lab; library services; nursing audiovisuals; remedial services; resume preparation assistance; skills, simulation, or other laboratory; tutoring; unpaid internships.

Library Facilities 39,020 volumes (3,450 in health, 1,100 in nursing); 40 periodical subscriptions (183 health-care related).

BACCALAUREATE PROGRAMS

Degree BSN

Available Programs Generic Baccalaureate.

Study Options Full-time and part-time.

Program Entrance Requirements Minimum overall college GPA of 3.0, transcript of college record, written essay, health exam, health insurance, high school chemistry, 2 years high school math, 2 years high school science, high school transcript, immunizations, interview, 2 letters of recommendation, minimum high school GPA of 3.0, minimum GPA in nursing prerequisites of 2.5, prerequisite course work. Transfer students are accepted. **Standardized tests** *Required:* SAT or ACT, TOEFL for international students. **Application** *Deadline:* 9/1 (freshmen), 9/1 (transfer). *Early decision:* 12/15. *Notification:* continuous (freshmen), 1/2 (early action). *Application fee:* $25.

Advanced Placement Credit by examination available. Credit given for nursing courses completed elsewhere dependent upon specific evaluations.

Expenses (2006–07) *Tuition:* full-time $11,520; part-time $384 per credit hour. *International tuition:* $11,520 full-time. *Room and board:* $6030; room only: $3150 per academic year. *Required fees:* full-time $267; part-time $134 per term.

Husson College (continued)

Financial Aid 86% of baccalaureate students in nursing programs received some form of financial aid in 2005–06. *Gift aid (need-based):* Federal Pell, FSEOG, state, private, college/university gift aid from institutional funds. *Loans:* FFEL (Subsidized and Unsubsidized Stafford PLUS), Perkins, alternative loans. *Work-Study:* Federal Work-Study. *Application deadline (priority):* 4/15.

Contact Dr. Ann P. Ellis, Director, Undergraduate Nursing Program, School of Nursing, Husson College, One College Circle, Bangor, ME 04401-2999. *Telephone:* 207-941-7050. *Fax:* 207-941-7198. *E-mail:* ellisa@husson.edu.

GRADUATE PROGRAMS

Expenses (2006–07) *Tuition:* full-time $4068; part-time $384 per credit hour. *International tuition:* $4068 full-time. *Required fees:* full-time $193; part-time $89 per term.

Financial Aid 71% of graduate students in nursing programs received some form of financial aid in 2005–06.

Contact Ms. Lisa P. Newman, Student Services Coordinator, School of Nursing, Husson College, One College Circle, Bangor, ME 04401. *Telephone:* 207-941-7001. *Fax:* 207-941-7198. *E-mail:* newmanL@husson.edu.

MASTER'S DEGREE PROGRAM

Degree MSN

Available Programs Master's; Master's for Nurses with Non-Nursing Degrees.

Concentrations Available *Clinical nurse specialist programs in:* psychiatric/mental health. *Nurse practitioner programs in:* family health.

Site Options *Distance Learning:* South Portland, ME; Caribou, ME.

Study Options Full-time and part-time.

Program Entrance Requirements Clinical experience, minimum overall college GPA of 3.0, transcript of college record, written essay, immunizations, interview, 3 letters of recommendation, physical assessment course, prerequisite course work, statistics course.

Advanced Placement Credit by examination available. Credit given for nursing courses completed elsewhere dependent upon specific evaluations.

Degree Requirements 43 total credit hours, thesis or project.

POST-MASTER'S PROGRAM

Areas of Study *Clinical nurse specialist programs in:* psychiatric/mental health. *Nurse practitioner programs in:* family health, psychiatric/mental health.

Saint Joseph's College of Maine
Department of Nursing
Standish, Maine

Founded in 1912

DEGREES • BSN • MSN • MSN/MS

Nursing Program Faculty 34 (11% with doctorates).

Baccalaureate Enrollment 487
Women 95% **Men** 5% **Minority** 1% **Part-time** 70%

Graduate Enrollment 271
Women 96% **Men** 4% **Minority** 3% **International** 1% **Part-time** 100%

Nursing Student Activities Sigma Theta Tau, Student Nurses' Association.

Nursing Student Resources Academic advising; academic or career counseling; assistance for students with disabilities; bookstore; campus computer network; computer lab; computer-assisted instruction; e-mail services; interactive nursing skills videos; Internet; learning resource lab; library services; nursing audiovisuals; remedial services; resume preparation assistance; skills, simulation, or other laboratory; tutoring.

Library Facilities 113,453 volumes (1,653 in health, 1,363 in nursing); 15,646 periodical subscriptions (2,271 health-care related).

BACCALAUREATE PROGRAMS

Degree BSN

Available Programs RN Baccalaureate; RPN to Baccalaureate.

Study Options Full-time and part-time.

Program Entrance Requirements Minimum overall college GPA of 2.0, transcript of college record, written essay, health exam, health insurance, high school biology, high school chemistry, 3 years high school math, 2 years high school science, high school transcript, immunizations, 1 letter of recommendation, minimum high school GPA of 2.0. **Standardized tests** *Required:* SAT or ACT, TOEFL for international students. **Application** *Deadline:* rolling (freshmen), rolling (transfer). *Early decision:* 11/15. *Notification:* continuous (freshmen), 12/15 (early action). *Application fee:* $50.

Advanced Placement Credit given for nursing courses completed elsewhere dependent upon specific evaluations.

Expenses (2006–07) *Tuition:* full-time $18,950; part-time $590 per credit hour. *Room and board:* $8160 per academic year. *Required fees:* full-time $250.

Financial Aid 98% of baccalaureate students in nursing programs received some form of financial aid in 2005–06. *Gift aid (need-based):* Federal Pell, FSEOG, state, private, college/university gift aid from institutional funds, Federal Nursing. *Loans:* Federal Nursing Student Loans, FFEL (Subsidized and Unsubsidized Stafford PLUS), Perkins, state. *Work-Study:* Federal Work-Study. *Application deadline (priority):* 3/1.

Contact Admissions Department, Department of Nursing, Saint Joseph's College of Maine, 278 Whites Bridge Road, Standish, ME 04084-5263. *Telephone:* 207-893-7830. *Fax:* 207-892-7423. *E-mail:* info@sjcme.edu.

GRADUATE PROGRAMS

Expenses (2006–07) *Tuition:* part-time $260 per credit hour.

Financial Aid 5% of graduate students in nursing programs received some form of financial aid in 2005–06. Institutionally sponsored loans available. Aid available to part-time students.

Contact Dr. Linda Conover, Director of Distance Nursing Education, Department of Nursing, Saint Joseph's College of Maine, 278 Whites Bridge Road, Standish, ME 04084-5263. *Telephone:* 207-893-7956. *Fax:* 207-893-7520. *E-mail:* lconover@sjcme.edu.

MASTER'S DEGREE PROGRAM

Degrees MSN; MSN/MS

Available Programs Master's; Master's for Nurses with Non-Nursing Degrees; RN to Master's.

Concentrations Available Nursing administration; nursing education.

Study Options Full-time and part-time.

Program Entrance Requirements Clinical experience, computer literacy, minimum overall college GPA of 3.0, transcript of college record, written essay, 3 letters of recommendation, prerequisite course work, resume, statistics course, MAT. *Application deadline:* Applications are processed on a rolling basis. *Application fee:* $50.

Advanced Placement Credit given for nursing courses completed elsewhere dependent upon specific evaluations.

Degree Requirements 42 total credit hours, thesis or project.

CONTINUING EDUCATION PROGRAM

Contact Dr. Linda Conover, Director of Distance Nursing Education, Department of Nursing, Saint Joseph's College of Maine, 278 Whites Bridge Road, Standish, ME 04084-5263. *Telephone:* 207-893-7956. *Fax:* 207-893-7520. *E-mail:* lconover@sjcme.edu.

University of Maine
School of Nursing
Orono, Maine

Founded in 1865

DEGREES • BSN • MSN

Nursing Program Faculty 20 (58% with doctorates).

Baccalaureate Enrollment 438
Women 87% **Men** 13% **Minority** 4% **International** 2% **Part-time** 9%

Graduate Enrollment 23
Women 89% **Men** 11% **Part-time** 50%

Nursing Student Activities Sigma Theta Tau, Student Nurses' Association.

Nursing Student Resources Academic advising; academic or career counseling; assistance for students with disabilities; bookstore; campus computer network; computer lab; daycare for children of students; e-mail services; employment services for current students; housing assistance; interactive nursing skills videos; Internet; learning resource lab; library services; nursing audiovisuals; skills, simulation, or other laboratory; tutoring.

Library Facilities 1 million volumes (826,648 in health); 13,041 periodical subscriptions (5,400 health-care related).

BACCALAUREATE PROGRAMS

Degree BSN

Available Programs Generic Baccalaureate; RN Baccalaureate.

Site Options *Distance Learning:* Augusta, ME; Waterville, ME; Belfast, ME.

Study Options Full-time and part-time.

Program Entrance Requirements Minimum overall college GPA of 2.6, transcript of college record, CPR certification, health exam, high school biology, high school chemistry, high school foreign language, 3 years high school math, 3 years high school science, high school transcript, immunizations, minimum high school rank 30%. Transfer students are accepted.

Standardized tests *Required:* SAT or ACT, TOEFL for international students. Application *Deadline:* rolling (freshmen), rolling (transfer). *Notification:* continuous (freshmen). *Application fee:* $40.

Advanced Placement Credit by examination available. Credit given for nursing courses completed elsewhere dependent upon specific evaluations.

Expenses (2006–07) *Tuition, area resident:* full-time $5970. *Tuition, nonresident:* full-time $16,920. *Room and board:* $7126; room only: $3594 per academic year. *Required fees:* full-time $1404.

Financial Aid 75% of baccalaureate students in nursing programs received some form of financial aid in 2005–06. *Gift aid (need-based):* Federal Pell, FSEOG, state, private, college/university gift aid from institutional funds. *Loans:* FFEL (Subsidized and Unsubsidized Stafford PLUS), Perkins, state, college/university. *Work-Study:* Federal Work-Study. *Application deadline (priority):* 3/1.

Contact Dr. Therese B. Shipps, Director, School of Nursing, University of Maine, 5724 Dunn Hall, Orono, ME 04469. *Telephone:* 207-581-2599. *Fax:* 207-581-2585. *E-mail:* therese.shipps@umit.maine.edu.

GRADUATE PROGRAMS

Expenses (2006–07) *Tuition, state resident:* full-time $5328; part-time $296 per credit. *Tuition, nonresident:* full-time $15,210; part-time $845 per credit. *Room and board:* $7126; room only: $3594 per academic year. *Required fees:* full-time $574; part-time $94 per term.

Financial Aid 100% of graduate students in nursing programs received some form of financial aid in 2005–06. Career-related internships or fieldwork, Federal Work-Study, institutionally sponsored loans, and tuition waivers (full and partial) available. Aid available to part-time students. *Financial aid application deadline:* 3/1.

Contact Dr. Carol Wood, Coordinator, School of Nursing, University of Maine, 218 Dunn Hall, Orono, ME 04469. *Telephone:* 207-581-2605. *Fax:* 207-581-2585. *E-mail:* carol_wood@umit.maine.edu.

MASTER'S DEGREE PROGRAM

Degree MSN

Available Programs Master's; RN to Master's.

Concentrations Available Health-care administration; nursing education. *Nurse practitioner programs in:* family health.

Study Options Full-time and part-time.

Program Entrance Requirements Clinical experience, minimum overall college GPA of 3.0, transcript of college record, CPR certification, written essay, immunizations, interview, 3 letters of recommendation, nursing research course, physical assessment course, statistics course, GRE General Test. *Application deadline:* Applications are processed on a rolling basis. *Application fee:* $50.

Advanced Placement Credit given for nursing courses completed elsewhere dependent upon specific evaluations.

Degree Requirements 47 total credit hours, thesis or project.

University of Maine at Fort Kent
Department of Nursing
Fort Kent, Maine

http://www.umfk.maine.edu/academics/ programs/nursing/

Founded in 1878

DEGREE • BSN

Nursing Program Faculty 5 (20% with doctorates).

Baccalaureate Enrollment 296
Women 90% Men 10% Minority 2% International 2% Part-time 63%

Nursing Student Activities Nursing Honor Society, Student Nurses' Association, nursing club.

Nursing Student Resources Academic advising; academic or career counseling; assistance for students with disabilities; bookstore; campus computer network; career placement assistance; computer lab; computer-assisted instruction; e-mail services; housing assistance; interactive nursing skills videos; Internet; learning resource lab; library services; nursing audiovisuals; remedial services; resume preparation assistance; skills, simulation, or other laboratory; tutoring; unpaid internships.

Library Facilities 69,189 volumes (3,386 in health, 2,425 in nursing); 335 periodical subscriptions (73 health-care related).

BACCALAUREATE PROGRAMS

Degree BSN

Available Programs Accelerated Baccalaureate; Generic Baccalaureate; RN Baccalaureate.

Study Options Full-time and part-time.

Program Entrance Requirements Minimum overall college GPA of 2.5, CPR certification, health exam, health insurance, high school transcript, immunizations, prerequisite course work. Transfer students are accepted.

Standardized tests *Required:* TOEFL for international students. *Recommended:* SAT and SAT Subject Tests or ACT. *Required for some:* SAT, SAT and SAT Subject Tests or ACT. Application *Deadline:* rolling (freshmen), rolling (transfer). *Notification:* continuous (freshmen). *Application fee:* $40.

Contact *Telephone:* 207-834-7586. *Fax:* 207-834-7577.

University of New England
Department of Nursing
Biddeford, Maine

http://www.une.edu/chp/nursing/

Founded in 1831

DEGREE • BSN

Nursing Program Faculty 17 (24% with doctorates).

Baccalaureate Enrollment 22
Women 73% Men 27%

Nursing Student Activities Nursing Honor Society, Sigma Theta Tau, Student Nurses' Association, nursing club.

Nursing Student Resources Academic advising; academic or career counseling; assistance for students with disabilities; bookstore; campus computer network; career placement assistance; computer lab; computer-assisted instruction; e-mail services; employment services for current students; housing assistance; interactive nursing skills videos; Internet; learning resource lab; library services; nursing audiovisuals; placement services for program completers; remedial services; resume preparation assistance; skills, simulation, or other laboratory; tutoring; unpaid internships.

Library Facilities 144,632 volumes (10,000 in health, 5,500 in nursing); 27,285 periodical subscriptions (1,300 health-care related).

BACCALAUREATE PROGRAMS

Degree BSN

Available Programs RN Baccalaureate.

Study Options Full-time and part-time.

University of New England (continued)

Program Entrance Requirements Minimum overall college GPA of 2.5, transcript of college record, CPR certification, health exam, health insurance, high school biology, high school chemistry, 2 years high school math, 2 years high school science, high school transcript, immunizations, minimum high school GPA of 2.5, professional liability insurance/malpractice insurance. Transfer students are accepted. **Standardized tests** *Required:* TOEFL for international students, SAT or ACT. **Application** *Deadline:* 2/15 (freshmen), rolling (transfer). *Notification:* continuous (freshmen). *Application fee:* $40.

Advanced Placement Credit by examination available. Credit given for nursing courses completed elsewhere dependent upon specific evaluations.

Expenses (2006–07) *Tuition:* full-time $24,440.

Financial Aid 88% of baccalaureate students in nursing programs received some form of financial aid in 2005–06. *Gift aid (need-based):* Federal Pell, FSEOG, state, private, college/university gift aid from institutional funds. *Loans:* Federal Nursing Student Loans, FFEL (Subsidized and Unsubsidized Stafford PLUS), Perkins, state, college/university. *Work-Study:* Federal Work-Study. *Application deadline (priority):* 5/1.

Contact Ms. Sharon Giles, Admissions, Department of Nursing, University of New England, 716 Stevens Avenue, Portland, ME 04103-7225. *Telephone:* 207-221-4354. *E-mail:* sgiles@une.edu.

CONTINUING EDUCATION PROGRAM

Contact Ms. Melissa DaDiego, Department of Nursing, University of New England, 716 Stevens Avenue, Portland, ME 04103. *Telephone:* 207-221-4343. *E-mail:* CPE@UNE.edu.

University of Southern Maine
College of Nursing and Health Professions
Portland, Maine

http://www.usm.maine.edu/conhp

Founded in 1878

DEGREES • BS • MS • MS/MBA

Nursing Program Faculty 62 (27% with doctorates).

Baccalaureate Enrollment 460
Women 90% **Men** 10% **Minority** 6% **Part-time** 32%

Graduate Enrollment 107
Women 96% **Men** 4% **Minority** 6% **Part-time** 49%

Nursing Student Activities Sigma Theta Tau, Student Nurses' Association.

Nursing Student Resources Academic advising; academic or career counseling; assistance for students with disabilities; bookstore; campus computer network; computer lab; computer-assisted instruction; daycare for children of students; e-mail services; interactive nursing skills videos; Internet; learning resource lab; library services; nursing audiovisuals; remedial services; resume preparation assistance; skills, simulation, or other laboratory; tutoring.

Library Facilities 545,246 volumes (18,042 in health, 622 in nursing); 2,585 periodical subscriptions (230 health-care related).

BACCALAUREATE PROGRAMS

Degree BS

Available Programs ADN to Baccalaureate; Accelerated Baccalaureate for Second Degree; Generic Baccalaureate.

Site Options Lewiston, ME.

Study Options Full-time and part-time.

Program Entrance Requirements Minimum overall college GPA of 2.75, transcript of college record, written essay, high school biology, high school chemistry, 3 years high school math, 2 years high school science, high school transcript, immunizations. Transfer students are accepted. **Standardized tests** *Required:* SAT or ACT, TOEFL for international students. **Application** *Deadline:* 2/15 (freshmen), 2/15 (transfer). *Notification:* continuous (freshmen). *Application fee:* $40.

Advanced Placement Credit by examination available. Credit given for nursing courses completed elsewhere dependent upon specific evaluations.

Expenses (2006–07) *Tuition, state resident:* full-time $5400; part-time $180 per credit hour. *Tuition, nonresident:* full-time $14,640; part-time $488 per credit hour. *International tuition:* $14,640 full-time. *Room and board:* $5639; room only: $3834 per academic year. *Required fees:* full-time $941; part-time $353 per term.

Financial Aid 96% of baccalaureate students in nursing programs received some form of financial aid in 2005–06. *Gift aid (need-based):* Federal Pell, FSEOG, state, college/university gift aid from institutional funds. *Loans:* Federal Nursing Student Loans, FFEL (Subsidized and Unsubsidized Stafford PLUS), Perkins, college/university. *Work-Study:* Federal Work-Study. *Application deadline (priority):* 2/15.

Contact Ms. Brenda Diane Webster, Coordinator of Nursing Student Services, College of Nursing and Health Professions, University of Southern Maine, PO Box 9300, Portland, ME 04104-9300. *Telephone:* 207-780-4802. *Fax:* 207-228-8177. *E-mail:* bwebster@usm.maine.edu.

GRADUATE PROGRAMS

Expenses (2006–07) *Tuition, state resident:* full-time $4860; part-time $270 per credit. *Tuition, nonresident:* full-time $13,572; part-time $754 per credit. *International tuition:* $13,572 full-time. *Room and board:* $5639; room only: $3834 per academic year. *Required fees:* full-time $561; part-time $222 per term.

Financial Aid 85% of graduate students in nursing programs received some form of financial aid in 2005–06. 5 research assistantships with tuition reimbursements available (averaging $3,375 per year), 7 teaching assistantships with tuition reimbursements available (averaging $3,375 per year) were awarded; career-related internships or fieldwork, Federal Work-Study, scholarships, traineeships, tuition waivers (full and partial), and unspecified assistantships also available. Aid available to part-time students. *Financial aid application deadline:* 2/15.

Contact Dr. Susan B. Sepples, Director, School of Nursing, College of Nursing and Health Professions, University of Southern Maine, PO Box 9300, Portland, ME 04104-9300. *Telephone:* 207-780-4082. *Fax:* 207-228-8177. *E-mail:* sepples@usm.maine.edu.

MASTER'S DEGREE PROGRAM

Degrees MS; MS/MBA

Available Programs Master's; Master's for Non-Nursing College Graduates; RN to Master's.

Concentrations Available *Clinical nurse specialist programs in:* medical-surgical, psychiatric/mental health. *Nurse practitioner programs in:* adult health, family health, psychiatric/mental health.

Study Options Full-time and part-time.

Program Entrance Requirements Minimum overall college GPA of 3.0, transcript of college record, written essay, immunizations, 2 letters of recommendation, physical assessment course, prerequisite course work, statistics course, GRE General Test or MAT. *Application deadline:* Applications are processed on a rolling basis. *Application fee:* $50.

Advanced Placement Credit given for nursing courses completed elsewhere dependent upon specific evaluations.

Degree Requirements 54 total credit hours.

POST-MASTER'S PROGRAM

Areas of Study *Clinical nurse specialist programs in:* medical-surgical, psychiatric/mental health. *Nurse practitioner programs in:* adult health, family health, psychiatric/mental health.

CONTINUING EDUCATION PROGRAM

Contact Ms. Molly Morrell, Senior Program Specialist, College of Nursing and Health Professions, University of Southern Maine, Center for Continuing Education, PO Box 9300, Portland, ME 04104-9300. *Telephone:* 207-780-5931. *Fax:* 207-780-5954. *E-mail:* mmorrell@usm.maine.edu.

MARYLAND

Bowie State University
Department of Nursing
Bowie, Maryland

http://www.bowiestate.edu/academics/nursing. htm

Founded in 1865

DEGREES • BSN • MSN

Nursing Program Faculty 13.
Nursing Student Activities Student Nurses' Association.
Nursing Student Resources Library services.
Library Facilities 331,640 volumes; 3,152 periodical subscriptions.

BACCALAUREATE PROGRAMS
Degree BSN

Available Programs RN Baccalaureate.
Study Options Full-time and part-time.
Program Entrance Requirements Minimum overall college GPA of 2.0, health exam, minimum high school GPA of 2.5, prerequisite course work, RN licensure. Transfer students are accepted. **Standardized tests** *Required:* SAT or ACT, TOEFL for international students. **Application** *Deadline:* 4/1 (freshmen), 4/1 (transfer). *Notification:* continuous (freshmen). *Application fee:* $40.
Advanced Placement Credit by examination available.
Contact *Telephone:* 301-860-3202. *Fax:* 301-860-3222.

GRADUATE PROGRAMS
Contact *Telephone:* 301-860-4000. *Fax:* 301-860-3222.

MASTER'S DEGREE PROGRAM
Degree MSN

Available Programs Master's.
Concentrations Available Nursing administration; nursing education. *Nurse practitioner programs in:* family health.
Program Entrance Requirements Clinical experience, minimum overall college GPA of 2.5, CPR certification, written essay, 3 letters of recommendation, physical assessment course, professional liability insurance/malpractice insurance, resume, statistics course. *Application deadline:* For fall admission, 5/15. Applications are processed on a rolling basis. *Application fee:* $40.
Advanced Placement Credit by examination available. Credit given for nursing courses completed elsewhere dependent upon specific evaluations.
Degree Requirements 47 total credit hours, thesis or project, comprehensive exam.

College of Notre Dame of Maryland
Department of Nursing
Baltimore, Maryland

http://206.205.71.30/academics/departments/ nd_aca_nursing.cfm

Founded in 1873

DEGREE • BS

Nursing Program Faculty 5 (60% with doctorates).
Nursing Student Resources Library services.
Library Facilities 400,000 volumes; 1,800 periodical subscriptions.

BACCALAUREATE PROGRAMS
Degree BS

Available Programs Accelerated RN Baccalaureate; RN Baccalaureate.
Site Options Frederick, MD; Aberdeen, MD.
Study Options Full-time and part-time.
Program Entrance Requirements Minimum overall college GPA of 2.5, transcript of college record, interview, minimum GPA in nursing prerequisites of 2.0, prerequisite course work, RN licensure. Transfer students are accepted. **Standardized tests** *Required:* SAT or ACT, TOEFL for international students. **Application** *Deadline:* 2/15 (freshmen), 2/15 (transfer). *Early decision:* 12/3. *Notification:* continuous until 6/30 (freshmen), 1/1 (early action). *Application fee:* $25.
Advanced Placement Credit by examination available. Credit given for nursing courses completed elsewhere dependent upon specific evaluations.
Contact *Telephone:* 410-532-5500.

Columbia Union College
Nursing Department
Takoma Park, Maryland

Founded in 1904

DEGREE • BS

Nursing Program Faculty 8 (14% with doctorates).
Baccalaureate Enrollment 240
Women 90% **Men** 10% **Minority** 75% **International** 1% **Part-time** 10%
Nursing Student Activities Student Nurses' Association, nursing club.
Nursing Student Resources Academic advising; academic or career counseling; bookstore; campus computer network; computer lab; e-mail services; externships; interactive nursing skills videos; Internet; learning resource lab; library services; nursing audiovisuals; remedial services; skills, simulation, or other laboratory; tutoring; unpaid internships.
Library Facilities 141,534 volumes; 9,000 periodical subscriptions.

BACCALAUREATE PROGRAMS
Degree BS

Available Programs Accelerated RN Baccalaureate; Generic Baccalaureate.
Study Options Full-time.
Program Entrance Requirements Minimum overall college GPA of 2.75, transcript of college record, CPR certification, written essay, health exam, immunizations, interview, 2 letters of recommendation, minimum GPA in nursing prerequisites of 2.75, prerequisite course work. Transfer students are accepted. **Standardized tests** *Required:* SAT or ACT, TOEFL for international students. **Application** *Deadline:* 8/1 (freshmen), 8/1 (transfer). *Notification:* continuous (freshmen). *Application fee:* $25.
Advanced Placement Credit given for nursing courses completed elsewhere dependent upon specific evaluations.
Expenses (2006–07) *Tuition:* full-time $17,339; part-time $725 per credit hour. *Room and board:* $6247 per academic year. *Required fees:* full-time $550; part-time $134 per term.
Financial Aid 95% of baccalaureate students in nursing programs received some form of financial aid in 2005–06.
Contact Ms. Letetia H.P. Edmonds, Office Manager, Nursing Department, Columbia Union College, 7600 Flower Avenue, Takoma Park, MD 20912-7796. *Telephone:* 301-891-4144. *Fax:* 301-891-4191. *E-mail:* ledmonds@ cuc.edu.

Coppin State University
Helene Fuld School of Nursing
Baltimore, Maryland

http://www.coppin.edu/nursing

Founded in 1900

Coppin State University (continued)
DEGREES • BSN • MSN

Nursing Program Faculty 15 (22% with doctorates).

Baccalaureate Enrollment 315
Women 96% **Men** 4% **Minority** 95% **International** 8% **Part-time** 6%

Graduate Enrollment 28
Women 93% **Men** 7% **Minority** 98% **International** 14% **Part-time** 35%

Nursing Student Activities Nursing Honor Society, Sigma Theta Tau, Student Nurses' Association.

Nursing Student Resources Academic advising; academic or career counseling; campus computer network; career placement assistance; computer lab; computer-assisted instruction; e-mail services; interactive nursing skills videos; Internet; learning resource lab; nursing audiovisuals; other; remedial services; skills, simulation, or other laboratory; tutoring.

Library Facilities 134,983 volumes (1,339 in health, 1,298 in nursing); 665 periodical subscriptions (132 health-care related).

BACCALAUREATE PROGRAMS

Degree BSN

Available Programs ADN to Baccalaureate; Accelerated RN Baccalaureate; Baccalaureate for Second Degree; Generic Baccalaureate; RN Baccalaureate.

Study Options Full-time.

Program Entrance Requirements Minimum overall college GPA of 2.5, transcript of college record, high school biology, high school chemistry, high school transcript, 3 letters of recommendation, minimum high school GPA of 2.5, minimum GPA in nursing prerequisites of 2.5. Transfer students are accepted. **Standardized tests** *Required:* SAT or ACT, TOEFL for international students. **Application** *Deadline:* 7/15 (freshmen), 7/15 (transfer). *Notification:* continuous (freshmen). *Application fee:* $35.

Expenses (2006–07) *Tuition, state resident:* full-time $4910; part-time $151 per credit hour. *Tuition, nonresident:* full-time $11,993; part-time $364 per credit hour. *International tuition:* $11,993 full-time. *Room and board:* $5269; room only: $3136 per academic year. *Required fees:* full-time $1383; part-time $692 per term.

Financial Aid 90% of baccalaureate students in nursing programs received some form of financial aid in 2005–06. *Gift aid (need-based):* Federal Pell, FSEOG, state, private, college/university gift aid from institutional funds, Federal Nursing. *Loans:* Federal Direct (Subsidized and Unsubsidized Stafford), FFEL, Perkins, alternative loans from lenders. *Work-Study:* Federal Work-Study. *Application deadline (priority):* 3/1.

Contact Mr. Darryl A. Boyd, Nursing Admissions Coordinator/Recruiter, Helene Fuld School of Nursing, Coppin State University, 2500 West North Avenue, Baltimore, MD 21216-3698. *Telephone:* 410-951-3988. *Fax:* 410-462-3032. *E-mail:* dboyd@coppin.edu.

GRADUATE PROGRAMS

Expenses (2006–07) *Tuition, state resident:* part-time $207 per credit hour. *Tuition, nonresident:* part-time $375 per credit hour. *Required fees:* full-time $407.

Financial Aid 70% of graduate students in nursing programs received some form of financial aid in 2005–06.

Contact Mr. Darryl A. Boyd, Nursing Admissions Coordinator/Recruiter, Helene Fuld School of Nursing, Coppin State University, 2500 West North Avenue, Baltimore, MD 21216-3698. *Telephone:* 410-951-3988. *Fax:* 410-462-3032. *E-mail:* dboyd@coppin.edu.

MASTER'S DEGREE PROGRAM

Degree MSN

Available Programs Master's.

Concentrations Available *Nurse practitioner programs in:* family health.

Study Options Full-time and part-time.

Program Entrance Requirements Clinical experience, computer literacy, minimum overall college GPA of 3.0, transcript of college record, CPR certification, written essay, immunizations, interview, 3 letters of recommendation, nursing research course, physical assessment course, statistics course.

Advanced Placement Credit given for nursing courses completed elsewhere dependent upon specific evaluations.

Degree Requirements 48 total credit hours, thesis or project, comprehensive exam.

POST-MASTER'S PROGRAM

Areas of Study *Nurse practitioner programs in:* family health.

The Johns Hopkins University
School of Nursing
Baltimore, Maryland

http://www.son.jhmi.edu

Founded in 1876

DEGREES • BS • MSN • MSN/MBA • MSN/MPH • MSN/PHD

Nursing Program Faculty 201.

Baccalaureate Enrollment 455
Women 90% **Men** 10% **Minority** 22% **International** 3% **Part-time** 1%

Graduate Enrollment 280
Women 95% **Men** 5% **Minority** 25% **International** 2% **Part-time** 55%

Nursing Student Activities Nursing Honor Society, Sigma Theta Tau, Student Nurses' Association, nursing club.

Nursing Student Resources Academic advising; academic or career counseling; assistance for students with disabilities; bookstore; campus computer network; career placement assistance; computer lab; computer-assisted instruction; e-mail services; externships; housing assistance; Internet; learning resource lab; library services; nursing audiovisuals; other; paid internships; resume preparation assistance; skills, simulation, or other laboratory; tutoring; unpaid internships.

Library Facilities 3.5 million volumes (370,000 in health, 40,000 in nursing); 30,023 periodical subscriptions (3,000 health-care related).

BACCALAUREATE PROGRAMS

Degree BS

Available Programs Accelerated Baccalaureate for Second Degree; Baccalaureate for Second Degree; Generic Baccalaureate; RN Baccalaureate.

Study Options Full-time and part-time.

Program Entrance Requirements Minimum overall college GPA of 3.0, transcript of college record, CPR certification, written essay, health exam, health insurance, immunizations, interview, 3 letters of recommendation, minimum GPA in nursing prerequisites of 3.0, prerequisite course work. Transfer students are accepted. **Standardized tests** *Required:* SAT or ACT, TOEFL for international students. *Recommended:* SAT Subject Tests. **Application** *Deadline:* 1/1 (freshmen), 3/15 (transfer). *Early decision:* 11/15. *Notification:* 4/1 (freshmen), 12/15 (out-of-state freshmen), 12/15 (early decision). *Application fee:* $60.

Advanced Placement Credit by examination available. Credit given for nursing courses completed elsewhere dependent upon specific evaluations.

Expenses (2006–07) *Tuition:* full-time $26,880; part-time $1120 per credit. *International tuition:* $26,880 full-time.

Financial Aid 90% of baccalaureate students in nursing programs received some form of financial aid in 2005–06. *Gift aid (need-based):* Federal Pell, FSEOG, state, private, college/university gift aid from institutional funds. *Loans:* Federal Direct (Subsidized and Unsubsidized Stafford), FFEL, Perkins, college/university. *Work-Study:* Federal Work-Study, part-time campus jobs. *Application deadline:* 2/15 (priority: 2/1).

Contact Office of Admissions and Student Services, School of Nursing, The Johns Hopkins University, 525 North Wolfe Street, Baltimore, MD 21205-2110. *Telephone:* 410-955-7548. *Fax:* 410-614-7086. *E-mail:* jhuson@son.jhmi.edu.

GRADUATE PROGRAMS

Expenses (2006–07) *Tuition:* full-time $26,712; part-time $1113 per credit. *International tuition:* $26,712 full-time.

Financial Aid 60% of graduate students in nursing programs received some form of financial aid in 2005–06. 6 fellowships with partial tuition reimbursements available (averaging $23,272 per year) were awarded; research assistantships with full tuition reimbursements available, teaching assistantships with full tuition reimbursements available, career-related internships or fieldwork, Federal Work-Study, institutionally sponsored loans, scholarships, traineeships, and tuition waivers (partial) also available. Aid available to part-time students. *Financial aid application deadline:* 3/15.

Contact Ms. Mary O'Rourke, Director of Admissions and Student Services, School of Nursing, The Johns Hopkins University, 525 North Wolfe Street, Suite 113, Baltimore, MD 21205-2110. *Telephone:* 410-955-7548. *Fax:* 410-614-7086. *E-mail:* jhuson@son.jhmi.edu.

MASTER'S DEGREE PROGRAM

Degrees MSN; MSN/MBA; MSN/MPH; MSN/PhD

Available Programs Master's.

Concentrations Available Nurse case management; nurse-midwifery; nursing administration. *Clinical nurse specialist programs in:* acute care, adult health, cardiovascular, community health, critical care, family health, forensic nursing, gerontology, maternity-newborn, medical-surgical, oncology, palliative care, parent-child, pediatric, perinatal, public health, women's health. *Nurse practitioner programs in:* acute care, adult health, community health, family health, pediatric.

Study Options Full-time and part-time.

Program Entrance Requirements Clinical experience, computer literacy, minimum overall college GPA of 3.0, transcript of college record, written essay, immunizations, interview, 3 letters of recommendation, nursing research course, physical assessment course, prerequisite course work, resume, statistics course, GRE. *Application deadline:* For fall admission, 3/1 (priority date); for winter and spring admission, 7/1 (priority date). Applications are processed on a rolling basis. *Application fee:* $75.

Advanced Placement Credit by examination available. Credit given for nursing courses completed elsewhere dependent upon specific evaluations.

Degree Requirements 36 total credit hours, thesis or project.

POST-MASTER'S PROGRAM

Areas of Study *Nurse practitioner programs in:* acute care, adult health, family health, pediatric.

DOCTORAL DEGREE PROGRAM

Degree PhD

Available Programs Doctorate.

Areas of Study Addiction/substance abuse, advanced practice nursing, aging, bio-behavioral research, biology of health and illness, clinical practice, community health, critical care, ethics, family health, forensic nursing, gerontology, health policy, health promotion/disease prevention, health-care systems, human health and illness, illness and transition, individualized study, maternity-newborn, nurse case management, nursing administration, nursing policy, nursing research, nursing science, oncology, urban health, women's health.

Program Entrance Requirements Clinical experience, minimum overall college GPA of 3.5, interview by faculty committee, 3 letters of recommendation, MSN or equivalent, scholarly papers, statistics course, vita, writing sample, GRE. *Application deadline:* For fall admission, 3/1 (priority date); for winter and spring admission, 7/1 (priority date). Applications are processed on a rolling basis. *Application fee:* $75.

Degree Requirements 63 total credit hours, dissertation, oral exam, written exam.

POSTDOCTORAL PROGRAM

Areas of Study Health promotion/disease prevention, vulnerable population.

Postdoctoral Program Contact Dr. Gayle Page, Director of Center for Nursing Research and Sponsored Projects, School of Nursing, The Johns Hopkins University, 525 North Wolfe Street, Baltimore, MD 21205-2110. *Telephone:* 410-955-7548. *Fax:* 410-614-7086. *E-mail:* gpage@son.jhmi.edu.

CONTINUING EDUCATION PROGRAM

Contact Jane Shivnan, Director, Institute for Johns Hopkins Nursing, School of Nursing, The Johns Hopkins University, 525 North Wolfe Street, Baltimore, MD 21205-2110. *Telephone:* 443-287-4745. *Fax:* 410-614-8972. *E-mail:* IJHN@son.jhmi.edu.

See full description on page 498.

Salisbury University
Program in Nursing
Salisbury, Maryland

http://www.ssu.edu/Schools/Henson/NursingDept.html

Founded in 1925

DEGREES • BS • MS

Nursing Program Faculty 18 (60% with doctorates).

Baccalaureate Enrollment 475
Women 90% **Men** 10% **Minority** 15% **International** 3% **Part-time** 10%

Graduate Enrollment 19
Women 90% **Men** 10% **Minority** 10% **International** 5% **Part-time** 85%

Nursing Student Activities Nursing Honor Society, Sigma Theta Tau, Student Nurses' Association.

Nursing Student Resources Academic advising; academic or career counseling; assistance for students with disabilities; bookstore; campus computer network; career placement assistance; computer lab; computer-assisted instruction; e-mail services; employment services for current students; externships; housing assistance; interactive nursing skills videos; Internet; learning resource lab; library services; nursing audiovisuals; paid internships; resume preparation assistance; skills, simulation, or other laboratory; tutoring; unpaid internships.

Library Facilities 269,550 volumes (6,850 in health, 1,025 in nursing); 1,235 periodical subscriptions (145 health-care related).

BACCALAUREATE PROGRAMS

Degree BS

Available Programs ADN to Baccalaureate; Accelerated Baccalaureate for Second Degree; Accelerated RN Baccalaureate; Generic Baccalaureate; RN Baccalaureate.

Study Options Full-time and part-time.

Program Entrance Requirements Minimum overall college GPA, transcript of college record, CPR certification, health exam, high school biology, high school chemistry, 2 years high school math, high school transcript, immunizations, minimum GPA in nursing prerequisites, prerequisite course work. Transfer students are accepted. **Standardized tests** *Required:* TOEFL for international students. *Required for some:* SAT and SAT Subject Tests or ACT. **Application** *Deadline:* 1/15 (freshmen), rolling (transfer). *Early decision:* 12/1. *Notification:* 3/15 (freshmen), 1/15 (early action). *Application fee:* $45.

Advanced Placement Credit given for nursing courses completed elsewhere dependent upon specific evaluations.

Expenses (2006–07) *Tuition, area resident:* full-time $4814; part-time $200 per credit hour. *Tuition, nonresident:* full-time $12,708; part-time $529 per credit hour. *International tuition:* $12,708 full-time. *Room and board:* $7000 per academic year. *Required fees:* full-time $1598; part-time $200 per credit.

Financial Aid 90% of baccalaureate students in nursing programs received some form of financial aid in 2005–06.

Contact Susan Battistoni, PhD, Chair, Department of Nursing, Program in Nursing, Salisbury University, 1101 Camden Avenue, Salisbury, MD 21801. *Telephone:* 410-543-6366. *Fax:* 410-548-3313. *E-mail:* sbbattistoni@salisbury.edu.

GRADUATE PROGRAMS

Expenses (2006–07) *Tuition, state resident:* full-time $4814; part-time $260 per credit hour. *Tuition, nonresident:* full-time $12,708; part-time $546 per credit hour. *International tuition:* $12,708 full-time. *Required fees:* full-time $1598; part-time $49 per credit.

Financial Aid 75% of graduate students in nursing programs received some form of financial aid in 2005–06. Career-related internships or fieldwork, scholarships, and unspecified assistantships available. Aid available to part-time students.

Contact Dr. Karin E. Johnson, RN, Director, Graduate Program, Program in Nursing, Salisbury University, 1101 Camden Avenue, Salisbury, MD 21801. *Telephone:* 410-543-6411. *Fax:* 410-548-3313. *E-mail:* kejohnson@salisbury.edu.

Salisbury University (continued)

MASTER'S DEGREE PROGRAM

Degree MS

Available Programs Master's.

Concentrations Available Health-care administration. *Nurse practitioner programs in:* family health.

Study Options Full-time and part-time.

Program Entrance Requirements Minimum overall college GPA of 3.0, transcript of college record, CPR certification, written essay, interview, 2 letters of recommendation, nursing research course, physical assessment course, resume, statistics course. *Application deadline:* For fall admission, 2/15; for spring admission, 10/15. Applications are processed on a rolling basis. *Application fee:* $45.

Advanced Placement Credit given for nursing courses completed elsewhere dependent upon specific evaluations.

Degree Requirements 43 total credit hours, thesis or project.

POST-MASTER'S PROGRAM

Areas of Study Health-care administration. *Nurse practitioner programs in:* family health.

Towson University
Department of Nursing
Towson, Maryland

http://www.towson.edu

Founded in 1866

DEGREES • BS • MS

Nursing Program Faculty 20 (75% with doctorates).

Baccalaureate Enrollment 190
Women 96% **Men** 4% **Minority** 24% **Part-time** 14%

Graduate Enrollment 24
Women 92% **Men** 8% **Minority** 21% **Part-time** 100%

Nursing Student Activities Sigma Theta Tau, Student Nurses' Association.

Nursing Student Resources Academic advising; academic or career counseling; assistance for students with disabilities; bookstore; campus computer network; career placement assistance; computer lab; computer-assisted instruction; daycare for children of students; e-mail services; employment services for current students; housing assistance; interactive nursing skills videos; Internet; learning resource lab; library services; nursing audiovisuals; remedial services; resume preparation assistance; skills, simulation, or other laboratory; tutoring.

Library Facilities 580,036 volumes (15,660 in health, 1,409 in nursing); 4,154 periodical subscriptions (550 health-care related).

BACCALAUREATE PROGRAMS

Degree BS

Available Programs Generic Baccalaureate; RN Baccalaureate; RPN to Baccalaureate.

Study Options Full-time and part-time.

Program Entrance Requirements Minimum overall college GPA of 2.5, transcript of college record, CPR certification, health exam, health insurance, immunizations, minimum GPA in nursing prerequisites, prerequisite course work. Transfer students are accepted. **Standardized tests** *Required:* SAT or ACT, TOEFL for international students. **Application Deadline:** 2/15 (freshmen), 2/15 (transfer). *Notification:* continuous (freshmen). *Application fee:* $45.

Advanced Placement Credit by examination available. Credit given for nursing courses completed elsewhere dependent upon specific evaluations.

Financial Aid 89% of baccalaureate students in nursing programs received some form of financial aid in 2004–05. *Gift aid (need-based):* Federal Pell, FSEOG, state, private, college/university gift aid from institutional funds. *Loans:* Federal Direct (Subsidized and Unsubsidized Stafford PLUS), Perkins. *Work-Study:* Federal Work-Study, part-time campus jobs. *Application deadline:* 3/1 (priority: 1/31).

Contact Ms. Brook R. Necker, Department of Nursing, Towson University, 8000 York Road, Towson, MD 21252-0001. *Telephone:* 410-704-4170. *E-mail:* bnecker@towson.edu.

GRADUATE PROGRAMS

Contact Dr. Marilyn Halstead, Graduate Program Director, Department of Nursing, Towson University, 8000 York Road, Towson, MD 21252-0001. *E-mail:* mhalstead@towson.edu.

MASTER'S DEGREE PROGRAM

Degree MS

Available Programs Master's.

Concentrations Available Health-care administration; nursing education.

Study Options Part-time.

Program Entrance Requirements Minimum overall college GPA of 3.0, transcript of college record, nursing research course, physical assessment course, resume, statistics course.

Degree Requirements 36 total credit hours.

University of Maryland, Baltimore
Master's Program in Nursing
Baltimore, Maryland

http://nursing.umaryland.edu

Founded in 1807

DEGREES • BSN • MS • MSN/MBA • MSN/MPH • MSN/PHD

Nursing Program Faculty 157 (63% with doctorates).

Baccalaureate Enrollment 727
Women 90% **Men** 10% **Minority** 42% **International** 2% **Part-time** 8%

Graduate Enrollment 571
Women 89% **Men** 11% **Minority** 39% **International** 3% **Part-time** 42%

Nursing Student Activities Nursing Honor Society, Sigma Theta Tau, Student Nurses' Association.

Nursing Student Resources Academic advising; academic or career counseling; assistance for students with disabilities; bookstore; campus computer network; career placement assistance; computer lab; computer-assisted instruction; e-mail services; housing assistance; interactive nursing skills videos; Internet; learning resource lab; library services; nursing audiovisuals; remedial services; skills, simulation, or other laboratory; tutoring.

Library Facilities 360,000 volumes in health, 60 volumes in nursing; 2,400 periodical subscriptions health-care related.

BACCALAUREATE PROGRAMS

Degree BSN

Available Programs Generic Baccalaureate; RN Baccalaureate.

Site Options *Distance Learning:* Shady Grove, MD; Cumberland, MD.

Study Options Full-time.

Program Entrance Requirements Minimum overall college GPA of 3.00, transcript of college record, written essay, health exam, letters of recommendation, minimum GPA in nursing prerequisites of 3.0, prerequisite course work. Transfer students are accepted.

Expenses (2006–07) *Tuition, area resident:* full-time $3445; part-time $301 per credit hour. *Tuition, nonresident:* full-time $9429; part-time $484 per credit hour. *Required fees:* full-time $1366; part-time $823 per term.

Financial Aid 90% of baccalaureate students in nursing programs received some form of financial aid in 2005–06.

Contact Ms. Amanda Barnes, Admissions Counselor, Master's Program in Nursing, University of Maryland, Baltimore, 655 West Lombard Street, Baltimore, MD 21201. *Telephone:* 410-706-0488. *Fax:* 410-706-7238. *E-mail:* winfield@son.umaryland.edu.

GRADUATE PROGRAMS

Expenses (2006–07) *Tuition, state resident:* full-time $429. *Tuition, nonresident:* full-time $767. *International tuition:* $767 full-time.

Financial Aid 50% of graduate students in nursing programs received some form of financial aid in 2005–06. Fellowships, research assistantships, teaching assistantships, career-related internships or fieldwork and traineeships available. Aid available to part-time students. *Financial aid application deadline:* 2/15.

Contact Ms. Marie-Anusche Chapman, Admissions Counselor, Master's Program in Nursing, University of Maryland, Baltimore, 655 West Lombard Street, Room 102, Baltimore, MD 21201-1579. *Telephone:* 410-706-8346. *Fax:* 410-706-7238. *E-mail:* Achap002@son.umaryland.edu.

MASTER'S DEGREE PROGRAM

Degrees MS; MSN/MBA; MSN/MPH; MSN/PhD

Available Programs Accelerated Master's for Non-Nursing College Graduates; Master's; Master's for Nurses with Non-Nursing Degrees; RN to Master's.

Concentrations Available Nurse anesthesia; nurse case management; nurse-midwifery; nursing administration; nursing informatics. *Clinical nurse specialist programs in:* acute care, community health, critical care, pediatric, psychiatric/mental health. *Nurse practitioner programs in:* acute care, family health, gerontology, oncology, pediatric, primary care, psychiatric/mental health.

Site Options *Distance Learning:* Shady Grove, MD; Cumberland, MD.

Program Entrance Requirements Minimum overall college GPA of 3.0, transcript of college record, immunizations, letters of recommendation, nursing research course, physical assessment course, resume, statistics course, GRE General Test. *Application fee:* $50.

Degree Requirements 38 total credit hours, comprehensive exam.

POST-MASTER'S PROGRAM

Areas of Study Nurse case management; nurse-midwifery; nursing administration; nursing education; nursing informatics. *Nurse practitioner programs in:* acute care, family health, gerontology, oncology, pediatric, primary care, psychiatric/mental health.

DOCTORAL DEGREE PROGRAM

Degree PhD

Available Programs Doctorate; Post-Baccalaureate Doctorate.

Areas of Study Addiction/substance abuse, aging, bio-behavioral research, biology of health and illness, community health, critical care, faculty preparation, family health, gerontology, health promotion/disease prevention, health-care systems, human health and illness, information systems, neuro-behavior, nursing administration, nursing education, nursing research, oncology.

Program Entrance Requirements Minimum overall college GPA of 3.0, interview by faculty committee, 3 letters of recommendation, MSN or equivalent, statistics course, vita. *Application fee:* $50.

Degree Requirements 60 total credit hours, written exam, residency.

CONTINUING EDUCATION PROGRAM

Contact Dr. Kathryn Montgomery, Associate Dean for Organizational Partnership and Outreach, Master's Program in Nursing, University of Maryland, Baltimore, 655 West Lombard Street, Baltimore, MD 21201-1579. *Telephone:* 410-706-8198. *Fax:* 410-706-0018. *E-mail:* Montgomery@son.umaryland.edu.

Villa Julie College
Nursing Division
Stevenson, Maryland

http://www4.vjc.edu/Nursing

Founded in 1952

DEGREE • BS

Nursing Program Faculty 46 (23% with doctorates).

Baccalaureate Enrollment 402

Women 95% **Men** 5% **Minority** 18% **Part-time** 49%

Nursing Student Activities Sigma Theta Tau, Student Nurses' Association.

Nursing Student Resources Academic advising; academic or career counseling; assistance for students with disabilities; bookstore; campus computer network; career placement assistance; computer lab; e-mail services; employment services for current students; Internet; learning resource lab; library services; nursing audiovisuals; placement services for program completers; remedial services; resume preparation assistance; skills, simulation, or other laboratory; tutoring.

Library Facilities 81,802 volumes (3,301 in health, 776 in nursing); 1,058 periodical subscriptions (635 health-care related).

■ The nursing curriculum builds on a foundation of liberal arts and science courses and provides graduates with the education to creatively meet the challenges and demands of nursing in the twenty-first century. A unique feature of the traditional baccalaureate program is that nursing courses begin in the first semester and continue throughout all four years. There is also an accelerated evening/weekend option for second bachelor's and adult students. The RN-B.S. option is also offered through an accelerated distance learning format. RN-B.S. classes are taught at seven community colleges around the state as well as on the main campus.

BACCALAUREATE PROGRAMS

Degree BS

Available Programs ADN to Baccalaureate; Accelerated Baccalaureate for Second Degree; Accelerated RN Baccalaureate; Generic Baccalaureate; RN Baccalaureate.

Site Options Westminster, MD. *Distance Learning:* Easton, MD; Arnold, MD.

Study Options Full-time and part-time.

Program Entrance Requirements Minimum overall college GPA of 3.0, transcript of college record, written essay, health exam, health insurance, high school biology, high school chemistry, 2 years high school math, high school transcript, immunizations, interview, minimum high school GPA of 3.0, minimum GPA in nursing prerequisites of 3.0. Transfer students are accepted. **Standardized tests** *Required:* SAT or ACT, TOEFL for international students. **Application** *Deadline:* 3/1 (freshmen), 3/1 (transfer). *Notification:* continuous (freshmen). *Application fee:* $25.

Advanced Placement Credit by examination available. Credit given for nursing courses completed elsewhere dependent upon specific evaluations.

Expenses (2006–07) *Tuition:* full-time $15,700; part-time $425 per credit. *International tuition:* $15,700 full-time. *Room and board:* $9188; room only: $6188 per academic year. *Required fees:* full-time $1070; part-time $75 per term.

Financial Aid 80% of baccalaureate students in nursing programs received some form of financial aid in 2005–06. *Gift aid (need-based):* Federal Pell, FSEOG, state, private, college/university gift aid from institutional funds. *Loans:* FFEL (Subsidized and Unsubsidized Stafford PLUS), Perkins. *Work-Study:* Federal Work-Study. *Application deadline (priority):* 2/15.

Contact Dr. Judith A. Feustle, Director, Nursing Division, Villa Julie College, 1525 Greenspring Valley Road, Stevenson, MD 21153-0641. *Telephone:* 443-334-2312. *Fax:* 443-334-2148. *E-mail:* fac-feus@mail.vjc.edu.

MASSACHUSETTS

American International College
Division of Nursing
Springfield, Massachusetts

http://www.aic.edu/pages/315.html

Founded in 1885

American International College (continued)
DEGREES • BSN • MSN

Nursing Program Faculty 11 (10% with doctorates).

Baccalaureate Enrollment 336
Women 92% **Men** 8% **Minority** 37% **International** 1% **Part-time** 5%

Graduate Enrollment 8
Women 100% **Minority** 13% **Part-time** 100%

Nursing Student Activities Nursing Honor Society, Student Nurses' Association.

Nursing Student Resources Academic advising; academic or career counseling; assistance for students with disabilities; bookstore; campus computer network; career placement assistance; computer lab; e-mail services; employment services for current students; externships; housing assistance; interactive nursing skills videos; Internet; learning resource lab; library services; nursing audiovisuals; other; placement services for program completers; resume preparation assistance; skills, simulation, or other laboratory; tutoring.

Library Facilities 118,000 volumes (750 in health, 275 in nursing); 390 periodical subscriptions (50 health-care related).

■ The American International College (AIC) B.S.N. program is accredited by the NLNAC. Nursing students are admitted directly into the program upon acceptance to the College. Clinical experiences start in the second semester of the sophomore year. Off-campus clinical sites include medical, surgical, maternity, pediatric, rehabilitation, and mental health units. One hundred percent of classes are faculty taught, with a student-faculty ratio of 12:1 in the classroom and 5:1 in clinical settings. Founded in 1885, AIC's campus is conveniently located in Springfield, Massachusetts, a metropolitan hub of a half-million people. It is 1½ hours from Boston and 2½ hours from New York City and is easily accessible by car, train, bus, or air service.

BACCALAUREATE PROGRAMS
Degree BSN

Available Programs Generic Baccalaureate; RN Baccalaureate.
Study Options Full-time and part-time.

Program Entrance Requirements Minimum overall college GPA of 2.75, transcript of college record, health exam, health insurance, high school biology, high school chemistry, 3 years high school math, 2 years high school science, high school transcript, immunizations, 1 letter of recommendation, minimum high school GPA of 2.5, minimum GPA in nursing prerequisites of 2.5, professional liability insurance/malpractice insurance. Transfer students are accepted. **Standardized tests** *Required:* SAT or ACT, TOEFL for international students. **Application** *Deadline:* rolling (freshmen), rolling (transfer). *Notification:* continuous (freshmen). *Application fee:* $20.

Advanced Placement Credit by examination available. Credit given for nursing courses completed elsewhere dependent upon specific evaluations.

Expenses (2006–07) *Tuition:* full-time $20,990; part-time $445 per credit. *International tuition:* $20,990 full-time. *Room and board:* $9270 per academic year. *Required fees:* full-time $150; part-time $75 per term.

Financial Aid 90% of baccalaureate students in nursing programs received some form of financial aid in 2005–06. *Gift aid (need-based):* Federal Pell, FSEOG, state, private, college/university gift aid from institutional funds. *Loans:* FFEL (Subsidized and Unsubsidized Stafford PLUS), Perkins, state, college/university, alternative loans. *Work-Study:* Federal Work-Study, part-time campus jobs. *Application deadline (priority):* 5/1.

Contact Mr. Peter Joseph Miller, Vice President for Admission Services, Division of Nursing, American International College, 1000 State Street, Springfield, MA 01109. *Telephone:* 413-205-3201. *Fax:* 413-205-3051. *E-mail:* peter.miller@aic.edu.

GRADUATE PROGRAMS
Expenses (2006–07) *Tuition:* part-time $565 per credit. *Room and board:* $9270 per academic year. *Required fees:* full-time $150; part-time $75 per term.

Financial Aid 50% of graduate students in nursing programs received some form of financial aid in 2005–06.

Contact Dr. Anne R. Glanovsky, Director, Division of Nursing, American International College, 1000 State Street, Springfield, MA 01109. *Telephone:* 413-205-3519. *Fax:* 413-205-3957. *E-mail:* anne.glanovsky@aic.edu.

MASTER'S DEGREE PROGRAM
Degree MSN

Available Programs Master's.
Concentrations Available Nursing administration; nursing education.
Study Options Part-time.

Program Entrance Requirements Clinical experience, minimum overall college GPA of 3.0, transcript of college record, CPR certification, immunizations, interview, 2 letters of recommendation, nursing research course, professional liability insurance/malpractice insurance, prerequisite course work, resume, statistics course.

Advanced Placement Credit given for nursing courses completed elsewhere dependent upon specific evaluations.

Degree Requirements 36 total credit hours, thesis or project.

Anna Maria College
Department of Nursing
Paxton, Massachusetts

http://www.annamaria.edu
Founded in 1946
DEGREE • BSN

Nursing Program Faculty 7 (14% with doctorates).

Baccalaureate Enrollment 44
Women 98% **Men** 2% **Minority** 4% **Part-time** 100%

Nursing Student Activities Sigma Theta Tau.

Nursing Student Resources Academic advising; academic or career counseling; assistance for students with disabilities; bookstore; campus computer network; career placement assistance; computer lab; e-mail services; employment services for current students; Internet; learning resource lab; library services; nursing audiovisuals; placement services for program completers; remedial services; resume preparation assistance; skills, simulation, or other laboratory; tutoring; unpaid internships.

Library Facilities 79,039 volumes (4,213 in health); 318 periodical subscriptions (44 health-care related).

BACCALAUREATE PROGRAMS
Degree BSN

Available Programs ADN to Baccalaureate; RN Baccalaureate.
Study Options Part-time.

Program Entrance Requirements Minimum overall college GPA of 2.5, transcript of college record, interview, 2 letters of recommendation, minimum high school GPA of 2.5, minimum GPA in nursing prerequisites of 2.5, RN licensure. Transfer students are accepted. **Standardized tests** *Required:* SAT or ACT, TOEFL for international students. **Application** *Deadline:* rolling (freshmen), rolling (transfer). *Notification:* continuous (freshmen). *Application fee:* $40.

Advanced Placement Credit by examination available. Credit given for nursing courses completed elsewhere dependent upon specific evaluations.

Expenses (2006–07) *Tuition:* part-time $250 per credit.

Financial Aid 4% of baccalaureate students in nursing programs received some form of financial aid in 2005–06. *Gift aid (need-based):* Federal Pell, FSEOG, state, private, college/university gift aid from institutional funds, United Negro College Fund, Federal Nursing. *Loans:* FFEL (Subsidized and Unsubsidized Stafford PLUS), Perkins, state, college/university. *Work-Study:* Federal Work-Study. *Application deadline:* Continuous.

Contact Dr. Audrey Marie Silveri, Director of Nursing Program, Department of Nursing, Anna Maria College, 50 Sunset Lane, Paxton, MA 01612-1198. *Telephone:* 508-829-3316 Ext. 316. *Fax:* 508-849-3343 Ext. 371. *E-mail:* asilveri@annamaria.edu.

Atlantic Union College
Department of Nursing
South Lancaster, Massachusetts

http://www.atlanticuc.edu

Founded in 1882

DEGREE • BSN

Nursing Program Faculty 14.

Baccalaureate Enrollment 32
Women 97% **Men** 3% **Minority** 53% **Part-time** 59%

Nursing Student Activities Nursing Honor Society, Sigma Theta Tau.

Nursing Student Resources Academic advising; academic or career counseling; bookstore; campus computer network; career placement assistance; computer lab; computer-assisted instruction; e-mail services; employment services for current students; housing assistance; interactive nursing skills videos; Internet; learning resource lab; library services; nursing audiovisuals; remedial services; resume preparation assistance; skills, simulation, or other laboratory; tutoring.

Library Facilities 135,694 volumes (1,478 in health, 892 in nursing); 533 periodical subscriptions (76 health-care related).

BACCALAUREATE PROGRAMS

Degree BSN

Available Programs ADN to Baccalaureate; RN Baccalaureate.

Study Options Full-time and part-time.

Program Entrance Requirements Minimum overall college GPA of 2.5, transcript of college record, CPR certification, written essay, health exam, health insurance, high school biology, high school chemistry, high school foreign language, 3 years high school math, 2 years high school science, high school transcript, immunizations, interview, 2 letters of recommendation, minimum high school GPA of 2.5, minimum GPA in nursing prerequisites of 2.5, professional liability insurance/malpractice insurance, prerequisite course work, RN licensure. Transfer students are accepted. **Standardized tests** *Required:* TOEFL for international students. *Placement: Required:* SAT or ACT. *Recommended:* SAT. **Application** *Deadline:* 8/1 (freshmen), 8/1 (transfer). *Application fee:* $25.

Advanced Placement Credit by examination available. Credit given for nursing courses completed elsewhere dependent upon specific evaluations.

Financial Aid 33% of baccalaureate students in nursing programs received some form of financial aid in 2005–06. *Gift aid (need-based):* Federal Pell, FSEOG, state, private, college/university gift aid from institutional funds. *Loans:* Federal Nursing Student Loans, FFEL (Subsidized and Unsubsidized Stafford PLUS), Perkins, state, college/university, TERI Loans, Signature Loans, Campus Door. *Work-Study:* Federal Work-Study, part-time campus jobs. *Application deadline (priority):* 4/15.

Contact Dr. Lenora D. Follett, Chairperson, Department of Nursing, Atlantic Union College, 338 Main Street, PO Box 1000, South Lancaster, MA 01561-1000. *Telephone:* 978-368-2401. *Fax:* 978-368-2518. *E-mail:* lenora.follett@auc.edu.

Boston College
William F. Connell School of Nursing
Chestnut Hill, Massachusetts

http://www.bc.edu/nursing

Founded in 1863

DEGREES • BS • MS • MS/MA • MS/MBA • MSN/PHD

Nursing Program Faculty 49 (91% with doctorates).

Baccalaureate Enrollment 376
Women 97% **Men** 3% **Minority** 21% **International** 1%

Graduate Enrollment 231
Women 95% **Men** 5% **Minority** 4% **International** 3% **Part-time** 40%

Nursing Student Activities Nursing Honor Society, Sigma Theta Tau, Student Nurses' Association.

Nursing Student Resources Academic advising; academic or career counseling; assistance for students with disabilities; bookstore; campus computer network; career placement assistance; computer lab; computer-assisted instruction; e-mail services; employment services for current students; externships; housing assistance; interactive nursing skills videos; Internet; learning resource lab; library services; nursing audiovisuals; other; paid internships; placement services for program completers; remedial services; resume preparation assistance; skills, simulation, or other laboratory; tutoring; unpaid internships.

Library Facilities 2.1 million volumes (60,186 in health, 18,289 in nursing); 52,338 periodical subscriptions (5,288 health-care related).

BACCALAUREATE PROGRAMS

Degree BS

Available Programs Generic Baccalaureate.

Study Options Full-time.

Program Entrance Requirements Transcript of college record, written essay, health exam, health insurance, high school biology, high school chemistry, high school foreign language, 4 years high school math, 3 years high school science, high school transcript, immunizations, 2 letters of recommendation. Transfer students are accepted. **Standardized tests** *Required:* SAT and SAT Subject Tests or ACT, TOEFL for international students. **Application** *Deadline:* 1/1 (freshmen), 4/1 (transfer). *Early decision:* 11/1. *Notification:* 4/15 (freshmen), 12/25 (early action). *Application fee:* $70.

Advanced Placement Credit given for nursing courses completed elsewhere dependent upon specific evaluations.

Expenses (2006–07) *Tuition:* full-time $33,000. *International tuition:* $33,000 full-time. *Room and board:* $11,690; room only: $7590 per academic year. *Required fees:* full-time $506.

Financial Aid 70% of baccalaureate students in nursing programs received some form of financial aid in 2005–06.

Contact Ms. Maureen Eldredge, Undergraduate Program Assistant, William F. Connell School of Nursing, Boston College, 140 Commonwealth Avenue, Cushing Hall 202D, Chestnut Hill, MA 02467-3812. *Telephone:* 617-552-4925. *Fax:* 617-552-0745. *E-mail:* eldredgm@bc.edu.

GRADUATE PROGRAMS

Expenses (2006–07) *Tuition:* full-time $11,064; part-time $922 per credit. *International tuition:* $11,064 full-time. *Room and board:* room only: $15,000 per academic year. *Required fees:* full-time $90.

Financial Aid 70% of graduate students in nursing programs received some form of financial aid in 2005–06. 15 fellowships with partial tuition reimbursements available (averaging $9,705 per year), 6 research assistantships (averaging $5,000 per year), 3 teaching assistantships (averaging $12,183 per year) were awarded; Federal Work-Study, institutionally sponsored loans, scholarships, traineeships, and tuition waivers (partial) also available. Aid available to part-time students. *Financial aid application deadline:* 3/2.

Contact Ms. Zanifer John-Bayard, Graduate Programs Office, William F. Connell School of Nursing, Boston College, 140 Commonwealth Avenue, Cushing Hall, Chestnut Hill, MA 02467-3812. *Telephone:* 617-552-4059. *Fax:* 617-552-2121. *E-mail:* johnza@bc.edu.

MASTER'S DEGREE PROGRAM

Degrees MS; MS/MA; MS/MBA; MSN/PhD

Available Programs Accelerated Master's for Non-Nursing College Graduates; Master's; RN to Master's.

Concentrations Available Nurse anesthesia. *Clinical nurse specialist programs in:* adult health, community health, gerontology, palliative care, psychiatric/mental health. *Nurse practitioner programs in:* adult health, family health, gerontology, pediatric, psychiatric/mental health, women's health.

Study Options Full-time and part-time.

Program Entrance Requirements Minimum overall college GPA of 3.0, transcript of college record, written essay, immunizations, 3 letters of recommendation, statistics course, GRE General Test. *Application deadline:* For fall admission, 10/15; for spring admission, 3/15. *Application fee:* $40.

Advanced Placement Credit given for nursing courses completed elsewhere dependent upon specific evaluations.

Degree Requirements 45 total credit hours, comprehensive exam.

Boston College (continued)

POST-MASTER'S PROGRAM

Areas of Study Nursing education. *Clinical nurse specialist programs in:* adult health, community health, gerontology, palliative care, psychiatric/mental health. *Nurse practitioner programs in:* adult health, family health, gerontology, pediatric, psychiatric/mental health, women's health.

DOCTORAL DEGREE PROGRAM

Degree PhD

Available Programs Doctorate.

Areas of Study Ethics, human health and illness, individualized study, nursing research, nursing science.

Program Entrance Requirements Minimum overall college GPA of 3.0, interview by faculty committee, interview, 3 letters of recommendation, MSN or equivalent, scholarly papers, statistics course, vita, writing sample, GRE General Test. *Application deadline:* For fall admission, 10/15; for spring admission, 3/15. *Application fee:* $40.

Degree Requirements 46 total credit hours, dissertation, oral exam, written exam.

CONTINUING EDUCATION PROGRAM

Contact Dr. Jean Weyman, Director of Continuing Education, William F. Connell School of Nursing, Boston College, 140 Commonwealth Avenue, Service Building 211F, Chestnut Hill, MA 02467-3812. *Telephone:* 617-552-4256. *Fax:* 617-552-0745. *E-mail:* jean.weyman@bc.edu.

See full description on page 460.

Curry College
Division of Nursing
Milton, Massachusetts

http://www.curry.edu
Founded in 1879

DEGREE • BS

Nursing Program Faculty 50 (25% with doctorates).

Baccalaureate Enrollment 594
Women 92% **Men** 8% **Minority** 16% **Part-time** 48%

Nursing Student Activities Sigma Theta Tau, Student Nurses' Association.

Nursing Student Resources Academic advising; academic or career counseling; assistance for students with disabilities; bookstore; campus computer network; career placement assistance; computer lab; computer-assisted instruction; daycare for children of students; e-mail services; employment services for current students; housing assistance; interactive nursing skills videos; Internet; learning resource lab; library services; nursing audiovisuals; placement services for program completers; remedial services; resume preparation assistance; skills, simulation, or other laboratory; tutoring.

Library Facilities 90,000 volumes (5,867 in health, 4,589 in nursing); 675 periodical subscriptions (162 health-care related).

BACCALAUREATE PROGRAMS

Degree BS

Available Programs Accelerated Baccalaureate for Second Degree; Generic Baccalaureate; RN Baccalaureate.
Site Options Plymouth, MA; Boston, MA.
Study Options Full-time and part-time.
Program Entrance Requirements Minimum overall college GPA of 2.0, CPR certification, written essay, health exam, health insurance, high school biology, high school chemistry, 3 years high school math, 2 years high school science, high school transcript, immunizations, minimum high school GPA of 2.0, minimum GPA in nursing prerequisites of 2.0. Transfer students are accepted. **Standardized tests** *Required:* TOEFL for international students. *Required for some:* SAT or ACT, Wechsler Adult Intelligence

Scale-Revised for PAL candidates. **Application** *Deadline:* 4/1 (freshmen), 7/1 (transfer). *Early decision:* 12/1. *Notification:* continuous (freshmen), 12/15 (out-of-state freshmen), 12/15 (early decision). *Application fee:* $40.

Advanced Placement Credit by examination available. Credit given for nursing courses completed elsewhere dependent upon specific evaluations.

Expenses (2006–07) *Tuition:* full-time $23,400; part-time $780 per credit. *International tuition:* $23,400 full-time. *Room and board:* $9400; room only: $5400 per academic year. *Required fees:* full-time $1337; part-time $650 per term.

Financial Aid 60% of baccalaureate students in nursing programs received some form of financial aid in 2005–06. *Gift aid (need-based):* Federal Pell, FSEOG, state, private, college/university gift aid from institutional funds. *Loans:* FFEL (Subsidized and Unsubsidized Stafford PLUS), Perkins, state. *Work-Study:* Federal Work-Study, part-time campus jobs. *Application deadline (priority):* 3/1.

Contact Miss Jane Fidler, Director of Admissions, Division of Nursing, Curry College, 1071 Blue Hill Avenue, Milton, MA 02186. *Telephone:* 800-669-0686. *Fax:* 617-333-2114. *E-mail:* jfidler0803@curry.edu.

Elms College
Division of Nursing
Chicopee, Massachusetts

Founded in 1928

DEGREE • BSC PN

Nursing Program Faculty 12 (25% with doctorates).

Baccalaureate Enrollment 180
Women 87% **Men** 13% **Minority** 11% **Part-time** 35%

Nursing Student Activities Sigma Theta Tau, Student Nurses' Association.

Nursing Student Resources Academic advising; academic or career counseling; assistance for students with disabilities; bookstore; campus computer network; career placement assistance; computer lab; computer-assisted instruction; e-mail services; employment services for current students; externships; interactive nursing skills videos; Internet; learning resource lab; library services; nursing audiovisuals; paid internships; remedial services; resume preparation assistance; skills, simulation, or other laboratory; tutoring.

Library Facilities 111,379 volumes (3,832 in health, 3,000 in nursing); 529 periodical subscriptions (130 health-care related).

BACCALAUREATE PROGRAMS

Degree BSc PN

Available Programs Generic Baccalaureate; RN Baccalaureate.
Study Options Full-time and part-time.
Program Entrance Requirements Minimum overall college GPA of 2.5, transcript of college record, CPR certification, written essay, health exam, health insurance, high school biology, high school chemistry, high school transcript, immunizations, interview, 2 letters of recommendation, minimum high school GPA of 3.3, minimum GPA in nursing prerequisites of 2.5, professional liability insurance/malpractice insurance. Transfer students are accepted. **Standardized tests** *Required:* SAT or ACT, TOEFL for international students. **Application** *Deadline:* rolling (freshmen), rolling (transfer). *Notification:* continuous (freshmen). *Application fee:* $30.

Advanced Placement Credit given for nursing courses completed elsewhere dependent upon specific evaluations.

Expenses (2006–07) *Tuition:* full-time $21,520; part-time $440 per credit hour. *Room and board:* $8400 per academic year. *Required fees:* full-time $1215.

Financial Aid 90% of baccalaureate students in nursing programs received some form of financial aid in 2005–06.

Contact Dr. Kathleen B. Scoble, RN, Director of Nursing Department/Chair of Health Sciences Division, Division of Nursing, Elms College, 291 Springfield Street, Chicopee, MA 01013. *Telephone:* 413-265-2237. *Fax:* 413-265-2335. *E-mail:* scoblek@elms.edu.

Emmanuel College
Department of Nursing
Boston, Massachusetts

http://www.emmanuel.edu/gradprof

Founded in 1919

DEGREE • BSN

Nursing Program Faculty 15 (20% with doctorates).

Baccalaureate Enrollment 139
Women 96% **Men** 4% **Minority** 20% **Part-time** 93%

Nursing Student Activities Sigma Theta Tau.

Nursing Student Resources Academic advising; academic or career counseling; assistance for students with disabilities; bookstore; campus computer network; computer lab; computer-assisted instruction; e-mail services; interactive nursing skills videos; Internet; learning resource lab; library services; nursing audiovisuals; skills, simulation, or other laboratory.

Library Facilities 3,148 volumes in health, 1,262 volumes in nursing; 92 periodical subscriptions health-care related.

■ The Emmanuel College CCNE-accredited Nursing Program is designed specifically for the registered nurse. The faculty members believe that baccalaureate education builds on the prior educational and practice experiences of the registered nurse. The Nursing Program prepares a professional who thinks critically, communicates effectively, appreciates the diversity of human experience, and uses personal and professional values and standards in responsible, ethical practice. Liberal transfer-credit policies, a strong advisement program, and outstanding individualized clinical placements ensure that the Nursing Program works for practicing nurses. Evening and Saturday courses on two campus locations underpin the commitment to adult learners. Graduates report career and educational advancement.

BACCALAUREATE PROGRAMS

Degree BSN

Available Programs RN Baccalaureate.
Site Options Woburn, MA.
Study Options Full-time and part-time.
Program Entrance Requirements Transcript of college record, written essay, interview, 2 letters of recommendation, RN licensure. Transfer students are accepted. **Standardized tests** *Required:* SAT or ACT, TOEFL for international students. **Application** *Deadline:* 3/1 (freshmen), 4/1 (transfer). *Early decision:* 11/1. *Notification:* 12/1 (freshmen), 12/1 (out-of-state freshmen), 12/1 (early decision). *Application fee:* $40.
Advanced Placement Credit given for nursing courses completed elsewhere dependent upon specific evaluations.
Expenses (2006–07) *Tuition:* part-time $1360 per course.
Financial Aid *Gift aid (need-based):* Federal Pell, FSEOG, state, private, college/university gift aid from institutional funds. *Loans:* FFEL (Subsidized and Unsubsidized Stafford PLUS), Perkins, state, alternative loans. *Work-Study:* Federal Work-Study, part-time campus jobs. *Application deadline (priority):* 4/1.
Contact Dr. Joan M. Riley, RN, Chair and Professor, Department of Nursing, Emmanuel College, 400 The Fenway, Boston, MA 02115. *Telephone:* 617-735-9935. *Fax:* 617-735-9797. *E-mail:* riley@emmanuel.edu.

Endicott College
Major in Nursing
Beverly, Massachusetts

http://www.endicott.edu

Founded in 1939

DEGREE • BS

Nursing Program Faculty 4.

Baccalaureate Enrollment 75
Women 95% **Men** 5% **Minority** 2%

Nursing Student Activities Student Nurses' Association.

Nursing Student Resources Academic advising; academic or career counseling; assistance for students with disabilities; bookstore; campus computer network; career placement assistance; computer lab; e-mail services; externships; interactive nursing skills videos; Internet; learning resource lab; library services; nursing audiovisuals; resume preparation assistance; skills, simulation, or other laboratory; tutoring; unpaid internships.

Library Facilities 121,000 volumes (2,828 in health, 624 in nursing); 3,500 periodical subscriptions (55 health-care related).

BACCALAUREATE PROGRAMS

Degree BS

Available Programs Generic Baccalaureate; RN Baccalaureate.
Site Options Beverly, MA.
Study Options Full-time.
Program Entrance Requirements Minimum overall college GPA of 2.5, transcript of college record, written essay, health exam, health insurance, high school biology, high school chemistry, 3 years high school math, 2 years high school science, high school transcript, immunizations, interview, 1 letter of recommendation, minimum high school GPA of 2.5, minimum high school rank 50%, minimum GPA in nursing prerequisites of 2.5. Transfer students are accepted. **Standardized tests** *Required:* SAT or ACT, TOEFL for international students. **Application** *Deadline:* 2/15 (freshmen), 2/15 (transfer). *Notification:* continuous (freshmen). *Application fee:* $40.
Advanced Placement Credit given for nursing courses completed elsewhere dependent upon specific evaluations.
Contact *Telephone:* 978-921-1000. *Fax:* 978-232-2500.

CONTINUING EDUCATION PROGRAM

Contact *Telephone:* 978-232-2328. *Fax:* 978-232-3100.

Fitchburg State College
Department of Nursing
Fitchburg, Massachusetts

http://www.fsc.edu/nursing/

Founded in 1894

DEGREES • BS • MS

Nursing Program Faculty 18 (28% with doctorates).

Baccalaureate Enrollment 269
Women 96% **Men** 4% **Minority** 13% **Part-time** 2%

Graduate Enrollment 34
Women 97% **Men** 3% **Minority** 5% **Part-time** 100%

Nursing Student Activities Sigma Theta Tau, Student Nurses' Association.

Nursing Student Resources Academic advising; academic or career counseling; assistance for students with disabilities; bookstore; campus computer network; career placement assistance; computer lab; computer-assisted instruction; e-mail services; employment services for current students; housing assistance; interactive nursing skills videos; Internet; learning resource lab; library services; nursing audiovisuals; remedial services; resume preparation assistance; skills, simulation, or other laboratory; tutoring; unpaid internships.

Library Facilities 242,418 volumes (111 in health, 74 in nursing); 2,208 periodical subscriptions (1,218 health-care related).

BACCALAUREATE PROGRAMS

Degree BS

Available Programs ADN to Baccalaureate; Generic Baccalaureate; RN Baccalaureate.
Study Options Full-time.

Fitchburg State College (continued)

Program Entrance Requirements Minimum overall college GPA of 2.5, transcript of college record, CPR certification, written essay, health exam, health insurance, high school biology, high school chemistry, 3 years high school math, 3 years high school science, high school transcript, immunizations, minimum high school GPA of 3.0, minimum GPA in nursing prerequisites of 2.5, prerequisite course work. Transfer students are accepted. **Standardized tests** *Required:* SAT or ACT, TOEFL for international students. **Application** *Notification:* continuous (freshmen). *Application fee:* $10.

Expenses (2006–07) *Tuition, state resident:* full-time $970; part-time $40 per credit. *Tuition, nonresident:* full-time $7050; part-time $294 per credit. *International tuition:* $7050 full-time. *Room and board:* $3340; room only: $2110 per academic year. *Required fees:* part-time $170 per credit; part-time $191 per term.

Financial Aid 41% of baccalaureate students in nursing programs received some form of financial aid in 2005–06.

Contact Office of Admissions, Department of Nursing, Fitchburg State College, 160 Pearl Street, Fitchburg, MA 01420-2697. *Telephone:* 978-665-3144. *Fax:* 978-665-4540. *E-mail:* admissions@fsc.edu.

GRADUATE PROGRAMS

Expenses (2006–07) *Tuition, state resident:* full-time $1800; part-time $150 per credit. *Tuition, nonresident:* full-time $1800; part-time $150 per credit. *International tuition:* $1800 full-time. *Required fees:* full-time $1080; part-time $90 per credit; part-time $540 per term.

Contact Dr. Rachel Boersma, RN, Chairperson, Department of Nursing, Fitchburg State College, 160 Pearl Street, Fitchburg, MA 01420-2697. *Telephone:* 978-665-3036. *Fax:* 978-665-3658. *E-mail:* rboersma@fsc.edu.

MASTER'S DEGREE PROGRAM

Degree MS

Available Programs Master's.

Concentrations Available *Clinical nurse specialist programs in:* forensic nursing.

Study Options Part-time.

Program Entrance Requirements Clinical experience, computer literacy, minimum overall college GPA of 2.8, transcript of college record, CPR certification, written essay, immunizations, 3 letters of recommendation, nursing research course, physical assessment course, prerequisite course work, resume, statistics course.

Degree Requirements 37 total credit hours, thesis or project.

Framingham State College
Department of Nursing
Framingham, Massachusetts

http://www.framingham.edu/nursing

Founded in 1839

DEGREE • BS

Nursing Program Faculty 5 (60% with doctorates).

Baccalaureate Enrollment 60
Women 90% **Men** 10% **Minority** 30% **Part-time** 90%

Nursing Student Activities Sigma Theta Tau.

Nursing Student Resources Academic advising; academic or career counseling; assistance for students with disabilities; bookstore; campus computer network; career placement assistance; computer lab; computer-assisted instruction; e-mail services; employment services for current students; housing assistance; interactive nursing skills videos; Internet; learning resource lab; library services; nursing audiovisuals; placement services for program completers; remedial services; resume preparation assistance; skills, simulation, or other laboratory; tutoring.

Library Facilities 165,219 volumes; 409 periodical subscriptions.

BACCALAUREATE PROGRAMS

Degree BS

Available Programs ADN to Baccalaureate.

Study Options Full-time and part-time.

Program Entrance Requirements Minimum overall college GPA, written essay, professional liability insurance/malpractice insurance, RN licensure. Transfer students are accepted. **Standardized tests** *Required:* SAT or ACT, TOEFL for international students. **Application** *Deadline:* 2/15 (freshmen), 2/15 (transfer). *Early decision:* 11/15. *Notification:* 3/31 (freshmen), 12/15 (early action). *Application fee:* $25.

Advanced Placement Credit by examination available. Credit given for nursing courses completed elsewhere dependent upon specific evaluations.

Expenses (2006–07) *Tuition, state resident:* full-time $1940; part-time $324 per course. *Tuition, nonresident:* full-time $14,100; part-time $2350 per course. *International tuition:* $14,100 full-time. *Room and board:* room only: $7994 per academic year. *Required fees:* part-time $336 per credit.

Financial Aid 60% of baccalaureate students in nursing programs received some form of financial aid in 2005–06.

Contact Dr. Susan L. Conrad, RN, Chairperson and Professor, Department of Nursing, Framingham State College, 100 State Street, H220, Framingham, MA 01701. *Telephone:* 508-626-4715. *Fax:* 508-626-4746. *E-mail:* sconrad@frc.mass.edu.

MGH Institute of Health Professions
Program in Nursing
Boston, Massachusetts

http://www.mghihp.edu

Founded in 1977

DEGREE • MS

Nursing Program Faculty 36 (64% with doctorates).

Graduate Enrollment 252
Women 89% **Men** 11% **Minority** 14% **International** 1% **Part-time** 17%

Nursing Student Activities Nursing Honor Society, Student Nurses' Association.

Nursing Student Resources Academic advising; academic or career counseling; assistance for students with disabilities; bookstore; career placement assistance; computer lab; e-mail services; Internet; learning resource lab; library services; nursing audiovisuals; resume preparation assistance; skills, simulation, or other laboratory; tutoring.

Library Facilities 31,843 volumes in health, 13,000 volumes in nursing; 1,737 periodical subscriptions health-care related.

GRADUATE PROGRAMS

Expenses (2006–07) *Tuition:* part-time $800 per credit. *Required fees:* full-time $800; part-time $400 per term.

Financial Aid 80% of graduate students in nursing programs received some form of financial aid in 2005–06. 1 research assistantship (averaging $1,200 per year), 2 teaching assistantships (averaging $1,200 per year) were awarded; career-related internships or fieldwork, scholarships, traineeships, tuition waivers (full and partial), and unspecified assistantships also available. Aid available to part-time students. *Financial aid application deadline:* 3/4.

Contact Office of Student Affairs, Program in Nursing, MGH Institute of Health Professions, PO Box 6357, Boston, MA 02114. *Telephone:* 617-726-3140. *Fax:* 617-726-8010. *E-mail:* admissions@mghihp.edu.

MASTER'S DEGREE PROGRAM

Degree MS

Available Programs Master's; Master's for Non-Nursing College Graduates; Master's for Nurses with Non-Nursing Degrees; RN to Master's.

Concentrations Available Nursing education. *Clinical nurse specialist programs in:* psychiatric/mental health. *Nurse practitioner programs in:* acute care, adult health, family health, gerontology, pediatric, primary care, psychiatric/mental health, women's health.

Site Options *Distance Learning:* Boston, MA.

Study Options Full-time and part-time.

Program Entrance Requirements Minimum overall college GPA of 3.0, transcript of college record, CPR certification, written essay, immunizations, 3 letters of recommendation, professional liability insurance/malpractice insurance, prerequisite course work, statistics course, GRE General Test. *Application deadline:* For fall admission, 1/10. *Application fee:* $50.

Advanced Placement Credit by examination available. Credit given for nursing courses completed elsewhere dependent upon specific evaluations.

Degree Requirements Thesis or project.

POST-MASTER'S PROGRAM

Areas of Study *Clinical nurse specialist programs in:* psychiatric/mental health. *Nurse practitioner programs in:* acute care, adult health, gerontology, pediatric, primary care, psychiatric/mental health, women's health.

CONTINUING EDUCATION PROGRAM

Contact Joan Blue, Program Manager, Program in Nursing, MGH Institute of Health Professions, Charlestown Navy Yard, 36 1st Avenue, Boston, MA 02129. *Telephone:* 617-726-8053. *Fax:* 617-726-3152. *E-mail:* jblue@mghihp.edu.

See full description on page 514.

Northeastern University
School of Nursing
Boston, Massachusetts

http://www.bouve.neu.edu/Nursing
Founded in 1898
DEGREES • BSN • MS • MSN/MBA

Nursing Program Faculty 26 (69% with doctorates).

Baccalaureate Enrollment 533
Women 94% **Men** 6% **Minority** 21%

Graduate Enrollment 246
Women 85% **Men** 15% **International** 2% **Part-time** 38%

Nursing Student Activities Sigma Theta Tau, Student Nurses' Association.

Nursing Student Resources Academic advising; academic or career counseling; assistance for students with disabilities; bookstore; campus computer network; career placement assistance; computer lab; computer-assisted instruction; e-mail services; employment services for current students; externships; housing assistance; interactive nursing skills videos; Internet; learning resource lab; library services; nursing audiovisuals; other; paid internships; placement services for program completers; resume preparation assistance; skills, simulation, or other laboratory; tutoring.

Library Facilities 994,122 volumes; 6,773 periodical subscriptions.

BACCALAUREATE PROGRAMS

Degree BSN

Available Programs Generic Baccalaureate; RN Baccalaureate.

Study Options Full-time.

Program Entrance Requirements Transcript of college record, written essay, health exam, high school biology, high school chemistry, high school math, 2 years high school science, high school transcript, immunizations, 2 letters of recommendation, prerequisite course work. Transfer students are accepted. **Standardized tests** *Required:* SAT or ACT, TOEFL for international students. **Application** *Deadline:* 1/15 (freshmen), 5/1 (transfer). *Notification:* continuous until 4/1 (freshmen). *Application fee:* $75.

Advanced Placement Credit given for nursing courses completed elsewhere dependent upon specific evaluations.

Expenses (2006–07) *Tuition:* full-time $29,910. *International tuition:* $29,910 full-time. *Room and board:* $5840; room only: $5130 per academic year. *Required fees:* full-time $399.

Financial Aid 64% of baccalaureate students in nursing programs received some form of financial aid in 2005–06. *Gift aid (need-based):* Federal Pell, FSEOG, state, private, college/university gift aid from institutional funds, Federal Nursing. *Loans:* Federal Nursing Student Loans, FFEL (Subsidized and Unsubsidized Stafford PLUS), Perkins, state, MEFA, TERI, Mass. No Interset Loan (NIL), CitiAssist. *Work-Study:* Federal Work-Study. *Application deadline (priority):* 2/15.

Contact Undergraduate Admissions, School of Nursing, Northeastern University, 150 Richards Hall, 360 Huntington Avenue, Boston, MA 02115. *Telephone:* 617-373-2200. *Fax:* 617-373-8780. *E-mail:* admissions@neu.edu.

GRADUATE PROGRAMS

Expenses (2006–07) *Tuition:* part-time $875 per credit hour. *Room and board:* $10,080; room only: $6130 per academic year.

Financial Aid 62% of graduate students in nursing programs received some form of financial aid in 2005–06. 2 research assistantships with full tuition reimbursements available (averaging $13,025 per year), 7 teaching assistantships with full tuition reimbursements available (averaging $13,025 per year) were awarded; fellowships, career-related internships or fieldwork, institutionally sponsored loans, tuition waivers (full and partial), and unspecified assistantships also available. Aid available to part-time students. *Financial aid application deadline:* 7/1.

Contact Ms. Molly Schnabel, Director of Graduate Admissions and Student Services, School of Nursing, Northeastern University, 123 Behrakis Health Sciences Building, 360 Huntington Avenue, Boston, MA 02115. *Telephone:* 617-373-3501. *Fax:* 617-373-4701. *E-mail:* bouvegrad@neu.edu.

MASTER'S DEGREE PROGRAM

Degrees MS; MSN/MBA

Available Programs Accelerated RN to Master's; Master's; Master's for Non-Nursing College Graduates; RN to Master's.

Concentrations Available Nurse anesthesia; nursing administration. *Clinical nurse specialist programs in:* psychiatric/mental health. *Nurse practitioner programs in:* acute care, adult health, family health, gerontology, neonatal health, pediatric, primary care, psychiatric/mental health.

Study Options Full-time and part-time.

Program Entrance Requirements Clinical experience, minimum overall college GPA of 3.0, transcript of college record, written essay, immunizations, 3 letters of recommendation, professional liability insurance/malpractice insurance, resume, statistics course, GRE General Test. *Application deadline:* Applications are processed on a rolling basis. *Application fee:* $50.

Advanced Placement Credit given for nursing courses completed elsewhere dependent upon specific evaluations.

Degree Requirements 43 total credit hours.

POST-MASTER'S PROGRAM

Areas of Study Nurse anesthesia; nursing administration. *Clinical nurse specialist programs in:* psychiatric/mental health. *Nurse practitioner programs in:* acute care, adult health, family health, gerontology, neonatal health, pediatric, primary care, psychiatric/mental health.

CONTINUING EDUCATION PROGRAM

Contact Ms. Lea Johnson, Director, Bouve Institute for Healthcare, School of Nursing, Northeastern University, 275 Ryder Hall, Boston, MA 02115. *Telephone:* 617-373-4237. *Fax:* 617-373-2325. *E-mail:* l.johnson@neu.edu.

See full description on page 522.

Regis College
Department of Nursing
Weston, Massachusetts

http://regisnet.regiscollege.edu/nursing/pro_ovrview.htm
Founded in 1927
DEGREES • BSN • DNP • MSN

Nursing Program Faculty 36 (75% with doctorates).

Baccalaureate Enrollment 69
Women 100%

Regis College (continued)
Graduate Enrollment 292
Women 91% **Men** 9% **Minority** 14% **Part-time** 70%
Nursing Student Activities Sigma Theta Tau, Student Nurses' Association.

Nursing Student Resources Academic advising; academic or career counseling; assistance for students with disabilities; bookstore; campus computer network; computer lab; e-mail services; Internet; learning resource lab; library services; nursing audiovisuals; resume preparation assistance; skills, simulation, or other laboratory; tutoring.

Library Facilities 139,837 volumes (6,300 in health, 4,700 in nursing); 787 periodical subscriptions (228 health-care related).

BACCALAUREATE PROGRAMS

Degree BSN

Available Programs ADN to Baccalaureate; Accelerated Baccalaureate; Accelerated Baccalaureate for Second Degree; Accelerated RN Baccalaureate; Baccalaureate for Second Degree; Generic Baccalaureate; RN Baccalaureate.

Site Options Brighton, MA; Medford, MA; Boston, MA.

Study Options Full-time.

Program Entrance Requirements Written essay, health exam, health insurance, high school foreign language, 3 years high school math, 2 years high school science, high school transcript, immunizations, 2 letters of recommendation, minimum high school GPA of 3.0, minimum high school rank 40%, minimum GPA in nursing prerequisites. Transfer students are accepted. **Standardized tests** *Required:* SAT or ACT. **Application** *Deadline:* rolling (freshmen), rolling (transfer). *Application fee:* $50.

Advanced Placement Credit by examination available. Credit given for nursing courses completed elsewhere dependent upon specific evaluations.

Expenses (2006–07) *Tuition:* full-time $23,680. *Room and board:* $10,560 per academic year.

Financial Aid 85% of baccalaureate students in nursing programs received some form of financial aid in 2005–06. *Gift aid (need-based):* Federal Pell, FSEOG, state, private, college/university gift aid from institutional funds. *Loans:* FFEL (Subsidized and Unsubsidized Stafford PLUS), Perkins, state. *Work-Study:* Federal Work-Study, part-time campus jobs. *Application deadline (priority):* 2/15.

Contact Dr. Antionette Hays, Center Director, Department of Nursing, Regis College, 235 Wellesley Street, Weston, MA 02493. *Telephone:* 781-768-7090. *Fax:* 781-768-7071. *E-mail:* antoinette.hays@regiscollege.edu.

GRADUATE PROGRAMS

Expenses (2006–07) *Tuition:* full-time $25,000; part-time $645 per credit. *Room and board:* $10,560 per academic year.

Financial Aid 52% of graduate students in nursing programs received some form of financial aid in 2005–06. 12 research assistantships (averaging $22,500 per year) were awarded; Federal Work-Study, scholarships, traineeships, and unspecified assistantships also available. Aid available to part-time students.

Contact Ms. Claudia C. Pouravelis, Assistant Director of Graduate Admission, Department of Nursing, Regis College, 235 Wellesley Street, Weston, MA 02493. *Telephone:* 781-768-7058. *Fax:* 781-768-7071. *E-mail:* claudia.pouravelis@regiscollege.edu.

MASTER'S DEGREE PROGRAM

Degree MSN

Available Programs Accelerated AD/RN to Master's; Accelerated Master's; Accelerated Master's for Non-Nursing College Graduates; Accelerated Master's for Nurses with Non-Nursing Degrees; Accelerated RN to Master's; Master's; Master's for Non-Nursing College Graduates; Master's for Nurses with Non-Nursing Degrees; RN to Master's.

Concentrations Available Health-care administration; nursing administration. *Clinical nurse specialist programs in:* acute care. *Nurse practitioner programs in:* adult health, family health, pediatric, primary care, psychiatric/mental health.

Site Options Brighton, MA; Medford, MA; Boston, MA.

Study Options Full-time.

Program Entrance Requirements Computer literacy, minimum overall college GPA of 3.0, transcript of college record, CPR certification, written essay, immunizations, interview, 3 letters of recommendation, physical assessment course, professional liability insurance/malpractice insurance, prerequisite course work, resume, statistics course, GRE General Test or MAT. *Application deadline:* Applications are processed on a rolling basis. *Application fee:* $40.

Advanced Placement Credit by examination available. Credit given for nursing courses completed elsewhere dependent upon specific evaluations.

Degree Requirements 44 total credit hours, thesis or project.

POST-MASTER'S PROGRAM

Areas of Study Health-care administration; nursing administration; nursing education. *Clinical nurse specialist programs in:* family health. *Nurse practitioner programs in:* adult health, family health, pediatric, primary care, psychiatric/mental health.

DOCTORAL DEGREE PROGRAM

Degree DNP

Available Programs Doctorate.

Areas of Study Family health.

Program Entrance Requirements Clinical experience, minimum overall college GPA of 3.0, interview by faculty committee, interview, 3 letters of recommendation, MSN or equivalent, statistics course, vita, writing sample. *Application deadline:* Applications are processed on a rolling basis. *Application fee:* $40.

CONTINUING EDUCATION PROGRAM

Contact Dr. Antoinette Hays, Center Director, Department of Nursing, Regis College, 235 Wellesley Street, Weston, MA 02493. *Telephone:* 781-768-7090. *Fax:* 781-768-7089. *E-mail:* antoinette.hays@regiscollege.edu.

See full description on page 526.

Salem State College
Program in Nursing
Salem, Massachusetts

http://www.salemstate.edu
Founded in 1854

DEGREES • BSN • MSN • MSN/MBA

Nursing Program Faculty 70 (25% with doctorates).

Nursing Student Activities Nursing Honor Society, Sigma Theta Tau, Student Nurses' Association.

Nursing Student Resources Academic advising; academic or career counseling; assistance for students with disabilities; bookstore; campus computer network; career placement assistance; computer lab; computer-assisted instruction; daycare for children of students; e-mail services; employment services for current students; externships; housing assistance; interactive nursing skills videos; Internet; learning resource lab; library services; nursing audiovisuals; paid internships; remedial services; resume preparation assistance; skills, simulation, or other laboratory; tutoring.

Library Facilities 217,842 volumes (2,000 in health, 1,600 in nursing); 1,914 periodical subscriptions (50 health-care related).

BACCALAUREATE PROGRAMS

Degree BSN

Available Programs ADN to Baccalaureate; Accelerated Baccalaureate for Second Degree; Generic Baccalaureate; International Nurse to Baccalaureate; LPN to Baccalaureate; LPN to RN Baccalaureate.

Site Options Haverhill, MA.

Study Options Full-time.

Program Entrance Requirements Minimum overall college GPA of 3.0, transcript of college record, CPR certification, health exam, health insurance, high school biology, high school chemistry, 3 years high school math, 2 years high school science, high school transcript, immunizations, interview, minimum high school GPA of 3.0, professional liability insurance/malpractice insurance. Transfer students are accepted. **Stan-**

dardized tests *Required:* SAT and SAT Subject Tests or ACT, TOEFL for international students. **Application** *Deadline:* rolling (freshmen), rolling (transfer). *Notification:* continuous (freshmen). *Application fee:* $25.

Advanced Placement Credit given for nursing courses completed elsewhere dependent upon specific evaluations.

Expenses (2006–07) *Tuition, state resident:* full-time $455; part-time $105 per credit hour. *Tuition, nonresident:* full-time $3525; part-time $140 per credit hour. *International tuition:* $3525 full-time. *Room and board:* $9600; room only: $7000 per academic year.

Financial Aid 60% of baccalaureate students in nursing programs received some form of financial aid in 2005–06.

Contact Mr. Nate Bryant, Assistant Dean of Admissions, Program in Nursing, Salem State College, 352 Lafayette Street, Salem, MA 01970. *Telephone:* 978-542-6200. *E-mail:* admissions@salemstate.edu.

GRADUATE PROGRAMS

Expenses (2006–07) *Tuition, state resident:* part-time $140 per credit hour. *Tuition, nonresident:* part-time $230 per credit hour. *Required fees:* part-time $97 per credit; part-time $300 per term.

Financial Aid 25% of graduate students in nursing programs received some form of financial aid in 2005–06.

Contact Dr. Kathleen Skrabut, Coordinator, Graduate Program, Program in Nursing, Salem State College, 352 Lafayette Street, Salem, MA 01970. *Telephone:* 978-542-7018. *Fax:* 978-542-2016. *E-mail:* kskrabut@salemstate.edu.

MASTER'S DEGREE PROGRAM

Degrees MSN; MSN/MBA

Available Programs Accelerated Master's for Non-Nursing College Graduates; Master's; Master's for Nurses with Non-Nursing Degrees; RN to Master's.

Concentrations Available Nursing administration; nursing education. *Clinical nurse specialist programs in:* adult health, community health, rehabilitation.

Site Options Burlington, MA.

Study Options Full-time and part-time.

Program Entrance Requirements Clinical experience, computer literacy, minimum overall college GPA of 3.0, transcript of college record, CPR certification, written essay, immunizations, interview, 3 letters of recommendation, professional liability insurance/malpractice insurance, resume, statistics course, GRE General Test, MAT. *Application deadline:* Applications are processed on a rolling basis. *Application fee:* $25.

Advanced Placement Credit given for nursing courses completed elsewhere dependent upon specific evaluations.

Degree Requirements 39 total credit hours, thesis or project.

CONTINUING EDUCATION PROGRAM

Contact Ms. Linda A. Frontiero, RN, Director of the Nursing Resource Center, Program in Nursing, Salem State College, 352 Lafayette Street, Salem, MA 01970. *Telephone:* 978-542-6849. *Fax:* 978-542-2016. *E-mail:* lfrontiero@salemstate.edu.

Simmons College
Department of Nursing
Boston, Massachusetts

http://www.simmons.edu/gsbs/nursing/

Founded in 1899

DEGREES • BS • MS • MSN/MS

Nursing Program Faculty 135 (15% with doctorates).

Baccalaureate Enrollment 438
Women 100% **Minority** 29% **Part-time** 53%

Graduate Enrollment 160
Women 95% **Men** 5% **Minority** 15% **Part-time** 28%

Nursing Student Activities Sigma Theta Tau, Student Nurses' Association, nursing club.

Nursing Student Resources Academic advising; academic or career counseling; assistance for students with disabilities; bookstore; campus computer network; career placement assistance; computer lab; computer-assisted instruction; e-mail services; employment services for current students; housing assistance; interactive nursing skills videos; Internet; learning resource lab; library services; nursing audiovisuals; paid internships; placement services for program completers; remedial services; resume preparation assistance; skills, simulation, or other laboratory; tutoring.

Library Facilities 243,161 volumes (5,005 in health, 1,562 in nursing); 1,696 periodical subscriptions (196 health-care related).

BACCALAUREATE PROGRAMS

Degree BS

Available Programs ADN to Baccalaureate; Accelerated Baccalaureate; Accelerated Baccalaureate for Second Degree; Baccalaureate for Second Degree; Generic Baccalaureate; LPN to Baccalaureate; RN Baccalaureate.

Site Options Quincy, MA; Winchester, MA.

Study Options Full-time and part-time.

Program Entrance Requirements Transcript of college record, written essay, health exam, health insurance, high school biology, high school chemistry, high school foreign language, 3 years high school math, 3 years high school science, high school transcript, immunizations, 2 letters of recommendation, minimum GPA in nursing prerequisites of 3.0, prerequisite course work. Transfer students are accepted. **Standardized tests** *Required:* SAT or ACT, TOEFL for international students. **Application** *Deadline:* 2/1 (freshmen), 4/1 (transfer). *Early decision:* 12/1. *Notification:* 4/15 (freshmen), 1/20 (early action). *Application fee:* $35.

Advanced Placement Credit given for nursing courses completed elsewhere dependent upon specific evaluations.

Expenses (2006–07) *Tuition:* full-time $25,914; part-time $809 per credit hour. *International tuition:* $25,914 full-time. *Room and board:* $10,710 per academic year. *Required fees:* full-time $794.

Financial Aid 75% of baccalaureate students in nursing programs received some form of financial aid in 2005–06. *Gift aid (need-based):* Federal Pell, FSEOG, state, private, college/university gift aid from institutional funds. *Loans:* FFEL (Subsidized and Unsubsidized Stafford PLUS), Perkins, state, college/university. *Work-Study:* Federal Work-Study. *Application deadline (priority):* 2/15.

Contact Ms. Catherine Capolupo, Director, Undergraduate Admission, Department of Nursing, Simmons College, 300 The Fenway, Boston, MA 02115. *Telephone:* 617-521-2057. *Fax:* 617-521-3190. *E-mail:* catherine.capolupo@simmons.edu.

GRADUATE PROGRAMS

Expenses (2006–07) *Tuition:* part-time $830 per credit hour. *Room and board:* $11,970 per academic year. *Required fees:* full-time $670.

Financial Aid 40% of graduate students in nursing programs received some form of financial aid in 2005–06.

Contact Dr. Judy Beal, Associate Dean, SHS/Chair, Department of Nursing, Simmons College, 300 The Fenway, Boston, MA 02115. *Telephone:* 617-521-2139. *Fax:* 617-521-3045. *E-mail:* judy.beal@simmons.edu.

MASTER'S DEGREE PROGRAM

Degrees MS; MSN/MS

Available Programs Accelerated AD/RN to Master's; Accelerated Master's; Accelerated Master's for Non-Nursing College Graduates; Accelerated Master's for Nurses with Non-Nursing Degrees; Accelerated RN to Master's; Master's; Master's for Non-Nursing College Graduates; Master's for Nurses with Non-Nursing Degrees; RN to Master's.

Concentrations Available Nursing education. *Nurse practitioner programs in:* adult health, family health, gerontology, pediatric, primary care, school health, women's health.

Site Options Quincy, MA; Winchester, MA.

Study Options Full-time.

Program Entrance Requirements Clinical experience, computer literacy, minimum overall college GPA of 3.0, transcript of college record, written essay, immunizations, 3 letters of recommendation, physical assessment course, professional liability insurance/malpractice insurance, prerequisite course work, resume, statistics course.

Degree Requirements 64 total credit hours, thesis or project.

Simmons College (continued)
POST-MASTER'S PROGRAM
Areas of Study Nursing education. *Nurse practitioner programs in:* adult health, family health, gerontology, occupational health, pediatric, primary care, school health, women's health.

CONTINUING EDUCATION PROGRAM
Contact Ms. Lauren Avalos, Assistant Director of Admission, Department of Nursing, Simmons College, Dix Scholar Program, 300 The Fenway, Boston, MA 02115. *Telephone:* 617-521-2052. *Fax:* 617-521-3190. *E-mail:* lauren.avalos@simmons.edu.

University of Massachusetts Amherst
School of Nursing
Amherst, Massachusetts

http://www.umass.edu/nursing
Founded in 1863
DEGREES • BS • MS • PHD

Nursing Program Faculty 82 (32% with doctorates).
Baccalaureate Enrollment 441
Women 92% **Men** 8% **Minority** 12% **International** .5%
Graduate Enrollment 98
Women 96% **Men** 4% **Minority** 13% **International** 3% **Part-time** 74%
Nursing Student Activities Nursing Honor Society, Sigma Theta Tau, Student Nurses' Association, nursing club.
Nursing Student Resources Academic advising; academic or career counseling; bookstore; campus computer network; career placement assistance; computer lab; computer-assisted instruction; e-mail services; employment services for current students; housing assistance; interactive nursing skills videos; Internet; learning resource lab; library services; nursing audiovisuals; resume preparation assistance; skills, simulation, or other laboratory; tutoring; unpaid internships.
Library Facilities 3.2 million volumes (276,952 in health, 31,238 in nursing); 37,716 periodical subscriptions (3,792 health-care related).

BACCALAUREATE PROGRAMS
Degree BS
Available Programs Accelerated Baccalaureate for Second Degree; Accelerated RN Baccalaureate; Generic Baccalaureate.
Study Options Full-time.
Program Entrance Requirements Minimum overall college GPA of 2.5, transcript of college record, CPR certification, written essay, health exam, health insurance, high school foreign language, 3 years high school math, 3 years high school science, high school transcript, immunizations, 1 letter of recommendation, minimum high school GPA of 3.5, minimum GPA in nursing prerequisites of 2.5, professional liability insurance/malpractice insurance, prerequisite course work. Transfer students are accepted. **Standardized tests** *Required:* SAT or ACT, TOEFL for international students. **Application** *Deadline:* 1/15 (freshmen), 4/15 (transfer). *Early decision:* 11/1. *Notification:* continuous (freshmen), 12/15 (early action). *Application fee:* $40.
Advanced Placement Credit given for nursing courses completed elsewhere dependent upon specific evaluations.
Expenses (2006–07) *Tuition, state resident:* full-time $1714; part-time $72 per credit. *Tuition, nonresident:* full-time $9936; part-time $414 per credit. *International tuition:* $9936 full-time. *Room and board:* $6989; room only: $3905 per academic year.
Financial Aid 78% of baccalaureate students in nursing programs received some form of financial aid in 2005–06.
Contact Miss Elizabeth Theroux, Academic Secretary, Office for the Advancement of Nursing Education, School of Nursing, University of Massachusetts Amherst, 219 Arnold House, 715 North Pleasant Street, Amherst, MA 01003-9304. *Telephone:* 413-545-5096. *Fax:* 413-577-2550. *E-mail:* etheroux@acad.umass.edu.

GRADUATE PROGRAMS
Expenses (2006–07) *Tuition, state resident:* part-time $567 per credit. *Tuition, nonresident:* part-time $567 per credit. *Required fees:* part-time $40 per term.
Financial Aid Fellowships (averaging $682 per year), research assistantships (averaging $14,200 per year), teaching assistantships (averaging $5,046 per year) were awarded; career-related internships or fieldwork, Federal Work-Study, scholarships, traineeships, tuition waivers (full), and unspecified assistantships also available.
Contact Mr. Scott Campbell, Graduate Programs Administrator, School of Nursing, University of Massachusetts Amherst, 216 Arnold House, 715 North Pleasant Street, Amherst, MA 01003-9304. *Telephone:* 413-545-0484. *Fax:* 413-577-2550. *E-mail:* scampbell@nursing.umass.edu.

MASTER'S DEGREE PROGRAM
Degree MS
Available Programs Master's; Master's for Nurses with Non-Nursing Degrees.
Concentrations Available Nurse-midwifery. *Clinical nurse specialist programs in:* psychiatric/mental health, public health, women's health. *Nurse practitioner programs in:* psychiatric/mental health, women's health.
Study Options Full-time and part-time.
Program Entrance Requirements Minimum overall college GPA of 3.0, transcript of college record, CPR certification, written essay, immunizations, interview, 2 letters of recommendation, physical assessment course, professional liability insurance/malpractice insurance, prerequisite course work, statistics course, GRE General Test. *Application deadline:* For fall admission, 2/1 (priority date); for spring admission, 10/1. Applications are processed on a rolling basis. *Application fee:* $40 ($65 for international students).
Advanced Placement Credit given for nursing courses completed elsewhere dependent upon specific evaluations.
Degree Requirements 37 total credit hours, thesis or project.

DOCTORAL DEGREE PROGRAM
Degree PhD
Available Programs Doctorate; Post-Baccalaureate Doctorate.
Areas of Study Advanced practice nursing, aging, clinical practice, community health, faculty preparation, family health, gerontology, health promotion/disease prevention, health-care systems, human health and illness, illness and transition, information systems, maternity-newborn, nursing education, nursing research, nursing science, oncology, urban health, women's health.
Program Entrance Requirements Minimum overall college GPA of 3.0, interview, 2 letters of recommendation, MSN or equivalent, scholarly papers, statistics course, vita, writing sample. *Application deadline:* For fall admission, 2/1 (priority date); for spring admission, 10/1. Applications are processed on a rolling basis. *Application fee:* $40 ($65 for international students).
Degree Requirements 57 total credit hours, dissertation, oral exam, written exam, residency.

CONTINUING EDUCATION PROGRAM
Contact Mr. Scott Campbell, Graduate Programs Administrator, School of Nursing, University of Massachusetts Amherst, 216 Arnold House, 715 North Pleasant Street, Amherst, MA 01003-9304. *Telephone:* 413-545-0484. *Fax:* 413-577-2550. *E-mail:* scampbell@nursing.umass.edu.

University of Massachusetts Boston
College of Nursing and Health Sciences
Boston, Massachusetts

http://www.cnhs.umb.edu/
Founded in 1964
DEGREES • BS • MS • PHD
Nursing Program Faculty 89 (34% with doctorates).

Baccalaureate Enrollment 694
Women 86.5% **Men** 13.5% **Minority** 39.2% **International** 1.6% **Part-time** 32.6%

Graduate Enrollment 140
Women 96.02% **Men** 3.98% **Minority** 11% **International** 1.3% **Part-time** 38.5%

Nursing Student Activities Nursing Honor Society, Sigma Theta Tau, Student Nurses' Association.

Nursing Student Resources Academic advising; academic or career counseling; assistance for students with disabilities; bookstore; campus computer network; career placement assistance; computer lab; computer-assisted instruction; daycare for children of students; e-mail services; employment services for current students; housing assistance; interactive nursing skills videos; Internet; learning resource lab; library services; nursing audiovisuals; other; remedial services; resume preparation assistance; skills, simulation, or other laboratory; tutoring.

Library Facilities 584,015 volumes (3,700 in health, 1,500 in nursing); 25,575 periodical subscriptions (5,000 health-care related).

BACCALAUREATE PROGRAMS

Degree BS

Available Programs Generic Baccalaureate; RN Baccalaureate.
Study Options Full-time.

Program Entrance Requirements Minimum overall college GPA of 2.75, transcript of college record, written essay, health insurance, high school biology, high school chemistry, 3 years high school math, high school transcript, immunizations, 3 letters of recommendation, minimum high school GPA of 2.75, minimum GPA in nursing prerequisites of 3.0. Transfer students are accepted. **Standardized tests** *Required:* SAT or ACT, TOEFL for international students. **Application** *Deadline:* 6/1 (freshmen), rolling (transfer). *Notification:* continuous (freshmen). *Application fee:* $40.

Advanced Placement Credit given for nursing courses completed elsewhere dependent upon specific evaluations.

Expenses (2006–07) *Tuition, state resident:* full-time $11,020; part-time $72 per credit. *Tuition, nonresident:* full-time $22,451; part-time $407 per credit. *International tuition:* $22,451 full-time. *Required fees:* full-time $6832; part-time $426 per credit; part-time $3408 per term.

Financial Aid 85% of baccalaureate students in nursing programs received some form of financial aid in 2005–06.

Contact Mr. Jon Hutton, Assistant Director of Enrollment Marketing and Information Service, College of Nursing and Health Sciences, University of Massachusetts Boston, 100 Morrissey Boulevard, Boston, MA 02125. *Telephone:* 617-287-6000. *Fax:* 617-265-7173. *E-mail:* enrollment. information@umb.edu.

GRADUATE PROGRAMS

Expenses (2006–07) *Tuition, state resident:* full-time $12,302; part-time $108 per credit. *Tuition, nonresident:* full-time $22,461; part-time $407 per credit. *International tuition:* $22,461 full-time.

Financial Aid 20% of graduate students in nursing programs received some form of financial aid in 2005–06. 3 research assistantships with full tuition reimbursements available (averaging $8,000 per year), 13 teaching assistantships with full tuition reimbursements available (averaging $5,000 per year) were awarded; career-related internships or fieldwork, Federal Work-Study, and unspecified assistantships also available. Aid available to part-time students. *Financial aid application deadline:* 3/1.

Contact Mr. Jon Hutton, Assistant Director of Enrollment Marketing and Information Service, College of Nursing and Health Sciences, University of Massachusetts Boston, 100 Morrissey Boulevard, Boston, MA 02125. *Telephone:* 617-287-6000. *Fax:* 617-265-7173. *E-mail:* enrollment. information@umb.edu.

MASTER'S DEGREE PROGRAM

Degree MS

Available Programs Master's.
Concentrations Available *Clinical nurse specialist programs in:* acute care, critical care. *Nurse practitioner programs in:* adult health, family health, gerontology.
Study Options Full-time and part-time.

Program Entrance Requirements Clinical experience, minimum overall college GPA of 2.75, transcript of college record, CPR certification, written essay, immunizations, 3 letters of recommendation, physical assessment course, prerequisite course work, statistics course. *Application deadline:* For fall admission, 3/1 (priority date); for spring admission, 11/1. *Application fee:* $25.

Advanced Placement Credit given for nursing courses completed elsewhere dependent upon specific evaluations.

Degree Requirements 48 total credit hours, thesis or project.

POST-MASTER'S PROGRAM

Areas of Study *Nurse practitioner programs in:* adult health, family health, gerontology.

DOCTORAL DEGREE PROGRAM

Degree PhD
Available Programs Doctorate.
Areas of Study Health policy.

Program Entrance Requirements Clinical experience, minimum overall college GPA of 3.3, interview by faculty committee, interview, 3 letters of recommendation, MSN or equivalent, statistics course, vita, writing sample, GRE General Test. *Application deadline:* For fall admission, 3/1 (priority date); for spring admission, 11/1. *Application fee:* $25.

Degree Requirements 60 total credit hours, dissertation, oral exam, written exam, residency.

CONTINUING EDUCATION PROGRAM

Contact Ms. Wanda Willard, Director of Credit Programs, College of Nursing and Health Sciences, University of Massachusetts Boston, 100 Morrissey Boulevard, Wheatley Building, 2nd Floor, Boston, MA 02125-3393. *Telephone:* 617-287-7874. *Fax:* 617-287-7922. *E-mail:* wanda. willard@umb.edu.

University of Massachusetts Dartmouth
College of Nursing
North Dartmouth, Massachusetts

http://www.umassd.edu/nursing
Founded in 1895
DEGREES • BSN • MS

Nursing Student Activities Sigma Theta Tau, nursing club.

Nursing Student Resources Academic advising; academic or career counseling; assistance for students with disabilities; bookstore; campus computer network; career placement assistance; computer lab; computer-assisted instruction; daycare for children of students; e-mail services; employment services for current students; externships; housing assistance; interactive nursing skills videos; Internet; learning resource lab; library services; nursing audiovisuals; placement services for program completers; resume preparation assistance; skills, simulation, or other laboratory; tutoring; unpaid internships.

Library Facilities 468,266 volumes; 2,800 periodical subscriptions.

■ Graduates of the University of Massachusetts Dartmouth College of Nursing receive a comprehensive education that combines knowledge with diverse clinical experiences in various health-care settings. Faculty members have advanced degrees and expertise in specific areas and are engaged in scholarly research. Students spend their senior semesters working side by side with a nurse mentor at a health-care site. UMass Dartmouth nursing graduates consistently score at the highest levels on the Massachusetts licensing exam.

BACCALAUREATE PROGRAMS

Degree BSN
Available Programs Generic Baccalaureate; RN Baccalaureate.

University of Massachusetts Dartmouth (continued)

Site Options Fall River, MA.

Study Options Full-time and part-time.

Program Entrance Requirements Transcript of college record, CPR certification, written essay, health exam, health insurance, high school biology, high school chemistry, high school foreign language, 3 years high school math, 3 years high school science, high school transcript, immunizations, letters of recommendation, minimum high school GPA of 3.0, minimum high school rank 66%, professional liability insurance/malpractice insurance. Transfer students are accepted. **Standardized tests** *Required:* SAT or ACT, TOEFL for international students. **Application** *Deadline:* rolling (freshmen), rolling (transfer). *Early decision:* 11/15. *Notification:* continuous (freshmen), 12/15 (out-of-state freshmen), 12/15 (early decision). *Application fee:* $40, $55 for non-residents.

Advanced Placement Credit by examination available. Credit given for nursing courses completed elsewhere dependent upon specific evaluations.

Contact Admissions Office, College of Nursing, University of Massachusetts Dartmouth, 285 Old Westport Road, North Dartmouth, MA 02747. *Telephone:* 508-999-8605. *Fax:* 508-999-8755. *E-mail:* admissions@umassd.edu.

GRADUATE PROGRAMS

Financial Aid 2 research assistantships (averaging $3,250 per year), 9 teaching assistantships (averaging $3,333 per year) were awarded; Federal Work-Study, scholarships, and unspecified assistantships also available.

Contact Prof. Jeanne Leffers, Director, Graduate Program, College of Nursing, University of Massachusetts Dartmouth, 285 Old Westport Road, North Dartmouth, MA 02747-2300. *Telephone:* 508-999-8581. *E-mail:* jleffers@umassd.edu.

MASTER'S DEGREE PROGRAM

Degree MS

Available Programs Master's.

Concentrations Available *Clinical nurse specialist programs in:* adult health, community health. *Nurse practitioner programs in:* adult health.

Study Options Full-time and part-time.

Program Entrance Requirements Clinical experience, computer literacy, minimum overall college GPA of 3.0, transcript of college record, CPR certification, written essay, immunizations, interview, 3 letters of recommendation, nursing research course, physical assessment course, professional liability insurance/malpractice insurance, statistics course, GRE General Test. *Application deadline:* For fall admission, 4/20; for spring admission, 11/15. *Application fee:* $35 ($55 for international students).

Advanced Placement Credit given for nursing courses completed elsewhere dependent upon specific evaluations.

Degree Requirements 39 total credit hours, thesis or project.

POST-MASTER'S PROGRAM

Areas of Study *Nurse practitioner programs in:* adult health.

CONTINUING EDUCATION PROGRAM

Contact Lorraine Fisher, Director, Division of Continuing Education, College of Nursing, University of Massachusetts Dartmouth, 285 Old Westport Road, North Dartmouth, MA 02747-2300. *Telephone:* 508-910-6929. *Fax:* 508-999-9127. *E-mail:* lfisher@umassd.edu.

University of Massachusetts Lowell

Department of Nursing
Lowell, Massachusetts

http://www.uml.edu/dept/nursing

Founded in 1894

DEGREES • BS • MS • PHD

Nursing Program Faculty 27 (95% with doctorates).

Baccalaureate Enrollment 298

Women 90% **Men** 10%

Graduate Enrollment 50

Women 90% **Men** 10%

Nursing Student Activities Sigma Theta Tau, Student Nurses' Association.

Nursing Student Resources Academic advising; academic or career counseling; assistance for students with disabilities; bookstore; campus computer network; career placement assistance; computer lab; computer-assisted instruction; e-mail services; employment services for current students; housing assistance; interactive nursing skills videos; Internet; learning resource lab; library services; nursing audiovisuals; placement services for program completers; resume preparation assistance; skills, simulation, or other laboratory; tutoring.

Library Facilities 517,960 volumes (29,100 in health, 4,465 in nursing); 12,300 periodical subscriptions (350 health-care related).

BACCALAUREATE PROGRAMS

Degree BS

Available Programs Generic Baccalaureate; RN Baccalaureate.

Study Options Full-time.

Program Entrance Requirements Minimum overall college GPA of 2.7, transcript of college record, CPR certification, health exam, health insurance, high school chemistry, high school foreign language, 3 years high school math, 3 years high school science, high school transcript, immunizations, minimum high school GPA of 3.25, minimum GPA in nursing prerequisites of 2.7, professional liability insurance/malpractice insurance. Transfer students are accepted. **Standardized tests** *Required:* SAT or ACT, TOEFL for international students. **Application** *Deadline:* rolling (freshmen), rolling (transfer). *Notification:* continuous (freshmen). *Application fee:* $40.

Advanced Placement Credit by examination available.

Expenses (2006–07) *Tuition, state resident:* full-time $8444. *Tuition, nonresident:* full-time $19,714. *Room and board:* $6520 per academic year.

Financial Aid 68% of baccalaureate students in nursing programs received some form of financial aid in 2005–06.

Contact Office of Undergraduate Admissions, Department of Nursing, University of Massachusetts Lowell, 883 Broadway Street, Suite 110, Lowell, MA 01854-5104. *Telephone:* 800-410-4607. *E-mail:* admissions@uml.edu.

GRADUATE PROGRAMS

Expenses (2006–07) *Tuition, area resident:* part-time $91 per credit. *Tuition, state resident:* full-time $7969; part-time $91 per credit. *Tuition, nonresident:* full-time $15,753; part-time $357 per credit. *Room and board:* $6520; room only: $3955 per academic year.

Financial Aid 50% of graduate students in nursing programs received some form of financial aid in 2005–06. 37 fellowships with tuition reimbursements available, 10 teaching assistantships with full tuition reimbursements available were awarded; research assistantships with full tuition reimbursements available, career-related internships or fieldwork, Federal Work-Study, institutionally sponsored loans, scholarships, and traineeships also available. Aid available to part-time students. *Financial aid application deadline:* 4/1.

Contact Dr. Susan Crocker Houde, Director of MS Program/Professor, Department of Nursing, University of Massachusetts Lowell, 3 Solomont Way, Suite 2, Lowell, MA 01854-5126. *Telephone:* 978-934-4426. *Fax:* 978-934-3006. *E-mail:* Susan_Houde@uml.edu.

MASTER'S DEGREE PROGRAM

Degree MS

Available Programs Accelerated Master's; Accelerated RN to Master's; Master's.

Concentrations Available *Clinical nurse specialist programs in:* psychiatric/mental health. *Nurse practitioner programs in:* family health, gerontology, psychiatric/mental health.

Study Options Full-time and part-time.

Program Entrance Requirements Computer literacy, minimum overall college GPA of 3.0, transcript of college record, CPR certification, written essay, immunizations, interview, 3 letters of recommendation, professional liability insurance/malpractice insurance, statistics course, GRE General Test. *Application deadline:* For fall admission, 4/1 (priority date); for spring admission, 10/1. Applications are processed on a rolling basis. *Application fee:* $20 ($35 for international students).

Advanced Placement Credit given for nursing courses completed elsewhere dependent upon specific evaluations.

Degree Requirements 42 total credit hours, thesis or project.

DOCTORAL DEGREE PROGRAM

Degree PhD

Available Programs Doctorate.

Areas of Study Health promotion/disease prevention.

Program Entrance Requirements Minimum overall college GPA of 3.4, interview by faculty committee, interview, 3 letters of recommendation, MSN or equivalent, scholarly papers, statistics course, writing sample, GRE General Test. *Application deadline:* For fall admission, 4/1 (priority date); for spring admission, 10/1. Applications are processed on a rolling basis. *Application fee:* $20 ($35 for international students).

Degree Requirements 60 total credit hours, dissertation, oral exam, written exam.

University of Massachusetts Worcester

Graduate School of Nursing
Worcester, Massachusetts

http://www.umassmed.edu/gsn/

Founded in 1962

DEGREES • MS • PHD

Nursing Program Faculty 48 (58% with doctorates).

Graduate Enrollment 181
Women 90% **Men** 10% **Minority** 12% **International** 1% **Part-time** 6%

Nursing Student Activities Sigma Theta Tau, nursing club.

Nursing Student Resources Academic advising; academic or career counseling; assistance for students with disabilities; bookstore; campus computer network; computer lab; computer-assisted instruction; e-mail services; interactive nursing skills videos; Internet; learning resource lab; library services; nursing audiovisuals; paid internships; remedial services; resume preparation assistance; skills, simulation, or other laboratory; tutoring; unpaid internships.

Library Facilities 258,800 volumes in health, 55,000 volumes in nursing; 20,000 periodical subscriptions health-care related.

GRADUATE PROGRAMS

Expenses (2006–07) *Tuition, state resident:* full-time $2640. *Tuition, nonresident:* full-time $9856.

Financial Aid 60% of graduate students in nursing programs received some form of financial aid in 2005–06. Scholarships and traineeships available. Aid available to part-time students. *Financial aid application deadline:* 3/22.

Contact Mr. Lawrence W. Shattuck, Director of Recruitment and Retention, Graduate School of Nursing, University of Massachusetts Worcester, 55 Lake Avenue North, Worcester, MA 01655-0115. *Telephone:* 508-856-3488. *Fax:* 508-856-5851. *E-mail:* GSNAdmissions@umassmed.edu.

MASTER'S DEGREE PROGRAM

Degree MS

Available Programs Master's; Master's for Non-Nursing College Graduates.

Concentrations Available Nursing education. *Nurse practitioner programs in:* acute care, adult health, community health, family health, gerontology, oncology, primary care, psychiatric/mental health.

Site Options Shrewsbury, MA. *Distance Learning:* Worcester, MA.

Study Options Full-time and part-time.

Program Entrance Requirements Clinical experience, computer literacy, minimum overall college GPA of 3.0, transcript of college record, CPR certification, written essay, immunizations, interview, 3 letters of recommendation, physical assessment course, professional liability insurance/malpractice insurance, prerequisite course work, resume, statistics course, GRE General Test. *Application deadline:* For fall admission, 3/15. Applications are processed on a rolling basis. *Application fee:* $25 ($50 for international students).

Degree Requirements 42 total credit hours, thesis or project.

POST-MASTER'S PROGRAM

Areas of Study Nursing education. *Nurse practitioner programs in:* acute care, adult health, community health, gerontology, primary care.

DOCTORAL DEGREE PROGRAM

Degree PhD

Available Programs Doctorate.

Areas of Study Nursing education, nursing research, nursing science.

Site Options *Distance Learning:* Worcester, MA.

Program Entrance Requirements Clinical experience, minimum overall college GPA of 3.0, interview by faculty committee, interview, 2 letters of recommendation, MSN or equivalent, scholarly papers, statistics course, vita, writing sample. *Application deadline:* For fall admission, 3/15. Applications are processed on a rolling basis. *Application fee:* $25 ($50 for international students).

Degree Requirements 54 total credit hours, dissertation, written exam, residency.

CONTINUING EDUCATION PROGRAM

Contact Mr. Lawrence W. Shattuck, Director of Recruitment and Retention, Graduate School of Nursing, University of Massachusetts Worcester, 55 Lake Avenue North, Worcester, MA 01655-0115. *Telephone:* 508-856-5801. *E-mail:* GSNAdmissions@umassmed.edu.

Worcester State College

Department of Nursing
Worcester, Massachusetts

http://www.worcester.edu

Founded in 1874

DEGREES • BS • MS

Nursing Program Faculty 17 (60% with doctorates).

Baccalaureate Enrollment 239
Women 92% **Men** 8% **Minority** 13% **International** 1%

Graduate Enrollment 23
Women 96% **Men** 4% **Minority** 17% **Part-time** 100%

Nursing Student Activities Sigma Theta Tau, Student Nurses' Association, nursing club.

Nursing Student Resources Academic advising; academic or career counseling; assistance for students with disabilities; bookstore; campus computer network; career placement assistance; computer lab; computer-assisted instruction; e-mail services; employment services for current students; housing assistance; interactive nursing skills videos; Internet; learning resource lab; library services; nursing audiovisuals; paid internships; remedial services; resume preparation assistance; skills, simulation, or other laboratory; tutoring; unpaid internships.

Library Facilities 197,235 volumes (5,400 in health, 500 in nursing); 568 periodical subscriptions (85 health-care related).

BACCALAUREATE PROGRAMS

Degree BS

Available Programs Accelerated RN Baccalaureate; Generic Baccalaureate.

Study Options Full-time.

Program Entrance Requirements Minimum overall college GPA of 3.0, CPR certification, written essay, health exam, health insurance, high school chemistry, high school foreign language, 1 year of high school math, 2 years high school science, high school transcript, immunizations, interview, minimum high school GPA of 3.0, minimum GPA in nursing prerequisites of 3.0, professional liability insurance/malpractice insurance, prerequisite course work, RN licensure. Transfer students are accepted.

Standardized tests *Required:* SAT or ACT, TOEFL for international students. *Required for some:* SAT Subject Tests. **Application** *Deadline:* 6/1 (freshmen), 6/1 (transfer). *Notification:* continuous (freshmen). *Application fee:* $20.

Advanced Placement Credit by examination available. Credit given for nursing courses completed elsewhere dependent upon specific evaluations.

Worcester State College (continued)

Expenses (2005–06) *Tuition, area resident:* full-time $970; part-time $40 per credit. *Tuition, state resident:* full-time $1455; part-time $61 per credit. *Tuition, nonresident:* full-time $7050; part-time $294 per credit. *International tuition:* $7050 full-time. *Room and board:* $7048; room only: $2950 per academic year. *Required fees:* full-time $3609; part-time $146 per credit; part-time $1805 per term.

Financial Aid 81% of baccalaureate students in nursing programs received some form of financial aid in 2004–05.

Contact Ms. Elizabeth Axelson, Associate Director, Admissions, Department of Nursing, Worcester State College, 486 Chandler Street, Worcester, MA 01602. *Telephone:* 508-929-8090. *Fax:* 508-929-8183. *E-mail:* baxelson@worcester.edu.

GRADUATE PROGRAMS

Financial Aid 40% of graduate students in nursing programs received some form of financial aid in 2004–05.

Contact Dr. Anne Marie Catalano, RN, Coordinator, Department of Nursing, Worcester State College, 486 Chandler Street, Worcester, MA 01602. *Telephone:* 508-929-8129. *Fax:* 508-929-8168. *E-mail:* acatalano@worcester.edu.

MASTER'S DEGREE PROGRAM

Degree MS

Available Programs Master's; Master's for Nurses with Non-Nursing Degrees.

Concentrations Available *Clinical nurse specialist programs in:* community health.

Study Options Part-time.

Program Entrance Requirements Clinical experience, minimum overall college GPA of 3.0, transcript of college record, CPR certification, immunizations, interview, 1 letter of recommendation, nursing research course, professional liability insurance/malpractice insurance, prerequisite course work, resume, statistics course.

Advanced Placement Credit by examination available.

Degree Requirements 42 total credit hours, comprehensive exam.

MICHIGAN

Andrews University
Department of Nursing
Berrien Springs, Michigan

Founded in 1874

DEGREES • BS • MS

Nursing Program Faculty 11 (50% with doctorates).

Baccalaureate Enrollment 106

Graduate Enrollment 10

Nursing Student Activities Nursing Honor Society, Sigma Theta Tau, Student Nurses' Association.

Nursing Student Resources Academic advising; academic or career counseling; assistance for students with disabilities; bookstore; campus computer network; career placement assistance; computer lab; computer-assisted instruction; daycare for children of students; e-mail services; employment services for current students; externships; housing assistance; interactive nursing skills videos; Internet; learning resource lab; library services; nursing audiovisuals; paid internships; placement services for program completers; remedial services; resume preparation assistance; skills, simulation, or other laboratory; tutoring; unpaid internships.

Library Facilities 512,100 volumes (77,000 in health, 500 in nursing); 3,032 periodical subscriptions (700 health-care related).

BACCALAUREATE PROGRAMS

Degree BS

Available Programs ADN to Baccalaureate; Generic Baccalaureate.

Study Options Full-time.

Program Entrance Requirements Minimum overall college GPA of 2.5, transcript of college record, health exam, high school transcript, immunizations, minimum GPA in nursing prerequisites of 2.5. Transfer students are accepted. **Standardized tests** *Required:* SAT or ACT. **Application** *Deadline:* rolling (freshmen), rolling (transfer). *Notification:* continuous (freshmen). *Application fee:* $32.

Contact *Telephone:* 269-471-3192. *Fax:* 269-471-3454.

GRADUATE PROGRAMS

Contact *Telephone:* 269-471-3337. *Fax:* 269-471-3454.

MASTER'S DEGREE PROGRAM

Degree MS

Available Programs Master's.

Concentrations Available Nursing education.

Study Options Part-time.

Program Entrance Requirements Minimum overall college GPA of 3.0, transcript of college record, CPR certification, immunizations, 3 letters of recommendation. *Application deadline:* Applications are processed on a rolling basis. *Application fee:* $43.

Degree Requirements 38 total credit hours, thesis or project.

POST-MASTER'S PROGRAM

Areas of Study Nursing education.

Calvin College
Department of Nursing
Grand Rapids, Michigan

Founded in 1876

DEGREE • BSN

Nursing Program Faculty 20 (20% with doctorates).

Baccalaureate Enrollment 120
Women 95% **Men** 5% **Minority** 10% **International** 10%

Nursing Student Activities Sigma Theta Tau, Student Nurses' Association, nursing club.

Nursing Student Resources Academic advising; academic or career counseling; assistance for students with disabilities; bookstore; campus computer network; career placement assistance; computer lab; computer-assisted instruction; e-mail services; employment services for current students; externships; housing assistance; interactive nursing skills videos; Internet; learning resource lab; library services; nursing audiovisuals; paid internships; placement services for program completers; remedial services; resume preparation assistance; skills, simulation, or other laboratory; tutoring.

Library Facilities 824,806 volumes; 14,464 periodical subscriptions.

BACCALAUREATE PROGRAMS

Degree BSN

Available Programs Generic Baccalaureate.

Site Options Grand Rapids, MI.

Study Options Full-time.

Program Entrance Requirements Minimum overall college GPA of 2.5, transcript of college record, CPR certification, health exam, health insurance, immunizations, 2 letters of recommendation, minimum GPA in nursing prerequisites of 2.5, professional liability insurance/malpractice insurance, prerequisite course work. Transfer students are accepted. **Standardized tests** *Required:* SAT and SAT Subject Tests or ACT, TOEFL for international students. **Application** *Deadline:* 8/15 (freshmen), rolling (transfer). *Notification:* continuous (freshmen). *Application fee:* $35.

Expenses (2006–07) *Tuition:* full-time $20,470. *Room and board:* $7040 per academic year. *Required fees:* full-time $1800.

Financial Aid 75% of baccalaureate students in nursing programs received some form of financial aid in 2005–06. *Gift aid (need-based):* Federal Pell, FSEOG, state, private, college/university gift aid from institutional funds. *Loans:* Federal Direct (Subsidized and Unsubsidized Stafford PLUS), Perkins, state, college/university, alternative loans. *Work-Study:* Federal Work-Study, part-time campus jobs. *Application deadline (priority):* 2/15.

Contact Dr. Mary Molewyk Doornbos, Chairperson and Professor, Department of Nursing, Calvin College, Science Building, 1734 Knollcrest Circle SE, Grand Rapids, MI 49546-4403. *Telephone:* 616-526-6268. *Fax:* 616-526-8567. *E-mail:* door@calvin.edu.

Eastern Michigan University
School of Nursing
Ypsilanti, Michigan

http://www.emich.edu/nursing

Founded in 1849

DEGREES • BSN • MSN

Nursing Program Faculty 44 (27% with doctorates).

Baccalaureate Enrollment 320
Women 88% **Men** 12% **Minority** 27% **International** 2% **Part-time** 57%

Graduate Enrollment 22
Women 100% **Minority** 41% **Part-time** 100%

Nursing Student Activities Sigma Theta Tau, Student Nurses' Association.

Nursing Student Resources Academic advising; academic or career counseling; assistance for students with disabilities; bookstore; campus computer network; career placement assistance; computer lab; computer-assisted instruction; daycare for children of students; e-mail services; employment services for current students; housing assistance; interactive nursing skills videos; Internet; learning resource lab; library services; nursing audiovisuals; placement services for program completers; remedial services; resume preparation assistance; skills, simulation, or other laboratory; tutoring.

Library Facilities 658,648 volumes (23,500 in health, 4,800 in nursing); 4,457 periodical subscriptions (825 health-care related).

BACCALAUREATE PROGRAMS

Degree BSN

Available Programs Baccalaureate for Second Degree; Generic Baccalaureate; RN Baccalaureate.

Site Options Jackson, MI; Brighton, MI; Detroit, MI; Livonia, MI; Monroe, MI.

Study Options Full-time and part-time.

Program Entrance Requirements Transcript of college record, CPR certification, health exam, health insurance, immunizations, minimum GPA in nursing prerequisites of 2.8, prerequisite course work, RN licensure. **Standardized tests** *Required:* TOEFL for international students. *Required for some:* ACT. **Application** *Deadline:* rolling (transfer). *Notification:* continuous (freshmen). *Application fee:* $30.

Advanced Placement Credit given for nursing courses completed elsewhere dependent upon specific evaluations.

Expenses (2006–07) *Tuition, state resident:* full-time $4668; part-time $285 per credit hour. *Tuition, nonresident:* full-time $13,752; part-time $664 per credit hour. *International tuition:* $13,752 full-time. *Room and board:* $6610; room only: $3104 per academic year. *Required fees:* full-time $2257; part-time $91 per credit; part-time $1128 per term.

Financial Aid 73% of baccalaureate students in nursing programs received some form of financial aid in 2005–06.

Contact Ms. Sheila Steiner, RN, BSN Coordinator, School of Nursing, Eastern Michigan University, 309 Marshall Building, Ypsilanti, MI 48197. *Telephone:* 734-487-2334. *Fax:* 734-487-6946. *E-mail:* sritonda@emich.edu.

GRADUATE PROGRAMS

Expenses (2006–07) *Tuition, state resident:* full-time $5448; part-time $443 per credit hour. *Tuition, nonresident:* full-time $10,736; part-time $773 per credit hour. *International tuition:* $10,736 full-time. *Room and board:* $6610; room only: $3104 per academic year. *Required fees:* full-time $1712; part-time $102 per credit; part-time $856 per term.

Financial Aid 41% of graduate students in nursing programs received some form of financial aid in 2005–06.

Contact Dr. Sandra Nelson, RN, Graduate Program Coordinator, School of Nursing, Eastern Michigan University, 311 Marshall Building, Ypsilanti, MI 48197. *Telephone:* 734-487-3267. *Fax:* 734-487-6946. *E-mail:* sandra.nelson@emich.edu.

MASTER'S DEGREE PROGRAM

Degree MSN

Available Programs Master's.

Concentrations Available *Clinical nurse specialist programs in:* adult health.

Site Options Livonia, MI; Monroe, MI.

Study Options Full-time and part-time.

Program Entrance Requirements Clinical experience, minimum overall college GPA of 2.5, transcript of college record, CPR certification, written essay, immunizations, interview, 3 letters of recommendation, physical assessment course, statistics course.

Advanced Placement Credit given for nursing courses completed elsewhere dependent upon specific evaluations.

Degree Requirements 40 total credit hours, thesis or project.

Ferris State University
School of Nursing
Big Rapids, Michigan

Founded in 1884

DEGREES • BSN • MSN • MSN/MBA

Nursing Program Faculty 12 (16% with doctorates).

Baccalaureate Enrollment 179
Women 93% **Men** 7% **Minority** 11% **Part-time** 89%

Graduate Enrollment 34
Women 95% **Men** 5% **Minority** 2% **Part-time** 100%

Nursing Student Activities Student Nurses' Association.

Nursing Student Resources Academic advising; academic or career counseling; assistance for students with disabilities; bookstore; campus computer network; career placement assistance; computer lab; computer-assisted instruction; daycare for children of students; e-mail services; employment services for current students; housing assistance; interactive nursing skills videos; Internet; library services; nursing audiovisuals; resume preparation assistance; tutoring.

Library Facilities 354,173 volumes (12,177 in health, 785 in nursing); 1,049 periodical subscriptions (515 health-care related).

BACCALAUREATE PROGRAMS

Degree BSN

Available Programs Accelerated Baccalaureate; Generic Baccalaureate; RN Baccalaureate.

Site Options *Distance Learning:* Traverse City, MI; Grand Rapids, MI; Flint, MI.

Study Options Full-time.

Program Entrance Requirements Minimum overall college GPA, transcript of college record, CPR certification, health insurance, high school biology, high school chemistry, high school transcript, immunizations, minimum GPA in nursing prerequisites, prerequisite course work. Transfer students are accepted. **Standardized tests** *Required:* SAT or ACT, TOEFL for international students. **Application** *Deadline:* 8/1 (freshmen), 7/1 (transfer). *Notification:* continuous (freshmen). *Application fee:* $30.

Advanced Placement Credit by examination available. Credit given for nursing courses completed elsewhere dependent upon specific evaluations.

Expenses (2006–07) *Tuition, state resident:* full-time $7200; part-time $270 per credit. *Tuition, nonresident:* full-time $14,640; part-time $530 per credit. *International tuition:* $14,640 full-time. *Room and board:* $3610; room only: $1834 per academic year.

Financial Aid 60% of baccalaureate students in nursing programs received some form of financial aid in 2005–06. *Gift aid (need-based):* Federal Pell, FSEOG, state, private, college/university gift aid from institutional funds. *Loans:* Federal Nursing Student Loans, Federal Direct (Subsidized and Unsubsidized Stafford PLUS), Perkins, college/university, alternative loans. *Work-Study:* Federal Work-Study, part-time campus jobs. *Application deadline (priority):* 3/1.

Contact Dr. Julie A. Coon, EdD, Director, School of Nursing, Ferris State University, 200 Ferris Drive, Room 400A, Big Rapids, MI 49307. *Telephone:* 231-591-2267. *Fax:* 231-591-2325. *E-mail:* coonj@ferris.edu.

Ferris State University (continued)

GRADUATE PROGRAMS

Expenses (2006–07) *Tuition, state resident:* part-time $355 per credit. *Tuition, nonresident:* part-time $687 per credit.

Financial Aid 3% of graduate students in nursing programs received some form of financial aid in 2005–06.

Contact Dr. Marietta Bell-Scriber, Program Coordinator, School of Nursing, Ferris State University, 200 Ferris Drive, Big Rapids, MI 49307. *Telephone:* 231-591-3987. *Fax:* 231-591-2325. *E-mail:* bellscri@ferris.edu.

MASTER'S DEGREE PROGRAM

Degrees MSN; MSN/MBA

Available Programs Master's.

Concentrations Available Nursing administration; nursing education; nursing informatics.

Study Options Full-time and part-time.

Program Entrance Requirements Clinical experience, minimum overall college GPA of 3.0, transcript of college record, written essay, 3 letters of recommendation, resume.

Advanced Placement Credit given for nursing courses completed elsewhere dependent upon specific evaluations.

Degree Requirements 36 total credit hours, thesis or project, comprehensive exam.

Grand Valley State University
Russell B. Kirkhof College of Nursing
Allendale, Michigan

http://www4.gvsu.edu/kson/

Founded in 1960

DEGREES • BSN • MSN • MSN/MBA

Nursing Program Faculty 66 (29% with doctorates).

Baccalaureate Enrollment 508
Women 90.4% **Men** 9.6% **Minority** 6.5% **International** .2% **Part-time** 39%

Graduate Enrollment 48
Women 92% **Men** 8% **Minority** 6% **Part-time** 93.7%

Nursing Student Activities Sigma Theta Tau, Student Nurses' Association.

Nursing Student Resources Academic advising; academic or career counseling; assistance for students with disabilities; bookstore; campus computer network; career placement assistance; computer lab; computer-assisted instruction; daycare for children of students; e-mail services; employment services for current students; housing assistance; interactive nursing skills videos; Internet; learning resource lab; library services; nursing audiovisuals; placement services for program completers; remedial services; resume preparation assistance; skills, simulation, or other laboratory; tutoring.

Library Facilities 634,000 volumes (29,315 in health, 1,888 in nursing); 5,000 periodical subscriptions (3,450 health-care related).

BACCALAUREATE PROGRAMS

Degree BSN

Available Programs ADN to Baccalaureate; Accelerated Baccalaureate; Accelerated Baccalaureate for Second Degree; Baccalaureate for Second Degree; Generic Baccalaureate; RN Baccalaureate.

Site Options *Distance Learning:* Holland, MI; Grand Rapids, MI.

Study Options Full-time and part-time.

Program Entrance Requirements Minimum overall college GPA of 2.8, transcript of college record, CPR certification, written essay, health exam, health insurance, immunizations, minimum GPA in nursing prerequisites, prerequisite course work. Transfer students are accepted. **Standardized tests** *Required:* SAT or ACT, TOEFL for international students. **Application** *Deadline:* 5/1 (freshmen), 7/28 (transfer). *Notification:* continuous until 5/1 (freshmen). *Application fee:* $30.

Advanced Placement Credit by examination available. Credit given for nursing courses completed elsewhere dependent upon specific evaluations.

Financial Aid 86% of baccalaureate students in nursing programs received some form of financial aid in 2005–06. *Gift aid (need-based):* Federal Pell, FSEOG, state, private, college/university gift aid from institutional funds, Federal Nursing. *Loans:* Federal Nursing Student Loans, Federal Direct (Subsidized and Unsubsidized Stafford PLUS), Perkins, state. *Work-Study:* Federal Work-Study, part-time campus jobs. *Application deadline (priority):* 2/15.

Contact Ms. Susan Baker-Clark, Student Services Coordinator, Russell B. Kirkhof College of Nursing, Grand Valley State University, Cook-DeVos Center for Health Sciences, 301 Michigan Street NE, Room 453, Grand Rapids, MI 49503-3314. *Telephone:* 616-331-2594. *Fax:* 616-331-2510. *E-mail:* bakercls@gvsu.edu.

GRADUATE PROGRAMS

Financial Aid 40% of graduate students in nursing programs received some form of financial aid in 2005–06. 6 research assistantships with full and partial tuition reimbursements available (averaging $8,000 per year) were awarded; career-related internships or fieldwork, Federal Work-Study, institutionally sponsored loans, and traineeships also available. *Financial aid application deadline:* 2/15.

Contact Dr. Jean Martin, Director of RN/BSN and MSN Programs/Assistant Professor of Nursing, Russell B. Kirkhof College of Nursing, Grand Valley State University, Cook-DeVos Center for Health Sciences, 301 Michigan Street NE, Grand Rapids, MI 49503-3314. *Telephone:* 616-331-3558. *Fax:* 616-331-2510.

MASTER'S DEGREE PROGRAM

Degrees MSN; MSN/MBA

Available Programs Master's for Nurses with Non-Nursing Degrees.

Concentrations Available Nurse case management; nursing administration; nursing education. *Clinical nurse specialist programs in:* adult health, family health, gerontology, pediatric, psychiatric/mental health, women's health. *Nurse practitioner programs in:* adult health, family health, gerontology, pediatric, primary care, psychiatric/mental health, women's health.

Site Options *Distance Learning:* Grand Rapids, MI.

Study Options Full-time and part-time.

Program Entrance Requirements Minimum overall college GPA of 3.0, transcript of college record, CPR certification, written essay, immunizations, 3 letters of recommendation, physical assessment course, statistics course, GRE. *Application deadline:* For fall admission, 3/15 (priority date). Applications are processed on a rolling basis. *Application fee:* $30.

Degree Requirements 43 total credit hours, thesis or project, comprehensive exam.

POST-MASTER'S PROGRAM

Areas of Study Nurse case management; nursing administration; nursing education. *Clinical nurse specialist programs in:* adult health, family health, gerontology, pediatric, women's health. *Nurse practitioner programs in:* adult health, family health, gerontology, pediatric, primary care, women's health.

CONTINUING EDUCATION PROGRAM

Contact Ms. Jan Coye, Academic Community Liaison, Russell B. Kirkhof College of Nursing, Grand Valley State University, Cook-DeVos Center for Health Sciences, 301 Michigan Street NE, Grand Rapids, MI 49503-3314. *Telephone:* 616-331-3558. *Fax:* 616-331-2510. *E-mail:* coyej@gvsu.edu.

Hope College
Department of Nursing
Holland, Michigan

Founded in 1866

DEGREE • BSN

Nursing Program Faculty 14.

Baccalaureate Enrollment 100

Nursing Student Activities Sigma Theta Tau, Student Nurses' Association.

Nursing Student Resources Academic advising; academic or career counseling; assistance for students with disabilities; bookstore; campus computer network; career placement assistance; computer lab; computer-assisted instruction; e-mail services; employment services for current students; externships; housing assistance; interactive nursing skills videos; Internet; learning resource lab; library services; nursing audiovisuals; remedial services; resume preparation assistance; skills, simulation, or other laboratory; tutoring; unpaid internships.

Library Facilities 358,329 volumes; 2,878 periodical subscriptions.

BACCALAUREATE PROGRAMS

Degree BSN

Available Programs Generic Baccalaureate.

Study Options Full-time and part-time.

Program Entrance Requirements Minimum overall college GPA of 2.9, transcript of college record, written essay, 2 letters of recommendation, minimum GPA in nursing prerequisites of 2.5. Transfer students are accepted. **Standardized tests** *Required:* SAT or ACT, TOEFL for international students. **Application** *Deadline:* rolling (freshmen), rolling (transfer). *Notification:* continuous (freshmen). *Application fee:* $35.

Contact Nursing Contact, Department of Nursing, Hope College, 35 East 12th Street, Holland, MI 49422-9000. *Telephone:* 616-395-7420. *Fax:* 616-395-7163. *E-mail:* nursing@hope.edu.

Lake Superior State University
Department of Nursing
Sault Sainte Marie, Michigan

http://www.lssu.edu/academics/science/schools/ nursing_health/nursdept/

Founded in 1946

DEGREE • BSN

Nursing Program Faculty 10 (20% with doctorates).

Baccalaureate Enrollment 115
Women 90% **Men** 10% **Minority** 10% **International** 3%

Nursing Student Activities Nursing Honor Society, Sigma Theta Tau, Student Nurses' Association.

Nursing Student Resources Academic advising; academic or career counseling; assistance for students with disabilities; bookstore; campus computer network; career placement assistance; computer lab; computer-assisted instruction; daycare for children of students; e-mail services; employment services for current students; interactive nursing skills videos; Internet; learning resource lab; library services; nursing audiovisuals; placement services for program completers; skills, simulation, or other laboratory; tutoring.

Library Facilities 200,449 volumes (5,114 in health); 850 periodical subscriptions (72 health-care related).

BACCALAUREATE PROGRAMS

Degree BSN

Available Programs ADN to Baccalaureate; Generic Baccalaureate; LPN to RN Baccalaureate; RN Baccalaureate; RPN to Baccalaureate.

Site Options *Distance Learning:* Petoskey, MI; Escanaba, MI.

Study Options Full-time and part-time.

Program Entrance Requirements Minimum overall college GPA of 2.5, transcript of college record, CPR certification, health exam, health insurance, high school biology, high school chemistry, high school transcript, immunizations, minimum high school GPA of 2.0, minimum GPA in nursing prerequisites of 2.5, professional liability insurance/malpractice insurance, prerequisite course work. Transfer students are accepted. **Standardized tests** *Required:* SAT or ACT, TOEFL for international students. **Application** *Deadline:* 8/15 (freshmen), rolling (transfer). *Notification:* continuous (freshmen). *Application fee:* $35.

Advanced Placement Credit given for nursing courses completed elsewhere dependent upon specific evaluations.

Expenses (2006–07) *Tuition, state resident:* full-time $6558; part-time $273 per credit. *Tuition, nonresident:* full-time $13,116; part-time $547 per credit. *International tuition:* $13,116 full-time. *Required fees:* full-time $750; part-time $25 per credit.

Financial Aid 76% of baccalaureate students in nursing programs received some form of financial aid in 2005–06.

Contact Dr. Steven E. Merrill, Dean of Nursing, Department of Nursing, Lake Superior State University, 650 West Easterday Avenue, Sault Sainte Marie, MI 49783. *Telephone:* 906-635-2446. *Fax:* 906-635-2266. *E-mail:* smerrill@lssu.edu.

Madonna University
College of Nursing and Health
Livonia, Michigan

http://www.madonna.edu

Founded in 1947

DEGREES • BSN • MSN • MSN/MBA

Nursing Program Faculty 55 (12% with doctorates).

Baccalaureate Enrollment 373
Women 90% **Men** 10% **Minority** 16% **International** 1% **Part-time** 25%

Graduate Enrollment 52
Women 94% **Men** 6% **Minority** 14% **International** 4% **Part-time** 94%

Nursing Student Activities Sigma Theta Tau, Student Nurses' Association.

Nursing Student Resources Academic advising; academic or career counseling; assistance for students with disabilities; bookstore; campus computer network; career placement assistance; computer lab; computer-assisted instruction; e-mail services; interactive nursing skills videos; Internet; learning resource lab; library services; nursing audiovisuals; remedial services; resume preparation assistance; skills, simulation, or other laboratory; tutoring.

Library Facilities 199,144 volumes (106,387 in health, 6,290 in nursing); 1,679 periodical subscriptions (891 health-care related).

BACCALAUREATE PROGRAMS

Degree BSN

Available Programs ADN to Baccalaureate; Baccalaureate for Second Degree; Generic Baccalaureate; LPN to Baccalaureate; RN Baccalaureate.

Site Options *Distance Learning:* Gaylord, MI; Orchard Lake, MI.

Study Options Full-time and part-time.

Program Entrance Requirements Minimum overall college GPA of 2.5, transcript of college record, CPR certification, health exam, high school biology, high school chemistry, 1 year of high school math, high school transcript, immunizations, minimum high school GPA of 2.75, professional liability insurance/malpractice insurance. Transfer students are accepted. **Standardized tests** *Required:* SAT or ACT, TOEFL for international students. **Application** *Deadline:* rolling (freshmen), rolling (transfer). *Notification:* continuous (freshmen). *Application fee:* $25.

Advanced Placement Credit by examination available. Credit given for nursing courses completed elsewhere dependent upon specific evaluations.

Expenses (2005–06) *Tuition:* full-time $10,200; part-time $385 per credit hour. *International tuition:* $12,750 full-time. *Room and board:* $5700; room only: $2600 per academic year. *Required fees:* full-time $250; part-time $125 per term.

Financial Aid 75% of baccalaureate students in nursing programs received some form of financial aid in 2004–05.

Contact Ms. Linda Smith, Nursing Admissions Counselor, College of Nursing and Health, Madonna University, 36600 Schoolcraft Road, Livonia, MI 48150-1173. *Telephone:* 734-432-5718. *Fax:* 734-432-5463. *E-mail:* lsmith@madonna.edu.

GRADUATE PROGRAMS

Expenses (2005–06) *Tuition:* full-time $7138; part-time $391 per credit hour. *International tuition:* $8923 full-time. *Room and board:* $5768; room only: $2600 per academic year. *Required fees:* full-time $150; part-time $50 per term.

Madonna University (continued)

Financial Aid 14% of graduate students in nursing programs received some form of financial aid in 2004–05.

Contact Dr. Nancy O'Connor, Chair of Graduate Nursing Program, College of Nursing and Health, Madonna University, 36600 Schoolcraft Road, Livonia, MI 48150-1173. *Telephone:* 734-432-5461. *Fax:* 734-432-5463. *E-mail:* noconnor@madonna.edu.

MASTER'S DEGREE PROGRAM

Degrees MSN; MSN/MBA

Available Programs Accelerated AD/RN to Master's; Accelerated RN to Master's; Master's.

Concentrations Available Nursing administration. *Nurse practitioner programs in:* adult health, primary care.

Site Options *Distance Learning:* Alpena, MI; Orchard Lake, MI.

Study Options Full-time and part-time.

Program Entrance Requirements Clinical experience, computer literacy, minimum overall college GPA of 3.0, transcript of college record, written essay, interview, 2 letters of recommendation, nursing research course, physical assessment course, resume, statistics course.

Advanced Placement Credit given for nursing courses completed elsewhere dependent upon specific evaluations.

Degree Requirements 48 total credit hours.

POST-MASTER'S PROGRAM

Areas of Study *Nurse practitioner programs in:* adult health, primary care.

CONTINUING EDUCATION PROGRAM

Contact Ms. Susan Hasenau, Coordinator of Nursing Continuing Education, College of Nursing and Health, Madonna University, 36600 Schoolcraft Road, Livonia, MI 48150-1173. *Telephone:* 734-432-5863. *Fax:* 734-432-5463. *E-mail:* shasenau@madonna.edu.

Michigan State University
College of Nursing
East Lansing, Michigan

http://www.nursing.msu.edu/

Founded in 1855

DEGREES • BSN • MSN • PHD

Nursing Program Faculty 77 (26% with doctorates).

Baccalaureate Enrollment 284
Women 87% **Men** 13% **Minority** 12% **Part-time** 90%

Graduate Enrollment 155
Women 91% **Men** 9% **Minority** 8% **Part-time** 4%

Nursing Student Activities Sigma Theta Tau, Student Nurses' Association.

Nursing Student Resources Academic advising; academic or career counseling; computer lab; Internet; library services; nursing audiovisuals; remedial services; skills, simulation, or other laboratory; tutoring.

Library Facilities 4.8 million volumes; 37,832 periodical subscriptions.

BACCALAUREATE PROGRAMS

Degree BSN

Available Programs Accelerated Baccalaureate for Second Degree; Generic Baccalaureate; RN Baccalaureate.

Program Entrance Requirements Minimum overall college GPA of 2.5, letters of recommendation, minimum GPA in nursing prerequisites of 2.2, prerequisite course work. Transfer students are accepted. **Standardized tests** *Required:* SAT or ACT, TOEFL for international students. **Application** *Deadline:* rolling (freshmen), rolling (transfer). *Notification:* continuous until 9/1 (freshmen). *Application fee:* $35.

Expenses (2005–06) *Tuition, area resident:* full-time $8020; part-time $259 per credit. *Tuition, nonresident:* full-time $20,057. *Room and board:* room only: $5744 per academic year.

Financial Aid *Gift aid (need-based):* Federal Pell, FSEOG, state, private, college/university gift aid from institutional funds, United Negro College Fund, Federal Nursing. *Loans:* Federal Nursing Student Loans, FFEL (Subsidized and Unsubsidized Stafford PLUS), Perkins, state, college/university. *Work-Study:* Federal Work-Study, part-time campus jobs. *Application deadline:* 6/30 (priority: 3/1).

Contact Sharon Graver, Undergraduate Adviser, College of Nursing, Michigan State University, A-117 Life Sciences Building, East Lansing, MI 48824-1317. *Telephone:* 517-353-4827. *Fax:* 517-432-8251. *E-mail:* graver@msu.edu.

GRADUATE PROGRAMS

Expenses (2005–06) *Tuition, area resident:* part-time $430 per credit. *Tuition, nonresident:* part-time $455 per credit. *Required fees:* full-time $1270.

Financial Aid 12 fellowships (averaging $9,805 per year), 5 research assistantships (averaging $12,883 per year) were awarded; Federal Work-Study, scholarships, and unspecified assistantships also available.

Contact Ms. Julie Roush, Program Advisor, College of Nursing, Michigan State University, A-117 Life Sciences Building, East Lansing, MI 48824-1317. *Telephone:* 517-353-4827. *E-mail:* roushjul@msu.edu.

MASTER'S DEGREE PROGRAM

Degree MSN

Available Programs Master's.

Concentrations Available Nursing education. *Nurse practitioner programs in:* adult health, family health, gerontology.

Study Options Part-time.

Program Entrance Requirements Minimum overall college GPA of 3.0, written essay, 3 letters of recommendation, resume, statistics course, GRE General Test. *Application deadline:* For fall admission, 11/1 (priority date). *Application fee:* $50.

Degree Requirements 47 total credit hours, comprehensive exam.

POST-MASTER'S PROGRAM

Areas of Study Nursing education. *Nurse practitioner programs in:* adult health, family health, gerontology.

DOCTORAL DEGREE PROGRAM

Degree PhD

Available Programs Doctorate; Post-Baccalaureate Doctorate.

Areas of Study Family health, health promotion/disease prevention, human health and illness, individualized study, nursing research.

Program Entrance Requirements Minimum overall college GPA of 3.5, interview by faculty committee, 3 letters of recommendation, statistics course, vita, GRE General Test. *Application deadline:* For fall admission, 11/1 (priority date). *Application fee:* $50.

Degree Requirements 61 total credit hours, dissertation, oral exam, written exam, residency.

POSTDOCTORAL PROGRAM

Areas of Study Nursing research.

Postdoctoral Program Contact Dr. Audrey G. Gift, Professor and Associate Dean for Research and Doctoral Program, College of Nursing, Michigan State University, A-212 Life Sciences Building, East Lansing, MI 48824-1317. *Telephone:* 517-432-6220. *E-mail:* agift@msu.edu.

CONTINUING EDUCATION PROGRAM

Contact Katie Kessler, Coordinator of Professional Education, College of Nursing, Michigan State University, A-112 Life Sciences Building, East Lansing, MI 48824-1317. *Telephone:* 517-355-8539. *Fax:* 517-432-8131. *E-mail:* kessle24@msu.edu.

Northern Michigan University
College of Nursing and Allied Health Science
Marquette, Michigan

http://www.nmu.edu/departments/nursing.html

Founded in 1899

DEGREES • BSN • MSN

Nursing Program Faculty 17 (50% with doctorates).

Baccalaureate Enrollment 189
Women 86% **Men** 14% **Minority** 4% **Part-time** 9%

Graduate Enrollment 15
Women 100% **Part-time** 100%

Nursing Student Activities Sigma Theta Tau, Student Nurses' Association.

Nursing Student Resources Academic advising; academic or career counseling; assistance for students with disabilities; bookstore; campus computer network; career placement assistance; computer lab; computer-assisted instruction; e-mail services; employment services for current students; housing assistance; interactive nursing skills videos; Internet; learning resource lab; library services; nursing audiovisuals; other; paid internships; remedial services; resume preparation assistance; skills, simulation, or other laboratory; tutoring.

Library Facilities 615,406 volumes (36,777 in health, 2,557 in nursing); 4,573 periodical subscriptions (306 health-care related).

BACCALAUREATE PROGRAMS

Degree BSN

Available Programs ADN to Baccalaureate; Accelerated Baccalaureate; Accelerated Baccalaureate for Second Degree; Accelerated LPN to Baccalaureate; Generic Baccalaureate; LPN to RN Baccalaureate.

Study Options Full-time and part-time.

Program Entrance Requirements Minimum overall college GPA of 2.75, transcript of college record, CPR certification, health exam, high school transcript, immunizations, minimum GPA in nursing prerequisites of 2.0, prerequisite course work. Transfer students are accepted. **Standardized tests** *Required:* SAT or ACT, TOEFL for international students. **Application** *Deadline:* rolling (freshmen), rolling (transfer). *Notification:* continuous (freshmen). *Application fee:* $30.

Advanced Placement Credit by examination available. Credit given for nursing courses completed elsewhere dependent upon specific evaluations.

Expenses (2005–06) *Tuition, area resident:* full-time $5328; part-time $222 per credit hour. *Tuition, state resident:* full-time $8872; part-time $378 per credit hour. *Tuition, nonresident:* full-time $8872; part-time $378 per credit hour. *Room and board:* $6482 per academic year. *Required fees:* full-time $470.

Financial Aid 85% of baccalaureate students in nursing programs received some form of financial aid in 2004–05.

Contact Dr. Kerri Durnell Schuiling, Associate Director of BSN/MSN Programs, College of Nursing and Allied Health Science, Northern Michigan University, 1401 Presque Isle Avenue, 2302 New Science Facility, Marquette, MI 49855. *Telephone:* 906-227-2834. *Fax:* 906-227-1658. *E-mail:* kschuili@nmu.edu.

GRADUATE PROGRAMS

Financial Aid 90% of graduate students in nursing programs received some form of financial aid in 2004–05. Career-related internships or fieldwork, Federal Work-Study, institutionally sponsored loans, and unspecified assistantships available. Aid available to part-time students. *Financial aid application deadline:* 3/1.

Contact Prof. Mary A. Wallace, Coordinator of MSN Program, College of Nursing and Allied Health Science, Northern Michigan University, 2310 New Science Facility, Marquette, MI 49855. *Telephone:* 906-227-2487. *Fax:* 906-227-1658. *E-mail:* mwallace@nmu.eduh.

MASTER'S DEGREE PROGRAM

Degree MSN

Available Programs Master's.

Concentrations Available *Nurse practitioner programs in:* family health.

Study Options Part-time.

Program Entrance Requirements Clinical experience, computer literacy, minimum overall college GPA of 3.0, transcript of college record, CPR certification, written essay, immunizations, 2 letters of recommendation, physical assessment course, professional liability insurance/malpractice insurance, GRE General Test. *Application deadline:* For spring admission, 11/1. Applications are processed on a rolling basis. *Application fee:* $25.

Advanced Placement Credit given for nursing courses completed elsewhere dependent upon specific evaluations.

Degree Requirements 45 total credit hours, thesis or project, comprehensive exam.

POST-MASTER'S PROGRAM

Areas of Study *Nurse practitioner programs in:* family health.

CONTINUING EDUCATION PROGRAM

Contact Dr. Cynthia A. Prosen, Dean of Graduate Studies and Research, College of Nursing and Allied Health Science, Northern Michigan University, 401 Cohodas Administration Center, Marquette, MI 49855. *Telephone:* 906-227-2300. *E-mail:* cprosen@nmu.edu.

Oakland University
School of Nursing
Rochester, Michigan

http://www2.oakland.edu/nursing

Founded in 1957

DEGREES • BSN • MSN

Nursing Program Faculty 44 (50% with doctorates).

Baccalaureate Enrollment 462
Women 89% **Men** 11% **Minority** 12% **Part-time** 29%

Graduate Enrollment 123
Women 79% **Men** 21% **Minority** 11% **International** 1% **Part-time** 35%

Nursing Student Activities Nursing Honor Society, Sigma Theta Tau, Student Nurses' Association.

Nursing Student Resources Academic advising; academic or career counseling; assistance for students with disabilities; bookstore; campus computer network; career placement assistance; computer lab; computer-assisted instruction; e-mail services; employment services for current students; externships; housing assistance; interactive nursing skills videos; Internet; learning resource lab; library services; nursing audiovisuals; paid internships; placement services for program completers; remedial services; resume preparation assistance; skills, simulation, or other laboratory; tutoring; unpaid internships.

Library Facilities 2.1 million volumes (12,652 in health, 2,780 in nursing); 11,896 periodical subscriptions (375 health-care related).

BACCALAUREATE PROGRAMS

Degree BSN

Available Programs Generic Baccalaureate; RN Baccalaureate.

Site Options Royal Oak, MI.

Study Options Full-time and part-time.

Program Entrance Requirements Minimum overall college GPA of 3.0, transcript of college record, CPR certification, health exam, high school biology, high school chemistry, 2 years high school math, 1 year of high school science, high school transcript, immunizations, minimum high school GPA of 3.0, minimum GPA in nursing prerequisites of 3.0, professional liability insurance/malpractice insurance, prerequisite course work. Transfer students are accepted. **Standardized tests** *Required:* TOEFL for international students. *Recommended:* SAT or ACT. **Application** *Deadline:* rolling (freshmen), rolling (out-of-state freshmen), rolling (transfer). *Notification:* continuous (freshmen), continuous (out-of-state freshmen). *Application fee:* $40.

Advanced Placement Credit given for nursing courses completed elsewhere dependent upon specific evaluations.

Contact *Telephone:* 248-370-4065. *Fax:* 248-370-4279.

GRADUATE PROGRAMS

Contact *Telephone:* 248-370-4082. *Fax:* 248-370-2996.

MASTER'S DEGREE PROGRAM

Degree MSN

Available Programs Master's.

Concentrations Available Nurse anesthesia; nursing education. *Nurse practitioner programs in:* adult health, family health, gerontology.

Oakland University (continued)
Site Options Royal Oak, MI.
Study Options Full-time and part-time.
Program Entrance Requirements Clinical experience, minimum overall college GPA of 3.0, transcript of college record, CPR certification, written essay, immunizations, interview, 2 letters of recommendation, professional liability insurance/malpractice insurance, prerequisite course work, GRE General Test. *Application fee:* $30.
Advanced Placement Credit given for nursing courses completed elsewhere dependent upon specific evaluations.
Degree Requirements 45 total credit hours, thesis or project.

POST-MASTER'S PROGRAM

Areas of Study Nurse anesthesia; nursing education. *Nurse practitioner programs in:* adult health, family health, gerontology.

CONTINUING EDUCATION PROGRAM

Contact *Telephone:* 248-370-4013. *Fax:* 248-370-4279.

Saginaw Valley State University
Crystal M. Lange College of Nursing and Health Sciences
University Center, Michigan

http://www.svsu.edu/acadprog/nhs/
Founded in 1963
DEGREES • BSN • MSN
Nursing Program Faculty 12 (50% with doctorates).
Nursing Student Activities Sigma Theta Tau, Student Nurses' Association.
Nursing Student Resources Academic advising; academic or career counseling; assistance for students with disabilities; bookstore; campus computer network; career placement assistance; computer lab; computer-assisted instruction; e-mail services; externships; interactive nursing skills videos; Internet; learning resource lab; library services; nursing audiovisuals; remedial services; resume preparation assistance; skills, simulation, or other laboratory; tutoring.
Library Facilities 641,190 volumes; 11,770 periodical subscriptions.

BACCALAUREATE PROGRAMS

Degree BSN
Available Programs Accelerated Baccalaureate for Second Degree; Baccalaureate for Second Degree; Generic Baccalaureate; RN Baccalaureate.
Site Options *Distance Learning:* Tawas, MI; Cass City, MI; Mt. Pleasant, MI.
Study Options Full-time and part-time.
Program Entrance Requirements Minimum overall college GPA of 2.5, transcript of college record, CPR certification, written essay, health exam, immunizations, interview, minimum GPA in nursing prerequisites of 2.5, professional liability insurance/malpractice insurance, prerequisite course work. Transfer students are accepted. **Standardized tests** *Required:* ACT, TOEFL for international students. **Application** *Deadline:* rolling (freshmen), rolling (transfer). *Notification:* continuous (freshmen). *Application fee:* $25.
Advanced Placement Credit by examination available. Credit given for nursing courses completed elsewhere dependent upon specific evaluations.
Contact *Telephone:* 989-964-4145 Ext. 4145. *Fax:* 989-964-4024.

GRADUATE PROGRAMS

Contact *Telephone:* 989-964-4145 Ext. 4145. *Fax:* 989-964-4024.

MASTER'S DEGREE PROGRAM

Degree MSN
Available Programs Master's; RN to Master's.
Concentrations Available Nursing administration; nursing education; nursing informatics. *Nurse practitioner programs in:* family health.

Study Options Full-time and part-time.
Program Entrance Requirements Clinical experience, minimum overall college GPA of 3.0, transcript of college record, written essay, interview, 3 letters of recommendation, professional liability insurance/malpractice insurance, resume, statistics course, GRE. *Application deadline:* Applications are processed on a rolling basis. *Application fee:* $25.
Advanced Placement Credit given for nursing courses completed elsewhere dependent upon specific evaluations.
Degree Requirements 39 total credit hours, thesis or project.

POST-MASTER'S PROGRAM

Areas of Study Nursing administration; nursing education; nursing informatics. *Nurse practitioner programs in:* family health.

CONTINUING EDUCATION PROGRAM

Contact *Telephone:* 989-964-4145.

Spring Arbor University
Program in Nursing
Spring Arbor, Michigan

http://www.arbor.edu/bsn
Founded in 1873
DEGREE • BSN
Nursing Program Faculty 21 (10% with doctorates).
Baccalaureate Enrollment 38
Nursing Student Resources Academic advising; campus computer network; Internet; library services; nursing audiovisuals; other.
Library Facilities 111,736 volumes (1,000 in health, 350 in nursing); 665 periodical subscriptions (25 health-care related).

BACCALAUREATE PROGRAMS

Degree BSN
Available Programs ADN to Baccalaureate.
Site Options Battle Creek, MI; Jackson, MI; Toledo, OH.
Program Entrance Requirements Minimum overall college GPA of 2.5, transcript of college record, written essay, high school biology, high school chemistry, 1 year of high school math, 2 years high school science, high school transcript, minimum GPA in nursing prerequisites of 2.5, RN licensure. **Standardized tests** *Required:* SAT or ACT, TOEFL for international students. *Recommended:* ACT. **Application** *Deadline:* 8/1 (freshmen), 8/1 (out-of-state freshmen), rolling (transfer). *Notification:* continuous (freshmen), continuous (out-of-state freshmen). *Application fee:* $30.
Contact *Telephone:* 517-750-6344. *Fax:* 517-750-6602.

University of Detroit Mercy
McAuley School of Nursing
Detroit, Michigan

http://www.udmercy.edu/healthprof/nursing/
Founded in 1877
DEGREES • BSN • MSN
Nursing Program Faculty 28.
Baccalaureate Enrollment 630
Women 93% **Men** 7% **Minority** 17% **International** 3% **Part-time** 76%
Graduate Enrollment 37
Women 97% **Men** 3% **Minority** 28% **Part-time** 89%
Nursing Student Activities Sigma Theta Tau, Student Nurses' Association.
Nursing Student Resources Academic advising; academic or career counseling; bookstore; campus computer network; career placement assistance; computer lab; computer-assisted instruction; e-mail services; Internet; learning resource lab; library services; nursing audiovisuals; other;

paid internships; placement services for program completers; remedial services; resume preparation assistance; skills, simulation, or other laboratory; tutoring.

Library Facilities 21,436 volumes in health, 3,100 volumes in nursing; 9,340 periodical subscriptions (585 health-care related).

BACCALAUREATE PROGRAMS

Degree BSN

Available Programs Generic Baccalaureate; RN Baccalaureate.

Site Options Dearborn, MI; Wayne, MI; Royal Oak, MI.

Study Options Full-time and part-time.

Program Entrance Requirements Minimum overall college GPA of 2.5, transcript of college record, CPR certification, health exam, health insurance, high school biology, high school chemistry, 2 years high school math, 2 years high school science, high school transcript, immunizations, minimum high school GPA of 2.5, minimum GPA in nursing prerequisites of 2.5, prerequisite course work. Transfer students are accepted. **Standardized tests** *Required:* SAT or ACT. **Application** *Deadline:* rolling (freshmen), rolling (transfer). *Notification:* continuous (freshmen). *Application fee:* $25.

Advanced Placement Credit given for nursing courses completed elsewhere dependent upon specific evaluations.

Expenses (2005–06) *Tuition:* full-time $21,900; part-time $535 per credit hour. *International tuition:* $21,900 full-time. *Room and board:* $7328; room only: $4288 per academic year. *Required fees:* full-time $570; part-time $185 per term.

Financial Aid 51% of baccalaureate students in nursing programs received some form of financial aid in 2004–05.

Contact Denise Williams, Admissions Office, McAuley School of Nursing, University of Detroit Mercy, 4001 West McNichols Road, Detroit, MI 48221-3038. *Telephone:* 313-993-1245. *Fax:* 313-993-3325. *E-mail:* admissions@udmercy.edu.

GRADUATE PROGRAMS

Expenses (2005–06) *Tuition:* full-time $14,670; part-time $815 per credit hour. *International tuition:* $14,670 full-time. *Room and board:* $7328; room only: $4288 per academic year. *Required fees:* full-time $570; part-time $185 per term.

Financial Aid 90% of graduate students in nursing programs received some form of financial aid in 2004–05.

Contact Janet Bairdi, McAuley School of Nursing, University of Detroit Mercy, 4001 West McNichols Road, Detroit, MI 48221-3038. *Telephone:* 313-993-6423. *Fax:* 313-993-6175. *E-mail:* baiardjm@udmercy.edu.

MASTER'S DEGREE PROGRAM

Degree MSN

Available Programs Accelerated AD/RN to Master's; Master's; Master's for Nurses with Non-Nursing Degrees.

Concentrations Available Nursing administration. *Nurse practitioner programs in:* family health.

Study Options Full-time and part-time.

Program Entrance Requirements Clinical experience, minimum overall college GPA of 3.0, transcript of college record, CPR certification, immunizations, interview, 3 letters of recommendation, resume.

Degree Requirements 50 total credit hours.

POST-MASTER'S PROGRAM

Areas of Study Nursing administration. *Nurse practitioner programs in:* family health.

University of Michigan
School of Nursing
Ann Arbor, Michigan

http://www.nursing.umich.edu

Founded in 1817

DEGREES • BSN • MS • MSN/MBA • MSN/MPH • PHD

Nursing Program Faculty 115 (38% with doctorates).

Baccalaureate Enrollment 610
Women 93% **Men** 7% **Minority** 12% **International** 1% **Part-time** 17%
Graduate Enrollment 245
Women 94.5% **Men** 5.5% **Minority** 23% **International** 7% **Part-time** 58%

Nursing Student Activities Nursing Honor Society, Sigma Theta Tau, Student Nurses' Association, nursing club.

Nursing Student Resources Academic advising; academic or career counseling; assistance for students with disabilities; bookstore; campus computer network; career placement assistance; computer lab; computer-assisted instruction; daycare for children of students; e-mail services; employment services for current students; externships; housing assistance; interactive nursing skills videos; Internet; learning resource lab; library services; nursing audiovisuals; paid internships; placement services for program completers; remedial services; resume preparation assistance; skills, simulation, or other laboratory; tutoring; unpaid internships.

Library Facilities 8 million volumes (1.2 million in nursing); 67,554 periodical subscriptions.

BACCALAUREATE PROGRAMS

Degree BSN

Available Programs Accelerated Baccalaureate for Second Degree; Generic Baccalaureate; RN Baccalaureate.

Site Options Kalamazoo, MI; Traverse City, MI.

Study Options Full-time and part-time.

Program Entrance Requirements Minimum overall college GPA of 3.0, transcript of college record, written essay, high school chemistry, 2 years high school math, 2 years high school science, high school transcript, minimum high school GPA of 3.0, prerequisite course work. Transfer students are accepted. **Standardized tests** *Required:* SAT or ACT, TOEFL for international students. *Required for some:* SAT Subject Tests. **Application** *Deadline:* 2/1 (freshmen), 3/1 (transfer). *Notification:* continuous until 4/1 (freshmen). *Application fee:* $40.

Advanced Placement Credit given for nursing courses completed elsewhere dependent upon specific evaluations.

Expenses (2006–07) *Tuition, area resident:* full-time $9534; part-time $710 per credit hour. *Tuition, state resident:* full-time $9534; part-time $369 per credit hour. *Tuition, nonresident:* full-time $28,942; part-time $762 per credit hour. *International tuition:* $28,942 full-time. *Required fees:* full-time $185.

Financial Aid 60% of baccalaureate students in nursing programs received some form of financial aid in 2005–06.

Contact Sheila Pantlind, Admissions Counselor, School of Nursing, University of Michigan, 1220 Student Activities Building, Ann Arbor, MI 48109. *Telephone:* 734-647-1443. *Fax:* 734-936-0740. *E-mail:* pantlin@umich.edu.

GRADUATE PROGRAMS

Expenses (2006–07) *Tuition, area resident:* full-time $15,266; part-time $1152 per credit hour. *Tuition, state resident:* full-time $15,266; part-time $811 per credit hour. *Tuition, nonresident:* full-time $30,898; part-time $2020 per credit hour. *International tuition:* $30,898 full-time. *Required fees:* full-time $180.

Financial Aid 80% of graduate students in nursing programs received some form of financial aid in 2005–06. 15 research assistantships with full and partial tuition reimbursements available, 28 teaching assistantships with full tuition reimbursements available were awarded; fellowships with full and partial tuition reimbursements available, Federal Work-Study, institutionally sponsored loans, scholarships, traineeships, and tuition waivers (partial) also available. Aid available to part-time students.

Contact Dr. Carol J. Loveland-Cherry, Professor and Executive Associate Dean, Academic Affairs, School of Nursing, University of Michigan, 400 North Ingalls Building, Room 1154, Ann Arbor, MI 48109-0482. *Telephone:* 734-764-7188. *Fax:* 734-647-1419. *E-mail:* loveland@umich.edu.

MASTER'S DEGREE PROGRAM

Degrees MS; MSN/MBA; MSN/MPH

Available Programs Accelerated RN to Master's; Master's; RN to Master's.

Concentrations Available Health-care administration; nurse-midwifery; nursing administration; nursing informatics. *Clinical nurse specialist programs in:* community health, gerontology, home health care, medical-surgical, occupational health, psychiatric/mental health. *Nurse practitioner programs in:* acute care, adult health, family health, gerontology, pediatric, primary care, psychiatric/mental health.

University of Michigan (continued)

Study Options Full-time and part-time.

Program Entrance Requirements Computer literacy, minimum overall college GPA of 3.0, transcript of college record, written essay, interview, 3 letters of recommendation, resume, GRE General Test. *Application deadline:* For fall admission, 2/1 (priority date); for winter admission, 5/1 (priority date); for spring admission, 11/1 (priority date). Applications are processed on a rolling basis. *Application fee:* $55.

Advanced Placement Credit given for nursing courses completed elsewhere dependent upon specific evaluations.

Degree Requirements 36 total credit hours, thesis or project.

POST-MASTER'S PROGRAM

Areas of Study Health-care administration; nurse-midwifery; nursing administration; nursing informatics. *Clinical nurse specialist programs in:* community health, gerontology, home health care, medical-surgical, occupational health, psychiatric/mental health, women's health. *Nurse practitioner programs in:* acute care, adult health, family health, gerontology, pediatric, primary care, psychiatric/mental health, women's health.

DOCTORAL DEGREE PROGRAM

Degree PhD

Available Programs Doctorate; Post-Baccalaureate Doctorate.

Areas of Study Advanced practice nursing, aging, bio-behavioral research, biology of health and illness, community health, critical care, ethics, family health, gerontology, health policy, health promotion/disease prevention, health-care systems, individualized study, information systems, neuro-behavior, nursing administration, nursing policy, nursing research, nursing science, women's health.

Program Entrance Requirements Minimum overall college GPA of 3.0, interview, 3 letters of recommendation, scholarly papers, vita, writing sample, GRE General Test. *Application deadline:* For fall admission, 2/1 (priority date); for winter admission, 5/1 (priority date); for spring admission, 11/1 (priority date). Applications are processed on a rolling basis. *Application fee:* $55.

Degree Requirements 50 total credit hours, dissertation, oral exam, written exam, residency.

POSTDOCTORAL PROGRAM

Areas of Study Addiction/substance abuse, aging, chronic illness, community health, family health, gerontology, health promotion/disease prevention, individualized study, information systems, neuro-behavior, nursing interventions, nursing research, nursing science, vulnerable population, women's health.

Postdoctoral Program Contact Dr. Richard Redman, Director, Doctoral and Postdoctoral Studies, School of Nursing, University of Michigan, 400 North Ingalls Building, Room 1305, Ann Arbor, MI 48109-0482. *Telephone:* 734-764-9454. *Fax:* 734-763-6668. *E-mail:* rwr@umich.edu.

See full description on page 546.

University of Michigan–Flint
Department of Nursing
Flint, Michigan

http://www.umflint.edu/nur

Founded in 1956

DEGREES • BSN • MSN

Nursing Program Faculty 54 (17% with doctorates).

Baccalaureate Enrollment 294

Women 92% **Men** 8% **Minority** 11% **Part-time** 26%

Graduate Enrollment 39

Women 99.97% **Men** .03% **Minority** 13% **Part-time** 100%

Nursing Student Activities Nursing Honor Society, Sigma Theta Tau, Student Nurses' Association.

Nursing Student Resources Academic advising; academic or career counseling; assistance for students with disabilities; bookstore; campus computer network; career placement assistance; computer lab; computer-assisted instruction; daycare for children of students; e-mail services;

employment services for current students; externships; interactive nursing skills videos; Internet; library services; nursing audiovisuals; remedial services; resume preparation assistance; skills, simulation, or other laboratory; tutoring.

Library Facilities 253,182 volumes (10,982 in health, 5,443 in nursing); 900 periodical subscriptions (210 health-care related).

BACCALAUREATE PROGRAMS

Degree BSN

Available Programs Baccalaureate for Second Degree; Generic Baccalaureate; RN Baccalaureate.

Site Options *Distance Learning:* Flint, MI.

Study Options Full-time.

Program Entrance Requirements Minimum overall college GPA of 2.75, transcript of college record, CPR certification, written essay, health exam, health insurance, immunizations, 2 letters of recommendation, minimum GPA in nursing prerequisites of 2.75, prerequisite course work. Transfer students are accepted. **Standardized tests** *Required:* SAT or ACT, TOEFL for international students. **Application** *Deadline:* 8/19 (transfer). *Notification:* continuous (freshmen). *Application fee:* $30.

Advanced Placement Credit given for nursing courses completed elsewhere dependent upon specific evaluations.

Expenses (2006–07) *Tuition, state resident:* full-time $6216; part-time $259 per credit. *Tuition, nonresident:* full-time $12,432; part-time $518 per credit. *International tuition:* $12,432 full-time. *Required fees:* full-time $334; part-time $258 per term.

Financial Aid 54% of baccalaureate students in nursing programs received some form of financial aid in 2005–06.

Contact Mrs. Carol Hall, Secretary, Nursing Development and Research, Department of Nursing, University of Michigan–Flint, 303 East Kearsley, Flint, MI 48502-1950. *Telephone:* 810-762-3420. *Fax:* 810-766-6851. *E-mail:* nursing@list.flint.umich.edu.

GRADUATE PROGRAMS

Expenses (2006–07) *Tuition, state resident:* part-time $377 per credit hour. *Tuition, nonresident:* part-time $566 per credit hour. *Required fees:* part-time $129 per term.

Financial Aid 39% of graduate students in nursing programs received some form of financial aid in 2005–06.

Contact Ms. Margaret A. Hathaway, Administrative Specialist, Department of Nursing, University of Michigan–Flint, 303 East Kearsley, Flint, MI 48502-1950. *Telephone:* 810-762-3420. *Fax:* 810-766-6851. *E-mail:* nursing@list.flint.umich.edu.

MASTER'S DEGREE PROGRAM

Degree MSN

Available Programs Master's; RN to Master's.

Concentrations Available *Nurse practitioner programs in:* adult health, family health, psychiatric/mental health.

Site Options *Distance Learning:* Flint, MI.

Study Options Part-time.

Program Entrance Requirements Minimum overall college GPA of 3.0, transcript of college record, CPR certification, written essay, immunizations, interview, 3 letters of recommendation, physical assessment course, professional liability insurance/malpractice insurance, prerequisite course work, resume, statistics course.

Advanced Placement Credit by examination available. Credit given for nursing courses completed elsewhere dependent upon specific evaluations.

Degree Requirements 40 total credit hours, thesis or project.

CONTINUING EDUCATION PROGRAM

Contact Mrs. Carol Hall, Secretary, Nursing Development and Research, Department of Nursing, University of Michigan–Flint, 303 East Kearsley, Flint, MI 48502-1950. *Telephone:* 810-762-3420. *Fax:* 810-766-6851. *E-mail:* nursing@list.flint.umich.edu.

University of Phoenix–Metro Detroit Campus

College of Health and Human Services
Southfield, Michigan

DEGREES • BSN • MSN • MSN/MBA • MSN/MHA

Nursing Program Faculty 86 (31% with doctorates).

Baccalaureate Enrollment 78
Women 93.59% **Men** 6.41% **Minority** 51.28%

Graduate Enrollment 112
Women 91.07% **Men** 8.93% **Minority** 53.57%

Nursing Student Activities Sigma Theta Tau.

Nursing Student Resources Academic advising; academic or career counseling; assistance for students with disabilities; bookstore; computer lab; library services.

Library Facilities 444 volumes; 666 periodical subscriptions.

BACCALAUREATE PROGRAMS

Degree BSN

Available Programs Accelerated Baccalaureate.

Site Options Ann Arbor, MI; Livonia, MI; Southfield, MI.

Study Options Full-time.

Program Entrance Requirements Transcript of college record, 1 letter of recommendation, RN licensure. Transfer students are accepted. **Standardized tests** *Required:* TOEFL for international students. **Application** *Deadline:* rolling (freshmen), rolling (transfer). *Application fee:* $110.

Advanced Placement Credit by examination available. Credit given for nursing courses completed elsewhere dependent upon specific evaluations.

Expenses (2006–07) *Tuition:* full-time $11,700. *International tuition:* $11,700 full-time. *Required fees:* full-time $750.

Contact Campus College Chair, Nursing, College of Health and Human Services, University of Phoenix–Metro Detroit Campus, 5480 Corporate Drive, Suite 240, Troy, MI 48098-2623. *Telephone:* 800-834-2438.

GRADUATE PROGRAMS

Expenses (2006–07) *Tuition:* full-time $11,880. *International tuition:* $11,880 full-time. *Required fees:* full-time $760.

Contact Campus College Chair, Nursing, College of Health and Human Services, University of Phoenix–Metro Detroit Campus, 5480 Corporate Drive, Suite 240, Troy, MI 48098-2623. *Telephone:* 800-834-2438.

MASTER'S DEGREE PROGRAM

Degrees MSN; MSN/MBA; MSN/MHA

Available Programs Master's.

Concentrations Available Health-care administration; nursing administration; nursing education.

Site Options Ann Arbor, MI; Livonia, MI; Southfield, MI.

Study Options Full-time.

Program Entrance Requirements Clinical experience, computer literacy, minimum overall college GPA of 2.5, transcript of college record. *Application deadline:* Applications are processed on a rolling basis. *Application fee:* $110.

Degree Requirements 39 total credit hours, thesis or project.

University of Phoenix–West Michigan Campus

College of Health and Human Services
Grand Rapids, Michigan

Founded in 2000

DEGREES • BSN • MSN

Nursing Program Faculty 37 (22% with doctorates).

Baccalaureate Enrollment 23
Women 100%

Graduate Enrollment 15
Women 86.67% **Men** 13.33% **Minority** 13.33%

Nursing Student Activities Sigma Theta Tau.

Nursing Student Resources Academic advising; academic or career counseling; assistance for students with disabilities; bookstore; computer lab; library services.

Library Facilities 444 volumes; 666 periodical subscriptions.

BACCALAUREATE PROGRAMS

Degree BSN

Available Programs Accelerated Baccalaureate.

Site Options Portage, MI; East Lansing, MI.

Study Options Full-time.

Program Entrance Requirements Transcript of college record, 1 letter of recommendation, RN licensure. Transfer students are accepted. **Standardized tests** *Required:* TOEFL for international students. **Application** *Deadline:* rolling (freshmen), rolling (transfer). *Application fee:* $110.

Advanced Placement Credit by examination available. Credit given for nursing courses completed elsewhere dependent upon specific evaluations.

Expenses (2006–07) *Tuition:* full-time $11,400. *International tuition:* $11,400 full-time. *Required fees:* full-time $750.

Contact Campus College Chair, Nursing, College of Health and Human Services, University of Phoenix–West Michigan Campus, 318 River Ridge Drive NW, Grand Rapids, MI 49544-1683. *Telephone:* 888-345-9699.

GRADUATE PROGRAMS

Expenses (2006–07) *Tuition:* full-time $11,640. *International tuition:* $11,640 full-time. *Required fees:* full-time $760.

Contact Campus College Chair, Nursing, College of Health and Human Services, University of Phoenix–West Michigan Campus, 318 River Ridge Drive NW, Grand Rapids, MI 49544-1683. *Telephone:* 888-345-9699.

MASTER'S DEGREE PROGRAM

Degree MSN

Available Programs Master's.

Concentrations Available Health-care administration; nursing administration.

Site Options Portage, MI; East Lansing, MI.

Study Options Full-time.

Program Entrance Requirements Clinical experience, computer literacy, minimum overall college GPA of 2.5, transcript of college record. *Application deadline:* Applications are processed on a rolling basis. *Application fee:* $110.

Advanced Placement Credit given for nursing courses completed elsewhere dependent upon specific evaluations.

Degree Requirements 39 total credit hours, thesis or project.

Wayne State University

College of Nursing
Detroit, Michigan

http://www.nursing.wayne.edu

Founded in 1868

DEGREES • BSN • MSN • PHD

Nursing Program Faculty 83 (39% with doctorates).

Baccalaureate Enrollment 420
Women 90% **Men** 10% **Minority** 39% **International** 1% **Part-time** 25%

Graduate Enrollment 160
Women 93% **Men** 7% **Minority** 23% **International** 10% **Part-time** 60%

Nursing Student Activities Nursing Honor Society, Sigma Theta Tau, Student Nurses' Association, nursing club.

Wayne State University (continued)

Nursing Student Resources Academic advising; academic or career counseling; bookstore; campus computer network; career placement assistance; computer lab; computer-assisted instruction; e-mail services; employment services for current students; interactive nursing skills videos; Internet; learning resource lab; library services; nursing audiovisuals; placement services for program completers; resume preparation assistance; skills, simulation, or other laboratory.

Library Facilities 1.9 million volumes (500,000 in health, 23,000 in nursing); 18,645 periodical subscriptions (5,000 health-care related).

BACCALAUREATE PROGRAMS

Degree BSN

Available Programs Accelerated Baccalaureate for Second Degree; Generic Baccalaureate; RN Baccalaureate.

Site Options Farmington Hills, MI. *Distance Learning:* Detroit, MI; Clinton Township, MI.

Study Options Full-time.

Program Entrance Requirements Minimum overall college GPA of 2.0, transcript of college record, written essay, high school transcript, minimum high school GPA of 2.8, minimum GPA in nursing prerequisites of 2.5, prerequisite course work. Transfer students are accepted. **Standardized tests** *Required:* SAT or ACT, TOEFL for international students. **Application** *Deadline:* 8/1 (freshmen), 8/1 (transfer). *Notification:* continuous until 9/1 (freshmen). *Application fee:* $30.

Expenses (2006–07) *Tuition, state resident:* full-time $4962; part-time $236 per credit hour. *Tuition, nonresident:* full-time $11,411; part-time $543 per credit hour. *International tuition:* $11,411 full-time. *Room and board:* $6680; room only: $4280 per academic year. *Required fees:* full-time $1150; part-time $75 per credit.

Financial Aid 80% of baccalaureate students in nursing programs received some form of financial aid in 2005–06. *Gift aid (need-based):* Federal Pell, FSEOG, state, private, college/university gift aid from institutional funds. *Loans:* Federal Nursing Student Loans, FFEL (Subsidized and Unsubsidized Stafford PLUS), Perkins, state, college/university. *Work-Study:* Federal Work-Study, part-time campus jobs. *Application deadline (priority):* 3/1.

Contact Ms. Moira A. Fracassa, Academic Services Officer, College of Nursing, Wayne State University, 10 Cohn Building, 5557 Cass Avenue, Detroit, MI 48202. *Telephone:* 313-577-4082. *Fax:* 313-577-6949. *E-mail:* moira.f@wayne.edu.

GRADUATE PROGRAMS

Expenses (2006–07) *Tuition, state resident:* full-time $6632; part-time $415 per credit. *Tuition, nonresident:* full-time $13,538; part-time $846 per credit. *International tuition:* $13,538 full-time. *Room and board:* $6680; room only: $4280 per academic year. *Required fees:* full-time $250; part-time $25 per credit.

Financial Aid 60% of graduate students in nursing programs received some form of financial aid in 2005–06. 2 fellowships with tuition reimbursements available, 6 research assistantships with tuition reimbursements available (averaging $14,773 per year), 1 teaching assistantship (averaging $14,998 per year) were awarded; Federal Work-Study, institutionally sponsored loans, scholarships, and traineeships also available. Aid available to part-time students. *Financial aid application deadline:* 7/1.

Contact Mr. Robert G. Hellar, Academic Advisor, College of Nursing, Wayne State University, 10 Cohn Building, 5557 Cass Avenue, Detroit, MI 48202. *Telephone:* 313-577-4082. *Fax:* 313-577-6949. *E-mail:* ac4659@wayne.edu.

MASTER'S DEGREE PROGRAM

Degree MSN

Available Programs Accelerated AD/RN to Master's; Master's.

Concentrations Available Nurse-midwifery. *Clinical nurse specialist programs in:* acute care, community health, psychiatric/mental health. *Nurse practitioner programs in:* acute care, gerontology, neonatal health, pediatric, primary care, women's health.

Site Options *Distance Learning:* Detroit, MI; Clinton Township, MI.

Study Options Full-time and part-time.

Program Entrance Requirements Minimum overall college GPA of 3.0, transcript of college record, written essay, 3 letters of recommendation, resume, GRE General Test. *Application deadline:* Applications are processed on a rolling basis. *Application fee:* $30 ($50 for international students).

Advanced Placement Credit given for nursing courses completed elsewhere dependent upon specific evaluations.

Degree Requirements 46 total credit hours.

POST-MASTER'S PROGRAM

Areas of Study Nurse-midwifery. *Clinical nurse specialist programs in:* psychiatric/mental health. *Nurse practitioner programs in:* acute care, gerontology, neonatal health, pediatric, primary care, psychiatric/mental health, women's health.

DOCTORAL DEGREE PROGRAM

Degree PhD

Available Programs Doctorate; Doctorate for Nurses with Non-Nursing Degrees; Post-Baccalaureate Doctorate.

Areas of Study Nursing research, nursing science, urban health.

Program Entrance Requirements Clinical experience, minimum overall college GPA of 3.3, interview by faculty committee, interview, 3 letters of recommendation, scholarly papers, vita, writing sample, GRE General Test. *Application deadline:* Applications are processed on a rolling basis. *Application fee:* $30 ($50 for international students).

Degree Requirements 90 total credit hours, dissertation, oral exam, written exam, residency.

POSTDOCTORAL PROGRAM

Areas of Study Self-care, vulnerable population.

Postdoctoral Program Contact Dr. Stephen Cavanagh, Associate Dean for Academic and Professional Affairs/Professor and Director of Doctoral and Postdoctoral Programs, College of Nursing, Wayne State University, 230 Cohn Building, 5557 Cass Avenue, Detroit, MI 48202. *Telephone:* 313-577-4138. *Fax:* 313-577-0414. *E-mail:* ad5949@wayne.edu.

CONTINUING EDUCATION PROGRAM

Contact Office of the Dean, College of Nursing, Wayne State University, 5557 Cass Avenue, Detroit, MI 48202. *Telephone:* 313-577-4070. *E-mail:* nursinginfo@wayne.edu.

See full description on page 576.

Western Michigan University
College of Health and Human Services
Kalamazoo, Michigan

Founded in 1903

DEGREE • BSN

Nursing Program Faculty 26 (31% with doctorates).

Baccalaureate Enrollment 377

Women 92% **Men** 8% **Minority** 9% **International** 1% **Part-time** 25%

Nursing Student Activities Nursing Honor Society, Student Nurses' Association.

Nursing Student Resources Academic advising; academic or career counseling; assistance for students with disabilities; bookstore; campus computer network; career placement assistance; computer lab; computer-assisted instruction; daycare for children of students; e-mail services; employment services for current students; externships; housing assistance; interactive nursing skills videos; Internet; learning resource lab; library services; nursing audiovisuals; placement services for program completers; remedial services; resume preparation assistance; skills, simulation, or other laboratory.

Library Facilities 4.5 million volumes (766 in nursing); 10,074 periodical subscriptions (362 health-care related).

BACCALAUREATE PROGRAMS

Degree BSN

Available Programs ADN to Baccalaureate; Baccalaureate for Second Degree; Generic Baccalaureate; RN Baccalaureate.

Site Options St. Joseph, MI.

Study Options Full-time and part-time.

Program Entrance Requirements Minimum overall college GPA of 2.8, transcript of college record, CPR certification, written essay, high school biology, high school chemistry, 3 years high school math, 2 years high school science, high school transcript, immunizations, minimum high school GPA of 2.8, minimum GPA in nursing prerequisites of 2.8, prerequisite course work. Transfer students are accepted. **Standardized tests** *Required:* SAT or ACT, TOEFL for international students. **Application** *Deadline:* rolling (freshmen), 8/1 (transfer). *Notification:* continuous (freshmen). *Application fee:* $35.

Advanced Placement Credit given for nursing courses completed elsewhere dependent upon specific evaluations.

Financial Aid 43% of baccalaureate students in nursing programs received some form of financial aid in 2005–06.

Contact Mrs. Marsha Ann Mahan, Student Advisor, College of Health and Human Services, Western Michigan University, 1903 West Michigan Avenue, Kalamazoo, MI 49008. *Telephone:* 269-387-8150. *Fax:* 269-387-8170. *E-mail:* marsha.mahan@wmich.edu.

MINNESOTA

Augsburg College
Program in Nursing
Minneapolis, Minnesota

http://www.augsburg.edu/nursing

Founded in 1869

DEGREES • BS • MA

Nursing Program Faculty 6 (50% with doctorates).

Baccalaureate Enrollment 169
Women 83% **Men** 17% **Part-time** 89%

Graduate Enrollment 42
Women 100% **Minority** 2% **Part-time** 90%

Nursing Student Resources Academic advising; academic or career counseling; assistance for students with disabilities; bookstore; campus computer network; computer lab; computer-assisted instruction; e-mail services; Internet; library services; tutoring.

Library Facilities 146,166 volumes (1,550 in health, 200 in nursing); 754 periodical subscriptions (70 health-care related).

BACCALAUREATE PROGRAMS

Degree BS

Available Programs ADN to Baccalaureate.

Site Options Rochester, MN; Saint Paul, MN.

Study Options Full-time and part-time.

Program Entrance Requirements Minimum overall college GPA of 2.5, transcript of college record, CPR certification, written essay, high school transcript, immunizations, letters of recommendation, professional liability insurance/malpractice insurance, prerequisite course work, RN licensure. Transfer students are accepted. **Standardized tests** *Required:* TOEFL for international students. *Recommended:* SAT or ACT. **Application** *Deadline:* 8/15 (freshmen), 8/15 (transfer). *Notification:* continuous (freshmen). *Application fee:* $25.

Contact Admissions Counselor, Program in Nursing, Augsburg College, 2211 Riverside Avenue South, CB 65, Minneapolis, MN 55454. *Telephone:* 612-330-1101. *Fax:* 612-330-1784. *E-mail:* wecinfo@augsburg.edu.

GRADUATE PROGRAMS

Contact Graduate Admissions Counselor, Program in Nursing, Augsburg College, 2211 Riverside Avenue South, CB 65, Minneapolis, MN 55454. *Telephone:* 612-330-1101. *Fax:* 612-330-1784. *E-mail:* manursing@augsburg.edu.

MASTER'S DEGREE PROGRAM

Degree MA

Available Programs Master's.

Concentrations Available *Clinical nurse specialist programs in:* community health.

Site Options Rochester, MN; Saint Paul, MN.

Study Options Full-time and part-time.

Program Entrance Requirements Computer literacy, minimum overall college GPA of 3.0, transcript of college record, written essay, immunizations, 3 letters of recommendation, professional liability insurance/malpractice insurance, prerequisite course work, statistics course.

Advanced Placement Credit given for nursing courses completed elsewhere dependent upon specific evaluations.

Degree Requirements 48 total credit hours, thesis or project.

Bemidji State University
Department of Nursing
Bemidji, Minnesota

Founded in 1919

DEGREE • BS

Nursing Program Faculty 4 (25% with doctorates).

Baccalaureate Enrollment 63
Women 95% **Men** 5% **Minority** 6% **Part-time** 87%

Nursing Student Resources Academic advising; academic or career counseling; assistance for students with disabilities; bookstore; campus computer network; career placement assistance; computer lab; computer-assisted instruction; daycare for children of students; e-mail services; employment services for current students; housing assistance; Internet; library services; nursing audiovisuals; remedial services.

Library Facilities 554,087 volumes (9,000 in health, 1,000 in nursing); 991 periodical subscriptions (300 health-care related).

BACCALAUREATE PROGRAMS

Degree BS

Available Programs RN Baccalaureate.

Site Options *Distance Learning:* Hibbing, MN; Duluth, MN; Brainerd, MN.

Study Options Full-time and part-time.

Program Entrance Requirements Minimum overall college GPA, transcript of college record, immunizations, professional liability insurance/malpractice insurance, RN licensure. Transfer students are accepted. **Standardized tests** *Required:* ACT, TOEFL for international students. **Application** *Deadline:* rolling (freshmen), rolling (transfer). *Notification:* continuous (freshmen). *Application fee:* $20.

Expenses (2006–07) *Tuition, state resident:* full-time $5500; part-time $230 per credit. *Tuition, nonresident:* full-time $5500; part-time $230 per credit. *International tuition:* $5500 full-time. *Room and board:* $5200; room only: $5200 per academic year. *Required fees:* full-time $770.

Financial Aid *Gift aid (need-based):* Federal Pell, FSEOG, state, private, college/university gift aid from institutional funds. *Loans:* Federal Direct (Subsidized and Unsubsidized Stafford PLUS), Perkins, state, Alaska Loans, Canada Student Loans, Norwest Collegiate Loans, CitiAssist Loans and other alternative loans. *Work-Study:* Federal Work-Study, part-time campus jobs. *Application deadline (priority):* 5/15.

Contact Ms. Jeanine E. Gangeness, Chair and Assistant Professor, Department of Nursing, Bemidji State University, Deputy Hall 105, #15, 1500 Birchmont Drive NE, Bemidji, MN 56601. *Telephone:* 218-755-3892. *Fax:* 218-755-4402. *E-mail:* jgangeness@bemidjistate.edu.

CONTINUING EDUCATION PROGRAM

Contact Ms. Jeanine E. Gangeness, Chair and Assistant Professor, Department of Nursing, Bemidji State University, Deputy Hall 105, #15, 1500 Birchmont Drive NE, Bemidji, MN 56601. *Telephone:* 218-755-3892. *Fax:* 218-755-4402. *E-mail:* jgangeness@bemidjistate.edu.

Bethel University
Department of Nursing
St. Paul, Minnesota

http://www.bethel.edu/college/dept/nursing/index.html

Founded in 1871

DEGREES • BSN • MA

Nursing Program Faculty 37 (30% with doctorates).

Baccalaureate Enrollment 255
Women 95.3% **Men** 4.7% **Minority** 11.3%

Graduate Enrollment 64
Women 99% **Men** 1% **Minority** 4.6%

Nursing Student Activities Sigma Theta Tau, nursing club.

Nursing Student Resources Academic advising; academic or career counseling; assistance for students with disabilities; bookstore; campus computer network; career placement assistance; computer lab; computer-assisted instruction; daycare for children of students; e-mail services; employment services for current students; interactive nursing skills videos; Internet; learning resource lab; library services; nursing audiovisuals; paid internships; placement services for program completers; remedial services; resume preparation assistance; skills, simulation, or other laboratory; tutoring.

Library Facilities 184,000 volumes (4,800 in nursing); 21,343 periodical subscriptions (110 health-care related).

BACCALAUREATE PROGRAMS
Degree BSN

Available Programs Generic Baccalaureate; RN Baccalaureate.
Site Options Brroklyn Park, MN.
Study Options Full-time and part-time.
Program Entrance Requirements Minimum overall college GPA of 2.5, transcript of college record, CPR certification, written essay, health exam, health insurance, high school transcript, immunizations, interview, 2 letters of recommendation, minimum GPA in nursing prerequisites of 2.5, professional liability insurance/malpractice insurance, prerequisite course work. Transfer students are accepted. **Standardized tests** *Required:* SAT or ACT, TOEFL for international students. **Application** *Deadline:* 8/1 (freshmen), 8/1 (transfer). *Early decision:* 11/1. *Notification:* continuous (freshmen), 12/15 (early action). *Application fee:* $25.
Advanced Placement Credit given for nursing courses completed elsewhere dependent upon specific evaluations.
Expenses (2006–07) *Tuition:* full-time $22,590; part-time $865 per credit. *Room and board:* $6260; room only: $4260 per academic year. *Required fees:* part-time $80 per term.
Financial Aid 80% of baccalaureate students in nursing programs received some form of financial aid in 2005–06. *Gift aid (need-based):* Federal Pell, FSEOG, state, private, college/university gift aid from institutional funds. *Loans:* FFEL (Subsidized and Unsubsidized Stafford PLUS), Perkins, state, alternative loans. *Work-Study:* Federal Work-Study, part-time campus jobs. *Application deadline (priority):* 4/15.
Contact Ms. Elizabeth A. Peterson, Director, Pre-Professional Program, Department of Nursing, Bethel University, 3900 Bethel Drive, St. Paul, MN 55112-6999. *Telephone:* 651-638-6455. *Fax:* 651-635-1965. *E-mail:* e-peterson@bethel.edu.

GRADUATE PROGRAMS
Expenses (2006–07) *Tuition:* part-time $395 per credit.
Financial Aid 30% of graduate students in nursing programs received some form of financial aid in 2005–06. Institutionally sponsored loans and scholarships available.
Contact Dr. Mary Alkire, EdD, Associate Professor, Department of Nursing, Bethel University, 3900 Bethel Drive, St. Paul, MN 55112. *Telephone:* 651-638-6189. *Fax:* 651-635-1965. *E-mail:* mary-reuland@bethel.edu.

MASTER'S DEGREE PROGRAM
Degree MA

Available Programs Master's.

Concentrations Available Nursing administration; nursing education.
Site Options *Distance Learning:* St. Paul, MN.
Study Options Full-time and part-time.
Program Entrance Requirements Clinical experience, computer literacy, minimum overall college GPA of 3.0, transcript of college record, written essay, immunizations, interview, 3 letters of recommendation, professional liability insurance/malpractice insurance, resume, statistics course, MAT. *Application deadline:* For fall admission, 3/20 (priority date). *Application fee:* $25.
Advanced Placement Credit given for nursing courses completed elsewhere dependent upon specific evaluations.
Degree Requirements 42 total credit hours, thesis or project.

CONTINUING EDUCATION PROGRAM
Contact Ms. Kaye Cusick, Professional Development Coordinator, Department of Nursing, Bethel University, 3900 Bethel Drive, St. Paul, MN 55112-6999. *Telephone:* 651-635-8013. *Fax:* 651-635-8004. *E-mail:* k-cusick@bethel.edu.

College of Saint Benedict
Department of Nursing
Saint Joseph, Minnesota

http://www.csbsju.edu/nursing/

Founded in 1887

DEGREE • BS

Nursing Program Faculty 18 (33% with doctorates).

Baccalaureate Enrollment 146
Women 86.4% **Men** 13.6% **Minority** 1% **Part-time** 2%

Nursing Student Activities Sigma Theta Tau, Student Nurses' Association, nursing club.

Nursing Student Resources Academic advising; academic or career counseling; assistance for students with disabilities; bookstore; campus computer network; career placement assistance; computer lab; computer-assisted instruction; e-mail services; interactive nursing skills videos; Internet; learning resource lab; library services; nursing audiovisuals; placement services for program completers; resume preparation assistance; skills, simulation, or other laboratory; tutoring.

Library Facilities 481,338 volumes (7,300 in health, 700 in nursing); 5,315 periodical subscriptions (335 health-care related).

BACCALAUREATE PROGRAMS
Degree BS

Available Programs Generic Baccalaureate.
Study Options Full-time.
Program Entrance Requirements Transcript of college record, CPR certification, written essay, health exam, health insurance, high school biology, high school chemistry, immunizations, 3 letters of recommendation, minimum GPA in nursing prerequisites of 2.5, professional liability insurance/malpractice insurance, prerequisite course work. **Standardized tests** *Required:* SAT or ACT, TOEFL for international students. **Application** *Deadline:* rolling (freshmen), rolling (transfer). *Notification:* continuous until 10/1 (freshmen).
Expenses (2006–07) *Tuition:* full-time $24,448; part-time $1020 per credit. *International tuition:* $24,448 full-time. *Room and board:* $6898; room only: $3546 per academic year. *Required fees:* full-time $691.
Financial Aid 90% of baccalaureate students in nursing programs received some form of financial aid in 2005–06. *Gift aid (need-based):* Federal Pell, FSEOG, state, private, college/university gift aid from institutional funds. *Loans:* FFEL (Subsidized and Unsubsidized Stafford PLUS), Perkins, state, alternative loans. *Work-Study:* Federal Work-Study, part-time campus jobs. *Application deadline (priority):* 3/15.
Contact Dr. Kathleen M. Twohy, Chairperson, Department of Nursing, College of Saint Benedict, 37 College Avenue South, St. Joseph, MN 56374. *Telephone:* 320-363-5404. *Fax:* 320-363-6099. *E-mail:* nursing@csbsju.edu.

College of St. Catherine
Department of Nursing
St. Paul, Minnesota

http://www.stkate.edu/offices/academic/nursing.nsf

Founded in 1905

DEGREES • BA • MA

Nursing Program Faculty 42 (43% with doctorates).

Baccalaureate Enrollment 258
Women 97% **Men** 3% **Minority** 22% **International** 2%

Graduate Enrollment 65
Women 100% **Minority** 15% **Part-time** 11%

Nursing Student Activities Nursing Honor Society, Sigma Theta Tau, Student Nurses' Association.

Nursing Student Resources Academic advising; academic or career counseling; assistance for students with disabilities; bookstore; campus computer network; career placement assistance; computer lab; computer-assisted instruction; daycare for children of students; e-mail services; employment services for current students; housing assistance; interactive nursing skills videos; Internet; learning resource lab; library services; nursing audiovisuals; remedial services; resume preparation assistance; skills, simulation, or other laboratory; tutoring; unpaid internships.

Library Facilities 263,495 volumes (71,172 in health, 17,920 in nursing); 1,141 periodical subscriptions (900 health-care related).

BACCALAUREATE PROGRAMS

Degree BA

Available Programs Baccalaureate for Second Degree; Generic Baccalaureate; RN Baccalaureate.

Site Options Minneapolis, MN.

Study Options Full-time.

Program Entrance Requirements Minimum overall college GPA of 2.75, transcript of college record, CPR certification, written essay, health insurance, immunizations, 2 letters of recommendation, minimum GPA in nursing prerequisites of 2.6, prerequisite course work. Transfer students are accepted. **Standardized tests** *Required:* SAT or ACT, TOEFL for international students. **Application** *Deadline:* rolling (freshmen), rolling (transfer). *Notification:* continuous (freshmen).

Expenses (2006–07) *Tuition:* full-time $24,128; part-time $754 per credit. *International tuition:* $24,128 full-time. *Room and board:* $6432; room only: $3592 per academic year. *Required fees:* full-time $260; part-time $130 per term.

Financial Aid 92% of baccalaureate students in nursing programs received some form of financial aid in 2005–06. *Gift aid (need-based):* Federal Pell, FSEOG, state, private, college/university gift aid from institutional funds, Federal Nursing. *Loans:* Federal Nursing Student Loans, FFEL (Subsidized and Unsubsidized Stafford PLUS), Perkins, state, alternative loans. *Work-Study:* Federal Work-Study, part-time campus jobs. *Application deadline (priority):* 4/15.

Contact Dr. Vicki Schug, Baccalaureate Program Director, Department of Nursing, College of St. Catherine, 2004 Randolph Avenue, St. Paul, MN 55105. *Telephone:* 651-690-6940. *Fax:* 651-690-6941. *E-mail:* vlschug@stkate.edu.

GRADUATE PROGRAMS

Expenses (2006–07) *Tuition:* part-time $608 per credit hour. *Room and board:* $6432; room only: $3592 per academic year. *Required fees:* full-time $60; part-time $30 per term.

Financial Aid 75% of graduate students in nursing programs received some form of financial aid in 2005–06.

Contact Dr. Jan S. Borman, Graduate Program Director, Department of Nursing, College of St. Catherine, 2004 Randolph Avenue, #4250, St. Paul, MN 55105. *Telephone:* 651-690-8817. *Fax:* 651-690-6941. *E-mail:* jsborman@stkate.edu.

MASTER'S DEGREE PROGRAM

Degree MA

Available Programs Master's.

Concentrations Available Nursing education. *Nurse practitioner programs in:* adult health, gerontology, neonatal health, pediatric.

Study Options Full-time and part-time.

Program Entrance Requirements Clinical experience, minimum overall college GPA of 3.0, transcript of college record, CPR certification, written essay, immunizations, interview, 3 letters of recommendation, professional liability insurance/malpractice insurance, statistics course.

Degree Requirements 40 total credit hours, thesis or project.

POST-MASTER'S PROGRAM

Areas of Study Nursing education. *Nurse practitioner programs in:* adult health, gerontology, neonatal health, pediatric.

The College of St. Scholastica
Department of Nursing
Duluth, Minnesota

http://www.css.edu

Founded in 1912

DEGREES • BA • MA

Nursing Program Faculty 29 (37% with doctorates).

Baccalaureate Enrollment 302
Women 89% **Men** 11% **Minority** 5% **Part-time** 14.5%

Graduate Enrollment 94
Women 97% **Men** 3% **Minority** 8% **International** 2% **Part-time** 83%

Nursing Student Activities Sigma Theta Tau, Student Nurses' Association.

Nursing Student Resources Academic advising; academic or career counseling; assistance for students with disabilities; bookstore; campus computer network; career placement assistance; computer lab; computer-assisted instruction; e-mail services; Internet; learning resource lab; library services; nursing audiovisuals; paid internships; placement services for program completers; resume preparation assistance; skills, simulation, or other laboratory; tutoring; unpaid internships.

Library Facilities 130,353 volumes (7,280 in health, 1,150 in nursing); 21,656 periodical subscriptions (291 health-care related).

BACCALAUREATE PROGRAMS

Degree BA

Available Programs Accelerated Baccalaureate for Second Degree; Accelerated RN Baccalaureate; Generic Baccalaureate.

Site Options Duluth, MN; St. Cloud, MN; Brainerd, MN.

Study Options Full-time and part-time.

Program Entrance Requirements Minimum overall college GPA of 3.0, transcript of college record, CPR certification, written essay, health exam, health insurance, high school transcript, immunizations, minimum GPA in nursing prerequisites of 2.0, prerequisite course work. Transfer students are accepted. **Standardized tests** *Required:* SAT or ACT, TOEFL for international students. **Application** *Deadline:* rolling (freshmen), rolling (transfer). *Notification:* continuous (freshmen). *Application fee:* $25.

Expenses (2006–07) *Tuition:* full-time $23,434. *International tuition:* $23,434 full-time. *Room and board:* $6514; room only: $4256 per academic year. *Required fees:* full-time $560; part-time $280 per term.

Financial Aid 98% of baccalaureate students in nursing programs received some form of financial aid in 2005–06. *Gift aid (need-based):* Federal Pell, FSEOG, state, private, college/university gift aid from institutional funds. *Loans:* Federal Nursing Student Loans, FFEL (Subsidized and Unsubsidized Stafford PLUS), Perkins, state, private supplemental loans. *Work-Study:* Federal Work-Study, part-time campus jobs. *Application deadline (priority):* 3/15.

Contact Ann Leja, RN, Chair, Department of Undergraduate Nursing, Department of Nursing, The College of St. Scholastica, 1200 Kenwood Avenue, Duluth, MN 55811. *Telephone:* 218-723-6020. *Fax:* 218-723-6472. *E-mail:* aleja@css.edu.

The College of St. Scholastica (continued)
GRADUATE PROGRAMS

Expenses (2006–07) *Tuition:* full-time $16,800; part-time $600 per credit. *International tuition:* $16,800 full-time. *Room and board:* $6514; room only: $4256 per academic year. *Required fees:* full-time $300; part-time $150 per term.

Financial Aid 90% of graduate students in nursing programs received some form of financial aid in 2005–06. Scholarships and traineeships available. Aid available to part-time students.

Contact Dr. Carleen Maynard, Chair, Graduate Nursing Department, Department of Nursing, The College of St. Scholastica, 1200 Kenwood Avenue, Duluth, MN 55811. *Telephone:* 218-723-6452. *Fax:* 218-723-6472. *E-mail:* cmaynard@css.edu.

MASTER'S DEGREE PROGRAM

Degree MA

Available Programs Master's.

Concentrations Available Nursing administration. *Clinical nurse specialist programs in:* adult health, gerontology. *Nurse practitioner programs in:* adult health, family health, gerontology, pediatric, psychiatric/mental health.

Site Options Duluth, MN.

Study Options Full-time and part-time.

Program Entrance Requirements Clinical experience, computer literacy, minimum overall college GPA of 3.0, transcript of college record, CPR certification, written essay, immunizations, interview, 3 letters of recommendation, nursing research course, physical assessment course, professional liability insurance/malpractice insurance, resume, statistics course, GRE General Test or MAT. *Application deadline:* For fall admission, 4/1 (priority date). Applications are processed on a rolling basis. *Application fee:* $50.

Advanced Placement Credit given for nursing courses completed elsewhere dependent upon specific evaluations.

Degree Requirements 47 total credit hours, thesis or project.

POST-MASTER'S PROGRAM

Areas of Study Nursing administration. *Clinical nurse specialist programs in:* adult health, gerontology. *Nurse practitioner programs in:* adult health, family health, gerontology, pediatric, psychiatric/mental health.

Concordia College
Department of Nursing
Moorhead, Minnesota

http://www.cord.edu/dept/nursing/index.htm
Founded in 1891
DEGREES • BA • MS

Nursing Program Faculty 6 (33% with doctorates).

Baccalaureate Enrollment 96
Women 94% **Men** 6% **Minority** 7%

Graduate Enrollment 2
Women 100%

Nursing Student Activities Sigma Theta Tau, Student Nurses' Association.

Nursing Student Resources Academic advising; academic or career counseling; assistance for students with disabilities; bookstore; campus computer network; career placement assistance; computer lab; computer-assisted instruction; e-mail services; employment services for current students; externships; Internet; learning resource lab; library services; nursing audiovisuals; paid internships; placement services for program completers; remedial services; resume preparation assistance; skills, simulation, or other laboratory; tutoring; unpaid internships.

Library Facilities 325,408 volumes (2,135 in health, 837 in nursing); 3,528 periodical subscriptions (81 health-care related).

BACCALAUREATE PROGRAMS

Degree BA

Available Programs Accelerated Baccalaureate for Second Degree; Generic Baccalaureate.

Study Options Full-time.

Program Entrance Requirements Minimum overall college GPA of 2.7, transcript of college record, written essay, health exam, health insurance, immunizations, 2 letters of recommendation, minimum GPA in nursing prerequisites of 2.7, prerequisite course work. Transfer students are accepted. **Standardized tests** *Required:* SAT or ACT, TOEFL for international students. **Application** *Deadline:* rolling (freshmen), rolling (transfer). *Application fee:* $20.

Advanced Placement Credit by examination available. Credit given for nursing courses completed elsewhere dependent upon specific evaluations.

Financial Aid 89% of baccalaureate students in nursing programs received some form of financial aid in 2004–05.

Contact Dr. Polly K. Kloster, Chair, Department of Nursing, Concordia College, 901 South 8th Street, Moorhead, MN 56562. *Telephone:* 218-299-4060. *Fax:* 218-299-4308. *E-mail:* kloster@cord.edu.

GRADUATE PROGRAMS

Financial Aid 100% of graduate students in nursing programs received some form of financial aid in 2004–05.

Contact Dr. Polly K. Kloster, Chair, Department of Nursing, Concordia College, 901 South 8th Street, Moorhead, MN 56562. *Telephone:* 218-299-4060. *Fax:* 218-299-4308. *E-mail:* kloster@cord.edu.

MASTER'S DEGREE PROGRAM

Degree MS

Available Programs Master's; Master's for Nurses with Non-Nursing Degrees.

Concentrations Available Nursing education. *Clinical nurse specialist programs in:* adult health. *Nurse practitioner programs in:* family health.

Study Options Full-time and part-time.

Program Entrance Requirements Computer literacy, minimum overall college GPA of 3.0, transcript of college record, written essay, interview, 3 letters of recommendation.

Advanced Placement Credit given for nursing courses completed elsewhere dependent upon specific evaluations.

Degree Requirements 36 total credit hours, thesis or project, comprehensive exam.

Gustavus Adolphus College
Department of Nursing
St. Peter, Minnesota

Founded in 1862
DEGREE • BA

Nursing Program Faculty 9 (20% with doctorates).

Baccalaureate Enrollment 76
Women 92% **Men** 8% **Minority** 8% **International** 4%

Nursing Student Activities Sigma Theta Tau, Student Nurses' Association.

Nursing Student Resources Academic advising; academic or career counseling; assistance for students with disabilities; bookstore; campus computer network; career placement assistance; computer lab; computer-assisted instruction; e-mail services; employment services for current students; housing assistance; interactive nursing skills videos; Internet; learning resource lab; library services; nursing audiovisuals; paid internships; remedial services; resume preparation assistance; skills, simulation, or other laboratory; tutoring; unpaid internships.

Library Facilities 297,861 volumes; 17,078 periodical subscriptions.

BACCALAUREATE PROGRAMS

Degree BA

Available Programs Generic Baccalaureate.

Study Options Full-time.

Program Entrance Requirements Minimum overall college GPA of 2.7, transcript of college record, written essay, high school transcript, immunizations, interview, minimum GPA in nursing prerequisites, prerequisite course work. Transfer students are accepted. **Standardized tests** *Required:* TOEFL for international students. **Application** *Deadline:* 4/1 (freshmen), 4/1 (transfer). *Early decision:* 11/1. *Notification:* continuous until 5/1 (freshmen), 11/20 (early action).

Expenses (2006–07) *Tuition:* full-time $26,310. *International tuition:* $10,000 full-time. *Room and board:* $6765; room only: $3400 per academic year. *Required fees:* full-time $1000.

Financial Aid 69% of baccalaureate students in nursing programs received some form of financial aid in 2005–06.

Contact Ms. Judith M. Gardner, RN, Associate Professor and Chair, Department of Nursing, Gustavus Adolphus College, 800 West College Avenue, St. Peter, MN 56082. *Telephone:* 507-933-6126. *Fax:* 507-933-6153. *E-mail:* jgardner@gustavus.edu.

Metropolitan State University
School of Nursing
St. Paul, Minnesota

http://www.metrostate.edu

Founded in 1971

DEGREES • BSN • MSN

Nursing Program Faculty 22 (18% with doctorates).

Baccalaureate Enrollment 230
Women 91% **Men** 9% **Minority** 9% **Part-time** 96%

Graduate Enrollment 40
Women 95% **Men** 5% **Minority** 8% **Part-time** 23%

Nursing Student Activities Sigma Theta Tau, Student Nurses' Association.

Nursing Student Resources Academic advising; academic or career counseling; assistance for students with disabilities; bookstore; campus computer network; computer lab; e-mail services; externships; Internet; library services; skills, simulation, or other laboratory.

Library Facilities 29,385 volumes; 385 periodical subscriptions.

BACCALAUREATE PROGRAMS

Degree BSN

Site Options Minneapolis, MN.

Study Options Full-time and part-time.

Program Entrance Requirements Minimum overall college GPA of 2.5, transcript of college record, health insurance, immunizations, minimum GPA in nursing prerequisites of 3.0, professional liability insurance/malpractice insurance, prerequisite course work. Transfer students are accepted. **Standardized tests** *Required:* TOEFL for international students. *Required for some:* SAT or ACT. **Application** *Deadline:* 6/15 (freshmen), 6/15 (transfer). *Application fee:* $20.

Advanced Placement Credit given for nursing courses completed elsewhere dependent upon specific evaluations.

Contact *Telephone:* 651-793-1379. *Fax:* 651-793-1382.

GRADUATE PROGRAMS

Contact *Telephone:* 651-793-1378. *Fax:* 651-793-1382.

MASTER'S DEGREE PROGRAM

Degree MSN

Available Programs Master's for Nurses with Non-Nursing Degrees; RN to Master's.

Concentrations Available Nursing administration. *Nurse practitioner programs in:* adult health, family health.

Study Options Full-time and part-time.

Program Entrance Requirements Clinical experience, computer literacy, minimum overall college GPA of 3.0, transcript of college record, written essay, immunizations, interview, 3 letters of recommendation, professional liability insurance/malpractice insurance, resume, statistics course, GRE General Test or MAT. *Application deadline:* For fall admission, 1/15. *Application fee:* $20.

Advanced Placement Credit given for nursing courses completed elsewhere dependent upon specific evaluations.

Degree Requirements 42 total credit hours, thesis or project.

POST-MASTER'S PROGRAM

Areas of Study *Nurse practitioner programs in:* adult health, family health.

Minnesota Intercollegiate Nursing Consortium
Minnesota Intercollegiate Nursing Consortium
Northfield, Minnesota

DEGREE • BA

Nursing Program Faculty 9 (22% with doctorates).

Baccalaureate Enrollment 96
Women 94% **Men** 6% **Minority** 8% **International** 2%

Nursing Student Activities Sigma Theta Tau, Student Nurses' Association.

Nursing Student Resources Academic advising; academic or career counseling; assistance for students with disabilities; bookstore; campus computer network; career placement assistance; computer lab; computer-assisted instruction; e-mail services; employment services for current students; externships; interactive nursing skills videos; Internet; learning resource lab; library services; nursing audiovisuals; paid internships; resume preparation assistance; skills, simulation, or other laboratory; tutoring; unpaid internships.

BACCALAUREATE PROGRAMS

Degree BA

Available Programs Generic Baccalaureate.

Site Options Northfield, MN; St. Peter, MN.

Study Options Full-time.

Program Entrance Requirements Minimum overall college GPA of 2.7, transcript of college record, CPR certification, written essay, high school transcript, immunizations, interview, minimum GPA in nursing prerequisites of 2.7, prerequisite course work. Transfer students are accepted.

Expenses (2006–07) *Required fees:* full-time $1000.

Contact Dr. Rita S. Glazebrook, Director, Minnesota Intercollegiate Nursing Consortium, 1520 St. Olaf Avenue, Northfield, MN 55057-1098. *Telephone:* 507-646-3265. *Fax:* 507-646-3733. *E-mail:* glazebro@stolaf.edu.

Minnesota State University Mankato
School of Nursing
Mankato, Minnesota

http://www.mnsu.edu/nursing/

Founded in 1868

DEGREES • BS • MSN • MSN/MS

Nursing Program Faculty 48 (21% with doctorates).

Baccalaureate Enrollment 292
Women 90% **Men** 10% **Minority** 9% **International** 1% **Part-time** 1%

Graduate Enrollment 44
Women 96% **Men** 4% **Part-time** 48%

Nursing Student Activities Nursing Honor Society, Sigma Theta Tau, Student Nurses' Association.

Nursing Student Resources Academic advising; academic or career counseling; assistance for students with disabilities; bookstore; campus computer network; career placement assistance; computer lab; computer-assisted instruction; daycare for children of students; e-mail services; employment services for current students; Internet; learning resource lab;

Minnesota State University Mankato (continued)
library services; nursing audiovisuals; paid internships; placement services for program completers; resume preparation assistance; skills, simulation, or other laboratory; tutoring.

Library Facilities 474,252 volumes (35,852 in health, 1,500 in nursing); 3,400 periodical subscriptions (156 health-care related).

BACCALAUREATE PROGRAMS

Degree BS

Available Programs Accelerated Baccalaureate for Second Degree; Generic Baccalaureate; RN Baccalaureate.

Study Options Full-time and part-time.

Program Entrance Requirements Minimum overall college GPA of 2.5, transcript of college record, health insurance, minimum GPA in nursing prerequisites of 2.0, prerequisite course work. Transfer students are accepted. **Standardized tests** *Required:* ACT, TOEFL for international students. **Application** *Deadline:* rolling (freshmen), rolling (transfer). *Notification:* continuous (freshmen). *Application fee:* $20.

Advanced Placement Credit by examination available. Credit given for nursing courses completed elsewhere dependent upon specific evaluations.

Expenses (2006–07) *Tuition, state resident:* full-time $5104; part-time $204 per credit. *Tuition, nonresident:* full-time $10,932; part-time $436 per credit. *International tuition:* $10,932 full-time. *Room and board:* $4910 per academic year. *Required fees:* full-time $736; part-time $31 per credit; part-time $368 per term.

Financial Aid 75% of baccalaureate students in nursing programs received some form of financial aid in 2005–06. *Gift aid (need-based):* Federal Pell, FSEOG, state, private, college/university gift aid from institutional funds. *Loans:* FFEL (Subsidized and Unsubsidized Stafford PLUS), Perkins, state, SELF Loans. *Work-Study:* Federal Work-Study, part-time campus jobs. *Application deadline (priority):* 3/15.

Contact Mrs. Julia Hebenstreit, Assistant Professor of Nursing, School of Nursing, Minnesota State University Mankato, 360 Wissink Hall, Mankato, MN 56001. *Telephone:* 507-389-6828. *Fax:* 507-389-6516. *E-mail:* julia. hebenstreit@mnsu.edu.

GRADUATE PROGRAMS

Expenses (2006–07) *Tuition, state resident:* full-time $4768; part-time $265 per credit. *Tuition, nonresident:* full-time $3924; part-time $436 per credit. *International tuition:* $3924 full-time. *Room and board:* $4910 per academic year. *Required fees:* full-time $736; part-time $31 per credit; part-time $368 per term.

Financial Aid 75% of graduate students in nursing programs received some form of financial aid in 2005–06.

Contact Dr. Sonja J. Meiers, Graduate Program Director, School of Nursing, Minnesota State University Mankato, 360 Wissink Hall, Mankato, MN 56001. *Telephone:* 507-389-1317. *Fax:* 507-389-6516. *E-mail:* sonja. meiers@mnsu.edu.

MASTER'S DEGREE PROGRAM

Degrees MSN; MSN/MS

Available Programs Master's; Master's for Nurses with Non-Nursing Degrees.

Concentrations Available Nursing education. *Clinical nurse specialist programs in:* family health. *Nurse practitioner programs in:* family health.

Study Options Full-time and part-time.

Program Entrance Requirements Clinical experience, computer literacy, minimum overall college GPA of 3.0, transcript of college record, CPR certification, written essay, immunizations, 3 letters of recommendation, nursing research course, professional liability insurance/malpractice insurance, prerequisite course work, resume, statistics course.

Advanced Placement Credit given for nursing courses completed elsewhere dependent upon specific evaluations.

Degree Requirements 53 total credit hours, thesis or project.

POST-MASTER'S PROGRAM

Areas of Study Nursing education. *Clinical nurse specialist programs in:* family health. *Nurse practitioner programs in:* family health.

CONTINUING EDUCATION PROGRAM

Contact Shirley Murray, Continuing Education Director, College of Allied Health and Nursing, School of Nursing, Minnesota State University Mankato, 360 Wissink Hall, Mankato, MN 56001. *Telephone:* 507-389-5194. *Fax:* 507-389-6516. *E-mail:* shirley.murray@mnsu.edu.

Minnesota State University Moorhead
Tri-College University Nursing Consortium
Moorhead, Minnesota

http://www.tri-college.org/nursing.htm
Founded in 1885

DEGREES • BSN • MS

Nursing Program Faculty 8 (50% with doctorates).

Baccalaureate Enrollment 118

Graduate Enrollment 20

Women 96% **Men** 4% **Minority** 7% **International** 7% **Part-time** 33%

Nursing Student Activities Sigma Theta Tau, Student Nurses' Association.

Nursing Student Resources Academic advising; academic or career counseling; assistance for students with disabilities; bookstore; campus computer network; career placement assistance; computer lab; computer-assisted instruction; daycare for children of students; e-mail services; employment services for current students; Internet; library services; nursing audiovisuals; remedial services; resume preparation assistance; tutoring; unpaid internships.

Library Facilities 367,334 volumes (5,405 in health, 716 in nursing); 1,539 periodical subscriptions (35 health-care related).

BACCALAUREATE PROGRAMS

Degree BSN

Available Programs Generic Baccalaureate; RN Baccalaureate.

Site Options *Distance Learning:* Alexandria, MN.

Study Options Full-time.

Program Entrance Requirements CPR certification, written essay, high school biology, high school chemistry, high school transcript, 2 letters of recommendation, minimum high school GPA of 3.25. Transfer students are accepted. **Standardized tests** *Required:* SAT or ACT, TOEFL for international students. **Application** *Deadline:* 8/7 (freshmen), 8/7 (transfer). *Notification:* continuous (freshmen). *Application fee:* $20.

Expenses (2006–07) *Tuition, state resident:* full-time $4888; part-time $163 per credit. *Tuition, nonresident:* full-time $4888; part-time $163 per credit. *International tuition:* $4888 full-time. *Room and board:* $5218; room only: $977 per academic year. *Required fees:* full-time $832; part-time $144 per credit; part-time $416 per term.

Financial Aid 60% of baccalaureate students in nursing programs received some form of financial aid in 2005–06.

Contact Dr. Barbara Matthees, Director, Tri-College University Nursing Consortium, Minnesota State University Moorhead, 1104 7th Avenue South, Moorhead, MN 56563. *Telephone:* 218-477-2695. *Fax:* 218-477-5990. *E-mail:* matthees@mnstate.edu.

GRADUATE PROGRAMS

Expenses (2006–07) *Tuition, state resident:* full-time $3132; part-time $348 per credit. *Tuition, nonresident:* full-time $3132; part-time $348 per credit. *International tuition:* $3132 full-time. *Room and board:* $4888; room only: $3891 per academic year. *Required fees:* full-time $243; part-time $27 per credit.

Financial Aid 66% of graduate students in nursing programs received some form of financial aid in 2005–06.

Contact Dr. Jane Giedt, Director, Graduate Program, Tri-College University Nursing Consortium, Minnesota State University Moorhead, 1104 7th Avenue South, Moorhead, MN 56563. *Telephone:* 218-477-4699. *Fax:* 218-477-5990. *E-mail:* giedt@mnstate.edu.

MASTER'S DEGREE PROGRAM

Degree MS

Available Programs Master's; Master's for Nurses with Non-Nursing Degrees.

Concentrations Available Nursing education. *Clinical nurse specialist programs in:* adult health. *Nurse practitioner programs in:* family health.

Site Options *Distance Learning:* Alexandria, MN.

Study Options Full-time and part-time.

Program Entrance Requirements Computer literacy, minimum overall college GPA of 3.0, transcript of college record, written essay, interview, 3 letters of recommendation.

Advanced Placement Credit given for nursing courses completed elsewhere dependent upon specific evaluations.

Degree Requirements 52 total credit hours, thesis or project.

St. Cloud State University
Department of Nursing Science
St. Cloud, Minnesota

Founded in 1869

DEGREE • BS

Nursing Program Faculty 12 (25% with doctorates).

Baccalaureate Enrollment 111

Nursing Student Activities Nursing club.

Nursing Student Resources Academic advising; academic or career counseling; assistance for students with disabilities; bookstore; campus computer network; career placement assistance; computer lab; computer-assisted instruction; daycare for children of students; e-mail services; interactive nursing skills videos; Internet; learning resource lab; library services; nursing audiovisuals; remedial services; resume preparation assistance; skills, simulation, or other laboratory; tutoring; unpaid internships.

Library Facilities 897,973 volumes (18,000 in health, 750 in nursing); 1,737 periodical subscriptions (100 health-care related).

BACCALAUREATE PROGRAMS

Degree BS

Available Programs Generic Baccalaureate.

Study Options Full-time.

Program Entrance Requirements Minimum overall college GPA of 2.75, transcript of college record, CPR certification, health exam, immunizations, 2 letters of recommendation, minimum GPA in nursing prerequisites of 2.75, prerequisite course work. **Standardized tests** *Required:* SAT or ACT, TOEFL for international students. **Application** *Deadline:* 6/1 (freshmen), 8/15 (transfer). *Notification:* continuous (freshmen). *Application fee:* $20.

Financial Aid 86% of baccalaureate students in nursing programs received some form of financial aid in 2004–05. *Gift aid (need-based):* Federal Pell, FSEOG, state, private, college/university gift aid from institutional funds. *Loans:* FFEL (Subsidized and Unsubsidized Stafford PLUS), Perkins, state. *Work-Study:* Federal Work-Study, part-time campus jobs. *Application deadline:* Continuous.

Contact Carrie M. Barth, Department of Nursing Science, Department of Nursing Science, St. Cloud State University, BH 228, 720 4th Avenue South, St. Cloud, MN 56301. *Telephone:* 320-308-1749. *E-mail:* nursing@stcloudstate.edu.

St. Olaf College
Department of Nursing
Northfield, Minnesota

Founded in 1874

DEGREE • BA

Nursing Program Faculty 5 (20% with doctorates).

Baccalaureate Enrollment 48

Women 90% **Men** 10% **Minority** 10%

Nursing Student Activities Sigma Theta Tau, Student Nurses' Association.

Nursing Student Resources Academic advising; academic or career counseling; assistance for students with disabilities; bookstore; campus computer network; career placement assistance; computer lab; computer-assisted instruction; e-mail services; employment services for current students; externships; interactive nursing skills videos; Internet; learning resource lab; library services; nursing audiovisuals; paid internships; placement services for program completers; remedial services; resume preparation assistance; skills, simulation, or other laboratory; tutoring; unpaid internships.

Library Facilities 1.1 million volumes; 2,319 periodical subscriptions.

BACCALAUREATE PROGRAMS

Degree BA

Available Programs Generic Baccalaureate.

Site Options Northfield, MN; St. Peter, MN.

Study Options Full-time.

Program Entrance Requirements Minimum overall college GPA of 2.7, transcript of college record, CPR certification, written essay, high school transcript, immunizations, interview, minimum GPA in nursing prerequisites of 2.7, prerequisite course work. Transfer students are accepted. **Standardized tests** *Required:* SAT or ACT, TOEFL for international students. **Application** *Deadline:* rolling (freshmen). *Early decision:* 11/1, 12/1. *Notification:* continuous (freshmen), 12/1 (out-of-state freshmen), 12/1 (early decision), 2/1 (early action). *Application fee:* $40.

Expenses (2006–07) *Tuition:* full-time $28,200; part-time $3525 per course. *International tuition:* $28,200 full-time. *Room and board:* $7400; room only: $3450 per academic year. *Required fees:* full-time $1000.

Contact Dr. Rita S. Glazebrook, Chair of the Department of Nursing, Department of Nursing, St. Olaf College, 1520 St. Olaf Avenue, Northfield, MN 55057-1098. *Telephone:* 507-646-3265. *Fax:* 507-646-3733. *E-mail:* glazebro@stolaf.edu.

University of Minnesota, Twin Cities Campus
School of Nursing
Minneapolis, Minnesota

http://www.nursing.umn.edu

Founded in 1851

DEGREES • BSN • MS • MS/MPH • PHD

Nursing Program Faculty 85 (90% with doctorates).

Baccalaureate Enrollment 392
Women 87% **Men** 13% **Minority** 12% **Part-time** 8%

Graduate Enrollment 343
Women 98% **Men** 2% **Minority** 12% **International** 5% **Part-time** 44%

Nursing Student Activities Nursing Honor Society, Sigma Theta Tau, Student Nurses' Association.

Nursing Student Resources Academic advising; academic or career counseling; assistance for students with disabilities; bookstore; campus computer network; computer lab; computer-assisted instruction; daycare for children of students; e-mail services; employment services for current students; housing assistance; Internet; learning resource lab; library services; skills, simulation, or other laboratory.

Library Facilities 5.7 million volumes (4,000 in health, 1,500 in nursing); 45,000 periodical subscriptions (4,800 health-care related).

BACCALAUREATE PROGRAMS

Degree BSN

Available Programs Generic Baccalaureate.

Site Options Rochester, MN.

Study Options Full-time.

Program Entrance Requirements Minimum overall college GPA of 2.8, transcript of college record, CPR certification, written essay, health exam, health insurance, immunizations, minimum GPA in nursing prerequisites of 2.8, prerequisite course work. Transfer students are accepted.

University of Minnesota, Twin Cities Campus (continued)

Standardized tests *Required:* SAT or ACT, TOEFL for international students. **Application** *Deadline:* rolling (freshmen), rolling (transfer). *Notification:* continuous (freshmen). *Application fee:* $45.

Financial Aid 73% of baccalaureate students in nursing programs received some form of financial aid in 2005–06. *Gift aid (need-based):* Federal Pell, FSEOG, state, private, college/university gift aid from institutional funds, Federal Nursing. *Loans:* Federal Nursing Student Loans, Federal Direct (Subsidized and Unsubsidized Stafford PLUS), Perkins, state, college/university, Health Professions Loans, alternative loans. *Work-Study:* Federal Work-Study, part-time campus jobs. *Application deadline (priority):* 1/15.

Contact Office of Student Services, School of Nursing, University of Minnesota, Twin Cities Campus, 5-160 Weaver-Densford Hall, 308 Harvard Street SE, Minneapolis, MN 55455-0213. *Telephone:* 612-625-7980. *Fax:* 612-625-7727. *E-mail:* sonstudentinfo@umn.edu.

GRADUATE PROGRAMS

Financial Aid Fellowships, research assistantships, teaching assistantships, career-related internships or fieldwork and traineeships available.

Contact Office of Student Services, School of Nursing, University of Minnesota, Twin Cities Campus, 5-160 Weaver-Densford Hall, 308 Harvard Street SE, Minneapolis, MN 55455-0213. *Telephone:* 612-625-7980. *Fax:* 612-625-7727. *E-mail:* sonstudentinfo@umn.edu.

MASTER'S DEGREE PROGRAM

Degrees MS; MS/MPH

Available Programs Master's.

Concentrations Available Nurse anesthesia; nurse-midwifery; nursing administration. *Clinical nurse specialist programs in:* adult health, gerontology, pediatric, psychiatric/mental health. *Nurse practitioner programs in:* family health, gerontology, pediatric, women's health.

Study Options Full-time and part-time.

Program Entrance Requirements Clinical experience, computer literacy, minimum overall college GPA of 3.0, transcript of college record, CPR certification, written essay, immunizations, interview, 2 letters of recommendation, statistics course. *Application fee:* $55 ($75 for international students).

Degree Requirements 33 total credit hours, thesis or project.

DOCTORAL DEGREE PROGRAM

Degree PhD

Available Programs Doctorate; Doctorate for Nurses with Non-Nursing Degrees; Post-Baccalaureate Doctorate.

Program Entrance Requirements Minimum overall college GPA of 3.0, interview by faculty committee, interview, 2 letters of recommendation, GRE General Test. *Application fee:* $55 ($75 for international students).

Degree Requirements 30 total credit hours, dissertation, oral exam, written exam, residency.

CONTINUING EDUCATION PROGRAM

Contact Office of Student Services, School of Nursing, University of Minnesota, Twin Cities Campus, 5-160 Weaver-Densford Hall, 308 Harvard Street SE, Minneapolis, MN 55455-0213. *Telephone:* 612-625-7980. *Fax:* 612-625-7727. *E-mail:* sonstudentinfo@umn.edu.

See full description on page 548.

Winona State University
College of Nursing
Winona, Minnesota

http://www.winona.edu/nursing/

Founded in 1858

DEGREES • BS • MS

Nursing Program Faculty 39 (50% with doctorates).

Baccalaureate Enrollment 350

Women 92% **Men** 8% **Minority** 3% **Part-time** 8%

Graduate Enrollment 130

Women 89% **Men** 11% **Minority** 4% **International** 1% **Part-time** 75%

Nursing Student Activities Sigma Theta Tau, Student Nurses' Association, nursing club.

Nursing Student Resources Academic advising; academic or career counseling; assistance for students with disabilities; bookstore; campus computer network; career placement assistance; computer lab; computer-assisted instruction; daycare for children of students; e-mail services; employment services for current students; externships; housing assistance; Internet; learning resource lab; library services; nursing audiovisuals; paid internships; placement services for program completers; remedial services; resume preparation assistance; skills, simulation, or other laboratory; tutoring.

Library Facilities 350,000 volumes (6,132 in health, 3,920 in nursing); 1,000 periodical subscriptions (413 health-care related).

BACCALAUREATE PROGRAMS

Degree BS

Available Programs Generic Baccalaureate; RN Baccalaureate.

Site Options *Distance Learning:* Rochester, MN.

Study Options Full-time and part-time.

Program Entrance Requirements Minimum overall college GPA of 3.00, transcript of college record, CPR certification, health exam, health insurance, immunizations, professional liability insurance/malpractice insurance, prerequisite course work. Transfer students are accepted. **Standardized tests** *Required:* SAT or ACT, TOEFL for international students. **Application** *Deadline:* rolling (freshmen), 8/1 (transfer). *Notification:* continuous (freshmen). *Application fee:* $20.

Expenses (2006–07) *Tuition, state resident:* full-time $6345. *Tuition, nonresident:* full-time $8420. *International tuition:* $8420 full-time. *Room and board:* $2870 per academic year. *Required fees:* full-time $1000.

Financial Aid 70% of baccalaureate students in nursing programs received some form of financial aid in 2005–06.

Contact Nursing Contact, College of Nursing, Winona State University, PO Box 5838, Winona, MN 55987-5838. *Telephone:* 507-457-5120. *Fax:* 507-457-5550. *E-mail:* nursing@winona.edu.

GRADUATE PROGRAMS

Expenses (2006–07) *Tuition, state resident:* part-time $273 per credit. *Tuition, nonresident:* part-time $411 per credit. *Required fees:* part-time $17 per credit.

Financial Aid 90% of graduate students in nursing programs received some form of financial aid in 2005–06. 3 research assistantships with partial tuition reimbursements available (averaging $6,000 per year) were awarded; Federal Work-Study, traineeships, and unspecified assistantships also available. Aid available to part-time students.

Contact Dr. William McBreen, Director, College of Nursing, Winona State University, 859 SE 30th Avenue, Rochester, MN 55904. *Telephone:* 507-285-7489. *Fax:* 507-292-5127. *E-mail:* wmcbreen@winona.msus.edu.

MASTER'S DEGREE PROGRAM

Degree MS

Available Programs Master's; RN to Master's.

Concentrations Available Nursing administration; nursing education. *Clinical nurse specialist programs in:* adult health. *Nurse practitioner programs in:* adult health, family health.

Site Options *Distance Learning:* Rochester, MN.

Study Options Full-time and part-time.

Program Entrance Requirements Clinical experience, computer literacy, minimum overall college GPA of 3.0, transcript of college record, written essay, immunizations, interview, 3 letters of recommendation, nursing research course, physical assessment course, professional liability insurance/malpractice insurance, statistics course. *Application deadline:* For fall admission, 2/1. *Application fee:* $20.

Advanced Placement Credit given for nursing courses completed elsewhere dependent upon specific evaluations.

Degree Requirements 43 total credit hours, thesis or project, comprehensive exam.

POST-MASTER'S PROGRAM

Areas of Study Nursing administration; nursing education. *Clinical nurse specialist programs in:* adult health. *Nurse practitioner programs in:* adult health, family health.

MISSISSIPPI

Alcorn State University
School of Nursing
Natchez, Mississippi

http://www.alcorn.edu/academic/academ/nurses.htm

Founded in 1871

DEGREES • BSN • MSN

Nursing Program Faculty 23 (33% with doctorates).

Baccalaureate Enrollment 63
Women 88.8% **Men** 11.2% **Minority** 42.8% **Part-time** 7.9%

Graduate Enrollment 56
Women 89.3% **Men** 10.7% **Minority** 35.7% **Part-time** 78.6%

Nursing Student Activities Nursing Honor Society, Sigma Theta Tau, Student Nurses' Association.

Nursing Student Resources Academic advising; computer lab; housing assistance; learning resource lab; library services; nursing audiovisuals; paid internships; skills, simulation, or other laboratory.

Library Facilities 229,238 volumes (2,082 in health, 1,385 in nursing); 1,046 periodical subscriptions (30 health-care related).

BACCALAUREATE PROGRAMS

Degree BSN

Available Programs Generic Baccalaureate; RN Baccalaureate.

Study Options Full-time and part-time.

Program Entrance Requirements Minimum overall college GPA of 2.5, transcript of college record, health exam, minimum high school GPA of 2.5, prerequisite course work. Transfer students are accepted. **Standardized tests** *Required:* SAT or ACT, TOEFL for international students. **Application** *Deadline:* rolling (freshmen), rolling (transfer). *Notification:* continuous (freshmen).

Advanced Placement Credit given for nursing courses completed elsewhere dependent upon specific evaluations.

Contact *Telephone:* 601-304-4305. *Fax:* 601-304-4398.

GRADUATE PROGRAMS

Contact *Telephone:* 601-304-4303. *Fax:* 601-304-4398.

MASTER'S DEGREE PROGRAM

Degree MSN

Available Programs Master's.

Concentrations Available Nursing education. *Nurse practitioner programs in:* family health.

Study Options Full-time and part-time.

Program Entrance Requirements Computer literacy, minimum overall college GPA of 3.0, transcript of college record, written essay, 2 letters of recommendation, statistics course. *Application deadline:* For fall admission, 7/15 (priority date); for spring admission, 11/25. Applications are processed on a rolling basis. *Application fee:* $10 for international students).

Advanced Placement Credit given for nursing courses completed elsewhere dependent upon specific evaluations.

Degree Requirements 43 total credit hours, thesis or project.

POST-MASTER'S PROGRAM

Areas of Study Nursing education. *Nurse practitioner programs in:* family health, gerontology.

Delta State University
School of Nursing
Cleveland, Mississippi

http://www.deltastate.edu

Founded in 1924

DEGREES • BSN • MSN

Nursing Program Faculty 17 (35% with doctorates).

Baccalaureate Enrollment 91
Women 82% **Men** 18% **Minority** 30% **Part-time** 3%

Graduate Enrollment 61
Women 97% **Men** 3% **Minority** 27% **Part-time** 36%

Nursing Student Activities Sigma Theta Tau, Student Nurses' Association.

Nursing Student Resources Academic advising; academic or career counseling; assistance for students with disabilities; bookstore; campus computer network; career placement assistance; computer lab; computer-assisted instruction; daycare for children of students; e-mail services; externships; housing assistance; interactive nursing skills videos; Internet; learning resource lab; library services; nursing audiovisuals; other; resume preparation assistance; skills, simulation, or other laboratory; tutoring.

Library Facilities 360,286 volumes (5,000 in health, 1,000 in nursing); 1,258 periodical subscriptions (120 health-care related).

BACCALAUREATE PROGRAMS

Degree BSN

Available Programs ADN to Baccalaureate; Generic Baccalaureate.

Site Options *Distance Learning:* Clarksdale, MS; Greenville, MS.

Study Options Full-time and part-time.

Program Entrance Requirements Transcript of college record, CPR certification, written essay, health exam, health insurance, immunizations, interview, 3 letters of recommendation, minimum GPA in nursing prerequisites of 2.5, professional liability insurance/malpractice insurance, prerequisite course work. Transfer students are accepted. **Standardized tests** *Required:* SAT or ACT, TOEFL for international students. **Application** *Deadline:* 8/1 (freshmen), 8/1 (transfer). *Notification:* continuous (freshmen). *Application fee:* $15.

Advanced Placement Credit given for nursing courses completed elsewhere dependent upon specific evaluations.

Expenses (2006–07) *Tuition, state resident:* full-time $4008; part-time $167 per credit hour. *Tuition, nonresident:* full-time $9574; part-time $566 per credit hour. *International tuition:* $9574 full-time. *Room and board:* $4574; room only: $2770 per academic year. *Required fees:* full-time $500; part-time $60 per credit; part-time $250 per term.

Financial Aid 95% of baccalaureate students in nursing programs received some form of financial aid in 2005–06.

Contact Mrs. Vicki L. Bingham, Chair of Academic Programs, School of Nursing, Delta State University, PO Box 3343, Cleveland, MS 38733. *Telephone:* 662-846-4255. *Fax:* 662-846-4267. *E-mail:* vbingham@deltastate.edu.

GRADUATE PROGRAMS

Expenses (2006–07) *Tuition, state resident:* full-time $2004; part-time $222 per credit hour. *Tuition, nonresident:* full-time $2004; part-time $222 per credit hour. *International tuition:* $2004 full-time. *Room and board:* $4574; room only: $2770 per academic year. *Required fees:* full-time $120; part-time $20 per credit; part-time $60 per term.

Financial Aid 70% of graduate students in nursing programs received some form of financial aid in 2005–06. Research assistantships, career-related internships or fieldwork, Federal Work-Study, and institutionally sponsored loans available. *Financial aid application deadline:* 6/1.

Contact Mrs. Vicki L. Bingham, Chair of Academic Programs, School of Nursing, Delta State University, PO Box 3343, Cleveland, MS 38733. *Telephone:* 662-846-4255. *Fax:* 662-846-4267. *E-mail:* vbingham@deltastate.edu.

MASTER'S DEGREE PROGRAM

Degree MSN

Available Programs Accelerated Master's for Nurses with Non-Nursing Degrees; Master's.

Delta State University (continued)

Concentrations Available Nursing administration; nursing education. *Nurse practitioner programs in:* family health.

Study Options Full-time and part-time.

Program Entrance Requirements Clinical experience, computer literacy, minimum overall college GPA of 3.0, transcript of college record, CPR certification, written essay, immunizations, interview, 3 letters of recommendation, physical assessment course, professional liability insurance/malpractice insurance, prerequisite course work, statistics course, GRE General Test. *Application deadline:* For fall admission, 8/1 (priority date); for spring admission, 12/1 (priority date). Applications are processed on a rolling basis.

Advanced Placement Credit given for nursing courses completed elsewhere dependent upon specific evaluations.

Degree Requirements 44 total credit hours, thesis or project, comprehensive exam.

POST-MASTER'S PROGRAM

Areas of Study Nursing education. *Nurse practitioner programs in:* family health.

Mississippi College
School of Nursing
Clinton, Mississippi

http://www.mc.edu
Founded in 1826
DEGREE • BSN

Nursing Program Faculty 20 (35% with doctorates).

Baccalaureate Enrollment 135
Women 85% **Men** 15% **Minority** 25% **Part-time** 8%

Nursing Student Activities Sigma Theta Tau, Student Nurses' Association, nursing club.

Nursing Student Resources Academic advising; academic or career counseling; assistance for students with disabilities; bookstore; campus computer network; career placement assistance; computer lab; computer-assisted instruction; e-mail services; employment services for current students; externships; housing assistance; interactive nursing skills videos; Internet; learning resource lab; library services; nursing audiovisuals; other; paid internships; placement services for program completers; remedial services; resume preparation assistance; skills, simulation, or other laboratory; tutoring; unpaid internships.

Library Facilities 370,404 volumes (40,000 in health, 8,000 in nursing); 4,742 periodical subscriptions (290 health-care related).

BACCALAUREATE PROGRAMS

Degree BSN

Available Programs Generic Baccalaureate; RN Baccalaureate.

Study Options Full-time and part-time.

Program Entrance Requirements Minimum overall college GPA of 2.5, transcript of college record, CPR certification, health exam, high school biology, high school chemistry, high school transcript, immunizations, 2 letters of recommendation, minimum GPA in nursing prerequisites of 2.5, prerequisite course work. Transfer students are accepted. **Standardized tests** *Required:* SAT or ACT. **Application** *Deadline:* rolling (freshmen), rolling (transfer). *Early decision:* 12/1. *Notification:* continuous (freshmen), 12/15 (out-of-state freshmen), 12/15 (early decision).

Advanced Placement Credit given for nursing courses completed elsewhere dependent upon specific evaluations.

Expenses (2006–07) *Tuition:* full-time $11,600; part-time $355 per contact hour. *International tuition:* $11,600 full-time. *Room and board:* $5700 per academic year. *Required fees:* full-time $600; part-time $500 per term.

Financial Aid 80% of baccalaureate students in nursing programs received some form of financial aid in 2005–06.

Contact Dr. Mary Jean Padgett, RN, Dean, School of Nursing, Mississippi College, Box 4037, 200 South Capitol Street, Clinton, MS 39058. *Telephone:* 601-925-3278. *Fax:* 601-925-3379. *E-mail:* padgett@mc.edu.

Mississippi University for Women
Division of Nursing
Columbus, Mississippi

http://www.muw.edu/nursing
Founded in 1884
DEGREES • BSN • MN

Nursing Program Faculty 37 (22% with doctorates).

Baccalaureate Enrollment 151
Women 90% **Men** 10% **Minority** 20%

Graduate Enrollment 36
Women 90% **Men** 10% **Minority** 20% **Part-time** 2%

Nursing Student Activities Sigma Theta Tau, Student Nurses' Association.

Nursing Student Resources Academic advising; academic or career counseling; assistance for students with disabilities; bookstore; campus computer network; career placement assistance; computer lab; computer-assisted instruction; e-mail services; externships; housing assistance; interactive nursing skills videos; Internet; learning resource lab; library services; nursing audiovisuals; paid internships; remedial services; resume preparation assistance; skills, simulation, or other laboratory; tutoring; unpaid internships.

Library Facilities 426,543 volumes (30,765 in health, 25,765 in nursing); 1,629 periodical subscriptions (215 health-care related).

BACCALAUREATE PROGRAMS

Degree BSN

Available Programs ADN to Baccalaureate; Generic Baccalaureate.

Site Options *Distance Learning:* Tupelo, MS.

Study Options Full-time.

Program Entrance Requirements Minimum overall college GPA of 2.0, transcript of college record, CPR certification, health exam, immunizations, minimum GPA in nursing prerequisites of 2.0, professional liability insurance/malpractice insurance, prerequisite course work. Transfer students are accepted. **Standardized tests** *Required:* TOEFL for international students. *Recommended:* SAT or ACT. *Required for some:* SAT or ACT. **Application** *Deadline:* rolling (freshmen), 9/6 (transfer). *Notification:* continuous (freshmen).

Advanced Placement Credit given for nursing courses completed elsewhere dependent upon specific evaluations.

Expenses (2006–07) *Tuition, state resident:* full-time $3933; part-time $164 per credit hour. *Tuition, nonresident:* full-time $9724; part-time $405 per credit hour. *International tuition:* $9724 full-time. *Room and board:* $4516 per academic year. *Required fees:* full-time $1000; part-time $100 per term.

Financial Aid 80% of baccalaureate students in nursing programs received some form of financial aid in 2005–06.

Contact Dr. Linda Cox, Program Director, Division of Nursing, Mississippi University for Women, 1100 College Street, MUW-910, Columbus, MS 39701-5800. *Telephone:* 662-329-7302. *Fax:* 662-329-8559. *E-mail:* lcox@muw.edu.

GRADUATE PROGRAMS

Expenses (2006–07) *Tuition, state resident:* full-time $3933; part-time $219 per credit hour. *Tuition, nonresident:* full-time $9724; part-time $540 per credit hour. *International tuition:* $9724 full-time. *Room and board:* $4516 per academic year. *Required fees:* full-time $1000.

Financial Aid 90% of graduate students in nursing programs received some form of financial aid in 2005–06. Fellowships, Federal Work-Study, institutionally sponsored loans, and traineeships available. *Financial aid application deadline:* 4/1.

Contact Dr. Patsy Smyth, DNS, Director of Graduate Nursing Program, Division of Nursing, Mississippi University for Women, 1100 College Street, MUW-910, Columbus, MS 39701-5800. *Telephone:* 662-329-7323. *Fax:* 662-329-7372. *E-mail:* psmyth@muw.edu.

MASTER'S DEGREE PROGRAM

Degree MN

Available Programs Master's.

Concentrations Available *Nurse practitioner programs in:* family health, pediatric.

Study Options Full-time.

Program Entrance Requirements Clinical experience, computer literacy, minimum overall college GPA of 3.0, transcript of college record, CPR certification, immunizations, interview, nursing research course, professional liability insurance/malpractice insurance, statistics course, GRE General Test. *Application deadline:* For fall admission, 4/1.

Advanced Placement Credit given for nursing courses completed elsewhere dependent upon specific evaluations.

Degree Requirements 39 total credit hours, thesis or project, comprehensive exam.

POST-MASTER'S PROGRAM

Areas of Study *Nurse practitioner programs in:* family health, pediatric.

University of Mississippi Medical Center
Program in Nursing
Jackson, Mississippi

http://son.umc.edu/

Founded in 1955

DEGREES • BSN • MSN • PHD

Nursing Program Faculty 51 (57% with doctorates).

Baccalaureate Enrollment 225
Women 88% **Men** 12% **Minority** 14% **Part-time** 12%

Graduate Enrollment 113
Women 86% **Men** 14% **Minority** 25% **Part-time** 48%

Nursing Student Activities Nursing Honor Society, Sigma Theta Tau, Student Nurses' Association, nursing club.

Nursing Student Resources Academic advising; academic or career counseling; assistance for students with disabilities; bookstore; campus computer network; computer lab; computer-assisted instruction; e-mail services; employment services for current students; externships; housing assistance; interactive nursing skills videos; Internet; learning resource lab; library services; nursing audiovisuals; remedial services; skills, simulation, or other laboratory; tutoring; unpaid internships.

Library Facilities 310,016 volumes (63,578 in health); 2,732 periodical subscriptions (150,333 health-care related).

BACCALAUREATE PROGRAMS

Degree BSN

Available Programs ADN to Baccalaureate; Accelerated Baccalaureate for Second Degree; Generic Baccalaureate.

Site Options *Distance Learning:* Oxford, MS; Southaven, MS.

Study Options Full-time and part-time.

Program Entrance Requirements Minimum overall college GPA of 2.5, transcript of college record, CPR certification, written essay, health exam, health insurance, immunizations, minimum GPA in nursing prerequisites of 2.5, professional liability insurance/malpractice insurance, prerequisite course work. Transfer students are accepted. **Application Deadline:** 2/15 (transfer). *Application fee:* $10.

Advanced Placement Credit given for nursing courses completed elsewhere dependent upon specific evaluations.

Expenses (2006–07) *Tuition, area resident:* full-time $4379; part-time $204 per credit hour. *Tuition, nonresident:* full-time $12,077; part-time $357 per credit hour. *Required fees:* full-time $1755.

Financial Aid 98% of baccalaureate students in nursing programs received some form of financial aid in 2005–06.

Contact Dr. Robin Wilkerson, Assistant Dean for Undergraduate Programs, Program in Nursing, University of Mississippi Medical Center, 2500 North State Street, Jackson, MS 39216-4505. *Telephone:* 601-984-6253. *Fax:* 601-984-6206. *E-mail:* rwilkerson@son.umsmed.edu.

GRADUATE PROGRAMS

Expenses (2006–07) *Tuition, state resident:* full-time $3407; part-time $189 per credit hour. *Tuition, nonresident:* full-time $7083; part-time $393 per credit hour. *Required fees:* full-time $1530.

Financial Aid 98% of graduate students in nursing programs received some form of financial aid in 2005–06. Institutionally sponsored loans and traineeships available. Aid available to part-time students. *Financial aid application deadline:* 4/1.

Contact Dr. Sharon Lobert, Associate Dean for Graduate Studies, Program in Nursing, University of Mississippi Medical Center, 2500 North State Street, Jackson, MS 39216-4505. *Telephone:* 601-984-6242. *Fax:* 601-984-6206. *E-mail:* slobert@son.umsmed.edu.

MASTER'S DEGREE PROGRAM

Degree MSN

Available Programs Accelerated AD/RN to Master's; Master's.

Concentrations Available Health-care administration; nursing administration; nursing education. *Nurse practitioner programs in:* acute care, family health, neonatal health, psychiatric/mental health.

Site Options *Distance Learning:* Southaven, MS.

Study Options Full-time and part-time.

Program Entrance Requirements Clinical experience, computer literacy, minimum overall college GPA of 3.0, transcript of college record, CPR certification, immunizations, interview, 3 letters of recommendation, professional liability insurance/malpractice insurance, prerequisite course work, resume, statistics course, GRE. *Application deadline:* Applications are processed on a rolling basis. *Application fee:* $10.

Advanced Placement Credit given for nursing courses completed elsewhere dependent upon specific evaluations.

Degree Requirements 40 total credit hours, thesis or project.

POST-MASTER'S PROGRAM

Areas of Study Nursing education. *Nurse practitioner programs in:* acute care, family health, neonatal health, psychiatric/mental health.

DOCTORAL DEGREE PROGRAM

Degree PhD

Available Programs Doctorate.

Areas of Study Bio-behavioral research, nursing research, nursing science.

Program Entrance Requirements Clinical experience, minimum overall college GPA of 3.0, interview by faculty committee, interview, letters of recommendation, MSN or equivalent, statistics course, vita, writing sample, GRE. *Application deadline:* Applications are processed on a rolling basis. *Application fee:* $10.

Degree Requirements 60 total credit hours, dissertation, oral exam, written exam, residency.

CONTINUING EDUCATION PROGRAM

Contact Dr. Renee Williams, Director of Continuing Education, Program in Nursing, University of Mississippi Medical Center, 2500 North State Street, Jackson, MS 39216-4505. *Telephone:* 601-984-6227. *Fax:* 601-984-6214. *E-mail:* rwilliams@son.umsmed.edu.

University of Southern Mississippi
School of Nursing
Hattiesburg, Mississippi

http://www.nursing.usm.edu

Founded in 1910

DEGREES • BSN • MSN • PHD

Nursing Program Faculty 48 (38% with doctorates).

Baccalaureate Enrollment 333
Women 77% **Men** 23% **Minority** 17% **Part-time** 3.6%

Graduate Enrollment 94
Women 89% **Men** 11% **Minority** 23% **Part-time** 62%

Nursing Student Activities Nursing Honor Society, Sigma Theta Tau, Student Nurses' Association.

University of Southern Mississippi (continued)

Nursing Student Resources Academic advising; academic or career counseling; assistance for students with disabilities; bookstore; campus computer network; career placement assistance; computer lab; computer-assisted instruction; e-mail services; externships; interactive nursing skills videos; Internet; learning resource lab; library services; nursing audiovisuals; remedial services; resume preparation assistance; skills, simulation, or other laboratory.

Library Facilities 1.5 million volumes; 37,095 periodical subscriptions (170 health-care related).

BACCALAUREATE PROGRAMS

Degree BSN

Available Programs ADN to Baccalaureate; Generic Baccalaureate.

Site Options Meridian, MS; Long Beach, MS.

Study Options Full-time and part-time.

Program Entrance Requirements Minimum overall college GPA of 2.5, transcript of college record, CPR certification, written essay, health exam, health insurance, high school transcript, immunizations, minimum GPA in nursing prerequisites of 2.5, professional liability insurance/malpractice insurance, prerequisite course work. Transfer students are accepted. **Standardized tests** *Required:* SAT or ACT, TOEFL for international students. *Required for some:* SAT and SAT Subject Tests or ACT. **Application** *Deadline:* rolling (freshmen), rolling (transfer). *Notification:* continuous (freshmen).

Expenses (2006–07) *Tuition, state resident:* full-time $4594; part-time $180 per credit hour. *Tuition, nonresident:* full-time $6028; part-time $227 per credit hour. *International tuition:* $6028 full-time. *Room and board:* $4300; room only: $3300 per academic year. *Required fees:* full-time $600; part-time $45 per credit.

Financial Aid 85% of baccalaureate students in nursing programs received some form of financial aid in 2005–06.

Contact Tara Burcham, Coordinator of Student Services, School of Nursing, University of Southern Mississippi, 118 College Drive, #5095, Hattiesburg, MS 39406-0001. *Telephone:* 601-266-5454. *Fax:* 601-266-5927. *E-mail:* tara.mccrink-burcham@usm.edu.

GRADUATE PROGRAMS

Expenses (2006–07) *Tuition, state resident:* full-time $3874; part-time $255 per credit hour. *Tuition, nonresident:* full-time $6313; part-time $590 per credit hour. *International tuition:* $6313 full-time. *Room and board:* $4660; room only: $2870 per academic year. *Required fees:* full-time $375.

Financial Aid 1 research assistantship (averaging $8,500 per year) was awarded; Federal Work-Study and traineeships also available.

Contact Ms. Rosalind Hawthorn, Program Contact, School of Nursing, University of Southern Mississippi, 118 College Drive, #5095, Hattiesburg, MS 39406-5095. *Telephone:* 601-266-5457. *Fax:* 601-266-5927. *E-mail:* rosalind.hawthorn@usm.edu.

MASTER'S DEGREE PROGRAM

Degree MSN

Available Programs Master's; RN to Master's.

Concentrations Available Nursing administration. *Clinical nurse specialist programs in:* adult health, community health, psychiatric/mental health. *Nurse practitioner programs in:* family health, psychiatric/mental health.

Site Options Meridian, MS; Long Beach, MS.

Study Options Full-time and part-time.

Program Entrance Requirements Minimum overall college GPA of 3.0, transcript of college record, CPR certification, immunizations, 3 letters of recommendation, professional liability insurance/malpractice insurance, statistics course, GRE General Test. *Application deadline:* For fall admission, 3/15 (priority date); for spring admission, 11/1 (priority date). Applications are processed on a rolling basis. *Application fee:* $25.

Degree Requirements 45 total credit hours, thesis or project, comprehensive exam.

POST-MASTER'S PROGRAM

Areas of Study Nursing administration. *Clinical nurse specialist programs in:* adult health, community health, psychiatric/mental health. *Nurse practitioner programs in:* family health, psychiatric/mental health.

DOCTORAL DEGREE PROGRAM

Degree PhD

Available Programs Doctorate.

Areas of Study Ethics, health policy, nursing administration, nursing education.

Program Entrance Requirements Clinical experience, minimum overall college GPA of 3.5, interview by faculty committee, 3 letters of recommendation, MSN or equivalent, statistics course, vita, writing sample, GRE General Test. *Application deadline:* For fall admission, 3/15 (priority date); for spring admission, 11/1 (priority date). Applications are processed on a rolling basis. *Application fee:* $25.

Degree Requirements 72 total credit hours, dissertation, written exam, residency.

William Carey College
School of Nursing
Hattiesburg, Mississippi

Founded in 1906

DEGREES • BSN • MSN

Nursing Program Faculty 21 (35% with doctorates).

Baccalaureate Enrollment 174
Women 93% **Men** 7% **Minority** 33% **Part-time** 7%

Graduate Enrollment 19
Women 100% **Minority** 26% **Part-time** 11%

Nursing Student Activities Sigma Theta Tau, Student Nurses' Association.

Nursing Student Resources Academic advising; academic or career counseling; assistance for students with disabilities; bookstore; campus computer network; computer lab; computer-assisted instruction; e-mail services; interactive nursing skills videos; Internet; learning resource lab; library services; nursing audiovisuals; resume preparation assistance; skills, simulation, or other laboratory; tutoring.

Library Facilities 98,139 volumes (450 in health, 450 in nursing); 472 periodical subscriptions (50 health-care related).

BACCALAUREATE PROGRAMS

Degree BSN

Available Programs ADN to Baccalaureate; Generic Baccalaureate.

Site Options Gulfport, MS; New Orleans, LA.

Study Options Full-time and part-time.

Program Entrance Requirements Minimum overall college GPA of 2.5, transcript of college record, CPR certification, health exam, high school transcript, immunizations, minimum GPA in nursing prerequisites of 3.0, prerequisite course work. Transfer students are accepted. **Standardized tests** *Required:* SAT or ACT, TOEFL for international students. **Application** *Deadline:* rolling (freshmen), rolling (transfer). *Notification:* continuous until 8/15 (freshmen). *Application fee:* $20.

Advanced Placement Credit given for nursing courses completed elsewhere dependent upon specific evaluations.

Expenses (2006–07) *Tuition:* full-time $10,000; part-time $280 per credit hour. *Room and board:* $2700; room only: $2000 per academic year. *Required fees:* full-time $800; part-time $200 per term.

Financial Aid 90% of baccalaureate students in nursing programs received some form of financial aid in 2005–06. *Gift aid (need-based):* Federal Pell, FSEOG, state, private, college/university gift aid from institutional funds. *Loans:* Federal Nursing Student Loans, FFEL (Subsidized and Unsubsidized Stafford PLUS), Perkins, college/university. *Work-Study:* Federal Work-Study, part-time campus jobs. *Application deadline (priority):* 4/1.

Contact Prof. Kay C. Cater, Director, BSN Programs, School of Nursing, William Carey College, 498 Tuscan Avenue, Hattiesburg, MS 39401. *Telephone:* 601-318-6147. *Fax:* 601-318-6446. *E-mail:* kay.cater@wmcarey.edu.

GRADUATE PROGRAMS

Expenses (2006–07) *Tuition:* full-time $7200; part-time $240 per credit hour. *Required fees:* full-time $100.

Financial Aid 50% of graduate students in nursing programs received some form of financial aid in 2005–06.

Contact Prof. Wanda Dubuisson, Director of MSN Program, School of Nursing, William Carey College, Gulfport Campus, 1856 Beach Drive, Gulfport, MS 39507. *Telephone:* 228-897-7200. *E-mail:* wanda.dubuisson@wmcarey.edu.

MASTER'S DEGREE PROGRAM

Degree MSN

Available Programs Master's.

Concentrations Available Nursing education.

Site Options Gulfport, MS.

Study Options Full-time and part-time.

Program Entrance Requirements Computer literacy, minimum overall college GPA of 3.0, transcript of college record, CPR certification, immunizations, nursing research course, professional liability insurance/malpractice insurance, prerequisite course work, statistics course.

Advanced Placement Credit given for nursing courses completed elsewhere dependent upon specific evaluations.

Degree Requirements 35 total credit hours, thesis or project.

MISSOURI

Avila University

School of Nursing
Kansas City, Missouri

http://www.avila.edu/catalog/degrees/nursing_.htm

Founded in 1916

DEGREE • BSN

Nursing Program Faculty 16 (15% with doctorates).

Baccalaureate Enrollment 75
Women 95% **Men** 5% **Minority** 17% **International** 4%

Nursing Student Activities Nursing Honor Society, Sigma Theta Tau, Student Nurses' Association.

Nursing Student Resources Academic advising; academic or career counseling; assistance for students with disabilities; bookstore; campus computer network; career placement assistance; computer lab; computer-assisted instruction; daycare for children of students; e-mail services; employment services for current students; externships; interactive nursing skills videos; Internet; learning resource lab; library services; nursing audiovisuals; remedial services; resume preparation assistance; skills, simulation, or other laboratory; tutoring.

Library Facilities 80,865 volumes (1,625 in health, 1,145 in nursing); 7,179 periodical subscriptions (100 health-care related).

BACCALAUREATE PROGRAMS

Degree BSN

Available Programs Generic Baccalaureate.

Study Options Full-time.

Program Entrance Requirements Minimum overall college GPA of 2.7, transcript of college record, CPR certification, written essay, health exam, health insurance, immunizations, interview, minimum GPA in nursing prerequisites of 2.0, prerequisite course work. Transfer students are accepted. **Standardized tests** *Required:* SAT or ACT, TOEFL for international students. **Application** *Deadline:* rolling (freshmen), rolling (transfer). *Notification:* continuous (freshmen).

Advanced Placement Credit given for nursing courses completed elsewhere dependent upon specific evaluations.

Expenses (2006–07) *Tuition:* full-time $17,300; part-time $455 per credit hour. *Room and board:* $5500 per academic year. *Required fees:* full-time $1105; part-time $15 per term.

Financial Aid 87% of baccalaureate students in nursing programs received some form of financial aid in 2005–06. *Gift aid (need-based):* Federal Pell, FSEOG, state, private, college/university gift aid from institutional funds. *Loans:* FFEL (Subsidized and Unsubsidized Stafford PLUS), Perkins. *Work-Study:* Federal Work-Study, part-time campus jobs. *Application deadline:* Continuous.

Contact Office of Admissions, School of Nursing, Avila University, 11901 Wornall Road, Kansas City, MO 64145-1698. *Telephone:* 816-501-2400. *Fax:* 816-501-2453. *E-mail:* admissions@avila.edu.

Barnes-Jewish College of Nursing and Allied Health

Division of Nursing
St. Louis, Missouri

Founded in 1902

DEGREES • BSN • MSN

Nursing Program Faculty 29 (40% with doctorates).

Baccalaureate Enrollment 101
Women 90% **Men** 10% **Minority** 20% **Part-time** 80%

Graduate Enrollment 60
Women 95% **Men** 5% **Minority** 10% **Part-time** 60%

Nursing Student Activities Nursing Honor Society, Sigma Theta Tau, Student Nurses' Association.

Nursing Student Resources Academic advising; assistance for students with disabilities; bookstore; campus computer network; career placement assistance; computer lab; e-mail services; employment services for current students; externships; housing assistance; Internet; library services; placement services for program completers; remedial services; skills, simulation, or other laboratory; tutoring.

Library Facilities 3,765 volumes (11,000 in health, 8,100 in nursing); 232 periodical subscriptions (225 health-care related).

BACCALAUREATE PROGRAMS

Degree BSN

Available Programs RN Baccalaureate.

Study Options Full-time and part-time.

Program Entrance Requirements Minimum overall college GPA of 2.75, transcript of college record, CPR certification, health exam, high school biology, high school chemistry, high school math, high school transcript, immunizations, 2 letters of recommendation, minimum high school GPA of 2.75, prerequisite course work, RN licensure. Transfer students are accepted. **Standardized tests** *Required:* SAT or ACT. **Application** *Deadline:* rolling (freshmen), rolling (transfer). *Application fee:* $25.

Advanced Placement Credit by examination available. Credit given for nursing courses completed elsewhere dependent upon specific evaluations.

Contact *Telephone:* 314-454-7064. *Fax:* 314-454-5239.

GRADUATE PROGRAMS

Contact *Telephone:* 314-454-7064. *Fax:* 314-454-5239.

MASTER'S DEGREE PROGRAM

Degree MSN

Available Programs Master's; RN to Master's.

Concentrations Available Nurse anesthesia; nursing education. *Nurse practitioner programs in:* adult health, gerontology, neonatal health, oncology.

Study Options Full-time and part-time.

Program Entrance Requirements Computer literacy, minimum overall college GPA of 3.0, transcript of college record, CPR certification, immunizations, 3 letters of recommendation, nursing research course, physical assessment course, resume, statistics course. *Application deadline:* Applications are processed on a rolling basis. *Application fee:* $25.

Degree Requirements 34 total credit hours, thesis or project.

Barnes-Jewish College of Nursing and Allied Health (continued)
POST-MASTER'S PROGRAM
Areas of Study *Nurse practitioner programs in:* adult health, gerontology, neonatal health, oncology.

Chamberlain College of Nursing
Chamberlain College of Nursing
St. Louis, Missouri

Founded in 1889
DEGREE • BSN

Nursing Program Faculty 14 (21% with doctorates).

Baccalaureate Enrollment 191
Women 96% **Men** 4% **Minority** 25%

Nursing Student Activities Student Nurses' Association.

Nursing Student Resources Academic advising; academic or career counseling; campus computer network; career placement assistance; computer lab; computer-assisted instruction; e-mail services; employment services for current students; housing assistance; Internet; learning resource lab; library services; nursing audiovisuals; placement services for program completers; skills, simulation, or other laboratory; tutoring.

Library Facilities 8,700 volumes (3,287 in health, 957 in nursing); 233 periodical subscriptions (182 health-care related).

BACCALAUREATE PROGRAMS
Degree BSN

Available Programs ADN to Baccalaureate; RN Baccalaureate; RPN to Baccalaureate.

Study Options Full-time and part-time.

Program Entrance Requirements Minimum overall college GPA of 2.5, transcript of college record, written essay, health exam, health insurance, high school biology, high school chemistry, 3 years high school math, 3 years high school science, high school transcript, immunizations, minimum high school GPA of 2.5, minimum high school rank 33%. Transfer students are accepted. **Standardized tests** *Required:* ACT, TOEFL for international students. **Application** *Deadline:* rolling (freshmen), rolling (transfer). *Notification:* continuous (freshmen). *Application fee:* $50.

Advanced Placement Credit by examination available. Credit given for nursing courses completed elsewhere dependent upon specific evaluations.

Contact *Telephone:* 800-942-4310 Ext. 1. *Fax:* 314-768-3044 Ext. 1.

Cox College of Nursing and Health Sciences
Department of Nursing
Springfield, Missouri

Founded in 1994
DEGREE • BSN

Nursing Program Faculty 20 (50% with doctorates).

Baccalaureate Enrollment 250
Women 95% **Men** 5% **Minority** 5% **International** 4% **Part-time** 80%

Nursing Student Activities Nursing Honor Society, Student Nurses' Association, nursing club.

Nursing Student Resources Academic advising; academic or career counseling; assistance for students with disabilities; bookstore; campus computer network; career placement assistance; computer lab; computer-assisted instruction; daycare for children of students; e-mail services; employment services for current students; externships; housing assistance; interactive nursing skills videos; Internet; learning resource lab; library services; nursing audiovisuals; placement services for program completers; remedial services; resume preparation assistance; skills, simulation, or other laboratory; tutoring.

Library Facilities 5,500 volumes in health, 1,900 volumes in nursing; 250 periodical subscriptions health-care related.

BACCALAUREATE PROGRAMS
Degree BSN

Available Programs ADN to Baccalaureate; Accelerated Baccalaureate; Accelerated Baccalaureate for Second Degree; Baccalaureate for Second Degree; Generic Baccalaureate; LPN to Baccalaureate; LPN to RN Baccalaureate; RN Baccalaureate.

Site Options Springfield, MO. *Distance Learning:* Springfield, MO.

Study Options Full-time and part-time.

Program Entrance Requirements Minimum overall college GPA of 3.0, transcript of college record, CPR certification, written essay, health exam, high school biology, high school chemistry, 2 years high school math, 2 years high school science, high school transcript, immunizations, interview, minimum high school GPA of 3.0, minimum GPA in nursing prerequisites of 3.0, prerequisite course work. Transfer students are accepted. **Standardized tests** *Recommended:* SAT or ACT. **Application** *Deadline:* 2/1 (freshmen), 8/1 (transfer). *Early decision:* 11/1. *Notification:* 3/1 (freshmen), 12/1 (out-of-state freshmen), 12/1 (early decision). *Application fee:* $30.

Advanced Placement Credit given for nursing courses completed elsewhere dependent upon specific evaluations.

Expenses (2005–06) *Tuition:* full-time $9240; part-time $308 per credit. *International tuition:* $9240 full-time. *Room and board:* room only: $2800 per academic year. *Required fees:* full-time $1050; part-time $35 per credit; part-time $150 per term.

Financial Aid 80% of baccalaureate students in nursing programs received some form of financial aid in 2004–05.

Contact Ms. Jennifer Plimmer, Admissions Coordinator, Department of Nursing, Cox College of Nursing and Health Sciences, 1423 North Jefferson Avenue, Springfield, MO 65802. *Telephone:* 417-269-3038. *E-mail:* jplimme@coxcollege.edu.

CONTINUING EDUCATION PROGRAM
Contact Dr. Susan Fairchild, Continuing Education Coordinator, Department of Nursing, Cox College of Nursing and Health Sciences, 1423 North Jefferson Avenue, Springfield, MO 65802. *Telephone:* 417-269-8450. *E-mail:* sfairc@coxcollege.edu.

Culver-Stockton College
Blessing–Rieman College of Nursing
Canton, Missouri

http://www.culver.edu/

See description of programs under Blessing–Rieman College of Nursing (Quincy, Illinois).

Graceland University
School of Nursing
Independence, Missouri

http://www.graceland.edu/show.cfm?durki=26

Founded in 1895
DEGREES • BSN • MSN

Nursing Program Faculty 22 (32% with doctorates).

Baccalaureate Enrollment 141
Women 92% **Men** 8% **Minority** 6% **Part-time** 52%

Graduate Enrollment 233
Women 85% **Men** 15% **Minority** 8% **Part-time** 64%

Nursing Student Activities Nursing Honor Society, Sigma Theta Tau, Student Nurses' Association, nursing club.

Nursing Student Resources Academic advising; academic or career counseling; bookstore; campus computer network; computer lab; computer-assisted instruction; e-mail services; housing assistance; interactive nursing skills videos; Internet; learning resource lab; library services; nursing audiovisuals; resume preparation assistance; skills, simulation, or other laboratory; tutoring.

Library Facilities 193,109 volumes (2,344 in health, 794 in nursing); 503 periodical subscriptions (1,381 health-care related).

BACCALAUREATE PROGRAMS

Degree BSN

Available Programs ADN to Baccalaureate; Accelerated Baccalaureate; Accelerated Baccalaureate for Second Degree; Accelerated RN Baccalaureate; Generic Baccalaureate; RN Baccalaureate.

Site Options *Distance Learning:* Independence, MO.

Study Options Full-time and part-time.

Program Entrance Requirements Minimum overall college GPA of 2.5, transcript of college record, written essay, health exam, high school chemistry, high school transcript, immunizations, 2 letters of recommendation, minimum high school GPA, minimum GPA in nursing prerequisites of 2.0, prerequisite course work. Transfer students are accepted. **Standardized tests** *Required:* SAT or ACT, TOEFL for international students. **Application** *Deadline:* rolling (freshmen), rolling (transfer). *Early decision:* 1/31. *Notification:* continuous (freshmen). *Application fee:* $50.

Advanced Placement Credit given for nursing courses completed elsewhere dependent upon specific evaluations.

Expenses (2006–07) *Tuition:* part-time $355 per credit hour. *Required fees:* full-time $500.

Financial Aid 67% of baccalaureate students in nursing programs received some form of financial aid in 2005–06. *Gift aid (need-based):* Federal Pell, FSEOG, state, private, college/university gift aid from institutional funds. *Loans:* Federal Direct (Subsidized and Unsubsidized Stafford PLUS), Perkins, state, college/university. *Work-Study:* Federal Work-Study, part-time campus jobs. *Application deadline:* Continuous.

Contact Mr. John D. Koehler, Manager of Recruiting, School of Nursing, Graceland University, 1401 West Truman Road, Independence, MO 64050-3434. *Telephone:* 800-833-0524 Ext. 4804. *Fax:* 816-833-2990. *E-mail:* jkoehler@graceland.edu.

GRADUATE PROGRAMS

Expenses (2006–07) *Tuition:* part-time $445 per credit hour. *Required fees:* full-time $1025.

Financial Aid 25% of graduate students in nursing programs received some form of financial aid in 2005–06.

Contact Mr. John D. Koehler, Manager of Recruiting, School of Nursing, Graceland University, 1401 West Truman Road, Independence, MO 64050-3434. *Telephone:* 816-833-0524 Ext. 4804. *Fax:* 816-833-2990. *E-mail:* jkoehler@graceland.edu.

MASTER'S DEGREE PROGRAM

Degree MSN

Available Programs Master's; RN to Master's.

Concentrations Available Health-care administration; nursing education. *Nurse practitioner programs in:* family health.

Site Options *Distance Learning:* Independence, MO.

Study Options Full-time and part-time.

Program Entrance Requirements Clinical experience, minimum overall college GPA of 3.0, transcript of college record, written essay, 3 letters of recommendation, nursing research course, physical assessment course, prerequisite course work, statistics course.

Advanced Placement Credit given for nursing courses completed elsewhere dependent upon specific evaluations.

Degree Requirements 43 total credit hours, thesis or project, comprehensive exam.

POST-MASTER'S PROGRAM

Areas of Study Health-care administration; nursing education. *Nurse practitioner programs in:* family health.

Lincoln University
Department of Nursing
Jefferson City, Missouri

Founded in 1866

DEGREE • BSN

Library Facilities 204,948 volumes; 368 periodical subscriptions.

BACCALAUREATE PROGRAMS

Degree BSN

Available Programs RN Baccalaureate.

Program Entrance Requirements **Standardized tests** *Required:* TOEFL for international students. **Application** *Deadline:* 7/15 (freshmen), 7/15 (out-of-state freshmen), 6/15 (transfer). *Notification:* continuous (freshmen), continuous (out-of-state freshmen). *Application fee:* $17.

Contact Connie Hamacher, PhD, Department Head of Nursing Science, Department of Nursing, Lincoln University, Elliff Hall, Room 100, 820 Chestnut Street, Jefferson City, MO 65101. *Telephone:* 573-681-5421. *E-mail:* nursing@lincolnu.edu.

Maryville University of Saint Louis
Nursing Program, School of Health Professions
St. Louis, Missouri

http://www.maryville.edu

Founded in 1872

DEGREES • BSN • MSN

Nursing Program Faculty 46 (17% with doctorates).

Baccalaureate Enrollment 412
Women 97% **Men** 3% **Minority** 10% **Part-time** 40%

Graduate Enrollment 93
Women 94% **Men** 6% **Minority** 10% **Part-time** 99%

Nursing Student Activities Sigma Theta Tau, Student Nurses' Association.

Nursing Student Resources Academic advising; academic or career counseling; assistance for students with disabilities; bookstore; campus computer network; computer lab; computer-assisted instruction; e-mail services; externships; interactive nursing skills videos; Internet; learning resource lab; library services; nursing audiovisuals; resume preparation assistance; skills, simulation, or other laboratory; tutoring.

Library Facilities 213,053 volumes (9,459 in health, 1,521 in nursing); 14,110 periodical subscriptions (2,500 health-care related).

BACCALAUREATE PROGRAMS

Degree BSN

Available Programs Accelerated Baccalaureate; Accelerated RN Baccalaureate; Generic Baccalaureate; LPN to Baccalaureate; RN Baccalaureate.

Study Options Full-time and part-time.

Program Entrance Requirements Minimum overall college GPA of 2.75, transcript of college record, health exam, high school transcript, immunizations, minimum high school GPA of 2.75, minimum GPA in nursing prerequisites of 2.75. Transfer students are accepted. **Standardized tests** *Required:* SAT or ACT, TOEFL for international students. **Application** *Deadline:* 8/15 (freshmen), rolling (transfer). *Notification:* continuous (freshmen). *Application fee:* $25.

Advanced Placement Credit given for nursing courses completed elsewhere dependent upon specific evaluations.

Expenses (2006–07) *Tuition:* full-time $17,800; part-time $540 per credit hour. *International tuition:* $17,800 full-time. *Room and board:* $7720; room only: $4246 per academic year. *Required fees:* full-time $320; part-time $80 per term.

Financial Aid 57% of baccalaureate students in nursing programs received some form of financial aid in 2005–06. *Gift aid (need-based):* Federal Pell, FSEOG, state, private, college/university gift aid from institutional funds. *Loans:* Federal Direct (Subsidized and Unsubsidized Stafford

Maryville University of Saint Louis (continued)

PLUS), Perkins, Sallie Mae Signature Loans, Keybank Loans, TERI Loans, CitiAssist Loans, MOHELA ED Cash Loans, Wells Fargo Loans, Nelnet. *Work-Study:* Federal Work-Study, part-time campus jobs. *Application deadline (priority):* 3/1.

Contact Dr. Mary Curtis, Director, Nursing Program, School of Health Professions, Maryville University of Saint Louis, 650 Maryville University Drive, St. Louis, MO 63141-7299. *Telephone:* 314-529-9478. *Fax:* 314-529-9139. *E-mail:* maryc@maryville.edu.

GRADUATE PROGRAMS

Expenses (2006–07) *Tuition:* full-time $17,800; part-time $555 per credit hour. *International tuition:* $17,800 full-time. *Room and board:* $7720; room only: $4246 per academic year. *Required fees:* full-time $1500; part-time $55 per term.

Financial Aid 29% of graduate students in nursing programs received some form of financial aid in 2005–06.

Contact Debbie Fritz, PhD, Coordinator of Graduate Program, Nursing Program, School of Health Professions, Maryville University of Saint Louis, 650 Maryville University Drive, St. Louis, MO 63141. *Telephone:* 314-529-9453. *Fax:* 314-529-9139. *E-mail:* fritz@maryville.edu.

MASTER'S DEGREE PROGRAM

Degree MSN

Available Programs Accelerated RN to Master's; Master's; RN to Master's.

Concentrations Available Nursing education. *Nurse practitioner programs in:* adult health, family health.

Study Options Full-time and part-time.

Program Entrance Requirements Minimum overall college GPA of 3.0, transcript of college record, 3 letters of recommendation, resume, statistics course.

Advanced Placement Credit by examination available. Credit given for nursing courses completed elsewhere dependent upon specific evaluations.

Degree Requirements 42 total credit hours, thesis or project.

Missouri Southern State University

Department of Nursing
Joplin, Missouri

http://www.mssu.edu/nursing/
Founded in 1937

DEGREE • BSN

Nursing Program Faculty 9 (25% with doctorates).

Baccalaureate Enrollment 99
Women 85% **Men** 15% **Minority** 3% **International** 1%

Nursing Student Activities Nursing Honor Society, Student Nurses' Association.

Nursing Student Resources Academic advising; academic or career counseling; assistance for students with disabilities; bookstore; campus computer network; career placement assistance; computer lab; computer-assisted instruction; daycare for children of students; e-mail services; employment services for current students; housing assistance; interactive nursing skills videos; Internet; learning resource lab; library services; nursing audiovisuals; remedial services; resume preparation assistance; skills, simulation, or other laboratory; tutoring.

Library Facilities 4,872 volumes in health, 4,470 volumes in nursing; 4,412 periodical subscriptions health-care related.

BACCALAUREATE PROGRAMS

Degree BSN

Available Programs ADN to Baccalaureate; Baccalaureate for Second Degree; Generic Baccalaureate; LPN to RN Baccalaureate; RN Baccalaureate.

Study Options Full-time.

Program Entrance Requirements Transcript of college record, CPR certification, health exam, health insurance, immunizations, minimum GPA in nursing prerequisites of 2.5, professional liability insurance/malpractice insurance, prerequisite course work. Transfer students are accepted.
Standardized tests *Required:* SAT or ACT, TOEFL for international students. *Recommended:* ACT. *Required for some:* Michigan Test of English Language Proficiency. **Application** *Deadline:* 8/1 (freshmen), 8/1 (transfer). *Notification:* continuous (freshmen). *Application fee:* $15.

Advanced Placement Credit by examination available. Credit given for nursing courses completed elsewhere dependent upon specific evaluations.

Financial Aid 83% of baccalaureate students in nursing programs received some form of financial aid in 2005–06.

Contact Dr. J. Mari Beth Linder, Director, Department of Nursing, Missouri Southern State University, Kuhn Hall, Room 210B, 3950 East Newman Road, Joplin, MO 64801-1595. *Telephone:* 417-625-9322. *Fax:* 417-625-3186. *E-mail:* linder-m@mssu.edu.

Missouri State University

Department of Nursing
Springfield, Missouri

http://www.smsu.edu/nursing
Founded in 1905

DEGREES • BSN • MSN

Nursing Program Faculty 13 (39% with doctorates).

Baccalaureate Enrollment 147
Women 90% **Men** 10% **Minority** 3% **International** 1% **Part-time** 42%

Graduate Enrollment 32
Women 94% **Men** 6% **Minority** 1%

Nursing Student Activities Sigma Theta Tau, Student Nurses' Association.

Nursing Student Resources Academic advising; academic or career counseling; assistance for students with disabilities; bookstore; campus computer network; career placement assistance; computer lab; computer-assisted instruction; daycare for children of students; e-mail services; employment services for current students; externships; housing assistance; interactive nursing skills videos; Internet; learning resource lab; library services; nursing audiovisuals; paid internships; placement services for program completers; remedial services; resume preparation assistance; skills, simulation, or other laboratory; tutoring; unpaid internships.

Library Facilities 1.7 million volumes (10,500 in health, 3,516 in nursing); 4,238 periodical subscriptions (370 health-care related).

BACCALAUREATE PROGRAMS

Degree BSN

Available Programs ADN to Baccalaureate; Baccalaureate for Second Degree; Generic Baccalaureate; LPN to Baccalaureate.

Site Options *Distance Learning:* Branson, MO; West Plains, MO.

Study Options Full-time.

Program Entrance Requirements Minimum overall college GPA of 2.75, transcript of college record, CPR certification, health insurance, immunizations, prerequisite course work. Transfer students are accepted.
Standardized tests *Required:* SAT or ACT, TOEFL for international students. **Application** *Deadline:* 7/20 (freshmen), 7/20 (transfer). *Notification:* continuous (freshmen). *Application fee:* $30.

Advanced Placement Credit given for nursing courses completed elsewhere dependent upon specific evaluations.

Expenses (2006–07) *Tuition, state resident:* part-time $173 per credit. *Tuition, nonresident:* part-time $337 per credit. *International tuition:* $360 full-time. *Room and board:* $6606; room only: $3600 per academic year. *Required fees:* full-time $5320.

Financial Aid 30% of baccalaureate students in nursing programs received some form of financial aid in 2005–06. *Gift aid (need-based):* Federal Pell, FSEOG, state, private, college/university gift aid from institutional funds. *Loans:* FFEL (Subsidized and Unsubsidized Stafford PLUS), Perkins, state, college/university. *Work-Study:* Federal Work-Study, part-time campus jobs. *Application deadline (priority):* 3/30.

Contact Dr. Kathryn L. Hope, Associate Professor, Department of Nursing, Missouri State University, 901 South National Avenue, Springfield, MO 65897. *Telephone:* 417-836-5310. *Fax:* 417-836-5484. *E-mail:* kathrynhope@missouristate.edu.

GRADUATE PROGRAMS

Expenses (2006–07) *International tuition:* $418 full-time. *Room and board:* $5178; room only: $3600 per academic year. *Required fees:* full-time $600; part-time $84 per credit; part-time $214 per term.

Financial Aid 25% of graduate students in nursing programs received some form of financial aid in 2005–06. Research assistantships with full tuition reimbursements available (averaging $6,575 per year), teaching assistantships with full tuition reimbursements available (averaging $6,575 per year) were awarded; Federal Work-Study and unspecified assistantships also available. *Financial aid application deadline:* 3/31.

Contact Dr. Kathryn L. Hope, Associate Professor, Department of Nursing, Missouri State University, 901 South National Avenue, Springfield, MO 65897. *Telephone:* 417-836-5310. *Fax:* 417-836-5484. *E-mail:* kathrynhope@missouristate.edu.

MASTER'S DEGREE PROGRAM

Degree MSN

Available Programs Accelerated AD/RN to Master's; Master's; RN to Master's.

Concentrations Available Nursing education. *Nurse practitioner programs in:* family health.

Study Options Full-time and part-time.

Program Entrance Requirements Computer literacy, minimum overall college GPA of 3.0, transcript of college record, written essay, immunizations, interview, 2 letters of recommendation, nursing research course, physical assessment course, professional liability insurance/malpractice insurance, statistics course, GRE General Test. *Application deadline:* For fall admission, 7/20 (priority date); for spring admission, 12/20 (priority date). Applications are processed on a rolling basis. *Application fee:* $30.

Advanced Placement Credit given for nursing courses completed elsewhere dependent upon specific evaluations.

Degree Requirements 51 total credit hours, thesis or project, comprehensive exam.

POST-MASTER'S PROGRAM

Areas of Study Nursing education. *Nurse practitioner programs in:* family health.

CONTINUING EDUCATION PROGRAM

Contact Virginia Cordova, Program Coordinator, Department of Nursing, Missouri State University, Department of Continuing Education, 901 South National, Springfield, MO 65897. *Telephone:* 417-836-6660. *Fax:* 417-836-7674. *E-mail:* virginiacordova@missouristate.edu.

Missouri Western State University
Department of Nursing
St. Joseph, Missouri

http://www.mwsc.edu/nursing
Founded in 1915
DEGREE • BSN

Nursing Program Faculty 14 (28% with doctorates).

Baccalaureate Enrollment 213
Women 85% **Men** 15% **Minority** 3% **Part-time** 3%

Nursing Student Activities Sigma Theta Tau, Student Nurses' Association.

Nursing Student Resources Academic advising; academic or career counseling; assistance for students with disabilities; bookstore; campus computer network; career placement assistance; computer lab; computer-assisted instruction; daycare for children of students; e-mail services; employment services for current students; interactive nursing skills videos;

Internet; library services; nursing audiovisuals; paid internships; remedial services; resume preparation assistance; skills, simulation, or other laboratory; tutoring; unpaid internships.

Library Facilities 147,509 volumes (8,607 in nursing); 1,068 periodical subscriptions (21 health-care related).

BACCALAUREATE PROGRAMS

Degree BSN

Available Programs Generic Baccalaureate; LPN to Baccalaureate; RN Baccalaureate.

Study Options Full-time and part-time.

Program Entrance Requirements Minimum overall college GPA of 2.5, transcript of college record, CPR certification, written essay, health exam, health insurance, high school transcript, immunizations, 3 letters of recommendation, minimum high school GPA of 2.5, minimum GPA in nursing prerequisites, prerequisite course work. Transfer students are accepted. **Standardized tests** *Required:* TOEFL for international students. **Application** *Deadline:* 6/1 (freshmen), 6/1 (transfer). *Notification:* continuous until 8/10 (freshmen). *Application fee:* $15.

Advanced Placement Credit by examination available. Credit given for nursing courses completed elsewhere dependent upon specific evaluations.

Contact *Telephone:* 816-271-4415. *Fax:* 816-271-5849.

CONTINUING EDUCATION PROGRAM

Contact *Telephone:* 816-271-4100.

Research College of Nursing
College of Nursing
Kansas City, Missouri

Founded in 1980
DEGREES • BSN • MSN

Nursing Program Faculty 45 (15% with doctorates).

Baccalaureate Enrollment 213
Women 98% **Men** 2% **Minority** 5% **International** 1% **Part-time** 4%

Graduate Enrollment 28
Women 95% **Men** 5% **Minority** 95% **International** 5% **Part-time** 96%

Nursing Student Activities Sigma Theta Tau, Student Nurses' Association.

Nursing Student Resources Academic advising; academic or career counseling; bookstore; campus computer network; career placement assistance; computer lab; computer-assisted instruction; daycare for children of students; e-mail services; housing assistance; Internet; learning resource lab; library services; resume preparation assistance; skills, simulation, or other laboratory; tutoring.

Library Facilities 150,000 volumes; 675 periodical subscriptions.

BACCALAUREATE PROGRAMS

Degree BSN

Available Programs Accelerated Baccalaureate; Accelerated Baccalaureate for Second Degree; Baccalaureate for Second Degree; Generic Baccalaureate.

Study Options Full-time.

Program Entrance Requirements Transcript of college record, high school chemistry, 3 years high school math, 2 years high school science, high school transcript, minimum high school rank 50%, minimum GPA in nursing prerequisites of 2.7. Transfer students are accepted. **Standardized tests** *Required:* SAT or ACT, TOEFL for international students. **Application** *Deadline:* 6/30 (freshmen), 2/15 (transfer). *Notification:* continuous until 8/15 (freshmen). *Application fee:* $20.

Advanced Placement Credit given for nursing courses completed elsewhere dependent upon specific evaluations.

Expenses (2006–07) *Tuition:* full-time $20,200; part-time $675 per credit hour. *International tuition:* $20,200 full-time. *Room and board:* $6200; room only: $3200 per academic year. *Required fees:* full-time $650; part-time $60 per term.

Research College of Nursing (continued)

Financial Aid   90% of baccalaureate students in nursing programs received some form of financial aid in 2005–06.

Contact   Leslie Mendenhall, Director of Transfer and Graduate Admissions, College of Nursing, Research College of Nursing, 2525 East Meyer Boulevard, Kansas City, MO 64132-1199. *Telephone:* 816-995-2820. *Fax:* 816-995-2813. *E-mail:* leslie.mendenhall@researchcollege.edu.

GRADUATE PROGRAMS

Expenses (2006–07)   *Tuition:* part-time $350 per credit hour. *Required fees:* part-time $25 per term.

Financial Aid   15% of graduate students in nursing programs received some form of financial aid in 2005–06.

Contact   Leslie Mendenhall, Director of Transfer and Graduate Admissions, College of Nursing, Research College of Nursing, 2525 East Meyer Boulevard, Kansas City, MO 64132-1199. *Telephone:* 816-995-2820. *Fax:* 816-995-2813. *E-mail:* leslie.mendenhall@researchcollege.edu.

MASTER'S DEGREE PROGRAM

Degree   MSN

Available Programs   Master's.

Concentrations Available   Nursing administration; nursing education. *Nurse practitioner programs in:* family health.

Study Options   Full-time and part-time.

Program Entrance Requirements   Minimum overall college GPA of 3.0, transcript of college record, CPR certification, written essay, immunizations, interview, 3 letters of recommendation, physical assessment course, professional liability insurance/malpractice insurance, resume, statistics course.

Advanced Placement   Credit given for nursing courses completed elsewhere dependent upon specific evaluations.

Degree Requirements   45 total credit hours, thesis or project.

Saint Louis University
School of Nursing
St. Louis, Missouri

http://www.slu.edu/colleges/NR

Founded in 1818

DEGREES • BSN • MSN • MSN/MPH • PHD

Nursing Program Faculty   54 (50% with doctorates).

Baccalaureate Enrollment   400
Women 93% **Men** 7% **Minority** 12% **Part-time** 5%

Graduate Enrollment   269
Women 94% **Men** 6% **Minority** 13% **International** 4% **Part-time** 89%

Nursing Student Activities   Sigma Theta Tau, Student Nurses' Association.

Nursing Student Resources   Academic advising; academic or career counseling; assistance for students with disabilities; bookstore; campus computer network; career placement assistance; computer lab; computer-assisted instruction; e-mail services; employment services for current students; housing assistance; interactive nursing skills videos; Internet; learning resource lab; library services; nursing audiovisuals; placement services for program completers; remedial services; resume preparation assistance; skills, simulation, or other laboratory; tutoring; unpaid internships.

Library Facilities   1.9 million volumes (112,581 in health, 41,034 in nursing); 14,395 periodical subscriptions (6,427 health-care related).

BACCALAUREATE PROGRAMS

Degree   BSN

Available Programs   Accelerated Baccalaureate; Accelerated Baccalaureate for Second Degree; Generic Baccalaureate; RN Baccalaureate.

Study Options   Full-time and part-time.

Program Entrance Requirements   Minimum overall college GPA of 3.0, transcript of college record, health exam, high school biology, high school chemistry, high school transcript, immunizations, minimum high school GPA of 3.0. Transfer students are accepted. **Standardized tests** *Required:* SAT or ACT. *Recommended:* TOEFL for international students. **Application** *Deadline:* 8/1 (freshmen), rolling (transfer). *Notification:* 10/1 (freshmen). *Application fee:* $25.

Advanced Placement   Credit by examination available. Credit given for nursing courses completed elsewhere dependent upon specific evaluations.

Financial Aid   75% of baccalaureate students in nursing programs received some form of financial aid in 2005–06. *Gift aid (need-based):* Federal Pell, FSEOG, state, private, college/university gift aid from institutional funds. *Loans:* Federal Nursing Student Loans, FFEL (Subsidized and Unsubsidized Stafford PLUS), Perkins. *Work-Study:* Federal Work-Study, part-time campus jobs. *Application deadline (priority):* 3/1.

Contact   Mrs. Sarah Calame, Director of Marketing and Recruitment, School of Nursing, Saint Louis University, 3525 Caroline Street, St. Louis, MO 63104. *Telephone:* 314-977-8995. *Fax:* 314-977-8949. *E-mail:* slunurse@slu.edu.

GRADUATE PROGRAMS

Financial Aid   50% of graduate students in nursing programs received some form of financial aid in 2005–06. 1 research assistantship with full tuition reimbursement available (averaging $10,000 per year), 6 teaching assistantships with full tuition reimbursements available (averaging $9,500 per year) were awarded; traineeships, tuition waivers (partial), and unspecified assistantships also available. *Financial aid application deadline:* 6/1.

Contact   Dr. Margie Edel, Chairperson, Master's Program in Nursing, School of Nursing, Saint Louis University, 3525 Caroline Mall, St. Louis, MO 63104. *Telephone:* 314-977-8931. *Fax:* 314-977-8949. *E-mail:* edele@slu.edu.

MASTER'S DEGREE PROGRAM

Degrees   MSN; MSN/MPH

Available Programs   Master's; Master's for Nurses with Non-Nursing Degrees; RN to Master's.

Concentrations Available   Nursing education. *Clinical nurse specialist programs in:* acute care, adult health, gerontology, pediatric, perinatal, psychiatric/mental health. *Nurse practitioner programs in:* acute care, adult health, family health, gerontology, pediatric, psychiatric/mental health.

Site Options   *Distance Learning:* St. Louis, MO.

Study Options   Full-time and part-time.

Program Entrance Requirements   Minimum overall college GPA of 3.0, transcript of college record, CPR certification, immunizations, 3 letters of recommendation, physical assessment course, resume, statistics course. *Application deadline:* For fall admission, 7/1; for spring admission, 11/1. Applications are processed on a rolling basis. *Application fee:* $40.

Advanced Placement   Credit given for nursing courses completed elsewhere dependent upon specific evaluations.

Degree Requirements   36 total credit hours.

POST-MASTER'S PROGRAM

Areas of Study   Nursing education. *Clinical nurse specialist programs in:* acute care, adult health, gerontology, pediatric, perinatal, psychiatric/mental health. *Nurse practitioner programs in:* acute care, adult health, family health, gerontology, pediatric, psychiatric/mental health.

DOCTORAL DEGREE PROGRAM

Degree   PhD

Available Programs   Doctorate.

Areas of Study   Faculty preparation, gerontology, health promotion/disease prevention, human health and illness, maternity-newborn, nursing education, nursing research, nursing science, women's health.

Program Entrance Requirements   Minimum overall college GPA of 3.25, 3 letters of recommendation, MSN or equivalent, statistics course, vita, writing sample, GRE General Test. *Application deadline:* For fall admission, 7/1; for spring admission, 11/1. Applications are processed on a rolling basis. *Application fee:* $40.

Degree Requirements   69 total credit hours, dissertation, oral exam, written exam, residency.

CONTINUING EDUCATION PROGRAM

Contact Ms. Kristine M. L'Ecuyer, Director, Continuing Education, School of Nursing, Saint Louis University, 3525 Caroline Mall, St. Louis, MO 63104. *Telephone:* 314-977-8975. *Fax:* 314-977-8949. *E-mail:* lecuyerk@slu.edu.

Saint Luke's College
Nursing College
Kansas City, Missouri

http://www.saintlukescollege.edu

Founded in 1903

DEGREE • BSN

Nursing Program Faculty 17 (18% with doctorates).

Baccalaureate Enrollment 115
Women 95% **Men** 5% **Minority** 10% **International** 1% **Part-time** 12%

Nursing Student Activities Student Nurses' Association.

Nursing Student Resources Academic advising; assistance for students with disabilities; bookstore; campus computer network; career placement assistance; computer lab; computer-assisted instruction; e-mail services; employment services for current students; interactive nursing skills videos; Internet; learning resource lab; library services; nursing audiovisuals; skills, simulation, or other laboratory; tutoring.

BACCALAUREATE PROGRAMS

Degree BSN

Available Programs Generic Baccalaureate.

Site Options Kansas City, MO.

Study Options Full-time and part-time.

Program Entrance Requirements Transcript of college record, CPR certification, written essay, health exam, health insurance, high school transcript, immunizations, interview, 3 letters of recommendation, minimum GPA in nursing prerequisites of 2.7, prerequisite course work. Transfer students are accepted. **Standardized tests** *Required:* TOEFL for international students. **Application** *Deadline:* 12/31 (transfer). *Application fee:* $20.

Advanced Placement Credit given for nursing courses completed elsewhere dependent upon specific evaluations.

Expenses (2005–06) *Tuition:* full-time $8850; part-time $295 per credit hour. *Required fees:* full-time $670.

Financial Aid 90% of baccalaureate students in nursing programs received some form of financial aid in 2004–05.

Contact Mr. Jeff Gannon, Director of Admissions, Nursing College, Saint Luke's College, 8320 Ward Parkway, Suite 300, Kansas City, MO 64114. *Telephone:* 816-932-2367. *Fax:* 816-932-9064. *E-mail:* slc-admissions@saint-lukes.org.

Southeast Missouri State University
Department of Nursing
Cape Girardeau, Missouri

http://www2.semo.edu/nursing

Founded in 1873

DEGREES • BSN • MSN

Nursing Program Faculty 24 (60% with doctorates).

Baccalaureate Enrollment 408
Women 95% **Men** 5% **Minority** 7% **Part-time** 20%

Graduate Enrollment 37
Women 80% **Men** 20% **Minority** 2% **Part-time** 65%

Nursing Student Activities Sigma Theta Tau, Student Nurses' Association.

Nursing Student Resources Academic advising; academic or career counseling; assistance for students with disabilities; bookstore; campus computer network; computer lab; computer-assisted instruction; daycare for children of students; e-mail services; employment services for current students; housing assistance; interactive nursing skills videos; Internet; learning resource lab; library services; nursing audiovisuals; remedial services; skills, simulation, or other laboratory; tutoring.

Library Facilities 429,108 volumes (450,750 in health, 16,145 in nursing); 32,455 periodical subscriptions (75 health-care related).

BACCALAUREATE PROGRAMS

Degree BSN

Available Programs Generic Baccalaureate; RN Baccalaureate.

Site Options *Distance Learning:* Poplar Bluff, MO; Kennett, MO.

Study Options Full-time.

Program Entrance Requirements Minimum overall college GPA of 2.5, transcript of college record, CPR certification, health exam, health insurance, high school transcript, immunizations, professional liability insurance/malpractice insurance, prerequisite course work. Transfer students are accepted. **Standardized tests** *Required:* SAT or ACT, TOEFL for international students. **Application** *Notification:* 10/1 (freshmen). *Application fee:* $20.

Contact *Telephone:* 573-651-2585. *Fax:* 573-651-2142.

GRADUATE PROGRAMS

Contact *Telephone:* 573-651-2871. *Fax:* 573-651-2142.

MASTER'S DEGREE PROGRAM

Degree MSN

Available Programs Master's.

Concentrations Available Nursing education. *Clinical nurse specialist programs in:* adult health. *Nurse practitioner programs in:* family health.

Site Options *Distance Learning:* Poplar Bluff, MO; Kennett, MO.

Study Options Full-time and part-time.

Program Entrance Requirements Clinical experience, minimum overall college GPA of 3.0, transcript of college record, CPR certification, written essay, immunizations, 2 letters of recommendation, physical assessment course, professional liability insurance/malpractice insurance, prerequisite course work, resume, statistics course. *Application deadline:* For fall admission, 8/1; for spring admission, 11/21. Applications are processed on a rolling basis. *Application fee:* $20 ($100 for international students).

Degree Requirements 45 total credit hours, thesis or project.

POST-MASTER'S PROGRAM

Areas of Study *Nurse practitioner programs in:* family health.

Southwest Baptist University
College of Nursing
Bolivar, Missouri

Founded in 1878

DEGREE • BSN

Nursing Program Faculty 8 (33% with doctorates).

Baccalaureate Enrollment 113
Women 95% **Men** 5% **Minority** 2% **Part-time** 85%

Nursing Student Activities Nursing Honor Society, Student Nurses' Association.

Nursing Student Resources Academic advising; bookstore; campus computer network; computer lab; computer-assisted instruction; e-mail services; interactive nursing skills videos; Internet; learning resource lab; library services; nursing audiovisuals; skills, simulation, or other laboratory.

Library Facilities 180,115 volumes; 22,080 periodical subscriptions.

BACCALAUREATE PROGRAMS

Degree BSN

Available Programs RN Baccalaureate.

Southwest Baptist University (continued)

Site Options Springfield, MO.

Study Options Full-time and part-time.

Program Entrance Requirements Minimum overall college GPA of 2.5, transcript of college record, CPR certification, health exam, high school transcript, immunizations, interview, minimum GPA in nursing prerequisites of 2.5, professional liability insurance/malpractice insurance, prerequisite course work, RN licensure. Transfer students are accepted. **Standardized tests** *Required:* SAT or ACT, TOEFL for international students. **Application** *Deadline:* rolling (freshmen), rolling (transfer). *Notification:* continuous (freshmen). *Application fee:* $30.

Advanced Placement Credit given for nursing courses completed elsewhere dependent upon specific evaluations.

Expenses (2006–07) *Tuition:* full-time $3840; part-time $160 per credit hour. *Required fees:* full-time $960; part-time $40 per credit.

Financial Aid 50% of baccalaureate students in nursing programs received some form of financial aid in 2005–06. *Gift aid (need-based):* Federal Pell, FSEOG, state, private, college/university gift aid from institutional funds. *Loans:* Federal Nursing Student Loans, FFEL (Subsidized and Unsubsidized Stafford PLUS), Perkins, state, alternative loans. *Work-Study:* Federal Work-Study. *Application deadline (priority):* 3/15.

Contact Dr. Martha C. Baker, Director, BSN Program, College of Nursing, Southwest Baptist University, 4431 South Fremont Avenue, Springfield, MO 65804. *Telephone:* 417-820-5058. *Fax:* 417-887-4847. *E-mail:* mbaker@sbuniv.edu.

Truman State University

Program in Nursing
Kirksville, Missouri

http://nursing.truman.edu

Founded in 1867

DEGREE • BSN

Nursing Program Faculty 12 (16% with doctorates).

Baccalaureate Enrollment 168
Women 94% **Men** 6% **Minority** 5% **International** 5% **Part-time** 1%

Nursing Student Activities Nursing Honor Society, Sigma Theta Tau, Student Nurses' Association, nursing club.

Nursing Student Resources Academic advising; academic or career counseling; assistance for students with disabilities; bookstore; campus computer network; career placement assistance; computer lab; computer-assisted instruction; e-mail services; employment services for current students; externships; interactive nursing skills videos; Internet; learning resource lab; library services; nursing audiovisuals; paid internships; remedial services; resume preparation assistance; skills, simulation, or other laboratory; tutoring; unpaid internships.

Library Facilities 499,536 volumes (6,923 in health, 1,654 in nursing); 3,340 periodical subscriptions (900 health-care related).

BACCALAUREATE PROGRAMS

Degree BSN

Available Programs Generic Baccalaureate.

Site Options St. Louis, MO.

Study Options Full-time.

Program Entrance Requirements Minimum overall college GPA of 2.75, transcript of college record, written essay, high school biology, high school chemistry, high school foreign language, 3 years high school math, 3 years high school science, high school transcript, minimum high school GPA of 3.30, minimum GPA in nursing prerequisites of 3.0. Transfer students are accepted. **Standardized tests** *Required:* SAT or ACT, TOEFL for international students. *Recommended:* ACT. **Application** *Deadline:* 3/1 (freshmen), rolling (transfer). *Early decision:* 11/15. *Notification:* continuous (freshmen), 12/15 (early action).

Expenses (2006–07) *Tuition, state resident:* full-time $5970; part-time $248 per credit hour. *Tuition, nonresident:* full-time $10,400; part-time $434 per credit hour. *International tuition:* $10,400 full-time. *Room and board:* $5790; room only: $5435 per academic year. *Required fees:* full-time $1000.

Financial Aid 75% of baccalaureate students in nursing programs received some form of financial aid in 2005–06. *Gift aid (need-based):* Federal Pell, FSEOG, state, private, college/university gift aid from institutional funds. *Loans:* Federal Nursing Student Loans, FFEL (Subsidized and Unsubsidized Stafford PLUS), Perkins, state, college/university. *Work-Study:* Federal Work-Study, part-time campus jobs. *Application deadline (priority):* 4/1.

Contact Dr. Stephanie A. Powelson, Nursing Program Director, Program in Nursing, Truman State University, 100 East Normal, Barnett 223, Kirksville, MO 63501. *Telephone:* 660-785-4557. *Fax:* 660-785-7424. *E-mail:* spowelso@truman.edu.

University of Central Missouri

Department of Nursing
Warrensburg, Missouri

http://www.ucmo.edu/extcamp

Founded in 1871

DEGREES • BS • MS

Nursing Program Faculty 17 (23% with doctorates).

Baccalaureate Enrollment 118
Women 94% **Men** 6% **Minority** 9% **International** 4%

Graduate Enrollment 45
Women 96% **Men** 4% **Minority** 4% **Part-time** 95%

Nursing Student Activities Nursing club.

Nursing Student Resources Academic advising; academic or career counseling; assistance for students with disabilities; bookstore; campus computer network; career placement assistance; computer lab; computer-assisted instruction; daycare for children of students; e-mail services; employment services for current students; externships; housing assistance; interactive nursing skills videos; Internet; learning resource lab; library services; nursing audiovisuals; placement services for program completers; remedial services; resume preparation assistance; skills, simulation, or other laboratory; tutoring.

Library Facilities 2.1 million volumes (17,000 in health, 860 in nursing); 1,703 periodical subscriptions (250 health-care related).

BACCALAUREATE PROGRAMS

Degree BS

Available Programs Generic Baccalaureate; RN Baccalaureate.

Site Options *Distance Learning:* North Kansas City, MO; Lee's Summit, MO; Warrensburg, MO.

Study Options Full-time.

Program Entrance Requirements Minimum overall college GPA of 2.5, health insurance, immunizations, 2 letters of recommendation, minimum GPA in nursing prerequisites of 2.0, prerequisite course work. Transfer students are accepted. **Standardized tests** *Required:* ACT, TOEFL for international students. **Application** *Deadline:* rolling (freshmen), rolling (transfer). *Notification:* continuous (freshmen). *Application fee:* $30.

Advanced Placement Credit by examination available. Credit given for nursing courses completed elsewhere dependent upon specific evaluations.

Expenses (2006–07) *Tuition, state resident:* full-time $5835; part-time $195 per credit hour. *Tuition, nonresident:* full-time $11,250; part-time $375 per credit hour. *Room and board:* $6612; room only: $4606 per academic year. *Required fees:* full-time $175.

Financial Aid 84% of baccalaureate students in nursing programs received some form of financial aid in 2005–06.

Contact Dr. Julie Ann Clawson, RN, Chair, Department of Nursing, University of Central Missouri, 600 South College, UHC 106A, Warrensburg, MO 64093. *Telephone:* 660-543-4775. *Fax:* 660-543-8304. *E-mail:* clawson@cmsu.edu.

GRADUATE PROGRAMS

Expenses (2006–07) *Tuition, state resident:* full-time $4336; part-time $241 per credit hour. *Tuition, nonresident:* full-time $8424; part-time $468 per credit hour. *Required fees:* part-time $60 per credit.

Financial Aid 61% of graduate students in nursing programs received some form of financial aid in 2005–06.

Contact Dr. Novella Perrin, Dean, Department of Nursing, University of Central Missouri, Graduate Studies, WDE 1800, Warrensburg, MO 64093. *Telephone:* 660-543-4621. *E-mail:* perrin@cmsu1.cmsu.edu.

MASTER'S DEGREE PROGRAM

Degree MS

Available Programs Master's.

Concentrations Available Nursing education. *Nurse practitioner programs in:* family health.

Site Options *Distance Learning:* Lee's Summit, MO; Warrensburg, MO.

Study Options Full-time and part-time.

Program Entrance Requirements Clinical experience, minimum overall college GPA of 3.0, transcript of college record, CPR certification, written essay, immunizations, 2 letters of recommendation, professional liability insurance/malpractice insurance.

Advanced Placement Credit given for nursing courses completed elsewhere dependent upon specific evaluations.

Degree Requirements 32 total credit hours, thesis or project.

POST-MASTER'S PROGRAM

Areas of Study Nursing education. *Nurse practitioner programs in:* family health.

University of Missouri–Columbia
Sinclair School of Nursing
Columbia, Missouri

http://www.muhealth.org/

Founded in 1839

DEGREES • BSN • MS • PHD

Nursing Program Faculty 62 (56% with doctorates).

Baccalaureate Enrollment 378
Women 90% **Men** 10% **Minority** 6% **International** 3% **Part-time** 31%
Graduate Enrollment 207
Women 95% **Men** 5% **Minority** 8% **International** 2% **Part-time** 77%

Nursing Student Activities Sigma Theta Tau, Student Nurses' Association, nursing club.

Nursing Student Resources Academic advising; academic or career counseling; campus computer network; computer lab; computer-assisted instruction; e-mail services; externships; interactive nursing skills videos; Internet; learning resource lab; library services; nursing audiovisuals; paid internships; resume preparation assistance; skills, simulation, or other laboratory; tutoring; unpaid internships.

Library Facilities 3.2 million volumes (253,271 in health); 36,244 periodical subscriptions.

BACCALAUREATE PROGRAMS

Degree BSN

Available Programs Accelerated Baccalaureate for Second Degree; Generic Baccalaureate; RN Baccalaureate.

Study Options Full-time and part-time.

Program Entrance Requirements Minimum overall college GPA of 2.5, transcript of college record, CPR certification, high school biology, high school chemistry, 4 years high school math, high school science, high school transcript, immunizations, minimum GPA in nursing prerequisites of 2.5, prerequisite course work. Transfer students are accepted. **Standardized tests** *Required:* SAT or ACT, TOEFL for international students. *Recommended:* ACT. **Application** *Deadline:* rolling (freshmen), rolling (transfer). *Notification:* continuous (freshmen). *Application fee:* $45.

Advanced Placement Credit by examination available. Credit given for nursing courses completed elsewhere dependent upon specific evaluations.

Expenses (2006–07) *Tuition, area resident:* full-time $6819; part-time $227 per credit hour. *Tuition, state resident:* full-time $6189; part-time $227 per credit hour. *Tuition, nonresident:* full-time $17,085; part-time $570 per credit hour. *International tuition:* $17,085 full-time. *Room and board:* $7000 per academic year.

Financial Aid 92% of baccalaureate students in nursing programs received some form of financial aid in 2005–06. *Gift aid (need-based):* Federal Pell, FSEOG, state, private, college/university gift aid from institutional funds, Federal Nursing. *Loans:* Federal Nursing Student Loans, Federal Direct (Subsidized and Unsubsidized Stafford PLUS), Perkins, state, college/university, Health Professions Loans, Primary Care Loans, alternative loans. *Work-Study:* Federal Work-Study. *Application deadline (priority):* 3/1.

Contact Ms. Jenette Hough, Undergraduate Academic Advisor, Sinclair School of Nursing, University of Missouri–Columbia, S235, Columbia, MO 65211. *Telephone:* 573-882-0277. *Fax:* 573-884-4544. *E-mail:* houghje@missouri.edu.

GRADUATE PROGRAMS

Expenses (2006–07) *Tuition, state resident:* full-time $6080; part-time $276 per credit hour. *Tuition, nonresident:* full-time $16,572; part-time $753 per credit hour. *International tuition:* $16,572 full-time.

Financial Aid 70% of graduate students in nursing programs received some form of financial aid in 2005–06. Fellowships, research assistantships, teaching assistantships, career-related internships or fieldwork, institutionally sponsored loans, traineeships, and tuition waivers (full) available.

Contact Ms. Nancy Lee Johnson, Coordinator of Student Services and Records, Sinclair School of Nursing, University of Missouri–Columbia, S235, Columbia, MO 65211. *Telephone:* 573-882-0277. *Fax:* 573-884-4544. *E-mail:* johnsonn@missouri.edu.

MASTER'S DEGREE PROGRAM

Degree MS

Available Programs Master's.

Concentrations Available Nursing administration; nursing education. *Clinical nurse specialist programs in:* adult health, gerontology, medical-surgical, pediatric, psychiatric/mental health, public health, women's health. *Nurse practitioner programs in:* family health, gerontology, pediatric, psychiatric/mental health.

Program Entrance Requirements Minimum overall college GPA of 3.0, transcript of college record, CPR certification, immunizations, interview, 2 letters of recommendation, statistics course, GRE General Test. *Application deadline:* For fall admission, 2/1 (priority date). Applications are processed on a rolling basis. *Application fee:* $45 ($60 for international students).

Degree Requirements 43 total credit hours, comprehensive exam.

POST-MASTER'S PROGRAM

Areas of Study Nursing administration; nursing education. *Clinical nurse specialist programs in:* adult health, gerontology, medical-surgical, pediatric, psychiatric/mental health, public health, women's health. *Nurse practitioner programs in:* family health, gerontology, pediatric, psychiatric/mental health.

DOCTORAL DEGREE PROGRAM

Degree PhD

Available Programs Doctorate; Post-Baccalaureate Doctorate.

Areas of Study Health promotion/disease prevention, health-care systems, nursing administration, nursing policy, nursing research, nursing science.

Program Entrance Requirements Minimum overall college GPA of 3.5, interview by faculty committee, interview, 3 letters of recommendation, vita, writing sample. *Application deadline:* For fall admission, 2/1 (priority date). Applications are processed on a rolling basis. *Application fee:* $45 ($60 for international students).

Degree Requirements 72 total credit hours, dissertation, oral exam, written exam, residency.

CONTINUING EDUCATION PROGRAM

Contact Dr. Shirley Farrah, Assistant Dean, Nursing Outreach and Distance Education, Sinclair School of Nursing, University of Missouri–Columbia, S266B, Columbia, MO 65211. *Telephone:* 573-882-0215. *Fax:* 573-884-4544. *E-mail:* farrahs@missouri.edu.

University of Missouri–Kansas City
School of Nursing
Kansas City, Missouri

Founded in 1929

DEGREES • BSN • MSN • PHD

Nursing Program Faculty 65 (26% with doctorates).

Baccalaureate Enrollment 265
Women 97% **Men** 3% **Minority** 24% **International** 2% **Part-time** 23%
Graduate Enrollment 248
Women 96% **Men** 4% **Minority** 10% **Part-time** 83%

Nursing Student Activities Sigma Theta Tau, Student Nurses' Association.

Nursing Student Resources Academic advising; academic or career counseling; assistance for students with disabilities; bookstore; campus computer network; career placement assistance; computer lab; computer-assisted instruction; e-mail services; housing assistance; interactive nursing skills videos; Internet; learning resource lab; library services; nursing audiovisuals; other; placement services for program completers; remedial services; resume preparation assistance; skills, simulation, or other laboratory; tutoring.

Library Facilities 1.3 million volumes (81,000 in health, 10,530 in nursing); 25,022 periodical subscriptions (796 health-care related).

BACCALAUREATE PROGRAMS

Degree BSN

Available Programs Generic Baccalaureate; RN Baccalaureate.
Study Options Full-time.
Program Entrance Requirements Minimum overall college GPA of 2.75, transcript of college record, CPR certification, written essay, health insurance, high school foreign language, 4 years high school math, 4 years high school science, high school transcript, immunizations, minimum GPA in nursing prerequisites of 2.75, prerequisite course work. Transfer students are accepted. **Standardized tests** *Required:* SAT or ACT, TOEFL for international students. **Application** *Deadline:* rolling (freshmen), rolling (transfer). *Notification:* continuous (freshmen). *Application fee:* $35.
Expenses (2006–07) *Tuition, state resident:* full-time $8183; part-time $227 per credit hour. *Tuition, nonresident:* full-time $19,915; part-time $553 per credit hour. *International tuition:* $19,915 full-time. *Required fees:* full-time $2336; part-time $65 per credit; part-time $1170 per term.
Financial Aid 75% of baccalaureate students in nursing programs received some form of financial aid in 2005–06. *Gift aid (need-based):* Federal Pell, FSEOG, state, private, college/university gift aid from institutional funds, United Negro College Fund, Federal Nursing. *Loans:* Federal Nursing Student Loans, FFEL (Subsidized and Unsubsidized Stafford PLUS), Perkins, state, college/university. *Work-Study:* Federal Work-Study. *Application deadline (priority):* 3/1.
Contact Ms. Judy A. Jellison, Manager, Student Services, School of Nursing, University of Missouri–Kansas City, 2220 Holmes Street, Kansas City, MO 64108. *Telephone:* 816-235-1740. *Fax:* 816-235-1701. *E-mail:* jellisonj@umkc.edu.

GRADUATE PROGRAMS

Expenses (2006–07) *Tuition, state resident:* full-time $7739; part-time $276 per credit hour. *Tuition, nonresident:* full-time $19,984; part-time $714 per credit hour. *International tuition:* $19,984 full-time. *Required fees:* full-time $1680.
Financial Aid 45% of graduate students in nursing programs received some form of financial aid in 2005–06. 2 fellowships (averaging $500 per year), 12 research assistantships (averaging $4,000 per year), 5 teaching assistantships with partial tuition reimbursements available (averaging $4,000 per year) were awarded; career-related internships or fieldwork, Federal Work-Study, institutionally sponsored loans, and tuition waivers (full and partial) also available. Aid available to part-time students. *Financial aid application deadline:* 6/30.
Contact Ms. Judy A. Jellison, Manager, Student Services, School of Nursing, University of Missouri–Kansas City, 2220 Holmes Street, Kansas City, MO 64108. *Telephone:* 816-235-1740. *Fax:* 816-235-1701. *E-mail:* jellisonj@umkc.edu.

MASTER'S DEGREE PROGRAM

Degree MSN

Available Programs Master's.
Concentrations Available Nursing administration; nursing education. *Clinical nurse specialist programs in:* pediatric. *Nurse practitioner programs in:* adult health, family health, neonatal health, pediatric, women's health.
Site Options *Distance Learning:* St. Joseph, MO; Joplin, MO.
Study Options Full-time and part-time.
Program Entrance Requirements Clinical experience, computer literacy, minimum overall college GPA of 3.2, transcript of college record, CPR certification, immunizations, physical assessment course, resume, statistics course, California Critical Thinking Skills Test. *Application deadline:* For fall admission, 2/1 (priority date); for spring admission, 9/15 (priority date). *Application fee:* $25.
Degree Requirements 42 total credit hours, thesis or project.

POST-MASTER'S PROGRAM

Areas of Study Nursing administration; nursing education. *Clinical nurse specialist programs in:* pediatric. *Nurse practitioner programs in:* adult health, family health, neonatal health, pediatric, women's health.

DOCTORAL DEGREE PROGRAM

Degree PhD

Available Programs Doctorate; Post-Baccalaureate Doctorate.
Areas of Study Health promotion/disease prevention, health-care systems.
Program Entrance Requirements Minimum overall college GPA of 3.5, interview by faculty committee, interview, 3 letters of recommendation, MSN or equivalent, vita, writing sample, GRE. *Application deadline:* For fall admission, 2/1 (priority date); for spring admission, 9/15 (priority date). *Application fee:* $25.
Degree Requirements 82 total credit hours, dissertation, oral exam, written exam, residency.

University of Missouri–St. Louis
College of Nursing
St. Louis, Missouri

Founded in 1963

DEGREES • BSN • MSN • PHD

Nursing Program Faculty 35 (54% with doctorates).

Baccalaureate Enrollment 507
Women 93% **Men** 7% **Minority** 19% **International** 1% **Part-time** 32%
Graduate Enrollment 177
Women 96% **Men** 4% **Minority** 21% **International** 2% **Part-time** 92%

Nursing Student Activities Sigma Theta Tau, Student Nurses' Association.

Nursing Student Resources Academic advising; academic or career counseling; assistance for students with disabilities; bookstore; campus computer network; career placement assistance; computer lab; computer-assisted instruction; daycare for children of students; e-mail services; employment services for current students; externships; interactive nursing skills videos; Internet; learning resource lab; library services; nursing audiovisuals; resume preparation assistance; skills, simulation, or other laboratory; tutoring; unpaid internships.

Library Facilities 1.2 million volumes (15,530 in health, 8,450 in nursing); 3,174 periodical subscriptions (485 health-care related).

BACCALAUREATE PROGRAMS
Degree BSN

Available Programs Accelerated Baccalaureate; Generic Baccalaureate; RN Baccalaureate.
Site Options *Distance Learning:* St. Charles, MO; Florissant.
Study Options Full-time and part-time.

Program Entrance Requirements Minimum overall college GPA of 2.5, transcript of college record, CPR certification, health exam, 4 years high school math, 3 years high school science, high school transcript, immunizations, minimum high school GPA of 2.5, minimum high school rank 67%. Transfer students are accepted. **Standardized tests** *Required:* SAT or ACT, TOEFL for international students. **Application** *Deadline:* rolling (freshmen), rolling (out-of-state freshmen), rolling (transfer). *Notification:* continuous (freshmen), continuous (out-of-state freshmen). *Application fee:* $35.

Advanced Placement Credit given for nursing courses completed elsewhere dependent upon specific evaluations.

Contact *Telephone:* 314-516-7087. *Fax:* 314-516-7519.

GRADUATE PROGRAMS

Contact *Telephone:* 314-516-7087. *Fax:* 314-516-7519.

MASTER'S DEGREE PROGRAM

Degree MSN

Available Programs RN to Master's.

Concentrations Available Nursing administration; nursing education. *Clinical nurse specialist programs in:* adult health, pediatric, women's health. *Nurse practitioner programs in:* adult health, family health, pediatric, women's health.

Site Options *Distance Learning:* Park Hill, MO; St. Charles, MO.

Study Options Full-time and part-time.

Program Entrance Requirements Clinical experience, minimum overall college GPA of 3.0, transcript of college record, CPR certification, immunizations, 2 letters of recommendation, physical assessment course, statistics course. *Application deadline:* Applications are processed on a rolling basis. *Application fee:* $35 ($40 for international students).

Advanced Placement Credit given for nursing courses completed elsewhere dependent upon specific evaluations.

Degree Requirements 36 total credit hours.

DOCTORAL DEGREE PROGRAM

Degree PhD

Available Programs Doctorate.

Areas of Study Nursing administration, nursing education, nursing policy, nursing research.

Program Entrance Requirements Minimum overall college GPA of 3.2, interview, 3 letters of recommendation, vita, writing sample, GRE General Test. *Application deadline:* Applications are processed on a rolling basis. *Application fee:* $35 ($40 for international students).

Degree Requirements 72 total credit hours, dissertation, oral exam, written exam, residency.

Webster University
Department of Nursing
St. Louis, Missouri

http://www.webster.edu/depts/artsci/nursing/nursing.html

Founded in 1915

DEGREES • BSN • MSN

Nursing Program Faculty 12 (72% with doctorates).

Baccalaureate Enrollment 150

Women 93% **Men** 7% **Minority** 14% **International** 1% **Part-time** 90%

Graduate Enrollment 75

Women 90% **Men** 10% **Minority** 20% **International** 10% **Part-time** 100%

Nursing Student Activities Nursing Honor Society, Sigma Theta Tau.

Nursing Student Resources Academic advising; academic or career counseling; assistance for students with disabilities; bookstore; campus computer network; career placement assistance; computer lab; e-mail services; employment services for current students; Internet; learning resource lab; library services; nursing audiovisuals; placement services for program completers; remedial services; resume preparation assistance; skills, simulation, or other laboratory; tutoring.

Library Facilities 283,742 volumes (7,030 in health, 3,114 in nursing); 2,429 periodical subscriptions (108 health-care related).

BACCALAUREATE PROGRAMS

Degree BSN

Available Programs ADN to Baccalaureate; RN Baccalaureate.

Site Options Kansas City, MO.

Program Entrance Requirements Minimum overall college GPA of 2.5, transcript of college record, immunizations, interview, prerequisite course work, RN licensure. Transfer students are accepted. **Standardized tests** *Required:* SAT or ACT, TOEFL for international students. **Application** *Deadline:* 6/1 (freshmen), 8/1 (transfer). *Notification:* continuous (freshmen). *Application fee:* $25.

Financial Aid 45% of baccalaureate students in nursing programs received some form of financial aid in 2005–06. *Gift aid (need-based):* Federal Pell, FSEOG, state, private, college/university gift aid from institutional funds. *Loans:* FFEL (Subsidized and Unsubsidized Stafford PLUS), Perkins. *Work-Study:* Federal Work-Study, part-time campus jobs. *Application deadline (priority):* 4/1.

Contact Ms. Kathy J. Halvachs, Administrative Assistant, Department of Nursing, Webster University, 470 East Lockwood Avenue, St. Louis, MO 63119-3194. *Telephone:* 314-968-7483. *Fax:* 314-963-6101. *E-mail:* halvackj@webster.edu.

GRADUATE PROGRAMS

Financial Aid 40% of graduate students in nursing programs received some form of financial aid in 2005–06. Federal Work-Study available. Aid available to part-time students. *Financial aid application deadline:* 4/1.

Contact Dr. Jennifer Broeder, Coordinator, MSN Program, Department of Nursing, Webster University, 470 East Lockwood Avenue, St. Louis, MO 63119-3194. *Telephone:* 314-968-7483. *Fax:* 314-963-6101. *E-mail:* jbroeder@webster.edu.

MASTER'S DEGREE PROGRAM

Degree MSN

Available Programs Master's; RN to Master's.

Concentrations Available Nursing administration; nursing education. *Clinical nurse specialist programs in:* family health.

Site Options Kansas City, MO.

Study Options Part-time.

Program Entrance Requirements Clinical experience, computer literacy, minimum overall college GPA of 3.0, transcript of college record, written essay, immunizations, interview, 3 letters of recommendation, nursing research course, physical assessment course, resume, statistics course. *Application deadline:* Applications are processed on a rolling basis. *Application fee:* $25 ($50 for international students).

Advanced Placement Credit given for nursing courses completed elsewhere dependent upon specific evaluations.

Degree Requirements 36 total credit hours, thesis or project.

William Jewell College
Department of Nursing
Liberty, Missouri

http://www.jewell.edu

Founded in 1849

DEGREE • BS

Nursing Program Faculty 36 (25% with doctorates).

Baccalaureate Enrollment 191

Women 89% **Men** 11% **Minority** 3% **International** 1%

Nursing Student Activities Nursing Honor Society, Sigma Theta Tau, Student Nurses' Association.

Nursing Student Resources Academic advising; academic or career counseling; assistance for students with disabilities; bookstore; campus computer network; career placement assistance; computer lab; computer-assisted instruction; e-mail services; employment services for current students; externships; housing assistance; interactive nursing skills videos; Internet; learning resource lab; library services; nursing audiovisuals; paid

William Jewell College (continued)

internships; placement services for program completers; resume preparation assistance; skills, simulation, or other laboratory; tutoring; unpaid internships.

Library Facilities 255,750 volumes (4,000 in health, 1,000 in nursing); 527 periodical subscriptions (250 health-care related).

BACCALAUREATE PROGRAMS

Degree BS

Available Programs Accelerated Baccalaureate; Generic Baccalaureate.

Study Options Full-time and part-time.

Program Entrance Requirements Minimum overall college GPA of 2.5, transcript of college record, CPR certification, written essay, health insurance, high school foreign language, high school transcript, immunizations, minimum high school GPA, minimum GPA in nursing prerequisites of 2.5, professional liability insurance/malpractice insurance, prerequisite course work. Transfer students are accepted. **Standardized tests** *Required:* SAT or ACT, TOEFL for international students. **Application** *Deadline:* 8/15 (freshmen), rolling (transfer). *Notification:* 10/1 (freshmen). *Application fee:* $25.

Expenses (2006–07) *Tuition:* full-time $20,150; part-time $675 per semester. *International tuition:* $20,150 full-time. *Room and board:* $5510; room only: $1160 per academic year.

Financial Aid 90% of baccalaureate students in nursing programs received some form of financial aid in 2005–06. *Gift aid (need-based):* Federal Pell, FSEOG, state, college/university gift aid from institutional funds. *Loans:* Federal Nursing Student Loans, FFEL (Subsidized and Unsubsidized Stafford PLUS), Perkins, non-Federal alternative loans (noncollege). *Work-Study:* Federal Work-Study, part-time campus jobs. *Application deadline (priority):* 3/1.

Contact Dr. Nelda S. Godfrey, Associate Professor and Chair, Department of Nursing, William Jewell College, 500 College Hill, Box 2002, Liberty, MO 64068. *Telephone:* 816-415-7605. *Fax:* 816-415-5024. *E-mail:* godfreyn@william.jewell.edu.

MONTANA

Carroll College
Department of Nursing
Helena, Montana

http://www.carroll.edu

Founded in 1909

DEGREE • BA

Nursing Program Faculty 18 (11% with doctorates).

Baccalaureate Enrollment 166

Women 90.7% **Men** 9.3% **Minority** 9.5% **International** .9% **Part-time** 9.6%

Nursing Student Activities Sigma Theta Tau, Student Nurses' Association.

Nursing Student Resources Academic advising; academic or career counseling; assistance for students with disabilities; bookstore; campus computer network; career placement assistance; computer lab; computer-assisted instruction; e-mail services; employment services for current students; externships; housing assistance; interactive nursing skills videos; Internet; learning resource lab; library services; nursing audiovisuals; paid internships; placement services for program completers; remedial services; resume preparation assistance; skills, simulation, or other laboratory; tutoring; unpaid internships.

Library Facilities 89,003 volumes (38,000 in health, 250 in nursing); 2,721 periodical subscriptions (152 health-care related).

BACCALAUREATE PROGRAMS

Degree BA

Available Programs Generic Baccalaureate; LPN to Baccalaureate.

Study Options Full-time and part-time.

Program Entrance Requirements Minimum overall college GPA of 2.75, transcript of college record, high school transcript, immunizations, minimum GPA in nursing prerequisites of 2.75, prerequisite course work. Transfer students are accepted. **Standardized tests** *Required:* SAT or ACT, TOEFL for international students. *Required for some:* SAT Subject Tests. **Application** *Deadline:* 6/1 (freshmen), 6/1 (transfer). *Notification:* continuous (freshmen). *Application fee:* $35.

Advanced Placement Credit given for nursing courses completed elsewhere dependent upon specific evaluations.

Expenses (2006–07) *Tuition:* full-time $18,105. *Room and board:* $3200; room only: $1600 per academic year. *Required fees:* full-time $200.

Financial Aid 97% of baccalaureate students in nursing programs received some form of financial aid in 2005–06. *Gift aid (need-based):* Federal Pell, FSEOG, state, private, college/university gift aid from institutional funds. *Loans:* FFEL (Subsidized and Unsubsidized Stafford PLUS), Perkins. *Work-Study:* Federal Work-Study, part-time campus jobs. *Application deadline:* Continuous.

Contact Dave Thorvilson, Associate Director, Admissions, Department of Nursing, Carroll College, 1601 North Benton Avenue, Helena, MT 59625. *Telephone:* 406-447-5481. *Fax:* 406-447-4533. *E-mail:* dthorvil@carroll.edu.

CONTINUING EDUCATION PROGRAM

Contact Dr. Cynthia Z. Gustafson, Chair, Department of Nursing, Department of Nursing, Carroll College, 1601 North Benton Avenue, Helena, MT 59625. *Telephone:* 406-447-5494. *Fax:* 406-447-5476. *E-mail:* cgustafs@carroll.edu.

Montana State University
College of Nursing
Bozeman, Montana

http://www.montana.edu/wwwnu/index.html

Founded in 1893

DEGREES • BSN • MN

Nursing Program Faculty 90 (22% with doctorates).

Baccalaureate Enrollment 774

Women 92.6% **Men** 7.4% **Minority** 6.3% **International** .25% **Part-time** 16.8%

Graduate Enrollment 34

Women 85.3% **Men** 14.7% **Minority** 2.94% **Part-time** 29.4%

Nursing Student Activities Sigma Theta Tau, Student Nurses' Association.

Nursing Student Resources Academic advising; academic or career counseling; assistance for students with disabilities; bookstore; campus computer network; career placement assistance; computer lab; computer-assisted instruction; daycare for children of students; e-mail services; employment services for current students; housing assistance; Internet; library services; nursing audiovisuals; placement services for program completers; remedial services; resume preparation assistance; skills, simulation, or other laboratory; tutoring; unpaid internships.

Library Facilities 712,241 volumes (80,389 in health, 11,535 in nursing); 8,757 periodical subscriptions (1,690 health-care related).

BACCALAUREATE PROGRAMS

Degree BSN

Available Programs Generic Baccalaureate; LPN to Baccalaureate.

Site Options *Distance Learning:* Billings, MT; Great Falls, MT; Missoula, MT.

Study Options Full-time and part-time.

Program Entrance Requirements Minimum overall college GPA of 2.5, transcript of college record, CPR certification, health exam, health insurance, high school transcript, immunizations, minimum high school GPA of 2.5, minimum high school rank 50%, minimum GPA in nursing prerequisites of 2.5, professional liability insurance/malpractice insurance, prerequisite course work. Transfer students are accepted. **Standardized tests** *Required:* SAT or ACT, TOEFL for international students. **Application** *Deadline:* rolling (freshmen), rolling (transfer). *Notification:* continuous (freshmen). *Application fee:* $30.

Advanced Placement Credit by examination available. Credit given for nursing courses completed elsewhere dependent upon specific evaluations.

Expenses (2006–07) *Tuition, state resident:* full-time $4559; part-time $190 per credit. *Tuition, nonresident:* full-time $14,322; part-time $597 per credit. *Room and board:* $6450 per academic year. *Required fees:* full-time $2575; part-time $95 per credit; part-time $1288 per term.

Financial Aid 70% of baccalaureate students in nursing programs received some form of financial aid in 2005–06.

Contact Ms. Patricia Hanson, Undergraduate Student Services Coordinator, College of Nursing, Montana State University, Sherrick Hall, PO Box 173560, Bozeman, MT 59717-3560. *Telephone:* 406-994-3783. *Fax:* 406-994-6020. *E-mail:* phanson@montana.edu.

GRADUATE PROGRAMS

Expenses (2006–07) *Tuition, state resident:* full-time $5471; part-time $228 per credit. *Tuition, nonresident:* full-time $15,234; part-time $635 per credit. *Required fees:* full-time $2575; part-time $95 per credit; part-time $1288 per term.

Financial Aid 70% of graduate students in nursing programs received some form of financial aid in 2005–06. 1 research assistantship, 405 teaching assistantships with partial tuition reimbursements available were awarded; institutionally sponsored loans, scholarships, traineeships, and unspecified assistantships also available. Aid available to part-time students. *Financial aid application deadline:* 3/1.

Contact Ms. Lynn Taylor, Graduate Program Administrative Assistant, College of Nursing, Montana State University, Sherrick Hall, PO Box 173560, Bozeman, MT 59717-3560. *Telephone:* 406-994-3500. *Fax:* 406-994-6020. *E-mail:* lynnt@montana.edu.

MASTER'S DEGREE PROGRAM

Degree MN

Available Programs Master's.

Concentrations Available Nursing education. *Clinical nurse specialist programs in:* medical-surgical. *Nurse practitioner programs in:* family health.

Site Options *Distance Learning:* Billings, MT; Great Falls, MT; Missoula, MT.

Study Options Full-time and part-time.

Program Entrance Requirements Computer literacy, minimum overall college GPA of 3.0, transcript of college record, CPR certification, written essay, immunizations, interview, 3 letters of recommendation, nursing research course, physical assessment course, professional liability insurance/malpractice insurance, prerequisite course work, statistics course, GRE General Test. *Application deadline:* For fall admission, 7/15 (priority date); for spring admission, 12/1 (priority date). Applications are processed on a rolling basis. *Application fee:* $30.

Advanced Placement Credit given for nursing courses completed elsewhere dependent upon specific evaluations.

Degree Requirements 63 total credit hours, thesis or project, comprehensive exam.

POST-MASTER'S PROGRAM

Areas of Study Nursing education. *Clinical nurse specialist programs in:* medical-surgical. *Nurse practitioner programs in:* family health.

Montana State University–Northern

College of Nursing
Havre, Montana

http://www.msun.edu/academics/nursing

Founded in 1929

DEGREE • BSN

Nursing Program Faculty 9.

Baccalaureate Enrollment 33
Women 100% **Part-time** 92%

Nursing Student Activities Nursing club.

Nursing Student Resources Academic advising; academic or career counseling; assistance for students with disabilities; bookstore; campus computer network; career placement assistance; computer lab; computer-assisted instruction; daycare for children of students; e-mail services; employment services for current students; housing assistance; interactive nursing skills videos; Internet; learning resource lab; library services; nursing audiovisuals; remedial services; resume preparation assistance; skills, simulation, or other laboratory; tutoring.

Library Facilities 128,000 volumes (2,600 in health, 2,600 in nursing); 1,729 periodical subscriptions (50 health-care related).

BACCALAUREATE PROGRAMS

Degree BSN

Available Programs ADN to Baccalaureate; RN Baccalaureate.

Site Options *Distance Learning:* Great Falls, MT; Lewistown, MT.

Study Options Full-time and part-time.

Program Entrance Requirements Minimum overall college GPA of 2.25, transcript of college record, CPR certification, health exam, health insurance, immunizations, professional liability insurance/malpractice insurance, prerequisite course work, RN licensure. Transfer students are accepted. **Standardized tests** *Required:* TOEFL for international students. *Placement: Required:* ACT. **Application** *Deadline:* rolling (freshmen), rolling (transfer). *Notification:* continuous (freshmen). *Application fee:* $30.

Advanced Placement Credit given for nursing courses completed elsewhere dependent upon specific evaluations.

Expenses (2005–06) *Tuition, state resident:* full-time $6267; part-time $706 per course. *Tuition, nonresident:* full-time $17,996; part-time $1653 per course. *International tuition:* $17,996 full-time. *Required fees:* full-time $1761; part-time $130 per credit; part-time $1091 per term.

Financial Aid 75% of baccalaureate students in nursing programs received some form of financial aid in 2004–05.

Contact Ms. Renae Munson, Administrative Associate II, College of Nursing, Montana State University–Northern, 2100 16th Avenue South, Great Falls, MT 59405. *Telephone:* 800-446-2698 Ext. 4437. *Fax:* 406-771-4340. *E-mail:* rmunson@msun.edu.

Salish Kootenai College

Nursing Department
Pablo, Montana

Founded in 1977

DEGREE • BS

Nursing Program Faculty 7.

Nursing Student Activities Nursing club.

Nursing Student Resources Academic advising; academic or career counseling; bookstore; computer lab; daycare for children of students; employment services for current students; Internet; library services.

Library Facilities 24,000 volumes; 200 periodical subscriptions.

BACCALAUREATE PROGRAMS

Degree BS

Available Programs RN Baccalaureate.

Study Options Full-time and part-time.

Program Entrance Requirements Transcript of college record, CPR certification, health exam, health insurance, high school biology, high school chemistry, 2 years high school math, 2 years high school science, high school transcript, immunizations, minimum high school GPA of 2.5, professional liability insurance/malpractice insurance, prerequisite course work, RN licensure. *Placement: Required:* TABE. **Application** *Deadline:* rolling (freshmen), rolling (transfer). *Notification:* continuous (freshmen).

Expenses (2006–07) *Tuition:* full-time $3276; part-time $91 per credit hour. *Required fees:* full-time $789; part-time $95 per credit; part-time $248 per term.

Contact Jacque Dolberry, Director, Nursing Department, Salish Kootenai College, 52000 Highway 93, PO Box 70, Pablo, MT 59855. *Telephone:* 406-275-4800. *E-mail:* jacque_dolberry@skc.edu.

NEBRASKA

Clarkson College
Department of Nursing
Omaha, Nebraska

http://www.clarksoncollege.edu

Founded in 1888

DEGREES • BSN • MSN

Nursing Program Faculty 39 (3% with doctorates).

Baccalaureate Enrollment 363
Women 94% **Men** 6% **Minority** 12% **Part-time** 19%

Graduate Enrollment 89
Women 93% **Men** 7% **Minority** 7% **Part-time** 100%

Nursing Student Activities Sigma Theta Tau, Student Nurses' Association.

Nursing Student Resources Academic advising; academic or career counseling; assistance for students with disabilities; bookstore; campus computer network; career placement assistance; computer lab; computer-assisted instruction; e-mail services; employment services for current students; interactive nursing skills videos; Internet; learning resource lab; library services; nursing audiovisuals; placement services for program completers; resume preparation assistance; skills, simulation, or other laboratory; tutoring.

Library Facilities 8,807 volumes (8,013 in health, 2,541 in nursing); 262 periodical subscriptions (583 health-care related).

BACCALAUREATE PROGRAMS

Degree BSN

Available Programs ADN to Baccalaureate; Accelerated RN Baccalaureate; LPN to RN Baccalaureate; RN Baccalaureate.

Study Options Full-time and part-time.

Program Entrance Requirements Minimum overall college GPA of 2.5, transcript of college record, CPR certification, written essay, health exam, health insurance, 2 years high school math, 2 years high school science, high school transcript, immunizations, minimum high school GPA of 2.5, minimum high school rank 50%. Transfer students are accepted. **Standardized tests** *Required for some:* SAT or ACT. **Application** *Deadline:* rolling (freshmen), rolling (transfer). *Notification:* continuous (freshmen). *Application fee:* $15.

Advanced Placement Credit given for nursing courses completed elsewhere dependent upon specific evaluations.

Expenses (2005–06) *Tuition:* part-time $345 per credit hour. *Room and board:* room only: $4400 per academic year. *Required fees:* part-time $37 per credit; part-time $280 per term.

Financial Aid 78% of baccalaureate students in nursing programs received some form of financial aid in 2004–05.

Contact Ms. Anne Folkers, Admissions Coordinator, Department of Nursing, Clarkson College, 101 South 42nd Street, Omaha, NE 68131-2739. *Telephone:* 402-552-3100. *Fax:* 402-552-6057. *E-mail:* folkers@clarksoncollege.edu.

GRADUATE PROGRAMS

Expenses (2005–06) *Tuition:* part-time $390 per credit hour. *Required fees:* full-time $680; part-time $37 per credit; part-time $340 per term.

Financial Aid 40% of graduate students in nursing programs received some form of financial aid in 2004–05. Federal Work-Study, institutionally sponsored loans, and scholarships available. Aid available to part-time students. *Financial aid application deadline:* 4/1.

Contact Ms. Anne Folkers, Admissions Coordinator, Department of Nursing, Clarkson College, 101 South 42nd Street, Omaha, NE 68131-2739. *Telephone:* 800-647-5500. *Fax:* 402-552-6057. *E-mail:* admiss@clarksoncollege.edu.

MASTER'S DEGREE PROGRAM

Degree MSN

Available Programs Master's; RN to Master's.

Concentrations Available Nursing administration; nursing education. *Nurse practitioner programs in:* adult health, family health.

Study Options Full-time and part-time.

Program Entrance Requirements Clinical experience, minimum overall college GPA of 3.0, transcript of college record, written essay, 2 letters of recommendation, resume. *Application deadline:* For fall admission, 7/13; for spring admission, 1/5. Applications are processed on a rolling basis. *Application fee:* $15.

Advanced Placement Credit given for nursing courses completed elsewhere dependent upon specific evaluations.

Degree Requirements Thesis or project.

POST-MASTER'S PROGRAM

Areas of Study Nursing administration; nursing education. *Nurse practitioner programs in:* adult health, family health.

CONTINUING EDUCATION PROGRAM

Contact Ms. Judi Dunn, Director, Professional Development, Department of Nursing, Clarkson College, 101 South 42nd Street, Omaha, NE 68131-2739. *Telephone:* 402-552-3100 Ext. 26123. *Fax:* 402-552-6058. *E-mail:* dunn@clarksoncollege.edu.

College of Saint Mary
Division of Health Care Professions
Omaha, Nebraska

Founded in 1923

DEGREE • BSN

Nursing Program Faculty 18 (6% with doctorates).

Baccalaureate Enrollment 45
Women 100% **Minority** 10% **Part-time** 65%

Graduate Enrollment 8

Nursing Student Activities Nursing Honor Society, Sigma Theta Tau, Student Nurses' Association, nursing club.

Nursing Student Resources Academic advising; academic or career counseling; bookstore; campus computer network; career placement assistance; computer lab; computer-assisted instruction; e-mail services; interactive nursing skills videos; Internet; learning resource lab; library services; nursing audiovisuals; other; placement services for program completers; resume preparation assistance; skills, simulation, or other laboratory; tutoring.

Library Facilities 77,246 volumes; 398 periodical subscriptions (100 health-care related).

BACCALAUREATE PROGRAMS

Degree BSN

Available Programs ADN to Baccalaureate; Generic Baccalaureate.

Study Options Full-time and part-time.

Program Entrance Requirements Minimum overall college GPA of 2.5, transcript of college record, CPR certification, health exam, immunizations, 2 letters of recommendation, minimum high school GPA, minimum GPA in nursing prerequisites of 2.5, prerequisite course work. Transfer students are accepted. **Standardized tests** *Required:* SAT or ACT, TOEFL for international students. **Application** *Deadline:* rolling (freshmen), rolling (transfer). *Notification:* continuous until 8/24 (freshmen). *Application fee:* $30.

Advanced Placement Credit given for nursing courses completed elsewhere dependent upon specific evaluations.

Financial Aid 81% of baccalaureate students in nursing programs received some form of financial aid in 2005–06. *Gift aid (need-based):* Federal Pell, FSEOG, state, college/university gift aid from institutional funds. *Loans:* Federal Nursing Student Loans, FFEL (Subsidized and Unsubsidized Stafford PLUS), Perkins. *Work-Study:* Federal Work-Study, part-time campus jobs. *Application deadline (priority):* 3/1.

Contact Dr. Peggy L. Hawkins, RN, Associate Dean, Division of Health Care Professions, College of Saint Mary, 7000 Mercy Road, Omaha, NE 68106. *Telephone:* 402-399-2658. *Fax:* 402-399-2654. *E-mail:* phawkins@csm.edu.

GRADUATE PROGRAMS

Financial Aid 100% of graduate students in nursing programs received some form of financial aid in 2005–06.

Contact Dr. Martin Larrey, Dean of Graduate Studies, Division of Health Care Professions, College of Saint Mary, 7000 Mercy Road, Omaha, NE 68106. *Telephone:* 402-399-2482. *Fax:* 402-399-2414. *E-mail:* mlarrey@csm. edu.

Creighton University
School of Nursing
Omaha, Nebraska

http://nursing.creighton.edu/

Founded in 1878

DEGREES • BSN • MS

Nursing Program Faculty 52 (30% with doctorates).

Baccalaureate Enrollment 464
Women 94% **Men** 6% **Minority** 10% **International** .2% **Part-time** 3.2%

Graduate Enrollment 70
Women 90% **Men** 10% **Minority** 5.7% **Part-time** 50%

Nursing Student Activities Nursing Honor Society, Sigma Theta Tau, Student Nurses' Association.

Nursing Student Resources Academic advising; academic or career counseling; assistance for students with disabilities; bookstore; campus computer network; career placement assistance; computer lab; computer-assisted instruction; daycare for children of students; e-mail services; employment services for current students; Internet; learning resource lab; library services; nursing audiovisuals; remedial services; resume preparation assistance; skills, simulation, or other laboratory; tutoring; unpaid internships.

Library Facilities 466,556 volumes (248,803 in health, 3,272 in nursing); 27,144 periodical subscriptions (3,185 health-care related).

BACCALAUREATE PROGRAMS

Degree BSN

Available Programs Accelerated Baccalaureate for Second Degree; Generic Baccalaureate; RN Baccalaureate.

Site Options *Distance Learning:* Hastings, NE.

Study Options Full-time and part-time.

Program Entrance Requirements Minimum overall college GPA of 2.0, transcript of college record, health exam, health insurance, high school chemistry, 3 years high school math, 2 years high school science, high school transcript, immunizations, 1 letter of recommendation, minimum high school GPA of 2.75, minimum high school rank 50%, minimum GPA in nursing prerequisites of 2.0. Transfer students are accepted. **Standardized tests** *Required:* SAT or ACT, TOEFL for international students. **Application** *Deadline:* 8/1 (freshmen), 8/1 (transfer). *Notification:* continuous (freshmen). *Application fee:* $40.

Advanced Placement Credit given for nursing courses completed elsewhere dependent upon specific evaluations.

Expenses (2006–07) *Tuition:* full-time $12,083; part-time $675 per credit hour. *International tuition:* $12,083 full-time. *Room and board:* $8200; room only: $5800 per academic year. *Required fees:* full-time $1464; part-time $258 per term.

Financial Aid 85% of baccalaureate students in nursing programs received some form of financial aid in 2005–06. *Gift aid (need-based):* Federal Pell, FSEOG, state, private, college/university gift aid from institutional funds, Federal Nursing. *Loans:* Federal Nursing Student Loans, FFEL (Subsidized and Unsubsidized Stafford PLUS), Perkins, college/university. *Work-Study:* Federal Work-Study. *Application deadline (priority):* 5/15.

Contact Dr. Linda L. Lazure, RN, Associate Dean for Student Affairs, School of Nursing, Creighton University, 2500 California Plaza, Omaha, NE 68178. *Telephone:* 402-280-2001. *Fax:* 402-280-2045. *E-mail:* llazure@creighton.edu.

GRADUATE PROGRAMS

Expenses (2006–07) *Tuition:* full-time $9520; part-time $595 per credit hour. *International tuition:* $9520 full-time. *Room and board:* $8200; room only: $5800 per academic year. *Required fees:* full-time $734; part-time $239 per term.

Financial Aid 85% of graduate students in nursing programs received some form of financial aid in 2005–06. Career-related internships or fieldwork, Federal Work-Study, institutionally sponsored loans, and traineeships available.

Contact Dr. Mary Kunes-Connell, RN, Associate Dean, School of Nursing, Creighton University, 2500 California Plaza, Omaha, NE 68178. *Telephone:* 402-280-2024. *Fax:* 402-280-2045. *E-mail:* mkc@creighton.edu.

MASTER'S DEGREE PROGRAM

Degree MS

Available Programs Master's.

Concentrations Available Nursing administration; nursing education. *Clinical nurse specialist programs in:* cardiovascular, community health, gerontology, psychiatric/mental health. *Nurse practitioner programs in:* adult health, family health, neonatal health.

Study Options Full-time and part-time.

Program Entrance Requirements Clinical experience, minimum overall college GPA of 3.0, transcript of college record, CPR certification, written essay, immunizations, 3 letters of recommendation, physical assessment course, prerequisite course work, resume, statistics course. *Application deadline:* For fall admission, 3/15 (priority date); for spring admission, 10/15 (priority date). Applications are processed on a rolling basis. *Application fee:* $40.

Advanced Placement Credit given for nursing courses completed elsewhere dependent upon specific evaluations.

Degree Requirements 43 total credit hours, thesis or project.

POST-MASTER'S PROGRAM

Areas of Study Nursing administration; nursing education. *Clinical nurse specialist programs in:* cardiovascular, community health, gerontology, psychiatric/mental health. *Nurse practitioner programs in:* adult health, family health, neonatal health.

Midland Lutheran College
Department of Nursing
Fremont, Nebraska

http://www.mlc.edu

Founded in 1883

DEGREE • BSN

Nursing Program Faculty 12 (25% with doctorates).

Baccalaureate Enrollment 70
Women 91% **Men** 9% **Minority** 3% **International** 1%

Nursing Student Activities Sigma Theta Tau, Student Nurses' Association.

Nursing Student Resources Academic advising; academic or career counseling; assistance for students with disabilities; bookstore; campus computer network; career placement assistance; computer lab; computer-assisted instruction; e-mail services; employment services for current students; housing assistance; interactive nursing skills videos; Internet; learning resource lab; library services; nursing audiovisuals; paid internships; placement services for program completers; remedial services; resume preparation assistance; skills, simulation, or other laboratory; tutoring; unpaid internships.

Library Facilities 110,000 volumes (3,600 in health, 1,900 in nursing); 900 periodical subscriptions (375 health-care related).

BACCALAUREATE PROGRAMS

Degree BSN

Available Programs ADN to Baccalaureate; Generic Baccalaureate; LPN to Baccalaureate; LPN to RN Baccalaureate; RN Baccalaureate.

Study Options Full-time and part-time.

Midland Lutheran College (continued)

Program Entrance Requirements Minimum overall college GPA of 2.5, transcript of college record, CPR certification, written essay, health exam, health insurance, high school foreign language, high school transcript, immunizations, interview, 2 letters of recommendation, minimum GPA in nursing prerequisites of 2.5, professional liability insurance/malpractice insurance, prerequisite course work. Transfer students are accepted. **Standardized tests** *Required:* SAT or ACT, TOEFL for international students. **Application** *Deadline:* rolling (freshmen), rolling (transfer). *Notification:* continuous until 9/1 (freshmen). *Application fee:* $30.

Advanced Placement Credit given for nursing courses completed elsewhere dependent upon specific evaluations.

Expenses (2006–07) *Tuition:* full-time $19,210. *Room and board:* $4950; room only: $2190 per academic year. *Required fees:* full-time $300.

Financial Aid 98% of baccalaureate students in nursing programs received some form of financial aid in 2005–06.

Contact Jeff LaFavor, Assistant Director of Admissions, Department of Nursing, Midland Lutheran College, 900 North Clarkson, Fremont, NE 68025. *Telephone:* 402-941-6203. *Fax:* 402-941-6513. *E-mail:* LaFavor@mlc.edu.

CONTINUING EDUCATION PROGRAM

Contact Dr. Nancy A. Harms, RN, Chair, Department of Nursing, Midland Lutheran College, 900 North Clarkson, Fremont, NE 68025. *Telephone:* 402-941-6280. *Fax:* 402-941-6279. *E-mail:* harms@mlc.edu.

Nebraska Methodist College

Department of Nursing
Omaha, Nebraska

http://www.methodistcollege.edu

Founded in 1891

DEGREES • BSN • MSN

Nursing Program Faculty 38 (19% with doctorates).

Baccalaureate Enrollment 327
Women 88% **Men** 12% **Minority** 5% **Part-time** 25%

Graduate Enrollment 26
Women 100%

Nursing Student Activities Nursing Honor Society, Sigma Theta Tau, Student Nurses' Association.

Nursing Student Resources Academic advising; academic or career counseling; assistance for students with disabilities; bookstore; campus computer network; career placement assistance; computer lab; computer-assisted instruction; e-mail services; employment services for current students; interactive nursing skills videos; learning resource lab; library services; nursing audiovisuals; remedial services; resume preparation assistance; skills, simulation, or other laboratory; tutoring.

Library Facilities 8,656 volumes (10,000 in health); 475 periodical subscriptions (640 health-care related).

BACCALAUREATE PROGRAMS

Degree BSN

Available Programs ADN to Baccalaureate; Accelerated Baccalaureate for Second Degree; Generic Baccalaureate; LPN to Baccalaureate.

Site Options *Distance Learning:* Omaha, NE.

Study Options Full-time and part-time.

Program Entrance Requirements Minimum overall college GPA of 2.0, transcript of college record, written essay, high school biology, high school chemistry, 2 years high school math, 2 years high school science, high school transcript, interview, 1 letter of recommendation, minimum high school GPA of 2.0, minimum GPA in nursing prerequisites of 2.0. Transfer students are accepted. **Standardized tests** *Required:* SAT or ACT, TOEFL for international students. **Application** *Deadline:* 4/1 (freshmen), 4/1 (transfer). *Notification:* 4/15 (freshmen). *Application fee:* $25.

Advanced Placement Credit given for nursing courses completed elsewhere dependent upon specific evaluations.

Expenses (2006–07) *Tuition:* full-time $11,340; part-time $378 per credit hour. *International tuition:* $11,340 full-time. *Required fees:* full-time $600; part-time $20 per credit; part-time $300 per term.

Financial Aid 90% of baccalaureate students in nursing programs received some form of financial aid in 2005–06.

Contact Dr. Marilyn Valerio, Chairperson, Department of Nursing, Nebraska Methodist College, 720 North 87th Street, Omaha, NE 68114-3426. *Telephone:* 402-354-7027. *Fax:* 402-354-7020. *E-mail:* Marilyn.Valerio@methodistcollege.edu.

GRADUATE PROGRAMS

Expenses (2006–07) *Tuition:* full-time $8225; part-time $457 per credit hour. *International tuition:* $8225 full-time. *Required fees:* full-time $450; part-time $25 per credit; part-time $225 per term.

Financial Aid 40% of graduate students in nursing programs received some form of financial aid in 2005–06.

Contact Dr. Linda Foley, Associate Chairperson, Department of Nursing, Nebraska Methodist College, 720 North 87th Street, Omaha, NE 68114-3426. *Telephone:* 402-354-7050. *Fax:* 402-354-7020. *E-mail:* Linda.Foley@methodistcollege.edu.

MASTER'S DEGREE PROGRAM

Degree MSN

Available Programs Master's.

Concentrations Available Nursing education.

Site Options *Distance Learning:* Omaha, NE.

Study Options Full-time and part-time.

Program Entrance Requirements Clinical experience, computer literacy, minimum overall college GPA of 3.0, transcript of college record, CPR certification, written essay, interview, 3 letters of recommendation, nursing research course, physical assessment course, prerequisite course work, statistics course.

Advanced Placement Credit given for nursing courses completed elsewhere dependent upon specific evaluations.

Degree Requirements 38 total credit hours, thesis or project.

POST-MASTER'S PROGRAM

Areas of Study Nursing education.

CONTINUING EDUCATION PROGRAM

Contact Ms. Phyllis Zimmerman, Coordinator, Nursing Programs, Department of Nursing, Nebraska Methodist College, 720 North 87th Street, Omaha, NE 68114. *Telephone:* 402-354-7109. *Fax:* 402-354-7020. *E-mail:* phyllis.zimmerman@methodistcollege.edu.

Nebraska Wesleyan University

Department of Nursing
Lincoln, Nebraska

http://www.nebrwesleyan.edu

Founded in 1887

DEGREES • BSN • MSN

Nursing Program Faculty 9 (50% with doctorates).

Baccalaureate Enrollment 86
Women 97% **Men** 3% **Minority** 2% **Part-time** 100%

Graduate Enrollment 52
Women 94% **Men** 6% **Minority** 2% **Part-time** 100%

Nursing Student Activities Sigma Theta Tau.

Nursing Student Resources Academic advising; academic or career counseling; assistance for students with disabilities; bookstore; campus computer network; career placement assistance; computer lab; e-mail services; employment services for current students; interactive nursing skills videos; Internet; library services; nursing audiovisuals; placement services for program completers; remedial services; resume preparation assistance; tutoring; unpaid internships.

Library Facilities 178,531 volumes (3,700 in health, 3,700 in nursing); 743 periodical subscriptions (38 health-care related).

BACCALAUREATE PROGRAMS

Degree BSN

Available Programs ADN to Baccalaureate; Accelerated RN Baccalaureate; International Nurse to Baccalaureate; RN Baccalaureate.

Site Options Omaha, NE.

Study Options Full-time and part-time.

Program Entrance Requirements Minimum overall college GPA of 2.5, transcript of college record, CPR certification, immunizations, interview, 3 letters of recommendation, minimum GPA in nursing prerequisites of 2.5, professional liability insurance/malpractice insurance, prerequisite course work, RN licensure. Transfer students are accepted. **Standardized tests** *Required:* SAT or ACT, TOEFL for international students. **Application** *Deadline:* 8/15 (freshmen), 8/15 (transfer). *Early decision:* 11/15. *Notification:* continuous (freshmen), 12/15 (out-of-state freshmen), 12/15 (early decision). *Application fee:* $20.

Advanced Placement Credit by examination available. Credit given for nursing courses completed elsewhere dependent upon specific evaluations.

Expenses (2005–06) *Tuition:* full-time $18,090; part-time $350 per hour. *International tuition:* $18,090 full-time. *Room and board:* $5200; room only: $3500 per academic year. *Required fees:* full-time $155.

Financial Aid 85% of baccalaureate students in nursing programs received some form of financial aid in 2004–05. *Gift aid (need-based):* Federal Pell, FSEOG, state, private, college/university gift aid from institutional funds. *Loans:* FFEL (Subsidized and Unsubsidized Stafford PLUS), Perkins. *Work-Study:* Federal Work-Study, part-time campus jobs. *Application deadline:* Continuous.

Contact Dr. Jeri L. Brandt, RN, Program Director, Department of Nursing, Nebraska Wesleyan University, 5000 St. Paul Avenue, Lincoln, NE 68504. *Telephone:* 800-541-3818 Ext. 2336. *Fax:* 402-465-2479. *E-mail:* jlb@nebrwesleyan.edu.

GRADUATE PROGRAMS

Expenses (2005–06) *Tuition:* part-time $350 per hour. *Room and board:* $5200; room only: $3500 per academic year.

Financial Aid 65% of graduate students in nursing programs received some form of financial aid in 2004–05.

Contact Dr. Jeri L. Brandt, RN, Program Director, Department of Nursing, Nebraska Wesleyan University, 5000 St. Paul Avenue, Lincoln, NE 68504. *Telephone:* 402-465-2336. *Fax:* 402-465-2179. *E-mail:* jlb@nebrwesleyan.edu.

MASTER'S DEGREE PROGRAM

Degree MSN

Available Programs Accelerated Master's; Master's.

Concentrations Available Nursing administration; nursing education.

Site Options Omaha, NE.

Study Options Full-time and part-time.

Program Entrance Requirements Minimum overall college GPA of 3.0, transcript of college record, written essay, 2 letters of recommendation, nursing research course, resume, statistics course.

Advanced Placement Credit given for nursing courses completed elsewhere dependent upon specific evaluations.

Degree Requirements 36 total credit hours, thesis or project.

POST-MASTER'S PROGRAM

Areas of Study Nursing administration; nursing education.

Union College
Division of Health Sciences
Lincoln, Nebraska

http://www.ucollege.edu

Founded in 1891

DEGREE • BSN

Nursing Program Faculty 10.

Baccalaureate Enrollment 135

Women 88% **Men** 12% **Minority** 10% **International** 10% **Part-time** 5%

Nursing Student Activities Sigma Theta Tau, nursing club.

Nursing Student Resources Academic advising; academic or career counseling; bookstore; campus computer network; career placement assistance; computer lab; computer-assisted instruction; e-mail services; externships; interactive nursing skills videos; Internet; learning resource lab; library services; nursing audiovisuals; placement services for program completers; resume preparation assistance; skills, simulation, or other laboratory; tutoring; unpaid internships.

Library Facilities 147,813 volumes (450 in health, 350 in nursing); 1,357 periodical subscriptions (50 health-care related).

BACCALAUREATE PROGRAMS

Degree BSN

Available Programs ADN to Baccalaureate; Generic Baccalaureate; LPN to Baccalaureate.

Study Options Full-time and part-time.

Program Entrance Requirements Minimum overall college GPA of 2.75, transcript of college record, CPR certification, written essay, health exam, health insurance, high school transcript, immunizations, 3 letters of recommendation, minimum GPA in nursing prerequisites of 2.75, professional liability insurance/malpractice insurance, prerequisite course work. Transfer students are accepted. **Standardized tests** *Required:* SAT or ACT. **Application** *Deadline:* rolling (freshmen), rolling (transfer). *Notification:* continuous (freshmen).

Advanced Placement Credit by examination available. Credit given for nursing courses completed elsewhere dependent upon specific evaluations.

Expenses (2006–07) *Tuition:* full-time $14,790; part-time $625 per hour. *Room and board:* $4898; room only: $2898 per academic year. *Required fees:* full-time $820; part-time $410 per term.

Financial Aid 83% of baccalaureate students in nursing programs received some form of financial aid in 2005–06.

Contact Ms. Aileen Schuh, Office Manager, Division of Health Sciences, Union College, Nursing Program, 3800 South 48th Street, Lincoln, NE 68506. *Telephone:* 402-486-2524. *Fax:* 402-486-2559. *E-mail:* aischuh@ucollege.edu.

University of Nebraska Medical Center
College of Nursing
Omaha, Nebraska

http://www.unmc.edu/nursing/

Founded in 1869

DEGREES • BSN • MSN • PHD

Nursing Program Faculty 112 (60% with doctorates).

Baccalaureate Enrollment 600

Graduate Enrollment 300

Nursing Student Activities Nursing Honor Society, Sigma Theta Tau, Student Nurses' Association, nursing club.

Nursing Student Resources Academic advising; academic or career counseling; assistance for students with disabilities; bookstore; campus computer network; career placement assistance; computer lab; computer-assisted instruction; daycare for children of students; e-mail services; employment services for current students; externships; housing assistance; interactive nursing skills videos; Internet; learning resource lab; library services; nursing audiovisuals; other; paid internships; placement services for program completers; remedial services; resume preparation assistance; skills, simulation, or other laboratory; tutoring.

Library Facilities 241,551 volumes (240,000 in health, 3,500 in nursing); 4,280 periodical subscriptions (2,200 health-care related).

BACCALAUREATE PROGRAMS

Degree BSN

University of Nebraska Medical Center (continued)

Available Programs ADN to Baccalaureate; Accelerated Baccalaureate; Accelerated Baccalaureate for Second Degree; Accelerated RN Baccalaureate; Baccalaureate for Second Degree; Generic Baccalaureate; International Nurse to Baccalaureate; LPN to Baccalaureate; LPN to RN Baccalaureate; RN Baccalaureate; RPN to Baccalaureate.

Site Options *Distance Learning:* Scottsbluff, NE; Kearney, NE; Lincoln, NE.

Study Options Full-time.

Program Entrance Requirements Minimum overall college GPA of 2.5, transcript of college record, CPR certification, health insurance, high school transcript, immunizations, 2 letters of recommendation, prerequisite course work. Transfer students are accepted. **Standardized tests** *Required:* TOEFL for international students. **Application** *Deadline:* rolling (transfer). *Application fee:* $45.

Advanced Placement Credit by examination available. Credit given for nursing courses completed elsewhere dependent upon specific evaluations.

Financial Aid 88% of baccalaureate students in nursing programs received some form of financial aid in 2004–05.

Contact Ms. Dani S. Eveloff, RN, Recruitment Coordinator, College of Nursing, University of Nebraska Medical Center, 985330 Nebraska Medical Center, Omaha, NE 68198-5330. *Telephone:* 402-559-5184. *E-mail:* develoff@unmc.edu.

GRADUATE PROGRAMS

Contact Ms. Dani Eveloff, RN, Recruitment Coordinator, College of Nursing, University of Nebraska Medical Center, 985330 Nebraska Medical Center, Omaha, NE 68198-5330. *Telephone:* 402-559-5184. *E-mail:* develoff@unmc.edu.

MASTER'S DEGREE PROGRAM

Degree MSN

Available Programs Master's; Master's for Non-Nursing College Graduates; RN to Master's.

Concentrations Available Health-care administration; nurse case management; nursing administration; nursing education; nursing informatics. *Clinical nurse specialist programs in:* acute care, adult health, cardiovascular, community health, critical care, family health, gerontology, maternity-newborn, medical-surgical, oncology, parent-child, pediatric, perinatal, psychiatric/mental health, public health, women's health. *Nurse practitioner programs in:* acute care, adult health, community health, family health, gerontology, neonatal health, oncology, pediatric, primary care, psychiatric/mental health, women's health.

Site Options *Distance Learning:* Scottsbluff, NE; Kearney, NE; Lincoln, NE.

Study Options Full-time and part-time.

Program Entrance Requirements Computer literacy, minimum overall college GPA of 3.0, transcript of college record, CPR certification, immunizations, interview, 3 letters of recommendation, nursing research course, statistics course.

Advanced Placement Credit given for nursing courses completed elsewhere dependent upon specific evaluations.

Degree Requirements 45 total credit hours.

POST-MASTER'S PROGRAM

Areas of Study Health-care administration; nurse case management; nursing administration; nursing education; nursing informatics. *Clinical nurse specialist programs in:* acute care, adult health, cardiovascular, community health, critical care, family health, gerontology, maternity-newborn, medical-surgical, oncology, parent-child, pediatric, perinatal, psychiatric/mental health, public health, women's health. *Nurse practitioner programs in:* acute care, adult health, community health, family health, gerontology, neonatal health, oncology, pediatric, primary care, psychiatric/mental health, women's health.

DOCTORAL DEGREE PROGRAM

Degree PhD

Available Programs Doctorate; Doctorate for Nurses with Non-Nursing Degrees; Post-Baccalaureate Doctorate.

Areas of Study Advanced practice nursing, aging, bio-behavioral research, biology of health and illness, clinical practice, community health, critical care, faculty preparation, family health, gerontology, health policy, health promotion/disease prevention, health-care systems, human health and illness, illness and transition, individualized study, information systems, maternity-newborn, neuro-behavior, nurse case management, nursing administration, nursing policy, nursing research, nursing science, oncology, women's health.

Site Options *Distance Learning:* Scottsbluff, NE; Kearney, NE; Lincoln, NE.

Program Entrance Requirements Minimum overall college GPA of 3.2, interview by faculty committee, interview, 3 letters of recommendation, scholarly papers, statistics course, vita, writing sample.

Degree Requirements Dissertation, oral exam, written exam.

POSTDOCTORAL PROGRAM

Postdoctoral Program Contact Dr. Margaret Wilson, Associate Dean for Graduate Programs, College of Nursing, University of Nebraska Medical Center, 985330 Nebraska Medical Center, Omaha, NE 68198-5330. *Telephone:* 402-559-7457. *Fax:* 410-706-0945. *E-mail:* mwilson@unmc.edu.

CONTINUING EDUCATION PROGRAM

Contact Ms. Rhonda Harnish, Program Associate, College of Nursing, University of Nebraska Medical Center, 985330 Nebraska Medical Center, Omaha, NE 68198-5330. *Telephone:* 402-559-7487. *E-mail:* cbevil@unmc.edu.

NEVADA

Nevada State College at Henderson
Nursing Program
Henderson, Nevada

Founded in 2002
DEGREE • BS

BACCALAUREATE PROGRAMS

Degree BS

Available Programs Generic Baccalaureate; RN Baccalaureate.

Program Entrance Requirements Standardized tests *Recommended:* SAT or ACT. **Application** *Deadline:* 8/20 (freshmen), 8/20 (transfer). *Notification:* continuous (freshmen). *Application fee:* $30.

Contact Office of Admissions and Financial Aid, Nursing Program, Nevada State College at Henderson, 1125 Nevada State Drive, Henderson, NV 89015. *Telephone:* 702-992-2000. *E-mail:* admissions@nsc.nevada.edu.

University of Nevada, Las Vegas
School of Nursing
Las Vegas, Nevada

Founded in 1957
DEGREES • BSN • MSN • PHD

Nursing Program Faculty 38 (55% with doctorates).

Baccalaureate Enrollment 190
Women 84% **Men** 16% **Minority** 37% **International** 9% **Part-time** 13%

Graduate Enrollment 132
Women 84% **Men** 16% **Minority** 13% **International** 44% **Part-time** 44%

Nursing Student Activities Sigma Theta Tau, Student Nurses' Association.

Nursing Student Resources Academic advising; academic or career counseling; assistance for students with disabilities; bookstore; campus computer network; career placement assistance; computer lab; computer-assisted instruction; daycare for children of students; e-mail services; employment services for current students; interactive nursing skills videos;

Internet; learning resource lab; library services; nursing audiovisuals; remedial services; resume preparation assistance; skills, simulation, or other laboratory; tutoring; unpaid internships.

Library Facilities 1 million volumes (35,800 in health, 12,000 in nursing); 9,536 periodical subscriptions (305 health-care related).

BACCALAUREATE PROGRAMS

Degree BSN

Available Programs Generic Baccalaureate.

Study Options Full-time and part-time.

Program Entrance Requirements Minimum overall college GPA of 3.0, transcript of college record, CPR certification, health exam, health insurance, high school biology, high school chemistry, 1 year of high school math, high school transcript, immunizations, minimum GPA in nursing prerequisites of 3.0, prerequisite course work. Transfer students are accepted. **Standardized tests** *Required:* TOEFL for international students. *Recommended:* SAT or ACT. *Required for some:* SAT or ACT. **Application** *Deadline:* 2/1 (freshmen), 4/1 (transfer). *Notification:* continuous (freshmen). *Application fee:* $60.

Advanced Placement Credit by examination available. Credit given for nursing courses completed elsewhere dependent upon specific evaluations.

Expenses (2006–07) *Tuition, state resident:* full-time $3158; part-time $105 per credit. *Tuition, nonresident:* full-time $6630; part-time $221 per credit. *International tuition:* $6830 full-time. *Room and board:* $8624; room only: $5600 per academic year. *Required fees:* full-time $454; part-time $4 per credit; part-time $108 per term.

Financial Aid 60% of baccalaureate students in nursing programs received some form of financial aid in 2005–06. *Gift aid (need-based):* Federal Pell, FSEOG, state, private, college/university gift aid from institutional funds. *Loans:* Federal Direct (Subsidized and Unsubsidized Stafford PLUS), Perkins, state, college/university. *Work-Study:* Federal Work-Study, part-time campus jobs. *Application deadline (priority):* 2/1.

Contact Dr. Susan Kowalski, RN, Undergraduate Coordinator, School of Nursing, University of Nevada, Las Vegas, 4505 Maryland Parkway, Las Vegas, NV 89154-3018. *Telephone:* 702-895-3360. *Fax:* 702-895-4807. *E-mail:* susan.kowalski@unlv.edu.

GRADUATE PROGRAMS

Expenses (2006–07) *Tuition, state resident:* full-time $3594; part-time $150 per credit. *Tuition, nonresident:* full-time $7774; part-time $315 per credit. *International tuition:* $7974 full-time. *Room and board:* $8624; room only: $5600 per academic year. *Required fees:* full-time $454; part-time $4 per credit; part-time $108 per term.

Financial Aid 40% of graduate students in nursing programs received some form of financial aid in 2005–06. Research assistantships with partial tuition reimbursements available, teaching assistantships with partial tuition reimbursements available, career-related internships or fieldwork, Federal Work-Study, institutionally sponsored loans, scholarships, and unspecified assistantships available. Aid available to part-time students. *Financial aid application deadline:* 3/1.

Contact Dr. Patricia Alpert, Coordinator, Graduate Programs, School of Nursing, University of Nevada, Las Vegas, Las Vegas, NV 89154-3018. *Telephone:* 702-895-3360. *Fax:* 702-895-4807. *E-mail:* patricia.alpert@unlv. edu.

MASTER'S DEGREE PROGRAM

Degree MSN

Available Programs Master's.

Concentrations Available Nursing education. *Nurse practitioner programs in:* family health, pediatric.

Study Options Full-time and part-time.

Program Entrance Requirements Clinical experience, computer literacy, minimum overall college GPA of 3.0, transcript of college record, CPR certification, written essay, immunizations, 2 letters of recommendation, nursing research course, physical assessment course, professional liability insurance/malpractice insurance, prerequisite course work, resume, statistics course, GRE General Test. *Application deadline:* For fall admission, 3/15. *Application fee:* $60 ($75 for international students).

Advanced Placement Credit given for nursing courses completed elsewhere dependent upon specific evaluations.

Degree Requirements 40 total credit hours, thesis or project, comprehensive exam.

POST-MASTER'S PROGRAM

Areas of Study Nursing education. *Nurse practitioner programs in:* family health, pediatric.

DOCTORAL DEGREE PROGRAM

Degree PhD

Available Programs Doctorate.

Areas of Study Nursing education.

Program Entrance Requirements Clinical experience, minimum overall college GPA of 3.0, interview by faculty committee, 2 letters of recommendation, MSN or equivalent, statistics course, vita, writing sample. *Application deadline:* For fall admission, 3/15. *Application fee:* $60 ($75 for international students).

Degree Requirements 60 total credit hours, dissertation, oral exam.

CONTINUING EDUCATION PROGRAM

Contact Mrs. Deborah Warner, RN, Continuing Education Coordinator, School of Nursing, University of Nevada, Las Vegas, 4505 Maryland Parkway, Las Vegas, NV 89154-3018. *Telephone:* 702-895-3360. *Fax:* 702-895-4807. *E-mail:* deborah.warner@unlv.edu.

University of Nevada, Reno
Orvis School of Nursing
Reno, Nevada

http://www.unr.edu/bcs/osn

Founded in 1874

DEGREES • BSN • MSN • MSN/MPH

Nursing Program Faculty 27 (40% with doctorates).

Baccalaureate Enrollment 149
Women 60% **Men** 40% **Minority** 16% **International** 5% **Part-time** 20%

Graduate Enrollment 35
Women 90% **Men** 10% **Minority** 1% **Part-time** 85%

Nursing Student Activities Sigma Theta Tau, Student Nurses' Association.

Nursing Student Resources Academic advising; academic or career counseling; assistance for students with disabilities; bookstore; campus computer network; computer lab; computer-assisted instruction; e-mail services; Internet; learning resource lab; library services; nursing audiovisuals; remedial services; skills, simulation, or other laboratory.

Library Facilities 1.2 million volumes (5,000 in health, 3,000 in nursing); 19,058 periodical subscriptions (172 health-care related).

BACCALAUREATE PROGRAMS

Degree BSN

Available Programs ADN to Baccalaureate; Accelerated Baccalaureate; Generic Baccalaureate; RN Baccalaureate.

Site Options *Distance Learning:* Reno, NV.

Study Options Full-time.

Program Entrance Requirements Transcript of college record, CPR certification, health exam, health insurance, immunizations, minimum GPA in nursing prerequisites of 3.0, professional liability insurance/malpractice insurance, prerequisite course work. Transfer students are accepted. **Standardized tests** *Required:* TOEFL for international students. **Application** *Deadline:* rolling (freshmen), rolling (transfer). *Early decision:* 11/15. *Notification:* continuous (freshmen). *Application fee:* $60.

Advanced Placement Credit given for nursing courses completed elsewhere dependent upon specific evaluations.

Expenses (2006–07) *Tuition, state resident:* full-time $3278; part-time $109 per credit hour. *Tuition, nonresident:* full-time $13,188; part-time $440 per credit hour. *International tuition:* $13,788 full-time. *Room and board:* $9780; room only: $5981 per academic year. *Required fees:* full-time $406; part-time $203 per term.

Financial Aid 50% of baccalaureate students in nursing programs received some form of financial aid in 2005–06.

University of Nevada, Reno (continued)

Contact Mary Ann Lambert, Coordinator, Undergraduate Program, Orvis School of Nursing, University of Nevada, Reno, Mail Stop 134, Reno, NV 89557. *Telephone:* 775-682-7150. *Fax:* 775-784-4262. *E-mail:* lambert@unr. edu.

GRADUATE PROGRAMS

Expenses (2006–07) *Tuition, state resident:* full-time $3690; part-time $154 per credit hour. *Tuition, nonresident:* full-time $13,601; part-time $567 per credit hour. *International tuition:* $13,601 full-time. *Room and board:* $9780; room only: $5981 per academic year. *Required fees:* full-time $412; part-time $206 per term.

Financial Aid 90% of graduate students in nursing programs received some form of financial aid in 2005–06. 3 research assistantships were awarded; teaching assistantships. *Financial aid application deadline:* 3/1.

Contact Alice Running, PhD, Coordinator, Graduate Program, Orvis School of Nursing, University of Nevada, Reno, Mail Stop 134, Reno, NV 89557. *Telephone:* 775-682-7148 Ext. 242. *Fax:* 775-784-4262. *E-mail:* running@unr.edu.

MASTER'S DEGREE PROGRAM

Degrees MSN; MSN/MPH

Available Programs Master's.

Concentrations Available Nursing education. *Clinical nurse specialist programs in:* school health. *Nurse practitioner programs in:* family health.

Site Options *Distance Learning:* Reno, NV.

Study Options Full-time and part-time.

Program Entrance Requirements Computer literacy, minimum overall college GPA of 3.0, transcript of college record, CPR certification, immunizations, 3 letters of recommendation, physical assessment course, professional liability insurance/malpractice insurance, statistics course, GRE General Test or MAT. *Application deadline:* For fall admission, 3/1 (priority date). Applications are processed on a rolling basis. *Application fee:* $60 ($95 for international students).

Advanced Placement Credit given for nursing courses completed elsewhere dependent upon specific evaluations.

Degree Requirements 58 total credit hours, thesis or project, comprehensive exam.

POST-MASTER'S PROGRAM

Areas of Study Nursing education. *Nurse practitioner programs in:* family health.

NEW HAMPSHIRE

Colby-Sawyer College
Department of Nursing
New London, New Hampshire

http://www.colby-sawyer.edu/academic/nursing
Founded in 1837

DEGREE • BS

Nursing Program Faculty 17 (6% with doctorates).

Baccalaureate Enrollment 112
Women 95% **Men** 5% **Minority** 3% **Part-time** 1%

Nursing Student Activities Nursing Honor Society, Student Nurses' Association.

Nursing Student Resources Academic advising; academic or career counseling; assistance for students with disabilities; bookstore; campus computer network; career placement assistance; computer lab; computer-assisted instruction; e-mail services; employment services for current students; housing assistance; interactive nursing skills videos; Internet; learning resource lab; library services; nursing audiovisuals; remedial services; resume preparation assistance; skills, simulation, or other laboratory; tutoring; unpaid internships.

Library Facilities 90,055 volumes (10,980 in health, 751 in nursing); 514 periodical subscriptions (104 health-care related).

BACCALAUREATE PROGRAMS

Degree BS

Available Programs Generic Baccalaureate.

Study Options Full-time and part-time.

Program Entrance Requirements Minimum overall college GPA of 2.5, transcript of college record, written essay, health exam, health insurance, high school foreign language, 3 years high school math, 2 years high school science, high school transcript, immunizations, 2 letters of recommendation, minimum GPA in nursing prerequisites of 2.3, prerequisite course work. Transfer students are accepted. **Standardized tests** *Required:* SAT or ACT, TOEFL for international students. **Application** *Deadline:* 4/1 (freshmen), 8/1 (transfer). *Notification:* 1/1 (freshmen). *Application fee:* $45.

Advanced Placement Credit by examination available. Credit given for nursing courses completed elsewhere dependent upon specific evaluations.

Expenses (2006–07) *Tuition:* full-time $26,350; part-time $880 per credit hour. *International tuition:* $26,350 full-time. *Room and board:* $9900; room only: $5600 per academic year.

Financial Aid 90% of baccalaureate students in nursing programs received some form of financial aid in 2005–06.

Contact Ellen Ceppetelli, Department of Nursing, Colby-Sawyer College, 541 Main Street, New London, NH 03257-7835. *Telephone:* 603-526-3646. *Fax:* 603-526-3452. *E-mail:* eceppetelli@colby-sawyer.edu.

Rivier College
Department of Nursing and Health Sciences
Nashua, New Hampshire

Founded in 1933

DEGREES • BS • MS • MS/MBA

Nursing Program Faculty 24 (25% with doctorates).

Baccalaureate Enrollment 250
Women 97% **Men** 3% **Minority** 3% **Part-time** 75%

Graduate Enrollment 43
Women 95% **Men** 5% **Minority** 3% **Part-time** 84%

Nursing Student Activities Nursing Honor Society, Student Nurses' Association.

Nursing Student Resources Academic advising; academic or career counseling; assistance for students with disabilities; bookstore; campus computer network; career placement assistance; computer lab; computer-assisted instruction; e-mail services; employment services for current students; externships; housing assistance; interactive nursing skills videos; Internet; learning resource lab; library services; nursing audiovisuals; other; placement services for program completers; remedial services; resume preparation assistance; skills, simulation, or other laboratory; tutoring.

Library Facilities 92,000 volumes (4,400 in health, 3,800 in nursing); 500 periodical subscriptions (275 health-care related).

BACCALAUREATE PROGRAMS

Degree BS

Available Programs ADN to Baccalaureate; RN Baccalaureate.

Site Options Lowell, MA; Manchester, NH.

Study Options Full-time and part-time.

Program Entrance Requirements Transcript of college record, written essay, health exam, health insurance, high school chemistry, high school foreign language, 2 years high school math, high school transcript, immunizations, 2 letters of recommendation, minimum high school GPA of 2.5, minimum high school rank 80%, prerequisite course work. Transfer students are accepted. **Standardized tests** *Required:* SAT or ACT, TOEFL for international students. *Required for some:* nursing exam. **Application** *Deadline:* rolling (freshmen), rolling (transfer). *Early decision:* 11/15. *Notification:* continuous (freshmen), 12/1 (early action). *Application fee:* $25.

Advanced Placement Credit by examination available. Credit given for nursing courses completed elsewhere dependent upon specific evaluations.

Contact *Telephone:* 603-897-8627. *Fax:* 603-897-8884.

GRADUATE PROGRAMS

Contact *Telephone:* 603-897-8627. *Fax:* 603-897-8884.

MASTER'S DEGREE PROGRAM

Degrees MS; MS/MBA

Available Programs Master's; Master's for Nurses with Non-Nursing Degrees.

Concentrations Available Health-care administration; nursing education. *Clinical nurse specialist programs in:* psychiatric/mental health. *Nurse practitioner programs in:* family health, psychiatric/mental health.

Study Options Full-time and part-time.

Program Entrance Requirements Clinical experience, transcript of college record, written essay, immunizations, interview, 2 letters of recommendation, resume, statistics course, GRE, MAT. *Application deadline:* Applications are processed on a rolling basis. *Application fee:* $25.

Advanced Placement Credit given for nursing courses completed elsewhere dependent upon specific evaluations.

Degree Requirements 43 total credit hours, thesis or project.

POST-MASTER'S PROGRAM

Areas of Study Nursing education. *Clinical nurse specialist programs in:* psychiatric/mental health. *Nurse practitioner programs in:* family health, psychiatric/mental health.

Saint Anselm College
Department of Nursing
Manchester, New Hampshire

Founded in 1889

DEGREE • BS

Nursing Program Faculty 23 (31% with doctorates).

Baccalaureate Enrollment 194
Women 96% **Men** 4% **Minority** 2% **International** 1% **Part-time** 1%

Nursing Student Activities Student Nurses' Association.

Nursing Student Resources Academic advising; academic or career counseling; assistance for students with disabilities; bookstore; campus computer network; career placement assistance; computer lab; computer-assisted instruction; e-mail services; employment services for current students; externships; housing assistance; interactive nursing skills videos; Internet; learning resource lab; library services; nursing audiovisuals; resume preparation assistance; skills, simulation, or other laboratory; tutoring.

Library Facilities 222,000 volumes (7,127 in health); 1,900 periodical subscriptions (292 health-care related).

BACCALAUREATE PROGRAMS

Degree BS

Available Programs RN Baccalaureate.

Study Options Full-time and part-time.

Program Entrance Requirements Minimum overall college GPA of 2.0, transcript of college record, written essay, health exam, health insurance, high school biology, high school chemistry, high school foreign language, 3 years high school math, 3 years high school science, high school transcript, immunizations, 2 letters of recommendation, professional liability insurance/malpractice insurance. Transfer students are accepted. **Standardized tests** *Required:* SAT or ACT, TOEFL for international students. **Application** *Deadline:* rolling (freshmen), rolling (transfer). *Early decision:* 11/15. *Notification:* continuous (freshmen), 12/1 (out-of-state freshmen), 12/1 (early decision). *Application fee:* $55.

Advanced Placement Credit by examination available. Credit given for nursing courses completed elsewhere dependent upon specific evaluations.

Expenses (2005–06) *Tuition:* full-time $23,990; part-time $2400 per course. *International tuition:* $23,990 full-time. *Room and board:* $9070 per academic year. *Required fees:* full-time $750.

Financial Aid 83% of baccalaureate students in nursing programs received some form of financial aid in 2004–05. *Gift aid (need-based):* Federal Pell, FSEOG, state, private, college/university gift aid from institutional funds. *Loans:* FFEL (Subsidized and Unsubsidized Stafford PLUS), Perkins, GATE Loans. *Work-Study:* Federal Work-Study, part-time campus jobs. *Application deadline:* 3/15 (priority: 3/15).

Contact Nancy Davis Griffin, Director of Admission, Department of Nursing, Saint Anselm College, 100 Saint Anselm Drive, Manchester, NH 03102-1310. *Telephone:* 603-641-7500. *Fax:* 603-641-7550. *E-mail:* ngriffin@anselm.edu.

CONTINUING EDUCATION PROGRAM

Contact Debra McLaughlin, Director, Continuing Nursing Education, Department of Nursing, Saint Anselm College, 100 Saint Anselm Drive, #1745, Manchester, NH 03102-1310. *Telephone:* 603-641-7083. *Fax:* 603-641-7089. *E-mail:* dmclauglin@anselm.edu.

University of New Hampshire
Department of Nursing
Durham, New Hampshire

http://www.unh.edu/ur-nurs.html

Founded in 1866

DEGREES • BS • MS

Nursing Program Faculty 13 (75% with doctorates).

Baccalaureate Enrollment 268
Women 91% **Men** 9% **Minority** 1%

Graduate Enrollment 54
Women 95% **Men** 5% **Minority** 1%

Nursing Student Activities Nursing Honor Society, Sigma Theta Tau, Student Nurses' Association.

Nursing Student Resources Academic advising; academic or career counseling; assistance for students with disabilities; bookstore; campus computer network; computer lab; computer-assisted instruction; daycare for children of students; e-mail services; housing assistance; interactive nursing skills videos; Internet; learning resource lab; nursing audiovisuals; paid internships; resume preparation assistance; skills, simulation, or other laboratory; tutoring.

Library Facilities 1.8 million volumes; 36,313 periodical subscriptions.

BACCALAUREATE PROGRAMS

Degree BS

Available Programs Generic Baccalaureate; RN Baccalaureate.

Study Options Full-time and part-time.

Program Entrance Requirements High school transcript, prerequisite course work. Transfer students are accepted. **Standardized tests** *Required:* SAT or ACT, TOEFL for international students. **Application** *Deadline:* 2/1 (freshmen), 3/1 (transfer). *Early decision:* 12/1. *Notification:* 4/15 (freshmen), 1/15 (early action). *Application fee:* $45.

Contact *Telephone:* 603-862-4715. *Fax:* 603-862-4771.

GRADUATE PROGRAMS

Contact *Telephone:* 603-862-2285. *Fax:* 603-862-4771.

MASTER'S DEGREE PROGRAM

Degree MS

Available Programs Master's; Master's for Nurses with Non-Nursing Degrees.

Concentrations Available *Clinical nurse specialist programs in:* adult health. *Nurse practitioner programs in:* adult health, family health.

Program Entrance Requirements GRE General Test or MAT. *Application deadline:* For fall admission, 4/1 (priority date); for winter admission, 12/1. Applications are processed on a rolling basis. *Application fee:* $50.

University of New Hampshire (continued)
Degree Requirements 45 total credit hours, thesis or project, comprehensive exam.

POST-MASTER'S PROGRAM

Areas of Study *Clinical nurse specialist programs in:* adult health. *Nurse practitioner programs in:* adult health, family health.

NEW JERSEY

Bloomfield College
Division of Nursing
Bloomfield, New Jersey

http://www.bloomfield.edu
Founded in 1868
DEGREE • BS

Nursing Program Faculty 20 (30% with doctorates).
Baccalaureate Enrollment 145
Women 85% **Men** 15% **Minority** 74% **International** 1% **Part-time** 21%
Nursing Student Activities Student Nurses' Association.
Nursing Student Resources Academic advising; academic or career counseling; assistance for students with disabilities; bookstore; campus computer network; career placement assistance; computer lab; computer-assisted instruction; e-mail services; employment services for current students; interactive nursing skills videos; Internet; learning resource lab; library services; nursing audiovisuals; placement services for program completers; remedial services; resume preparation assistance; skills, simulation, or other laboratory; tutoring.
Library Facilities 64,700 volumes (1,500 in health, 1,500 in nursing); 456 periodical subscriptions (44 health-care related).

BACCALAUREATE PROGRAMS

Degree BS

Available Programs Generic Baccalaureate; RN Baccalaureate.
Site Options Manahawkin, NJ. *Distance Learning:* Toms River, NJ.
Study Options Full-time and part-time.
Program Entrance Requirements Transcript of college record, CPR certification, health exam, minimum GPA in nursing prerequisites of 2.5, prerequisite course work. Transfer students are accepted. **Standardized tests** *Required:* SAT or ACT, TOEFL for international students. **Application** *Deadline:* 7/1 (freshmen), 8/1 (transfer). *Early decision:* 1/7. *Notification:* continuous (freshmen), 1/21 (early action). *Application fee:* $40.
Advanced Placement Credit given for nursing courses completed elsewhere dependent upon specific evaluations.
Expenses (2006–07) *Tuition:* full-time $16,100; part-time $1650 per course. *International tuition:* $16,100 full-time. *Room and board:* $9100; room only: $4050 per academic year. *Required fees:* full-time $300; part-time $50 per term.
Financial Aid 77% of baccalaureate students in nursing programs received some form of financial aid in 2005–06. *Gift aid (need-based):* Federal Pell, FSEOG, state, private, college/university gift aid from institutional funds. *Loans:* FFEL (Subsidized and Unsubsidized Stafford PLUS). *Work-Study:* Federal Work-Study, part-time campus jobs. *Application deadline:* 10/1 (priority: 3/15).
Contact Ms. Lourdes Delgado, Vice President of Enrollment Management/Dean of Admission, Division of Nursing, Bloomfield College, 1 Park Place, Bloomfield, NJ 07003. *Telephone:* 973-748-9000 Ext. 392. *Fax:* 973-748-0916. *E-mail:* lourdes_delgado@bloomfield.edu.

The College of New Jersey
School of Nursing
Ewing, New Jersey

http://www.tcnj.edu/~nursing
Founded in 1855
DEGREES • BSN • MSN

Nursing Program Faculty 15 (60% with doctorates).
Baccalaureate Enrollment 273
Women 93% **Men** 7% **Minority** 34% **Part-time** 1%
Graduate Enrollment 47
Women 98% **Men** 2% **Minority** 23% **Part-time** 2%
Nursing Student Activities Sigma Theta Tau, Student Nurses' Association.
Nursing Student Resources Academic advising; academic or career counseling; assistance for students with disabilities; bookstore; campus computer network; career placement assistance; computer lab; computer-assisted instruction; daycare for children of students; e-mail services; employment services for current students; externships; interactive nursing skills videos; Internet; learning resource lab; library services; nursing audiovisuals; paid internships; resume preparation assistance; skills, simulation, or other laboratory; tutoring; unpaid internships.
Library Facilities 662,152 volumes (30,000 in health, 18,800 in nursing); 429,632 periodical subscriptions (228 health-care related).

BACCALAUREATE PROGRAMS

Degree BSN

Available Programs Generic Baccalaureate.
Study Options Full-time and part-time.
Program Entrance Requirements Written essay, health exam, high school transcript, immunizations. Transfer students are accepted. **Standardized tests** *Required:* SAT, TOEFL for international students. **Application** *Deadline:* 2/15 (freshmen), 2/15 (transfer). *Early decision:* 11/15. *Notification:* continuous until 4/1 (freshmen), 12/15 (out-of-state freshmen), 12/15 (early decision). *Application fee:* $60.
Advanced Placement Credit by examination available. Credit given for nursing courses completed elsewhere dependent upon specific evaluations.
Expenses (2005–06) *Tuition, state resident:* full-time $7051; part-time $250 per credit hour. *Tuition, nonresident:* full-time $12,315; part-time $436 per credit hour. *International tuition:* $12,315 full-time. *Room and board:* $8807 per academic year. *Required fees:* full-time $2806.
Financial Aid 42% of baccalaureate students in nursing programs received some form of financial aid in 2004–05. *Gift aid (need-based):* Federal Pell, FSEOG, state, private, college/university gift aid from institutional funds, Federal Nursing. *Loans:* Federal Nursing Student Loans, FFEL (Subsidized and Unsubsidized Stafford PLUS), Perkins, state. *Work-Study:* Federal Work-Study, part-time campus jobs. *Application deadline:* 10/1 (priority: 3/1).
Contact Mr. Patrick Roger-Gordon, Assistant Dean for Student Services, School of Nursing, The College of New Jersey, PO Box 7718, 2000 Pennington Road, Ewing, NJ 08628-0718. *Telephone:* 609-771-2669. *Fax:* 609-637-5159. *E-mail:* roger@tcnj.edu.

GRADUATE PROGRAMS

Expenses (2005–06) *Tuition, state resident:* full-time $12,314; part-time $487 per credit hour. *Tuition, nonresident:* full-time $16,322; part-time $681 per credit hour. *International tuition:* $16,322 full-time. *Required fees:* full-time $2154.
Financial Aid 8% of graduate students in nursing programs received some form of financial aid in 2004–05. Unspecified assistantships available. *Financial aid application deadline:* 5/1.
Contact Dr. Claire Lindberg, Chair, Division of Advanced Nursing Education and Practice, School of Nursing, The College of New Jersey, PO Box 7718, 2000 Pennington Road, Ewing, NJ 08628-0718. *Telephone:* 609-771-2591. *Fax:* 609-637-5159. *E-mail:* lindberg@tcnj.edu.

MASTER'S DEGREE PROGRAM
Degree MSN

Available Programs Master's; Master's for Nurses with Non-Nursing Degrees; RN to Master's.

Concentrations Available Nursing administration. *Clinical nurse specialist programs in:* adult health. *Nurse practitioner programs in:* family health, neonatal health.

Study Options Full-time and part-time.

Program Entrance Requirements Computer literacy, minimum overall college GPA of 3.0, transcript of college record, written essay, immunizations, interview, 3 letters of recommendation, physical assessment course, statistics course, GRE General Test. *Application deadline:* For fall admission, 3/15. *Application fee:* $50.

Advanced Placement Credit given for nursing courses completed elsewhere dependent upon specific evaluations.

Degree Requirements 47 total credit hours, comprehensive exam.

POST-MASTER'S PROGRAM

Areas of Study Nursing administration. *Clinical nurse specialist programs in:* adult health. *Nurse practitioner programs in:* family health, neonatal health.

College of Saint Elizabeth
Department of Nursing
Morristown, New Jersey

http://www.cse.edu/sgcs_continuingstudies.btm
Founded in 1899
DEGREE • BSN

Nursing Program Faculty 13 (25% with doctorates).

Baccalaureate Enrollment 231
Women 95% **Men** 5% **Minority** 48% **Part-time** 99%

Nursing Student Activities Nursing Honor Society, Sigma Theta Tau, nursing club.

Nursing Student Resources Academic advising; academic or career counseling; assistance for students with disabilities; bookstore; campus computer network; career placement assistance; computer lab; computer-assisted instruction; e-mail services; employment services for current students; interactive nursing skills videos; Internet; learning resource lab; library services; nursing audiovisuals; other; remedial services; resume preparation assistance; skills, simulation, or other laboratory; tutoring.

Library Facilities 109,352 volumes (4,246 in health, 702 in nursing); 561 periodical subscriptions (194 health-care related).

BACCALAUREATE PROGRAMS
Degree BSN

Available Programs ADN to Baccalaureate; Accelerated RN Baccalaureate; International Nurse to Baccalaureate; RN Baccalaureate.

Site Options Randolph, NJ; Elizabeth, NJ; Hoboken, NJ.

Study Options Part-time.

Program Entrance Requirements Minimum overall college GPA of 2.0, transcript of college record, CPR certification, health exam, immunizations, prerequisite course work, RN licensure. Transfer students are accepted. **Standardized tests** *Required:* SAT or ACT, TOEFL for international students. **Application** *Deadline:* 8/15 (freshmen), rolling (transfer). *Notification:* 11/15 (freshmen). *Application fee:* $35.

Advanced Placement Credit by examination available. Credit given for nursing courses completed elsewhere dependent upon specific evaluations.

Expenses (2006–07) *Tuition:* part-time $623 per credit. *Required fees:* part-time $280 per term.

Financial Aid 75% of baccalaureate students in nursing programs received some form of financial aid in 2005–06.

Contact Dr. Ellen G. Ehrlich, Chairperson, Department of Nursing, College of Saint Elizabeth, 2 Convent Road, Morristown, NJ 07960-6989. *Telephone:* 973-290-4056. *Fax:* 973-290-4177. *E-mail:* eehrlich@cse.edu.

CONTINUING EDUCATION PROGRAM

Contact Dr. Eileen Specchio, Associate Professor, Department of Nursing, College of Saint Elizabeth, 2 Convent Road, Morristown, NJ 07960-6989. *Telephone:* 973-290-4073. *Fax:* 973-290-4177. *E-mail:* especchio@cse.edu.

Fairleigh Dickinson University, Metropolitan Campus
Henry P. Becton School of Nursing and Allied Health
Teaneck, New Jersey

http://fduinfo.com/depts/ucnab.pbp
Founded in 1942
DEGREES • BSN • DNP • MSN

Nursing Program Faculty 14 (42% with doctorates).

Baccalaureate Enrollment 220
Women 90% **Men** 10% **Minority** 67.7% **International** 3.6% **Part-time** 22.7%

Graduate Enrollment 69
Women 96.6% **Men** 3.4% **Minority** 29% **Part-time** 100%

Nursing Student Activities Nursing Honor Society, Sigma Theta Tau, Student Nurses' Association.

Nursing Student Resources Academic advising; academic or career counseling; assistance for students with disabilities; bookstore; campus computer network; career placement assistance; computer lab; computer-assisted instruction; e-mail services; employment services for current students; externships; housing assistance; interactive nursing skills videos; Internet; learning resource lab; library services; nursing audiovisuals; other; remedial services; resume preparation assistance; skills, simulation, or other laboratory; tutoring.

Library Facilities 371,900 volumes (2,166 in nursing); 1,690 periodical subscriptions (104 health-care related).

BACCALAUREATE PROGRAMS
Degree BSN

Available Programs Accelerated Baccalaureate for Second Degree; Generic Baccalaureate; RN Baccalaureate.

Site Options *Distance Learning:* Sewell, NJ; Morristown, NJ; Westwood, NJ.

Study Options Full-time and part-time.

Program Entrance Requirements Minimum overall college GPA of 3.0, transcript of college record, health exam, health insurance, high school biology, high school chemistry, 2 years high school math, 2 years high school science, high school transcript, immunizations, 2 letters of recommendation. Transfer students are accepted. **Standardized tests** *Required:* SAT or ACT, TOEFL for international students. **Application** *Deadline:* rolling (freshmen). *Notification:* continuous (freshmen). *Application fee:* $40.

Advanced Placement Credit given for nursing courses completed elsewhere dependent upon specific evaluations.

Expenses (2006–07) *Tuition:* full-time $24,072; part-time $772 per credit. *Room and board:* $8540; room only: $5198 per academic year. *Required fees:* full-time $1000; part-time $137 per term.

Financial Aid 85% of baccalaureate students in nursing programs received some form of financial aid in 2005–06.

Contact Prof. Carol Jasko, Associate Director, Undergraduate Nursing, Henry P. Becton School of Nursing and Allied Health, Fairleigh Dickinson University, Metropolitan Campus, 1000 River Road, H-DH4-02, Teaneck, NJ 07666-1914. *Telephone:* 201-692-2880. *Fax:* 201-692-2388. *E-mail:* clj@fdu.edu.

GRADUATE PROGRAMS

Expenses (2006–07) *Tuition:* part-time $839 per credit. *Room and board:* $8540; room only: $5198 per academic year. *Required fees:* full-time $1000; part-time $135 per term.

Fairleigh Dickinson University, Metropolitan Campus (continued)

Contact Dr. Elizabeth S. Parietti, Associate Director of Graduate Programs, Henry P. Becton School of Nursing and Allied Health, Fairleigh Dickinson University, Metropolitan Campus, 1000 River Road, H-DH4-02, H4444, Teaneck, NJ 07666-1914. *Telephone:* 201-692-2881. *Fax:* 201-692-2388. *E-mail:* parietti@fdu.edu.

MASTER'S DEGREE PROGRAM

Degree MSN

Available Programs Accelerated RN to Master's; Master's; Master's for Nurses with Non-Nursing Degrees; RN to Master's.

Concentrations Available Nursing administration; nursing education; nursing informatics. *Clinical nurse specialist programs in:* forensic nursing. *Nurse practitioner programs in:* adult health, psychiatric/mental health.

Site Options *Distance Learning:* Sewell, NJ; Morristown, NJ; Westwood, NJ.

Study Options Full-time and part-time.

Program Entrance Requirements Computer literacy, minimum overall college GPA of 3.0, transcript of college record, CPR certification, written essay, immunizations, 2 letters of recommendation, nursing research course, physical assessment course, professional liability insurance/malpractice insurance, statistics course.

Advanced Placement Credit given for nursing courses completed elsewhere dependent upon specific evaluations.

Degree Requirements 28 total credit hours, thesis or project.

POST-MASTER'S PROGRAM

Areas of Study Nursing administration; nursing education; nursing informatics. *Clinical nurse specialist programs in:* forensic nursing. *Nurse practitioner programs in:* adult health, psychiatric/mental health.

DOCTORAL DEGREE PROGRAM

Degree DNP

Available Programs Doctorate.

Areas of Study Advanced practice nursing, nursing administration, nursing education.

Program Entrance Requirements Minimum overall college GPA of 3.0, interview by faculty committee, 3 letters of recommendation, MSN or equivalent.

Degree Requirements 40 total credit hours, residency.

CONTINUING EDUCATION PROGRAM

Contact Corinne Ellis, RN, Lecturer, Henry P. Becton School of Nursing and Allied Health, Fairleigh Dickinson University, Metropolitan Campus, 1000 River Road, H-DH4-02, Teaneck, NJ 07666-1914. *Telephone:* 201-692-2343. *Fax:* 201-692-2388. *E-mail:* cellis@fdu.edu.

See full description on page 482.

Felician College
Department of Professional Nursing–BSN
Lodi, New Jersey

http://www.felician.edu/academics/nahp/nursing.asp

Founded in 1942

DEGREES • BSN • MA/MSM • MSN

Nursing Program Faculty 17 (30% with doctorates).

Baccalaureate Enrollment 411
Women 92% **Men** 8% **Minority** 42% **Part-time** 10%

Graduate Enrollment 20
Women 99% **Men** 1% **Minority** 60% **Part-time** 99%

Nursing Student Activities Nursing Honor Society, Sigma Theta Tau, Student Nurses' Association.

Nursing Student Resources Academic advising; academic or career counseling; assistance for students with disabilities; bookstore; campus computer network; career placement assistance; computer lab; computer-assisted instruction; daycare for children of students; e-mail services; interactive nursing skills videos; Internet; learning resource lab; library services; nursing audiovisuals; remedial services; resume preparation assistance; skills, simulation, or other laboratory; tutoring.

Library Facilities 101,040 volumes (12,519 in health, 12,519 in nursing); 563 periodical subscriptions (21 health-care related).

BACCALAUREATE PROGRAMS

Degree BSN

Available Programs Accelerated RN Baccalaureate; Generic Baccalaureate; RN Baccalaureate.

Study Options Full-time and part-time.

Program Entrance Requirements Minimum overall college GPA of 3.0, transcript of college record, CPR certification, written essay, health exam, health insurance, high school biology, high school chemistry, 2 years high school math, 2 years high school science, high school transcript, immunizations, 2 letters of recommendation, minimum high school GPA of 2.75, minimum GPA in nursing prerequisites of 3.0, professional liability insurance/malpractice insurance. Transfer students are accepted. **Standardized tests** *Required:* SAT or ACT, TOEFL for international students. *Required for some:* ACT, SAT Subject Tests. **Application** *Deadline:* rolling (freshmen), rolling (transfer). *Notification:* continuous (freshmen). *Application fee:* $30.

Advanced Placement Credit given for nursing courses completed elsewhere dependent upon specific evaluations.

Expenses (2006–07) *Tuition:* full-time $18,900; part-time $625 per credit. *Room and board:* $8500 per academic year. *Required fees:* full-time $1588.

Contact Office of Undergraduate Admissions, Department of Professional Nursing–BSN, Felician College, 262 South Main Street, Lodi, NJ 07644-2117. *Telephone:* 201-559-6131. *Fax:* 201-559-6138. *E-mail:* admissions@felician.edu.

GRADUATE PROGRAMS

Expenses (2006–07) *Tuition:* part-time $675 per credit.

Financial Aid 3% of graduate students in nursing programs received some form of financial aid in 2005–06.

Contact Mr. Rajeev Pahuja, Associate Director of Adult and Graduate Admissions, Department of Professional Nursing–BSN, Felician College, 262 South Main Street, Lodi, NJ 07644-2117. *Telephone:* 201-559-6051. *Fax:* 201-559-6138. *E-mail:* pahujar@felician.edu.

MASTER'S DEGREE PROGRAM

Degrees MA/MSM; MSN

Available Programs Master's.

Concentrations Available *Nurse practitioner programs in:* adult health, family health.

Study Options Full-time and part-time.

Program Entrance Requirements Computer literacy, minimum overall college GPA of 3.0, transcript of college record, CPR certification, written essay, immunizations, 2 letters of recommendation, nursing research course, physical assessment course, professional liability insurance/malpractice insurance, prerequisite course work, statistics course.

Advanced Placement Credit given for nursing courses completed elsewhere dependent upon specific evaluations.

Degree Requirements 46 total credit hours, thesis or project.

POST-MASTER'S PROGRAM

Areas of Study *Nurse practitioner programs in:* adult health, family health.

Kean University
Department of Nursing
Union, New Jersey

http://www.kean.edu/~nursing/

Founded in 1855

DEGREES • BSN • MSN • MSN/MPA

Nursing Program Faculty 18 (88% with doctorates).

Baccalaureate Enrollment 174
Women 93% **Men** 7% **Minority** 60% **Part-time** 90%

Graduate Enrollment 103
Women 93% **Men** 7% **Minority** 62% **Part-time** 87%

Nursing Student Activities Nursing Honor Society, Sigma Theta Tau, nursing club.

Nursing Student Resources Academic advising; academic or career counseling; assistance for students with disabilities; bookstore; campus computer network; career placement assistance; computer lab; computer-assisted instruction; daycare for children of students; e-mail services; employment services for current students; housing assistance; Internet; learning resource lab; library services; nursing audiovisuals; placement services for program completers; remedial services; resume preparation assistance; skills, simulation, or other laboratory; tutoring; unpaid internships.

Library Facilities 321,261 volumes; 2,790 periodical subscriptions.

BACCALAUREATE PROGRAMS

Degree BSN

Available Programs ADN to Baccalaureate; RN Baccalaureate.

Site Options Raritan, NJ; Plainfield, NJ; Perth Amboy, NJ.

Study Options Full-time and part-time.

Program Entrance Requirements Minimum overall college GPA of 2.0, written essay, 2 letters of recommendation, prerequisite course work, RN licensure. Transfer students are accepted. **Standardized tests** *Required:* SAT or ACT. **Application** *Deadline:* 5/31 (freshmen), 8/1 (transfer). *Notification:* continuous (freshmen). *Application fee:* $50.

Advanced Placement Credit by examination available. Credit given for nursing courses completed elsewhere dependent upon specific evaluations.

Contact *Telephone:* 908-737-3385. *Fax:* 908-737-3393.

GRADUATE PROGRAMS

Contact *Telephone:* 908-737-3386. *Fax:* 908-737-3393.

MASTER'S DEGREE PROGRAM

Degrees MSN; MSN/MPA

Available Programs Accelerated Master's for Nurses with Non-Nursing Degrees; Master's; Master's for Nurses with Non-Nursing Degrees.

Concentrations Available Health-care administration; nursing administration. *Clinical nurse specialist programs in:* community health, school health.

Study Options Full-time and part-time.

Program Entrance Requirements Clinical experience, computer literacy, minimum overall college GPA of 3.0, transcript of college record, written essay, immunizations, interview, 2 letters of recommendation, nursing research course, professional liability insurance/malpractice insurance, statistics course. *Application deadline:* For fall admission, 6/1; for spring admission, 11/1. *Application fee:* $60 ($150 for international students).

Advanced Placement Credit given for nursing courses completed elsewhere dependent upon specific evaluations.

Degree Requirements 36 total credit hours, thesis or project.

CONTINUING EDUCATION PROGRAM

Contact *Telephone:* 908-737-3385. *Fax:* 908-737-3393.

Monmouth University
Marjorie K. Unterberg School of Nursing
West Long Branch, New Jersey

http://www.monmouth.edu

Founded in 1933

DEGREES • BSN • MSN

Nursing Program Faculty 15 (65% with doctorates).

Baccalaureate Enrollment 52
Women 99% **Men** 1% **Minority** 25% **Part-time** 99%

Graduate Enrollment 191
Women 98% **Men** 2% **Minority** 25% **Part-time** 97%

Nursing Student Activities Sigma Theta Tau, Student Nurses' Association.

Nursing Student Resources Academic advising; academic or career counseling; assistance for students with disabilities; bookstore; campus computer network; career placement assistance; computer lab; computer-assisted instruction; e-mail services; employment services for current students; interactive nursing skills videos; Internet; learning resource lab; library services; nursing audiovisuals; paid internships; resume preparation assistance; skills, simulation, or other laboratory; tutoring.

Library Facilities 280,000 volumes (250,000 in health); 25,196 periodical subscriptions (98 health-care related).

BACCALAUREATE PROGRAMS

Degree BSN

Available Programs ADN to Baccalaureate; RN Baccalaureate.

Site Options Freehold, NJ.

Study Options Full-time and part-time.

Program Entrance Requirements Transcript of college record, health exam, immunizations, 2 letters of recommendation, minimum GPA in nursing prerequisites of 2.0, professional liability insurance/malpractice insurance, prerequisite course work, RN licensure. Transfer students are accepted. **Standardized tests** *Required:* SAT or ACT, TOEFL for international students. **Application** *Deadline:* 3/1 (freshmen), 7/15 (transfer). *Early decision:* 12/1, 12/15. *Notification:* 4/1 (freshmen), 1/1 (out-of-state freshmen), 1/1 (early decision), 1/15 (early action). *Application fee:* $50.

Advanced Placement Credit by examination available. Credit given for nursing courses completed elsewhere dependent upon specific evaluations.

Expenses (2006–07) *Tuition:* part-time $610 per credit. *Room and board:* $8700; room only: $5000 per academic year. *Required fees:* full-time $600; part-time $310 per term.

Financial Aid 80% of baccalaureate students in nursing programs received some form of financial aid in 2005–06. *Gift aid (need-based):* Federal Pell, FSEOG, state, private, college/university gift aid from institutional funds, Federal Nursing. *Loans:* Federal Direct (Subsidized and Unsubsidized Stafford PLUS), FFEL, Perkins, state, college/university. *Work-Study:* Federal Work-Study. *Application deadline:* Continuous.

Contact Dr. Cira Fraser, Associate Professor, Marjorie K. Unterberg School of Nursing, Monmouth University, West Long Branch, NJ 07764. *Telephone:* 732-571-3443. *Fax:* 732-263-5131. *E-mail:* cfraser@monmouth.edu.

GRADUATE PROGRAMS

Expenses (2006–07) *Tuition:* part-time $673 per credit. *Room and board:* $8700; room only: $5000 per academic year. *Required fees:* full-time $600; part-time $300 per term.

Financial Aid 80% of graduate students in nursing programs received some form of financial aid in 2005–06.

Contact Dr. Janet Mahoney, Director of MSN Program/Associate Dean, Marjorie K. Unterberg School of Nursing, Monmouth University, West Long Branch, NJ 07764. *Telephone:* 732-571-3443. *Fax:* 732-263-5131. *E-mail:* jmahoney@monmouth.edu.

MASTER'S DEGREE PROGRAM

Degree MSN

Available Programs Master's; Master's for Nurses with Non-Nursing Degrees.

Concentrations Available Nursing administration; nursing education. *Nurse practitioner programs in:* adult health, family health, psychiatric/mental health, school health.

Study Options Full-time and part-time.

Program Entrance Requirements Minimum overall college GPA of 2.75, transcript of college record, immunizations, 2 letters of recommendation, physical assessment course, professional liability insurance/malpractice insurance.

Advanced Placement Credit given for nursing courses completed elsewhere dependent upon specific evaluations.

Degree Requirements 40 total credit hours.

Monmouth University (continued)
POST-MASTER'S PROGRAM
Areas of Study Nursing administration; nursing education. *Nurse practitioner programs in:* adult health, family health, psychiatric/mental health, school health.

CONTINUING EDUCATION PROGRAM
Contact Ms. Barbara Paskewich, RN, Special Projects Coordinator, Marjorie K. Unterberg School of Nursing, Monmouth University, 400 Cedar Avenue, West Long Branch, NJ 07764. *Telephone:* 732-571-3694. *Fax:* 732-263-5131. *E-mail:* bpaskewi@monmouth.edu.

New Jersey City University
Department of Nursing
Jersey City, New Jersey

http://www.njcu.edu/dept/ProfStudies/nursing2/rnbsn.htm

Founded in 1927
DEGREES • BSN • MS
Nursing Program Faculty 4 (75% with doctorates).
Baccalaureate Enrollment 110
Women 90% **Men** 10% **Minority** 75% **Part-time** 90%
Graduate Enrollment 36
Women 95% **Men** 5% **Minority** 15% **Part-time** 100%
Nursing Student Activities Nursing Honor Society, Sigma Theta Tau, Student Nurses' Association.
Nursing Student Resources Academic advising; academic or career counseling; bookstore; campus computer network; computer lab; computer-assisted instruction; daycare for children of students; e-mail services; interactive nursing skills videos; Internet; learning resource lab; library services; nursing audiovisuals.
Library Facilities 212,786 volumes; 1,260 periodical subscriptions.

BACCALAUREATE PROGRAMS
Degree BSN
Available Programs RN Baccalaureate.
Site Options Montclair, NJ; East Orange, NJ; Newark, NJ.
Program Entrance Requirements Transfer students are accepted. **Standardized tests** *Required:* SAT, SAT or ACT, TOEFL for international students. **Application** *Deadline:* 4/1 (freshmen), rolling (transfer). *Notification:* continuous (freshmen). *Application fee:* $35.
Contact *Telephone:* 201-200-3157. *Fax:* 201-200-3222.

GRADUATE PROGRAMS
Contact *Telephone:* 201-200-3157. *Fax:* 201-200-3222.

MASTER'S DEGREE PROGRAM
Degree MS
Study Options Part-time.
Program Entrance Requirements Minimum overall college GPA of 3.3, transcript of college record, interview, 2 letters of recommendation.
Degree Requirements 36 total credit hours, thesis or project.

The Richard Stockton College of New Jersey
Program in Nursing
Pomona, New Jersey

http://talon.stockton.edu/eyos/page.cfm?siteID=14&pageID=48

Founded in 1969

DEGREES • BSN • MSN
Nursing Program Faculty 6 (66% with doctorates).
Baccalaureate Enrollment 69
Women 98% **Men** 2% **Minority** 10% **Part-time** 80%
Graduate Enrollment 20
Women 90% **Men** 10% **Minority** 15% **Part-time** 95%
Nursing Student Activities Sigma Theta Tau.
Nursing Student Resources Academic advising; academic or career counseling; assistance for students with disabilities; bookstore; campus computer network; computer lab; computer-assisted instruction; daycare for children of students; e-mail services; housing assistance; Internet; learning resource lab; library services; nursing audiovisuals; resume preparation assistance; skills, simulation, or other laboratory; tutoring.
Library Facilities 258,822 volumes (9,761 in health, 1,258 in nursing); 16,826 periodical subscriptions (83 health-care related).

BACCALAUREATE PROGRAMS
Degree BSN
Available Programs RN Baccalaureate.
Site Options *Distance Learning:* Vineland, NJ.
Study Options Full-time and part-time.
Program Entrance Requirements Transfer students are accepted. **Standardized tests** *Required:* SAT or ACT, TOEFL for international students. **Application** *Deadline:* 5/1 (freshmen), 6/1 (transfer). *Notification:* continuous until 5/15 (freshmen). *Application fee:* $50.
Advanced Placement Credit given for nursing courses completed elsewhere dependent upon specific evaluations.
Contact *Telephone:* 609-652-4837.

GRADUATE PROGRAMS
Contact *Telephone:* 609-652-4501.

MASTER'S DEGREE PROGRAM
Degree MSN
Concentrations Available *Nurse practitioner programs in:* adult health.
Study Options Full-time and part-time.
Program Entrance Requirements Clinical experience, computer literacy, minimum overall college GPA of 3.0, transcript of college record, CPR certification, written essay, immunizations, 2 letters of recommendation, nursing research course, physical assessment course, professional liability insurance/malpractice insurance, statistics course, GRE General Test. *Application deadline:* For fall admission, 6/1. Applications are processed on a rolling basis. *Application fee:* $35.
Advanced Placement Credit given for nursing courses completed elsewhere dependent upon specific evaluations.
Degree Requirements 42 total credit hours, thesis or project.

Rutgers, The State University of New Jersey, Camden College of Arts and Sciences
Department of Nursing
Camden, New Jersey

Founded in 1927
DEGREES • BS • DNP • MS
Nursing Program Faculty 10 (50% with doctorates).
Baccalaureate Enrollment 95
Women 90% **Men** 10% **Minority** 25%
Nursing Student Activities Sigma Theta Tau, Student Nurses' Association.
Nursing Student Resources Academic advising; academic or career counseling; bookstore; campus computer network; career placement assistance; computer lab; computer-assisted instruction; e-mail services; employment services for current students; externships; housing assistance;

interactive nursing skills videos; Internet; learning resource lab; library services; nursing audiovisuals; placement services for program completers; remedial services; resume preparation assistance; skills, simulation, or other laboratory; tutoring.

Library Facilities 6.4 million volumes; 28,934 periodical subscriptions.

BACCALAUREATE PROGRAMS

Degree BS

Available Programs Accelerated RN Baccalaureate; Baccalaureate for Second Degree; Generic Baccalaureate.

Study Options Full-time.

Program Entrance Requirements CPR certification, health exam, immunizations, professional liability insurance/malpractice insurance, prerequisite course work. Transfer students are accepted. **Standardized tests** *Required:* SAT or ACT, TOEFL for international students. *Required for some:* SAT Subject Tests. **Application** *Deadline:* 12/15 (freshmen), 3/1 (transfer). *Notification:* continuous until 2/27 (freshmen). *Application fee:* $50.

Financial Aid 75% of baccalaureate students in nursing programs received some form of financial aid in 2005–06.

Contact Dr. Kathleen C. Ashton, RN, Clinical Associate Professor and Acting Chair, Department of Nursing, Rutgers, The State University of New Jersey, Camden College of Arts and Sciences, 311 North Fifth Street, Camden, NJ 08102. *Telephone:* 856-225-6226. *Fax:* 856-225-6250. *E-mail:* romeo@camden.rutgers.edu.

GRADUATE PROGRAMS

Contact Dr. Wendy Nehring, RN, Associate Dean for Academic Affairs, Department of Nursing, Rutgers, The State University of New Jersey, Camden College of Arts and Sciences, 180 University Avenue, Newark, NJ 07102-1803. *Telephone:* 973-353-5293 Ext. 606. *Fax:* 973-353-1277. *E-mail:* nehring@nightingale.rutgers.edu.

MASTER'S DEGREE PROGRAM

Degree MS

Available Programs Master's.

DOCTORAL DEGREE PROGRAM

Available Programs Doctorate.

Degree Requirements 36 total credit hours, dissertation.

Rutgers, The State University of New Jersey, College of Nursing

Rutgers, The State University of New Jersey, College of Nursing
Newark, New Jersey

http://www.rutgers.edu/
Founded in 1956

DEGREES • BS • MS • MS/MPH • PHD

Nursing Program Faculty 35 (80% with doctorates).

Baccalaureate Enrollment 540
Women 90% **Men** 10% **Minority** 52% **International** 1% **Part-time** 20%

Graduate Enrollment 265
Women 98% **Men** 2% **Minority** 20% **Part-time** 90%

Nursing Student Activities Sigma Theta Tau, Student Nurses' Association, nursing club.

Nursing Student Resources Academic advising; academic or career counseling; assistance for students with disabilities; bookstore; campus computer network; career placement assistance; computer lab; computer-assisted instruction; e-mail services; employment services for current students; externships; housing assistance; interactive nursing skills videos; Internet; learning resource lab; library services; nursing audiovisuals; paid internships; resume preparation assistance; skills, simulation, or other laboratory; tutoring; unpaid internships.

Library Facilities 6.4 million volumes; 28,934 periodical subscriptions.

BACCALAUREATE PROGRAMS

Degree BS

Available Programs Accelerated Baccalaureate for Second Degree; Baccalaureate for Second Degree; Generic Baccalaureate; RN Baccalaureate.

Site Options New Brunswick, NJ. *Distance Learning:* Freehold, NJ.

Study Options Full-time and part-time.

Program Entrance Requirements Minimum overall college GPA of 3.0, transcript of college record, health exam, high school biology, high school chemistry, 3 years high school math, 2 years high school science, high school transcript, immunizations, minimum high school GPA of 3.0, minimum high school rank 20%. Transfer students are accepted. **Standardized tests** *Required:* SAT or ACT, TOEFL for international students. *Required for some:* SAT Subject Tests. **Application** *Deadline:* 12/15 (freshmen), 3/1 (transfer). *Notification:* continuous until 2/27 (freshmen). *Application fee:* $50.

Advanced Placement Credit by examination available. Credit given for nursing courses completed elsewhere dependent upon specific evaluations.

Expenses (2006–07) *Tuition, state resident:* full-time $7923. *Tuition, nonresident:* full-time $16,428. *Room and board:* $9042 per academic year. *Required fees:* full-time $2035.

Financial Aid 80% of baccalaureate students in nursing programs received some form of financial aid in 2005–06.

Contact Ms. Christina Godino, Senior Admissions Officer, Rutgers, The State University of New Jersey, College of Nursing, 249 University Avenue, Newark, NJ 07102-1803. *Telephone:* 973-353-5205. *E-mail:* godino@ugadm.rutgers.edu.

GRADUATE PROGRAMS

Expenses (2006–07) *Tuition, area resident:* full-time $12,723. *Tuition, state resident:* part-time $530 per credit hour. *Tuition, nonresident:* full-time $18,652; part-time $778 per credit hour. *International tuition:* $18,652 full-time. *Required fees:* part-time $216 per term.

Financial Aid 15% of graduate students in nursing programs received some form of financial aid in 2005–06.

Contact Dr. Wendy Nehring, RN, Associate Dean for Academic Affairs, Rutgers, The State University of New Jersey, College of Nursing, 180 University Avenue, Newark, NJ 07102-1803. *Telephone:* 973-353-5293. *Fax:* 973-353-1277. *E-mail:* nehring@rutgers.edu.

MASTER'S DEGREE PROGRAM

Degrees MS; MS/MPH

Available Programs Master's.

Concentrations Available *Clinical nurse specialist programs in:* community health, psychiatric/mental health. *Nurse practitioner programs in:* acute care, adult health, family health, pediatric, women's health.

Site Options *Distance Learning:* Camden, NJ; Freehold, NJ.

Study Options Full-time and part-time.

Program Entrance Requirements Computer literacy, minimum overall college GPA of 3.0, transcript of college record, written essay, immunizations, 3 letters of recommendation, physical assessment course, professional liability insurance/malpractice insurance, resume, statistics course.

Advanced Placement Credit given for nursing courses completed elsewhere dependent upon specific evaluations.

Degree Requirements 42 total credit hours.

POST-MASTER'S PROGRAM

Areas of Study Nursing administration; nursing education; nursing informatics. *Clinical nurse specialist programs in:* community health, psychiatric/mental health. *Nurse practitioner programs in:* acute care, family health, pediatric, women's health.

DOCTORAL DEGREE PROGRAM

Degree PhD

Available Programs Doctorate.

Areas of Study Nursing research.

Program Entrance Requirements Minimum overall college GPA of 3.2, interview by faculty committee, 3 letters of recommendation, MSN or equivalent, scholarly papers, statistics course, vita, writing sample.

Rutgers, The State University of New Jersey, College of Nursing (continued)

Degree Requirements 59 total credit hours, dissertation, oral exam, written exam, residency.

CONTINUING EDUCATION PROGRAM

Contact Dr. Gayle Pearson, Assistant Dean, Center for Professional Development, Rutgers, The State University of New Jersey, College of Nursing, 175 University Avenue, Newark, NJ 07102. *Telephone:* 973-353-5895. *Fax:* 973-353-1700. *E-mail:* gaylep@rutgers.edu.

Saint Peter's College
Nursing Program
Jersey City, New Jersey

Founded in 1872

DEGREES • BSN • MSN

Nursing Program Faculty 15 (73% with doctorates).

Baccalaureate Enrollment 129
Women 98% **Men** 2% **Minority** 40%

Graduate Enrollment 55
Women 99% **Men** 1% **Minority** 45%

Nursing Student Activities Nursing Honor Society, Sigma Theta Tau, Student Nurses' Association.

Nursing Student Resources Academic advising; academic or career counseling; assistance for students with disabilities; bookstore; campus computer network; career placement assistance; computer lab; computer-assisted instruction; e-mail services; interactive nursing skills videos; Internet; learning resource lab; library services; nursing audiovisuals; remedial services; resume preparation assistance; skills, simulation, or other laboratory; tutoring.

Library Facilities 178,587 volumes (7,200 in health); 1,741 periodical subscriptions (1,586 health-care related).

BACCALAUREATE PROGRAMS

Degree BSN

Available Programs ADN to Baccalaureate; Generic Baccalaureate; RN Baccalaureate.

Site Options Englewood Cliffs, NJ.

Study Options Full-time.

Program Entrance Requirements Minimum overall college GPA, transcript of college record, written essay, high school biology, high school chemistry, high school foreign language, high school math, high school science, high school transcript, immunizations, minimum high school GPA. Transfer students are accepted. **Standardized tests** *Required:* SAT or ACT, TOEFL for international students. **Application** *Deadline:* rolling (freshmen), 8/1 (transfer). *Notification:* continuous (freshmen). *Application fee:* $40.

Financial Aid 70% of baccalaureate students in nursing programs received some form of financial aid in 2005–06.

Contact Ms. MaryAnn Mattson, Admissions Counselor, Nursing Program, Saint Peter's College, 2641 Kennedy Boulevard, Jersey City, NJ 07306. *Telephone:* 888-772-9933. *Fax:* 201-432-5860. *E-mail:* mmattson@spc.edu.

GRADUATE PROGRAMS

Financial Aid 25% of graduate students in nursing programs received some form of financial aid in 2005–06. 2 research assistantships with partial tuition reimbursements available were awarded.

Contact Dr. Ann Tritak, Associate Dean of Nursing, Nursing Program, Saint Peter's College, Hudson Terrace, Englewood Cliffs, NJ 07632. *Telephone:* 201-568-5208. *Fax:* 201-569-1254. *E-mail:* atritak@spc.edu.

MASTER'S DEGREE PROGRAM

Degree MSN

Available Programs Master's; Master's for Nurses with Non-Nursing Degrees.

Concentrations Available Nurse case management; nursing administration. *Nurse practitioner programs in:* adult health.

Site Options Englewood Cliffs, NJ.

Study Options Part-time.

Program Entrance Requirements Clinical experience, minimum overall college GPA of 3.0, transcript of college record, written essay, immunizations, 3 letters of recommendation, nursing research course, physical assessment course, professional liability insurance/malpractice insurance, statistics course, GRE or MAT. *Application deadline:* For fall admission, 8/1 (priority date). Applications are processed on a rolling basis. *Application fee:* $20.

Degree Requirements 39 total credit hours.

POST-MASTER'S PROGRAM

Areas of Study *Nurse practitioner programs in:* adult health.

Seton Hall University
College of Nursing
South Orange, New Jersey

http://nursing.shu.edu/

Founded in 1856

DEGREES • BSN • MSN • MSN/MA • MSN/MBA • PHD

Nursing Program Faculty 48 (65% with doctorates).

Baccalaureate Enrollment 500

Graduate Enrollment 210

Nursing Student Activities Sigma Theta Tau, Student Nurses' Association.

Nursing Student Resources Academic advising; academic or career counseling; assistance for students with disabilities; bookstore; campus computer network; computer lab; computer-assisted instruction; e-mail services; housing assistance; interactive nursing skills videos; Internet; learning resource lab; library services; nursing audiovisuals; paid internships; remedial services; resume preparation assistance; skills, simulation, or other laboratory; tutoring.

Library Facilities 506,042 volumes; 1,475 periodical subscriptions.

BACCALAUREATE PROGRAMS

Degree BSN

Available Programs Accelerated Baccalaureate for Second Degree; Baccalaureate for Second Degree; Generic Baccalaureate; RN Baccalaureate.

Site Options *Distance Learning:* Lakewood, NJ; Camden, NJ; Brick/Toms River, NJ.

Study Options Full-time and part-time.

Program Entrance Requirements Minimum overall college GPA of 2.5, transcript of college record, written essay, high school biology, high school chemistry, high school foreign language, 3 years high school math, 2 years high school science, high school transcript, minimum high school GPA of 2.5, minimum high school rank 50%. Transfer students are accepted. **Standardized tests** *Required:* SAT or ACT, TOEFL for international students. **Application** *Deadline:* 3/1 (freshmen), 6/1 (transfer). *Notification:* continuous until 12/1 (freshmen). *Application fee:* $55.

Expenses (2006–07) *Tuition:* full-time $22,770; part-time $759 per credit. *Required fees:* full-time $2050; part-time $385 per term.

Financial Aid 75% of baccalaureate students in nursing programs received some form of financial aid in 2005–06.

Contact Mary Jo Bugel, RN, Director of Recruitment, College of Nursing, Seton Hall University, South Orange, NJ 07079-2697. *Telephone:* 973-761-9285. *Fax:* 973-761-9607. *E-mail:* bugelmar@shu.edu.

GRADUATE PROGRAMS

Expenses (2006–07) *Tuition:* part-time $787 per credit. *Required fees:* part-time $185 per term.

Financial Aid 68% of graduate students in nursing programs received some form of financial aid in 2005–06. Institutionally sponsored loans, traineeships, tuition waivers (partial), and unspecified assistantships available. Aid available to part-time students. *Financial aid application deadline:* 7/15.

Contact Mary Jo Bugel, RN, Director of Recruitment, College of Nursing, Seton Hall University, South Orange, NJ 07079-2697. *Telephone:* 973-761-9285. *Fax:* 973-761-9607. *E-mail:* bugelmar@shu.edu.

MASTER'S DEGREE PROGRAM

Degrees MSN; MSN/MA; MSN/MBA

Available Programs Master's; Master's for Non-Nursing College Graduates; Master's for Nurses with Non-Nursing Degrees; RN to Master's.

Concentrations Available Health-care administration; nurse case management; nursing administration; nursing education. *Clinical nurse specialist programs in:* school health. *Nurse practitioner programs in:* acute care, adult health, gerontology, pediatric, primary care, women's health.

Study Options Full-time and part-time.

Program Entrance Requirements Minimum overall college GPA of 3.0, transcript of college record, CPR certification, written essay, 2 letters of recommendation, nursing research course, physical assessment course, professional liability insurance/malpractice insurance, resume, statistics course, GRE or MAT. *Application deadline:* For fall admission, 6/15 (priority date). Applications are processed on a rolling basis. *Application fee:* $50.

Degree Requirements 43 total credit hours, thesis or project.

POST-MASTER'S PROGRAM

Areas of Study Health-care administration; nurse case management; nursing administration; nursing education. *Nurse practitioner programs in:* acute care, adult health, gerontology, pediatric, primary care, women's health.

DOCTORAL DEGREE PROGRAM

Degree PhD

Available Programs Doctorate.

Areas of Study Nursing research.

Program Entrance Requirements Clinical experience, minimum overall college GPA of 3.0, 2 letters of recommendation, MSN or equivalent, statistics course, vita, writing sample, GRE. *Application deadline:* For fall admission, 6/15 (priority date). Applications are processed on a rolling basis. *Application fee:* $50.

Degree Requirements 46 total credit hours, dissertation.

CONTINUING EDUCATION PROGRAM

Contact Mary Jo Bugel, Director of Recruitment, College of Nursing, Seton Hall University, South Orange, NJ 07079-2697. *Telephone:* 973-761-9285. *Fax:* 973-761-9607. *E-mail:* bugelmar@shu.edu.

See full description on page 530.

Thomas Edison State College
School of Nursing
Trenton, New Jersey

http://www.tesc.edu/nursing

Nursing program started in 1983

DEGREES • RN to BSN, RN to BSN/MSN, BSN to MSN

Nursing Student Resources Students in the School of Nursing have the opportunity to earn degrees through traditional and nontraditional methods, which take into consideration the individual needs and interests of each student. All nursing courses are designed and delivered as mentored, independent study courses via the Internet using MyEdison, the College's online course management system that utilizes the Blackboard platform. Students in these courses communicate with mentors and fellow students using e-mail and submit assignments to mentors through the Internet. Students may earn credit toward a degree by demonstrating college-level knowledge through testing and assessment of prior learning; by transfer credit for courses taken through other regionally accredited institutions; through the College's *e-Pack*® courses; and for licenses, certificates, and courses taken at work or through military training, if approved and recommended for academic credit.

School of Nursing Faculty The School utilizes off-site nurse educators from a variety of nursing education and service settings to develop, implement, and evaluate the program. All nurse educators have a minimum of a master's degree in nursing, with approximately 85 percent prepared

at the doctoral level and many tenured at their home institution. With its courses offered by distance learning, the School has the opportunity to draw nurse educators from throughout the United States, resulting in a very diverse and experienced group of online nurse educators. The BSN program is accredited by the New Jersey Board of Nursing and the National League for Nursing Accrediting Commission (NLNAC). A letter of support to develop the RN to BSN/MSN degree program is on file from NLNAC; accreditation will be sought in accordance with accreditation guidelines.

BACCALAUREATE AND MASTER'S DEGREE PROGRAMS

Degrees RN to BSN, RN to BSN/MSN, BSN to MSN

Study Options Self-paced programs; nursing courses offered quarterly online; multiple options for credit earning; no time limit for degree completion; no residency requirement with maximum flexibility in transfer credit.

Program Entrance Requirements Admission is open and rolling; RNs can enroll any day of the year. In addition to the submission of a notarized copy of their current RN license, valid in the U.S., all applicants must submit a completed School of Nursing application with a $75 fee and have transcripts of completed course work sent to the Office of the Registrar. Applicants to the RN to BSN and RN to BSN/MSN degree programs must also submit a BSN Credential Review fee of $300. All RNs will have 20 credits applied from previous nursing course work toward the 48-credit nursing requirement in the BSN degree. A total of 80 credits may be accepted from a community college, and up to 60 credits, including the 20 credits used in the nursing requirement, will be awarded to diploma graduates based on current licensure. There is no age restriction on credits transferred in to meet general education requirements or lower-division nursing requirements. All upper-division nursing credits must be from an accredited baccalaureate or higher degree nursing program and newer than 10 years if completed prior to application to the School of Nursing. All credits used in the nursing requirement must have a grade equivalent of "C" or better. All previously completed credits transferred in to meet MSN degree requirements must be newer than 10 years at the time of application to the School, have a grade equivalent of "B" or better, and be from an accredited graduate nursing degree program.

Expenses (2006–07) $286 per credit for New Jersey residents; $335 per credit for out-of-state residents for the BSN degree program; $433 for the MSN program.

Financial Aid Two percent of the RNs in the baccalaureate nursing program received some form of financial aid in 2005–06.

Contact Thomas Edison State College, 101 West State Street, Trenton, NJ 08608-1176. *Telephone:* (888) 442-8372. *E-mail:* nursinginfo@tesc.edu.

See full description on page 532.

University of Medicine and Dentistry of New Jersey
School of Nursing
Newark, New Jersey

http://sn.umdnj.edu/

Founded in 1970

DEGREES • BSN • DNP • MSN

Nursing Program Faculty 72.

Baccalaureate Enrollment 540
Women 81% **Men** 19% **Minority** 51% **International** 4%

Graduate Enrollment 435
Women 89% **Men** 11% **Minority** 49% **Part-time** 75%

Nursing Student Activities Sigma Theta Tau, Student Nurses' Association.

Nursing Student Resources Academic advising; academic or career counseling; assistance for students with disabilities; bookstore; campus computer network; computer lab; computer-assisted instruction; daycare for children of students; e-mail services; housing assistance; interactive nursing skills videos; Internet; learning resource lab; library services; nursing audiovisuals; skills, simulation, or other laboratory; tutoring.

University of Medicine and Dentistry of New Jersey (continued)
Library Facilities 91,446 volumes in health, 3,273 volumes in nursing; 5,567 periodical subscriptions health-care related.

BACCALAUREATE PROGRAMS

Degree BSN

Available Programs Accelerated Baccalaureate for Second Degree; Generic Baccalaureate; RN Baccalaureate.
Site Options Glassboro, NJ. *Distance Learning:* Mahwah, NJ; Stratford, NJ.
Study Options Full-time and part-time.
Program Entrance Requirements Minimum overall college GPA of 3.0, transcript of college record, CPR certification, written essay, health exam, health insurance, high school transcript, immunizations, 3 letters of recommendation, minimum high school rank 40%, prerequisite course work, RN licensure. Transfer students are accepted.
Advanced Placement Credit given for nursing courses completed elsewhere dependent upon specific evaluations.
Financial Aid 99% of baccalaureate students in nursing programs received some form of financial aid in 2005–06.
Contact Mr. Victor Marques, Marketing Representative/Recruiter, School of Nursing, University of Medicine and Dentistry of New Jersey, 65 Bergen Street, Newark, NJ 07101. *Telephone:* 973-972-7445. *Fax:* 973-972-7453. *E-mail:* marquevm@umdnj.edu.

GRADUATE PROGRAMS

Expenses (2006–07) *Tuition, state resident:* part-time $410 per course. *Tuition, nonresident:* part-time $582 per course.
Financial Aid 50% of graduate students in nursing programs received some form of financial aid in 2005–06. Teaching assistantships, institutionally sponsored loans and scholarships available. Aid available to part-time students. *Financial aid application deadline:* 5/1.
Contact Mr. Victor Marques, Marketing Representative/Recruiter, School of Nursing, University of Medicine and Dentistry of New Jersey, 65 Bergen Street, Newark, NJ 07101. *Telephone:* 973-972-7445. *Fax:* 973-972-7453. *E-mail:* marquevm@umdnj.edu.

MASTER'S DEGREE PROGRAM

Degree MSN

Available Programs Master's; RN to Master's.
Concentrations Available Nurse anesthesia; nurse-midwifery; nursing education; nursing informatics. *Clinical nurse specialist programs in:* psychiatric/mental health. *Nurse practitioner programs in:* acute care, adult health, family health, gerontology, oncology, psychiatric/mental health, women's health.
Site Options *Distance Learning:* Mahwah, NJ; Stratford, NJ.
Study Options Full-time and part-time.
Program Entrance Requirements Clinical experience, minimum overall college GPA of 3.0, transcript of college record, CPR certification, immunizations, 3 letters of recommendation, physical assessment course, prerequisite course work, statistics course, GRE. *Application deadline:* For fall admission, 4/1; for spring admission, 10/1. Applications are processed on a rolling basis. *Application fee:* $50.
Advanced Placement Credit given for nursing courses completed elsewhere dependent upon specific evaluations.
Degree Requirements 40 total credit hours.

POST-MASTER'S PROGRAM

Areas of Study Nurse anesthesia; nursing education; nursing informatics. *Clinical nurse specialist programs in:* psychiatric/mental health. *Nurse practitioner programs in:* acute care, adult health, family health, gerontology, oncology, psychiatric/mental health, women's health.

DOCTORAL DEGREE PROGRAM

Available Programs Doctorate.
Program Entrance Requirements Clinical experience, minimum overall college GPA of 3.0, interview by faculty committee, 3 letters of recommendation, MSN or equivalent, statistics course, vita. *Application deadline:* For fall admission, 4/1; for spring admission, 10/1. Applications are processed on a rolling basis. *Application fee:* $50.
Degree Requirements 32 total credit hours, residency.

CONTINUING EDUCATION PROGRAM

Contact Dr. Mary Kamienski, Director of Continuing Education, School of Nursing, University of Medicine and Dentistry of New Jersey, 65 Bergen Street, Room 1132-B, Newark, NJ 07101-1709. *Telephone:* 973-972-7451. *Fax:* 973-972-3225. *E-mail:* kamienma@umdnj.edu.

William Paterson University of New Jersey
Department of Nursing
Wayne, New Jersey

http://www.wpunj.edu/cos/nursing/
Founded in 1855

DEGREES • BSN • MSN

Nursing Program Faculty 38 (40% with doctorates).
Baccalaureate Enrollment 450
Women 90% **Men** 10% **Minority** 51% **International** 5% **Part-time** 25%
Graduate Enrollment 40
Women 98% **Men** 2% **Minority** 30% **Part-time** 92%
Nursing Student Activities Sigma Theta Tau, Student Nurses' Association.
Nursing Student Resources Academic advising; academic or career counseling; assistance for students with disabilities; bookstore; campus computer network; career placement assistance; computer lab; computer-assisted instruction; daycare for children of students; e-mail services; employment services for current students; housing assistance; interactive nursing skills videos; Internet; learning resource lab; library services; nursing audiovisuals; placement services for program completers; remedial services; resume preparation assistance; skills, simulation, or other laboratory; tutoring.
Library Facilities 305,155 volumes (15,000 in health, 12,700 in nursing); 4,112 periodical subscriptions (120 health-care related).

BACCALAUREATE PROGRAMS

Degree BSN

Available Programs ADN to Baccalaureate; Accelerated Baccalaureate for Second Degree; Generic Baccalaureate; LPN to Baccalaureate; RN Baccalaureate.
Study Options Full-time and part-time.
Program Entrance Requirements Minimum overall college GPA of 2.5, transcript of college record, CPR certification, health exam, health insurance, high school biology, high school chemistry, 1 year of high school math, 2 years high school science, high school transcript, immunizations, minimum GPA in nursing prerequisites of 3.0. Transfer students are accepted. **Standardized tests** *Required:* SAT or ACT, TOEFL for international students. **Application** *Deadline:* 5/1 (freshmen), 5/1 (transfer). *Notification:* continuous (freshmen). *Application fee:* $50.
Expenses (2006–07) *Tuition, state resident:* full-time $9422; part-time $303 per credit. *Tuition, nonresident:* full-time $15,370; part-time $497 per credit. *Room and board:* $8220; room only: $6750 per academic year. *Required fees:* full-time $200.
Financial Aid *Gift aid (need-based):* Federal Pell, FSEOG, state, college/university gift aid from institutional funds. *Loans:* FFEL (Subsidized and Unsubsidized Stafford PLUS), Perkins. *Work-Study:* Federal Work-Study, part-time campus jobs. *Application deadline:* 4/1 (priority: 4/1).
Contact Dr. Julie Bliss, Chairperson, Department of Nursing, William Paterson University of New Jersey, 300 Pompton Road, W106, Wayne, NJ 07470. *Telephone:* 973-720-2673. *Fax:* 973-720-2668. *E-mail:* blissj@wpunj.edu.

GRADUATE PROGRAMS

Expenses (2006–07) *Tuition, state resident:* part-time $514 per credit. *Tuition, nonresident:* part-time $799 per credit. *Required fees:* full-time $200.
Financial Aid 8% of graduate students in nursing programs received some form of financial aid in 2005–06. Research assistantships with tuition reimbursements available, unspecified assistantships available. *Financial aid application deadline:* 4/1.

Contact Dr. Kem Louie, Director, Graduate Program, Department of Nursing, William Paterson University of New Jersey, 300 Pompton Road, W240, Wayne, NJ 07470. *Telephone:* 973-720-3511. *Fax:* 973-720-3517. *E-mail:* louiek@wpunj.edu.

MASTER'S DEGREE PROGRAM

Degree MSN

Available Programs Master's; Master's for Nurses with Non-Nursing Degrees.

Concentrations Available Nursing administration; nursing education. *Clinical nurse specialist programs in:* community health. *Nurse practitioner programs in:* adult health.

Study Options Full-time and part-time.

Program Entrance Requirements Computer literacy, minimum overall college GPA of 3.0, transcript of college record, CPR certification, written essay, 3 letters of recommendation, nursing research course, physical assessment course, professional liability insurance/malpractice insurance, resume, statistics course, GRE General Test. *Application deadline:* Applications are processed on a rolling basis. *Application fee:* $50.

Advanced Placement Credit given for nursing courses completed elsewhere dependent upon specific evaluations.

Degree Requirements 36 total credit hours, thesis or project.

POST-MASTER'S PROGRAM

Areas of Study *Clinical nurse specialist programs in:* school health. *Nurse practitioner programs in:* adult health.

NEW MEXICO

Eastern New Mexico University
Department of Allied Health–Nursing
Portales, New Mexico

http://www.enmu.edu/academics/undergrad/ colleges/las/disorders-nursing

Founded in 1934

DEGREE • BSN

Nursing Program Faculty 6.

Nursing Student Resources Academic advising; academic or career counseling; assistance for students with disabilities; bookstore; campus computer network; computer lab; computer-assisted instruction; daycare for children of students; e-mail services; housing assistance; interactive nursing skills videos; Internet; learning resource lab; library services; nursing audiovisuals; other; resume preparation assistance; skills, simulation, or other laboratory; tutoring.

Library Facilities 305,108 volumes (100 in health, 50 in nursing); 7,621 periodical subscriptions (15 health-care related).

BACCALAUREATE PROGRAMS

Degree BSN

Available Programs RN Baccalaureate.

Site Options *Distance Learning:* Hobbs, NM.

Study Options Full-time and part-time.

Program Entrance Requirements Minimum overall college GPA of 2.0, transcript of college record, CPR certification, written essay, high school biology, high school chemistry, 2 years high school math, 2 years high school science, high school transcript, immunizations, interview, 3 letters of recommendation, minimum high school GPA of 2.5, minimum GPA in nursing prerequisites of 2.0, professional liability insurance/malpractice insurance, prerequisite course work, RN licensure. Transfer students are accepted. **Standardized tests** *Required:* SAT or ACT, TOEFL for international students. **Application** *Deadline:* rolling (freshmen), rolling (transfer).

Advanced Placement Credit given for nursing courses completed elsewhere dependent upon specific evaluations.

Expenses (2006–07) *Tuition, area resident:* full-time $1482; part-time $124 per credit hour. *Tuition, nonresident:* full-time $4260; part-time $355 per credit hour. *Room and board:* $2078 per academic year.

Financial Aid 2% of baccalaureate students in nursing programs received some form of financial aid in 2005–06.

Contact Ms. Irma Lorraine Goodrich, RN, Interim Program Director, Department of Allied Health–Nursing, Eastern New Mexico University, 1500 South Avenue K, Station 12, Portales, NM 88130. *Telephone:* 505-562-2403. *Fax:* 505-562-2293. *E-mail:* lorraine.goodrich@enmu.edu.

New Mexico State University
Department of Nursing
Las Cruces, New Mexico

http://www.nmsu.edu/~nursing

Founded in 1888

DEGREES • BSN • MSN

Nursing Program Faculty 36 (37% with doctorates).

Baccalaureate Enrollment 292
Women 84% **Men** 16% **Minority** 49% **International** 1% **Part-time** 15%

Graduate Enrollment 42
Women 88% **Men** 12% **Minority** 24% **International** 1% **Part-time** 69%

Nursing Student Activities Sigma Theta Tau, Student Nurses' Association.

Nursing Student Resources Academic advising; academic or career counseling; assistance for students with disabilities; bookstore; campus computer network; computer lab; computer-assisted instruction; daycare for children of students; e-mail services; housing assistance; interactive nursing skills videos; Internet; learning resource lab; library services; nursing audiovisuals; paid internships; remedial services; skills, simulation, or other laboratory; tutoring.

Library Facilities 1.7 million volumes (33,000 in health, 17,500 in nursing); 2,890 periodical subscriptions (620 health-care related).

BACCALAUREATE PROGRAMS

Degree BSN

Available Programs Accelerated Baccalaureate for Second Degree; Generic Baccalaureate; RN Baccalaureate.

Site Options *Distance Learning:* Carlsbad, NM; Alamagordo, NM.

Study Options Full-time.

Program Entrance Requirements Minimum overall college GPA of 3.0, transcript of college record, CPR certification, immunizations, minimum GPA in nursing prerequisites of 2.0, prerequisite course work. Transfer students are accepted. **Standardized tests** *Required:* SAT or ACT, TOEFL for international students. **Application** *Deadline:* 8/19 (freshmen), 8/14 (transfer). *Notification:* continuous (freshmen). *Application fee:* $15.

Advanced Placement Credit given for nursing courses completed elsewhere dependent upon specific evaluations.

Financial Aid 82% of baccalaureate students in nursing programs received some form of financial aid in 2005–06. *Gift aid (need-based):* Federal Pell, FSEOG, state, private, college/university gift aid from institutional funds. *Loans:* FFEL (Subsidized and Unsubsidized Stafford PLUS), Perkins, state. *Work-Study:* Federal Work-Study, part-time campus jobs. *Application deadline (priority):* 3/1.

Contact Lissa Kirby, Advising Coordinator, Department of Nursing, New Mexico State University, PO Box 30001, MSC 3446, Las Cruces, NM 88003-8001. *Telephone:* 505-646-3534. *Fax:* 505-646-6166. *E-mail:* lkirby@nmsu.edu.

GRADUATE PROGRAMS

Financial Aid 73% of graduate students in nursing programs received some form of financial aid in 2005–06. 2 teaching assistantships were awarded; fellowships, research assistantships, career-related internships or fieldwork, Federal Work-Study, scholarships, and traineeships also available. *Financial aid application deadline:* 3/1.

Contact Dr. Kathleen M. Huttlinger, Interim Associate Director for Graduate Studies, Department of Nursing, New Mexico State University, PO Box 30001, Department 3185, Las Cruces, NM 88003-8001. *Telephone:* 505-646-8170. *Fax:* 505-646-2167. *E-mail:* huttlin@nmsu.edu.

New Mexico State University (continued)

MASTER'S DEGREE PROGRAM

Degree MSN

Available Programs Master's.

Concentrations Available Nursing administration. *Clinical nurse specialist programs in:* community health, medical-surgical, psychiatric/mental health. *Nurse practitioner programs in:* psychiatric/mental health.

Study Options Full-time and part-time.

Program Entrance Requirements Minimum overall college GPA of 3.0, transcript of college record, CPR certification, written essay, immunizations, 3 letters of recommendation, resume, statistics course. *Application deadline:* For fall admission, 7/1 (priority date); for spring admission, 11/1 (priority date). Applications are processed on a rolling basis. *Application fee:* $30 ($50 for international students).

Advanced Placement Credit given for nursing courses completed elsewhere dependent upon specific evaluations.

Degree Requirements 50 total credit hours, comprehensive exam.

CONTINUING EDUCATION PROGRAM

Contact Dr. Mary H. Sizemore, Local Monitoring Program Chair, Department of Nursing, New Mexico State University, PO Box 30001, MSC-3185, Las Cruces, NM 88003-8001. *Telephone:* 505-646-3812. *Fax:* 505-646-2167. *E-mail:* masizemo@nmsu.edu.

University of New Mexico
College of Nursing
Albuquerque, New Mexico

http://hsc.unm.edu/consg/

Founded in 1889

DEGREES • BSN • MSN • MSN/MALAS • MSN/MPA • MSN/MPH • PHD

Nursing Program Faculty 55 (50% with doctorates).

Baccalaureate Enrollment 337
Women 91.7% **Men** 8.3% **Minority** 43% **Part-time** 21%

Graduate Enrollment 209
Women 94% **Men** 6% **Minority** 39% **Part-time** 69%

Nursing Student Activities Sigma Theta Tau, Student Nurses' Association.

Nursing Student Resources Academic advising; assistance for students with disabilities; bookstore; campus computer network; career placement assistance; computer lab; computer-assisted instruction; daycare for children of students; e-mail services; housing assistance; interactive nursing skills videos; Internet; learning resource lab; library services; nursing audiovisuals; remedial services; skills, simulation, or other laboratory.

Library Facilities 2.7 million volumes (176,055 in health, 5,081 in nursing); 592,243 periodical subscriptions (1,567 health-care related).

BACCALAUREATE PROGRAMS

Degree BSN

Available Programs Accelerated Baccalaureate for Second Degree; Generic Baccalaureate; RN Baccalaureate.

Site Options Taos, NM; Los Lunas, NM.

Study Options Full-time.

Program Entrance Requirements Minimum overall college GPA of 2.5, transcript of college record, written essay, minimum GPA in nursing prerequisites of 2.5, prerequisite course work. Transfer students are accepted. **Standardized tests** *Required:* SAT or ACT, TOEFL for international students. **Application** *Deadline:* 6/15 (freshmen), 6/15 (transfer). *Notification:* continuous (freshmen). *Application fee:* $20.

Advanced Placement Credit given for nursing courses completed elsewhere dependent upon specific evaluations.

Expenses (2006–07) *Tuition, state resident:* full-time $5400; part-time $180 per credit hour. *Tuition, nonresident:* full-time $15,176; part-time $180 per credit hour. *International tuition:* $15,176 full-time. *Room and board:* $10,500; room only: $6600 per academic year. *Required fees:* full-time $900; part-time $300 per term.

Financial Aid 70% of baccalaureate students in nursing programs received some form of financial aid in 2005–06.

Contact Ms. Ann Marie Oechsler, Director of Student Services, College of Nursing, University of New Mexico, MSCS09 5350, 1 University of New Mexico, Albuquerque, NM 87131-0001. *Telephone:* 505-272-4223. *Fax:* 505-272-3970. *E-mail:* aoechsler@salud.unm.edu.

GRADUATE PROGRAMS

Expenses (2006–07) *Tuition, state resident:* full-time $4600; part-time $200 per credit. *Tuition, nonresident:* full-time $12,000; part-time $200 per credit. *International tuition:* $12,000 full-time. *Room and board:* $10,500; room only: $6600 per academic year. *Required fees:* full-time $750; part-time $250 per term.

Financial Aid 40% of graduate students in nursing programs received some form of financial aid in 2005–06. 1 research assistantship (averaging $3,000 per year), 12 teaching assistantships with partial tuition reimbursements available (averaging $5,400 per year) were awarded; scholarships, traineeships, tuition waivers (full), and stipends also available. *Financial aid application deadline:* 3/1.

Contact Ms. Elizabeth Rowe, Senior Academic Advisor, College of Nursing, University of New Mexico, MSC09 5350, NRPH Building, Room 152, 1 University of New Mexico, Albuquerque, NM 87131-0001. *Telephone:* 505-272-4223. *Fax:* 505-272-3970. *E-mail:* erowe@salud.unm.edu.

MASTER'S DEGREE PROGRAM

Degrees MSN; MSN/MALAS; MSN/MPA; MSN/MPH

Available Programs Master's; Master's for Nurses with Non-Nursing Degrees.

Concentrations Available Nurse-midwifery; nursing administration; nursing education. *Nurse practitioner programs in:* acute care, family health, pediatric.

Study Options Full-time and part-time.

Program Entrance Requirements Clinical experience, minimum overall college GPA of 3.0, transcript of college record, 3 letters of recommendation, resume, GRE General Test. *Application deadline:* For fall admission, 3/15; for spring admission, 10/15. *Application fee:* $50.

Advanced Placement Credit by examination available. Credit given for nursing courses completed elsewhere dependent upon specific evaluations.

Degree Requirements 30 total credit hours, thesis or project, comprehensive exam.

POST-MASTER'S PROGRAM

Areas of Study Nurse-midwifery; nursing administration; nursing education. *Nurse practitioner programs in:* acute care, family health, pediatric.

DOCTORAL DEGREE PROGRAM

Degree PhD

Available Programs Doctorate.

Areas of Study Family health, nursing research, women's health.

Program Entrance Requirements Clinical experience, minimum overall college GPA of 3.0, interview by faculty committee, 3 letters of recommendation, MSN or equivalent, scholarly papers, vita. *Application deadline:* For fall admission, 3/15; for spring admission, 10/15. *Application fee:* $50.

Degree Requirements 66 total credit hours, dissertation.

University of Phoenix–New Mexico Campus
College of Health and Human Services
Albuquerque, New Mexico

DEGREES • BSN • MSN • MSN/MBA • MSN/MHA

Nursing Program Faculty 75 (23% with doctorates).

Baccalaureate Enrollment 53
Women 92.45% **Men** 7.55% **Minority** 1.89%

Graduate Enrollment 37
Women 78.38% **Men** 21.62% **Minority** 5.41%

Nursing Student Activities Sigma Theta Tau.

Nursing Student Resources Academic advising; academic or career counseling; assistance for students with disabilities; bookstore; computer lab; library services.

Library Facilities 444 volumes; 666 periodical subscriptions.

BACCALAUREATE PROGRAMS

Degree BSN

Available Programs Accelerated Baccalaureate.

Site Options Santa Fe, NM; Santa Teresa, NM.

Study Options Full-time.

Program Entrance Requirements Transcript of college record, 1 letter of recommendation, RN licensure. Transfer students are accepted. **Standardized tests** *Required:* TOEFL for international students. **Application** *Deadline:* rolling (freshmen), rolling (transfer). *Application fee:* $110.

Advanced Placement Credit by examination available. Credit given for nursing courses completed elsewhere dependent upon specific evaluations.

Expenses (2006–07) *Tuition:* full-time $9750. *International tuition:* $9750 full-time. *Required fees:* full-time $750.

Contact Campus College Chair, Nursing, College of Health and Human Services, University of Phoenix–New Mexico Campus, 7471 Pan American Freeway NE, Albuquerque, NM 87109-4645. *Telephone:* 505-821-4800.

GRADUATE PROGRAMS

Expenses (2006–07) *Tuition:* full-time $9005. *International tuition:* $9005 full-time. *Required fees:* full-time $760.

Contact Campus College Chair, Nursing, College of Health and Human Services, University of Phoenix–New Mexico Campus, 7471 Pan American Freeway NE, Albuquerque, NM 87109-4645. *Telephone:* 505-821-4800.

MASTER'S DEGREE PROGRAM

Degrees MSN; MSN/MBA; MSN/MHA

Available Programs Master's.

Concentrations Available Health-care administration; nursing administration; nursing education.

Site Options Santa Fe, NM; Santa Teresa, NM.

Study Options Full-time.

Program Entrance Requirements Clinical experience, computer literacy, minimum overall college GPA of 2.5, transcript of college record. *Application deadline:* Applications are processed on a rolling basis. *Application fee:* $110.

Advanced Placement Credit given for nursing courses completed elsewhere dependent upon specific evaluations.

Degree Requirements 39 total credit hours, thesis or project.

NEW YORK

Adelphi University
School of Nursing
Garden City, New York

Founded in 1896

DEGREES • BS • MS • MS/MBA • PHD

Nursing Program Faculty 161 (18% with doctorates).

Baccalaureate Enrollment 1,100
Women 90% **Men** 10% **Minority** 43% **International** 1.5% **Part-time** 30%

Graduate Enrollment 169
Women 97% **Men** 3% **Minority** 30% **Part-time** 100%

Nursing Student Activities Nursing Honor Society, Sigma Theta Tau, Student Nurses' Association, nursing club.

Nursing Student Resources Academic advising; academic or career counseling; assistance for students with disabilities; bookstore; campus computer network; career placement assistance; computer lab; computer-assisted instruction; e-mail services; employment services for current students; externships; housing assistance; interactive nursing skills videos; Internet; learning resource lab; library services; nursing audiovisuals; paid internships; remedial services; resume preparation assistance; skills, simulation, or other laboratory; tutoring; unpaid internships.

Library Facilities 667,293 volumes (29,918 in health, 2,666 in nursing); 28,856 periodical subscriptions (364 health-care related).

BACCALAUREATE PROGRAMS

Degree BS

Available Programs Accelerated Baccalaureate; Accelerated Baccalaureate for Second Degree; Baccalaureate for Second Degree; Generic Baccalaureate; LPN to Baccalaureate; RN Baccalaureate.

Site Options Forest Hills, NY; Glen Cove, NY.

Study Options Full-time and part-time.

Program Entrance Requirements Minimum overall college GPA of 3.0, transcript of college record, written essay, health exam, high school foreign language, 3 years high school math, 3 years high school science, high school transcript, immunizations, interview, 2 letters of recommendation, minimum high school GPA of 3.0. Transfer students are accepted. **Standardized tests** *Required:* SAT or ACT, TOEFL for international students. **Application** *Deadline:* rolling (freshmen), rolling (transfer). *Early decision:* 12/1. *Notification:* continuous (freshmen), 12/31 (early action). *Application fee:* $35.

Advanced Placement Credit by examination available.

Expenses (2006–07) *Tuition:* full-time $20,900; part-time $650 per credit hour. *Room and board:* $8020 per academic year. *Required fees:* full-time $650; part-time $275 per term.

Financial Aid 90% of baccalaureate students in nursing programs received some form of financial aid in 2005–06.

Contact Mr. Joseph Posillico, Director of Admissions, School of Nursing, Adelphi University, One South Avenue, Levermore Hall, Garden City, NY 11530. *Telephone:* 516-877-3052. *Fax:* 516-877-3052. *E-mail:* posillic@adelphi.edu.

GRADUATE PROGRAMS

Expenses (2006–07) *Tuition:* part-time $690 per credit hour. *International tuition:* $16,960 full-time. *Room and board:* $8550 per academic year. *Required fees:* full-time $400; part-time $225 per term.

Financial Aid 15% of graduate students in nursing programs received some form of financial aid in 2005–06. 1 research assistantship with full and partial tuition reimbursement available (averaging $1,180 per year) was awarded; teaching assistantships, career-related internships or fieldwork, unspecified assistantships, and graduate achievement awards also available. Aid available to part-time students. *Financial aid application deadline:* 2/15.

Contact Mr. Joseph Posillico, Director of Admissions, School of Nursing, Adelphi University, One South Avenue, Levermore Hall, Garden City, NY 11530. *Telephone:* 516-877-3052. *Fax:* 516-877-3039. *E-mail:* posillic@adelphi.edu.

MASTER'S DEGREE PROGRAM

Degrees MS; MS/MBA

Available Programs Master's; Master's for Nurses with Non-Nursing Degrees.

Concentrations Available Nursing administration; nursing education. *Nurse practitioner programs in:* adult health.

Site Options Glen Cove, NY; West Islip, NY.

Study Options Full-time and part-time.

Program Entrance Requirements Clinical experience, minimum overall college GPA of 3.0, transcript of college record, CPR certification, written essay, immunizations, interview, 2 letters of recommendation, professional liability insurance/malpractice insurance, resume, statistics course. *Application deadline:* Applications are processed on a rolling basis. *Application fee:* $50.

Advanced Placement Credit by examination available. Credit given for nursing courses completed elsewhere dependent upon specific evaluations.

Degree Requirements 39 total credit hours, thesis or project.

Adelphi University (continued)
POST-MASTER'S PROGRAM

Areas of Study Nursing administration; nursing education. *Nurse practitioner programs in:* adult health.

DOCTORAL DEGREE PROGRAM

Degree PhD

Available Programs Doctorate.

Areas of Study Nursing research.

Program Entrance Requirements Minimum overall college GPA of 3.5, interview by faculty committee, interview, 2 letters of recommendation, MSN or equivalent, statistics course, vita, writing sample. *Application deadline:* Applications are processed on a rolling basis. *Application fee:* $50.

Degree Requirements 54 total credit hours, dissertation, oral exam, written exam.

CONTINUING EDUCATION PROGRAM

Contact Karen Pappas, Director, Professional Development and Lifelong Learning, School of Nursing, Adelphi University, One South Avenue, Garden City, NY 11530. *Telephone:* 516-877-4554. *Fax:* 516-877-4558. *E-mail:* pappas@adelphi.edu.

College of Mount Saint Vincent
Department of Nursing
Riverdale, New York

http://www.mountsaintvincent.edu/academics/ majors_and_programs/nursing2/nursing.htm

Founded in 1911

DEGREES • BS • MSN

Nursing Program Faculty 30 (90% with doctorates).

Baccalaureate Enrollment 400
Women 80% **Men** 20% **Minority** 80% **International** 10% **Part-time** 10%

Graduate Enrollment 80
Women 90% **Men** 10% **Minority** 80% **International** 10% **Part-time** 100%

Nursing Student Activities Sigma Theta Tau, Student Nurses' Association.

Nursing Student Resources Academic advising; academic or career counseling; bookstore; campus computer network; computer lab; computer-assisted instruction; e-mail services; employment services for current students; housing assistance; interactive nursing skills videos; Internet; learning resource lab; library services; nursing audiovisuals; resume preparation assistance; skills, simulation, or other laboratory; tutoring.

Library Facilities 160,696 volumes (5,304 in nursing); 362 periodical subscriptions.

BACCALAUREATE PROGRAMS

Degree BS

Available Programs ADN to Baccalaureate; Baccalaureate for Second Degree; Generic Baccalaureate; RN Baccalaureate.

Site Options Manhattan, NY.

Study Options Full-time and part-time.

Program Entrance Requirements Minimum overall college GPA of 2.5, transcript of college record, CPR certification, written essay, health exam, health insurance, high school biology, high school chemistry, high school foreign language, 3 years high school math, 3 years high school science, high school transcript, immunizations, 1 letter of recommendation, minimum high school GPA of 2.5, minimum GPA in nursing prerequisites of 3.0, prerequisite course work. Transfer students are accepted. **Standardized tests** *Required:* SAT or ACT, TOEFL for international students. **Application** *Deadline:* rolling (freshmen), rolling (transfer). *Early decision:* 11/15. *Notification:* continuous (freshmen), 12/1 (early action). *Application fee:* $35.

Expenses (2006–07) *Tuition:* full-time $21,000; part-time $700 per credit. *Room and board:* $8500 per academic year. *Required fees:* part-time $700 per credit.

Financial Aid 90% of baccalaureate students in nursing programs received some form of financial aid in 2005–06.

Contact Ms. Harriet Rothman, RN, Recruitment and Advisement Coordinator, Department of Nursing, College of Mount Saint Vincent, 6301 Riverdale Avenue, Riverdale, NY 10471. *Telephone:* 718-405-3365. *Fax:* 718-405-3286. *E-mail:* nursing@mountsaintvincent.edu.

GRADUATE PROGRAMS

Expenses (2006–07) *Tuition:* part-time $625 per credit.

Financial Aid 90% of graduate students in nursing programs received some form of financial aid in 2005–06. Career-related internships or fieldwork available. *Financial aid application deadline:* 6/1.

Contact Dr. Carol Vicino, Chairperson, Graduate Program of Nursing, Department of Nursing, College of Mount Saint Vincent, 6301 Riverdale Avenue, Riverdale, NY 10471-1093. *Telephone:* 718-405-3362. *Fax:* 718-405-3286. *E-mail:* carol.vicino@mountsaintvincent.edu.

MASTER'S DEGREE PROGRAM

Degree MSN

Available Programs Master's; Master's for Nurses with Non-Nursing Degrees.

Concentrations Available Nursing administration. *Clinical nurse specialist programs in:* adult health, gerontology. *Nurse practitioner programs in:* adult health, family health.

Study Options Part-time.

Program Entrance Requirements Clinical experience, computer literacy, minimum overall college GPA of 3.0, transcript of college record, CPR certification, written essay, immunizations, interview, 2 letters of recommendation, nursing research course, physical assessment course, professional liability insurance/malpractice insurance, prerequisite course work, statistics course. *Application deadline:* For fall admission, 6/1; for spring admission, 11/1. Applications are processed on a rolling basis. *Application fee:* $50.

Degree Requirements 45 total credit hours, thesis or project.

POST-MASTER'S PROGRAM

Areas of Study Nursing education. *Nurse practitioner programs in:* adult health, family health.

The College of New Rochelle
School of Nursing
New Rochelle, New York

Founded in 1904

DEGREES • BSN • MS

Nursing Program Faculty 65 (12% with doctorates).

Baccalaureate Enrollment 512
Women 95% **Men** 5% **Minority** 67% **International** 1% **Part-time** 60%

Graduate Enrollment 112
Women 95% **Men** 5% **Minority** 18% **International** 1% **Part-time** 100%

Nursing Student Activities Nursing Honor Society, Sigma Theta Tau, Student Nurses' Association, nursing club.

Nursing Student Resources Academic advising; academic or career counseling; assistance for students with disabilities; bookstore; campus computer network; career placement assistance; computer lab; computer-assisted instruction; e-mail services; housing assistance; interactive nursing skills videos; Internet; learning resource lab; library services; nursing audiovisuals; other; remedial services; resume preparation assistance; skills, simulation, or other laboratory; tutoring.

Library Facilities 220,000 volumes (8,700 in health, 8,700 in nursing); 1,450 periodical subscriptions (165 health-care related).

BACCALAUREATE PROGRAMS

Degree BSN

Available Programs Accelerated Baccalaureate for Second Degree; Accelerated RN Baccalaureate; Baccalaureate for Second Degree; Generic Baccalaureate; RN Baccalaureate.

Study Options Full-time and part-time.

Program Entrance Requirements Transcript of college record, CPR certification, written essay, health exam, health insurance, high school biology, high school chemistry, high school transcript, immunizations. Transfer students are accepted. **Standardized tests** *Required:* SAT or ACT, TOEFL for international students. **Application** *Deadline:* rolling (freshmen), rolling (transfer). *Early decision:* 11/1. *Notification:* continuous (freshmen), 12/15 (out-of-state freshmen), 12/15 (early decision). *Application fee:* $20.

Advanced Placement Credit by examination available. Credit given for nursing courses completed elsewhere dependent upon specific evaluations.

Expenses (2006–07) *Tuition:* full-time $21,460; part-time $722 per credit. *Room and board:* $8200 per academic year. *Required fees:* full-time $21,460; part-time $722 per credit.

Financial Aid 80% of baccalaureate students in nursing programs received some form of financial aid in 2005–06.

Contact Dr. Mary Alice Donius, Dean, School of Nursing, The College of New Rochelle, 29 Castle Place, New Rochelle, NY 10805-2308. *Telephone:* 914-654-5803. *Fax:* 914-654-5994. *E-mail:* mdonius@cnr.edu.

GRADUATE PROGRAMS

Expenses (2006–07) *Tuition:* part-time $590 per credit.

Financial Aid 75% of graduate students in nursing programs received some form of financial aid in 2005–06.

Contact Dr. Mary Alice Donius, Dean, School of Nursing, The College of New Rochelle, 29 Castle Place, New Rochelle, NY 10805-2308. *Telephone:* 914-654-5803. *Fax:* 914-654-5994. *E-mail:* mdonius@cnr.edu.

MASTER'S DEGREE PROGRAM

Degree MS

Available Programs Master's; RN to Master's.

Concentrations Available Health-care administration; nursing administration; nursing education. *Nurse practitioner programs in:* family health.

Site Options New Rochelle, NY; Bronx, NY.

Study Options Full-time and part-time.

Program Entrance Requirements Clinical experience, minimum overall college GPA of 3.0, transcript of college record, written essay, immunizations, interview, 2 letters of recommendation, physical assessment course, professional liability insurance/malpractice insurance, resume, statistics course.

Advanced Placement Credit given for nursing courses completed elsewhere dependent upon specific evaluations.

Degree Requirements 40 total credit hours, thesis or project.

POST-MASTER'S PROGRAM

Areas of Study Health-care administration; nursing administration; nursing education. *Clinical nurse specialist programs in:* palliative care. *Nurse practitioner programs in:* family health.

See full description on page 462.

College of Staten Island of the City University of New York
Department of Nursing
Staten Island, New York

http://www.csi.cuny.edu/nursing
Founded in 1955
DEGREES • BS • MS

Nursing Program Faculty 40 (50% with doctorates).
Baccalaureate Enrollment 90
Women 83% **Men** 17% **Minority** 32% **International** 5% **Part-time** 90%
Graduate Enrollment 40
Women 98% **Men** 2% **Minority** 35% **International** 5% **Part-time** 99%
Nursing Student Activities Nursing Honor Society, Sigma Theta Tau, Student Nurses' Association, nursing club.

Nursing Student Resources Academic advising; academic or career counseling; assistance for students with disabilities; bookstore; campus computer network; career placement assistance; computer lab; computer-assisted instruction; daycare for children of students; e-mail services; employment services for current students; externships; interactive nursing skills videos; Internet; learning resource lab; library services; nursing audiovisuals; placement services for program completers; remedial services; resume preparation assistance; skills, simulation, or other laboratory; tutoring.

Library Facilities 229,000 volumes; 25,000 periodical subscriptions.

BACCALAUREATE PROGRAMS

Degree BS
Available Programs ADN to Baccalaureate; RN Baccalaureate.
Site Options Brooklyn, NY.
Study Options Full-time and part-time.
Program Entrance Requirements Minimum overall college GPA of 2.0, transcript of college record, CPR certification, health exam, health insurance, high school transcript, immunizations, minimum GPA in nursing prerequisites, professional liability insurance/malpractice insurance, prerequisite course work, RN licensure. Transfer students are accepted. **Standardized tests** *Required:* TOEFL for international students. *Recommended:* SAT or ACT. **Application** *Deadline:* rolling (freshmen), rolling (transfer). *Notification:* 12/15 (freshmen). *Application fee:* $65.
Advanced Placement Credit by examination available. Credit given for nursing courses completed elsewhere dependent upon specific evaluations.
Expenses (2006–07) *Tuition, area resident:* full-time $2000; part-time $170 per credit. *Tuition, state resident:* part-time $360 per credit. *Tuition, nonresident:* part-time $360 per credit. *Required fees:* full-time $700; part-time $112 per credit; part-time $112 per term.
Financial Aid 40% of baccalaureate students in nursing programs received some form of financial aid in 2005–06. *Gift aid (need-based):* Federal Pell, FSEOG, state, private, college/university gift aid from institutional funds, Federal Nursing. *Loans:* Federal Direct (Subsidized and Unsubsidized Stafford PLUS), Perkins. *Work-Study:* Federal Work-Study. *Application deadline (priority):* 3/31.
Contact Prof. Mary E. O'Donnell, RN, Chairperson, Department of Nursing, College of Staten Island of the City University of New York, 2800 Victory Boulevard, Marcus Hall, 5S-213, Staten Island, NY 10314. *Telephone:* 718-982-3810. *Fax:* 718-982-3813. *E-mail:* odonnellm@mail.csi.cuny.edu.

GRADUATE PROGRAMS

Expenses (2006–07) *Tuition, area resident:* part-time $270 per credit. *Tuition, state resident:* part-time $500 per credit. *Tuition, nonresident:* part-time $500 per credit. *Required fees:* full-time $700; part-time $200 per credit; part-time $200 per term.
Financial Aid 20% of graduate students in nursing programs received some form of financial aid in 2005–06.
Contact Dr. Margaret Lunney, Director, Graduate Program, Department of Nursing, College of Staten Island of the City University of New York, 2800 Victory Boulevard, Staten Island, NY 10314. *Telephone:* 718-982-3845. *Fax:* 718-982-3813. *E-mail:* lunney@mail.csi.cuny.edu.

MASTER'S DEGREE PROGRAM

Degree MS
Available Programs Master's.
Concentrations Available *Clinical nurse specialist programs in:* adult health. *Nurse practitioner programs in:* adult health, gerontology.
Site Options Brooklyn, NY.
Study Options Full-time and part-time.
Program Entrance Requirements Clinical experience, minimum overall college GPA of 3.0, transcript of college record, written essay, immunizations, interview, 2 letters of recommendation, nursing research course, physical assessment course, professional liability insurance/malpractice insurance, prerequisite course work, statistics course.
Advanced Placement Credit given for nursing courses completed elsewhere dependent upon specific evaluations.
Degree Requirements 48 total credit hours, thesis or project.

POST-MASTER'S PROGRAM

Areas of Study *Nurse practitioner programs in:* adult health, gerontology.

Columbia University
School of Nursing
New York, New York

http://www.nursing.hs.columbia.edu

Founded in 1754

DEGREES • BS • DN SC • MS • MS/MBA • MS/MPH

Nursing Program Faculty 80 (61% with doctorates).

Baccalaureate Enrollment 161
Women 90% **Men** 10% **Minority** 24% **International** 1%

Graduate Enrollment 332
Women 93% **Men** 7% **Minority** 20% **International** 1% **Part-time** 62%

Nursing Student Activities Sigma Theta Tau.

Nursing Student Resources Academic advising; academic or career counseling; assistance for students with disabilities; bookstore; campus computer network; career placement assistance; computer lab; computer-assisted instruction; daycare for children of students; e-mail services; employment services for current students; housing assistance; interactive nursing skills videos; Internet; learning resource lab; library services; resume preparation assistance; skills, simulation, or other laboratory.

Library Facilities 469,000 volumes in health; 4,352 periodical subscriptions health-care related.

BACCALAUREATE PROGRAMS

Degree BS

Available Programs Accelerated Baccalaureate for Second Degree.
Study Options Full-time.

Program Entrance Requirements Transcript of college record, CPR certification, written essay, health exam, immunizations, 3 letters of recommendation, prerequisite course work.

Advanced Placement Credit by examination available. Credit given for nursing courses completed elsewhere dependent upon specific evaluations.

Expenses (2006–07) *Tuition:* full-time $60,455; part-time $991 per credit.

Financial Aid 90% of baccalaureate students in nursing programs received some form of financial aid in 2005–06.

Contact Office of Admissions, School of Nursing, Columbia University, 630 West 168th Street, Box 6, New York, NY 10032. *Telephone:* 212-305-5756. *Fax:* 212-305-3680. *E-mail:* nursing@columbia.edu.

GRADUATE PROGRAMS

Expenses (2006–07) *Tuition:* part-time $991 per credit.

Financial Aid 70% of graduate students in nursing programs received some form of financial aid in 2005–06. Research assistantships, teaching assistantships, Federal Work-Study and institutionally sponsored loans available. Aid available to part-time students.

Contact Office of Admissions, School of Nursing, Columbia University, 630 West 168th Street, Box 6, New York, NY 10032. *Telephone:* 212-305-5756. *Fax:* 212-305-3680. *E-mail:* nursing@columbia.edu.

MASTER'S DEGREE PROGRAM

Degrees MS; MS/MBA; MS/MPH

Available Programs Accelerated AD/RN to Master's; Accelerated Master's for Non-Nursing College Graduates; Accelerated Master's for Nurses with Non-Nursing Degrees; Master's; Master's for Non-Nursing College Graduates.

Concentrations Available Nurse anesthesia; nurse-midwifery. *Nurse practitioner programs in:* acute care, adult health, family health, gerontology, neonatal health, oncology, pediatric, psychiatric/mental health, women's health.

Study Options Full-time and part-time.

Program Entrance Requirements Clinical experience, computer literacy, transcript of college record, CPR certification, written essay, immunizations, 3 letters of recommendation, physical assessment course, professional liability insurance/malpractice insurance, prerequisite course work, resume, statistics course, GRE General Test. *Application deadline:* Applications are processed on a rolling basis. *Application fee:* $90.

Advanced Placement Credit by examination available. Credit given for nursing courses completed elsewhere dependent upon specific evaluations.

Degree Requirements 45 total credit hours, thesis or project, comprehensive exam.

POST-MASTER'S PROGRAM

Areas of Study Nurse anesthesia. *Nurse practitioner programs in:* acute care, adult health, family health, gerontology, neonatal health, oncology, pediatric, psychiatric/mental health, women's health.

DOCTORAL DEGREE PROGRAM

Degree DN Sc

Available Programs Doctorate; Doctorate for Nurses with Non-Nursing Degrees; Post-Baccalaureate Doctorate.

Areas of Study Information systems, nursing policy, nursing research, nursing science.

Program Entrance Requirements Clinical experience, interview by faculty committee, interview, 3 letters of recommendation, MSN or equivalent, scholarly papers, statistics course, vita, writing sample, GRE General Test. *Application deadline:* Applications are processed on a rolling basis. *Application fee:* $90.

Degree Requirements 45 total credit hours, dissertation, oral exam, written exam.

CONTINUING EDUCATION PROGRAM

Contact Sarah Cook, Vice Dean, School of Nursing, Columbia University, 630 West 168th Street, Box 6, New York, NY 10032. *Telephone:* 212-305-3582. *Fax:* 212-305-1116. *E-mail:* ssc3@columbia.edu.

See full description on page 466.

Daemen College
Department of Nursing
Amherst, New York

http://www.daemen.edu

Founded in 1947

DEGREES • BS • MS

Nursing Program Faculty 15 (60% with doctorates).

Baccalaureate Enrollment 200
Women 96% **Men** 4% **Minority** 3% **International** 2% **Part-time** 15%

Graduate Enrollment 75
Women 96% **Men** 4% **Minority** 8% **International** 6% **Part-time** 90%

Nursing Student Activities Sigma Theta Tau, nursing club.

Nursing Student Resources Academic advising; academic or career counseling; assistance for students with disabilities; bookstore; campus computer network; career placement assistance; computer lab; computer-assisted instruction; e-mail services; Internet; learning resource lab; library services; nursing audiovisuals; placement services for program completers; remedial services; resume preparation assistance; skills, simulation, or other laboratory; tutoring.

Library Facilities 127,232 volumes (10,000 in health, 4,000 in nursing); 889 periodical subscriptions (250 health-care related).

BACCALAUREATE PROGRAMS

Degree BS

Available Programs ADN to Baccalaureate; Accelerated RN Baccalaureate; International Nurse to Baccalaureate; RN Baccalaureate.

Site Options *Distance Learning:* Poswell Park Cancer Institute, NY; Jamestown, NY; Olean, NY.

Program Entrance Requirements Minimum overall college GPA of 2.0, transcript of college record, high school transcript, immunizations. Transfer students are accepted. **Standardized tests** *Required:* SAT or ACT, TOEFL for international students. **Application** *Deadline:* rolling (freshmen), rolling (transfer). *Early decision:* 8/30. *Notification:* continuous (freshmen), 9/1 (early action). *Application fee:* $25.

Expenses (2006–07) *Tuition:* full-time $4310; part-time $288 per credit hour. *International tuition:* $4310 full-time. *Required fees:* full-time $110; part-time $2 per credit; part-time $34 per term.

Financial Aid 100% of baccalaureate students in nursing programs received some form of financial aid in 2005–06. *Gift aid (need-based):* Federal Pell, FSEOG, state, private, college/university gift aid from institutional funds. *Loans:* FFEL (Subsidized and Unsubsidized Stafford PLUS), Perkins, college/university, alternative loans. *Work-Study:* Federal Work-Study, part-time campus jobs. *Application deadline (priority):* 2/15.

Contact Dr. Mary Lou Rusin, Professor and Chair, Department of Nursing, Daemen College, 4380 Main Street, Amherst, NY 14226. *Telephone:* 716-839-8387. *Fax:* 716-839-8403. *E-mail:* mrusin@daemen.edu.

GRADUATE PROGRAMS

Expenses (2006–07) *Tuition:* part-time $650 per credit hour. *Required fees:* part-time $15 per credit.

Financial Aid 75% of graduate students in nursing programs received some form of financial aid in 2005–06. Institutionally sponsored loans and scholarships available. *Financial aid application deadline:* 2/15.

Contact Dr. Mary Lou Rusin, Professor and Chair, Department of Nursing, Daemen College, 4380 Main Street, Amherst, NY 14226. *Telephone:* 716-839-8387. *Fax:* 716-839-8403. *E-mail:* mrusin@daemen.edu.

MASTER'S DEGREE PROGRAM

Degree MS

Available Programs Accelerated AD/RN to Master's; Accelerated RN to Master's; Master's; RN to Master's.

Concentrations Available Health-care administration; nursing education. *Clinical nurse specialist programs in:* palliative care. *Nurse practitioner programs in:* adult health.

Study Options Full-time and part-time.

Program Entrance Requirements Clinical experience, minimum overall college GPA of 3.25, transcript of college record, written essay, immunizations, interview, 3 letters of recommendation, statistics course. *Application deadline:* For fall admission, 3/1 (priority date); for spring admission, 10/1 (priority date). Applications are processed on a rolling basis. *Application fee:* $25.

Advanced Placement Credit given for nursing courses completed elsewhere dependent upon specific evaluations.

Degree Requirements 30 total credit hours, thesis or project.

POST-MASTER'S PROGRAM

Areas of Study Health-care administration; nursing education. *Clinical nurse specialist programs in:* palliative care. *Nurse practitioner programs in:* adult health.

Dominican College
Department of Nursing
Orangeburg, New York

Founded in 1952

DEGREES • BSN • M SC N

Nursing Program Faculty 14 (21% with doctorates).

Baccalaureate Enrollment 182
Women 87% **Men** 13% **Minority** 44% **International** 40% **Part-time** 43%

Graduate Enrollment 37
Women 100% **Minority** 66% **International** 60% **Part-time** 100%

Nursing Student Activities Nursing Honor Society, Sigma Theta Tau, Student Nurses' Association.

Nursing Student Resources Academic advising; academic or career counseling; assistance for students with disabilities; bookstore; campus computer network; career placement assistance; computer lab; computer-assisted instruction; e-mail services; externships; Internet; learning resource lab; library services; nursing audiovisuals; paid internships; remedial services; resume preparation assistance; skills, simulation, or other laboratory; tutoring.

Library Facilities 103,350 volumes (5,650 in health); 650 periodical subscriptions (235 health-care related).

BACCALAUREATE PROGRAMS

Degree BSN

Available Programs Accelerated Baccalaureate for Second Degree; Accelerated LPN to Baccalaureate; Accelerated RN Baccalaureate; Generic Baccalaureate; LPN to Baccalaureate; RN Baccalaureate.

Study Options Full-time and part-time.

Program Entrance Requirements Minimum overall college GPA of 2.7, transcript of college record, CPR certification, health exam, health insurance, high school transcript, immunizations, minimum GPA in nursing prerequisites of 2.0, professional liability insurance/malpractice insurance, prerequisite course work. Transfer students are accepted. **Standardized tests** *Required:* SAT or ACT, TOEFL for international students. **Application** *Deadline:* rolling (freshmen), rolling (transfer). *Notification:* continuous (freshmen). *Application fee:* $35.

Advanced Placement Credit by examination available. Credit given for nursing courses completed elsewhere dependent upon specific evaluations.

Expenses (2006–07) *Tuition:* full-time $17,930; part-time $536 per credit. *International tuition:* $17,930 full-time. *Room and board:* $8960; room only: $6780 per academic year. *Required fees:* full-time $680; part-time $165 per term.

Financial Aid 95% of baccalaureate students in nursing programs received some form of financial aid in 2005–06. *Gift aid (need-based):* Federal Pell, FSEOG, state, private, college/university gift aid from institutional funds. *Loans:* Federal Nursing Student Loans, FFEL (Subsidized and Unsubsidized Stafford PLUS), Perkins. *Work-Study:* Federal Work-Study, part-time campus jobs. *Application deadline (priority):* 2/15.

Contact Dr. Nancy Ann DiDona, Acting Director, Division of Nursing, Department of Nursing, Dominican College, 470 Western Highway, Orangeburg, NY 10962. *Telephone:* 845-848-6051. *Fax:* 845-398-4891. *E-mail:* nancy.didona@dc.edu.

GRADUATE PROGRAMS

Expenses (2006–07) *Tuition:* full-time $24,040; part-time $585 per credit. *International tuition:* $24,040 full-time. *Room and board:* $8960; room only: $6780 per academic year. *Required fees:* full-time $680; part-time $165 per term.

Financial Aid 70% of graduate students in nursing programs received some form of financial aid in 2005–06.

Contact Miss Lynne Weissman, Coordinator of Family Nurse Practitioner Program, Department of Nursing, Dominican College, 470 Western Highway, Orangeburg, NY 10962. *Telephone:* 845-848-6026. *Fax:* 845-398-4891. *E-mail:* lynne.weissman@dc.edu.

MASTER'S DEGREE PROGRAM

Degree M Sc N

Available Programs Master's.

Concentrations Available *Nurse practitioner programs in:* family health.

Study Options Full-time and part-time.

Program Entrance Requirements Clinical experience, minimum overall college GPA of 3.0, transcript of college record, written essay, immunizations, 3 letters of recommendation, nursing research course, physical assessment course, professional liability insurance/malpractice insurance, prerequisite course work, statistics course. *Application deadline:* Applications are processed on a rolling basis. *Application fee:* $50.

Degree Requirements 42 total credit hours, thesis or project.

D'Youville College
Department of Nursing
Buffalo, New York

Founded in 1908

DEGREES • BSN • MS

Nursing Program Faculty 37 (5% with doctorates).

Baccalaureate Enrollment 430
Women 90% **Men** 10% **Minority** 10% **International** 5% **Part-time** 30%

Graduate Enrollment 108
Women 97% **Men** 3% **Minority** 10% **International** 35% **Part-time** 40%

D'Youville College (continued)

Nursing Student Activities Sigma Theta Tau, Student Nurses' Association.

Nursing Student Resources Academic advising; academic or career counseling; assistance for students with disabilities; bookstore; campus computer network; career placement assistance; computer lab; computer-assisted instruction; e-mail services; interactive nursing skills videos; Internet; learning resource lab; library services; nursing audiovisuals; paid internships; placement services for program completers; remedial services; resume preparation assistance; skills, simulation, or other laboratory; tutoring.

Library Facilities 122,057 volumes (100,000 in health, 17,000 in nursing); 665 periodical subscriptions (171 health-care related).

■ A current worldwide shortage in nursing leaves the door wide open for qualified nurses. D'Youville College has been educating nurses since 1942, and its nursing program is one of the largest four-year, private-college nursing programs in the country. The faculty members are hardworking and dedicated. Classes are small, which permits much individualized attention. Baccalaureate graduates who wish to continue their education can choose from three master's programs at D'Youville College. Registered nurses enrolled in the B.S.N. program have the option of completing some of their major courses via distance learning. D'Youville also offers a combined bachelor's/master's program for RNs and traditional students.

BACCALAUREATE PROGRAMS

Degree BSN

Available Programs ADN to Baccalaureate; Generic Baccalaureate; RN Baccalaureate.

Site Options *Distance Learning:* Buffalo, NY.

Study Options Full-time and part-time.

Program Entrance Requirements Minimum overall college GPA of 2.5, transcript of college record, health exam, health insurance, high school biology, high school chemistry, 1 year of high school math, 1 year of high school science, high school transcript, immunizations, minimum high school GPA of 2.0, minimum high school rank 50%, minimum GPA in nursing prerequisites of 2.0, professional liability insurance/malpractice insurance, prerequisite course work. Transfer students are accepted. **Standardized tests** *Required:* SAT or ACT, TOEFL for international students. **Application** *Deadline:* rolling (freshmen), rolling (transfer). *Notification:* continuous (freshmen). *Application fee:* $25.

Advanced Placement Credit given for nursing courses completed elsewhere dependent upon specific evaluations.

Expenses (2006–07) *Tuition:* full-time $16,600; part-time $460 per credit hour. *International tuition:* $16,600 full-time. *Room and board:* $8300; room only: $6800 per academic year. *Required fees:* full-time $200; part-time $64 per term.

Financial Aid *Gift aid (need-based):* Federal Pell, FSEOG, state, private, college/university gift aid from institutional funds. *Loans:* Federal Nursing Student Loans, FFEL (Subsidized and Unsubsidized Stafford PLUS), Perkins, college/university. *Work-Study:* Federal Work-Study, part-time campus jobs. *Application deadline (priority):* 3/1.

Contact Mr. Ron Dannecker, Director of Admissions, Department of Nursing, D'Youville College, 320 Porter Avenue, Buffalo, NY 14201. *Telephone:* 716-881-7600. *Fax:* 716-515-0679. *E-mail:* admiss@dyc.edu.

GRADUATE PROGRAMS

Expenses (2006–07) *Tuition:* part-time $600 per credit hour. *Room and board:* $8300; room only: $6400 per academic year. *Required fees:* full-time $200; part-time $64 per term.

Financial Aid 1 research assistantship (averaging $3,000 per year) was awarded; Federal Work-Study and scholarships also available.

Contact Miss Linda Fisher, Director of Graduate Admissions, Department of Nursing, D'Youville College, 320 Porter Avenue, Buffalo, NY 14201. *Telephone:* 716-881-7744. *Fax:* 716-515-0679. *E-mail:* fisherl@dyc.edu.

MASTER'S DEGREE PROGRAM

Degree MS

Available Programs Accelerated AD/RN to Master's; Master's; RN to Master's.

Concentrations Available Nursing education. *Clinical nurse specialist programs in:* community health. *Nurse practitioner programs in:* family health.

Study Options Full-time and part-time.

Program Entrance Requirements Clinical experience, computer literacy, minimum overall college GPA of 3.0, transcript of college record, CPR certification, written essay, immunizations, interview, 2 letters of recommendation, nursing research course, physical assessment course, professional liability insurance/malpractice insurance, prerequisite course work, resume, statistics course. *Application deadline:* Applications are processed on a rolling basis. *Application fee:* $25.

Advanced Placement Credit given for nursing courses completed elsewhere dependent upon specific evaluations.

Degree Requirements 39 total credit hours, thesis or project.

POST-MASTER'S PROGRAM

Areas of Study *Nurse practitioner programs in:* family health.

See full description on page 476.

Elmira College
Program in Nursing Education
Elmira, New York

Founded in 1855

DEGREE • BS

Nursing Program Faculty 13 (98% with doctorates).

Baccalaureate Enrollment 101

Women 97% **Men** 3% **Minority** 5% **Part-time** 29%

Nursing Student Activities Sigma Theta Tau, nursing club.

Nursing Student Resources Academic advising; academic or career counseling; assistance for students with disabilities; bookstore; campus computer network; career placement assistance; computer lab; computer-assisted instruction; e-mail services; housing assistance; interactive nursing skills videos; Internet; learning resource lab; library services; nursing audiovisuals; placement services for program completers; resume preparation assistance; skills, simulation, or other laboratory; tutoring; unpaid internships.

Library Facilities 391,038 volumes (7,461 in health, 5,200 in nursing); 859 periodical subscriptions (72 health-care related).

■ Many features distinguish the Elmira College nursing program from other nursing programs. Students in the Elmira College nursing program begin clinical experiences of 6 to 17 hours per week in the sophomore year. Students are admitted directly to the nursing program and do not have to qualify again. Clinical nursing experiences take place in a variety of community-based health-care agencies as well as in acute-care hospitals. Curriculum emphasis is on health maintenance within the community. Extracurricular activities and intercollegiate athletic participation are encouraged by the nursing faculty. A strong liberal arts component and a required community service experience ensure a well-rounded graduate.

BACCALAUREATE PROGRAMS

Degree BS

Available Programs ADN to Baccalaureate; Generic Baccalaureate; RN Baccalaureate.

Study Options Full-time and part-time.

Program Entrance Requirements Minimum overall college GPA of 2.0, transcript of college record, written essay, health exam, health insurance, high school biology, high school chemistry, 3 years high school math, 3 years high school science, high school transcript, immunizations, 2 letters of recommendation, minimum high school GPA of 2.5. Transfer students are accepted. **Standardized tests** *Required:* SAT or ACT, TOEFL for international students. **Application** *Deadline:* 4/15 (freshmen). *Early decision:* 11/15 (for plan 1), 1/15 (for plan 2). *Notification:* continuous until 4/30 (freshmen), 12/15 (out-of-state freshmen), 12/15 (early decision plan 1), 2/1 (early decision plan 2). *Application fee:* $50.

Advanced Placement Credit by examination available. Credit given for nursing courses completed elsewhere dependent upon specific evaluations.

Expenses (2006–07) *Tuition:* full-time $29,000. *International tuition:* $29,000 full-time. *Room and board:* $9100 per academic year. *Required fees:* full-time $1050.

Financial Aid 88% of baccalaureate students in nursing programs received some form of financial aid in 2005–06. *Gift aid (need-based):* Federal Pell, FSEOG, state, private, college/university gift aid from institutional funds. *Loans:* FFEL (Subsidized and Unsubsidized Stafford PLUS), Perkins, college/university, GATE Loans, alternative loans. *Work-Study:* Federal Work-Study, part-time campus jobs. *Application deadline (priority):* 2/1.

Contact Mr. Gary Fallis, Dean of Admissions, Program in Nursing Education, Elmira College, One Park Place, Elmira, NY 14901. *Telephone:* 607-735-1724. *Fax:* 607-735-1718. *E-mail:* gfallis@elmira.edu.

CONTINUING EDUCATION PROGRAM

Contact Dr. Lois Schoener, Professor of Nursing/Director of Nurse Education, Program in Nursing Education, Elmira College, One Park Place, Elmira, NY 14901. *Telephone:* 607-735-1890. *Fax:* 607-735-1758. *E-mail:* lschoener@elmira.edu.

Excelsior College
School of Health Sciences
Albany, New York

http://www.excelsior.edu

Founded in 1970

DEGREES • BSN • MS

Nursing Program Faculty 41 (64% with doctorates).

Baccalaureate Enrollment 1,103
Women 85% **Men** 15% **Minority** 25% **Part-time** 100%

Graduate Enrollment 334
Women 85% **Men** 15% **Minority** 23% **International** 1% **Part-time** 100%

Nursing Student Activities Sigma Theta Tau.

Nursing Student Resources Academic advising; academic or career counseling; assistance for students with disabilities; bookstore; computer-assisted instruction; e-mail services; Internet; learning resource lab; library services; nursing audiovisuals; other; resume preparation assistance; skills, simulation, or other laboratory; tutoring.

BACCALAUREATE PROGRAMS

Degree BSN

Available Programs RN Baccalaureate.

Site Options *Distance Learning:* Albany, NY.

Study Options Part-time.

Program Entrance Requirements Transcript of college record, high school transcript, RN licensure. Transfer students are accepted. **Application** *Deadline:* rolling (freshmen), rolling (transfer). *Notification:* continuous (freshmen). *Application fee:* $75.

Advanced Placement Credit by examination available. Credit given for nursing courses completed elsewhere dependent upon specific evaluations.

Expenses (2006–07) *Tuition:* part-time $275 per credit. *Required fees:* part-time $275 per credit.

Financial Aid 10% of baccalaureate students in nursing programs received some form of financial aid in 2005–06.

Contact Admissions Office, School of Health Sciences, Excelsior College, 7 Columbia Circle, Albany, NY 12203. *Telephone:* 518-464-8500. *Fax:* 518-464-8777. *E-mail:* admissions@excelsior.edu.

GRADUATE PROGRAMS

Expenses (2006–07) *Tuition:* part-time $385 per credit.

Financial Aid Scholarships available.

Contact Patricia Edwards, EdD, Director, Master of Science in Nursing, School of Health Sciences, Excelsior College, 7 Columbia Circle, Albany, NY 12203. *Telephone:* 518-464-8500. *Fax:* 518-464-8777. *E-mail:* msn@excelsior.edu.

MASTER'S DEGREE PROGRAM

Degree MS

Available Programs Master's; RN to Master's.

Concentrations Available Health-care administration; nursing education; nursing informatics.

Site Options *Distance Learning:* Albany, NY.

Study Options Full-time and part-time.

Program Entrance Requirements Computer literacy, minimum overall college GPA of 3.0, transcript of college record, written essay, resume. *Application deadline:* Applications are processed on a rolling basis. *Application fee:* $100.

Advanced Placement Credit given for nursing courses completed elsewhere dependent upon specific evaluations.

Degree Requirements 44 total credit hours, thesis or project.

See full description on page 480.

Hartwick College
Department of Nursing
Oneonta, New York

http://www.hartwick.edu

Founded in 1797

DEGREE • BS

Nursing Program Faculty 11 (9% with doctorates).

Baccalaureate Enrollment 128
Women 93% **Men** 7% **Minority** 12% **Part-time** 20%

Nursing Student Activities Sigma Theta Tau, Student Nurses' Association.

Nursing Student Resources Academic advising; academic or career counseling; assistance for students with disabilities; bookstore; campus computer network; career placement assistance; computer lab; computer-assisted instruction; e-mail services; employment services for current students; externships; housing assistance; interactive nursing skills videos; Internet; learning resource lab; library services; nursing audiovisuals; placement services for program completers; remedial services; resume preparation assistance; skills, simulation, or other laboratory; tutoring; unpaid internships.

Library Facilities 311,063 volumes (5,691 in health, 1,152 in nursing); 720 periodical subscriptions (184 health-care related).

BACCALAUREATE PROGRAMS

Degree BS

Available Programs Accelerated Baccalaureate; Accelerated Baccalaureate for Second Degree; Generic Baccalaureate; RN Baccalaureate.

Site Options Albany, NY; Cooperstown, NY.

Study Options Full-time and part-time.

Program Entrance Requirements Minimum overall college GPA of 2.0, CPR certification, written essay, health exam, high school biology, high school chemistry, high school foreign language, 3 years high school math, 2 years high school science, high school transcript, immunizations, 2 letters of recommendation, minimum GPA in nursing prerequisites of 2.0, professional liability insurance/malpractice insurance. Transfer students are accepted. **Standardized tests** *Required:* TOEFL for international students. **Application** *Deadline:* 2/15 (freshmen), 8/1 (transfer). *Early decision:* 11/15. *Notification:* 3/5 (freshmen). *Application fee:* $35.

Advanced Placement Credit given for nursing courses completed elsewhere dependent upon specific evaluations.

Expenses (2006–07) *Tuition:* full-time $27,450; part-time $915 per credit. *Room and board:* $7910; room only: $4080 per academic year. *Required fees:* full-time $2455.

Hartwick College (continued)

Financial Aid 90% of baccalaureate students in nursing programs received some form of financial aid in 2005–06.

Contact Mrs. Sharon D. Dettenrieder, RN, Professor and Chair, Department of Nursing, Hartwick College, Johnstone Science Center, 1 Hartwick Drive, Oneonta, NY 13820. *Telephone:* 607-431-4780. *Fax:* 607-431-4850. *E-mail:* dettenriedes@hartwick.edu.

Hunter College of the City University of New York
Hunter-Bellevue School of Nursing
New York, New York

http://www.hunter.cuny.edu/schoolhp/nursing

Founded in 1870

DEGREES • BS • MS • MS/MPH

Nursing Program Faculty 22 (56% with doctorates).

Nursing Student Activities Sigma Theta Tau.

Nursing Student Resources Academic advising; academic or career counseling; assistance for students with disabilities; bookstore; campus computer network; computer lab; computer-assisted instruction; e-mail services; interactive nursing skills videos; Internet; learning resource lab; library services; nursing audiovisuals.

Library Facilities 789,718 volumes (39,245 in health, 4,295 in nursing); 4,282 periodical subscriptions (375 health-care related).

BACCALAUREATE PROGRAMS

Degree BS

Available Programs Generic Baccalaureate; RN Baccalaureate.

Study Options Full-time.

Program Entrance Requirements Minimum overall college GPA of 2.5, CPR certification, health exam, immunizations, professional liability insurance/malpractice insurance, prerequisite course work. Transfer students are accepted. **Standardized tests** *Required:* SAT or ACT, TOEFL for international students. **Application** *Deadline:* 3/15 (freshmen), 3/15 (transfer). *Notification:* continuous until 1/3 (freshmen). *Application fee:* $65.

Contact *Telephone:* 212-481-7598. *Fax:* 212-481-4427.

GRADUATE PROGRAMS

Contact *Telephone:* 212-481-4465. *Fax:* 212-481-4427.

MASTER'S DEGREE PROGRAM

Degrees MS; MS/MPH

Available Programs Master's.

Concentrations Available *Clinical nurse specialist programs in:* community health, medical-surgical, parent-child, psychiatric/mental health. *Nurse practitioner programs in:* adult health, gerontology, pediatric.

Study Options Full-time and part-time.

Program Entrance Requirements Clinical experience, minimum overall college GPA of 3.0, transcript of college record, written essay, immunizations, 2 letters of recommendation, resume, statistics course. *Application deadline:* For fall admission, 4/1; for spring admission, 11/1. Applications are processed on a rolling basis. *Application fee:* $125.

Degree Requirements 42 total credit hours, thesis or project.

POST-MASTER'S PROGRAM

Areas of Study *Nurse practitioner programs in:* pediatric.

CONTINUING EDUCATION PROGRAM

Contact *Telephone:* 212-650-3850. *Fax:* 212-772-3402.

Keuka College
Division of Nursing
Keuka Park, New York

http://www.keuka.edu/asap/nursing.htm

Founded in 1890

DEGREE • BS

Nursing Program Faculty 5 (40% with doctorates).

Baccalaureate Enrollment 184
Women 94% **Men** 6% **Minority** 4%

Nursing Student Activities Nursing Honor Society.

Nursing Student Resources Academic advising; assistance for students with disabilities; bookstore; campus computer network; computer lab; computer-assisted instruction; e-mail services; interactive nursing skills videos; Internet; learning resource lab; library services; nursing audiovisuals; tutoring.

Library Facilities 112,541 volumes (986 in health, 532 in nursing); 384 periodical subscriptions (48 health-care related).

BACCALAUREATE PROGRAMS

Degree BS

Available Programs Accelerated RN Baccalaureate.

Site Options Rochester, NY. *Distance Learning:* Geneva, NY; Canandaigua, NY.

Program Entrance Requirements Minimum overall college GPA of 2.5, transcript of college record, CPR certification, health exam, immunizations, minimum GPA in nursing prerequisites of 2.5, prerequisite course work, RN licensure. Transfer students are accepted. **Standardized tests** *Required:* TOEFL for international students. *Recommended:* SAT or ACT. **Application** *Deadline:* rolling (freshmen), rolling (transfer). *Application fee:* $30.

Advanced Placement Credit by examination available. Credit given for nursing courses completed elsewhere dependent upon specific evaluations.

Expenses (2006–07) *Tuition:* full-time $15,130. *International tuition:* $15,130 full-time. *Required fees:* full-time $100.

Financial Aid 100% of baccalaureate students in nursing programs received some form of financial aid in 2005–06. *Gift aid (need-based):* Federal Pell, FSEOG, state, private, college/university gift aid from institutional funds. *Loans:* FFEL (Subsidized and Unsubsidized Stafford PLUS), Perkins. *Work-Study:* Federal Work-Study, part-time campus jobs. *Application deadline (priority):* 3/15.

Contact Linda R. Rossi, EdD, Chair, Division of Nursing, Keuka College, 141 Central Avenue, Keuka Park, NY 14478. *Telephone:* 315-536-5273. *Fax:* 315-531-5660. *E-mail:* lrrossi@mail.keuka.edu.

Lehman College of the City University of New York
Department of Nursing
Bronx, New York

http://www.lehman.cuny.edu/departments/

Founded in 1931

DEGREES • BS • MS

Nursing Program Faculty 43 (35% with doctorates).

Baccalaureate Enrollment 342
Women 80% **Men** 20% **Minority** 85% **International** 40%

Graduate Enrollment 120
Women 90% **Men** 10% **Minority** 75% **Part-time** 75%

Nursing Student Activities Sigma Theta Tau, Student Nurses' Association, nursing club.

Nursing Student Resources Academic advising; academic or career counseling; assistance for students with disabilities; bookstore; campus computer network; career placement assistance; computer lab; computer-assisted instruction; daycare for children of students; e-mail services;

externships; interactive nursing skills videos; Internet; learning resource lab; library services; nursing audiovisuals; paid internships; placement services for program completers; resume preparation assistance; skills, simulation, or other laboratory; tutoring; unpaid internships.

Library Facilities 592,698 volumes; 5,950 periodical subscriptions.

BACCALAUREATE PROGRAMS

Degree BS

Available Programs Baccalaureate for Second Degree; Generic Baccalaureate; International Nurse to Baccalaureate; RN Baccalaureate.

Site Options Queens, NY.

Study Options Full-time.

Program Entrance Requirements Minimum overall college GPA of 2.0, transcript of college record, high school transcript, immunizations, minimum GPA in nursing prerequisites of 2.75, prerequisite course work. Transfer students are accepted. **Standardized tests** *Required:* SAT or ACT, TOEFL for international students. **Application** *Deadline:* rolling (freshmen), rolling (transfer). *Notification:* continuous (freshmen). *Application fee:* $65.

Advanced Placement Credit given for nursing courses completed elsewhere dependent upon specific evaluations.

Expenses (2006–07) *Tuition, area resident:* full-time $2145; part-time $170 per credit. *Tuition, state resident:* full-time $2145; part-time $360 per credit. *Tuition, nonresident:* part-time $360 per credit. *Required fees:* full-time $75.

Financial Aid 60% of baccalaureate students in nursing programs received some form of financial aid in 2005–06. *Gift aid (need-based):* Federal Pell, FSEOG, state, college/university gift aid from institutional funds. *Loans:* Federal Direct (Subsidized and Unsubsidized Stafford PLUS), Perkins. *Work-Study:* Federal Work-Study. *Application deadline:* Continuous.

Contact Director of Undergraduate Programs, Department of Nursing, Lehman College of the City University of New York, 250 Bedford Park Boulevard West, Bronx, NY 10468. *Telephone:* 718-960-8214. *Fax:* 718-960-8488.

GRADUATE PROGRAMS

Expenses (2006–07) *Tuition, state resident:* full-time $2780; part-time $230 per credit. *Tuition, nonresident:* full-time $455.

Financial Aid 25% of graduate students in nursing programs received some form of financial aid in 2005–06. Career-related internships or fieldwork, Federal Work-Study, and tuition waivers (partial) available. Aid available to part-time students. *Financial aid application deadline:* 5/15.

Contact Graduate Program, Department of Nursing, Lehman College of the City University of New York, 250 Bedford Park Boulevard West, Bronx, NY 10468. *Telephone:* 718-960-8373. *Fax:* 718-960-8488.

MASTER'S DEGREE PROGRAM

Degree MS

Available Programs Master's; Master's for Nurses with Non-Nursing Degrees.

Concentrations Available Nursing administration; nursing education. *Clinical nurse specialist programs in:* adult health, gerontology, parent-child. *Nurse practitioner programs in:* pediatric.

Site Options New York, NY.

Study Options Full-time and part-time.

Program Entrance Requirements Clinical experience, minimum overall college GPA of 3.0, transcript of college record, written essay, immunizations, interview, 2 letters of recommendation, prerequisite course work. *Application deadline:* For fall admission, 4/1; for spring admission, 11/1. Applications are processed on a rolling basis. *Application fee:* $50.

Advanced Placement Credit given for nursing courses completed elsewhere dependent upon specific evaluations.

Degree Requirements 43 total credit hours.

Long Island University, Brooklyn Campus
School of Nursing
Brooklyn, New York

http://www.liunet.edu

Founded in 1926

DEGREES • BS • MS

Nursing Program Faculty 54 (25% with doctorates).

Baccalaureate Enrollment 900
Women 94% **Men** 6% **Minority** 85% **Part-time** 20%

Graduate Enrollment 200
Women 90% **Men** 10% **Minority** 85% **Part-time** 83%

Nursing Student Activities Nursing Honor Society, Student Nurses' Association.

Nursing Student Resources Academic advising; academic or career counseling; assistance for students with disabilities; bookstore; campus computer network; computer lab; daycare for children of students; e-mail services; employment services for current students; interactive nursing skills videos; Internet; learning resource lab; library services; nursing audiovisuals; paid internships; remedial services; skills, simulation, or other laboratory; tutoring.

Library Facilities 11,000 volumes in health, 850 volumes in nursing; 230 periodical subscriptions health-care related.

BACCALAUREATE PROGRAMS

Degree BS

Available Programs Generic Baccalaureate; International Nurse to Baccalaureate; RN Baccalaureate.

Study Options Full-time and part-time.

Program Entrance Requirements Minimum overall college GPA of 2.75, transcript of college record, CPR certification, health exam, health insurance, high school biology, high school chemistry, 2 years high school math, 2 years high school science, high school transcript, immunizations, interview, minimum high school GPA of 3.0, minimum GPA in nursing prerequisites of 2.75, professional liability insurance/malpractice insurance, prerequisite course work. Transfer students are accepted. **Standardized tests** *Required:* TOEFL for international students. *Required for some:* SAT or ACT. **Application** *Deadline:* rolling (freshmen), rolling (transfer). *Application fee:* $30.

Advanced Placement Credit given for nursing courses completed elsewhere dependent upon specific evaluations.

Expenses (2006–07) *Tuition:* full-time $21,870; part-time $729 per credit. *International tuition:* $21,870 full-time. *Room and board:* $9000 per academic year. *Required fees:* full-time $1500; part-time $250 per credit; part-time $400 per term.

Financial Aid 94% of baccalaureate students in nursing programs received some form of financial aid in 2005–06. *Gift aid (need-based):* Federal Pell, FSEOG, state, private, college/university gift aid from institutional funds, Scholarships for Disadvantaged Students (Nursing and Pharmacy). *Loans:* Federal Direct (Subsidized and Unsubsidized Stafford PLUS), Perkins, Federal Health Professions Student Loans, alternative loans. *Work-Study:* Federal Work-Study, part-time campus jobs. *Application deadline:* Continuous.

Contact Prof. Dawn F. Kilts, Dean, School of Nursing, Long Island University, Brooklyn Campus, 1 University Plaza, Brooklyn, NY 11201. *Telephone:* 718-488-1509. *Fax:* 718-780-4019. *E-mail:* Dawn.Kilts@liu.edu.

GRADUATE PROGRAMS

Expenses (2006–07) *Tuition:* full-time $8480; part-time $790 per credit. *International tuition:* $8480 full-time. *Room and board:* $9000 per academic year. *Required fees:* full-time $1500; part-time $250 per credit; part-time $400 per term.

Financial Aid 75% of graduate students in nursing programs received some form of financial aid in 2005–06. Scholarships and unspecified assistantships available. Aid available to part-time students.

Contact Prof. Susanne Flower, Director, School of Nursing, Long Island University, Brooklyn Campus, 1 University Plaza, Brooklyn, NY 11201. *Telephone:* 718-488-1059. *Fax:* 718-780-4019. *E-mail:* Susanne.Flower@liu.edu.

Long Island University, Brooklyn Campus (continued)

MASTER'S DEGREE PROGRAM

Degree MS

Available Programs Master's; RN to Master's.

Concentrations Available Nursing administration; nursing education. *Nurse practitioner programs in:* adult health, family health, gerontology.

Study Options Full-time and part-time.

Program Entrance Requirements Clinical experience, minimum overall college GPA of 3.0, transcript of college record, immunizations, interview, 3 letters of recommendation, nursing research course, physical assessment course, professional liability insurance/malpractice insurance, prerequisite course work, resume, statistics course. *Application deadline:* Applications are processed on a rolling basis. *Application fee:* $30.

Degree Requirements 43 total credit hours, thesis or project.

POST-MASTER'S PROGRAM

Areas of Study *Nurse practitioner programs in:* adult health, family health, gerontology.

See full description on page 506.

Long Island University, C.W. Post Campus

Department of Nursing
Brookville, New York

http://www.cwpost.liu.edu/cwis/cwp/health/ nursing

Founded in 1954

DEGREES • BS • MS

Nursing Program Faculty 11 (55% with doctorates).

Baccalaureate Enrollment 101
Women 96% **Men** 4% **Minority** 12% **International** 6% **Part-time** 100%

Graduate Enrollment 53
Women 94% **Men** 6% **Minority** 23% **International** 11% **Part-time** 100%

Nursing Student Activities Student Nurses' Association.

Nursing Student Resources Academic advising; academic or career counseling; assistance for students with disabilities; bookstore; campus computer network; career placement assistance; computer lab; computer-assisted instruction; e-mail services; employment services for current students; housing assistance; interactive nursing skills videos; Internet; library services; nursing audiovisuals; placement services for program completers; remedial services; resume preparation assistance; skills, simulation, or other laboratory; tutoring.

Library Facilities 20,000 volumes in health, 15,000 volumes in nursing; 3,100 periodical subscriptions health-care related.

BACCALAUREATE PROGRAMS

Degree BS

Available Programs RN Baccalaureate.

Site Options Manhasset, NY.

Study Options Part-time.

Program Entrance Requirements Minimum overall college GPA of 2.5, transcript of college record, health exam, health insurance, immunizations, minimum GPA in nursing prerequisites of 2.5, professional liability insurance/malpractice insurance, prerequisite course work, RN licensure. Transfer students are accepted. **Standardized tests** *Required:* SAT or ACT, TOEFL for international students. **Application** *Deadline:* rolling (freshmen), rolling (transfer). *Notification:* continuous (freshmen). *Application fee:* $30.

Advanced Placement Credit by examination available. Credit given for nursing courses completed elsewhere dependent upon specific evaluations.

Expenses (2006–07) *Tuition:* full-time $10,498; part-time $729 per credit. *International tuition:* $10,498 full-time. *Room and board:* $7643; room only: $6020 per academic year. *Required fees:* part-time $105 per credit; part-time $500 per term.

Financial Aid 10% of baccalaureate students in nursing programs received some form of financial aid in 2005–06.

Contact Dr. Minna Kapp, Chair, Department of Nursing, Long Island University, C.W. Post Campus, Life Science/Room 270, 720 Northern Boulevard, Brookville, NY 11548-1300. *Telephone:* 516-299-2320. *Fax:* 516-299-2352. *E-mail:* minna.kapp@liu.edu.

GRADUATE PROGRAMS

Expenses (2006–07) *Tuition:* full-time $12,113; part-time $790 per credit. *International tuition:* $12,113 full-time. *Room and board:* $7643; room only: $6020 per academic year. *Required fees:* part-time $105 per credit; part-time $500 per term.

Financial Aid 10% of graduate students in nursing programs received some form of financial aid in 2005–06. Federal Work-Study and unspecified assistantships available. Aid available to part-time students. *Financial aid application deadline:* 5/15.

Contact Dr. Minna Kapp, Chair, Department of Nursing, Long Island University, C.W. Post Campus, Life Science/Room 270, 720 Northern Boulevard, Brookville, NY 11548-1300. *Telephone:* 516-299-2320. *Fax:* 516-299-2352. *E-mail:* minna.kapp@liu.edu.

MASTER'S DEGREE PROGRAM

Degree MS

Available Programs Master's; Master's for Nurses with Non-Nursing Degrees.

Concentrations Available Nursing education. *Clinical nurse specialist programs in:* adult health, medical-surgical, parent-child. *Nurse practitioner programs in:* family health.

Site Options Manhasset, NY.

Study Options Part-time.

Program Entrance Requirements Clinical experience, minimum overall college GPA of 3.0, transcript of college record, written essay, immunizations, interview, 2 letters of recommendation, physical assessment course, professional liability insurance/malpractice insurance, prerequisite course work. *Application deadline:* Applications are processed on a rolling basis. *Application fee:* $30.

Degree Requirements 46 total credit hours.

POST-MASTER'S PROGRAM

Areas of Study Nursing education. *Nurse practitioner programs in:* family health.

Medgar Evers College of the City University of New York

Department of Nursing
Brooklyn, New York

http://www.mec.cuny.edu/academic_affairs/ science_tech_school/nursing/nurse_home.htm

Founded in 1969

DEGREE • BSN

Nursing Program Faculty 7 (85% with doctorates).

Baccalaureate Enrollment 60
Women 98% **Men** 2% **Minority** 99% **Part-time** 90%

Nursing Student Activities Student Nurses' Association, nursing club.

Nursing Student Resources Academic advising; academic or career counseling; assistance for students with disabilities; bookstore; campus computer network; computer lab; computer-assisted instruction; daycare for children of students; e-mail services; interactive nursing skills videos; Internet; learning resource lab; library services; nursing audiovisuals; remedial services; resume preparation assistance; skills, simulation, or other laboratory; tutoring; unpaid internships.

Library Facilities 111,000 volumes; 24,410 periodical subscriptions.

BACCALAUREATE PROGRAMS

Degree BSN

Available Programs ADN to Baccalaureate; Accelerated RN Baccalaureate.

Study Options Full-time and part-time.

Program Entrance Requirements Minimum overall college GPA of 2.5, transcript of college record, CPR certification, health exam, health insurance, immunizations, professional liability insurance/malpractice insurance, prerequisite course work, RN licensure. Transfer students are accepted. **Standardized tests** *Required:* TOEFL for international students. *Recommended:* SAT and SAT Subject Tests or ACT. **Application** *Deadline:* rolling (freshmen), rolling (transfer). *Notification:* continuous (freshmen). *Application fee:* $60.

Advanced Placement Credit given for nursing courses completed elsewhere dependent upon specific evaluations.

Expenses (2006–07) *Tuition, state resident:* part-time $170 per credit. *Tuition, nonresident:* part-time $230 per credit. *Required fees:* full-time $340; part-time $340 per term.

Financial Aid *Gift aid (need-based):* Federal Pell, FSEOG, state, private, college/university gift aid from institutional funds. *Loans:* Federal Direct (Subsidized and Unsubsidized Stafford PLUS), FFEL (Subsidized and Unsubsidized Stafford PLUS), Perkins. *Work-Study:* Federal Work-Study. *Application deadline (priority):* 4/1.

Contact Dr. Eileen McCarroll, Chair, Department of Nursing BSN, Department of Nursing, Medgar Evers College of the City University of New York, 1150 Carroll Street, Room M-20, Brooklyn, NY 11225. *Telephone:* 718-270-6230. *Fax:* 718-270-6235. *E-mail:* emccarroll@mec.cuny.edu.

Mercy College
Program in Nursing
Dobbs Ferry, New York

Founded in 1951

DEGREES • BS • MS

Nursing Program Faculty 12.

Baccalaureate Enrollment 200
Women 96% **Men** 4% **Minority** 75% **International** 1% **Part-time** 88%

Graduate Enrollment 100
Women 99% **Men** 1% **Minority** 50% **International** 10% **Part-time** 75%

Nursing Student Activities Sigma Theta Tau, Student Nurses' Association.

Nursing Student Resources Academic advising; academic or career counseling; assistance for students with disabilities; bookstore; campus computer network; career placement assistance; computer lab; computer-assisted instruction; e-mail services; employment services for current students; Internet; learning resource lab; library services; nursing audiovisuals; remedial services; resume preparation assistance; skills, simulation, or other laboratory; tutoring.

Library Facilities 322,610 volumes (10,000 in health, 550 in nursing); 1,765 periodical subscriptions (180 health-care related).

BACCALAUREATE PROGRAMS

Degree BS

Available Programs Accelerated RN Baccalaureate; RN Baccalaureate.

Site Options *Distance Learning:* Manhattan, NY; Dobbs Ferry, NY.

Study Options Full-time and part-time.

Program Entrance Requirements Transfer students are accepted. **Standardized tests** *Recommended:* SAT, TOEFL for international students. **Application** *Deadline:* rolling (freshmen), rolling (transfer). *Notification:* continuous (freshmen). *Application fee:* $37.

Expenses (2006–07) *Tuition:* part-time $520 per credit.

Financial Aid 10% of baccalaureate students in nursing programs received some form of financial aid in 2005–06.

Contact Dr. Mary McGuinness, Director, Program in Nursing, Mercy College, 555 Broadway, Dobbs Ferry, NY 10522. *Telephone:* 914-674-7862. *Fax:* 914-674-7623. *E-mail:* mmcguiness@mercy.edu.

GRADUATE PROGRAMS

Expenses (2006–07) *Tuition:* part-time $630 per credit.

Financial Aid 75% of graduate students in nursing programs received some form of financial aid in 2005–06. Career-related internships or fieldwork, Federal Work-Study, and institutionally sponsored loans available. Aid available to part-time students.

Contact Prof. Miriam Ford, RN, Associate Director, Program in Nursing, Mercy College, 555 Broadway, Dobbs Ferry, NY 10522. *Telephone:* 914-674-7867. *Fax:* 914-674-7623. *E-mail:* mford@mercy.edu.

MASTER'S DEGREE PROGRAM

Degree MS

Available Programs Accelerated Master's for Non-Nursing College Graduates; Accelerated Master's for Nurses with Non-Nursing Degrees; Master's; Master's for Non-Nursing College Graduates; Master's for Nurses with Non-Nursing Degrees.

Concentrations Available Health-care administration; nursing administration; nursing education.

Site Options *Distance Learning:* Dobbs Ferry, NY.

Study Options Full-time and part-time.

Program Entrance Requirements Clinical experience, minimum overall college GPA of 3.0, transcript of college record, written essay, immunizations, interview, 2 letters of recommendation, professional liability insurance/malpractice insurance, resume, GRE General Test or MAT. *Application deadline:* For fall admission, 8/15 (priority date); for spring admission, 2/15. Applications are processed on a rolling basis. *Application fee:* $62.

Advanced Placement Credit given for nursing courses completed elsewhere dependent upon specific evaluations.

Degree Requirements 36 total credit hours, thesis or project.

POST-MASTER'S PROGRAM

Areas of Study Nursing administration; nursing education.

CONTINUING EDUCATION PROGRAM

Contact Prof. Miriam Ford, RN, Associate Director, Program in Nursing, Mercy College, 555 Broadway, Dobbs Ferry, NY 10522. *Telephone:* 914-674-7867. *Fax:* 914-674-7623. *E-mail:* mford@mercy.edu.

Molloy College
Department of Nursing
Rockville Centre, New York

Founded in 1955

DEGREES • BS • MS

Nursing Program Faculty 111.

Nursing Student Activities Sigma Theta Tau, Student Nurses' Association.

Nursing Student Resources Academic advising; academic or career counseling; assistance for students with disabilities; bookstore; campus computer network; computer lab; computer-assisted instruction; e-mail services; interactive nursing skills videos; Internet; learning resource lab; library services; nursing audiovisuals; tutoring.

Library Facilities 135,000 volumes.

■ Undergraduate programs in nursing are designed to prepare the nurse generalist for practice in a variety of health-care settings. Eligible students may pursue one of the following options: baccalaureate degree in nursing, registered nurse baccalaureate completion program, LPN degree completion, and dual-degree programs for both second-degree students and registered nurse students. The Master of Science degree program combines academic, clinical, and research activities that educate graduate nurses for advanced clinical practice and role functions. Preparation as adult, pediatric, psychiatric, and family nurse practitioner is offered in both the master's and post-master's certificate programs. In addition, the post-master's program is available for role functions in education or administration.

Molloy College (continued)

BACCALAUREATE PROGRAMS

Degree BS

Available Programs Accelerated RN Baccalaureate; Baccalaureate for Second Degree; Generic Baccalaureate; LPN to Baccalaureate; RN Baccalaureate.

Site Options Plainview, NY; New Hyde Park, NY.

Study Options Full-time and part-time.

Program Entrance Requirements Minimum overall college GPA of 3.0, transcript of college record, written essay, high school biology, high school chemistry, 3 years high school math, high school transcript, immunizations, minimum high school GPA of 3.0, minimum high school rank 40%. Transfer students are accepted. **Standardized tests** *Required:* SAT or ACT, TOEFL for international students. **Application** *Deadline:* rolling (freshmen), rolling (transfer). *Early decision:* 11/1. *Notification:* continuous (freshmen), 12/1 (out-of-state freshmen), 12/1 (early decision). *Application fee:* $30.

Advanced Placement Credit given for nursing courses completed elsewhere dependent upon specific evaluations.

Expenses (2006–07) *Tuition:* full-time $16,560; part-time $550 per credit. *Required fees:* full-time $1035; part-time $75 per credit.

Contact Marguerite Lane, Director of Admissions, Department of Nursing, Molloy College, 1000 Hempstead Avenue, PO Box 5002, Rockville Centre, NY 11571-5002. *Telephone:* 516-678-5000 Ext. 6233. *E-mail:* mlane@molloy.edu.

GRADUATE PROGRAMS

Expenses (2006–07) *Tuition:* part-time $635 per credit. *Required fees:* part-time $75 per credit.

Financial Aid 1 research assistantship was awarded; teaching assistantships, institutionally sponsored loans, scholarships, and unspecified assistantships also available.

Contact Dr. Jeannine Muldoon, Associate Dean, Graduate Program, Department of Nursing, Molloy College, 1000 Hempstead Avenue, PO Box 5002, Rockville Centre, NY 11571-5002. *Telephone:* 516-678-5000 Ext. 6310. *E-mail:* jmuldoon@molloy.edu.

MASTER'S DEGREE PROGRAM

Degree MS

Available Programs Master's.

Concentrations Available Nursing administration; nursing education; nursing informatics. *Clinical nurse specialist programs in:* adult health. *Nurse practitioner programs in:* adult health, family health, pediatric, psychiatric/mental health.

Site Options Farmingdale, NY; Plainview, NY; New Hyde Park, NY.

Study Options Full-time and part-time.

Program Entrance Requirements Clinical experience, minimum overall college GPA of 3.0, transcript of college record, written essay, interview, 3 letters of recommendation, nursing research course, prerequisite course work, statistics course. *Application deadline:* For fall admission, 9/2 (priority date); for spring admission, 1/20 (priority date). Applications are processed on a rolling basis. *Application fee:* $60.

Degree Requirements 49 total credit hours, thesis or project.

POST-MASTER'S PROGRAM

Areas of Study Nursing administration; nursing education; nursing informatics. *Clinical nurse specialist programs in:* adult health. *Nurse practitioner programs in:* adult health, family health, pediatric, psychiatric/mental health.

CONTINUING EDUCATION PROGRAM

Contact Anna Jansson, RN, Associate Director, Continuing Education, Department of Nursing, Molloy College, 1000 Hempstead Avenue, Rockville Centre, NY 11570. *Telephone:* 516-678-5000 Ext. 6106. *Fax:* 516-678-7295. *E-mail:* ajansson@molloy.edu.

Mount Saint Mary College
Division of Nursing
Newburgh, New York

Founded in 1960

DEGREES • BSN • MS

Nursing Program Faculty 36 (50% with doctorates).

Nursing Student Activities Sigma Theta Tau, Student Nurses' Association, nursing club.

Nursing Student Resources Academic advising; academic or career counseling; assistance for students with disabilities; bookstore; campus computer network; career placement assistance; computer lab; computer-assisted instruction; e-mail services; employment services for current students; externships; housing assistance; interactive nursing skills videos; Internet; learning resource lab; library services; nursing audiovisuals; paid internships; remedial services; resume preparation assistance; skills, simulation, or other laboratory; tutoring.

Library Facilities 118,207 volumes (2,443 in health, 1,723 in nursing); 317 periodical subscriptions (114 health-care related).

BACCALAUREATE PROGRAMS

Degree BSN

Available Programs Accelerated Baccalaureate; Accelerated RN Baccalaureate; Generic Baccalaureate; RN Baccalaureate.

Study Options Full-time and part-time.

Program Entrance Requirements Minimum overall college GPA of 2.75, transcript of college record, CPR certification, health exam, high school biology, high school chemistry, 3 years high school math, high school transcript, immunizations, interview. Transfer students are accepted. **Standardized tests** *Required:* SAT or ACT, TOEFL for international students. **Application** *Deadline:* rolling (freshmen), rolling (transfer). *Notification:* continuous (freshmen). *Application fee:* $35.

Advanced Placement Credit by examination available. Credit given for nursing courses completed elsewhere dependent upon specific evaluations.

Expenses (2006–07) *Tuition:* full-time $17,730; part-time $591 per credit hour. *Room and board:* $9646; room only: $5650 per academic year. *Required fees:* full-time $780.

Contact J. Randall Ognibene, Director, Admissions, Division of Nursing, Mount Saint Mary College, 330 Powell Avenue, Newburgh, NY 12550. *Telephone:* 845-569-3248. *Fax:* 845-562-6762. *E-mail:* admissions@msmc.edu.

GRADUATE PROGRAMS

Expenses (2006–07) *Tuition:* full-time $15,840; part-time $660 per credit. *Required fees:* full-time $130.

Financial Aid 100% of graduate students in nursing programs received some form of financial aid in 2005–06. Unspecified assistantships and nursing lab assistant available. *Financial aid application deadline:* 3/15.

Contact Dr. Karen Baldwin, Associate Professor and Coordinator, Graduate Nursing Program, Division of Nursing, Mount Saint Mary College, 330 Powell Avenue, Newburgh, NY 12550. *Telephone:* 845-569-3138. *Fax:* 845-569-3360. *E-mail:* Baldwin@msmc.edu.

MASTER'S DEGREE PROGRAM

Degree MS

Available Programs Master's.

Concentrations Available *Clinical nurse specialist programs in:* adult health. *Nurse practitioner programs in:* adult health.

Study Options Full-time and part-time.

Program Entrance Requirements Clinical experience, computer literacy, minimum overall college GPA of 3.0, transcript of college record, written essay, immunizations, interview, 3 letters of recommendation, nursing research course, physical assessment course, professional liability insurance/malpractice insurance, resume, statistics course. *Application deadline:* For fall admission, 6/3 (priority date); for spring admission, 10/31 (priority date). Applications are processed on a rolling basis. *Application fee:* $35.

Degree Requirements 42 total credit hours, thesis or project.

POST-MASTER'S PROGRAM

Areas of Study Nursing administration; nursing education.

See full description on page 518.

Nazareth College of Rochester
Department of Nursing
Rochester, New York

http://www.naz.edu
Founded in 1924
DEGREES • BS • MS

Nursing Program Faculty 20 (30% with doctorates).
Baccalaureate Enrollment 173
Women 92% **Men** 8% **Minority** 11% **Part-time** 22%
Graduate Enrollment 20
Women 95% **Men** 5% **Minority** 10% **Part-time** 90%
Nursing Student Activities Nursing Honor Society, Sigma Theta Tau, nursing club.
Nursing Student Resources Academic advising; academic or career counseling; assistance for students with disabilities; bookstore; campus computer network; career placement assistance; computer lab; computer-assisted instruction; daycare for children of students; e-mail services; employment services for current students; externships; housing assistance; interactive nursing skills videos; Internet; learning resource lab; library services; nursing audiovisuals; resume preparation assistance; skills, simulation, or other laboratory; tutoring.
Library Facilities 162,593 volumes; 1,888 periodical subscriptions.

■ Nazareth College in Rochester, New York, offers a four-year B.S. in nursing, an RN-B.S., and an LPN-B.S. program. At the graduate level, Nazareth College offers a Gerontological Nurse Practitioner (GNP) program, a post-master's certificate GNP, and a post-master's certificate in nursing education. The mission of the Department of Nursing is to educate students in the profession within a transcultural context and to advance students' abilities to integrate the liberal arts and sciences within the discipline. The faculty members are committed to preparing students for culturally competent nursing practice, leadership in service to the community, and commitment to a life informed by intellectual, ethical, and aesthetic values.

BACCALAUREATE PROGRAMS
Degree BS
Available Programs Generic Baccalaureate; LPN to Baccalaureate; RN Baccalaureate.
Site Options *Distance Learning:* Geneva, NY; Rochester, NY.
Study Options Full-time and part-time.
Program Entrance Requirements Minimum overall college GPA of 2.5, transcript of college record, written essay, health exam, high school chemistry, high school transcript, immunizations, minimum high school GPA of 2.5, minimum GPA in nursing prerequisites of 2.5, prerequisite course work. Transfer students are accepted. **Standardized tests** *Required:* SAT or ACT, TOEFL for international students. **Application** *Deadline:* 2/15 (freshmen), 5/15 (transfer). *Early decision:* 11/15, 12/15. *Notification:* continuous (freshmen), 12/15 (out-of-state freshmen), 12/15 (early decision), 1/15 (early action). *Application fee:* $40.
Advanced Placement Credit by examination available. Credit given for nursing courses completed elsewhere dependent upon specific evaluations.
Expenses (2006–07) *Tuition:* full-time $20,656; part-time $493 per credit. *International tuition:* $20,656 full-time. *Room and board:* $8160; room only: $4960 per academic year. *Required fees:* full-time $502; part-time $35 per credit; part-time $435 per term.
Financial Aid 95% of baccalaureate students in nursing programs received some form of financial aid in 2005–06. *Gift aid (need-based):* Federal Pell, FSEOG, state, private, college/university gift aid from institutional funds. *Loans:* FFEL (Subsidized and Unsubsidized Stafford PLUS), Perkins. *Work-Study:* Federal Work-Study. *Application deadline:* 5/1 (priority: 2/15).
Contact Admissions Office, Department of Nursing, Nazareth College of Rochester, 4245 East Avenue, Rochester, NY 14618-3790. *Telephone:* 585-389-2865. *E-mail:* admissions@naz.edu.

GRADUATE PROGRAMS
Expenses (2006–07) *Tuition:* full-time $10,620; part-time $590 per credit. *International tuition:* $10,620 full-time. *Room and board:* $8980; room only: $5960 per academic year. *Required fees:* full-time $315; part-time $35 per credit; part-time $35 per term.
Financial Aid 100% of graduate students in nursing programs received some form of financial aid in 2005–06. Research assistantships with partial tuition reimbursements available, career-related internships or fieldwork available. Aid available to part-time students.
Contact Dr. Linda M. Janelli, Director, Masters Nursing Program, Department of Nursing, Nazareth College of Rochester, 4245 East Avenue, Rochester, NY 14618-3790. *Telephone:* 585-389-2713. *Fax:* 585-389-2714. *E-mail:* lmjanell@naz.edu.

MASTER'S DEGREE PROGRAM
Degree MS
Available Programs Master's.
Concentrations Available *Nurse practitioner programs in:* gerontology.
Site Options *Distance Learning:* Rochester, NY.
Study Options Full-time and part-time.
Program Entrance Requirements Minimum overall college GPA of 3.0, transcript of college record, written essay, immunizations, interview, 2 letters of recommendation, physical assessment course, statistics course. *Application deadline:* For fall admission, 4/1 (priority date); for spring admission, 10/1. Applications are processed on a rolling basis. *Application fee:* $40.
Advanced Placement Credit given for nursing courses completed elsewhere dependent upon specific evaluations.
Degree Requirements 42 total credit hours, thesis or project.

POST-MASTER'S PROGRAM
Areas of Study Nursing education. *Nurse practitioner programs in:* gerontology.

CONTINUING EDUCATION PROGRAM
Contact Mrs. Helene Lovett, Secretary, Department of Nursing, Nazareth College of Rochester, 4245 East Avenue, Rochester, NY 14618-3790. *Telephone:* 585-389-2709. *Fax:* 585-389-2714. *E-mail:* hlovett8@naz.edu.

New York University
College of Nursing
New York, New York

http://www.nyu.edu/education/nursing
Founded in 1831
DEGREES • BS • MA • MS/MA • PHD

Nursing Program Faculty 25 (75% with doctorates).
Baccalaureate Enrollment 514
Women 94% **Men** 6% **Minority** 38% **International** 2% **Part-time** 20%
Graduate Enrollment 461
Women 95% **Men** 5% **Minority** 35% **International** 3% **Part-time** 95%
Nursing Student Activities Sigma Theta Tau, Student Nurses' Association, nursing club.
Nursing Student Resources Academic advising; academic or career counseling; assistance for students with disabilities; bookstore; campus computer network; computer lab; computer-assisted instruction; e-mail services; employment services for current students; housing assistance; interactive nursing skills videos; Internet; learning resource lab; library services; nursing audiovisuals; resume preparation assistance; skills, simulation, or other laboratory; tutoring.
Library Facilities 5.2 million volumes (102,448 in health, 62,781 in nursing); 48,958 periodical subscriptions (4,658 health-care related).

BACCALAUREATE PROGRAMS
Degree BS

New York University (continued)

Available Programs Accelerated Baccalaureate; Accelerated Baccalaureate for Second Degree; Baccalaureate for Second Degree; Generic Baccalaureate; RN Baccalaureate.

Study Options Full-time and part-time.

Program Entrance Requirements Transcript of college record, written essay, health exam, high school biology, high school chemistry, 3 years high school math, 3 years high school science, high school transcript, immunizations, 2 letters of recommendation, minimum high school GPA of 2.8. Transfer students are accepted. **Standardized tests** *Required:* SAT or ACT, TOEFL for international students. *Recommended:* SAT Subject Tests. *Required for some:* SAT Subject Tests. **Application** *Deadline:* 1/15 (freshmen), 4/1 (transfer). *Early decision:* 11/1. *Notification:* 4/1 (freshmen), 12/15 (out-of-state freshmen), 12/15 (early decision). *Application fee:* $65.

Advanced Placement Credit by examination available. Credit given for nursing courses completed elsewhere dependent upon specific evaluations.

Financial Aid 79% of baccalaureate students in nursing programs received some form of financial aid in 2004–05. *Gift aid (need-based):* Federal Pell, FSEOG, state, private, college/university gift aid from institutional funds. *Loans:* Federal Nursing Student Loans, FFEL (Subsidized and Unsubsidized Stafford PLUS), Perkins. *Work-Study:* Federal Work-Study. *Application deadline (priority):* 2/15.

Contact Ms. Temi S. Pedro, Undergraduate Recruitment Coordinator, College of Nursing, New York University, 246 Greene Street, New York, NY 10003-6677. *Telephone:* 212-998-5336. *Fax:* 212-995-4302. *E-mail:* tp18@nyu.edu.

GRADUATE PROGRAMS

Financial Aid 30% of graduate students in nursing programs received some form of financial aid in 2004–05. 2 research assistantships with full and partial tuition reimbursements available were awarded; fellowships with full and partial tuition reimbursements available, career-related internships or fieldwork, Federal Work-Study, institutionally sponsored loans, scholarships, and tuition waivers (partial) also available. Aid available to part-time students. *Financial aid application deadline:* 2/1.

Contact Mrs. Vida Samuel-Wheeler, Graduate and Doctoral Recruitment Coordinator, College of Nursing, New York University, 246 Greene Street, New York, NY 10003-6677. *Telephone:* 212-992-9418. *Fax:* 212-995-4302. *E-mail:* nursing.programs@nyu.edu.

MASTER'S DEGREE PROGRAM

Degrees MA; MS/MA

Available Programs Master's; RN to Master's.

Concentrations Available Nurse-midwifery; nursing administration; nursing education; nursing informatics. *Clinical nurse specialist programs in:* acute care, adult health, critical care, gerontology, home health care, pediatric, psychiatric/mental health. *Nurse practitioner programs in:* acute care, adult health, gerontology, pediatric, primary care, psychiatric/mental health.

Study Options Full-time and part-time.

Program Entrance Requirements Minimum overall college GPA of 3.0, transcript of college record, written essay, 2 letters of recommendation, resume, statistics course. *Application deadline:* For fall admission, 1/15 (priority date); for spring admission, 11/1. Applications are processed on a rolling basis. *Application fee:* $50 ($60 for international students).

Advanced Placement Credit given for nursing courses completed elsewhere dependent upon specific evaluations.

Degree Requirements Comprehensive exam.

POST-MASTER'S PROGRAM

Areas of Study Nurse-midwifery; nursing administration; nursing education; nursing informatics. *Clinical nurse specialist programs in:* acute care, adult health, critical care, gerontology, home health care, pediatric, psychiatric/mental health. *Nurse practitioner programs in:* acute care, adult health, gerontology, pediatric, primary care, psychiatric/mental health.

DOCTORAL DEGREE PROGRAM

Degree PhD

Available Programs Doctorate.

Areas of Study Nursing research.

Program Entrance Requirements Minimum overall college GPA of 3.0, interview, 3 letters of recommendation, MSN or equivalent, vita, writing sample, GRE General Test. *Application deadline:* For fall admission, 1/15 (priority date); for spring admission, 11/1. Applications are processed on a rolling basis. *Application fee:* $50 ($60 for international students).

Degree Requirements Dissertation, oral exam.

CONTINUING EDUCATION PROGRAM

Contact Dr. Hila Richardson, Continuing Education Director, College of Nursing, New York University, 246 Greene Street, New York, NY 10003-6677. *Telephone:* 212-998-5329. *E-mail:* nursing.programs@nyu.edu.

See full description on page 520.

Pace University
Lienhard School of Nursing
New York, New York

http://appserv.pace.edu/execute/page.cfm?doc_id=558

Founded in 1906

DEGREES • BS • MS

Nursing Program Faculty 71 (30% with doctorates).

Baccalaureate Enrollment 511
Women 88% **Men** 12% **Minority** 43% **International** 2% **Part-time** 22%

Graduate Enrollment 191
Women 91% **Men** 9% **Minority** 50% **International** 3% **Part-time** 90%

Nursing Student Activities Nursing Honor Society, Sigma Theta Tau, Student Nurses' Association.

Nursing Student Resources Academic advising; academic or career counseling; assistance for students with disabilities; bookstore; campus computer network; career placement assistance; computer lab; computer-assisted instruction; e-mail services; employment services for current students; housing assistance; interactive nursing skills videos; Internet; learning resource lab; library services; nursing audiovisuals; placement services for program completers; resume preparation assistance; skills, simulation, or other laboratory.

Library Facilities 824,533 volumes (4,025 in health, 2,585 in nursing); 4,151 periodical subscriptions (190 health-care related).

BACCALAUREATE PROGRAMS

Degree BS

Available Programs Accelerated Baccalaureate for Second Degree; Accelerated RN Baccalaureate; Generic Baccalaureate; RN Baccalaureate.

Site Options *Distance Learning:* Pleasantville, NY.

Study Options Full-time and part-time.

Program Entrance Requirements Transcript of college record, CPR certification, written essay, health exam, health insurance, high school biology, high school chemistry, high school foreign language, 4 years high school math, 2 years high school science, high school transcript, immunizations, 2 letters of recommendation, minimum GPA in nursing prerequisites of 2.75. Transfer students are accepted. **Standardized tests** *Required:* SAT or ACT, TOEFL for international students. **Application** *Deadline:* 3/1 (freshmen), rolling (transfer). *Early decision:* 11/1. *Notification:* continuous (freshmen), 12/15 (early action). *Application fee:* $45.

Advanced Placement Credit by examination available. Credit given for nursing courses completed elsewhere dependent upon specific evaluations.

Expenses (2006–07) *Tuition:* full-time $29,454; part-time $845 per credit. *International tuition:* $29,454 full-time. *Room and board:* $9570 per academic year. *Required fees:* full-time $632.

Financial Aid 79% of baccalaureate students in nursing programs received some form of financial aid in 2005–06.

Contact Dr. Donna Hallas, Chairperson, Lienhard School of Nursing, Pace University, 861 Bedford Road, Pleasantville, NY 10570. *Telephone:* 914-773-3323. *Fax:* 914-773-3345. *E-mail:* dhallas@pace.edu.

GRADUATE PROGRAMS

Expenses (2006–07) *Tuition:* part-time $734 per credit. *Room and board:* $9570 per academic year. *Required fees:* full-time $480.

Financial Aid 29% of graduate students in nursing programs received some form of financial aid in 2005–06. Research assistantships, career-related internships or fieldwork, Federal Work-Study, and tuition waivers (partial) available. Aid available to part-time students.

Contact Dr. Marie Truglio-Londrigan, Chairperson, Lienhard School of Nursing, Pace University, 861 Bedford Road, Pleasantville, NY 10570. *Telephone:* 914-773-3709. *Fax:* 914-773-3345. *E-mail:* mlondrigan@pace.edu.

MASTER'S DEGREE PROGRAM

Degree MS

Available Programs Accelerated AD/RN to Master's; Accelerated RN to Master's; Master's; Master's for Nurses with Non-Nursing Degrees; RN to Master's.

Concentrations Available Nursing administration; nursing education; nursing informatics. *Nurse practitioner programs in:* family health, women's health.

Site Options *Distance Learning:* Pleasantville, NY.

Study Options Full-time and part-time.

Program Entrance Requirements Computer literacy, minimum overall college GPA of 3.0, transcript of college record, CPR certification, immunizations, 2 letters of recommendation, nursing research course, professional liability insurance/malpractice insurance, resume, statistics course, GRE General Test or MAT. *Application deadline:* For fall admission, 7/31 (priority date); for spring admission, 11/30. Applications are processed on a rolling basis. *Application fee:* $65.

Advanced Placement Credit by examination available. Credit given for nursing courses completed elsewhere dependent upon specific evaluations.

Degree Requirements 42 total credit hours, comprehensive exam.

POST-MASTER'S PROGRAM

Areas of Study Nursing administration; nursing education; nursing informatics. *Nurse practitioner programs in:* family health.

CONTINUING EDUCATION PROGRAM

Contact Director, Lienhard School of Nursing, Pace University, 861 Bedford Road, Pleasantville, NY 10570. *Telephone:* 914-773-3358. *Fax:* 914-773-3376. *E-mail:* cenurse@pace.edu.

Roberts Wesleyan College
Division of Nursing
Rochester, New York

http://www.roberts.edu/Nursing/

Founded in 1866

DEGREES • BSCN • M SC N

Nursing Program Faculty 13 (31% with doctorates).

Baccalaureate Enrollment 207
Women 90% **Men** 10% **Minority** 5%

Graduate Enrollment 19
Women 100% **Minority** 10%

Nursing Student Activities Sigma Theta Tau, nursing club.

Nursing Student Resources Academic advising; academic or career counseling; assistance for students with disabilities; bookstore; campus computer network; career placement assistance; computer lab; computer-assisted instruction; e-mail services; employment services for current students; externships; housing assistance; interactive nursing skills videos; Internet; learning resource lab; library services; nursing audiovisuals; placement services for program completers; remedial services; resume preparation assistance; skills, simulation, or other laboratory; tutoring.

Library Facilities 123,434 volumes (6,749 in health, 1,850 in nursing); 1,057 periodical subscriptions (1,750 health-care related).

BACCALAUREATE PROGRAMS

Degree BScN

Available Programs Accelerated RN Baccalaureate; Generic Baccalaureate; RN Baccalaureate.

Site Options Weedsport, NY; Buffalo, NY; Dansville, NY.

Study Options Full-time and part-time.

Program Entrance Requirements Minimum overall college GPA of 2.5, transcript of college record, CPR certification, written essay, health exam, health insurance, high school biology, high school chemistry, high school transcript, immunizations, 2 letters of recommendation, minimum high school GPA of 2.8, minimum GPA in nursing prerequisites of 2.5, prerequisite course work. Transfer students are accepted. **Standardized tests** *Required:* SAT or ACT, TOEFL for international students. **Application** *Deadline:* 2/1 (freshmen), rolling (transfer). *Application fee:* $35.

Advanced Placement Credit by examination available. Credit given for nursing courses completed elsewhere dependent upon specific evaluations.

Expenses (2006–07) *Tuition:* full-time $19,264; part-time $422 per credit hour. *International tuition:* $19,264 full-time. *Room and board:* $7448; room only: $5280 per academic year. *Required fees:* full-time $250.

Financial Aid 91% of baccalaureate students in nursing programs received some form of financial aid in 2005–06. *Gift aid (need-based):* Federal Pell, FSEOG, state, private, college/university gift aid from institutional funds. *Loans:* FFEL (Subsidized and Unsubsidized Stafford PLUS), Perkins. *Work-Study:* Federal Work-Study, part-time campus jobs. *Application deadline (priority):* 3/15.

Contact Mr. Kirk Kettinger, Director of Admissions, Division of Nursing, Roberts Wesleyan College, Office of Admissions, 2301 Westside Drive, Rochester, NY 14624. *Telephone:* 585-594-6400. *Fax:* 585-549-6371. *E-mail:* admissions@roberts.edu.

GRADUATE PROGRAMS

Expenses (2006–07) *Tuition:* full-time $25,610. *International tuition:* $25,610 full-time.

Financial Aid 91% of graduate students in nursing programs received some form of financial aid in 2005–06.

Contact Laurie J. DeSormeau, Assistant to the Chairperson of Division, Division of Nursing, Roberts Wesleyan College, 2301 Westside Drive, Rochester, NY 14624. *Telephone:* 585-594-6686. *Fax:* 585-594-6593. *E-mail:* desormeau_laurie@roberts.edu.

MASTER'S DEGREE PROGRAM

Degree M Sc N

Available Programs Accelerated Master's; Master's for Nurses with Non-Nursing Degrees.

Concentrations Available Nursing administration.

Study Options Part-time.

Program Entrance Requirements Clinical experience, computer literacy, minimum overall college GPA of 3.0, transcript of college record, written essay, immunizations, interview, 2 letters of recommendation, nursing research course, prerequisite course work, resume, statistics course.

Advanced Placement Credit given for nursing courses completed elsewhere dependent upon specific evaluations.

Degree Requirements 39 total credit hours, thesis or project.

CONTINUING EDUCATION PROGRAM

Contact Dr. Susanne M. Mohnkern, RN, Chairperson and Professor, Division of Nursing, Division of Nursing, Roberts Wesleyan College, 2301 Westside Drive, Rochester, NY 14624-1997. *Telephone:* 585-594-6686. *Fax:* 585-594-6599. *E-mail:* mohnkerns@roberts.edu.

The Sage Colleges
Division of Nursing
Troy, New York

http://www.sage.edu/departments/nur

DEGREES • BS • MS • MS/MBA

Nursing Student Resources Library services.

The Sage Colleges (continued)

Library Facilities 4,003 volumes in health, 2,516 volumes in nursing; 400 periodical subscriptions health-care related.

BACCALAUREATE PROGRAMS

Degree BS

Available Programs Generic Baccalaureate; RN Baccalaureate.

Study Options Full-time and part-time.

Program Entrance Requirements Minimum overall college GPA of 2.5, transcript of college record, written essay, health exam, high school biology, high school chemistry, high school foreign language, 3 years high school math, 3 years high school science, high school transcript, immunizations, interview, 2 letters of recommendation, minimum high school GPA of 3.0, professional liability insurance/malpractice insurance. Transfer students are accepted.

Advanced Placement Credit by examination available. Credit given for nursing courses completed elsewhere dependent upon specific evaluations.

Contact *Telephone:* 518-244-2231. *Fax:* 518-244-2009.

GRADUATE PROGRAMS

Contact *Telephone:* 518-244-2384. *Fax:* 518-244-2009.

MASTER'S DEGREE PROGRAM

Degrees MS; MS/MBA

Concentrations Available *Clinical nurse specialist programs in:* psychiatric/mental health. *Nurse practitioner programs in:* acute care, adult health, community health, family health, gerontology, psychiatric/mental health.

Study Options Full-time and part-time.

Program Entrance Requirements Minimum overall college GPA of 2.75, transcript of college record, CPR certification, written essay, 2 letters of recommendation, physical assessment course, professional liability insurance/malpractice insurance, resume. *Application fee:* $40.

Degree Requirements Thesis or project.

POST-MASTER'S PROGRAM

Areas of Study *Nurse practitioner programs in:* acute care, adult health, community health, family health, gerontology.

St. Francis College
Department of Nursing
Brooklyn Heights, New York

Founded in 1884

DEGREE • BS

Nursing Program Faculty 6.

Baccalaureate Enrollment 76

Women 98% **Men** 2% **Minority** 63% **International** 25% **Part-time** 56%

Nursing Student Resources Academic advising; academic or career counseling; assistance for students with disabilities; bookstore; campus computer network; career placement assistance; computer lab; computer-assisted instruction; e-mail services; employment services for current students; interactive nursing skills videos; learning resource lab; library services; nursing audiovisuals; placement services for program completers; remedial services; resume preparation assistance; skills, simulation, or other laboratory; tutoring.

Library Facilities 120,000 volumes (5,531 in health, 186 in nursing); 571 periodical subscriptions (558 health-care related).

BACCALAUREATE PROGRAMS

Degree BS

Available Programs ADN to Baccalaureate; International Nurse to Baccalaureate; RPN to Baccalaureate.

Site Options Brooklyn, NY; New York, NY; Brooklyn, NY.

Study Options Full-time and part-time.

Program Entrance Requirements Minimum overall college GPA of 2.0, transcript of college record, written essay, health exam, health insurance, high school transcript, immunizations, interview, 2 letters of recommendation, professional liability insurance/malpractice insurance, prerequisite course work, RN licensure. Transfer students are accepted. **Standardized tests** *Required:* SAT, TOEFL for international students. **Application** *Deadline:* rolling (freshmen), rolling (transfer). *Notification:* continuous (freshmen). *Application fee:* $35.

Advanced Placement Credit by examination available. Credit given for nursing courses completed elsewhere dependent upon specific evaluations.

Expenses (2006–07) *Tuition:* full-time $13,500; part-time $480 per contact hour. *International tuition:* $13,500 full-time. *Required fees:* full-time $260; part-time $140 per term.

Financial Aid *Gift aid (need-based):* Federal Pell, FSEOG, state, college/university gift aid from institutional funds. *Loans:* FFEL (Subsidized and Unsubsidized Stafford PLUS), Perkins. *Work-Study:* Federal Work-Study. *Application deadline (priority):* 2/15.

Contact Dr. Susan Saladino, Chairperson, Department of Nursing, St. Francis College, 180 Remsen Street, Brooklyn, NY 11201. *Telephone:* 718-489-5267 Ext. 5267. *Fax:* 718-489-5408. *E-mail:* ssaladino@stfranciscollege.edu.

St. John Fisher College
Advanced Practice Nursing Program
Rochester, New York

http://www.sjfc.edu

Founded in 1948

DEGREES • BS • MS

Nursing Program Faculty 40 (12% with doctorates).

Baccalaureate Enrollment 295

Women 89% **Men** 11% **Minority** 12% **Part-time** 15%

Graduate Enrollment 76

Women 97% **Men** 3% **Minority** 5% **Part-time** 95%

Nursing Student Activities Sigma Theta Tau, Student Nurses' Association.

Nursing Student Resources Academic advising; academic or career counseling; assistance for students with disabilities; bookstore; campus computer network; career placement assistance; computer lab; computer-assisted instruction; daycare for children of students; e-mail services; employment services for current students; interactive nursing skills videos; Internet; learning resource lab; library services; nursing audiovisuals; resume preparation assistance; skills, simulation, or other laboratory; tutoring.

Library Facilities 190,903 volumes (30,000 in health, 5,000 in nursing); 8,964 periodical subscriptions (200 health-care related).

BACCALAUREATE PROGRAMS

Degree BS

Available Programs ADN to Baccalaureate; Baccalaureate for Second Degree; Generic Baccalaureate; RN Baccalaureate.

Site Options Geneva, NY; Rochester, NY.

Study Options Full-time and part-time.

Program Entrance Requirements Minimum overall college GPA of 2.75, transcript of college record, CPR certification, written essay, health exam, health insurance, high school chemistry, 1 year of high school math, high school transcript, immunizations, 2 letters of recommendation, minimum high school GPA of 2.0, minimum GPA in nursing prerequisites of 2.75, prerequisite course work. Transfer students are accepted. **Standardized tests** *Required:* SAT or ACT, TOEFL for international students. **Application** *Deadline:* rolling (freshmen), rolling (transfer). *Early decision:* 12/1. *Notification:* continuous until 9/1 (freshmen), 12/15 (out-of-state freshmen), 12/15 (early decision). *Application fee:* $30.

Advanced Placement Credit by examination available. Credit given for nursing courses completed elsewhere dependent upon specific evaluations.

Expenses (2006–07) *Tuition:* full-time $20,450; part-time $555 per credit hour. *International tuition:* $20,450 full-time. *Room and board:* $8880; room only: $5720 per academic year. *Required fees:* full-time $260; part-time $50 per credit.

Financial Aid 95% of baccalaureate students in nursing programs received some form of financial aid in 2005–06. *Gift aid (need-based):* Federal Pell, FSEOG, state, private, college/university gift aid from institutional funds, Federal Nursing. *Loans:* FFEL (Subsidized and Unsubsidized Stafford PLUS), Perkins. *Work-Study:* Federal Work-Study. *Application deadline (priority):* 2/15.

Contact Dr. Marilyn Dollinger, DNS, Chairperson, Advanced Practice Nursing Program, St. John Fisher College, 3690 East Avenue, Rochester, NY 14618. *Telephone:* 585-385-8241. *Fax:* 585-385-8466. *E-mail:* mdollinger@sjfc.edu.

GRADUATE PROGRAMS

Expenses (2006–07) *Tuition:* full-time $11,070; part-time $615 per credit hour. *International tuition:* $11,070 full-time. *Required fees:* full-time $100.

Financial Aid 20% of graduate students in nursing programs received some form of financial aid in 2005–06. Federal Work-Study, scholarships, and traineeships available. *Financial aid application deadline:* 2/15.

Contact Dr. Cynthia Ricci McCloskey, DNS, Graduate Program Director, Advanced Practice Nursing Program, St. John Fisher College, 3690 East Avenue, Rochester, NY 14618. *Telephone:* 585-385-8471. *Fax:* 585-385-8466. *E-mail:* cmccloskey@sjfc.edu.

MASTER'S DEGREE PROGRAM

Degree MS

Available Programs Master's; RN to Master's.

Concentrations Available Nursing education. *Clinical nurse specialist programs in:* adult health, gerontology, pediatric, women's health. *Nurse practitioner programs in:* family health.

Study Options Full-time and part-time.

Program Entrance Requirements Computer literacy, minimum overall college GPA of 3.0, transcript of college record, CPR certification, written essay, immunizations, 2 letters of recommendation, nursing research course, physical assessment course, resume, statistics course. *Application deadline:* For fall admission, 7/1; for spring admission, 10/30. Applications are processed on a rolling basis. *Application fee:* $30.

Advanced Placement Credit given for nursing courses completed elsewhere dependent upon specific evaluations.

Degree Requirements 46 total credit hours, thesis or project.

POST-MASTER'S PROGRAM

Areas of Study Nursing education. *Nurse practitioner programs in:* family health.

St. Joseph's College, New York
Department of Nursing
Brooklyn, New York

http://www.sjcny.edu
Founded in 1916

DEGREES • BSN • MS

Nursing Program Faculty 16 (44% with doctorates).

Baccalaureate Enrollment 271
Women 96% **Men** 4% **Minority** 50% **International** 2% **Part-time** 94%

Graduate Enrollment 57
Women 98% **Men** 2% **Minority** 50% **Part-time** 100%

Nursing Student Activities Nursing Honor Society, nursing club.

Nursing Student Resources Academic advising; academic or career counseling; assistance for students with disabilities; bookstore; campus computer network; computer lab; computer-assisted instruction; e-mail services; Internet; learning resource lab; library services; nursing audiovisuals; remedial services; resume preparation assistance; skills, simulation, or other laboratory; tutoring.

Library Facilities 100,000 volumes (10,000 in health, 4,750 in nursing); 432 periodical subscriptions (750 health-care related).

BACCALAUREATE PROGRAMS

Degree BSN

Available Programs RN Baccalaureate.

Site Options Patchogue, NY.

Study Options Full-time and part-time.

Program Entrance Requirements Minimum overall college GPA of 2.5, transcript of college record, CPR certification, written essay, health exam, health insurance, immunizations, 2 letters of recommendation, minimum GPA in nursing prerequisites of 2.5, professional liability insurance/malpractice insurance, prerequisite course work, RN licensure. Transfer students are accepted. **Standardized tests** *Required:* SAT or ACT, TOEFL for international students. **Application** *Deadline:* 8/15 (freshmen), 8/15 (transfer). *Notification:* continuous until 8/30 (freshmen). *Application fee:* $25.

Advanced Placement Credit by examination available. Credit given for nursing courses completed elsewhere dependent upon specific evaluations.

Expenses (2006–07) *Tuition:* full-time $13,168; part-time $426 per credit. *International tuition:* $13,186 full-time. *Required fees:* full-time $610; part-time $42 per credit; part-time $305 per term.

Financial Aid 15% of baccalaureate students in nursing programs received some form of financial aid in 2005–06. *Gift aid (need-based):* Federal Pell, FSEOG, state, private, college/university gift aid from institutional funds. *Loans:* FFEL (Subsidized and Unsubsidized Stafford PLUS), Perkins. *Work-Study:* Federal Work-Study, part-time campus jobs. *Application deadline (priority):* 2/25.

Contact Dr. Barbara L. Sands, Director, Department of Nursing, St. Joseph's College, New York, 245 Clinton Avenue, Brooklyn, NY 11205-3688. *Telephone:* 718-399-0185. *Fax:* 718-638-8839. *E-mail:* bsands@sjcny.edu.

GRADUATE PROGRAMS

Expenses (2006–07) *Tuition:* full-time $10,070; part-time $530 per credit. *International tuition:* $10,070 full-time. *Required fees:* full-time $554; part-time $53 per credit; part-time $282 per term.

Financial Aid 23% of graduate students in nursing programs received some form of financial aid in 2005–06.

Contact Dr. Barbara L. Sands, Director, Department of Nursing, St. Joseph's College, New York, 245 Clinton Avenue, Brooklyn, NY 11205-3688. *Telephone:* 718-399-0185. *Fax:* 718-638-8839. *E-mail:* bsands@sjcny.edu.

MASTER'S DEGREE PROGRAM

Degree MS

Available Programs Master's.

Concentrations Available Nursing education. *Clinical nurse specialist programs in:* adult health.

Site Options Patchogue, NY.

Study Options Part-time.

Program Entrance Requirements Clinical experience, minimum overall college GPA of 3.0, transcript of college record, CPR certification, written essay, immunizations, interview, 2 letters of recommendation, nursing research course, physical assessment course, professional liability insurance/malpractice insurance, prerequisite course work, resume, statistics course.

Advanced Placement Credit given for nursing courses completed elsewhere dependent upon specific evaluations.

Degree Requirements 38 total credit hours, comprehensive exam.

State University of New York at Binghamton
Decker School of Nursing
Binghamton, New York

http://dson.binghamton.edu
Founded in 1946

DEGREES • BS • MS • PHD

Nursing Program Faculty 43 (40% with doctorates).

State University of New York at Binghamton (continued)

Baccalaureate Enrollment 300

Graduate Enrollment 150

Nursing Student Activities Sigma Theta Tau, Student Nurses' Association.

Nursing Student Resources Campus computer network; computer lab; skills, simulation, or other laboratory.

Library Facilities 2.3 million volumes (7,000 in health); 41,985 periodical subscriptions (9,300 health-care related).

BACCALAUREATE PROGRAMS

Degree BS

Available Programs Accelerated RN Baccalaureate; Generic Baccalaureate.

Study Options Full-time and part-time.

Program Entrance Requirements Minimum overall college GPA of 2.7, transcript of college record, CPR certification, written essay, health exam, high school biology, high school chemistry, high school foreign language, 3 years high school math, 2 years high school science, high school transcript, minimum high school GPA of 3.0, prerequisite course work. Transfer students are accepted. **Standardized tests** *Required:* SAT or ACT, TOEFL for international students. **Application** *Deadline:* rolling (freshmen), rolling (transfer). *Early decision:* 11/15. *Notification:* continuous (freshmen), 1/1 (early action). *Application fee:* $40.

Advanced Placement Credit by examination available. Credit given for nursing courses completed elsewhere dependent upon specific evaluations.

Contact *Telephone:* 607-777-4954. *Fax:* 607-777-4440.

GRADUATE PROGRAMS

Contact *Telephone:* 607-777-4964. *Fax:* 607-777-4440.

MASTER'S DEGREE PROGRAM

Degree MS

Available Programs Master's.

Concentrations Available Nursing administration; nursing education. *Clinical nurse specialist programs in:* community health, family health, gerontology. *Nurse practitioner programs in:* community health, family health, gerontology, primary care.

Study Options Full-time and part-time.

Program Entrance Requirements Minimum overall college GPA of 3.0, transcript of college record, written essay, 2 letters of recommendation, statistics course, GRE General Test. *Application deadline:* For fall admission, 4/15 (priority date); for spring admission, 11/1. Applications are processed on a rolling basis.

Advanced Placement Credit given for nursing courses completed elsewhere dependent upon specific evaluations.

Degree Requirements 48 total credit hours, thesis or project, comprehensive exam.

POST-MASTER'S PROGRAM

Areas of Study *Nurse practitioner programs in:* community health, family health, gerontology.

DOCTORAL DEGREE PROGRAM

Degree PhD

Available Programs Doctorate.

Program Entrance Requirements Clinical experience, interview by faculty committee, interview, 3 letters of recommendation, MSN or equivalent, scholarly papers, statistics course, vita, writing sample. *Application deadline:* For fall admission, 4/15 (priority date); for spring admission, 11/1. Applications are processed on a rolling basis.

Degree Requirements 66 total credit hours, dissertation, written exam.

CONTINUING EDUCATION PROGRAM

Contact *Telephone:* 607-777-4954. *Fax:* 607-777-4440.

State University of New York at New Paltz
Department of Nursing
New Paltz, New York

http://www.newpaltz.edu/nursing

Founded in 1828

DEGREES • BSN • MSN

Nursing Program Faculty 10 (90% with doctorates).

Nursing Student Activities Nursing Honor Society, Sigma Theta Tau, Student Nurses' Association.

Nursing Student Resources Academic advising; academic or career counseling; assistance for students with disabilities; bookstore; campus computer network; computer lab; computer-assisted instruction; daycare for children of students; e-mail services; interactive nursing skills videos; Internet; learning resource lab; library services; nursing audiovisuals; remedial services; resume preparation assistance; skills, simulation, or other laboratory; tutoring.

Library Facilities 532,381 volumes; 1,515 periodical subscriptions.

BACCALAUREATE PROGRAMS

Degree BSN

Available Programs ADN to Baccalaureate; Generic Baccalaureate; RN Baccalaureate.

Site Options Middletown, NY; Suffern, NY.

Study Options Full-time and part-time.

Program Entrance Requirements Transcript of college record, written essay, health exam, immunizations, 3 letters of recommendation, professional liability insurance/malpractice insurance, prerequisite course work. Transfer students are accepted. **Standardized tests** *Required:* SAT or ACT, TOEFL for international students. **Application** *Deadline:* 4/1 (freshmen), 4/1 (transfer). *Early decision:* 11/15. *Notification:* continuous until 1/1 (freshmen), 1/1 (early action). *Application fee:* $40.

Contact *Telephone:* 845-257-2963. *Fax:* 845-257-2926.

GRADUATE PROGRAMS

Contact *Telephone:* 845-257-2949. *Fax:* 845-257-2926.

MASTER'S DEGREE PROGRAM

Degree MSN

Concentrations Available *Clinical nurse specialist programs in:* family health, gerontology.

Program Entrance Requirements Clinical experience, minimum overall college GPA of 3.0, transcript of college record, 2 letters of recommendation, nursing research course, physical assessment course, resume, GRE General Test. *Application deadline:* For fall admission, 5/15 (priority date); for spring admission, 11/15 (priority date). Applications are processed on a rolling basis. *Application fee:* $50.

Degree Requirements 42 total credit hours, thesis or project.

State University of New York at Plattsburgh
Department of Nursing
Plattsburgh, New York

http://www.plattsburgh.edu/nursing

Founded in 1889

DEGREE • BS

Nursing Program Faculty 9 (50% with doctorates).

Baccalaureate Enrollment 215

Women 95% **Men** 5%

Nursing Student Activities Nursing Honor Society, Sigma Theta Tau, Student Nurses' Association.

Nursing Student Resources Academic advising; academic or career counseling; assistance for students with disabilities; bookstore; campus computer network; career placement assistance; computer lab; computer-assisted instruction; e-mail services; employment services for current students; Internet; learning resource lab; library services; nursing audio-visuals; remedial services; resume preparation assistance; skills, simulation, or other laboratory; tutoring.

Library Facilities 1.6 million volumes (19,450 in health, 200 in nursing); 4,238 periodical subscriptions (174 health-care related).

BACCALAUREATE PROGRAMS

Degree BS

Available Programs ADN to Baccalaureate; Generic Baccalaureate; RN Baccalaureate.

Site Options *Distance Learning:* Glens Falls, NY; Johnstown, NY; Potsdam, NY.

Study Options Full-time and part-time.

Program Entrance Requirements Minimum overall college GPA of 2.5, transcript of college record, CPR certification, health exam, high school biology, high school chemistry, high school math, high school transcript, immunizations, minimum GPA in nursing prerequisites of 2.5. Transfer students are accepted. **Standardized tests** *Required:* SAT or ACT, TOEFL for international students. **Application** *Deadline:* 3/1 (freshmen), rolling (transfer). *Early decision:* 11/15. *Notification:* continuous (freshmen), 12/15 (out-of-state freshmen), 12/15 (early decision). *Application fee:* $40.

Advanced Placement Credit given for nursing courses completed elsewhere dependent upon specific evaluations.

Contact *Telephone:* 518-564-4245. *Fax:* 518-564-3100.

CONTINUING EDUCATION PROGRAM

Contact *Telephone:* 518-564-4245. *Fax:* 518-564-3100.

State University of New York College at Brockport
Department of Nursing
Brockport, New York

http://www.brockport.edu

Founded in 1867

DEGREE • BSN

Nursing Program Faculty 21 (20% with doctorates).

Baccalaureate Enrollment 121
Women 94% **Men** 6% **Minority** 17% **Part-time** 9%

Nursing Student Activities Nursing Honor Society, Sigma Theta Tau, Student Nurses' Association.

Nursing Student Resources Academic advising; academic or career counseling; assistance for students with disabilities; bookstore; campus computer network; career placement assistance; computer lab; computer-assisted instruction; e-mail services; interactive nursing skills videos; Internet; learning resource lab; library services; nursing audiovisuals; remedial services; resume preparation assistance.

Library Facilities 995,618 volumes (18,952 in health, 1,065 in nursing); 26,769 periodical subscriptions (257 health-care related).

BACCALAUREATE PROGRAMS

Degree BSN

Available Programs ADN to Baccalaureate; Baccalaureate for Second Degree; Generic Baccalaureate; LPN to Baccalaureate; RN Baccalaureate.

Study Options Full-time and part-time.

Program Entrance Requirements Minimum overall college GPA of 2.5, transcript of college record, CPR certification, written essay, health exam, high school foreign language, high school transcript, immunizations, 3 letters of recommendation, minimum GPA in nursing prerequisites of 2.5, professional liability insurance/malpractice insurance, prerequisite course work. Transfer students are accepted. **Standardized tests** *Required:* SAT or ACT, TOEFL for international students. **Application** *Deadline:* rolling (freshmen), 8/1 (transfer). *Notification:* continuous (freshmen). *Application fee:* $40.

Advanced Placement Credit by examination available. Credit given for nursing courses completed elsewhere dependent upon specific evaluations.

Contact *Telephone:* 585-395-2355. *Fax:* 585-395-5312.

State University of New York Downstate Medical Center
College of Nursing
Brooklyn, New York

http://sls.downstate.edu/admissions/nursing/index.html

Founded in 1858

DEGREES • BS • MS • MS/MPH

Nursing Program Faculty 17 (53% with doctorates).

Baccalaureate Enrollment 133
Women 93% **Men** 7% **Minority** 80% **Part-time** 77%

Graduate Enrollment 192
Women 83% **Men** 17% **Minority** 79% **Part-time** 74%

Nursing Student Activities Student Nurses' Association, nursing club.

Nursing Student Resources Academic advising; academic or career counseling; assistance for students with disabilities; bookstore; campus computer network; computer lab; computer-assisted instruction; e-mail services; housing assistance; interactive nursing skills videos; Internet; learning resource lab; library services; nursing audiovisuals; paid internships; skills, simulation, or other laboratory.

Library Facilities 357,209 volumes (357,209 in health, 2,679 in nursing); 2,104 periodical subscriptions (619 health-care related).

BACCALAUREATE PROGRAMS

Degree BS

Available Programs Accelerated Baccalaureate for Second Degree; RN Baccalaureate.

Study Options Full-time.

Program Entrance Requirements Minimum overall college GPA of 3.0, transcript of college record, written essay, health exam, 2 letters of recommendation, professional liability insurance/malpractice insurance, prerequisite course work. Transfer students are accepted. **Application** *Deadline:* 5/1 (transfer). *Application fee:* $30.

Expenses (2006–07) *Tuition, area resident:* part-time $181 per credit. *Tuition, state resident:* full-time $2175; part-time $181 per credit. *Tuition, nonresident:* full-time $5305; part-time $442 per credit. *Room and board:* room only: $2134 per academic year.

Contact Dr. Nellie Bailey, Associate Dean, College of Nursing, State University of New York Downstate Medical Center, 450 Clarkson Avenue, Box 22, Brooklyn, NY 11203. *Telephone:* 718-270-7617. *Fax:* 718-270-7641. *E-mail:* nellie.bailey@downstate.edu.

GRADUATE PROGRAMS

Expenses (2006–07) *Tuition, state resident:* full-time $8342; part-time $288 per credit. *Tuition, nonresident:* full-time $15,195; part-time $455 per credit.

Financial Aid Traineeships and health workforce retraining available.

Contact Dr. Laila N. Sedhom, Associate Dean, College of Nursing, State University of New York Downstate Medical Center, 450 Clarkson Avenue, Box 22, Brooklyn, NY 11203-2098. *Telephone:* 718-270-7605. *Fax:* 718-270-7636. *E-mail:* laila.sedhom@downstate.edu.

MASTER'S DEGREE PROGRAM

Degrees MS; MS/MPH

Available Programs Master's.

Concentrations Available Nurse anesthesia; nurse-midwifery. *Clinical nurse specialist programs in:* adult health, maternity-newborn. *Nurse practitioner programs in:* family health, women's health.

Study Options Full-time and part-time.

State University of New York Downstate Medical Center (continued)

Program Entrance Requirements Clinical experience, minimum overall college GPA of 3.0, transcript of college record, CPR certification, written essay, interview, 2 letters of recommendation, nursing research course, physical assessment course, professional liability insurance/malpractice insurance, prerequisite course work, resume, statistics course, GRE. *Application deadline:* For fall admission, 4/1 (priority date). Applications are processed on a rolling basis. *Application fee:* $35.

Advanced Placement Credit by examination available. Credit given for nursing courses completed elsewhere dependent upon specific evaluations.

Degree Requirements Thesis or project.

POST-MASTER'S PROGRAM

Areas of Study *Nurse practitioner programs in:* family health, women's health.

CONTINUING EDUCATION PROGRAM

Contact Ms. Edna Lewis, Director of Continuing Education, College of Nursing, State University of New York Downstate Medical Center, 450 Clarkson Avenue, Box 22, Brooklyn, NY 11203. *Telephone:* 718-270-7616. *Fax:* 718-270-7641. *E-mail:* edna.lewis@downstate.edu.

State University of New York Institute of Technology
School of Nursing and Health Systems
Utica, New York

http://www.sunyit.edu

Founded in 1966

DEGREES • BS • MS

Nursing Program Faculty 8 (70% with doctorates).

Baccalaureate Enrollment 280
Women 96% **Men** 4% **Minority** 5% **Part-time** 82%

Graduate Enrollment 36
Women 96.5% **Men** 3.5% **Minority** 10% **Part-time** 70%

Nursing Student Activities Nursing Honor Society, Sigma Theta Tau, Student Nurses' Association, nursing club.

Nursing Student Resources Academic advising; academic or career counseling; assistance for students with disabilities; bookstore; campus computer network; career placement assistance; computer lab; computer-assisted instruction; e-mail services; employment services for current students; externships; housing assistance; interactive nursing skills videos; Internet; learning resource lab; library services; nursing audiovisuals; other; placement services for program completers; remedial services; resume preparation assistance; skills, simulation, or other laboratory; tutoring; unpaid internships.

Library Facilities 193,682 volumes (14,000 in health, 8,500 in nursing); 1,090 periodical subscriptions (335 health-care related).

BACCALAUREATE PROGRAMS

Degree BS

Available Programs ADN to Baccalaureate; Accelerated RN Baccalaureate; RN Baccalaureate.

Site Options *Distance Learning:* Albany, NY.

Study Options Full-time and part-time.

Program Entrance Requirements Minimum overall college GPA of 2.0, transcript of college record, CPR certification, minimum GPA in nursing prerequisites of 2.0, prerequisite course work. Transfer students are accepted. **Standardized tests** *Required:* TOEFL for international students. **Application** *Deadline:* rolling (freshmen), rolling (transfer). *Notification:* continuous until 1/15 (freshmen). *Application fee:* $40.

Advanced Placement Credit given for nursing courses completed elsewhere dependent upon specific evaluations.

Financial Aid 33% of baccalaureate students in nursing programs received some form of financial aid in 2004–05. *Gift aid (need-based):* Federal Pell, FSEOG, state. *Loans:* Federal Nursing Student Loans, Federal Direct (Subsidized and Unsubsidized Stafford PLUS), Perkins. *Work-Study:* Federal Work-Study. *Application deadline:* Continuous.

Contact Marybeth Lyons, Director of Admissions, School of Nursing and Health Systems, State University of New York Institute of Technology, PO Box 3050, Utica, NY 13504-3050. *Telephone:* 315-792-7500. *Fax:* 315-792-7837. *E-mail:* admissions@sunyit.edu.

GRADUATE PROGRAMS

Financial Aid 60% of graduate students in nursing programs received some form of financial aid in 2004–05. Federal Work-Study, scholarships, and unspecified assistantships available.

Contact Ms. Christine Paye, Staff Assistant, School of Nursing and Health Systems, State University of New York Institute of Technology, PO Box 3050, Utica, NY 13504-3050. *Telephone:* 315-792-7297. *Fax:* 315-792-7555. *E-mail:* payec@sunyit.edu.

MASTER'S DEGREE PROGRAM

Degree MS

Available Programs Accelerated AD/RN to Master's; Accelerated RN to Master's; Master's.

Concentrations Available Nursing administration. *Nurse practitioner programs in:* adult health, family health.

Site Options *Distance Learning:* Albany, NY.

Study Options Full-time and part-time.

Program Entrance Requirements Clinical experience, computer literacy, minimum overall college GPA of 3.0, transcript of college record, written essay, interview, 2 letters of recommendation, nursing research course, physical assessment course, prerequisite course work, statistics course, GRE General Test. *Application deadline:* For fall admission, 6/15 (priority date). Applications are processed on a rolling basis. *Application fee:* $50.

Advanced Placement Credit given for nursing courses completed elsewhere dependent upon specific evaluations.

Degree Requirements 45 total credit hours, thesis or project, comprehensive exam.

POST-MASTER'S PROGRAM

Areas of Study Nursing administration. *Nurse practitioner programs in:* adult health, family health.

CONTINUING EDUCATION PROGRAM

Contact Dr. Esther G. Bankert, Dean, School of Nursing and Health Systems, State University of New York Institute of Technology, PO Box 3050, Utica, NY 13504-3050. *Telephone:* 315-792-7295. *Fax:* 315-792-7555. *E-mail:* fegb@suny.edu.

State University of New York Upstate Medical University
College of Nursing
Syracuse, New York

http://www.upstate.edu/con

Founded in 1950

DEGREES • BS • MS

Nursing Program Faculty 12 (30% with doctorates).

Baccalaureate Enrollment 124
Women 99% **Men** 1% **Minority** 1% **Part-time** 80%

Graduate Enrollment 96
Women 99% **Men** 1% **Minority** 1% **Part-time** 80%

Nursing Student Activities Sigma Theta Tau, Student Nurses' Association.

Nursing Student Resources Academic advising; academic or career counseling; assistance for students with disabilities; bookstore; campus computer network; computer lab; computer-assisted instruction; daycare for children of students; e-mail services; Internet; learning resource lab; library services; skills, simulation, or other laboratory; tutoring.

Library Facilities 132,500 volumes (220,382 in health, 1,241 in nursing); 1,800 periodical subscriptions (4,928 health-care related).

BACCALAUREATE PROGRAMS

Degree BS

Available Programs ADN to Baccalaureate.

Program Entrance Requirements Transcript of college record, CPR certification, written essay, health exam, health insurance, immunizations, 2 letters of recommendation, prerequisite course work, RN licensure. **Standardized tests** *Recommended:* TOEFL for international students. **Application** *Deadline:* rolling (transfer). *Application fee:* $40.

Expenses (2006–07) *Tuition, state resident:* full-time $4350; part-time $181 per credit hour. *Tuition, nonresident:* full-time $10,610; part-time $442 per credit hour. *International tuition:* $10,610 full-time. *Room and board:* room only: $5000 per academic year. *Required fees:* full-time $25; part-time $1 per credit.

Financial Aid 35% of baccalaureate students in nursing programs received some form of financial aid in 2005–06.

Contact Mrs. Debora E. Kirsch, Director, Undergraduate Program, College of Nursing, State University of New York Upstate Medical University, 750 East Adams Street, Syracuse, NY 13210. *Telephone:* 315-464-4276. *Fax:* 315-464-5168. *E-mail:* kirschde@upstate.edu.

GRADUATE PROGRAMS

Expenses (2006–07) *Tuition, state resident:* full-time $6900; part-time $288 per credit hour. *Tuition, nonresident:* full-time $10,920; part-time $455 per credit hour. *International tuition:* $10,920 full-time. *Room and board:* room only: $5000 per academic year. *Required fees:* full-time $25; part-time $1 per credit.

Financial Aid 30% of graduate students in nursing programs received some form of financial aid in 2005–06. Federal Work-Study, institutionally sponsored loans, and scholarships available. Aid available to part-time students. *Financial aid application deadline:* 3/1.

Contact Dr. Carol Gavan, Associate Professor/Associate Dean and Director, Graduate Program, College of Nursing, State University of New York Upstate Medical University, 750 East Adams Street, Syracuse, NY 13210. *Telephone:* 315-464-4276. *Fax:* 315-464-5168. *E-mail:* gavanc@upstate.edu.

MASTER'S DEGREE PROGRAM

Degree MS

Available Programs Master's; Master's for Nurses with Non-Nursing Degrees.

Concentrations Available *Clinical nurse specialist programs in:* medical-surgical. *Nurse practitioner programs in:* adult health, family health, pediatric.

Program Entrance Requirements Clinical experience, minimum overall college GPA of 3.0, transcript of college record, CPR certification, written essay, immunizations, 3 letters of recommendation, nursing research course, physical assessment course, statistics course, GRE General Test, GRE Subject Test. *Application deadline:* For fall admission, 3/15 (priority date). Applications are processed on a rolling basis. *Application fee:* $40.

Degree Requirements 47 total credit hours, comprehensive exam.

POST-MASTER'S PROGRAM

Areas of Study *Clinical nurse specialist programs in:* medical-surgical. *Nurse practitioner programs in:* adult health, family health, pediatric.

CONTINUING EDUCATION PROGRAM

Contact Ms. Barbara A. Black, Director, Continuing Nursing Education, College of Nursing, State University of New York Upstate Medical University, 750 East Adams Street, Syracuse, NY 13210. *Telephone:* 315-464-4276. *Fax:* 315-464-5168. *E-mail:* blackb@upstate.edu.

Stony Brook University, State University of New York

School of Nursing
Stony Brook, New York

Founded in 1957

DEGREES • BS • MS

Nursing Program Faculty 79 (50% with doctorates).

Baccalaureate Enrollment 246
Women 82% **Men** 18% **Minority** 44% **International** 17% **Part-time** 57%

Graduate Enrollment 503
Women 91% **Men** 9% **Minority** 25% **International** 9%

Nursing Student Activities Nursing Honor Society, Sigma Theta Tau, Student Nurses' Association, nursing club.

Nursing Student Resources Academic advising; academic or career counseling; assistance for students with disabilities; bookstore; campus computer network; career placement assistance; computer lab; computer-assisted instruction; daycare for children of students; e-mail services; employment services for current students; housing assistance; interactive nursing skills videos; Internet; learning resource lab; library services; nursing audiovisuals; placement services for program completers; resume preparation assistance; skills, simulation, or other laboratory.

Library Facilities 1.9 million volumes; 29,275 periodical subscriptions.

BACCALAUREATE PROGRAMS

Degree BS

Available Programs Accelerated Baccalaureate; Accelerated RN Baccalaureate; RN Baccalaureate.

Study Options Full-time and part-time.

Program Entrance Requirements Minimum overall college GPA of 2.5, transcript of college record, CPR certification, written essay, health insurance, immunizations, 3 letters of recommendation, minimum GPA in nursing prerequisites of 2.5, professional liability insurance/malpractice insurance. Transfer students are accepted. **Standardized tests** *Required:* SAT or ACT, TOEFL for international students. *Recommended:* SAT Subject Tests. **Application** *Deadline:* 3/1 (freshmen), 4/15 (transfer). *Early decision:* 11/15. *Notification:* continuous (freshmen), 1/1 (early action). *Application fee:* $40.

Advanced Placement Credit by examination available. Credit given for nursing courses completed elsewhere dependent upon specific evaluations.

Expenses (2006–07) *Tuition, state resident:* full-time $8700; part-time $181 per credit. *Tuition, nonresident:* full-time $21,200; part-time $442 per credit. *Room and board:* $9014; room only: $6154 per academic year.

Financial Aid 85% of baccalaureate students in nursing programs received some form of financial aid in 2005–06.

Contact Health Sciences Center, School of Nursing, Stony Brook University, State University of New York, Stony Brook, NY 11974-8240. *Telephone:* 631-444-3200. *Fax:* 631-444-6628.

GRADUATE PROGRAMS

Expenses (2006–07) *Tuition, state resident:* full-time $13,800; part-time $288 per credit. *Tuition, nonresident:* full-time $21,840; part-time $455 per credit. *Room and board:* $9014; room only: $6154 per academic year.

Financial Aid 85% of graduate students in nursing programs received some form of financial aid in 2005–06. Fellowships, research assistantships, teaching assistantships, career-related internships or fieldwork, Federal Work-Study, institutionally sponsored loans, and traineeships available. *Financial aid application deadline:* 3/15.

Contact Office of Student Affairs, School of Nursing, Stony Brook University, State University of New York, Health Sciences Center, Stony Brook, NY 11794-8240. *Telephone:* 631-444-3200. *Fax:* 631-444-6628.

MASTER'S DEGREE PROGRAM

Degree MS

Available Programs Master's; RN to Master's.

Concentrations Available Nurse-midwifery. *Clinical nurse specialist programs in:* adult health, community health, critical care, family health, parent-child, pediatric, perinatal, psychiatric/mental health, women's health. *Nurse practitioner programs in:* adult health, family health, neonatal health, pediatric, psychiatric/mental health, women's health.

Study Options Full-time and part-time.

Program Entrance Requirements Clinical experience, computer literacy, minimum overall college GPA of 3.0, transcript of college record, CPR certification, written essay, immunizations, interview, 3 letters of recommendation, physical assessment course, professional liability insurance/malpractice insurance, prerequisite course work, resume, statistics course. *Application deadline:* For fall admission, 1/15. *Application fee:* $50.

Stony Brook University, State University of New York (continued)

Advanced Placement Credit given for nursing courses completed elsewhere dependent upon specific evaluations.

Degree Requirements 45 total credit hours.

POST-MASTER'S PROGRAM

Areas of Study Nurse-midwifery. *Clinical nurse specialist programs in:* adult health, community health, critical care, family health, parent-child, pediatric, perinatal, psychiatric/mental health, women's health. *Nurse practitioner programs in:* adult health, family health, neonatal health, pediatric, psychiatric/mental health, women's health.

CONTINUING EDUCATION PROGRAM

Contact Mrs. Valerie R. DiGiovanni, Assistant to the Dean for Records and Registration, School of Nursing, Stony Brook University, State University of New York, Health Sciences Center, Level 2, Room 216, Stony Brook, NY 11794-8240. *Telephone:* 631-444-3481. *Fax:* 631-444-6628. *E-mail:* valerie. digiovanni@sunysb.edu.

Teachers College Columbia University

Department of Health and Behavioral Studies

New York, New York

http://www.tc.edu/academic/hbs/nurseed

Founded in 1887

DEGREE • EDD

Nursing Program Faculty 5 (100% with doctorates).

Graduate Enrollment 18
Women 89% **Men** 11% **Minority** 33% **Part-time** 89%

Nursing Student Activities Sigma Theta Tau.

Nursing Student Resources Academic advising; assistance for students with disabilities; bookstore; campus computer network; computer lab; e-mail services; employment services for current students; housing assistance; Internet; library services.

GRADUATE PROGRAMS

Expenses (2006–07) *Tuition:* full-time $29,250; part-time $975 per credit hour. *Room and board:* room only: $6200 per academic year. *Required fees:* full-time $640; part-time $320 per term.

Financial Aid 70% of graduate students in nursing programs received some form of financial aid in 2005–06. Fellowships, research assistantships, teaching assistantships, career-related internships or fieldwork, Federal Work-Study, institutionally sponsored loans, and tuition waivers (full and partial) available. Aid available to part-time students. *Financial aid application deadline:* 2/1.

Contact Dr. Kathleen A. O'Connell, Isabel Maitland Stewart Professor of Nursing Education, Department of Health and Behavioral Studies, Teachers College Columbia University, Box 35, 525 West 120th Street, New York, NY 10027. *Telephone:* 212-678-3120. *Fax:* 212-678-4048. *E-mail:* oconnell@tc. columbia.edu.

MASTER'S DEGREE PROGRAM

Program Entrance Requirements *Application deadline:* For fall admission, 5/15. *Application fee:* $50.

DOCTORAL DEGREE PROGRAM

Degree EdD

Available Programs Doctorate; Doctorate for Nurses with Non-Nursing Degrees.

Areas of Study Addiction/substance abuse, bio-behavioral research, faculty preparation, health promotion/disease prevention, human health and illness, nursing research, women's health.

Program Entrance Requirements Minimum overall college GPA of 3.4, interview, 2 letters of recommendation, MSN or equivalent, vita, writing sample. *Application deadline:* For fall admission, 5/15. *Application fee:* $50.

Degree Requirements 90 total credit hours, dissertation, written exam.

University at Buffalo, the State University of New York

School of Nursing

Buffalo, New York

http://nursing.buffalo.edu

Founded in 1846

DEGREES • BS • MS • PHD

Nursing Program Faculty 47 (70% with doctorates).

Baccalaureate Enrollment 392
Women 92% **Men** 8% **Minority** 25% **International** 3% **Part-time** 10%

Graduate Enrollment 203
Women 86% **Men** 14% **Minority** 15% **International** 10% **Part-time** 35%

Nursing Student Activities Sigma Theta Tau, Student Nurses' Association, nursing club.

Nursing Student Resources Academic advising; academic or career counseling; assistance for students with disabilities; bookstore; campus computer network; career placement assistance; computer lab; computer-assisted instruction; daycare for children of students; e-mail services; employment services for current students; housing assistance; interactive nursing skills videos; Internet; learning resource lab; library services; nursing audiovisuals; paid internships; placement services for program completers; remedial services; resume preparation assistance; skills, simulation, or other laboratory; tutoring.

Library Facilities 3.4 million volumes (250,000 in health, 25,000 in nursing); 34,126 periodical subscriptions (2,500 health-care related).

BACCALAUREATE PROGRAMS

Degree BS

Available Programs ADN to Baccalaureate; Accelerated Baccalaureate for Second Degree; Baccalaureate for Second Degree; Generic Baccalaureate; International Nurse to Baccalaureate.

Study Options Full-time.

Program Entrance Requirements Minimum overall college GPA of 3.0, transcript of college record, CPR certification, health exam, health insurance, high school chemistry, high school transcript, immunizations, minimum high school GPA of 3.0, minimum GPA in nursing prerequisites of 3.0, prerequisite course work. Transfer students are accepted. **Standardized tests** *Required:* SAT or ACT, TOEFL for international students. **Application** *Early decision:* 11/1. *Notification:* continuous (freshmen), 12/15 (out-of-state freshmen), 12/15 (early decision). *Application fee:* $40.

Advanced Placement Credit by examination available. Credit given for nursing courses completed elsewhere dependent upon specific evaluations.

Expenses (2006–07) *Tuition, state resident:* full-time $4350; part-time $181 per credit. *Tuition, nonresident:* full-time $5305; part-time $442 per credit. *International tuition:* $5305 full-time. *Room and board:* $7526; room only: $4636 per academic year. *Required fees:* full-time $1779; part-time $78 per credit.

Financial Aid 92% of baccalaureate students in nursing programs received some form of financial aid in 2005–06. *Gift aid (need-based):* Federal Pell, FSEOG, state, private, college/university gift aid from institutional funds, Federal Nursing. *Loans:* Federal Nursing Student Loans, Federal Direct (Subsidized and Unsubsidized Stafford PLUS), Perkins, college/university. *Work-Study:* Federal Work-Study, part-time campus jobs. *Application deadline (priority):* 3/1.

Contact Dr. Elaine R. Cusker, Assistant Dean, School of Nursing, University at Buffalo, the State University of New York, 1040 Kimball Tower, Buffalo, NY 14214-3079. *Telephone:* 716-829-2537. *Fax:* 716-829-2021. *E-mail:* nurse-studentaffairs@buffalo.edu.

GRADUATE PROGRAMS

Expenses (2006–07) *Tuition, state resident:* full-time $7900; part-time $288 per credit. *Tuition, nonresident:* full-time $10,920; part-time $455 per credit. *International tuition:* $10,920 full-time. *Room and board:* $9581; room only: $6438 per academic year. *Required fees:* full-time $1319; part-time $103 per credit.

Financial Aid 69% of graduate students in nursing programs received some form of financial aid in 2005–06. 10 fellowships with full tuition reimbursements available (averaging $7,300 per year), 4 research assistantships with tuition reimbursements available (averaging $17,445 per year), 19 teaching assistantships with full tuition reimbursements available (averaging $10,921 per year) were awarded; Federal Work-Study, scholarships, traineeships, and unspecified assistantships also available. *Financial aid application deadline:* 3/15.

Contact Dr. Elaine R. Cusker, Assistant Dean, School of Nursing, University at Buffalo, the State University of New York, 1040 Kimball Tower, Buffalo, NY 14214-3079. *Telephone:* 716-829-2537. *Fax:* 716-829-2021. *E-mail:* nurse-studentaffairs@buffalo.edu.

MASTER'S DEGREE PROGRAM

Degree MS

Available Programs Master's.

Concentrations Available Nurse anesthesia; nursing education; nursing informatics. *Clinical nurse specialist programs in:* adult health, gerontology, medical-surgical. *Nurse practitioner programs in:* adult health, family health, gerontology, neonatal health, pediatric, psychiatric/mental health, women's health.

Site Options *Distance Learning:* Syracuse, NY.

Study Options Full-time and part-time.

Program Entrance Requirements Computer literacy, minimum overall college GPA of 3.0, transcript of college record, CPR certification, written essay, immunizations, interview, 3 letters of recommendation, physical assessment course, statistics course, GRE General Test (if overall GPA is below 3.0). *Application deadline:* For fall admission, 8/1 (priority date). Applications are processed on a rolling basis. *Application fee:* $35.

Advanced Placement Credit given for nursing courses completed elsewhere dependent upon specific evaluations.

Degree Requirements Thesis or project, comprehensive exam.

POST-MASTER'S PROGRAM

Areas of Study *Nurse practitioner programs in:* adult health, family health, gerontology, neonatal health, pediatric, psychiatric/mental health, women's health.

DOCTORAL DEGREE PROGRAM

Degree PhD

Available Programs Doctorate; Post-Baccalaureate Doctorate.

Areas of Study Addiction/substance abuse, advanced practice nursing, aging, clinical practice, critical care, ethics, faculty preparation, family health, gerontology, health policy, health promotion/disease prevention, health-care systems, individualized study, information systems, maternity-newborn, nurse case management, nursing administration, nursing education, nursing policy, nursing research, nursing science, oncology, women's health.

Program Entrance Requirements Minimum overall college GPA of 3.25, interview by faculty committee, interview, 3 letters of recommendation, statistics course, vita, writing sample, GRE General Test. *Application deadline:* For fall admission, 8/1 (priority date). Applications are processed on a rolling basis. *Application fee:* $35.

Degree Requirements 60 total credit hours, dissertation, written exam, residency.

University of Rochester
School of Nursing
Rochester, New York

http://www.urmc.rochester.edu/son
Founded in 1850

DEGREES • BS • MS • MSN/PHD

Nursing Program Faculty 67 (43% with doctorates).

Baccalaureate Enrollment 201
Women 90% **Men** 10% **Minority** 16% **International** 1% **Part-time** 14%

Graduate Enrollment 191
Women 87% **Men** 13% **Minority** 16% **International** 1% **Part-time** 79%

Nursing Student Activities Sigma Theta Tau, Student Nurses' Association.

Nursing Student Resources Academic advising; academic or career counseling; assistance for students with disabilities; bookstore; campus computer network; career placement assistance; computer lab; computer-assisted instruction; e-mail services; housing assistance; interactive nursing skills videos; Internet; learning resource lab; library services; nursing audiovisuals; resume preparation assistance; skills, simulation, or other laboratory.

Library Facilities 3 million volumes (240,000 in health); 11,254 periodical subscriptions (2,000 health-care related).

BACCALAUREATE PROGRAMS

Degree BS

Available Programs ADN to Baccalaureate; Accelerated Baccalaureate for Second Degree; Accelerated RN Baccalaureate; Baccalaureate for Second Degree; RN Baccalaureate.

Study Options Full-time and part-time.

Program Entrance Requirements Transcript of college record, CPR certification, written essay, health exam, health insurance, immunizations, 2 letters of recommendation, prerequisite course work. **Application Deadline:** 1/15 (freshmen), rolling (transfer). *Application fee:* $50.

Advanced Placement Credit by examination available.

Expenses (2006–07) *Tuition:* full-time $30,000; part-time $950 per credit hour. *International tuition:* $30,000 full-time. *Room and board:* $9000; room only: $7000 per academic year. *Required fees:* full-time $800; part-time $100 per term.

Financial Aid 95% of baccalaureate students in nursing programs received some form of financial aid in 2005–06. *Gift aid (need-based):* Federal Pell, FSEOG, state, college/university gift aid from institutional funds. *Loans:* Federal Nursing Student Loans, Federal Direct (Subsidized and Unsubsidized Stafford PLUS), Perkins, college/university, alternative loans. *Work-Study:* Federal Work-Study. *Application deadline (priority):* 2/1.

Contact Ms. Elaine M. Andolina, MS, RN, Director of Admissions, School of Nursing, University of Rochester, Box SON, 601 Elmwood Avenue, Rochester, NY 14642. *Telephone:* 585-275-2375. *Fax:* 585-756-8299. *E-mail:* son_admissions@urmc.rochester.edu.

GRADUATE PROGRAMS

Expenses (2006–07) *Tuition:* full-time $19,000; part-time $950 per credit hour. *International tuition:* $19,000 full-time. *Room and board:* $8000; room only: $6000 per academic year. *Required fees:* full-time $300; part-time $100 per term.

Financial Aid 95% of graduate students in nursing programs received some form of financial aid in 2005–06. 13 fellowships with full and partial tuition reimbursements available (averaging $13,900 per year), 4 research assistantships (averaging $10,000 per year), 3 teaching assistantships with full and partial tuition reimbursements available (averaging $2,800 per year) were awarded; scholarships, traineeships, tuition waivers (partial), and unspecified assistantships also available. Aid available to part-time students. *Financial aid application deadline:* 6/30.

Contact Ms. Elaine M. Andolina, MS, RN, Director of Admissions, School of Nursing, University of Rochester, Box SON, 601 Elmwood Avenue, Rochester, NY 14642. *Telephone:* 585-275-2375. *Fax:* 585-756-8299. *E-mail:* son_admissions@urmc.rochester.edu.

MASTER'S DEGREE PROGRAM

Degrees MS; MSN/PhD

Available Programs Accelerated AD/RN to Master's; Accelerated Master's for Non-Nursing College Graduates; Master's.

Concentrations Available Health-care administration. *Nurse practitioner programs in:* acute care, adult health, family health, gerontology, neonatal health, pediatric, psychiatric/mental health.

Study Options Full-time and part-time.

Program Entrance Requirements Minimum overall college GPA of 3.0, transcript of college record, CPR certification, written essay, immunizations, interview, 2 letters of recommendation, statistics course. *Application deadline:* For fall admission, 11/1 (priority date). *Application fee:* $25.

University of Rochester (continued)

Advanced Placement Credit given for nursing courses completed elsewhere dependent upon specific evaluations.

Degree Requirements 40 total credit hours, comprehensive exam.

POST-MASTER'S PROGRAM

Areas of Study *Nurse practitioner programs in:* acute care, adult health, family health, gerontology, neonatal health, pediatric, psychiatric/mental health.

DOCTORAL DEGREE PROGRAM

Degree PhD

Available Programs Doctorate; Post-Baccalaureate Doctorate.

Areas of Study Nursing research.

Program Entrance Requirements Minimum overall college GPA of 3.5, interview, 3 letters of recommendation, MSN or equivalent, statistics course, vita, writing sample, GRE General Test. *Application deadline:* For fall admission, 11/1 (priority date). *Application fee:* $25.

Degree Requirements 60 total credit hours, dissertation, oral exam, written exam, residency.

POSTDOCTORAL PROGRAM

Areas of Study Addiction/substance abuse, adolescent health, aging, cancer care, chronic illness, community health, family health, gerontology, individualized study, nursing interventions, nursing research, outcomes, vulnerable population.

Postdoctoral Program Contact Dr. Harriet Kitzman, Associate Dean for Research, School of Nursing, University of Rochester, Box SON, 601 Elmwood Avenue, Rochester, NY 14642. *Telephone:* 585-275-8874. *Fax:* 585-273-1258. *E-mail:* harriet_kitzman@urmc.rochester.edu.

CONTINUING EDUCATION PROGRAM

Contact Ms. Pamela Smith, RN, Director, Center for Lifelong Learning, School of Nursing, University of Rochester, Box SON, 601 Elmwood Avenue, Rochester, NY 14642. *Telephone:* 585-273-5456. *Fax:* 585-461-4488. *E-mail:* pamela_smith@urmc.rochester.edu.

Utica College
Department of Nursing
Utica, New York

http://www.utica.edu
Founded in 1946

DEGREE • BS

Nursing Program Faculty 17 (2% with doctorates).

Baccalaureate Enrollment 134
Women 89% **Men** 11% **Minority** 33%

Nursing Student Activities Student Nurses' Association.

Nursing Student Resources Academic advising; academic or career counseling; assistance for students with disabilities; bookstore; campus computer network; career placement assistance; computer lab; computer-assisted instruction; e-mail services; employment services for current students; externships; housing assistance; interactive nursing skills videos; Internet; learning resource lab; library services; nursing audiovisuals; paid internships; placement services for program completers; remedial services; resume preparation assistance; skills, simulation, or other laboratory; tutoring; unpaid internships.

Library Facilities 184,918 volumes (2,652 in health, 1,122 in nursing); 1,249 periodical subscriptions (118 health-care related).

BACCALAUREATE PROGRAMS

Degree BS

Available Programs Generic Baccalaureate; RN Baccalaureate.
Site Options Syracuse, NY.
Study Options Full-time and part-time.

Program Entrance Requirements Minimum overall college GPA of 2.5, transcript of college record, written essay, health exam, health insurance, high school biology, high school chemistry, 3 years high school math, 3 years high school science, high school transcript, immunizations, 3 letters of recommendation, minimum high school GPA of 2.5, minimum high school rank 25%, minimum GPA in nursing prerequisites of 2.0. Transfer students are accepted. **Standardized tests** *Required:* TOEFL for international students. *Recommended:* SAT or ACT. *Required for some:* SAT or ACT. **Application** *Deadline:* rolling (freshmen), rolling (out-of-state freshmen), rolling (transfer). *Notification:* 9/1 (freshmen), 1/9 (out-of-state freshmen). *Application fee:* $40.

Advanced Placement Credit by examination available. Credit given for nursing courses completed elsewhere dependent upon specific evaluations.

Expenses (2006–07) *Tuition:* full-time $22,030; part-time $750 per credit hour. *International tuition:* $22,030 full-time. *Room and board:* $10,250 per academic year. *Required fees:* full-time $400; part-time $105 per term.

Financial Aid 97% of baccalaureate students in nursing programs received some form of financial aid in 2005–06. *Gift aid (need-based):* Federal Pell, FSEOG, state, private, college/university gift aid from institutional funds, Federal Nursing. *Loans:* Federal Direct (Subsidized and Unsubsidized Stafford PLUS), Perkins, GATE Loans. *Work-Study:* Federal Work-Study, part-time campus jobs. *Application deadline (priority):* 2/15.

Contact Mr. Patrick A. Quinn, Vice President for Enrollment Management, Department of Nursing, Utica College, 1600 Burrstone Road, Utica, NY 13502-4892. *Telephone:* 315-792-3006. *Fax:* 315-792-3003. *E-mail:* pquinn@utica.edu.

CONTINUING EDUCATION PROGRAM

Contact Ms. Evelyn Fazekas, Director of Credit Programs, Continuing Education, Department of Nursing, Utica College, 1600 Burrstone Road, Utica, NY 13502-4892. *Telephone:* 315-792-3001. *Fax:* 315-792-3292. *E-mail:* efazekas@utica.edu.

Wagner College
Department of Nursing
Staten Island, New York

http://www.wagner.edu/programs/nursing.html
Founded in 1883

DEGREES • BS • MSN

Nursing Program Faculty 17 (90% with doctorates).

Baccalaureate Enrollment 60
Women 82% **Men** 18% **Minority** 20% **International** 10% **Part-time** 5%

Graduate Enrollment 63
Women 90% **Men** 10% **Minority** 10% **Part-time** 95%

Nursing Student Activities Nursing Honor Society, Sigma Theta Tau, Student Nurses' Association.

Nursing Student Resources Academic advising; academic or career counseling; assistance for students with disabilities; bookstore; campus computer network; career placement assistance; computer lab; computer-assisted instruction; e-mail services; externships; housing assistance; interactive nursing skills videos; Internet; learning resource lab; library services; nursing audiovisuals; remedial services; skills, simulation, or other laboratory; tutoring; unpaid internships.

Library Facilities 310,000 volumes (4,505 in health, 859 in nursing); 1,000 periodical subscriptions (87 health-care related).

BACCALAUREATE PROGRAMS

Degree BS

Available Programs Baccalaureate for Second Degree; Generic Baccalaureate.

Study Options Full-time.

Program Entrance Requirements Minimum overall college GPA of 3.0, written essay, health exam, health insurance, high school chemistry, high school transcript, immunizations, letters of recommendation, minimum high school GPA of 2.7, minimum GPA in nursing prerequisites of 3.0, prerequisite course work. Transfer students are accepted. **Standardized**

tests *Required:* SAT or ACT, TOEFL for international students. **Application** *Deadline:* rolling (freshmen), rolling (transfer). *Notification:* continuous (freshmen), continuous (early decision). *Application fee:* $50.

Advanced Placement Credit by examination available. Credit given for nursing courses completed elsewhere dependent upon specific evaluations.

Contact *Telephone:* 718-390-3452. *Fax:* 718-420-4009.

GRADUATE PROGRAMS

Contact *Telephone:* 718-390-3444. *Fax:* 718-420-4009.

MASTER'S DEGREE PROGRAM

Degree MSN

Concentrations Available Nursing education. *Nurse practitioner programs in:* family health.

Study Options Full-time and part-time.

Program Entrance Requirements Clinical experience, minimum overall college GPA of 2.7, transcript of college record, CPR certification, immunizations, interview, 2 letters of recommendation, nursing research course, professional liability insurance/malpractice insurance, resume. *Application deadline:* For fall admission, 8/1 (priority date); for spring admission, 12/10. Applications are processed on a rolling basis. *Application fee:* $50 ($85 for international students).

Degree Requirements 44 total credit hours.

POST-MASTER'S PROGRAM

Areas of Study *Nurse practitioner programs in:* family health.

York College of the City University of New York
Program in Nursing
Jamaica, New York

http://www.york.cuny.edu/~healthsci/nuprogram. html

Founded in 1967

DEGREE • BS

Nursing Program Faculty 5 (60% with doctorates).

Library Facilities 182,141 volumes (8,714 in health, 567 in nursing); 1,978 periodical subscriptions.

BACCALAUREATE PROGRAMS

Degree BS

Available Programs ADN to Baccalaureate; RN Baccalaureate.

Program Entrance Requirements Minimum overall college GPA of 2.5, transcript of college record, CPR certification, health exam, immunizations, minimum GPA in nursing prerequisites, professional liability insurance/malpractice insurance, prerequisite course work, RN licensure. Transfer students are accepted. **Standardized tests** *Required:* SAT or ACT, TOEFL for international students. *Required for some:* SAT, ACT. **Application** *Deadline:* rolling (freshmen), rolling (transfer). *Notification:* continuous (freshmen). *Application fee:* $65.

Advanced Placement Credit by examination available. Credit given for nursing courses completed elsewhere dependent upon specific evaluations.

Contact *Telephone:* 718-262-2165.

NORTH CAROLINA

Barton College
School of Nursing
Wilson, North Carolina

http://www.barton.edu/nursing

Founded in 1902

DEGREE • BSN

Nursing Program Faculty 10 (90% with doctorates).

Baccalaureate Enrollment 120
Women 90% **Men** 10% **Minority** 20% **International** 2% **Part-time** 5%

Nursing Student Activities Nursing Honor Society, Sigma Theta Tau, Student Nurses' Association.

Nursing Student Resources Academic advising; academic or career counseling; assistance for students with disabilities; bookstore; campus computer network; career placement assistance; computer lab; computer-assisted instruction; e-mail services; externships; interactive nursing skills videos; Internet; learning resource lab; library services; nursing audiovisuals; paid internships; placement services for program completers; remedial services; resume preparation assistance; skills, simulation, or other laboratory; tutoring; unpaid internships.

Library Facilities 193,672 volumes (3,500 in health, 2,250 in nursing); 16,866 periodical subscriptions (100 health-care related).

BACCALAUREATE PROGRAMS

Degree BSN

Available Programs Generic Baccalaureate.

Site Options Smithfield, NC; Goldsboro, NC; Raleigh, NC.

Study Options Full-time and part-time.

Program Entrance Requirements Minimum overall college GPA of 2.5, transcript of college record, CPR certification, health exam, health insurance, high school chemistry, immunizations, minimum GPA in nursing prerequisites of 2.5, professional liability insurance/malpractice insurance, prerequisite course work. Transfer students are accepted. **Standardized tests** *Required:* SAT or ACT, TOEFL for international students. **Application** *Deadline:* rolling (freshmen), rolling (transfer). *Notification:* continuous (freshmen). *Application fee:* $25.

Advanced Placement Credit given for nursing courses completed elsewhere dependent upon specific evaluations.

Expenses (2006–07) *Tuition:* full-time $16,352; part-time $696 per credit hour. *International tuition:* $16,352 full-time. *Room and board:* $5200; room only: $2173 per academic year. *Required fees:* full-time $850; part-time $650 per term.

Financial Aid 90% of baccalaureate students in nursing programs received some form of financial aid in 2005–06. *Gift aid (need-based):* Federal Pell, FSEOG, state, private, college/university gift aid from institutional funds, Federal Nursing. *Loans:* FFEL (Subsidized and Unsubsidized Stafford PLUS), Perkins, alternative loans. *Work-Study:* Federal Work-Study. *Application deadline (priority):* 4/1.

Contact Dr. Nancy West Simeonsson, Dean, School of Nursing, Barton College, PO Box 5000, Wilson, NC 27893-7000. *Telephone:* 252-399-6400 Ext. 6401. *Fax:* 252-399-6416. *E-mail:* simeonsson@barton.edu.

Cabarrus College of Health Sciences
Louise Harkey School of Nursing
Concord, North Carolina

http://www.cabarruscollege.edu

Founded in 1942

DEGREE • BSN

Nursing Program Faculty 3 (50% with doctorates).

Cabarrus College of Health Sciences (continued)
Baccalaureate Enrollment 22
Women 100% **Minority** 2% **Part-time** 98%
Nursing Student Activities Nursing Honor Society, Student Nurses' Association, nursing club.
Nursing Student Resources Academic advising; academic or career counseling; assistance for students with disabilities; bookstore; campus computer network; career placement assistance; computer lab; computer-assisted instruction; e-mail services; externships; interactive nursing skills videos; Internet; library services; skills, simulation, or other laboratory; unpaid internships.
Library Facilities 7,676 volumes (500 in health, 300 in nursing); 2,127 periodical subscriptions (300 health-care related).

BACCALAUREATE PROGRAMS

Degree BSN

Available Programs RN Baccalaureate.
Program Entrance Requirements Transcript of college record, CPR certification, health exam, immunizations, 2 letters of recommendation, RN licensure. Transfer students are accepted. **Standardized tests** *Required:* SAT or ACT. *Required for some:* ACT ASSET. **Application** *Deadline:* 3/1 (freshmen), 3/1 (transfer). *Notification:* 4/15 (freshmen). *Application fee:* $35.
Contact *Telephone:* 704-783-1756. *Fax:* 704-783-2077.

Duke University
School of Nursing
Durham, North Carolina

http://www.nursing.duke.edu
Founded in 1838
DEGREES • BSN • MSN • MSN/MBA • MSN/MCM • PHD

Nursing Program Faculty 45 (71% with doctorates).
Baccalaureate Enrollment 113
Women 91% **Men** 9% **Minority** 18%
Graduate Enrollment 360
Women 92% **Men** 8% **Minority** 13% **International** 1% **Part-time** 59%
Nursing Student Activities Sigma Theta Tau, Student Nurses' Association.
Nursing Student Resources Academic advising; academic or career counseling; assistance for students with disabilities; bookstore; campus computer network; career placement assistance; computer lab; computer-assisted instruction; e-mail services; Internet; library services; nursing audiovisuals; skills, simulation, or other laboratory.
Library Facilities 5.6 million volumes (272,767 in health, 40,915 in nursing); 31,892 periodical subscriptions (2,781 health-care related).

BACCALAUREATE PROGRAMS

Degree BSN

Available Programs Accelerated Baccalaureate for Second Degree.
Site Options Durham, NC.
Study Options Full-time.
Program Entrance Requirements Minimum overall college GPA of 3.0, transcript of college record, CPR certification, written essay, health exam, health insurance, immunizations, interview, 3 letters of recommendation, prerequisite course work. **Standardized tests** *Required:* SAT and SAT Subject Tests or ACT, TOEFL for international students. **Application** *Deadline:* 1/2 (freshmen), 3/15 (transfer). *Early decision:* 11/1. *Notification:* 4/1 (freshmen), 12/15 (out-of-state freshmen), 12/15 (early decision). *Application fee:* $75.
Advanced Placement Credit by examination available.
Expenses (2006–07) *Tuition:* full-time $28,609. *International tuition:* $28,609 full-time. *Room and board:* $11,880; room only: $6960 per academic year. *Required fees:* part-time $619 per credit; part-time $1615 per term.

Financial Aid 88% of baccalaureate students in nursing programs received some form of financial aid in 2005–06. *Gift aid (need-based):* Federal Pell, FSEOG, state, private, college/university gift aid from institutional funds. *Loans:* FFEL (Subsidized and Unsubsidized Stafford PLUS), Perkins, college/university, alternative loans. *Work-Study:* Federal Work-Study, part-time campus jobs. *Application deadline:* 2/1.
Contact Mrs. Melissa Ziberna, Admissions Officer, School of Nursing, Duke University, DUMC 3322 Trent Drive, Durham, NC 27710. *Telephone:* 919-684-9161. *Fax:* 919-668-4693. *E-mail:* ziber001@mc.duke.edu.

GRADUATE PROGRAMS

Expenses (2006–07) *Tuition:* full-time $21,195; part-time $14,130 per semester. *International tuition:* $21,195 full-time. *Room and board:* $11,880; room only: $6960 per academic year. *Required fees:* part-time $785 per credit; part-time $1460 per term.
Financial Aid 73% of graduate students in nursing programs received some form of financial aid in 2005–06. Career-related internships or fieldwork, institutionally sponsored loans, scholarships, traineeships, and tuition waivers (partial) available. Aid available to part-time students. *Financial aid application deadline:* 3/1.
Contact Mrs. Benet Bondi, Admissions Officer, School of Nursing, Duke University, Box 3322, Durham, NC 27710. *Telephone:* 919-684-9163. *Fax:* 919-668-4693. *E-mail:* bondi001@mc.duke.edu.

MASTER'S DEGREE PROGRAM

Degrees MSN; MSN/MBA; MSN/MCM

Available Programs Master's; RN to Master's.
Concentrations Available Health-care administration; nurse anesthesia; nurse case management; nursing administration; nursing education; nursing informatics. *Clinical nurse specialist programs in:* cardiovascular, critical care, gerontology, maternity-newborn, oncology, pediatric. *Nurse practitioner programs in:* acute care, adult health, family health, gerontology, neonatal health, oncology, pediatric, primary care.
Site Options *Distance Learning:* Durham, NC.
Study Options Full-time and part-time.
Program Entrance Requirements Clinical experience, computer literacy, minimum overall college GPA of 3.0, transcript of college record, CPR certification, written essay, immunizations, interview, 3 letters of recommendation, prerequisite course work, resume, statistics course, GRE General Test or MAT. *Application deadline:* For fall admission, 8/1 (priority date); for spring admission, 12/20 (priority date). Applications are processed on a rolling basis. *Application fee:* $50.
Advanced Placement Credit given for nursing courses completed elsewhere dependent upon specific evaluations.
Degree Requirements 39 total credit hours, thesis or project.

POST-MASTER'S PROGRAM

Areas of Study Health-care administration; nurse anesthesia; nurse case management; nursing administration; nursing education; nursing informatics. *Clinical nurse specialist programs in:* cardiovascular, critical care, gerontology, maternity-newborn, oncology, pediatric. *Nurse practitioner programs in:* acute care, adult health, family health, gerontology, neonatal health, oncology, pediatric, primary care.

DOCTORAL DEGREE PROGRAM

Degree PhD

Available Programs Doctorate.
Areas of Study Health-care systems, illness and transition, information systems, nursing education, nursing research, nursing science.
Site Options Durham, NC.
Program Entrance Requirements Minimum overall college GPA of 3.5, interview by faculty committee, interview, 3 letters of recommendation, MSN or equivalent, statistics course, vita. *Application deadline:* For fall admission, 8/1 (priority date); for spring admission, 12/20 (priority date). Applications are processed on a rolling basis. *Application fee:* $50.
Degree Requirements 54 total credit hours, dissertation, oral exam.

See full description on page 472.

East Carolina University
School of Nursing
Greenville, North Carolina

Founded in 1907

DEGREES • BSN • MSN • PHD

Nursing Program Faculty 85 (35% with doctorates).

Baccalaureate Enrollment 532
Women 88% **Men** 12% **Minority** 19% **Part-time** 18%

Graduate Enrollment 290
Women 90% **Men** 10% **Minority** 7% **Part-time** 47%

Nursing Student Activities Sigma Theta Tau, Student Nurses' Association.

Nursing Student Resources Academic advising; academic or career counseling; assistance for students with disabilities; bookstore; campus computer network; career placement assistance; computer lab; computer-assisted instruction; e-mail services; employment services for current students; externships; housing assistance; interactive nursing skills videos; Internet; learning resource lab; library services; nursing audiovisuals; paid internships; remedial services; resume preparation assistance; skills, simulation, or other laboratory.

Library Facilities 2 million volumes (67,627 in health, 6,692 in nursing); 252,699 periodical subscriptions (848 health-care related).

BACCALAUREATE PROGRAMS

Degree BSN

Available Programs ADN to Baccalaureate; Accelerated RN Baccalaureate; Baccalaureate for Second Degree; Generic Baccalaureate; RN Baccalaureate.

Study Options Full-time and part-time.

Program Entrance Requirements Minimum overall college GPA of 2.5, transcript of college record, CPR certification, health exam, health insurance, immunizations, professional liability insurance/malpractice insurance, prerequisite course work. Transfer students are accepted. **Standardized tests** *Required:* SAT or ACT. **Application** *Deadline:* 3/15 (freshmen). *Notification:* continuous (freshmen). *Application fee:* $60.

Advanced Placement Credit given for nursing courses completed elsewhere dependent upon specific evaluations.

Expenses (2006–07) *Tuition, state resident:* full-time $2335. *Tuition, nonresident:* full-time $12,849. *International tuition:* $12,849 full-time. *Room and board:* $8300; room only: $4150 per academic year. *Required fees:* full-time $2008.

Financial Aid 60% of baccalaureate students in nursing programs received some form of financial aid in 2005–06. *Gift aid (need-based):* Federal Pell, FSEOG, state, private, college/university gift aid from institutional funds. *Loans:* Federal Nursing Student Loans, FFEL (Subsidized and Unsubsidized Stafford PLUS), Perkins. *Work-Study:* Federal Work-Study, part-time campus jobs. *Application deadline (priority):* 4/15.

Contact Karen Krupa, RN, Director of Student Services, School of Nursing, East Carolina University, Health Sciences Building, Suite 2150, Greenville, NC 27858-4353. *Telephone:* 252-744-6477. *Fax:* 252-744-6391. *E-mail:* krupak@ecu.edu.

GRADUATE PROGRAMS

Expenses (2006–07) *Tuition, state resident:* full-time $2816. *Tuition, nonresident:* full-time $13,132. *International tuition:* $13,132 full-time. *Room and board:* $8300; room only: $4150 per academic year. *Required fees:* full-time $250; part-time $125 per term.

Financial Aid 49% of graduate students in nursing programs received some form of financial aid in 2005–06. Research assistantships with partial tuition reimbursements available, teaching assistantships with partial tuition reimbursements available, Federal Work-Study available. Aid available to part-time students. *Financial aid application deadline:* 6/1.

Contact Dr. Sylvia T. Brown, Associate Dean, School of Nursing, East Carolina University, Health Sciences Building, Room 3166B, Greenville, NC 27858-4353. *Telephone:* 252-744-6422. *Fax:* 252-744-6536. *E-mail:* brownsy@ecu.edu.

MASTER'S DEGREE PROGRAM

Degree MSN

Available Programs Master's; Master's for Nurses with Non-Nursing Degrees; RN to Master's.

Concentrations Available Nurse anesthesia; nurse-midwifery; nursing administration; nursing education. *Clinical nurse specialist programs in:* adult health, community health, medical-surgical. *Nurse practitioner programs in:* adult health, family health, neonatal health.

Study Options Full-time.

Program Entrance Requirements Clinical experience, computer literacy, minimum overall college GPA of 3.0, transcript of college record, CPR certification, written essay, immunizations, interview, 3 letters of recommendation, nursing research course, professional liability insurance/malpractice insurance, statistics course, GRE General Test or MAT. *Application deadline:* For fall admission, 6/1 (priority date). Applications are processed on a rolling basis. *Application fee:* $50.

Advanced Placement Credit by examination available. Credit given for nursing courses completed elsewhere dependent upon specific evaluations.

Degree Requirements 36 total credit hours, comprehensive exam.

POST-MASTER'S PROGRAM

Areas of Study Nurse anesthesia; nurse-midwifery; nursing education. *Clinical nurse specialist programs in:* adult health, medical-surgical. *Nurse practitioner programs in:* family health, neonatal health.

DOCTORAL DEGREE PROGRAM

Degree PhD

Available Programs Doctorate.

Areas of Study Nursing science.

Program Entrance Requirements Minimum overall college GPA of 3.2, interview by faculty committee, 3 letters of recommendation, MSN or equivalent, scholarly papers, statistics course, vita, writing sample. *Application deadline:* For fall admission, 6/1 (priority date). Applications are processed on a rolling basis. *Application fee:* $50.

Degree Requirements 54 total credit hours, dissertation, oral exam, written exam.

Fayetteville State University
Program in Nursing
Fayetteville, North Carolina

Founded in 1867

DEGREE • BS

Library Facilities 311,016 volumes; 2,712 periodical subscriptions.

BACCALAUREATE PROGRAMS

Degree BS

Available Programs Generic Baccalaureate; RN Baccalaureate.

Program Entrance Requirements Standardized tests *Required:* SAT or ACT, TOEFL for international students. **Application** *Deadline:* 7/1 (freshmen), 7/1 (transfer). *Notification:* continuous (freshmen). *Application fee:* $25.

Contact Nursing Department, Program in Nursing, Fayetteville State University, 1200 Murchison Road, Fayetteville, NC 28301-4298. *Telephone:* 910-672-1924. *E-mail:* sasmith@uncfsu.edu.

Gardner-Webb University
School of Nursing
Boiling Springs, North Carolina

http://www.nursing.gardner-webb.edu/index.html

Founded in 1905

DEGREES • BSN • MSN • MSN/MBA

Nursing Student Activities Nursing Honor Society, Student Nurses' Association.

Library Facilities 236,000 volumes; 15,000 periodical subscriptions.

Gardner-Webb University (continued)
BACCALAUREATE PROGRAMS
Degree BSN

Available Programs RN Baccalaureate.

Site Options Statesville, NC; Charlotte, NC; Cabarrus, NC.

Study Options Full-time and part-time.

Program Entrance Requirements Minimum overall college GPA of 2.5, transcript of college record, minimum GPA in nursing prerequisites of 2.5, prerequisite course work, RN licensure. Transfer students are accepted. **Standardized tests** *Required:* SAT or ACT, TOEFL for international students. **Application** *Deadline:* rolling (freshmen), rolling (transfer). *Application fee:* $40.

Contact *Telephone:* 704-406-4360. *Fax:* 704-406-3919.

GRADUATE PROGRAMS
Contact *Telephone:* 704-406-4358. *Fax:* 704-406-3919.

MASTER'S DEGREE PROGRAM
Degrees MSN; MSN/MBA

Available Programs Master's; RN to Master's.

Concentrations Available Nursing administration; nursing education.

Program Entrance Requirements Minimum overall college GPA of 2.7, transcript of college record, immunizations, 3 letters of recommendation, statistics course.

Degree Requirements 30 total credit hours.

Lees-McRae College
Nursing Program
Banner Elk, North Carolina

*http://www.lmc.edu/lmcAcademics/Outreach/
OffCampusPrograms/Mayland_Nursing.htm*

Founded in 1900

DEGREE • BSN

Nursing Program Faculty 3.

Baccalaureate Enrollment 39

Women 87% **Men** 13%

Nursing Student Resources Academic advising; academic or career counseling; bookstore; computer lab; computer-assisted instruction; e-mail services; Internet; learning resource lab; library services; nursing audiovisuals; skills, simulation, or other laboratory.

Library Facilities 88,756 volumes; 429 periodical subscriptions.

BACCALAUREATE PROGRAMS
Degree BSN

Available Programs ADN to Baccalaureate.

Site Options Spruce Pine, NC.

Study Options Full-time.

Program Entrance Requirements Transcript of college record, immunizations, 2 letters of recommendation, prerequisite course work, RN licensure. Transfer students are accepted. **Standardized tests** *Required:* SAT or ACT. **Application** *Deadline:* 8/1 (freshmen), 8/1 (transfer). *Notification:* continuous until 8/15 (freshmen). *Application fee:* $25.

Contact Ms. Martha P. Hartley, RN, Director of RN to BSN Completion Program, Nursing Program, Lees-McRae College, 375 College Drive, PO Box 128, Banner Elk, NC 28604. *Telephone:* 828-765-2667. *Fax:* 828-898-8814. *E-mail:* Hartley@lmc.edu.

Lenoir-Rhyne College
Program in Nursing
Hickory, North Carolina

http://www.lrc.edu

Founded in 1891

DEGREE • BS

Nursing Program Faculty 23 (17% with doctorates).

Baccalaureate Enrollment 224

Women 92% **Men** 8% **Minority** 8% **International** 3% **Part-time** 4%

Nursing Student Activities Sigma Theta Tau, Student Nurses' Association.

Nursing Student Resources Academic advising; academic or career counseling; assistance for students with disabilities; bookstore; campus computer network; career placement assistance; computer lab; computer-assisted instruction; e-mail services; employment services for current students; externships; housing assistance; interactive nursing skills videos; Internet; learning resource lab; library services; nursing audiovisuals; placement services for program completers; remedial services; resume preparation assistance; skills, simulation, or other laboratory; tutoring; unpaid internships.

Library Facilities 275,961 volumes (5,000 in health, 4,200 in nursing); 445 periodical subscriptions (220 health-care related).

BACCALAUREATE PROGRAMS
Degree BS

Available Programs ADN to Baccalaureate; Generic Baccalaureate.

Study Options Full-time and part-time.

Program Entrance Requirements Minimum overall college GPA of 2.5, transcript of college record, health exam, high school chemistry, 3 years high school math, high school transcript, immunizations, minimum high school GPA of 3.0, minimum GPA in nursing prerequisites of 2.5. Transfer students are accepted. **Standardized tests** *Required:* SAT or ACT, TOEFL for international students. **Application** *Deadline:* rolling (freshmen), 9/1 (transfer). *Notification:* continuous (freshmen), 9/1 (early action). *Application fee:* $25.

Advanced Placement Credit by examination available. Credit given for nursing courses completed elsewhere dependent upon specific evaluations.

Expenses (2006–07) *Tuition:* full-time $19,350; part-time $806 per credit hour. *International tuition:* $19,350 full-time. *Room and board:* $7130; room only: $3630 per academic year. *Required fees:* full-time $930.

Financial Aid 100% of baccalaureate students in nursing programs received some form of financial aid in 2005–06.

Contact Dr. Linda W. Reece, Head, Program in Nursing, Lenoir-Rhyne College, PO Box 7292, Hickory, NC 28603. *Telephone:* 828-328-7282. *Fax:* 828-328-7284. *E-mail:* reecel@lrc.edu.

North Carolina Agricultural and Technical State University
School of Nursing
Greensboro, North Carolina

http://www.ncat.edu/~nursing/index.html

Founded in 1891

DEGREE • BSN

Nursing Program Faculty 23 (30% with doctorates).

Baccalaureate Enrollment 418

Women 99% **Men** 1% **Minority** 91% **Part-time** 1%

Nursing Student Activities Nursing Honor Society, Sigma Theta Tau, Student Nurses' Association, nursing club.

Nursing Student Resources Academic advising; academic or career counseling; assistance for students with disabilities; bookstore; campus computer network; career placement assistance; computer lab; computer-assisted instruction; e-mail services; employment services for current students; externships; housing assistance; interactive nursing skills videos; Internet; learning resource lab; library services; nursing audiovisuals; other; paid internships; placement services for program completers; remedial services; resume preparation assistance; skills, simulation, or other laboratory; tutoring; unpaid internships.

Library Facilities 541,403 volumes (14,200 in health, 3,045 in nursing); 31,674 periodical subscriptions (85 health-care related).

BACCALAUREATE PROGRAMS

Degree BSN

Available Programs Generic Baccalaureate; LPN to Baccalaureate; RN Baccalaureate.

Site Options *Distance Learning:* Greensboro, NC; High Point, NC; Salisbury, NC.

Study Options Full-time and part-time.

Program Entrance Requirements Minimum overall college GPA of 2.6, transcript of college record, CPR certification, written essay, health exam, health insurance, 3 years high school math, 3 years high school science, high school transcript, immunizations, 3 letters of recommendation, minimum high school GPA of 3.0, minimum GPA in nursing prerequisites of 2.6, professional liability insurance/malpractice insurance, prerequisite course work. Transfer students are accepted. **Standardized tests** *Required:* TOEFL for international students. *Recommended:* SAT or ACT. **Application** *Deadline:* rolling (freshmen), rolling (transfer). *Notification:* continuous (freshmen). *Application fee:* $45.

Advanced Placement Credit by examination available. Credit given for nursing courses completed elsewhere dependent upon specific evaluations.

Expenses (2006–07) *Tuition, state resident:* full-time $1770; part-time $221 per credit hour. *Tuition, nonresident:* full-time $11,212; part-time $1402 per credit hour. *International tuition:* $11,212 full-time. *Room and board:* $7380; room only: $5080 per academic year. *Required fees:* full-time $1346; part-time $149 per credit; part-time $673 per term.

Financial Aid 97% of baccalaureate students in nursing programs received some form of financial aid in 2005–06. *Gift aid (need-based):* Federal Pell, FSEOG, state, private, college/university gift aid from institutional funds, United Negro College Fund. *Loans:* Federal Direct (Subsidized and Unsubsidized Stafford PLUS), Perkins, state, Alternative Loans. *Work-Study:* Federal Work-Study, part-time campus jobs. *Application deadline (priority):* 3/15.

Contact Ms. Dawn F. Murphy, Student Services Director, School of Nursing, North Carolina Agricultural and Technical State University, Noble Hall, 1601 East Market Street, Greensboro, NC 27411. *Telephone:* 336-334-7752. *Fax:* 336-334-7637. *E-mail:* dmurphy@ncat.edu.

North Carolina Central University
Department of Nursing
Durham, North Carolina

http://www.nccu.edu/artsci/nursing/

Founded in 1910

DEGREE • BSN

Nursing Program Faculty 30 (4% with doctorates).

Nursing Student Activities Sigma Theta Tau.

Nursing Student Resources Academic advising; academic or career counseling; assistance for students with disabilities; bookstore; campus computer network; career placement assistance; computer lab; computer-assisted instruction; e-mail services; employment services for current students; externships; housing assistance; interactive nursing skills videos; Internet; learning resource lab; library services; nursing audiovisuals; paid internships; placement services for program completers; resume preparation assistance; skills, simulation, or other laboratory; tutoring.

Library Facilities 500,712 volumes; 1,934 periodical subscriptions.

BACCALAUREATE PROGRAMS

Degree BSN

Available Programs Generic Baccalaureate.

Site Options *Distance Learning:* Henderson, NC.

Study Options Full-time.

Program Entrance Requirements Minimum overall college GPA of 2.0, transcript of college record, health exam, immunizations, minimum GPA in nursing prerequisites of 2.5, professional liability insurance/malpractice insurance, prerequisite course work. Transfer students are accepted. **Standardized tests** *Required:* SAT or ACT, TOEFL for international students. **Application** *Deadline:* 8/1 (freshmen), 8/1 (transfer). *Notification:* continuous until 10/15 (freshmen). *Application fee:* $30.

Advanced Placement Credit given for nursing courses completed elsewhere dependent upon specific evaluations.

Contact *Telephone:* 919-530-5336. *Fax:* 919-530-5343.

Queens University of Charlotte
Division of Nursing
Charlotte, North Carolina

http://www.queens.edu

Founded in 1857

DEGREES • BSN • MSN • MSN/MBA

Nursing Program Faculty 13 (33% with doctorates).

Baccalaureate Enrollment 100
Women 96% **Men** 4% **Minority** 12% **International** 2% **Part-time** 30%

Graduate Enrollment 20
Women 95% **Men** 5% **Minority** 15% **Part-time** 90%

Nursing Student Activities Sigma Theta Tau, Student Nurses' Association.

Nursing Student Resources Academic advising; academic or career counseling; assistance for students with disabilities; bookstore; campus computer network; career placement assistance; computer lab; computer-assisted instruction; e-mail services; employment services for current students; housing assistance; interactive nursing skills videos; Internet; learning resource lab; library services; nursing audiovisuals; placement services for program completers; resume preparation assistance; skills, simulation, or other laboratory; tutoring; unpaid internships.

Library Facilities 126,242 volumes (6,000 in health, 1,000 in nursing); 592 periodical subscriptions (500 health-care related).

BACCALAUREATE PROGRAMS

Degree BSN

Available Programs ADN to Baccalaureate; Baccalaureate for Second Degree; Generic Baccalaureate; LPN to Baccalaureate; RN Baccalaureate.

Study Options Full-time and part-time.

Program Entrance Requirements Minimum overall college GPA of 2.5, transcript of college record, CPR certification, health exam, health insurance, high school transcript, immunizations, minimum GPA in nursing prerequisites of 2.5, prerequisite course work. Transfer students are accepted. **Standardized tests** *Required:* SAT or ACT, TOEFL for international students. **Application** *Deadline:* rolling (freshmen), rolling (transfer). *Notification:* continuous (freshmen). *Application fee:* $40.

Advanced Placement Credit given for nursing courses completed elsewhere dependent upon specific evaluations.

Expenses (2005–06) *Tuition:* full-time $18,028; part-time $290 per credit hour. *International tuition:* $18,028 full-time. *Room and board:* $6500 per academic year. *Required fees:* full-time $200; part-time $100 per term.

Financial Aid 85% of baccalaureate students in nursing programs received some form of financial aid in 2004–05.

Contact Dr. Joan S. McGill, RN, Chair and Professor, Division of Nursing, Queens University of Charlotte, 1900 Selwyn Avenue, Charlotte, NC 28274. *Telephone:* 704-337-2276. *Fax:* 704-337-2477. *E-mail:* mcgillj@queens.edu.

GRADUATE PROGRAMS

Expenses (2005–06) *Tuition:* full-time $2610; part-time $290 per credit hour. *International tuition:* $2610 full-time.

Financial Aid 70% of graduate students in nursing programs received some form of financial aid in 2004–05.

Contact Dr. Susan Harvey, RN, Chair and Professor, Division of Nursing, Queens University of Charlotte, 1900 Selwyn Avenue, Charlotte, NC 28274. *Telephone:* 704-337-2292. *Fax:* 704-337-2477. *E-mail:* harveys@queens.edu.

MASTER'S DEGREE PROGRAM

Degrees MSN; MSN/MBA

Available Programs Accelerated RN to Master's; Master's; RN to Master's.

Concentrations Available Nursing administration.

Queens University of Charlotte (continued)

Study Options Full-time and part-time.

Program Entrance Requirements Minimum overall college GPA of 3.0, transcript of college record, 2 letters of recommendation, resume. *Application deadline:* Applications are processed on a rolling basis. *Application fee:* $40.

Advanced Placement Credit given for nursing courses completed elsewhere dependent upon specific evaluations.

Degree Requirements 39 total credit hours, thesis or project.

POST-MASTER'S PROGRAM

Areas of Study Nursing administration.

The University of North Carolina at Chapel Hill
School of Nursing
Chapel Hill, North Carolina

http://nursing.unc.edu/

Founded in 1789

DEGREES • BSN • MSN • MSN/MS • PHD

Nursing Program Faculty 112 (70% with doctorates).

Baccalaureate Enrollment 307
Women 92% **Men** 8% **Minority** 11%

Graduate Enrollment 174
Women 90% **Men** 10% **Minority** 20%

Nursing Student Activities Nursing Honor Society, Sigma Theta Tau, Student Nurses' Association, nursing club.

Nursing Student Resources Academic advising; academic or career counseling; assistance for students with disabilities; bookstore; campus computer network; career placement assistance; computer lab; computer-assisted instruction; e-mail services; employment services for current students; housing assistance; interactive nursing skills videos; Internet; learning resource lab; library services; nursing audiovisuals; other; remedial services; resume preparation assistance; skills, simulation, or other laboratory; tutoring.

Library Facilities 5.7 million volumes (315,000 in health); 53,444 periodical subscriptions (4,000 health-care related).

BACCALAUREATE PROGRAMS

Degree BSN

Available Programs ADN to Baccalaureate; Accelerated Baccalaureate for Second Degree; Generic Baccalaureate; RN Baccalaureate.

Site Options *Distance Learning:* Smithfield, NC; High Point, NC.

Study Options Full-time.

Program Entrance Requirements Minimum overall college GPA of 2.0, transcript of college record, CPR certification, written essay, health exam, health insurance, high school transcript, immunizations, 2 letters of recommendation, minimum GPA in nursing prerequisites of 2.0, prerequisite course work. Transfer students are accepted. **Standardized tests** *Required:* SAT or ACT, TOEFL for international students. **Application** *Deadline:* 1/15 (freshmen), 3/1 (transfer). *Early decision:* 11/1. *Notification:* 3/31 (freshmen), 1/31 (early action). *Application fee:* $70.

Advanced Placement Credit by examination available. Credit given for nursing courses completed elsewhere dependent upon specific evaluations.

Contact *Telephone:* 919-966-4260. *Fax:* 919-966-3540.

GRADUATE PROGRAMS

Contact *Telephone:* 919-966-4260. *Fax:* 919-966-3540.

MASTER'S DEGREE PROGRAM

Degrees MSN; MSN/MS

Available Programs Master's for Nurses with Non-Nursing Degrees; RN to Master's.

Concentrations Available Nurse case management; nursing administration; nursing education; nursing informatics. *Clinical nurse specialist programs in:* maternity-newborn, pediatric, psychiatric/mental health, women's health. *Nurse practitioner programs in:* adult health, family health, neonatal health, pediatric, primary care, psychiatric/mental health, women's health.

Study Options Full-time and part-time.

Program Entrance Requirements Clinical experience, minimum overall college GPA of 3.0, transcript of college record, CPR certification, written essay, immunizations, 3 letters of recommendation, physical assessment course, professional liability insurance/malpractice insurance, resume, statistics course, GRE General Test. *Application deadline:* For fall admission, 3/31; for spring admission, 10/15. *Application fee:* $55.

Advanced Placement Credit given for nursing courses completed elsewhere dependent upon specific evaluations.

Degree Requirements 40 total credit hours, thesis or project, comprehensive exam.

POST-MASTER'S PROGRAM

Areas of Study Nurse case management; nursing administration; nursing education; nursing informatics. *Clinical nurse specialist programs in:* maternity-newborn, pediatric, psychiatric/mental health, women's health. *Nurse practitioner programs in:* adult health, family health, neonatal health, pediatric, primary care, psychiatric/mental health, women's health.

DOCTORAL DEGREE PROGRAM

Degree PhD

Available Programs Doctorate.

Areas of Study Nursing research.

Program Entrance Requirements Minimum overall college GPA of 3.0, interview by faculty committee, 3 letters of recommendation, scholarly papers, statistics course, vita, writing sample, GRE General Test. *Application deadline:* For fall admission, 3/31; for spring admission, 10/15. *Application fee:* $55.

Degree Requirements 48 total credit hours, dissertation, oral exam, written exam, residency.

POSTDOCTORAL PROGRAM

Areas of Study Adolescent health, aging, cancer care, chronic illness, community health, family health, gerontology, health promotion/disease prevention, individualized study, information systems, neuro-behavior, nursing informatics, nursing interventions, nursing research, nursing science, outcomes, self-care, vulnerable population, women's health.

Postdoctoral Program Contact *Telephone:* 919-966-5294. *Fax:* 919-966-3540.

CONTINUING EDUCATION PROGRAM

Contact *Telephone:* 919-966-3638. *Fax:* 919-966-7298.

The University of North Carolina at Charlotte
School of Nursing
Charlotte, North Carolina

http://www.health.uncc.edu

Founded in 1946

DEGREES • BSN • MSN • MSN/MHA

Nursing Program Faculty 45 (53% with doctorates).

Baccalaureate Enrollment 260
Women 90% **Men** 10% **Minority** 15%

Graduate Enrollment 177
Women 80% **Men** 20% **Minority** 10% **Part-time** 75%

Nursing Student Activities Sigma Theta Tau, Student Nurses' Association.

Nursing Student Resources Academic advising; academic or career counseling; assistance for students with disabilities; bookstore; campus computer network; career placement assistance; computer lab; computer-assisted instruction; e-mail services; externships; interactive nursing skills videos; Internet; learning resource lab; library services; nursing audiovisuals; skills, simulation, or other laboratory.

Library Facilities 969,680 volumes (39,000 in health, 2,400 in nursing); 32,486 periodical subscriptions (160 health-care related).

BACCALAUREATE PROGRAMS

Degree BSN

Available Programs ADN to Baccalaureate; Generic Baccalaureate; RN Baccalaureate.

Study Options Full-time.

Program Entrance Requirements Minimum overall college GPA of 2.5, transcript of college record, CPR certification, health exam, health insurance, high school biology, high school chemistry, high school foreign language, 3 years high school math, 3 years high school science, high school transcript, immunizations, minimum GPA in nursing prerequisites of 2.5, prerequisite course work. Transfer students are accepted. **Standardized tests** *Required:* SAT or ACT, TOEFL for international students. **Application** *Deadline:* 7/1 (freshmen), 7/1 (transfer). *Early decision:* 10/15. *Notification:* continuous (freshmen). *Application fee:* $50.

Contact *Telephone:* 704-687-4682. *Fax:* 704-687-3180.

GRADUATE PROGRAMS

Contact *Telephone:* 704-687-4682. *Fax:* 704-687-3180.

MASTER'S DEGREE PROGRAM

Degrees MSN; MSN/MHA

Available Programs Master's; RN to Master's.

Concentrations Available Health-care administration; nurse anesthesia. *Clinical nurse specialist programs in:* adult health, community health, psychiatric/mental health. *Nurse practitioner programs in:* adult health, family health.

Site Options *Distance Learning:* Gastonia, NC; Salisbury, NC.

Program Entrance Requirements Clinical experience, computer literacy, minimum overall college GPA of 3.0, transcript of college record, CPR certification, written essay, immunizations, interview, 3 letters of recommendation, nursing research course, professional liability insurance/malpractice insurance, resume, statistics course.

POST-MASTER'S PROGRAM

Areas of Study Nurse anesthesia; nursing administration. *Nurse practitioner programs in:* family health.

CONTINUING EDUCATION PROGRAM

Contact *Telephone:* 704-687-4675. *Fax:* 704-687-3180.

The University of North Carolina at Greensboro
School of Nursing
Greensboro, North Carolina

http://www.uncg.edu/nur/

Founded in 1891

DEGREES • BSN • MSN • MSN/MBA • PHD

Nursing Program Faculty 60 (60% with doctorates).

Baccalaureate Enrollment 1,138
Women 93% **Men** 7% **Minority** 29% **International** 4% **Part-time** 33%

Graduate Enrollment 275
Women 80% **Men** 20% **Minority** 18% **International** 4% **Part-time** 30%

Nursing Student Activities Nursing Honor Society, Sigma Theta Tau, Student Nurses' Association.

Nursing Student Resources Academic advising; academic or career counseling; assistance for students with disabilities; bookstore; campus computer network; career placement assistance; computer lab; computer-assisted instruction; e-mail services; externships; Internet; learning resource lab; library services; nursing audiovisuals; paid internships; placement services for program completers; remedial services; resume preparation assistance; skills, simulation, or other laboratory; tutoring; unpaid internships.

Library Facilities 844,448 volumes; 8,714 periodical subscriptions.

BACCALAUREATE PROGRAMS

Degree BSN

Available Programs ADN to Baccalaureate; Baccalaureate for Second Degree; Generic Baccalaureate; LPN to Baccalaureate; LPN to RN Baccalaureate; RN Baccalaureate.

Site Options Hickory, NC; Greensboro, NC.

Study Options Full-time.

Program Entrance Requirements Minimum overall college GPA of 2.7, transcript of college record, CPR certification, health exam, immunizations, minimum GPA in nursing prerequisites of 3.0, professional liability insurance/malpractice insurance, prerequisite course work. Transfer students are accepted. **Standardized tests** *Required:* SAT or ACT, TOEFL for international students. **Application** *Deadline:* 3/1 (freshmen), 8/1 (transfer). *Notification:* continuous (freshmen). *Application fee:* $45.

Expenses (2006–07) *Tuition, state resident:* full-time $2308; part-time $289 per credit hour. *Tuition, nonresident:* full-time $13,576; part-time $1697 per credit hour. *Room and board:* $5760; room only: $3200 per academic year. *Required fees:* full-time $2268; part-time $162 per credit; part-time $162 per term.

Financial Aid 80% of baccalaureate students in nursing programs received some form of financial aid in 2005–06. *Gift aid (need-based):* Federal Pell, FSEOG, state, private, college/university gift aid from institutional funds. *Loans:* FFEL (Subsidized and Unsubsidized Stafford PLUS), Perkins, college/university. *Work-Study:* Federal Work-Study. *Application deadline (priority):* 3/1.

Contact Virginia B. Karb, PhD, Associate Dean, School of Nursing, The University of North Carolina at Greensboro, PO Box 26170, Greensboro, NC 27402-6170. *Telephone:* 336-334-5280. *Fax:* 336-334-3628. *E-mail:* virginia_karb@uncg.edu.

GRADUATE PROGRAMS

Expenses (2006–07) *Tuition, state resident:* full-time $2018; part-time $673 per course. *Tuition, nonresident:* full-time $10,304; part-time $3435 per course. *Required fees:* full-time $650; part-time $162 per credit; part-time $162 per term.

Financial Aid 80% of graduate students in nursing programs received some form of financial aid in 2005–06. Research assistantships with full tuition reimbursements available, career-related internships or fieldwork, Federal Work-Study, scholarships, and traineeships available. Aid available to part-time students.

Contact Eileen Kohlenberg, Associate Dean and Director of Graduate Studies, School of Nursing, The University of North Carolina at Greensboro, PO Box 26170, Greensboro, NC 27402-6170. *Telephone:* 336-334-5561. *Fax:* 336-334-3628. *E-mail:* eileen_kohlenberg@uncg.edu.

MASTER'S DEGREE PROGRAM

Degrees MSN; MSN/MBA

Available Programs Master's.

Concentrations Available Nurse anesthesia; nursing administration; nursing education. *Nurse practitioner programs in:* adult health, gerontology.

Site Options Hickory, NC.

Study Options Full-time and part-time.

Program Entrance Requirements Clinical experience, minimum overall college GPA of 3.0, transcript of college record, CPR certification, immunizations, 3 letters of recommendation, physical assessment course, professional liability insurance/malpractice insurance, prerequisite course work, statistics course, GRE General Test or MAT. *Application fee:* $45.

Advanced Placement Credit given for nursing courses completed elsewhere dependent upon specific evaluations.

Degree Requirements 36 total credit hours, thesis or project, comprehensive exam.

POST-MASTER'S PROGRAM

Areas of Study Nurse anesthesia. *Nurse practitioner programs in:* adult health, gerontology.

DOCTORAL DEGREE PROGRAM

Degree PhD

Available Programs Doctorate.

The University of North Carolina at Greensboro (continued)

Areas of Study Aging, faculty preparation, gerontology, health policy, health promotion/disease prevention, nursing administration, nursing education, nursing research, nursing science, women's health.

Program Entrance Requirements Minimum overall college GPA of 3.0, interview by faculty committee, interview, 3 letters of recommendation, MSN or equivalent, writing sample. *Application fee:* $45.

Degree Requirements 57 total credit hours, dissertation, oral exam, written exam, residency.

The University of North Carolina at Pembroke
Nursing Program
Pembroke, North Carolina

Founded in 1887

DEGREE • BSN

Library Facilities 342,723 volumes; 113,823 periodical subscriptions.

BACCALAUREATE PROGRAMS

Degree BSN

Available Programs RN Baccalaureate.

Program Entrance Requirements Standardized tests *Required:* SAT or ACT, TOEFL for international students. **Application** *Deadline:* rolling (freshmen), rolling (transfer). *Notification:* continuous (freshmen). *Application fee:* $40.

Contact Department of Nursing, Nursing Program, The University of North Carolina at Pembroke, PO Box 1510, Pembroke, NC 28372-1510. *Telephone:* 910-521-6522. *Fax:* 910-521-6178. *E-mail:* nursing@uncp.edu.

The University of North Carolina Wilmington
School of Nursing
Wilmington, North Carolina

http://www.uncwil.edu/inside

Founded in 1947

DEGREES • BS • MSN

Nursing Program Faculty 31 (40% with doctorates).

Baccalaureate Enrollment 212
Women 92% **Men** 8% **Minority** 6% **Part-time** 3%

Graduate Enrollment 20
Women 85% **Men** 15% **Part-time** 60%

Nursing Student Activities Sigma Theta Tau, Student Nurses' Association.

Nursing Student Resources Academic advising; academic or career counseling; assistance for students with disabilities; bookstore; campus computer network; career placement assistance; computer lab; computer-assisted instruction; e-mail services; employment services for current students; externships; housing assistance; interactive nursing skills videos; Internet; learning resource lab; library services; nursing audiovisuals; placement services for program completers; remedial services; resume preparation assistance; skills, simulation, or other laboratory; tutoring; unpaid internships.

Library Facilities 553,391 volumes (15,000 in health, 9,000 in nursing); 22,218 periodical subscriptions (600 health-care related).

BACCALAUREATE PROGRAMS

Degree BS

Available Programs Generic Baccalaureate; RN Baccalaureate.

Site Options *Distance Learning:* Jacksonville, Whiteville, Supply, Elizabethtown, NC; Kenansville, NC; Burgaw, MP.

Study Options Full-time.

Program Entrance Requirements Minimum overall college GPA of 2.5, transcript of college record, CPR certification, written essay, health exam, health insurance, immunizations, minimum GPA in nursing prerequisites of 2.0, professional liability insurance/malpractice insurance, prerequisite course work. Transfer students are accepted. **Standardized tests** *Required:* SAT or ACT, TOEFL for international students. **Application** *Deadline:* 2/1 (freshmen), 3/15 (transfer). *Early decision:* 11/1. *Notification:* 4/1 (freshmen), 1/20 (early action). *Application fee:* $45.

Advanced Placement Credit given for nursing courses completed elsewhere dependent upon specific evaluations.

Expenses (2006–07) *Tuition, state resident:* full-time $2221. *Tuition, nonresident:* full-time $12,156. *Room and board:* $6200 per academic year. *Required fees:* full-time $1939.

Financial Aid 70% of baccalaureate students in nursing programs received some form of financial aid in 2005–06. *Gift aid (need-based):* Federal Pell, FSEOG, state, private, college/university gift aid from institutional funds. *Loans:* Federal Direct (Subsidized and Unsubsidized Stafford PLUS), Perkins, state, college/university. *Work-Study:* Federal Work-Study. *Application deadline:* Continuous.

Contact Dr. Deborah Pollard, Assistant Professor, School of Nursing, The University of North Carolina Wilmington, 601 South College Road, Wilmington, NC 28403-5995. *Telephone:* 910-962-4121. *Fax:* 910-962-4921. *E-mail:* pollardd@uncw.edu.

GRADUATE PROGRAMS

Expenses (2006–07) *Tuition, state resident:* full-time $2522. *Tuition, nonresident:* full-time $12,359. *Room and board:* $6200 per academic year. *Required fees:* full-time $1939.

Financial Aid 88% of graduate students in nursing programs received some form of financial aid in 2005–06. 2 teaching assistantships were awarded. *Financial aid application deadline:* 3/15.

Contact Dr. Julie S. Taylor, Graduate Coordinator, School of Nursing, The University of North Carolina Wilmington, 601 South College Road, Wilmington, NC 28403-5995. *Telephone:* 910-962-7927. *Fax:* 910-962-4921. *E-mail:* taylorjs@uncw.edu.

MASTER'S DEGREE PROGRAM

Degree MSN

Available Programs Master's; RN to Master's.

Concentrations Available Nursing education. *Nurse practitioner programs in:* family health.

Site Options *Distance Learning:* Jacksonville, Whiteville, Supply, Elizabethtown, NC; Kenansville, NC; Burgaw, MP.

Study Options Full-time and part-time.

Program Entrance Requirements Clinical experience, computer literacy, minimum overall college GPA of 3.0, transcript of college record, CPR certification, written essay, immunizations, 3 letters of recommendation, nursing research course, physical assessment course, professional liability insurance/malpractice insurance, prerequisite course work, resume, statistics course, GRE General Test. *Application deadline:* For fall admission, 3/1. Applications are processed on a rolling basis. *Application fee:* $45.

Advanced Placement Credit given for nursing courses completed elsewhere dependent upon specific evaluations.

Degree Requirements 47 total credit hours, thesis or project, comprehensive exam.

Western Carolina University
Department of Nursing
Cullowhee, North Carolina

Founded in 1889

DEGREES • BSN • MSN

Nursing Program Faculty 18 (45% with doctorates).

Baccalaureate Enrollment 114
Women 97% **Men** 3% **Minority** 2%

Graduate Enrollment 30
Women 100%

Nursing Student Activities Sigma Theta Tau, Student Nurses' Association.

Nursing Student Resources Academic advising; academic or career counseling; assistance for students with disabilities; bookstore; campus computer network; career placement assistance; computer lab; computer-assisted instruction; daycare for children of students; e-mail services; externships; housing assistance; interactive nursing skills videos; Internet; learning resource lab; library services; nursing audiovisuals; resume preparation assistance; skills, simulation, or other laboratory; tutoring.

Library Facilities 692,253 volumes (10,000 in health, 900 in nursing); 33,950 periodical subscriptions (70 health-care related).

BACCALAUREATE PROGRAMS

Degree BSN

Available Programs Generic Baccalaureate; RN Baccalaureate.

Site Options *Distance Learning:* Enka, NC.

Study Options Full-time.

Program Entrance Requirements Transcript of college record, CPR certification, written essay, health exam, immunizations, minimum GPA in nursing prerequisites of 2.0, professional liability insurance/malpractice insurance, prerequisite course work. Transfer students are accepted. **Standardized tests** *Required:* SAT or ACT, TOEFL for international students. **Application** *Deadline:* 8/1 (freshmen), 8/1 (transfer). *Notification:* continuous (freshmen). *Application fee:* $40.

Advanced Placement Credit given for nursing courses completed elsewhere dependent upon specific evaluations.

Contact *Telephone:* 828-227-7467. *Fax:* 828-227-7052.

GRADUATE PROGRAMS

Contact *Telephone:* 828-670-8810 Ext. 222. *Fax:* 828-670-8807.

MASTER'S DEGREE PROGRAM

Degree MSN

Available Programs Master's.

Concentrations Available Nursing education. *Nurse practitioner programs in:* family health.

Site Options *Distance Learning:* Enka, NC.

Study Options Full-time and part-time.

Program Entrance Requirements Minimum overall college GPA of 3.0, transcript of college record, CPR certification, immunizations, 2 letters of recommendation, physical assessment course, professional liability insurance/malpractice insurance, statistics course.

Advanced Placement Credit given for nursing courses completed elsewhere dependent upon specific evaluations.

Degree Requirements Thesis or project, comprehensive exam.

POST-MASTER'S PROGRAM

Areas of Study Nursing education. *Nurse practitioner programs in:* family health.

POSTDOCTORAL PROGRAM

Postdoctoral Program Contact *Telephone:* 828-227-7467. *Fax:* 828-227-7071.

Winston-Salem State University
Department of Nursing
Winston-Salem, North Carolina

http://www.wssu.edu

Founded in 1892

DEGREES • BSN • MSN

Nursing Program Faculty 25 (24% with doctorates).

Baccalaureate Enrollment 229

Women 77% **Men** 23% **Minority** 75% **Part-time** 17%

Graduate Enrollment 15

Nursing Student Activities Nursing Honor Society, Sigma Theta Tau, Student Nurses' Association.

Nursing Student Resources Academic advising; campus computer network; computer lab; interactive nursing skills videos; learning resource lab; nursing audiovisuals; skills, simulation, or other laboratory.

Library Facilities 197,765 volumes (10,664 in nursing); 1,010 periodical subscriptions (182 health-care related).

BACCALAUREATE PROGRAMS

Degree BSN

Available Programs ADN to Baccalaureate; Accelerated RN Baccalaureate; Baccalaureate for Second Degree; Generic Baccalaureate; LPN to Baccalaureate; RN Baccalaureate.

Site Options *Distance Learning:* Boone, NC; Wilkesboro, NC; Salisbury, NC.

Study Options Full-time.

Program Entrance Requirements Minimum overall college GPA of 2.6, transcript of college record, CPR certification, health exam, immunizations, professional liability insurance/malpractice insurance, prerequisite course work. Transfer students are accepted. **Standardized tests** *Required:* SAT or ACT, TOEFL for international students. **Application** *Deadline:* 7/15 (freshmen), rolling (transfer). *Application fee:* $40.

Advanced Placement Credit by examination available. Credit given for nursing courses completed elsewhere dependent upon specific evaluations.

Financial Aid 80% of baccalaureate students in nursing programs received some form of financial aid in 2004–05.

Contact Ms. Charlena Garrison, Director of Student Affairs, Division of Nursing, Department of Nursing, Winston-Salem State University, 601 Martin Luther King Jr. Drive, Winston-Salem, NC 27110. *Telephone:* 336-750-2560. *Fax:* 336-750-2599. *E-mail:* garrisonc@wssn.edu.

GRADUATE PROGRAMS

Financial Aid 40% of graduate students in nursing programs received some form of financial aid in 2004–05.

Contact Dr. Lenora Campbell, RN, Interim Chair, MSN Program, Department of Nursing, Winston-Salem State University, 601 Martin Luther King Jr. Drive, Winston-Salem, NC 27110. *Telephone:* 336-750-2577. *Fax:* 336-750-2599. *E-mail:* campbellr@wssu.edu.

MASTER'S DEGREE PROGRAM

Degree MSN

Available Programs Master's.

Concentrations Available *Nurse practitioner programs in:* family health, psychiatric/mental health.

Study Options Full-time and part-time.

Program Entrance Requirements Clinical experience, transcript of college record, CPR certification, immunizations, interview, 3 letters of recommendation, nursing research course, physical assessment course, professional liability insurance/malpractice insurance, resume, statistics course.

Advanced Placement Credit given for nursing courses completed elsewhere dependent upon specific evaluations.

Degree Requirements 50 total credit hours, thesis or project.

CONTINUING EDUCATION PROGRAM

Contact Dr. Cecil Holland, Director of Special Projects, Department of Nursing, Winston-Salem State University, 601 Martin Luther King Jr. Drive, Winston-Salem, NC 27110. *Telephone:* 336-750-2560. *Fax:* 336-750-2599. *E-mail:* hollandc@wssu.edu.

NORTH DAKOTA

Dickinson State University
Department of Nursing
Dickinson, North Dakota

http://www.dsu.nodak.edu/Catalog/nursing.htm

Founded in 1918

Dickinson State University (continued)
DEGREE • BSN

Nursing Program Faculty 6.
Baccalaureate Enrollment 52
Women 96% **Men** 4% **Minority** 7% **International** 2% **Part-time** 15%
Nursing Student Activities Student Nurses' Association.

Nursing Student Resources Academic advising; academic or career counseling; assistance for students with disabilities; bookstore; campus computer network; career placement assistance; computer lab; computer-assisted instruction; e-mail services; employment services for current students; externships; housing services; Internet; learning resource lab; library services; nursing audiovisuals; placement services for program completers; remedial services; resume preparation assistance; skills, simulation, or other laboratory; tutoring.

Library Facilities 105,713 volumes (16,500 in health, 1,350 in nursing); 823 periodical subscriptions (10,000 health-care related).

BACCALAUREATE PROGRAMS

Degree BSN

Available Programs ADN to Baccalaureate; LPN to Baccalaureate; RN Baccalaureate.
Study Options Full-time and part-time.
Program Entrance Requirements Minimum overall college GPA of 2.5, transcript of college record, health exam, immunizations, minimum GPA in nursing prerequisites of 2.5, prerequisite course work. Transfer students are accepted. **Standardized tests** *Required:* SAT or ACT, TOEFL for international students. **Application** *Deadline:* rolling (freshmen), rolling (transfer). *Notification:* continuous (freshmen). *Application fee:* $35.
Advanced Placement Credit given for nursing courses completed elsewhere dependent upon specific evaluations.
Expenses (2006–07) *Tuition, state resident:* full-time $4470; part-time $187 per credit hour. *Tuition, nonresident:* full-time $10,560; part-time $440 per credit hour. *International tuition:* $10,560 full-time. *Room and board:* $3690; room only: $1390 per academic year. *Required fees:* full-time $1140; part-time $35 per credit; part-time $150 per term.
Financial Aid 64% of baccalaureate students in nursing programs received some form of financial aid in 2005–06.
Contact Dr. Mary Anne Marsh, Chair, Department of Nursing, Dickinson State University, 291 Campus Drive, Dickinson, ND 58601-4896. *Telephone:* 800-279-4295 Ext. 2133. *Fax:* 701-483-2524. *E-mail:* maryanne.marsh@dsu.nodak.edu.

Jamestown College
Department of Nursing
Jamestown, North Dakota

Founded in 1883
DEGREE • BSN

Nursing Program Faculty 11 (9% with doctorates).
Baccalaureate Enrollment 80
Nursing Student Activities Sigma Theta Tau, Student Nurses' Association.
Nursing Student Resources Academic advising; academic or career counseling; bookstore; campus computer network; computer lab; computer-assisted instruction; e-mail services; externships; interactive nursing skills videos; Internet; learning resource lab; library services; nursing audiovisuals; resume preparation assistance; skills, simulation, or other laboratory; tutoring.

Library Facilities 121,382 volumes (990 in health, 983 in nursing); 630 periodical subscriptions (163 health-care related).

BACCALAUREATE PROGRAMS

Degree BSN

Study Options Full-time and part-time.

Program Entrance Requirements Minimum overall college GPA of 3.0, transcript of college record, written essay, high school transcript, immunizations, prerequisite course work. Transfer students are accepted. **Standardized tests** *Required:* TOEFL for international students. *Recommended:* SAT or ACT. **Application** *Deadline:* rolling (freshmen), rolling (transfer). *Application fee:* $20.
Advanced Placement Credit given for nursing courses completed elsewhere dependent upon specific evaluations.
Contact *Telephone:* 701-252-3467 Ext. 2562. *Fax:* 701-253-4318.

Medcenter One College of Nursing
Medcenter One College of Nursing
Bismarck, North Dakota

http://www.college.medcenterone.com
Founded in 1988
DEGREE • BSN

Nursing Program Faculty 12 (8% with doctorates).
Baccalaureate Enrollment 93
Women 85% **Men** 15% **Part-time** 1%
Nursing Student Activities Sigma Theta Tau, Student Nurses' Association.

Nursing Student Resources Academic advising; assistance for students with disabilities; bookstore; computer lab; computer-assisted instruction; e-mail services; Internet; library services; nursing audiovisuals; placement services for program completers; resume preparation assistance; skills, simulation, or other laboratory; tutoring.

Library Facilities 28,470 volumes (4,717 in health, 2,217 in nursing); 331 periodical subscriptions (498 health-care related).

BACCALAUREATE PROGRAMS

Degree BSN

Available Programs ADN to Baccalaureate; RN Baccalaureate.
Study Options Full-time and part-time.
Program Entrance Requirements Minimum overall college GPA of 2.5, transcript of college record, CPR certification, written essay, health exam, high school transcript, immunizations, interview, minimum GPA in nursing prerequisites of 2.5, prerequisite course work. Transfer students are accepted. **Application** *Deadline:* 11/7 (transfer). *Application fee:* $40.
Advanced Placement Credit given for nursing courses completed elsewhere dependent upon specific evaluations.
Expenses (2006–07) *Tuition:* full-time $8652; part-time $361 per credit. *Required fees:* full-time $759; part-time $15 per credit; part-time $198 per term.
Financial Aid 89% of baccalaureate students in nursing programs received some form of financial aid in 2005–06. *Gift aid (need-based):* Federal Pell, FSEOG, state, private, college/university gift aid from institutional funds. *Loans:* Federal Nursing Student Loans, FFEL (Subsidized and Unsubsidized Stafford PLUS), Perkins, college/university. *Work-Study:* Federal Work-Study. *Application deadline (priority):* 3/15.
Contact Ms. Mary Smith, RN, Director of Student Services, Medcenter One College of Nursing, 512 North 7th Street, Bismarck, ND 58501. *Telephone:* 701-323-6271. *Fax:* 701-323-6289. *E-mail:* msmith@mohs.org.

Minot State University
Department of Nursing
Minot, North Dakota

http://www.minotstateu.edu/nursing/index.html
Founded in 1913
DEGREE • BSN

Nursing Program Faculty 21 (13% with doctorates).

Baccalaureate Enrollment 120
Women 94% **Men** 6% **Minority** 10% **International** 78% **Part-time** 22%
Nursing Student Activities Sigma Theta Tau, Student Nurses' Association.

Nursing Student Resources Academic advising; academic or career counseling; assistance for students with disabilities; bookstore; campus computer network; career placement assistance; computer lab; computer-assisted instruction; e-mail services; housing assistance; interactive nursing skills videos; Internet; learning resource lab; library services; nursing audiovisuals; paid internships; resume preparation assistance; skills, simulation, or other laboratory; tutoring.

Library Facilities 420,971 volumes (6,926 in health, 1,385 in nursing); 752 periodical subscriptions (56 health-care related).

BACCALAUREATE PROGRAMS

Degree BSN

Available Programs Generic Baccalaureate; LPN to Baccalaureate; RN Baccalaureate.

Study Options Full-time.

Program Entrance Requirements Minimum overall college GPA of 2.75, transcript of college record, CPR certification, immunizations, minimum GPA in nursing prerequisites of 2.8, prerequisite course work. Transfer students are accepted. **Standardized tests** *Required:* SAT or ACT, TOEFL for international students. **Application** *Deadline:* rolling (freshmen), rolling (transfer). *Notification:* continuous (freshmen). *Application fee:* $35.

Advanced Placement Credit given for nursing courses completed elsewhere dependent upon specific evaluations.

Financial Aid *Gift aid (need-based):* Federal Pell, FSEOG, state, private, college/university gift aid from institutional funds, Federal Nursing. *Loans:* Federal Nursing Student Loans, FFEL (Subsidized and Unsubsidized Stafford PLUS), Perkins, college/university. *Work-Study:* Federal Work-Study. *Application deadline (priority):* 3/15.

Contact Ms. Mary Smith, RN, Interim Department Chair, Department of Nursing, Minot State University, 500 University Avenue West, Minot, ND 58707-0002. *Telephone:* 701-858-3101. *Fax:* 701-858-4309. *E-mail:* mary.smith@minotstateu.edu.

North Dakota State University
Tri-College University Nursing Consortium
Fargo, North Dakota

http://www.ndsu.nodak.edu/instruct/nysveen/nursing

Founded in 1890

DEGREES • BSN • DNP • MS

Nursing Program Faculty 15 (49% with doctorates).
Baccalaureate Enrollment 200
Women 90% **Men** 10% **Minority** 5% **International** 2% **Part-time** 12%
Graduate Enrollment 24
Women 95% **Men** 5% **Minority** 1% **Part-time** 45%
Nursing Student Activities Sigma Theta Tau, Student Nurses' Association.

Nursing Student Resources Academic advising; academic or career counseling; assistance for students with disabilities; bookstore; campus computer network; career placement assistance; computer lab; computer-assisted instruction; daycare for children of students; e-mail services; employment services for current students; externships; interactive nursing skills videos; Internet; learning resource lab; library services; nursing audiovisuals; paid internships; placement services for program completers; remedial services; resume preparation assistance; skills, simulation, or other laboratory; tutoring; unpaid internships.

Library Facilities 303,274 volumes (8,631 in health, 1,841 in nursing); 2,499 periodical subscriptions (121 health-care related).

BACCALAUREATE PROGRAMS

Degree BSN

Available Programs ADN to Baccalaureate; Generic Baccalaureate; LPN to Baccalaureate.

Study Options Full-time.

Program Entrance Requirements Minimum overall college GPA of 3.0, transcript of college record, 2 letters of recommendation, minimum GPA in nursing prerequisites of 3.0, prerequisite course work. Transfer students are accepted. **Standardized tests** *Required:* SAT or ACT, TOEFL for international students. **Application** *Deadline:* 8/15 (freshmen), 8/15 (transfer). *Notification:* continuous (freshmen). *Application fee:* $35.

Advanced Placement Credit by examination available. Credit given for nursing courses completed elsewhere dependent upon specific evaluations.

Expenses (2006–07) *Tuition, area resident:* full-time $4774; part-time $199 per credit. *Tuition, state resident:* full-time $5142; part-time $214 per credit. *Tuition, nonresident:* full-time $12,747; part-time $531 per credit. *International tuition:* $12,747 full-time. *Room and board:* $5477; room only: $3877 per academic year. *Required fees:* full-time $600; part-time $300 per term.

Financial Aid 85% of baccalaureate students in nursing programs received some form of financial aid in 2005–06.

Contact Ms. Gloria J. Nysveen, Administrative Secretary, Tri-College University Nursing Consortium, North Dakota State University, PO Box 5055/136 Sudro Hall, Fargo, ND 58105-5055. *Telephone:* 701-231-7395. *Fax:* 701-231-7606. *E-mail:* gloria.nysveen@ndsu.edu.

GRADUATE PROGRAMS

Expenses (2006–07) *Tuition, area resident:* full-time $3840; part-time $213 per credit. *Tuition, state resident:* full-time $4712; part-time $261 per credit. *Tuition, nonresident:* full-time $10,252; part-time $569 per credit. *International tuition:* $10,254 full-time. *Room and board:* $5477; room only: $3877 per academic year. *Required fees:* full-time $1530; part-time $79 per credit.

Financial Aid 35% of graduate students in nursing programs received some form of financial aid in 2005–06.

Contact Dr. Jane Giedt, Director, Graduate Program, Tri-College University Nursing Consortium, North Dakota State University, 1104 7th Avenue South, Moorhead, MN 56563. *Telephone:* 218-477-4699. *Fax:* 218-477-5990. *E-mail:* giedt@mnstate.edu.

MASTER'S DEGREE PROGRAM

Degree MS

Available Programs Master's.

Concentrations Available Nursing education. *Clinical nurse specialist programs in:* adult health. *Nurse practitioner programs in:* family health.

Site Options *Distance Learning:* Moorhead, MN.

Study Options Full-time and part-time.

Program Entrance Requirements Computer literacy, minimum overall college GPA of 3.0, transcript of college record, CPR certification, immunizations, interview, 3 letters of recommendation, nursing research course, physical assessment course, professional liability insurance/malpractice insurance, resume, statistics course.

Advanced Placement Credit given for nursing courses completed elsewhere dependent upon specific evaluations.

Degree Requirements Thesis or project, comprehensive exam.

DOCTORAL DEGREE PROGRAM

Degree DNP

Available Programs Post-Baccalaureate Doctorate.

Areas of Study Advanced practice nursing, family health.

Program Entrance Requirements Clinical experience, minimum overall college GPA of 3.0, interview by faculty committee, 2 letters of recommendation, statistics course, vita, writing sample.

Degree Requirements 86 total credit hours, dissertation, oral exam.

University of Mary
Division of Nursing
Bismarck, North Dakota

http://www.umary.edu/AcadInfo/NurDiv

Founded in 1959

University of Mary (continued)

DEGREES • BSN • MSN

Nursing Program Faculty 21 (10% with doctorates).

Baccalaureate Enrollment 166
Women 93% **Men** 7% **Minority** 3% **Part-time** 2%

Graduate Enrollment 50
Women 98% **Men** 2% **Minority** 6% **International** 2% **Part-time** 44%

Nursing Student Activities Sigma Theta Tau, Student Nurses' Association.

Nursing Student Resources Academic advising; academic or career counseling; assistance for students with disabilities; bookstore; campus computer network; career placement assistance; computer lab; computer-assisted instruction; e-mail services; employment services for current students; externships; housing assistance; interactive nursing skills videos; Internet; library services; nursing audiovisuals; placement services for program completers; resume preparation assistance; skills, simulation, or other laboratory; unpaid internships.

Library Facilities 78,137 volumes (10,425 in health, 3,000 in nursing); 567 periodical subscriptions (125 health-care related).

BACCALAUREATE PROGRAMS

Degree BSN

Available Programs Generic Baccalaureate; LPN to Baccalaureate; RN Baccalaureate.

Study Options Full-time and part-time.

Program Entrance Requirements Minimum overall college GPA of 2.5, transcript of college record, CPR certification, health exam, high school transcript, immunizations, interview, 2 letters of recommendation, minimum GPA in nursing prerequisites of 2.0, professional liability insurance/malpractice insurance, prerequisite course work. Transfer students are accepted. **Standardized tests** *Required:* SAT or ACT, TOEFL for international students. **Application** *Deadline:* rolling (freshmen), rolling (transfer). *Application fee:* $25.

Advanced Placement Credit by examination available. Credit given for nursing courses completed elsewhere dependent upon specific evaluations.

Expenses (2006–07) *Tuition:* full-time $11,100; part-time $350 per credit. *International tuition:* $11,100 full-time. *Room and board:* $4000; room only: $2000 per academic year. *Required fees:* full-time $600; part-time $25 per credit.

Financial Aid 100% of baccalaureate students in nursing programs received some form of financial aid in 2005–06.

Contact Admissions Office, Division of Nursing, University of Mary, 7500 University Drive, Bismarck, ND 58504. *Telephone:* 701-255-7500. *Fax:* 701-255-7687.

GRADUATE PROGRAMS

Expenses (2006–07) *Tuition:* full-time $8010; part-time $445 per credit. *International tuition:* $8010 full-time. *Required fees:* full-time $750; part-time $125 per credit.

Financial Aid 95% of graduate students in nursing programs received some form of financial aid in 2005–06. 14 fellowships with partial tuition reimbursements available, 3 teaching assistantships with partial tuition reimbursements available were awarded; institutionally sponsored loans also available. Aid available to part-time students. *Financial aid application deadline:* 7/1.

Contact Prof. Mariah Dietz, DNS, Graduate Program Director, Division of Nursing, University of Mary, 7500 University Drive, Bismarck, ND 58504. *Telephone:* 701-355-8041. *Fax:* 701-255-7687. *E-mail:* mdietz@umary.edu.

MASTER'S DEGREE PROGRAM

Degree MSN

Available Programs Master's; RN to Master's.

Concentrations Available Nursing administration; nursing education. *Nurse practitioner programs in:* family health.

Study Options Full-time and part-time.

Program Entrance Requirements Clinical experience, minimum overall college GPA of 3.0, transcript of college record, CPR certification, written essay, immunizations, interview, 3 letters of recommendation, physical assessment course, statistics course. *Application deadline:* For fall admission, 4/15 (priority date). Applications are processed on a rolling basis. *Application fee:* $40.

Degree Requirements 39 total credit hours, thesis or project, comprehensive exam.

University of North Dakota
College of Nursing
Grand Forks, North Dakota

http://www.und.nodak.edu/dept/nursing

Founded in 1883

DEGREES • BSN • MS • PHD

Nursing Program Faculty 54 (33% with doctorates).

Baccalaureate Enrollment 303
Women 91% **Men** 9% **Minority** 11% **International** 1% **Part-time** 22%

Graduate Enrollment 75
Women 90% **Men** 10% **Minority** 7% **International** 3% **Part-time** 60%

Nursing Student Activities Sigma Theta Tau, Student Nurses' Association.

Nursing Student Resources Academic advising; academic or career counseling; assistance for students with disabilities; bookstore; campus computer network; career placement assistance; computer lab; computer-assisted instruction; daycare for children of students; e-mail services; employment services for current students; externships; housing assistance; interactive nursing skills videos; Internet; learning resource lab; library services; nursing audiovisuals; paid internships; remedial services; resume preparation assistance; skills, simulation, or other laboratory; tutoring.

Library Facilities 1.5 million volumes (83,000 in health, 2,368 in nursing); 16,153 periodical subscriptions (1,074 health-care related).

BACCALAUREATE PROGRAMS

Degree BSN

Available Programs ADN to Baccalaureate; Generic Baccalaureate; LPN to Baccalaureate; LPN to RN Baccalaureate; RN Baccalaureate.

Site Options *Distance Learning:* Grand Forks, ND.

Study Options Full-time and part-time.

Program Entrance Requirements Minimum overall college GPA of 2.5, transcript of college record, CPR certification, written essay, health insurance, high school math, immunizations, minimum GPA in nursing prerequisites of 2.5, prerequisite course work. Transfer students are accepted. **Standardized tests** *Required:* SAT or ACT, TOEFL for international students. *Recommended:* ACT. **Application** *Deadline:* rolling (transfer). *Application fee:* $35.

Advanced Placement Credit by examination available. Credit given for nursing courses completed elsewhere dependent upon specific evaluations.

Expenses (2005–06) *Tuition, state resident:* full-time $5327; part-time $241 per credit. *Tuition, nonresident:* full-time $12,659; part-time $546 per credit. *International tuition:* $12,659 full-time. *Room and board:* $4787 per academic year. *Required fees:* full-time $300; part-time $13 per credit; part-time $150 per term.

Financial Aid 89% of baccalaureate students in nursing programs received some form of financial aid in 2004–05.

Contact Ms. Marlys K. Escobar, Director of Student and Alumni Affairs, College of Nursing, University of North Dakota, PO Box 9025, Grand Forks, ND 58202-9025. *Telephone:* 701-777-4548. *Fax:* 701-777-4096. *E-mail:* marlysescobar@mail.und.nodak.edu.

GRADUATE PROGRAMS

Expenses (2005–06) *Tuition, area resident:* full-time $5659; part-time $255 per contact hour. *Tuition, state resident:* full-time $6761; part-time $301 per contact hour. *Tuition, nonresident:* full-time $13,547; part-time $583 per contact hour. *International tuition:* $13,547 full-time. *Room and board:* $5545; room only: $4000 per academic year. *Required fees:* full-time $1000; part-time $42 per credit; part-time $500 per term.

Financial Aid 85% of graduate students in nursing programs received some form of financial aid in 2004–05. 2 research assistantships (averaging $10,498 per year), 6 teaching assistantships with full tuition reimbursements available (averaging $10,669 per year) were awarded; fellowships, Federal

Work-Study, institutionally sponsored loans, scholarships, traineeships, and tuition waivers (full and partial) also available. Aid available to part-time students. *Financial aid application deadline:* 3/15.

Contact Dr. Ginny W. Guido, Director of Graduate Studies, College of Nursing, University of North Dakota, PO Box 9025, Grand Forks, ND 58202-9025. *Telephone:* 701-777-4552. *Fax:* 701-777-4096. *E-mail:* ginnyguido@mail.und.edu.

MASTER'S DEGREE PROGRAM

Degree MS

Available Programs Master's.

Concentrations Available Nurse anesthesia; nursing administration; nursing education. *Clinical nurse specialist programs in:* acute care, adult health, community health, family health, gerontology, home health care, psychiatric/mental health. *Nurse practitioner programs in:* family health, psychiatric/mental health.

Site Options *Distance Learning:* Grand Forks, ND.

Study Options Full-time and part-time.

Program Entrance Requirements Clinical experience, minimum overall college GPA of 3.0, transcript of college record, CPR certification, written essay, immunizations, interview, 3 letters of recommendation, prerequisite course work, resume, statistics course. *Application deadline:* For fall admission, 12/1. *Application fee:* $35.

Advanced Placement Credit given for nursing courses completed elsewhere dependent upon specific evaluations.

Degree Requirements 37 total credit hours, thesis or project.

POST-MASTER'S PROGRAM

Areas of Study Nurse anesthesia; nursing education. *Clinical nurse specialist programs in:* psychiatric/mental health. *Nurse practitioner programs in:* family health, psychiatric/mental health.

DOCTORAL DEGREE PROGRAM

Degree PhD

Available Programs Doctorate.

Areas of Study Faculty preparation, health promotion/disease prevention, nursing research.

Site Options *Distance Learning:* Grand Forks, ND.

Program Entrance Requirements Minimum overall college GPA of 3.5, interview by faculty committee, interview, 3 letters of recommendation, MSN or equivalent, statistics course, vita, GRE or MAT. *Application deadline:* For fall admission, 12/1. *Application fee:* $35.

Degree Requirements 90 total credit hours, dissertation, oral exam, written exam, residency.

OHIO

Ashland University
Department of Nursing
Ashland, Ohio

http://www.ashland.edu
Founded in 1878

DEGREE • BSN

Nursing Program Faculty 2 (50% with doctorates).

Baccalaureate Enrollment 50
Women 96% **Men** 4% **Minority** 12% **Part-time** 96%

Nursing Student Activities Sigma Theta Tau.

Nursing Student Resources Academic advising; academic or career counseling; assistance for students with disabilities; bookstore; campus computer network; career placement assistance; computer lab; computer-assisted instruction; e-mail services; Internet; library services; nursing audiovisuals; remedial services; resume preparation assistance; skills, simulation, or other laboratory; tutoring; unpaid internships.

Library Facilities 205,200 volumes; 1,625 periodical subscriptions.

BACCALAUREATE PROGRAMS

Degree BSN

Available Programs ADN to Baccalaureate; Accelerated RN Baccalaureate; Baccalaureate for Second Degree; RN Baccalaureate.

Site Options *Distance Learning:* Medina, OH; Canton, OH; Mansfield, OH.

Study Options Full-time and part-time.

Program Entrance Requirements Minimum overall college GPA of 2.0, transcript of college record, minimum GPA in nursing prerequisites of 2.0, prerequisite course work. Transfer students are accepted. **Standardized tests** *Required:* SAT or ACT, TOEFL for international students. **Application** *Deadline:* rolling (freshmen), rolling (transfer). *Notification:* continuous (freshmen). *Application fee:* $25.

Advanced Placement Credit by examination available. Credit given for nursing courses completed elsewhere dependent upon specific evaluations.

Expenses (2006–07) *Tuition:* part-time $403 per credit hour. *Required fees:* part-time $60 per term.

Financial Aid 80% of baccalaureate students in nursing programs received some form of financial aid in 2005–06. *Gift aid (need-based):* Federal Pell, FSEOG, state, private. *Loans:* Federal Direct (Subsidized and Unsubsidized Stafford PLUS), Perkins, college/university. *Work-Study:* Federal Work-Study. *Application deadline:* Continuous.

Contact Dr. Lori Brohm, Administrator, Department of Nursing, Ashland University, 401 College Avenue, Ashland, OH 44805. *Telephone:* 419-289-5242. *Fax:* 419-289-5989. *E-mail:* lbrohm@ashland.edu.

Capital University
School of Nursing
Columbus, Ohio

http://www.capital.edu/nursing/nurshome.shtml
Founded in 1830

DEGREES • BSN • MN/MBA • MSN • MSN/JD • MS/MTS

Nursing Program Faculty 35 (40% with doctorates).

Baccalaureate Enrollment 420
Women 90% **Men** 10% **Minority** 6% **International** 2% **Part-time** 30%
Graduate Enrollment 80
Women 92% **Men** 8% **Minority** 4% **International** 12.5% **Part-time** 75%

Nursing Student Activities Sigma Theta Tau, Student Nurses' Association.

Nursing Student Resources Academic advising; academic or career counseling; assistance for students with disabilities; bookstore; campus computer network; computer lab; computer-assisted instruction; e-mail services; interactive nursing skills videos; Internet; learning resource lab; library services; nursing audiovisuals; resume preparation assistance; skills, simulation, or other laboratory; tutoring; unpaid internships.

Library Facilities 196,000 volumes (6,209 in health); 7,055 periodical subscriptions (82 health-care related).

BACCALAUREATE PROGRAMS

Degree BSN

Available Programs ADN to Baccalaureate; Accelerated Baccalaureate for Second Degree; Generic Baccalaureate; RN Baccalaureate.

Study Options Full-time.

Program Entrance Requirements Minimum overall college GPA of 3.0, transcript of college record, health exam, high school biology, high school chemistry, high school foreign language, 3 years high school math, 3 years high school science, high school transcript, immunizations, minimum high school GPA of 3.3. Transfer students are accepted. **Standardized tests** *Required:* SAT or ACT, TOEFL for international students. **Application** *Deadline:* 4/1 (freshmen), rolling (transfer). *Notification:* 9/19 (freshmen). *Application fee:* $25.

Advanced Placement Credit by examination available. Credit given for nursing courses completed elsewhere dependent upon specific evaluations.

Financial Aid 95% of baccalaureate students in nursing programs received some form of financial aid in 2005–06.

Capital University (continued)

Contact Dr. Elaine F. Haynes, Dean and Professor, School of Nursing, Capital University, 1 College and Main, Columbus, OH 43209-2394. *Telephone:* 614-236-6703. *Fax:* 614-236-6157. *E-mail:* ehaynes@capital.edu.

GRADUATE PROGRAMS

Financial Aid 1 teaching assistantship was awarded; career-related internships or fieldwork and traineeships also available.

Contact Mrs. Connie Sasser, Program Coordinator, School of Nursing, Capital University, 1 College and Main, Columbus, OH 43209-2394. *Telephone:* 614-236-6703. *Fax:* 614-236-6703. *E-mail:* csasser@capital.edu.

MASTER'S DEGREE PROGRAM

Degrees MN/MBA; MSN; MSN/JD; MS/MTS

Available Programs Master's; RN to Master's.

Concentrations Available Health-care administration; nursing administration; nursing education.

Study Options Full-time and part-time.

Program Entrance Requirements Computer literacy, minimum overall college GPA of 3.0, transcript of college record, CPR certification, written essay, immunizations, 3 letters of recommendation, nursing research course, physical assessment course, professional liability insurance/malpractice insurance, prerequisite course work, resume, statistics course. *Application deadline:* For fall admission, 8/1 (priority date); for spring admission, 12/1. Applications are processed on a rolling basis. *Application fee:* $25.

Advanced Placement Credit given for nursing courses completed elsewhere dependent upon specific evaluations.

Degree Requirements 36 total credit hours, thesis or project.

POST-MASTER'S PROGRAM

Areas of Study Nursing education.

CONTINUING EDUCATION PROGRAM

Contact Dr. Elaine F. Haynes, Dean and Professor, School of Nursing, Capital University, 1 College and Main, Columbus, OH 43209-2394. *Telephone:* 614-236-6703. *Fax:* 614-236-6157. *E-mail:* ehaynes@capital.edu.

Case Western Reserve University
Frances Payne Bolton School of Nursing
Cleveland, Ohio

http://fpb.case.edu

Founded in 1826

DEGREES • BSN • MSN • MSN/MA • MSN/MBA • MSN/MPH • MSN/PHD

Nursing Program Faculty 105 (43% with doctorates).

Baccalaureate Enrollment 264
Women 91% **Men** 9% **Minority** 28%

Graduate Enrollment 526
Women 88% **Men** 12% **Minority** 24% **International** 9% **Part-time** 55%

Nursing Student Activities Nursing Honor Society, Sigma Theta Tau, Student Nurses' Association.

Nursing Student Resources Academic advising; academic or career counseling; assistance for students with disabilities; bookstore; campus computer network; career placement assistance; computer lab; computer-assisted instruction; e-mail services; employment services for current students; housing assistance; interactive nursing skills videos; Internet; learning resource lab; library services; nursing audiovisuals; placement services for program completers; remedial services; resume preparation assistance; skills, simulation, or other laboratory; tutoring.

Library Facilities 2.5 million volumes (475,000 in health); 20,265 periodical subscriptions (2,500 health-care related).

BACCALAUREATE PROGRAMS

Degree BSN

Available Programs ADN to Baccalaureate; Generic Baccalaureate; RN Baccalaureate.

Study Options Full-time.

Program Entrance Requirements Transcript of college record, CPR certification, written essay, high school biology, high school chemistry, high school foreign language, 2 years high school science, high school transcript, immunizations, 2 letters of recommendation, minimum high school GPA of 3.0, professional liability insurance/malpractice insurance. Transfer students are accepted. **Standardized tests** *Required:* SAT or ACT, TOEFL for international students. **Application** *Deadline:* 1/15 (freshmen), 5/15 (transfer). *Early decision:* 11/1. *Notification:* 4/1 (freshmen), 1/1 (early action).

Advanced Placement Credit given for nursing courses completed elsewhere dependent upon specific evaluations.

Expenses (2005–06) *Tuition:* full-time $28,400; part-time $1184 per credit hour. *International tuition:* $28,400 full-time. *Room and board:* $8559; room only: $6000 per academic year. *Required fees:* part-time $475 per term.

Financial Aid 100% of baccalaureate students in nursing programs received some form of financial aid in 2004–05. *Gift aid (need-based):* Federal Pell, FSEOG, state, private, college/university gift aid from institutional funds. *Loans:* Federal Nursing Student Loans, FFEL (Subsidized and Unsubsidized Stafford PLUS), Perkins, state, college/university, alternative loans-Custom Signature. *Work-Study:* Federal Work-Study. *Application deadline (priority):* 2/15.

Contact Office of Student Services, Frances Payne Bolton School of Nursing, Case Western Reserve University, 10900 Euclid Avenue, Cleveland, OH 44106-4904. *Telephone:* 216-368-2529. *Fax:* 216-368-0124. *E-mail:* admissions@fpb.case.edu.

GRADUATE PROGRAMS

Expenses (2005–06) *Tuition:* part-time $1184 per credit hour. *Required fees:* part-time $20 per term.

Financial Aid 90% of graduate students in nursing programs received some form of financial aid in 2004–05. 5 research assistantships, 7 teaching assistantships were awarded; fellowships, Federal Work-Study, institutionally sponsored loans, scholarships, and tuition waivers (partial) also available. Aid available to part-time students. *Financial aid application deadline:* 6/30.

Contact Office of Student Services, Frances Payne Bolton School of Nursing, Case Western Reserve University, 10900 Euclid Avenue, Cleveland, OH 44106-4904. *Telephone:* 216-368-2529. *Fax:* 216-368-0124. *E-mail:* admissions@fbp.case.edu.

MASTER'S DEGREE PROGRAM

Degrees MSN; MSN/MA; MSN/MBA; MSN/MPH; MSN/PhD

Available Programs Accelerated AD/RN to Master's; Accelerated Master's for Non-Nursing College Graduates; Accelerated Master's for Nurses with Non-Nursing Degrees; Master's; Master's for Non-Nursing College Graduates; Master's for Nurses with Non-Nursing Degrees; RN to Master's.

Concentrations Available Nurse anesthesia; nurse-midwifery; nursing informatics. *Clinical nurse specialist programs in:* acute care, cardiovascular, community health, critical care, gerontology, medical-surgical, oncology, pediatric, psychiatric/mental health. *Nurse practitioner programs in:* acute care, adult health, family health, gerontology, neonatal health, pediatric, psychiatric/mental health, women's health.

Study Options Full-time and part-time.

Program Entrance Requirements Minimum overall college GPA of 3.0, transcript of college record, CPR certification, written essay, immunizations, 3 letters of recommendation, nursing research course, professional liability insurance/malpractice insurance, resume, statistics course, MAT or GRE General Test. *Application deadline:* Applications are processed on a rolling basis. *Application fee:* $75.

Advanced Placement Credit given for nursing courses completed elsewhere dependent upon specific evaluations.

Degree Requirements 40 total credit hours.

POST-MASTER'S PROGRAM

Areas of Study Nurse anesthesia; nurse-midwifery; nursing informatics. *Clinical nurse specialist programs in:* acute care, cardiovascular, community health, critical care, medical-surgical, oncology, pediatric, psychiatric/mental health. *Nurse practitioner programs in:* acute care, adult health, family health, gerontology, neonatal health, pediatric, psychiatric/mental health, women's health.

DOCTORAL DEGREE PROGRAM

Degree PhD

Available Programs Doctorate; Doctorate for Nurses with Non-Nursing Degrees; Post-Baccalaureate Doctorate.

Areas of Study Aging, bio-behavioral research, community health, critical care, ethics, faculty preparation, family health, gerontology, health policy, health promotion/disease prevention, human health and illness, illness and transition, individualized study, maternity-newborn, nursing education, nursing research, nursing science, oncology, women's health.

Site Options Riverside, CA; Greenwich, CT; St Petersburg, FL.

Program Entrance Requirements Minimum overall college GPA of 3.0, interview by faculty committee, interview, 3 letters of recommendation, statistics course, writing sample, GRE General Test, MAT (ND). *Application deadline:* Applications are processed on a rolling basis. *Application fee:* $75.

Degree Requirements 54 total credit hours, dissertation, oral exam, residency.

POSTDOCTORAL PROGRAM

Areas of Study Aging, cancer care, chronic illness, community health, family health, gerontology, health promotion/disease prevention, individualized study, information systems, nursing interventions, nursing research, nursing science, outcomes, self-care, vulnerable population, women's health.

Postdoctoral Program Contact Dr. Shirley M. Moore, Professor and Associate Dean for Research, Frances Payne Bolton School of Nursing, Case Western Reserve University, 10900 Euclid Avenue, Cleveland, OH 44106-4904. *Telephone:* 216-368-5978. *Fax:* 216-368-3542. *E-mail:* shirley.moore@case.edu.

CONTINUING EDUCATION PROGRAM

Contact Dr. Noreen Brady, RN, Assistant Professor of Nursing, Frances Payne Bolton School of Nursing, Case Western Reserve University, 10900 Euclid Avenue, Cleveland, OH 44106-4904. *Telephone:* 216-368-6303. *Fax:* 216-368-5303. *E-mail:* Noreen.Brady@case.edu.

Cedarville University
Department of Nursing
Cedarville, Ohio

Founded in 1887

DEGREE • BSN

Nursing Program Faculty 19 (47% with doctorates).

Baccalaureate Enrollment 332
Women 93% **Men** 7%

Nursing Student Activities Nursing Honor Society, Sigma Theta Tau, Student Nurses' Association.

Nursing Student Resources Academic advising; academic or career counseling; assistance for students with disabilities; bookstore; campus computer network; career placement assistance; computer lab; computer-assisted instruction; e-mail services; housing assistance; interactive nursing skills videos; Internet; library services; nursing audiovisuals; paid internships; resume preparation assistance; skills, simulation, or other laboratory.

Library Facilities 170,561 volumes; 6,400 periodical subscriptions.

BACCALAUREATE PROGRAMS

Degree BSN

Available Programs RN Baccalaureate.

Study Options Full-time.

Program Entrance Requirements Minimum overall college GPA of 2.5, transcript of college record, CPR certification, written essay, health exam, health insurance, high school biology, high school chemistry, high school foreign language, 4 years high school math, 4 years high school science, high school transcript, immunizations, 1 letter of recommendation, minimum high school GPA of 3.0, minimum high school rank 50%, minimum GPA in nursing prerequisites of 2.5, professional liability insurance/malpractice insurance, prerequisite course work. Transfer students are accepted. **Standardized tests** *Required:* SAT or ACT, TOEFL for international students. *Recommended:* SAT and SAT Subject Tests or ACT.

Application *Deadline:* rolling (freshmen), rolling (transfer). *Notification:* continuous (freshmen). *Application fee:* $30.

Advanced Placement Credit given for nursing courses completed elsewhere dependent upon specific evaluations.

Expenses (2006–07) *Tuition:* full-time $18,400; part-time $575 per credit hour. *Room and board:* $5010; room only: $2684 per academic year.

Financial Aid 91% of baccalaureate students in nursing programs received some form of financial aid in 2005–06.

Contact Mr. Roscoe Smith, Admissions, Department of Nursing, Cedarville University, 251 North Main Street, Cedarville, OH 45314-0601. *Telephone:* 800-233-2784. *Fax:* 937-766-7575. *E-mail:* admissions@cedarville.edu.

Cleveland State University
Department of Nursing
Cleveland, Ohio

http://www.csuohio.edu

Founded in 1964

DEGREES • BSN • MSN • MSN/MBA

Nursing Program Faculty 24 (25% with doctorates).

Baccalaureate Enrollment 250
Women 85% **Men** 15% **Minority** 20% **International** 1% **Part-time** 1%

Graduate Enrollment 30
Women 88% **Men** 12% **Minority** 10% **Part-time** 80%

Nursing Student Activities Sigma Theta Tau, Student Nurses' Association.

Nursing Student Resources Academic advising; bookstore; campus computer network; computer lab; e-mail services; interactive nursing skills videos; Internet; learning resource lab; nursing audiovisuals; skills, simulation, or other laboratory.

Library Facilities 484,914 volumes (6,000 in health, 70 in nursing); 6,186 periodical subscriptions (70 health-care related).

BACCALAUREATE PROGRAMS

Degree BSN

Available Programs ADN to Baccalaureate; Accelerated Baccalaureate; Accelerated Baccalaureate for Second Degree; Generic Baccalaureate; RN Baccalaureate.

Site Options Kirkland, OH.

Study Options Full-time.

Program Entrance Requirements Minimum overall college GPA of 2.5, transcript of college record, CPR certification, written essay, health exam, health insurance, high school transcript, immunizations, minimum GPA in nursing prerequisites of 2.75, professional liability insurance/malpractice insurance, prerequisite course work. Transfer students are accepted. **Standardized tests** *Required:* SAT or ACT, TOEFL for international students. **Application** *Deadline:* rolling (freshmen), 7/18 (transfer). *Notification:* continuous (freshmen). *Application fee:* $30.

Advanced Placement Credit given for nursing courses completed elsewhere dependent upon specific evaluations.

Financial Aid 80% of baccalaureate students in nursing programs received some form of financial aid in 2004–05. *Gift aid (need-based):* Federal Pell, FSEOG, state, private, college/university gift aid from institutional funds. *Loans:* FFEL (Subsidized and Unsubsidized Stafford PLUS), Perkins, state, alternative loans. *Work-Study:* Federal Work-Study, part-time campus jobs. *Application deadline (priority):* 2/15.

Contact Mr. Ronald Mickler, Jr., Recruiter and Advisor, Department of Nursing, Cleveland State University, 2121 Euclid Avenue, RT 915, Cleveland, OH 44115. *Telephone:* 216-687-3810. *Fax:* 216-687-3556. *E-mail:* nurse.adviser@csuohio.edu.

GRADUATE PROGRAMS

Expenses (2005–06) *Tuition, area resident:* full-time $4626; part-time $385 per credit hour. *Tuition, nonresident:* full-time $6615. *International tuition:* $6615 full-time. *Room and board:* $6810; room only: $4210 per academic year. *Required fees:* full-time $100.

Financial Aid 50% of graduate students in nursing programs received some form of financial aid in 2004–05.

Cleveland State University (continued)

Contact Dr. Sharon Radzyminski, Graduate Program Director, Department of Nursing, Cleveland State University, 2121 Euclid Avenue, RT 915, Cleveland, OH 44115. *Telephone:* 216-687-3558. *Fax:* 216-687-3556. *E-mail:* s.radzyminski@csuohio.edu.

MASTER'S DEGREE PROGRAM

Degrees MSN; MSN/MBA

Available Programs Master's.

Concentrations Available Health-care administration.

Study Options Full-time and part-time.

Program Entrance Requirements Clinical experience, computer literacy, minimum overall college GPA of 3.0, transcript of college record, CPR certification, written essay, immunizations, 2 letters of recommendation, nursing research course, professional liability insurance/malpractice insurance, resume, statistics course.

Advanced Placement Credit given for nursing courses completed elsewhere dependent upon specific evaluations.

Degree Requirements 38 total credit hours, thesis or project.

CONTINUING EDUCATION PROGRAM

Contact Dr. Vida Svarcas, Director, Nursing and Health Science Continuing Education, Department of Nursing, Cleveland State University, Euclid Building 103, 1824 East 24th Street, Cleveland, OH 44115. *Telephone:* 216-687-4843. *Fax:* 216-687-9399. *E-mail:* v.svarcas@csuohio.edu.

College of Mount St. Joseph
Department of Nursing
Cincinnati, Ohio

Founded in 1920

DEGREES • BSN • MN

Nursing Program Faculty 32 (18% with doctorates).

Baccalaureate Enrollment 240
Women 90% **Men** 10% **Minority** 20% **International** 2% **Part-time** 35%

Graduate Enrollment 31
Women 93% **Men** 7% **Minority** 25% **International** 10%

Nursing Student Activities Nursing Honor Society, Sigma Theta Tau, Student Nurses' Association.

Nursing Student Resources Academic advising; academic or career counseling; assistance for students with disabilities; bookstore; campus computer network; career placement assistance; computer lab; computer-assisted instruction; daycare for children of students; e-mail services; employment services for current students; externships; housing assistance; interactive nursing skills videos; Internet; learning resource lab; library services; nursing audiovisuals; paid internships; placement services for program completers; remedial services; resume preparation assistance; skills, simulation, or other laboratory; tutoring.

Library Facilities 97,172 volumes (2,700 in health, 2,100 in nursing); 9,000 periodical subscriptions (1,800 health-care related).

BACCALAUREATE PROGRAMS

Degree BSN

Available Programs Accelerated RN Baccalaureate; Generic Baccalaureate.

Site Options Cincinnati, OH.

Study Options Full-time and part-time.

Program Entrance Requirements Minimum overall college GPA of 2.5, transcript of college record, CPR certification, health exam, health insurance, high school chemistry, 2 years high school math, 2 years high school science, high school transcript, immunizations, interview, minimum high school GPA of 2.25, minimum high school rank 60%, minimum GPA in nursing prerequisites of 2.5, professional liability insurance/malpractice insurance, prerequisite course work. Transfer students are accepted. **Standardized tests** *Required:* SAT or ACT, TOEFL for international students. **Application** *Deadline:* 8/15 (freshmen), 8/1 (transfer). *Notification:* continuous (freshmen). *Application fee:* $25.

Advanced Placement Credit by examination available. Credit given for nursing courses completed elsewhere dependent upon specific evaluations.

Expenses (2005–06) *Tuition:* full-time $18,400; part-time $430 per credit hour. *Room and board:* $5870; room only: $3000 per academic year. *Required fees:* full-time $1390; part-time $165 per term.

Financial Aid 85% of baccalaureate students in nursing programs received some form of financial aid in 2004–05. *Gift aid (need-based):* Federal Pell, FSEOG, state, private, college/university gift aid from institutional funds. *Loans:* Federal Nursing Student Loans, FFEL (Subsidized and Unsubsidized Stafford PLUS), Perkins, state. *Work-Study:* Federal Work-Study, part-time campus jobs. *Application deadline (priority):* 3/1.

Contact Dr. Darla Vale, Chairperson, Department of Nursing, College of Mount St. Joseph, 5701 Delhi Road, Cincinnati, OH 45233-1670. *Telephone:* 513-244-4511. *Fax:* 513-451-2547. *E-mail:* darla_vale@mail.msj.edu.

GRADUATE PROGRAMS

Expenses (2005–06) *Tuition:* full-time $24,000. *Room and board:* $5879; room only: $3000 per academic year.

Financial Aid 15% of graduate students in nursing programs received some form of financial aid in 2004–05.

Contact Dr. Darla Vale, Chairperson, Department of Nursing, College of Mount St. Joseph, 5701 Delhi Road, Cincinnati, OH 45233. *Telephone:* 513-244-4322. *Fax:* 513-451-2547. *E-mail:* darla_vale@mail.msj.edu.

MASTER'S DEGREE PROGRAM

Degree MN

Available Programs Accelerated Master's; Accelerated Master's for Nurses with Non-Nursing Degrees.

Study Options Full-time.

Program Entrance Requirements Minimum overall college GPA of 3.0, transcript of college record, CPR certification, written essay, immunizations, interview, prerequisite course work, statistics course.

Advanced Placement Credit by examination available. Credit given for nursing courses completed elsewhere dependent upon specific evaluations.

Degree Requirements 64 total credit hours, thesis or project.

Franciscan University of Steubenville
Department of Nursing
Steubenville, Ohio

Founded in 1946

DEGREES • BSN • MSN

Nursing Program Faculty 15 (20% with doctorates).

Baccalaureate Enrollment 177
Women 91% **Men** 9% **Minority** 5% **International** 1% **Part-time** 5%

Graduate Enrollment 23
Women 78% **Men** 22% **Minority** 4% **Part-time** 83%

Nursing Student Activities Student Nurses' Association.

Nursing Student Resources Academic advising; academic or career counseling; assistance for students with disabilities; bookstore; campus computer network; computer lab; e-mail services; Internet; learning resource lab; library services; resume preparation assistance; tutoring.

Library Facilities 231,176 volumes (29,761 in health, 8,946 in nursing); 578 periodical subscriptions (178 health-care related).

BACCALAUREATE PROGRAMS

Degree BSN

Available Programs Generic Baccalaureate; RN Baccalaureate; RPN to Baccalaureate.

Study Options Full-time and part-time.

Program Entrance Requirements Minimum overall college GPA of 2.5, transcript of college record, health exam, health insurance, high school biology, high school chemistry, 2 years high school science, high school transcript, immunizations, 2 letters of recommendation, minimum high school GPA of 2.4, minimum GPA in nursing prerequisites of 2.5, professional liability insurance/malpractice insurance, prerequisite course work. Transfer students are accepted. **Standardized tests** *Required:* SAT or ACT, TOEFL for international students. **Application** *Deadline:* rolling (transfer). *Notification:* continuous (freshmen). *Application fee:* $20.

Advanced Placement Credit by examination available. Credit given for nursing courses completed elsewhere dependent upon specific evaluations.

Contact *Telephone:* 740-283-6324. *Fax:* 740-283-6449.

GRADUATE PROGRAMS

Contact *Telephone:* 740-284-7245. *Fax:* 740-283-6449.

MASTER'S DEGREE PROGRAM

Degree MSN

Available Programs Master's; RN to Master's.

Concentrations Available Nursing education. *Nurse practitioner programs in:* family health.

Study Options Full-time and part-time.

Program Entrance Requirements Clinical experience, minimum overall college GPA of 3.0, transcript of college record, interview, 2 letters of recommendation, nursing research course, physical assessment course, professional liability insurance/malpractice insurance, prerequisite course work, statistics course.

Advanced Placement Credit given for nursing courses completed elsewhere dependent upon specific evaluations.

Degree Requirements 48 total credit hours, thesis or project.

Kent State University
College of Nursing
Kent, Ohio

http://www.kent.edu/nursing

Founded in 1910

DEGREES • BSN • MSN • MSN/MBA • MSN/MPA • PHD

Nursing Program Faculty 111 (20% with doctorates).

Baccalaureate Enrollment 898
Women 97.4% **Men** 2.6% **Minority** 2.6% **International** .4% **Part-time** 19.52%

Graduate Enrollment 179
Women 92% **Men** 8% **Minority** 8% **International** 2% **Part-time** 82%

Nursing Student Activities Nursing Honor Society, Sigma Theta Tau, Student Nurses' Association.

Nursing Student Resources Academic advising; academic or career counseling; assistance for students with disabilities; bookstore; campus computer network; career placement assistance; computer lab; computer-assisted instruction; e-mail services; employment services for current students; externships; housing assistance; interactive nursing skills videos; Internet; learning resource lab; library services; nursing audiovisuals; other; placement services for program completers; remedial services; resume preparation assistance; skills, simulation, or other laboratory; tutoring.

Library Facilities 2.3 million volumes; 12,000 periodical subscriptions (300 health-care related).

BACCALAUREATE PROGRAMS

Degree BSN

Available Programs ADN to Baccalaureate; Accelerated Baccalaureate; Accelerated Baccalaureate for Second Degree; Accelerated RN Baccalaureate; Baccalaureate for Second Degree; Generic Baccalaureate; LPN to Baccalaureate; RN Baccalaureate.

Site Options *Distance Learning:* Warren, OH; Canton, OH; Salem, OH; Burton, OH.

Study Options Full-time and part-time.

Program Entrance Requirements Transcript of college record, written essay, high school biology, high school transcript, immunizations, interview, 2 letters of recommendation, minimum high school GPA of 2.5, minimum GPA in nursing prerequisites of 2.5. Transfer students are accepted. **Standardized tests** *Required:* SAT or ACT, TOEFL for international students. **Application** *Deadline:* 5/1 (freshmen). *Application fee:* $30.

Advanced Placement Credit given for nursing courses completed elsewhere dependent upon specific evaluations.

Expenses (2006–07) *Tuition, state resident:* part-time $384 per credit hour. *Tuition, nonresident:* part-time $722 per credit hour. *Room and board:* $6880; room only: $4200 per academic year.

Financial Aid 85% of baccalaureate students in nursing programs received some form of financial aid in 2005–06. *Gift aid (need-based):* Federal Pell, FSEOG, state, private, college/university gift aid from institutional funds. *Loans:* Federal Nursing Student Loans, Federal Direct (Subsidized and Unsubsidized Stafford PLUS), Perkins, state, college/university, alternative loans. *Work-Study:* Federal Work-Study. *Application deadline (priority):* 3/1.

Contact Mr. Curtis Good, Director of Student Services, College of Nursing, Kent State University, Henderson Hall, Kent, OH 44242-0001. *Telephone:* 330-672-9972. *Fax:* 330-672-7911. *E-mail:* cjgood@kent.edu.

GRADUATE PROGRAMS

Expenses (2006–07) *Tuition, state resident:* part-time $408 per credit hour. *Tuition, nonresident:* part-time $728 per credit hour. *Room and board:* $6880; room only: $4200 per academic year.

Financial Aid 85% of graduate students in nursing programs received some form of financial aid in 2005–06. 10 research assistantships with full tuition reimbursements available, 10 teaching assistantships with full tuition reimbursements available were awarded; Federal Work-Study, institutionally sponsored loans, traineeships, tuition waivers (full), and unspecified assistantships also available. *Financial aid application deadline:* 2/1.

Contact Dr. Karen Budd, Director, Graduate Programs, College of Nursing, Kent State University, PO Box 5190, Kent, OH 44242-0001. *Telephone:* 330-672-8776. *Fax:* 330-672-5003. *E-mail:* kbudd@kent.edu.

MASTER'S DEGREE PROGRAM

Degrees MSN; MSN/MBA; MSN/MPA

Available Programs Accelerated RN to Master's; Master's.

Concentrations Available Health-care administration; nurse case management; nursing administration; nursing education. *Clinical nurse specialist programs in:* acute care, adult health, cardiovascular, critical care, gerontology, maternity-newborn, medical-surgical, oncology, parent-child, pediatric, psychiatric/mental health, school health, women's health. *Nurse practitioner programs in:* acute care, adult health, family health, gerontology, pediatric, primary care, psychiatric/mental health, women's health.

Study Options Full-time and part-time.

Program Entrance Requirements Computer literacy, minimum overall college GPA of 3.0, transcript of college record, CPR certification, written essay, immunizations, interview, letters of recommendation, nursing research course, professional liability insurance/malpractice insurance, statistics course, GRE if undergraduate GPA is less than 3.0. *Application deadline:* For fall admission, 7/12; for spring admission, 11/29. Applications are processed on a rolling basis. *Application fee:* $30.

Advanced Placement Credit given for nursing courses completed elsewhere dependent upon specific evaluations.

Degree Requirements 36 total credit hours.

POST-MASTER'S PROGRAM

Areas of Study Nursing education. *Nurse practitioner programs in:* adult health, family health, gerontology, pediatric, primary care, psychiatric/mental health, women's health.

DOCTORAL DEGREE PROGRAM

Degree PhD

Available Programs Doctorate.

Areas of Study Aging, clinical practice, ethics, gerontology, health policy, health promotion/disease prevention, maternity-newborn, nurse case management, nursing administration, nursing education, nursing research, nursing science, women's health.

Kent State University (continued)

Program Entrance Requirements Minimum overall college GPA of 3.0, interview, 3 letters of recommendation, MSN or equivalent, scholarly papers, statistics course, writing sample, GRE. *Application deadline:* For fall admission, 7/12; for spring admission, 11/29. Applications are processed on a rolling basis. *Application fee:* $30.

Degree Requirements 72 total credit hours, dissertation, residency.

CONTINUING EDUCATION PROGRAM

Contact Betty Freund, Coordinator of Continuing Nursing Education, College of Nursing, Kent State University, PO Box 5190, Kent, OH 44242-0001. *Telephone:* 330-672-8810. *Fax:* 330-672-2433. *E-mail:* bfreund@kent.edu.

See full description on page 502.

Kettering College of Medical Arts
Division of Nursing
Kettering, Ohio

http://www.kcma.edu

Founded in 1967

DEGREE • BSN

Nursing Program Faculty 5 (40% with doctorates).

Baccalaureate Enrollment 15
Women 100% **Part-time** 100%

Nursing Student Resources Academic advising; academic or career counseling; assistance for students with disabilities; bookstore; campus computer network; computer lab; computer-assisted instruction; e-mail services; Internet; learning resource lab; library services; nursing audiovisuals; remedial services; resume preparation assistance; skills, simulation, or other laboratory; tutoring.

Library Facilities 29,390 volumes (4,060 in health, 1,073 in nursing); 266 periodical subscriptions (173 health-care related).

BACCALAUREATE PROGRAMS

Degree BSN

Available Programs RN Baccalaureate.
Study Options Full-time and part-time.
Program Entrance Requirements Transcript of college record, health exam, immunizations, 3 letters of recommendation, RN licensure. Transfer students are accepted. **Standardized tests** *Required:* ACT, TOEFL for international students. *Recommended:* SAT. **Application** *Deadline:* rolling (freshmen), rolling (transfer). *Notification:* continuous (freshmen). *Application fee:* $25.
Advanced Placement Credit given for nursing courses completed elsewhere dependent upon specific evaluations.
Contact *Telephone:* 937-395-8642. *Fax:* 937-395-8810.

Lourdes College
Nursing Department
Sylvania, Ohio

http://www.lourdes.edu

Founded in 1958

DEGREE • BSN

Nursing Program Faculty 15 (20% with doctorates).

Baccalaureate Enrollment 298
Women 95% **Men** 5% **Minority** 17% **Part-time** 24%

Nursing Student Activities Sigma Theta Tau, Student Nurses' Association.

Nursing Student Resources Academic advising; academic or career counseling; assistance for students with disabilities; bookstore; campus computer network; computer lab; computer-assisted instruction; e-mail services; employment services for current students; interactive nursing skills videos; Internet; learning resource lab; library services; nursing audiovisuals; remedial services; resume preparation assistance; skills, simulation, or other laboratory; tutoring.

Library Facilities 62,222 volumes (1,200 in health, 700 in nursing); 6,200 periodical subscriptions (101 health-care related).

BACCALAUREATE PROGRAMS

Degree BSN

Available Programs Generic Baccalaureate; LPN to Baccalaureate; RN Baccalaureate.
Site Options Sandusky, OH.
Study Options Full-time and part-time.
Program Entrance Requirements Minimum overall college GPA of 2.0, transcript of college record, CPR certification, health exam, health insurance, high school biology, high school chemistry, high school transcript, immunizations, 3 letters of recommendation, minimum GPA in nursing prerequisites of 2.5, professional liability insurance/malpractice insurance, prerequisite course work. Transfer students are accepted.
Standardized tests *Required:* TOEFL for international students. *Required for some:* SAT or ACT. **Application** *Deadline:* rolling (freshmen), rolling (out-of-state freshmen), rolling (transfer). *Notification:* continuous (freshmen), continuous (out-of-state freshmen). *Application fee:* $25.
Advanced Placement Credit by examination available. Credit given for nursing courses completed elsewhere dependent upon specific evaluations.
Contact *Telephone:* 419-824-3793. *Fax:* 419-824-3985.

Malone College
School of Nursing
Canton, Ohio

http://www.malone.edu

Founded in 1892

DEGREES • BSN • MSN

Nursing Program Faculty 30 (20% with doctorates).

Baccalaureate Enrollment 300
Women 87% **Men** 13% **Minority** 6% **International** .3% **Part-time** 27%
Graduate Enrollment 44
Women 95% **Men** 5% **Minority** 5%

Nursing Student Activities Nursing Honor Society, Sigma Theta Tau, Student Nurses' Association.

Nursing Student Resources Academic advising; academic or career counseling; assistance for students with disabilities; bookstore; campus computer network; career placement assistance; computer lab; computer-assisted instruction; e-mail services; employment services for current students; interactive nursing skills videos; Internet; learning resource lab; library services; nursing audiovisuals; placement services for program completers; remedial services; resume preparation assistance; skills, simulation, or other laboratory; tutoring.

Library Facilities 245,530 volumes (4,405 in health, 3,960 in nursing); 6,869 periodical subscriptions (85 health-care related).

BACCALAUREATE PROGRAMS

Degree BSN

Available Programs Generic Baccalaureate; LPN to RN Baccalaureate; RN Baccalaureate.
Study Options Full-time and part-time.
Program Entrance Requirements Minimum overall college GPA of 2.0, transcript of college record, CPR certification, written essay, health exam, health insurance, high school biology, high school chemistry, 3 years high school math, 3 years high school science, high school transcript, immunizations, minimum high school GPA of 2.5, professional liability insurance/malpractice insurance, prerequisite course work. Transfer stu-

dents are accepted. **Standardized tests** *Required:* SAT or ACT, TOEFL for international students. **Application** *Deadline:* 7/1 (freshmen), 7/1 (transfer). *Notification:* continuous (freshmen). *Application fee:* $20.

Advanced Placement Credit by examination available. Credit given for nursing courses completed elsewhere dependent upon specific evaluations.

Expenses (2006–07) *Tuition:* full-time $17,520; part-time $330 per credit hour. *International tuition:* $17,520 full-time. *Room and board:* $6400; room only: $3300 per academic year. *Required fees:* full-time $250.

Financial Aid 83% of baccalaureate students in nursing programs received some form of financial aid in 2005–06. *Gift aid (need-based):* Federal Pell, FSEOG, state, private, college/university gift aid from institutional funds. *Loans:* FFEL (Subsidized and Unsubsidized Stafford PLUS), Perkins, state, college/university, alternative loans. *Work-Study:* Federal Work-Study, part-time campus jobs. *Application deadline:* 7/31 (priority: 3/1).

Contact Mr. John Chopka, Dean of Admissions, School of Nursing, Malone College, 515 25th Street NW, Canton, OH 44709. *Telephone:* 330-471-8145. *Fax:* 330-471-8149. *E-mail:* admissions@malone.edu.

GRADUATE PROGRAMS

Expenses (2006–07) *Tuition:* full-time $13,185. *Required fees:* full-time $1766.

Financial Aid 89% of graduate students in nursing programs received some form of financial aid in 2005–06.

Contact Dr. Loretta M. Reinhart, RN, Dean and Professor, School of Nursing, Malone College, 515 25th Street NW, Canton, OH 44709. *Telephone:* 330-471-8366. *Fax:* 330-471-8607. *E-mail:* lreinhart2@malone.edu.

MASTER'S DEGREE PROGRAM

Degree MSN

Available Programs Master's.

Concentrations Available *Clinical nurse specialist programs in:* adult health, medical-surgical. *Nurse practitioner programs in:* family health.

Study Options Full-time.

Program Entrance Requirements Clinical experience, computer literacy, minimum overall college GPA of 3.0, transcript of college record, CPR certification, written essay, immunizations, interview, 2 letters of recommendation, nursing research course, physical assessment course, professional liability insurance/malpractice insurance, resume.

Degree Requirements 56 total credit hours, thesis or project.

CONTINUING EDUCATION PROGRAM

Contact Dr. Loretta M. Reinhart, RN, Dean and Professor, School of Nursing, Malone College, 515 25th Street NW, Canton, OH 44709. *Telephone:* 330-471-8366. *Fax:* 330-471-8607. *E-mail:* lreinhart2@malone.edu.

MedCentral College of Nursing
MedCentral College of Nursing
Mansfield, Ohio

Founded in 1996
DEGREE • BS

BACCALAUREATE PROGRAMS

Degree BS

Available Programs Accelerated Baccalaureate; LPN to Baccalaureate; RN Baccalaureate.

Program Entrance Requirements **Standardized tests** *Required:* SAT or ACT. **Application** *Deadline:* 8/1 (freshmen), 8/1 (transfer). *Notification:* continuous until 8/15 (freshmen). *Application fee:* $40.

Contact Nursing Program, MedCentral College of Nursing, 335 Glessner Avenue, Mansfield, OH 44903. *Telephone:* 419-520-2600.

Mercy College of Northwest Ohio
Division of Nursing
Toledo, Ohio

Founded in 1993
DEGREE • BSN

Library Facilities 6,400 volumes; 172 periodical subscriptions.

BACCALAUREATE PROGRAMS

Degree BSN

Available Programs Generic Baccalaureate; RN Baccalaureate.

Program Entrance Requirements Minimum overall college GPA of 2.5, immunizations, minimum high school GPA of 2.5, RN licensure. **Standardized tests** *Recommended:* SAT or ACT. *Required for some:* SAT or ACT. **Application** *Deadline:* rolling (freshmen), rolling (transfer). *Notification:* continuous (freshmen). *Application fee:* $25.

Contact *Telephone:* 888-806-3729. *Fax:* 419-251-1313.

Miami University
Department of Nursing
Hamilton, Ohio

http://www.ham.muohio.edu/nursing/
Founded in 1809
DEGREE • BSN

Nursing Program Faculty 6 (75% with doctorates).

Baccalaureate Enrollment 69
Women 98% **Men** 2% **Minority** 7% **Part-time** 56%

Nursing Student Activities Sigma Theta Tau.

Nursing Student Resources Academic advising; academic or career counseling; assistance for students with disabilities; bookstore; campus computer network; computer lab; daycare for children of students; e-mail services; interactive nursing skills videos; Internet; learning resource lab; library services; nursing audiovisuals; resume preparation assistance; tutoring.

Library Facilities 2.7 million volumes (29,000 in nursing); 14,089 periodical subscriptions (852 health-care related).

BACCALAUREATE PROGRAMS

Degree BSN

Available Programs ADN to Baccalaureate; LPN to Baccalaureate; RN Baccalaureate.

Site Options Middletown, OH; Hamilton, OH.

Study Options Full-time and part-time.

Program Entrance Requirements Minimum overall college GPA of 2.5, transcript of college record, health exam, health insurance, immunizations, professional liability insurance/malpractice insurance, prerequisite course work, RN licensure. Transfer students are accepted. **Standardized tests** *Required:* SAT or ACT, TOEFL for international students. **Application** *Deadline:* 1/31 (freshmen), 5/1 (transfer). *Early decision:* 11/1. *Notification:* 3/15 (freshmen), 12/15 (out-of-state freshmen), 12/15 (early decision). *Application fee:* $45.

Advanced Placement Credit given for nursing courses completed elsewhere dependent upon specific evaluations.

Financial Aid 40% of baccalaureate students in nursing programs received some form of financial aid in 2004–05. *Gift aid (need-based):* Federal Pell, FSEOG, state, private, college/university gift aid from institutional funds. *Loans:* Federal Nursing Student Loans, Federal Direct (Subsidized and Unsubsidized Stafford PLUS), Perkins, college/university, bank alternative loans. *Work-Study:* Federal Work-Study. *Application deadline (priority):* 2/15.

Contact Paulette Worcester, PhD, Interim Chair, Department of Nursing, Miami University, University Hall 151, Hamilton, OH 45011. *Telephone:* 513-785-7751. *Fax:* 513-785-7767. *E-mail:* worcesp@muohio.edu.

Mount Carmel College of Nursing
Nursing Programs
Columbus, Ohio

http://www.mccn.edu/index.html

Founded in 1903

DEGREES • BSN • MS

Nursing Program Faculty 62 (11% with doctorates).

Baccalaureate Enrollment 601
Women 91% **Men** 9% **Minority** 11% **Part-time** 20%

Graduate Enrollment 28
Women 100% **Minority** 11% **Part-time** 93%

Nursing Student Activities Sigma Theta Tau, Student Nurses' Association.

Nursing Student Resources Academic advising; academic or career counseling; assistance for students with disabilities; bookstore; campus computer network; computer lab; computer-assisted instruction; e-mail services; interactive nursing skills videos; Internet; learning resource lab; library services; nursing audiovisuals; resume preparation assistance; skills, simulation, or other laboratory; tutoring.

Library Facilities 8,000 volumes in health, 1,600 volumes in nursing; 3,425 periodical subscriptions health-care related.

BACCALAUREATE PROGRAMS

Degree BSN

Available Programs Accelerated Baccalaureate for Second Degree; Generic Baccalaureate; RN Baccalaureate.

Study Options Full-time and part-time.

Program Entrance Requirements Minimum overall college GPA of 2.75, transcript of college record, written essay, health exam, high school biology, high school chemistry, high school foreign language, 3 years high school math, 3 years high school science, high school transcript, immunizations, minimum high school GPA of 2.75. Transfer students are accepted. **Application** *Deadline:* rolling (freshmen). *Application fee:* $30.

Advanced Placement Credit given for nursing courses completed elsewhere dependent upon specific evaluations.

Expenses (2006–07) *Tuition:* full-time $14,994. *Room and board:* room only: $1928 per academic year. *Required fees:* full-time $312; part-time $156 per term.

Financial Aid 88% of baccalaureate students in nursing programs received some form of financial aid in 2005–06.

Contact Ms. Kim M. Campbell, Director of Admissions and Recruitment, Nursing Programs, Mount Carmel College of Nursing, 127 South Davis Avenue, Columbus, OH 43222-1504. *Telephone:* 614-234-5144. *Fax:* 614-234-2875. *E-mail:* kcampbell@mchs.com.

GRADUATE PROGRAMS

Expenses (2006–07) *Tuition:* full-time $7287. *Room and board:* room only: $1928 per academic year.

Financial Aid 20% of graduate students in nursing programs received some form of financial aid in 2005–06.

Contact Ms. Kip Sexton, MS Program Coordinator, Nursing Programs, Mount Carmel College of Nursing, 127 South Davis Avenue, Columbus, OH 43222. *Telephone:* 614-234-5800. *Fax:* 614-234-2875. *E-mail:* esexton@mchs.com.

MASTER'S DEGREE PROGRAM

Degree MS

Available Programs Master's.

Concentrations Available Nursing education. *Clinical nurse specialist programs in:* adult health.

Study Options Full-time and part-time.

Program Entrance Requirements Minimum overall college GPA of 3.0, transcript of college record, CPR certification, written essay, immunizations, 3 letters of recommendation, professional liability insurance/malpractice insurance, resume.

Degree Requirements 42 total credit hours, thesis or project.

POST-MASTER'S PROGRAM

Areas of Study Nursing education.

See full description on page 516.

The Ohio State University
College of Nursing
Columbus, Ohio

http://www.nursing.osu.edu

Founded in 1870

DEGREES • BSN • MS • PHD

Nursing Program Faculty 79 (38% with doctorates).

Baccalaureate Enrollment 503
Women 89% **Men** 11% **Minority** 13% **Part-time** 24%

Graduate Enrollment 234
Women 93% **Men** 7% **Minority** 8% **International** 1% **Part-time** 27%

Nursing Student Activities Nursing Honor Society, Sigma Theta Tau, Student Nurses' Association, nursing club.

Nursing Student Resources Academic advising; academic or career counseling; assistance for students with disabilities; bookstore; campus computer network; career placement assistance; computer lab; computer-assisted instruction; daycare for children of students; e-mail services; employment services for current students; externships; housing assistance; interactive nursing skills videos; Internet; learning resource lab; library services; nursing audiovisuals; other; paid internships; placement services for program completers; remedial services; resume preparation assistance; skills, simulation, or other laboratory; tutoring; unpaid internships.

Library Facilities 5.9 million volumes (188,602 in health, 4,198 in nursing); 43,086 periodical subscriptions (5,060 health-care related).

BACCALAUREATE PROGRAMS

Degree BSN

Available Programs Accelerated RN Baccalaureate; Generic Baccalaureate.

Site Options *Distance Learning:* Newark, OH; Marion, OH; Lima, OH.

Study Options Full-time and part-time.

Program Entrance Requirements Minimum overall college GPA of 2.75, transcript of college record, CPR certification, written essay, health insurance, high school biology, high school chemistry, high school foreign language, 3 years high school math, 2 years high school science, high school transcript, immunizations, minimum GPA in nursing prerequisites of 2.75, professional liability insurance/malpractice insurance, prerequisite course work. Transfer students are accepted. **Standardized tests** *Required:* SAT or ACT, TOEFL for international students. **Application** *Deadline:* 2/1 (freshmen), 2/1 (out-of-state freshmen), 6/25 (transfer). *Notification:* continuous (freshmen), continuous (out-of-state freshmen). *Application fee:* $40.

Advanced Placement Credit by examination available. Credit given for nursing courses completed elsewhere dependent upon specific evaluations.

Expenses (2006–07) *Tuition, state resident:* full-time $8967; part-time $1538 per quarter. *Tuition, nonresident:* full-time $20,862; part-time $1983 per quarter. *International tuition:* $20,862 full-time. *Room and board:* $7236; room only: $5100 per academic year. *Required fees:* full-time $3500; part-time $1500 per term.

Financial Aid 70% of baccalaureate students in nursing programs received some form of financial aid in 2005–06. *Gift aid (need-based):* Federal Pell, FSEOG, state, private, college/university gift aid from institutional funds. *Loans:* Federal Nursing Student Loans, Federal Direct (Subsidized and Unsubsidized Stafford PLUS), Perkins, college/university. *Work-Study:* Federal Work-Study. *Application deadline (priority):* 3/1.

Contact Steven Mousetes, Coordinator of FYE and Academic Advisor, College of Nursing, The Ohio State University, 240 Newton Hall, 1585 Neil Avenue, Columbus, OH 43210-1289. *Telephone:* 614-292-4041. *Fax:* 614-292-9399. *E-mail:* mousetes.1@osu.edu.

GRADUATE PROGRAMS

Expenses (2006–07) *Tuition, state resident:* full-time $11,672; part-time $5836 per quarter. *Tuition, nonresident:* full-time $29,476; part-time $14,740 per quarter. *International tuition:* $29,476 full-time. *Room and board:* $11,288; room only: $7728 per academic year. *Required fees:* full-time $278; part-time $183 per term.

Financial Aid 70% of graduate students in nursing programs received some form of financial aid in 2005–06. Fellowships, research assistantships, teaching assistantships, Federal Work-Study, institutionally sponsored loans, and unspecified assistantships available. Aid available to part-time students.

Contact Ms. Jackie Min, Graduate Outreach Coordinator, College of Nursing, The Ohio State University, 1585 Neil Avenue, Columbus, OH 43210-1289. *Telephone:* 614-688-8145. *Fax:* 614-292-9399. *E-mail:* Min.37@osu.edu.

MASTER'S DEGREE PROGRAM

Degree MS

Available Programs Accelerated AD/RN to Master's; Accelerated Master's; Accelerated Master's for Non-Nursing College Graduates; Master's; Master's for Non-Nursing College Graduates.

Concentrations Available Nurse-midwifery; nursing administration. *Clinical nurse specialist programs in:* adult health, cardiovascular, community health, oncology, parent-child, perinatal, psychiatric/mental health, public health, women's health. *Nurse practitioner programs in:* adult health, family health, neonatal health, pediatric, primary care, psychiatric/mental health, school health, women's health.

Study Options Full-time and part-time.

Program Entrance Requirements Minimum overall college GPA of 3.0, transcript of college record, CPR certification, written essay, immunizations, 3 letters of recommendation, nursing research course, resume, GRE General Test. *Application deadline:* For fall admission, 8/15 (priority date); for winter admission, 12/1 (priority date); for spring admission, 3/1 (priority date). Applications are processed on a rolling basis. *Application fee:* $40 ($50 for international students).

Advanced Placement Credit given for nursing courses completed elsewhere dependent upon specific evaluations.

Degree Requirements 45 total credit hours, thesis or project, comprehensive exam.

POST-MASTER'S PROGRAM

Areas of Study Nurse-midwifery; nursing administration. *Clinical nurse specialist programs in:* adult health, cardiovascular, community health, oncology, parent-child, psychiatric/mental health, public health, women's health. *Nurse practitioner programs in:* adult health, family health, neonatal health, pediatric, primary care, psychiatric/mental health, school health, women's health.

DOCTORAL DEGREE PROGRAM

Degree PhD

Available Programs Doctorate.

Areas of Study Addiction/substance abuse, aging, bio-behavioral research, biology of health and illness, clinical practice, community health, critical care, ethics, family health, gerontology, health policy, health promotion/disease prevention, health-care systems, illness and transition, individualized study, maternity-newborn, neuro-behavior, nursing policy, nursing research, nursing science, oncology, women's health.

Program Entrance Requirements Minimum overall college GPA of 3.3, 3 letters of recommendation, MSN or equivalent, statistics course, vita, writing sample, GRE General Test. *Application deadline:* For fall admission, 8/15 (priority date); for winter admission, 12/1 (priority date); for spring admission, 3/1 (priority date). Applications are processed on a rolling basis. *Application fee:* $40 ($50 for international students).

Degree Requirements 90 total credit hours, dissertation, oral exam, written exam, residency.

Ohio University
School of Nursing
Athens, Ohio

http://www.ohio.edu/nursing/

Founded in 1804

DEGREES • BSN • MSN

Nursing Program Faculty 9 (89% with doctorates).

Nursing Student Activities Nursing Honor Society, Sigma Theta Tau.

Nursing Student Resources Academic or career counseling; career placement assistance; computer lab; e-mail services; Internet; library services.

Library Facilities 2.7 million volumes; 27,606 periodical subscriptions.

BACCALAUREATE PROGRAMS

Degree BSN

Available Programs RN Baccalaureate.

Study Options Full-time and part-time.

Program Entrance Requirements Minimum overall college GPA of 2.0, transcript of college record, CPR certification, high school transcript, immunizations, professional liability insurance/malpractice insurance, prerequisite course work. Transfer students are accepted. **Standardized tests** *Required:* SAT or ACT. **Application** *Deadline:* 2/1 (freshmen), 5/15 (transfer). *Notification:* continuous (freshmen). *Application fee:* $45.

Advanced Placement Credit by examination available. Credit given for nursing courses completed elsewhere dependent upon specific evaluations.

Contact *Telephone:* 740-593-4494. *Fax:* 740-593-0286.

GRADUATE PROGRAMS

Contact *Telephone:* 740-593-4494. *Fax:* 740-593-0144.

MASTER'S DEGREE PROGRAM

Degree MSN

Concentrations Available Nursing administration; nursing education. *Nurse practitioner programs in:* family health.

Study Options Full-time and part-time.

Program Entrance Requirements Minimum overall college GPA of 3.0, transcript of college record, written essay, 3 letters of recommendation, resume, statistics course.

Advanced Placement Credit given for nursing courses completed elsewhere dependent upon specific evaluations.

Degree Requirements 55 total credit hours.

Otterbein College
Department of Nursing
Westerville, Ohio

http://www.otterbein.edu/dept/NURS

Founded in 1847

DEGREES • BSN • MSN

Nursing Student Activities Nursing Honor Society, Sigma Theta Tau.

Library Facilities 182,629 volumes; 1,012 periodical subscriptions.

BACCALAUREATE PROGRAMS

Degree BSN

Available Programs Accelerated RN Baccalaureate; Generic Baccalaureate; LPN to Baccalaureate; RN Baccalaureate.

Site Options *Distance Learning:* Newark, OH; Nelsonville, OH.

Program Entrance Requirements Transfer students are accepted. **Standardized tests** *Required:* SAT or ACT, TOEFL for international students. **Application** *Deadline:* 3/1 (freshmen), rolling (transfer). *Notification:* continuous (freshmen). *Application fee:* $25.

Advanced Placement Credit by examination available. Credit given for nursing courses completed elsewhere dependent upon specific evaluations.

Contact *Telephone:* 614-823-1614. *Fax:* 614-823-3131.

GRADUATE PROGRAMS

Contact *Telephone:* 614-823-1614.

Otterbein College (continued)
MASTER'S DEGREE PROGRAM

Degree MSN

Available Programs Master's.

Concentrations Available Nursing administration; nursing education. *Clinical nurse specialist programs in:* adult health. *Nurse practitioner programs in:* adult health, family health.

Site Options *Distance Learning:* Newark, OH; Nelsonville, OH; Hillsboro, OH.

Study Options Part-time.

Program Entrance Requirements *Application deadline:* Applications are processed on a rolling basis.

POST-MASTER'S PROGRAM

Areas of Study Nursing education. *Nurse practitioner programs in:* adult health, family health.

CONTINUING EDUCATION PROGRAM

Contact *Telephone:* 614-823-1614.

Shawnee State University
Department of Nursing
Portsmouth, Ohio

http://www.shawnee.edu/acadamics/hsc/nurs/index.html
Founded in 1986
DEGREE • BSN

Nursing Program Faculty 9.

Nursing Student Activities Student Nurses' Association.

Nursing Student Resources Academic advising; academic or career counseling; assistance for students with disabilities; bookstore; campus computer network; career placement assistance; computer lab; computer-assisted instruction; daycare for children of students; e-mail services; employment services for current students; housing assistance; interactive nursing skills videos; Internet; learning resource lab; library services; nursing audiovisuals; other; placement services for program completers; remedial services; resume preparation assistance; skills, simulation, or other laboratory; tutoring.

Library Facilities 150,957 volumes (8,273 in health, 870 in nursing); 56,172 periodical subscriptions (1,798 health-care related).

BACCALAUREATE PROGRAMS

Degree BSN

Available Programs ADN to Baccalaureate; RN Baccalaureate.

Study Options Full-time and part-time.

Program Entrance Requirements Minimum overall college GPA of 2.5, transcript of college record, CPR certification, health exam, health insurance, high school transcript, immunizations, professional liability insurance/malpractice insurance, prerequisite course work, RN licensure. Transfer students are accepted. **Standardized tests** *Required:* TOEFL for international students. *Recommended:* ACT. *Required for some:* ACT. **Application** *Deadline:* rolling (freshmen), rolling (transfer). *Notification:* continuous (freshmen).

Advanced Placement Credit given for nursing courses completed elsewhere dependent upon specific evaluations.

Contact *Telephone:* 740-351-3378. *Fax:* 740-351-3354.

CONTINUING EDUCATION PROGRAM

Contact *Telephone:* 740-351-3281.

The University of Akron
College of Nursing
Akron, Ohio

http://www.uakron.edu/nursing
Founded in 1870
DEGREES • BSN • MSN • PHD

Nursing Program Faculty 92 (27% with doctorates).

Baccalaureate Enrollment 595
Women 90% **Men** 10% **Minority** 11% **Part-time** 8%

Graduate Enrollment 224
Women 84% **Men** 16% **Minority** 29% **Part-time** 75%

Nursing Student Activities Sigma Theta Tau, Student Nurses' Association, nursing club.

Nursing Student Resources Academic advising; academic or career counseling; assistance for students with disabilities; bookstore; campus computer network; career placement assistance; computer lab; computer-assisted instruction; daycare for children of students; e-mail services; employment services for current students; interactive nursing skills videos; Internet; learning resource lab; library services; nursing audiovisuals; remedial services; resume preparation assistance; skills, simulation, or other laboratory; tutoring.

Library Facilities 1.3 million volumes (32,000 in health, 7,286 in nursing); 13,677 periodical subscriptions (1,662 health-care related).

■ A joint Ph.D. in nursing is offered in conjunction with Kent State University for those students interested in becoming nurse scholars. The RN to Master of Science in Nursing program meets the needs of registered nurses whose goal is graduate study for advanced practice. The accelerated B.S.N. program provides the opportunity for postbaccalaureate students from other majors to earn a nursing degree in fifteen months. Postbaccalaureate certificate programs in nursing education and in nursing management and business are also available.

BACCALAUREATE PROGRAMS

Degree BSN

Available Programs ADN to Baccalaureate; Accelerated Baccalaureate for Second Degree; Generic Baccalaureate; LPN to Baccalaureate; RN Baccalaureate.

Site Options *Distance Learning:* Orville, OH; Lorain, OH.

Study Options Full-time and part-time.

Program Entrance Requirements Transcript of college record, CPR certification, health exam, immunizations, minimum GPA in nursing prerequisites of 2.75, prerequisite course work. Transfer students are accepted. **Standardized tests** *Required:* SAT or ACT, TOEFL for international students. **Application** *Deadline:* 8/1 (freshmen), rolling (transfer). *Early decision:* 11/15. *Notification:* continuous (freshmen). *Application fee:* $30.

Advanced Placement Credit given for nursing courses completed elsewhere dependent upon specific evaluations.

Expenses (2006–07) *Tuition, area resident:* full-time $8497; part-time $349 per credit hour. *Tuition, nonresident:* full-time $15,895; part-time $658 per degree program. *Room and board:* $7200; room only: $4764 per academic year. *Required fees:* full-time $412.

Financial Aid 80% of baccalaureate students in nursing programs received some form of financial aid in 2005–06. *Gift aid (need-based):* Federal Pell, FSEOG. *Loans:* Federal Nursing Student Loans, FFEL (Subsidized and Unsubsidized Stafford PLUS), Perkins, college/university. *Work-Study:* Federal Work-Study, part-time campus jobs. *Application deadline (priority):* 2/1.

Contact Rita A. Klein, EdD, Director of Student Affairs, Nursing, College of Nursing, The University of Akron, Akron, OH 44325-3701. *Telephone:* 330-972-5103. *Fax:* 330-972-5493. *E-mail:* rklein1@uakron.edu.

GRADUATE PROGRAMS

Expenses (2006–07) *Tuition, area resident:* full-time $8915; part-time $367 per credit hour. *Tuition, nonresident:* full-time $14,795; part-time $612 per credit hour.

Financial Aid 80% of graduate students in nursing programs received some form of financial aid in 2005–06. 9 fellowships with full tuition reimbursements available, 15 research assistantships with full tuition reimbursements available, 10 teaching assistantships with full tuition reimbursements available were awarded; career-related internships or fieldwork, Federal Work-Study, and tuition waivers (full) also available.

Contact Dr. Marlene Huff, Coordinator, Masters Program, College of Nursing, The University of Akron, Akron, OH 44325-3701. *Telephone:* 330-972-5930. *Fax:* 330-972-5737. *E-mail:* mhuff@uakron.edu.

MASTER'S DEGREE PROGRAM

Degree MSN

Available Programs Master's; RN to Master's.

Concentrations Available Nurse anesthesia; nursing administration. *Clinical nurse specialist programs in:* adult health, gerontology, pediatric, psychiatric/mental health. *Nurse practitioner programs in:* adult health, gerontology, pediatric, psychiatric/mental health.

Site Options *Distance Learning:* Orville, OH; Lorain, OH.

Study Options Full-time and part-time.

Program Entrance Requirements Clinical experience, computer literacy, minimum overall college GPA of 3.0, transcript of college record, CPR certification, written essay, immunizations, interview, 3 letters of recommendation, physical assessment course, professional liability insurance/malpractice insurance, resume, statistics course, GRE or MAT. *Application deadline:* For fall admission, 8/15. Applications are processed on a rolling basis. *Application fee:* $30 ($40 for international students).

Advanced Placement Credit given for nursing courses completed elsewhere dependent upon specific evaluations.

Degree Requirements 37 total credit hours.

POST-MASTER'S PROGRAM

Areas of Study Nurse anesthesia. *Clinical nurse specialist programs in:* adult health, gerontology, pediatric, psychiatric/mental health. *Nurse practitioner programs in:* adult health, gerontology, pediatric, psychiatric/mental health.

DOCTORAL DEGREE PROGRAM

Degree PhD

Available Programs Doctorate.

Areas of Study Aging, ethics, gerontology, health policy, health promotion/disease prevention, health-care systems, human health and illness, illness and transition, individualized study, nursing administration, nursing policy, nursing research, nursing science, women's health.

Program Entrance Requirements Minimum overall college GPA of 3.0, interview, 3 letters of recommendation, MSN or equivalent, vita, writing sample, GRE. *Application deadline:* For fall admission, 8/15. Applications are processed on a rolling basis. *Application fee:* $30 ($40 for international students).

Degree Requirements 72 total credit hours, dissertation, oral exam, written exam, residency.

CONTINUING EDUCATION PROGRAM

Contact Dr. Marlene Huff, Coordinator, Educational Progression Program, College of Nursing, The University of Akron, Akron, OH 44325-3701. *Telephone:* 330-972-5930. *Fax:* 330-972-5737. *E-mail:* mhuff@uakron.edu.

See full description on page 536.

University of Cincinnati
College of Nursing
Cincinnati, Ohio

http://www.nursing.uc.edu
Founded in 1819

DEGREES • BSN • MSN • MSN/MBA • PHD

Nursing Program Faculty 143 (31% with doctorates).

Baccalaureate Enrollment 631
Women 90% **Men** 10% **Minority** 14% **Part-time** 13%

Graduate Enrollment 360
Women 86% **Men** 14% **Minority** 14% **International** 2%

Nursing Student Activities Sigma Theta Tau, Student Nurses' Association.

Nursing Student Resources Academic advising; academic or career counseling; assistance for students with disabilities; bookstore; campus computer network; computer lab; computer-assisted instruction; e-mail services; employment services for current students; externships; housing assistance; interactive nursing skills videos; Internet; learning resource lab; library services; nursing audiovisuals; paid internships; remedial services; resume preparation assistance; skills, simulation, or other laboratory; tutoring; unpaid internships.

Library Facilities 3 million volumes (221,630 in health, 21,306 in nursing); 16,560 periodical subscriptions (2,384 health-care related).

BACCALAUREATE PROGRAMS

Degree BSN

Available Programs Generic Baccalaureate; RN Baccalaureate.

Site Options Cincinnati, OH.

Study Options Full-time and part-time.

Program Entrance Requirements Minimum overall college GPA of 2.5, transcript of college record, CPR certification, health insurance, high school biology, high school chemistry, 3 years high school math, high school transcript, immunizations, minimum GPA in nursing prerequisites of 2.5, prerequisite course work. Transfer students are accepted. **Standardized tests** *Required:* SAT or ACT, TOEFL for international students. **Application** *Deadline:* rolling (freshmen), rolling (transfer). *Notification:* continuous until 11/1 (freshmen). *Application fee:* $40.

Advanced Placement Credit by examination available. Credit given for nursing courses completed elsewhere dependent upon specific evaluations.

Expenses (2006–07) *Tuition, area resident:* full-time $9399; part-time $262 per credit hour. *Tuition, nonresident:* full-time $23,922; part-time $665 per credit hour. *International tuition:* $23,922 full-time. *Room and board:* $8286 per academic year. *Required fees:* full-time $1251; part-time $417 per term.

Financial Aid 65% of baccalaureate students in nursing programs received some form of financial aid in 2005–06. *Gift aid (need-based):* Federal Pell, FSEOG, state, private, college/university gift aid from institutional funds, Federal Nursing. *Loans:* Federal Nursing Student Loans, Federal Direct (Subsidized and Unsubsidized Stafford PLUS), FFEL (Subsidized and Unsubsidized Stafford PLUS), Perkins, state, college/university. *Work-Study:* Federal Work-Study. *Application deadline:* Continuous.

Contact Mr. Aaron Price, Baccalaureate Academic Advisor, College of Nursing, University of Cincinnati, Office of Student Affairs, PO Box 210038, Cincinnati, OH 45221-0038. *Telephone:* 513-558-5070. *Fax:* 513-558-7523. *E-mail:* aaron.price@uc.edu.

GRADUATE PROGRAMS

Expenses (2006–07) *Tuition, area resident:* full-time $11,661; part-time $389 per credit hour. *Tuition, state resident:* full-time $11,664; part-time $389 per credit hour. *Tuition, nonresident:* full-time $21,495; part-time $717 per credit hour. *International tuition:* $21,495 full-time. *Room and board:* $8286 per academic year. *Required fees:* full-time $1251; part-time $417 per term.

Financial Aid 70% of graduate students in nursing programs received some form of financial aid in 2005–06. 7 fellowships with full tuition reimbursements available (averaging $10,629 per year), 16 research assistantships with full tuition reimbursements available (averaging $12,375 per year), 6 teaching assistantships with full tuition reimbursements available (averaging $12,000 per year) were awarded; Federal Work-Study, scholarships, traineeships, tuition waivers (partial), and unspecified assistantships also available. Aid available to part-time students. *Financial aid application deadline:* 5/1.

Contact Mr. Loren Carter, Graduate Academic Advisor, College of Nursing, University of Cincinnati, PO Box 210038, Cincinnati, OH 45221-0038. *Telephone:* 513-558-5072. *Fax:* 513-558-7523. *E-mail:* loren.carter@uc.edu.

University of Cincinnati (continued)

MASTER'S DEGREE PROGRAM

Degrees MSN; MSN/MBA

Available Programs Accelerated Master's for Non-Nursing College Graduates; Accelerated RN to Master's; Master's.

Concentrations Available Nurse anesthesia; nurse-midwifery; nursing administration. *Clinical nurse specialist programs in:* acute care, adult health, community health, occupational health. *Nurse practitioner programs in:* acute care, adult health, family health, gerontology, neonatal health, pediatric, psychiatric/mental health, women's health.

Site Options *Distance Learning:* Cincinnati, OH.

Study Options Full-time and part-time.

Program Entrance Requirements Clinical experience, computer literacy, minimum overall college GPA of 3.0, transcript of college record, CPR certification, written essay, immunizations, interview, 3 letters of recommendation, physical assessment course, professional liability insurance/malpractice insurance, resume, statistics course, GRE General Test. *Application deadline:* For fall admission, 2/1 (priority date). Applications are processed on a rolling basis. *Application fee:* $40.

Advanced Placement Credit given for nursing courses completed elsewhere dependent upon specific evaluations.

Degree Requirements 60 total credit hours, thesis or project.

POST-MASTER'S PROGRAM

Areas of Study *Nurse practitioner programs in:* acute care, adult health, family health, gerontology, neonatal health, pediatric, psychiatric/mental health, women's health.

DOCTORAL DEGREE PROGRAM

Degree PhD

Available Programs Doctorate; Post-Baccalaureate Doctorate.

Areas of Study Addiction/substance abuse, community health, critical care, ethics, faculty preparation, family health, health promotion/disease prevention, health-care systems, human health and illness, illness and transition, individualized study, maternity-newborn, nursing administration, nursing research, nursing science, oncology, women's health.

Program Entrance Requirements Minimum overall college GPA of 3.0, interview, 3 letters of recommendation, statistics course, vita, writing sample, GRE General Test. *Application deadline:* For fall admission, 2/1 (priority date). Applications are processed on a rolling basis. *Application fee:* $40.

Degree Requirements 135 total credit hours, dissertation, written exam, residency.

CONTINUING EDUCATION PROGRAM

Contact Ms. Elizabeth Karle, Program Coordinator, Continuing Education, College of Nursing, University of Cincinnati, PO Box 210038, Cincinnati, OH 45221-0038. *Telephone:* 513-558-5311. *Fax:* 513-558-5054. *E-mail:* elizabeth.karle@uc.edu.

See full description on page 540.

University of Phoenix–Cleveland Campus

College of Health and Human Services
Independence, Ohio

Founded in 2000

DEGREES • BSN • MSN • MSN/MBA

Nursing Program Faculty 29 (28% with doctorates).

Baccalaureate Enrollment 41

Women 97.56% **Men** 2.44% **Minority** 26.83%

Graduate Enrollment 23

Women 100% **Minority** 39.13%

Nursing Student Activities Sigma Theta Tau.

Nursing Student Resources Academic advising; academic or career counseling; assistance for students with disabilities; bookstore; computer lab; library services; remedial services.

Library Facilities 444 volumes; 666 periodical subscriptions.

BACCALAUREATE PROGRAMS

Degree BSN

Available Programs Accelerated Baccalaureate.

Site Options Beachwood, OH.

Study Options Full-time.

Program Entrance Requirements Transcript of college record, 1 letter of recommendation, RN licensure. Transfer students are accepted. **Standardized tests** *Required:* TOEFL for international students. **Application** *Deadline:* rolling (freshmen), rolling (transfer). *Application fee:* $110.

Advanced Placement Credit by examination available. Credit given for nursing courses completed elsewhere dependent upon specific evaluations.

Expenses (2006–07) *Tuition:* full-time $11,910. *International tuition:* $11,910 full-time. *Required fees:* full-time $750.

Contact Campus College Chair, Nursing, College of Health and Human Services, University of Phoenix–Cleveland Campus, 5005 Rockside Road, Suite 130, Independence, OH 44131. *Telephone:* 216-447-8807.

GRADUATE PROGRAMS

Expenses (2006–07) *Tuition:* full-time $11,832. *International tuition:* $11,832 full-time. *Required fees:* full-time $760.

Contact Campus College Chair, Nursing, College of Health and Human Services, University of Phoenix–Cleveland Campus, 5005 Rockside Road, Suite 130, Independence, OH 44131. *Telephone:* 216-447-8807.

MASTER'S DEGREE PROGRAM

Degrees MSN; MSN/MBA

Available Programs Master's; Master's for Non-Nursing College Graduates.

Concentrations Available Nursing administration.

Site Options Beachwood, OH.

Study Options Full-time.

Program Entrance Requirements Clinical experience, computer literacy, minimum overall college GPA of 2.5, transcript of college record. *Application deadline:* Applications are processed on a rolling basis. *Application fee:* $110.

Advanced Placement Credit given for nursing courses completed elsewhere dependent upon specific evaluations.

Degree Requirements 39 total credit hours.

The University of Toledo

College of Nursing
Toledo, Ohio

http://www.mco.edu/snur/index.html

Founded in 1872

DEGREES • BSN • MSN

Nursing Program Faculty 60 (42% with doctorates).

Baccalaureate Enrollment 415

Women 90% **Men** 10% **Minority** 9% **International** 1% **Part-time** 15%

Graduate Enrollment 171

Women 94% **Men** 6% **Minority** 3% **Part-time** 63%

Nursing Student Activities Sigma Theta Tau, Student Nurses' Association, nursing club.

Nursing Student Resources Academic advising; academic or career counseling; assistance for students with disabilities; bookstore; campus computer network; computer lab; computer-assisted instruction; daycare for children of students; e-mail services; interactive nursing skills videos; Internet; learning resource lab; library services; nursing audiovisuals; resume preparation assistance; skills, simulation, or other laboratory; tutoring.

Library Facilities 1.8 million volumes (154,000 in health, 15,000 in nursing); 6,500 periodical subscriptions (2,400 health-care related).

BACCALAUREATE PROGRAMS

Degree BSN

Available Programs ADN to Baccalaureate; Generic Baccalaureate.

Site Options *Distance Learning:* Huron, OH; Lima, OH; Archbold, OH.

Study Options Full-time and part-time.

Program Entrance Requirements Minimum overall college GPA of 2.5, transcript of college record, CPR certification, health exam, health insurance, high school biology, high school chemistry, high school foreign language, 3 years high school math, 3 years high school science, high school transcript, immunizations, minimum high school GPA of 2.5, minimum GPA in nursing prerequisites of 2.0, professional liability insurance/malpractice insurance, prerequisite course work. Transfer students are accepted. **Standardized tests** *Required:* SAT or ACT. *Recommended:* TOEFL for international students. **Application** *Deadline:* rolling (freshmen), rolling (transfer). *Notification:* continuous (freshmen). *Application fee:* $40.

Advanced Placement Credit given for nursing courses completed elsewhere dependent upon specific evaluations.

Expenses (2006–07) *Tuition, state resident:* full-time $7814; part-time $271 per credit hour. *Tuition, nonresident:* full-time $15,628; part-time $639 per credit hour. *Required fees:* full-time $1112; part-time $47 per credit.

Financial Aid 60% of baccalaureate students in nursing programs received some form of financial aid in 2005–06. *Gift aid (need-based):* Federal Pell, FSEOG, state, private, college/university gift aid from institutional funds. *Loans:* Federal Direct (Subsidized and Unsubsidized Stafford PLUS), Perkins, alternative loans. *Work-Study:* Federal Work-Study. *Application deadline (priority):* 4/1.

Contact Paula Ballmer, RN, Admissions Representative, College of Nursing, The University of Toledo, Health Science Campus, 3000 Arlington Avenue, Mail Stop 1026, Toledo, OH 43614-2598. *Telephone:* 419-383-5839. *Fax:* 419-383-5894. *E-mail:* paula.ballmer@utoledo.edu.

GRADUATE PROGRAMS

Expenses (2006–07) *Tuition, state resident:* full-time $10,927; part-time $348 per credit hour. *Tuition, nonresident:* full-time $24,920; part-time $795 per credit hour. *Required fees:* full-time $1333; part-time $47 per credit; part-time $560 per term.

Financial Aid 60% of graduate students in nursing programs received some form of financial aid in 2005–06. Federal Work-Study, institutionally sponsored loans, and scholarships available.

Contact Ms. Kathleen Mitchell, RN, Graduate Nursing Advisor, College of Nursing, The University of Toledo, 3000 Arlington Avenue, Toledo, OH 43614-2598. *Telephone:* 419-383-5820. *Fax:* 419-383-5894. *E-mail:* kathleen.mitchell@utoledo.edu.

MASTER'S DEGREE PROGRAM

Degree MSN

Available Programs Master's; Master's for Non-Nursing College Graduates; Master's for Nurses with Non-Nursing Degrees.

Concentrations Available Nursing education. *Clinical nurse specialist programs in:* adult health, psychiatric/mental health. *Nurse practitioner programs in:* adult health, family health, pediatric.

Study Options Full-time and part-time.

Program Entrance Requirements Computer literacy, minimum overall college GPA of 3.0, transcript of college record, written essay, 2 letters of recommendation, resume, GRE General Test. *Application deadline:* For fall admission, 5/1; for spring admission, 9/1. *Application fee:* $45.

Advanced Placement Credit given for nursing courses completed elsewhere dependent upon specific evaluations.

Degree Requirements 55 total credit hours, thesis or project, comprehensive exam.

POST-MASTER'S PROGRAM

Areas of Study Nursing education. *Clinical nurse specialist programs in:* psychiatric/mental health. *Nurse practitioner programs in:* adult health, family health, pediatric.

CONTINUING EDUCATION PROGRAM

Contact Ms. Deborah Mattin, RN, Director, Continuing Nursing Education, College of Nursing, The University of Toledo, 3000 Arlington Avenue, Toledo, OH 43614-2598. *Telephone:* 419-383-5812. *Fax:* 419-383-5894. *E-mail:* deborah.mattin@utoledo.edu.

Ursuline College
The Breen School of Nursing
Pepper Pike, Ohio

http://www.ursuline.edu

Founded in 1871

DEGREES • BSN • MSN

Nursing Program Faculty 25 (28% with doctorates).

Baccalaureate Enrollment 475
Women 90% **Men** 10% **Minority** 25%

Graduate Enrollment 92
Women 95% **Men** 5% **Minority** 20% **International** 2% **Part-time** 40%

Nursing Student Activities Sigma Theta Tau, Student Nurses' Association.

Nursing Student Resources Academic advising; academic or career counseling; assistance for students with disabilities; bookstore; campus computer network; career placement assistance; computer lab; computer-assisted instruction; e-mail services; employment services for current students; externships; housing assistance; interactive nursing skills videos; Internet; learning resource lab; library services; nursing audiovisuals; placement services for program completers; remedial services; resume preparation assistance; skills, simulation, or other laboratory; tutoring.

Library Facilities 129,621 volumes; 14,198 periodical subscriptions.

BACCALAUREATE PROGRAMS

Degree BSN

Available Programs Accelerated Baccalaureate for Second Degree; Accelerated LPN to Baccalaureate; Accelerated RN Baccalaureate; Generic Baccalaureate.

Site Options Cleveland, OH.

Study Options Full-time and part-time.

Program Entrance Requirements Minimum overall college GPA of 2.5, transcript of college record, written essay, health exam, health insurance, high school biology, high school chemistry, 2 years high school math, 2 years high school science, high school transcript, immunizations, 1 letter of recommendation, minimum high school GPA of 2.75, minimum GPA in nursing prerequisites of 2.75. Transfer students are accepted. **Standardized tests** *Required:* SAT or ACT, TOEFL for international students. **Application** *Deadline:* rolling (freshmen), rolling (transfer). *Early decision:* 11/15. *Notification:* continuous (freshmen), 2/15 (early action). *Application fee:* $25.

Advanced Placement Credit given for nursing courses completed elsewhere dependent upon specific evaluations.

Expenses (2006–07) *Tuition:* part-time $662 per credit hour. *Room and board:* $3342 per academic year. *Required fees:* full-time $150.

Financial Aid 90% of baccalaureate students in nursing programs received some form of financial aid in 2005–06.

Contact Jackie Cannarella, Coordinator of Nursing Enrollment Management, The Breen School of Nursing, Ursuline College, 2550 Lander Road, Pepper Pike, OH 44124-4398. *Telephone:* 440-449-8171. *Fax:* 440-449-4267. *E-mail:* jcannarella@ursuline.edu.

GRADUATE PROGRAMS

Expenses (2006–07) *Tuition:* part-time $705 per credit hour.

Financial Aid 20% of graduate students in nursing programs received some form of financial aid in 2005–06.

Contact Dr. M. Murray Mayo, Director, Graduate Nursing, The Breen School of Nursing, Ursuline College, 2550 Lander Road, Pepper Pike, OH 44124. *Telephone:* 440-449-8172. *Fax:* 440-449-4267. *E-mail:* mmayo@ursuline.edu.

MASTER'S DEGREE PROGRAM

Degree MSN

Available Programs Accelerated Master's; Master's.

Concentrations Available Nurse case management. *Clinical nurse specialist programs in:* adult health, palliative care. *Nurse practitioner programs in:* adult health, family health.

Study Options Full-time and part-time.

Ursuline College (continued)

Program Entrance Requirements Clinical experience, minimum overall college GPA of 3.0, transcript of college record, CPR certification, immunizations, 3 letters of recommendation.

Advanced Placement Credit given for nursing courses completed elsewhere dependent upon specific evaluations.

Degree Requirements 39 total credit hours.

POST-MASTER'S PROGRAM

Areas of Study Nurse case management. *Clinical nurse specialist programs in:* adult health, palliative care. *Nurse practitioner programs in:* adult health, family health.

See full description on page 568.

Walsh University
Department of Nursing
North Canton, Ohio

http://www.walsh.edu/
Founded in 1958
DEGREE • BSN

Nursing Program Faculty 7 (12% with doctorates).
Baccalaureate Enrollment 263
Women 90% **Men** 10% **Minority** 6% **Part-time** 10%
Nursing Student Activities Nursing Honor Society, Student Nurses' Association.

Nursing Student Resources Academic advising; academic or career counseling; assistance for students with disabilities; bookstore; campus computer network; career placement assistance; computer lab; computer-assisted instruction; e-mail services; housing assistance; Internet; learning resource lab; library services; nursing audiovisuals; placement services for program completers; resume preparation assistance; skills, simulation, or other laboratory; tutoring.

Library Facilities 199,543 volumes (4,000 in health, 2,000 in nursing); 5,586 periodical subscriptions (114 health-care related).

BACCALAUREATE PROGRAMS

Degree BSN

Available Programs Accelerated RN Baccalaureate; Generic Baccalaureate.
Site Options Akron, OH; Canton, OH.
Study Options Full-time and part-time.
Program Entrance Requirements Minimum overall college GPA of 2.0, transcript of college record, CPR certification, high school foreign language, 3 years high school math, 3 years high school science, high school transcript, immunizations, minimum high school GPA of 2.0, professional liability insurance/malpractice insurance. Transfer students are accepted. **Standardized tests** *Required:* SAT or ACT, TOEFL for international students. **Application** *Deadline:* rolling (freshmen), rolling (out-of-state freshmen), rolling (transfer). *Notification:* continuous (freshmen), continuous (out-of-state freshmen). *Application fee:* $25.
Advanced Placement Credit by examination available.
Expenses (2005–06) *Tuition:* full-time $16,000; part-time $450 per credit hour. *International tuition:* $16,000 full-time. *Room and board:* $8200; room only: $6200 per academic year. *Required fees:* full-time $350; part-time $17 per credit; part-time $125 per term.
Financial Aid 94% of baccalaureate students in nursing programs received some form of financial aid in 2004–05.
Contact Dr. Janis M. Campbell, RN, Chair, Department of Nursing, Walsh University, 2020 East Maple Street, North Canton, OH 44720-3336. *Telephone:* 330-490-7250. *Fax:* 330-490-7206. *E-mail:* jcampbell@walsh.edu.

Wright State University
College of Nursing and Health
Dayton, Ohio

http://www.nursing.wright.edu
Founded in 1964
DEGREES • BSN • MS • MS/MBA

Nursing Program Faculty 68 (33% with doctorates).
Baccalaureate Enrollment 689
Women 88% **Men** 12% **Minority** 13% **International** 1% **Part-time** 23%
Graduate Enrollment 203
Women 92% **Men** 8% **Minority** 9% **International** 1% **Part-time** 78%
Nursing Student Activities Nursing Honor Society, Sigma Theta Tau, Student Nurses' Association, nursing club.

Nursing Student Resources Academic advising; academic or career counseling; assistance for students with disabilities; bookstore; campus computer network; career placement assistance; computer lab; computer-assisted instruction; daycare for children of students; e-mail services; employment services for current students; externships; housing assistance; interactive nursing skills videos; Internet; learning resource lab; library services; nursing audiovisuals; remedial services; resume preparation assistance; skills, simulation, or other laboratory; tutoring.

Library Facilities 703,000 volumes (111,826 in health, 7,646 in nursing); 443,200 periodical subscriptions (1,279 health-care related).

BACCALAUREATE PROGRAMS

Degree BSN

Available Programs Accelerated Baccalaureate for Second Degree; Baccalaureate for Second Degree; Generic Baccalaureate; RN Baccalaureate.
Site Options *Distance Learning:* Celina, OH; Dayton, OH.
Study Options Full-time and part-time.
Program Entrance Requirements Minimum overall college GPA of 2.5, transcript of college record, written essay, high school transcript, minimum GPA in nursing prerequisites of 2.5, prerequisite course work. Transfer students are accepted. **Standardized tests** *Required:* SAT or ACT, TOEFL for international students. **Application** *Deadline:* rolling (freshmen), rolling (transfer). *Notification:* continuous (freshmen). *Application fee:* $30.
Advanced Placement Credit by examination available. Credit given for nursing courses completed elsewhere dependent upon specific evaluations.
Expenses (2006–07) *Tuition, state resident:* full-time $7278; part-time $219 per quarter hour. *Tuition, nonresident:* full-time $14,004; part-time $425 per quarter hour. *International tuition:* $14,058 full-time. *Room and board:* $7180; room only: $3850 per academic year. *Required fees:* full-time $700.
Financial Aid 83% of baccalaureate students in nursing programs received some form of financial aid in 2005–06.
Contact Ms. Theresa A. Haghnazarian, Director, Student and Alumni Affairs, College of Nursing and Health, Wright State University, 3640 Colonel Glenn Highway, Dayton, OH 45435. *Telephone:* 937-775-3132. *Fax:* 937-775-4571. *E-mail:* theresa.haghnazarian@wright.edu.

GRADUATE PROGRAMS

Expenses (2006–07) *Tuition, state resident:* full-time $12,960; part-time $298 per quarter hour. *Tuition, nonresident:* full-time $21,928; part-time $507 per quarter hour. *International tuition:* $21,928 full-time.
Financial Aid 39% of graduate students in nursing programs received some form of financial aid in 2005–06. 15 fellowships with full tuition reimbursements available were awarded; research assistantships, teaching assistantships, Federal Work-Study, institutionally sponsored loans, and unspecified assistantships also available. Aid available to part-time students. *Financial aid application deadline:* 6/1.
Contact Ms. Theresa A. Haghnazarian, Director, Student and Alumni Affairs, College of Nursing and Health, Wright State University, 3640 Colonel Glenn Highway, Dayton, OH 45435. *Telephone:* 937-775-3132. *Fax:* 937-775-4571. *E-mail:* theresa.haghnazarian@wright.edu.

MASTER'S DEGREE PROGRAM

Degrees MS; MS/MBA

Available Programs Master's; Master's for Nurses with Non-Nursing Degrees.

Concentrations Available Health-care administration; nursing administration. *Clinical nurse specialist programs in:* adult health, community health, pediatric, public health, school health. *Nurse practitioner programs in:* acute care, family health, pediatric.

Study Options Full-time and part-time.

Program Entrance Requirements Clinical experience, computer literacy, minimum overall college GPA of 3.0, transcript of college record, written essay, interview, physical assessment course, statistics course, GRE General Test. *Application deadline:* For fall admission, 4/15 (priority date). *Application fee:* $25.

Advanced Placement Credit given for nursing courses completed elsewhere dependent upon specific evaluations.

Degree Requirements 48 total credit hours, thesis or project.

POST-MASTER'S PROGRAM

Areas of Study Nursing education. *Clinical nurse specialist programs in:* school health. *Nurse practitioner programs in:* acute care, family health, pediatric.

CONTINUING EDUCATION PROGRAM

Contact Ms. Shari Domico, Office Assistant, College of Nursing and Health, Wright State University, 3640 Colonel Glenn Highway, Dayton, OH 45435. *Telephone:* 937-775-3577. *Fax:* 937-775-4571. *E-mail:* shari.domico@wright.edu.

See full description on page 580.

Xavier University
Department of Nursing
Cincinnati, Ohio

Founded in 1831

DEGREES • BSN • MSN • MSN/MBA

Nursing Program Faculty 43 (14% with doctorates).

Baccalaureate Enrollment 228
Women 92% **Men** 8% **Minority** 14% **Part-time** 4%

Graduate Enrollment 168
Women 93% **Men** 7% **Minority** 21% **International** 15% **Part-time** 65%

Nursing Student Activities Sigma Theta Tau, nursing club.

Nursing Student Resources Academic advising; academic or career counseling; assistance for students with disabilities; bookstore; campus computer network; career placement assistance; computer lab; computer-assisted instruction; e-mail services; employment services for current students; externships; housing assistance; interactive nursing skills videos; Internet; learning resource lab; library services; nursing audiovisuals; paid internships; resume preparation assistance; skills, simulation, or other laboratory; tutoring.

Library Facilities 227,200 volumes (8,900 in health, 1,160 in nursing); 21,650 periodical subscriptions (200 health-care related).

BACCALAUREATE PROGRAMS

Degree BSN

Available Programs Generic Baccalaureate.

Study Options Full-time and part-time.

Program Entrance Requirements Minimum overall college GPA of 2.5, transcript of college record, written essay, high school chemistry, high school foreign language, 3 years high school math, 2 years high school science, high school transcript, minimum high school GPA of 2.8. Transfer students are accepted. **Standardized tests** *Required:* SAT or ACT, TOEFL for international students. **Application** *Deadline:* 2/1 (freshmen), rolling (transfer). *Early decision:* 12/1. *Notification:* 3/15 (freshmen), 1/15 (early action). *Application fee:* $35.

Advanced Placement Credit given for nursing courses completed elsewhere dependent upon specific evaluations.

Expenses (2006–07) *Tuition:* full-time $23,270; part-time $446 per credit hour. *Room and board:* $8710; room only: $4710 per academic year. *Required fees:* full-time $200; part-time $60 per credit.

Financial Aid 85% of baccalaureate students in nursing programs received some form of financial aid in 2005–06. *Gift aid (need-based):* Federal Pell, FSEOG, state, private, college/university gift aid from institutional funds. *Loans:* FFEL (Subsidized and Unsubsidized Stafford PLUS), Perkins. *Work-Study:* Federal Work-Study, part-time campus jobs. *Application deadline (priority):* 2/15.

Contact Ms. Marilyn Volk Gomez, Director of Nursing Student Services, Department of Nursing, Xavier University, 3800 Victory Parkway, Cincinnati, OH 45207-7351. *Telephone:* 513-745-4392. *Fax:* 513-745-1087. *E-mail:* gomez@xavier.edu.

GRADUATE PROGRAMS

Expenses (2006–07) *Tuition:* part-time $515 per credit hour. *Required fees:* full-time $200; part-time $100 per credit.

Financial Aid 30% of graduate students in nursing programs received some form of financial aid in 2005–06. Scholarships, traineeships, and unspecified assistantships available. Aid available to part-time students. *Financial aid application deadline:* 4/1.

Contact Ms. Marilyn Volk Gomez, Director of Nursing Student Services, Department of Nursing, Xavier University, 3800 Victory Parkway, Cincinnati, OH 45207-7351. *Telephone:* 513-745-4392. *Fax:* 513-745-1087. *E-mail:* gomez@xavier.edu.

MASTER'S DEGREE PROGRAM

Degrees MSN; MSN/MBA

Available Programs Master's; Master's for Nurses with Non-Nursing Degrees; RN to Master's.

Concentrations Available Nursing administration; nursing education.

Study Options Full-time and part-time.

Program Entrance Requirements Minimum overall college GPA of 2.8, transcript of college record, written essay, 3 letters of recommendation, statistics course, GMAT, GRE General Test. *Application deadline:* For fall admission, 8/28 (priority date). Applications are processed on a rolling basis. *Application fee:* $35.

Degree Requirements 36 total credit hours, thesis or project.

Youngstown State University
Department of Nursing
Youngstown, Ohio

Founded in 1908

DEGREES • BSN • MSN

Nursing Program Faculty 22 (18% with doctorates).

Baccalaureate Enrollment 22

Graduate Enrollment 24
Women 75% **Men** 25% **Minority** 13%

Nursing Student Activities Sigma Theta Tau, Student Nurses' Association.

Nursing Student Resources Academic advising; academic or career counseling; assistance for students with disabilities; bookstore; campus computer network; career placement assistance; computer lab; computer-assisted instruction; e-mail services; housing assistance; interactive nursing skills videos; Internet; learning resource lab; library services; nursing audiovisuals; placement services for program completers; resume preparation assistance; skills, simulation, or other laboratory; tutoring.

Library Facilities 868,835 volumes; 22,277 periodical subscriptions.

BACCALAUREATE PROGRAMS

Degree BSN

Site Options Boardman, OH.

Study Options Full-time.

Program Entrance Requirements Minimum overall college GPA of 2.0, transcript of college record, CPR certification, health exam, health insurance, high school biology, high school chemistry, high school foreign language, 3 years high school math, 3 years high school science, high school transcript, immunizations, minimum high school GPA, minimum high school rank, minimum GPA in nursing prerequisites of 2.5, prerequisite course work. Transfer students are accepted. **Standardized tests**

Youngstown State University (continued)

Required: SAT or ACT, TOEFL for international students. **Application Deadline:** 8/15 (freshmen), 8/15 (transfer). *Early decision:* 2/15. *Notification:* continuous (freshmen), 2/15 (early action). *Application fee:* $30.

Advanced Placement   Credit by examination available. Credit given for nursing courses completed elsewhere dependent upon specific evaluations.

Contact   *Telephone:* 330-941-2328. *Fax:* 330-941-2309.

GRADUATE PROGRAMS

Contact   *Telephone:* 330-941-1796. *Fax:* 330-941-2309.

MASTER'S DEGREE PROGRAM

Degree MSN

Concentrations Available   Nurse anesthesia; nursing education.

Study Options   Full-time and part-time.

Program Entrance Requirements   Clinical experience, computer literacy, transcript of college record, CPR certification, written essay, immunizations, nursing research course, physical assessment course, prerequisite course work, resume, GRE General Test. *Application deadline:* For fall admission, 7/15 (priority date); for spring admission, 12/15 (priority date). Applications are processed on a rolling basis. *Application fee:* $30 ($75 for international students).

Advanced Placement   Credit given for nursing courses completed elsewhere dependent upon specific evaluations.

Degree Requirements   Thesis or project.

OKLAHOMA

Bacone College
Department of Nursing
Muskogee, Oklahoma

Founded in 1880

DEGREE • BSN

Nursing Program Faculty 8.

Baccalaureate Enrollment 16
Women 100% **Minority** 65%

Nursing Student Activities Student Nurses' Association, nursing club.

Nursing Student Resources Academic advising; bookstore; campus computer network; computer lab; computer-assisted instruction; interactive nursing skills videos; Internet; learning resource lab; library services; nursing audiovisuals; remedial services; skills, simulation, or other laboratory.

Library Facilities 34,564 volumes; 121 periodical subscriptions.

BACCALAUREATE PROGRAMS

Degree BSN

Available Programs   Accelerated RN Baccalaureate.

Program Entrance Requirements   Transcript of college record, CPR certification, health exam, health insurance, immunizations, 2 letters of recommendation, minimum GPA in nursing prerequisites of 2.5, prerequisite course work, RN licensure. **Standardized tests** *Required:* SAT or ACT, TOEFL for international students. *Recommended:* ACT. **Application** *Deadline:* rolling (freshmen), rolling (transfer). *Notification:* continuous (freshmen). *Application fee:* $25.

Contact   *Telephone:* 888-682-5514.

East Central University
Department of Nursing
Ada, Oklahoma

http://www.ecok.edu/dept/nursing

Founded in 1909

DEGREE • BS

Nursing Program Faculty 17 (29% with doctorates).

Baccalaureate Enrollment 493
Women 86% **Men** 14% **Minority** 44% **International** 1% **Part-time** 14%

Nursing Student Activities Student Nurses' Association, nursing club.

Nursing Student Resources Academic advising; academic or career counseling; assistance for students with disabilities; bookstore; campus computer network; career placement assistance; computer lab; computer-assisted instruction; daycare for children of students; e-mail services; employment services for current students; externships; housing assistance; interactive nursing skills videos; Internet; learning resource lab; library services; nursing audiovisuals; other; placement services for program completers; resume preparation assistance; skills, simulation, or other laboratory; tutoring.

Library Facilities 182,126 volumes (2,236 in health, 893 in nursing); 25,076 periodical subscriptions (26 health-care related).

BACCALAUREATE PROGRAMS

Degree BS

Available Programs   ADN to Baccalaureate; Generic Baccalaureate.

Site Options   *Distance Learning:* McAlester, OK; Durant, OK; Ardmore, OK.

Study Options   Full-time and part-time.

Program Entrance Requirements   Minimum overall college GPA of 2.5, transcript of college record, CPR certification, health exam, immunizations, minimum GPA in nursing prerequisites of 2.5, professional liability insurance/malpractice insurance, prerequisite course work. Transfer students are accepted. **Standardized tests** *Required:* SAT or ACT, TOEFL for international students. *Recommended:* ACT. **Application** *Notification:* continuous (freshmen). *Application fee:* $20.

Advanced Placement   Credit given for nursing courses completed elsewhere dependent upon specific evaluations.

Expenses (2006–07) *Tuition, state resident:* full-time $3200; part-time $109 per credit hour. *Tuition, nonresident:* full-time $10,000; part-time $300 per credit hour. *International tuition:* $10,000 full-time. *Room and board:* $1300; room only: $1000 per academic year. *Required fees:* full-time $940; part-time $100 per credit; part-time $450 per term.

Financial Aid   63% of baccalaureate students in nursing programs received some form of financial aid in 2005–06. *Gift aid (need-based):* Federal Pell, FSEOG, state, private, college/university gift aid from institutional funds. *Loans:* FFEL (Subsidized and Unsubsidized Stafford PLUS), Perkins, college/university. *Work-Study:* Federal Work-Study, part-time campus jobs. *Application deadline (priority):* 3/1.

Contact   Dr. Joseph T. Catalano, Chair, Department of Nursing, East Central University, 1100 East 14th Street, Ada, OK 74820. *Telephone:* 580-310-5434. *Fax:* 580-310-5785. *E-mail:* jcatalan@mailclerk.ecok.edu.

Langston University
School of Nursing and Health Professions
Langston, Oklahoma

http://www.lunet.ed/nurs5.html

Founded in 1897

DEGREE • BSN

Nursing Program Faculty 16 (13% with doctorates).

Nursing Student Activities Student Nurses' Association, nursing club.

Nursing Student Resources Academic advising; academic or career counseling; assistance for students with disabilities; bookstore; campus computer network; career placement assistance; computer lab; computer-assisted instruction; daycare for children of students; e-mail services; housing assistance; interactive nursing skills videos; Internet; learning resource lab; library services; nursing audiovisuals; remedial services; resume preparation assistance; skills, simulation, or other laboratory; tutoring.

Library Facilities 97,565 volumes (35,397 in health, 2,664 in nursing); 1,235 periodical subscriptions (978 health-care related).

BACCALAUREATE PROGRAMS

Degree BSN

Available Programs Generic Baccalaureate; LPN to Baccalaureate; RN Baccalaureate.

Site Options Tulsa, OK.

Study Options Full-time and part-time.

Program Entrance Requirements Minimum overall college GPA of 2.5, transcript of college record, written essay, health exam, immunizations, minimum GPA in nursing prerequisites of 2.5, professional liability insurance/malpractice insurance, prerequisite course work. Transfer students are accepted. **Standardized tests** *Required:* SAT or ACT, TOEFL for international students. **Placement:** *Required:* SAT or ACT. **Application** *Deadline:* rolling (freshmen), rolling (transfer).

Advanced Placement Credit by examination available. Credit given for nursing courses completed elsewhere dependent upon specific evaluations.

Contact *Telephone:* 405-466-3411. *Fax:* 405-466-2195.

Northeastern State University

Department of Nursing
Tahlequah, Oklahoma

http://arapaho.nsuok.edu/~nursing

Founded in 1846

DEGREE • BSN

Nursing Program Faculty 4 (25% with doctorates).

Baccalaureate Enrollment 86
Women 93% **Men** 7% **Minority** 23% **Part-time** 94%

Nursing Student Activities Sigma Theta Tau, Student Nurses' Association.

Nursing Student Resources Academic advising; academic or career counseling; assistance for students with disabilities; bookstore; campus computer network; career placement assistance; computer lab; computer-assisted instruction; e-mail services; employment services for current students; housing assistance; Internet; library services; nursing audiovisuals; placement services for program completers; resume preparation assistance; tutoring.

Library Facilities 466,526 volumes (13,300 in health, 7,200 in nursing); 17,570 periodical subscriptions (200 health-care related).

BACCALAUREATE PROGRAMS

Degree BSN

Available Programs Accelerated RN Baccalaureate; RN Baccalaureate.

Site Options *Distance Learning:* Ponca City, OK; Broken Arrow, OK; Miami, OK.

Program Entrance Requirements Minimum overall college GPA of 2.0, transcript of college record, CPR certification, health exam, immunizations, 3 letters of recommendation, minimum GPA in nursing prerequisites of 2.0, professional liability insurance/malpractice insurance, prerequisite course work, RN licensure. Transfer students are accepted. **Standardized tests** *Required:* ACT, TOEFL for international students. **Application** *Deadline:* 8/1 (freshmen), 8/1 (transfer). *Notification:* continuous (freshmen).

Expenses (2006–07) *Tuition, state resident:* full-time $3339; part-time $111 per credit hour. *Tuition, nonresident:* full-time $9414; part-time $314 per credit hour. *Room and board:* $2800; room only: $1800 per academic year. *Required fees:* full-time $1389; part-time $46 per credit.

Financial Aid 70% of baccalaureate students in nursing programs received some form of financial aid in 2005–06.

Contact Dr. Joyce A. Van Nostrand, Chair, Nursing Program and Department of Health Professions, Department of Nursing, Northeastern State University, PO Box 549, Muskogee, OK 74402-0549. *Telephone:* 918-781-5410. *Fax:* 918-781-5411. *E-mail:* vannostr@nsuok.edu.

Northwestern Oklahoma State University

Division of Nursing
Alva, Oklahoma

http://www.nwosu.edu/nursing

Founded in 1897

DEGREE • BSN

Nursing Program Faculty 10 (10% with doctorates).

Baccalaureate Enrollment 42
Women 95% **Men** 5% **Minority** 5% **International** 2%

Nursing Student Activities Student Nurses' Association.

Nursing Student Resources Academic advising; academic or career counseling; assistance for students with disabilities; bookstore; campus computer network; career placement assistance; computer lab; computer-assisted instruction; e-mail services; housing assistance; Internet; learning resource lab; library services; remedial services; skills, simulation, or other laboratory.

Library Facilities 344,640 volumes; 3,990 periodical subscriptions (59 health-care related).

BACCALAUREATE PROGRAMS

Degree BSN

Site Options *Distance Learning:* Enid, OK; Woodward, OK.

Study Options Full-time and part-time.

Program Entrance Requirements Minimum overall college GPA of 2.5, transcript of college record, CPR certification, health exam, high school transcript, immunizations, 3 letters of recommendation, minimum high school GPA of 2.5, minimum GPA in nursing prerequisites of 2.5, professional liability insurance/malpractice insurance, prerequisite course work. Transfer students are accepted. **Standardized tests** *Required:* SAT or ACT, TOEFL for international students. **Placement:** *Required:* SAT or ACT. **Application** *Deadline:* rolling (freshmen), rolling (transfer). *Notification:* continuous (freshmen). *Application fee:* $15.

Advanced Placement Credit by examination available. Credit given for nursing courses completed elsewhere dependent upon specific evaluations.

Contact *Telephone:* 580-327-8489. *Fax:* 580-327-8434.

Oklahoma Baptist University

School of Nursing
Shawnee, Oklahoma

Founded in 1910

DEGREE • BSN

Nursing Program Faculty 15 (2.6% with doctorates).

Baccalaureate Enrollment 203
Women 94% **Men** 6% **Minority** 7% **International** 1% **Part-time** 5%

Nursing Student Activities Sigma Theta Tau, Student Nurses' Association.

Nursing Student Resources Academic advising; academic or career counseling; assistance for students with disabilities; bookstore; campus computer network; computer lab; computer-assisted instruction; e-mail services; externships; Internet; learning resource lab; library services; nursing audiovisuals; remedial services; resume preparation assistance; skills, simulation, or other laboratory; tutoring; unpaid internships.

Library Facilities 230,000 volumes (10,000 in health, 5,500 in nursing); 1,800 periodical subscriptions (60 health-care related).

BACCALAUREATE PROGRAMS

Degree BSN

Available Programs ADN to Baccalaureate; Baccalaureate for Second Degree; Generic Baccalaureate; LPN to Baccalaureate; RN Baccalaureate.

Study Options Full-time and part-time.

Oklahoma Baptist University (continued)

Program Entrance Requirements Minimum overall college GPA of 2.25, transcript of college record, CPR certification, health exam, high school transcript, immunizations, minimum GPA in nursing prerequisites of 2.3, prerequisite course work. Transfer students are accepted. **Standardized tests** *Required:* SAT or ACT, TOEFL for international students. **Application** *Deadline:* rolling (freshmen), 8/1 (transfer). *Notification:* continuous until 9/1 (freshmen). *Application fee:* $25.

Expenses (2006–07) *Tuition:* full-time $13,654; part-time $4447 per credit hour. *International tuition:* $13,654 full-time. *Room and board:* $4340; room only: $2040 per academic year. *Required fees:* full-time $360; part-time $20 per credit; part-time $60 per term.

Financial Aid 93% of baccalaureate students in nursing programs received some form of financial aid in 2005–06. *Gift aid (need-based):* Federal Pell, FSEOG, state, private, college/university gift aid from institutional funds. *Loans:* FFEL (Subsidized and Unsubsidized Stafford PLUS), Perkins. *Work-Study:* Federal Work-Study, part-time campus jobs. *Application deadline (priority):* 3/1.

Contact Dr. Lana Bolhouse, Dean, School of Nursing, Oklahoma Baptist University, 500 West University, Shawnee, OK 74804. *Telephone:* 405-878-2081. *Fax:* 405-878-2083. *E-mail:* lana.bolhouse@okbu.edu.

Oklahoma City University
Kramer School of Nursing
Oklahoma City, Oklahoma

http://www.okcu.edu ursing

Founded in 1904

DEGREES • BSN • MSN • MSN/MBA

Nursing Program Faculty 23 (26% with doctorates).

Baccalaureate Enrollment 141
Women 85% **Men** 15% **Minority** 43% **International** 2% **Part-time** 8%

Graduate Enrollment 35
Women 92% **Men** 8% **Minority** 17%

Nursing Student Activities Sigma Theta Tau, Student Nurses' Association.

Nursing Student Resources Academic advising; academic or career counseling; assistance for students with disabilities; bookstore; campus computer network; career placement assistance; computer lab; e-mail services; housing assistance; interactive nursing skills videos; Internet; learning resource lab; library services; nursing audiovisuals; skills, simulation, or other laboratory; tutoring.

Library Facilities 520,953 volumes (519 in health, 410 in nursing); 14,000 periodical subscriptions (62 health-care related).

BACCALAUREATE PROGRAMS
Degree BSN

Available Programs ADN to Baccalaureate; Accelerated Baccalaureate for Second Degree; Generic Baccalaureate.

Study Options Full-time.

Program Entrance Requirements Minimum overall college GPA of 3.0, transcript of college record, CPR certification, high school transcript, immunizations, minimum GPA in nursing prerequisites of 2.5, professional liability insurance/malpractice insurance, prerequisite course work. Transfer students are accepted. **Standardized tests** *Required:* SAT or ACT, TOEFL for international students. **Application** *Deadline:* 8/20 (freshmen), rolling (transfer). *Notification:* continuous (freshmen). *Application fee:* $30.

Advanced Placement Credit given for nursing courses completed elsewhere dependent upon specific evaluations.

Expenses (2006–07) *Tuition:* full-time $17,900; part-time $610 per credit hour. *International tuition:* $17,900 full-time. *Room and board:* $6560 per academic year. *Required fees:* full-time $4000; part-time $2000 per term.

Financial Aid 90% of baccalaureate students in nursing programs received some form of financial aid in 2005–06.

Contact Ms. Sherri Christian, Student Services Assistant, Kramer School of Nursing, Oklahoma City University, 2501 North Blackwelder, Oklahoma City, OK 73106. *Telephone:* 405-208-5901. *Fax:* 405-208-5914. *E-mail:* schristian@okcu.edu.

GRADUATE PROGRAMS

Expenses (2006–07) *Tuition:* full-time $15,660; part-time $870 per credit hour. *International tuition:* $15,660 full-time. *Room and board:* $6560 per academic year. *Required fees:* full-time $2400; part-time $1000 per term.

Financial Aid 90% of graduate students in nursing programs received some form of financial aid in 2005–06.

Contact Dr. Susan Barnes, Assistant Professor, Kramer School of Nursing, Oklahoma City University, 2501 North Blackwelder, Oklahoma City, OK 73106. *Telephone:* 405-208-5917. *Fax:* 405-208-5914. *E-mail:* sbarnes@ okcu.edu.

MASTER'S DEGREE PROGRAM

Degrees MSN; MSN/MBA

Available Programs Master's.

Study Options Full-time and part-time.

Program Entrance Requirements Minimum overall college GPA of 3.0, transcript of college record.

Degree Requirements 39 total credit hours, thesis or project.

CONTINUING EDUCATION PROGRAM

Contact Mrs. Julia Prasse, Clinical Instructor, Kramer School of Nursing, Oklahoma City University, 2501 North Blackwelder, Oklahoma City, OK 73106. *Telephone:* 405-208-5904. *Fax:* 405-208-5914. *E-mail:* jprasse@okcu. edu.

Oklahoma Panhandle State University
Bachelor of Science in Nursing Program
Goodwell, Oklahoma

http://www.opsu.edu

Founded in 1909

DEGREE • BSN

Nursing Program Faculty 4.

Baccalaureate Enrollment 46
Women 96% **Men** 4% **Minority** 15% **Part-time** 76%

Nursing Student Activities Student Nurses' Association.

Nursing Student Resources Academic advising; academic or career counseling; assistance for students with disabilities; bookstore; campus computer network; e-mail services; Internet; library services.

Library Facilities 1,019 volumes in health, 380 volumes in nursing; 14 periodical subscriptions health-care related.

BACCALAUREATE PROGRAMS
Degree BSN

Available Programs ADN to Baccalaureate.

Program Entrance Requirements Minimum overall college GPA of 2.0, transcript of college record, CPR certification, immunizations, minimum GPA in nursing prerequisites of 2.0, professional liability insurance/malpractice insurance, RN licensure. Transfer students are accepted. **Standardized tests** *Required:* TOEFL for international students. *Required for some:* SAT or ACT. **Application** *Deadline:* rolling (freshmen), rolling (out-of-state freshmen), rolling (transfer).

Advanced Placement Credit given for nursing courses completed elsewhere dependent upon specific evaluations.

Expenses (2006–07) *Tuition, state resident:* part-time $76 per credit hour. *Tuition, nonresident:* part-time $76 per credit hour. *Room and board:* $3500; room only: $2200 per academic year. *Required fees:* part-time $38 per credit; part-time $5 per term.

Financial Aid 50% of baccalaureate students in nursing programs received some form of financial aid in 2005–06.

Contact Lynna Brakhage, RN, Director, RN-BSN Program, Bachelor of Science in Nursing Program, Oklahoma Panhandle State University, PO Box 430, Goodwell, OK 73939. *Telephone:* 580-349-1520. *Fax:* 580-349-1529. *E-mail:* nursing@opsu.edu.

Oklahoma Wesleyan University
Division of Nursing
Bartlesville, Oklahoma

http://nursing.okwu.edu

Founded in 1909

DEGREE • BSN

Nursing Program Faculty 31 (35% with doctorates).

Baccalaureate Enrollment 140
Women 96% **Men** 4% **Minority** 23%

Nursing Student Resources Academic advising; academic or career counseling; assistance for students with disabilities; bookstore; campus computer network; computer lab; computer-assisted instruction; interactive nursing skills videos; Internet; learning resource lab; library services; nursing audiovisuals; skills, simulation, or other laboratory.

Library Facilities 124,722 volumes (946 in health, 483 in nursing); 300 periodical subscriptions (40 health-care related).

BACCALAUREATE PROGRAMS

Degree BSN

Available Programs ADN to Baccalaureate; Accelerated RN Baccalaureate; Baccalaureate for Second Degree; Generic Baccalaureate; International Nurse to Baccalaureate; LPN to Baccalaureate; RN Baccalaureate.

Site Options *Distance Learning:* McAlester, OK; Oklahoma City, OK; Tulsa, OK.

Study Options Full-time.

Program Entrance Requirements Minimum overall college GPA of 2.3, transcript of college record, CPR certification, health exam, health insurance, immunizations, 2 letters of recommendation, minimum GPA in nursing prerequisites of 2.75, professional liability insurance/malpractice insurance, prerequisite course work, RN licensure. Transfer students are accepted. **Standardized tests** *Required:* SAT or ACT. *Recommended:* TOEFL for international students. **Application** *Deadline:* rolling (freshmen), rolling (transfer). *Application fee:* $25.

Advanced Placement Credit by examination available. Credit given for nursing courses completed elsewhere dependent upon specific evaluations.

Contact *Telephone:* 918-335-6254. *Fax:* 918-335-6204.

Oral Roberts University
Anna Vaughn School of Nursing
Tulsa, Oklahoma

http://www.oru.edu

Founded in 1963

DEGREE • BSN

Nursing Program Faculty 13.

Baccalaureate Enrollment 56
Women 96% **Men** 4% **Minority** 14% **International** 2%

Nursing Student Activities Nursing Honor Society, Sigma Theta Tau, Student Nurses' Association.

Nursing Student Resources Academic advising; academic or career counseling; assistance for students with disabilities; bookstore; campus computer network; computer lab; computer-assisted instruction; e-mail services; employment services for current students; externships; housing assistance; interactive nursing skills videos; Internet; learning resource lab; library services; nursing audiovisuals; remedial services; resume preparation assistance; skills, simulation, or other laboratory; tutoring.

Library Facilities 216,691 volumes (8,980 in health, 2,143 in nursing); 600 periodical subscriptions (31,399 health-care related).

BACCALAUREATE PROGRAMS

Degree BSN

Available Programs ADN to Baccalaureate; Generic Baccalaureate.

Study Options Full-time and part-time.

Program Entrance Requirements Minimum overall college GPA of 2.5, transcript of college record, CPR certification, health exam, high school chemistry, 2 years high school math, 2 years high school science, high school transcript, immunizations, minimum high school GPA of 2.5, minimum GPA in nursing prerequisites of 2.5. Transfer students are accepted. **Standardized tests** *Required:* SAT or ACT, TOEFL for international students. **Application** *Deadline:* rolling (freshmen), rolling (transfer). *Early decision:* 9/1. *Notification:* continuous (freshmen), 9/1 (early action). *Application fee:* $35.

Contact *Telephone:* 918-495-6198. *Fax:* 918-495-6020.

Southern Nazarene University
School of Nursing
Bethany, Oklahoma

http://www.snu.edu

Founded in 1899

DEGREES • BS • MS

Nursing Program Faculty 27 (18% with doctorates).

Baccalaureate Enrollment 84
Women 90% **Men** 10% **Minority** 26% **International** 2%

Graduate Enrollment 15
Women 100% **Minority** 10% **International** 1%

Nursing Student Activities Sigma Theta Tau, Student Nurses' Association.

Nursing Student Resources Academic advising; academic or career counseling; assistance for students with disabilities; bookstore; campus computer network; career placement assistance; computer lab; computer-assisted instruction; e-mail services; employment services for current students; externships; housing assistance; interactive nursing skills videos; Internet; learning resource lab; library services; nursing audiovisuals; paid internships; remedial services; skills, simulation, or other laboratory; tutoring.

Library Facilities 95,535 volumes; 225 periodical subscriptions.

BACCALAUREATE PROGRAMS

Degree BS

Available Programs ADN to Baccalaureate; Generic Baccalaureate.

Study Options Full-time.

Program Entrance Requirements Minimum overall college GPA of 2.75, transcript of college record, CPR certification, written essay, health exam, health insurance, high school transcript, immunizations, 2 letters of recommendation, minimum GPA in nursing prerequisites of 2.75, professional liability insurance/malpractice insurance, prerequisite course work. Transfer students are accepted. **Standardized tests** *Required:* TOEFL for international students. **Application** *Deadline:* 8/15 (freshmen), 8/15 (transfer). *Notification:* continuous (freshmen). *Application fee:* $25.

Advanced Placement Credit by examination available. Credit given for nursing courses completed elsewhere dependent upon specific evaluations.

Financial Aid 80% of baccalaureate students in nursing programs received some form of financial aid in 2005–06.

Contact Dr. Carol Jean Dorough, Chair, School of Nursing, Southern Nazarene University, 6729 NW 39th Expressway, Bethany, OK 73008. *Telephone:* 405-717-6217. *Fax:* 405-717-6264. *E-mail:* cdorough@snu.edu.

GRADUATE PROGRAMS

Financial Aid 85% of graduate students in nursing programs received some form of financial aid in 2005–06.

Contact Dr. Carol Jean Dorough, Chair, School of Nursing, Southern Nazarene University, 6729 NW 39th Expressway, Bethany, OK 73008. *Telephone:* 405-717-6217. *Fax:* 405-717-6264. *E-mail:* cdorough@snu.edu.

MASTER'S DEGREE PROGRAM

Degree MS

Available Programs Accelerated Master's.

Concentrations Available Nursing administration; nursing education.

Study Options Full-time.

Southern Nazarene University (continued)

Program Entrance Requirements Computer literacy, minimum overall college GPA of 3.0, transcript of college record, 3 letters of recommendation, resume, statistics course.

Degree Requirements 39 total credit hours, thesis or project.

Southwestern Oklahoma State University
Division of Nursing
Weatherford, Oklahoma

http://www.swosu.edu/academic/nurse

Founded in 1901

DEGREE • BSN

Nursing Program Faculty 8.

Baccalaureate Enrollment 64
Women 90% **Men** 10% **Minority** 12% **International** 2%

Nursing Student Activities Sigma Theta Tau, Student Nurses' Association, nursing club.

Nursing Student Resources Academic advising; academic or career counseling; assistance for students with disabilities; bookstore; campus computer network; computer lab; computer-assisted instruction; e-mail services; interactive nursing skills videos; Internet; learning resource lab; library services; nursing audiovisuals; remedial services; skills, simulation, or other laboratory; tutoring.

Library Facilities 217,051 volumes; 1,230 periodical subscriptions (284 health-care related).

BACCALAUREATE PROGRAMS

Degree BSN

Available Programs ADN to Baccalaureate; Generic Baccalaureate.
Study Options Full-time.
Program Entrance Requirements Minimum overall college GPA of 2.25, transcript of college record, CPR certification, health exam, high school transcript, immunizations, 3 letters of recommendation, minimum GPA in nursing prerequisites of 2.25, professional liability insurance/malpractice insurance, prerequisite course work. Transfer students are accepted. **Standardized tests** *Required:* ACT, TOEFL for international students. **Application** *Notification:* continuous (freshmen). *Application fee:* $15.

Advanced Placement Credit given for nursing courses completed elsewhere dependent upon specific evaluations.

Financial Aid 50% of baccalaureate students in nursing programs received some form of financial aid in 2005–06.

Contact Ms. Marilyn Thigpen, Administrative Assistant, Division of Nursing, Southwestern Oklahoma State University, 100 Campus Drive, Weatherford, OK 73096-3098. *Telephone:* 580-774-3261. *Fax:* 580-774-7075. *E-mail:* marilyn.thigpen@swosu.edu.

University of Central Oklahoma
Department of Nursing
Edmond, Oklahoma

http://nursing.ucok.edu

Founded in 1890

DEGREE • BSN

Nursing Program Faculty 29 (17% with doctorates).

Baccalaureate Enrollment 214
Women 95% **Men** 5% **Minority** 11% **International** 10% **Part-time** 1%

Nursing Student Activities Nursing Honor Society, Sigma Theta Tau, Student Nurses' Association.

Nursing Student Resources Academic advising; academic or career counseling; assistance for students with disabilities; bookstore; campus computer network; career placement assistance; computer lab; computer-assisted instruction; e-mail services; externships; interactive nursing skills videos; Internet; library services; nursing audiovisuals; skills, simulation, or other laboratory.

Library Facilities 582,547 volumes (2,831 in health, 1,733 in nursing); 3,130 periodical subscriptions.

BACCALAUREATE PROGRAMS

Degree BSN

Available Programs Generic Baccalaureate; LPN to Baccalaureate; RN Baccalaureate.
Site Options Oklahoma City, OK; Midwest City, OK.
Study Options Full-time and part-time.
Program Entrance Requirements Minimum overall college GPA of 2.5, transcript of college record, CPR certification, high school math, immunizations, 3 letters of recommendation, professional liability insurance/malpractice insurance, prerequisite course work. Transfer students are accepted. **Standardized tests** *Required:* SAT or ACT, TOEFL for international students. *Recommended:* ACT. **Application** *Deadline:* rolling (freshmen), rolling (out-of-state freshmen), rolling (transfer). *Notification:* continuous (freshmen), continuous (out-of-state freshmen). *Application fee:* $25.

Advanced Placement Credit given for nursing courses completed elsewhere dependent upon specific evaluations.

Expenses (2006–07) *Tuition, state resident:* full-time $2831; part-time $118 per credit hour. *Tuition, nonresident:* full-time $7139; part-time $297 per credit hour. *International tuition:* $7139 full-time. *Room and board:* $6100 per academic year. *Required fees:* full-time $806; part-time $34 per credit.

Financial Aid 35% of baccalaureate students in nursing programs received some form of financial aid in 2005–06.

Contact Vicki Addison, Administrative Secretary, Department of Nursing, University of Central Oklahoma, 100 North University Drive, Edmond, OK 73034-5209. *Telephone:* 405-974-5000. *E-mail:* vaddison@ucok.edu.

University of Oklahoma Health Sciences Center
College of Nursing
Oklahoma City, Oklahoma

http://nursing.oubsc.edu/

Founded in 1890

DEGREES • BSN • MS

Nursing Program Faculty 92 (30% with doctorates).

Baccalaureate Enrollment 667
Women 86% **Men** 14% **Minority** 35% **International** 2% **Part-time** 8%
Graduate Enrollment 258
Women 86% **Men** 14% **Minority** 22% **International** 2% **Part-time** 7%

Nursing Student Activities Sigma Theta Tau, Student Nurses' Association.

Nursing Student Resources Academic advising; academic or career counseling; assistance for students with disabilities; bookstore; campus computer network; computer lab; computer-assisted instruction; e-mail services; employment services for current students; housing assistance; Internet; learning resource lab; library services; nursing audiovisuals; skills, simulation, or other laboratory; tutoring.

Library Facilities 300,260 volumes; 4,028 periodical subscriptions.

BACCALAUREATE PROGRAMS

Degree BSN

Available Programs ADN to Baccalaureate; Accelerated Baccalaureate for Second Degree; Generic Baccalaureate; LPN to Baccalaureate.
Site Options *Distance Learning:* Lawton, OK; Ardmore, OK; Tulsa, OK.
Study Options Full-time and part-time.

Program Entrance Requirements Minimum overall college GPA of 2.5, transcript of college record, high school transcript, minimum high school GPA of 2.5, minimum GPA in nursing prerequisites of 2.0, prerequisite course work. Transfer students are accepted. **Standardized tests** *Required:* TOEFL for international students. **Application** *Deadline:* rolling (transfer).

Advanced Placement Credit by examination available. Credit given for nursing courses completed elsewhere dependent upon specific evaluations.

Expenses (2006–07) *Tuition, state resident:* full-time $3006; part-time $1503 per semester. *Tuition, nonresident:* full-time $11,295; part-time $5647 per semester. *International tuition:* $11,295 full-time. *Required fees:* part-time $150 per credit; part-time $447 per term.

Financial Aid 87% of baccalaureate students in nursing programs received some form of financial aid in 2005–06. *Loans:* Federal Nursing Student Loans, Perkins, college/university.

Contact Rosalyn Alexander, Admissions Coordinator, College of Nursing, University of Oklahoma Health Sciences Center, PO Box 26901, 1100 North Stonewall Avenue, Oklahoma City, OK 73190. *Telephone:* 405-271-2128. *Fax:* 405-271-7341. *E-mail:* Rosalyn-Alexander@ouhsc.edu.

GRADUATE PROGRAMS

Expenses (2006–07) *Tuition, state resident:* full-time $2385; part-time $795 per semester. *Tuition, nonresident:* full-time $8510; part-time $2836 per semester. *International tuition:* $8510 full-time. *Required fees:* part-time $155 per credit; part-time $254 per term.

Financial Aid 87% of graduate students in nursing programs received some form of financial aid in 2005–06. 6 research assistantships (averaging $6,000 per year) were awarded; teaching assistantships, institutionally sponsored loans, scholarships, and traineeships also available. Aid available to part-time students. *Financial aid application deadline:* 8/1.

Contact Rosalyn Alexander, Admissions Coordinator, College of Nursing, University of Oklahoma Health Sciences Center, PO Box 26901, 1100 North Stonewall Avenue, Oklahoma City, OK 73190. *Telephone:* 405-271-2128. *Fax:* 405-271-7341. *E-mail:* Rosalyn-Alexander@ouhsc.edu.

MASTER'S DEGREE PROGRAM

Degree MS

Available Programs Master's; Master's for Non-Nursing College Graduates.

Concentrations Available Health-care administration; nursing education. *Clinical nurse specialist programs in:* acute care, gerontology. *Nurse practitioner programs in:* adult health, family health, neonatal health, pediatric.

Site Options *Distance Learning:* Lawton, OK; Ardmore, OK; Tulsa, OK.
Study Options Full-time and part-time.

Program Entrance Requirements Computer literacy, minimum overall college GPA of 3.0, transcript of college record, 3 letters of recommendation, nursing research course, professional liability insurance/malpractice insurance, prerequisite course work, statistics course. *Application deadline:* For fall admission, 6/1; for winter admission, 4/1; for spring admission, 11/1. Applications are processed on a rolling basis. *Application fee:* $50.

Advanced Placement Credit given for nursing courses completed elsewhere dependent upon specific evaluations.

Degree Requirements 38 total credit hours, thesis or project, comprehensive exam.

POST-MASTER'S PROGRAM

Areas of Study *Nurse practitioner programs in:* adult health, family health, neonatal health, pediatric.

CONTINUING EDUCATION PROGRAM

Contact Dr. Beverly Bowers, Assistant Dean for Faculty Development and Professional Continuing Education, College of Nursing, University of Oklahoma Health Sciences Center, PO Box 26901, 1100 North Stonewall Avenue, Oklahoma City, OK 73190. *Telephone:* 405-271-2428. *Fax:* 405-271-7341. *E-mail:* Beverly-Bowers@ouhsc.edu.

University of Phoenix–Oklahoma City Campus
College of Health and Human Services
Oklahoma City, Oklahoma

Founded in 1976

DEGREES • BSN • MSN

Nursing Program Faculty 21.

Baccalaureate Enrollment 7
Women 100%

Graduate Enrollment 7
Women 85.71% **Men** 14.29% **Minority** 14.29%

Nursing Student Activities Sigma Theta Tau.

Nursing Student Resources Academic advising; academic or career counseling; assistance for students with disabilities; computer lab; library services.

Library Facilities 444 volumes; 666 periodical subscriptions.

BACCALAUREATE PROGRAMS

Degree BSN

Available Programs Accelerated Baccalaureate.
Site Options Norman, OK.
Study Options Full-time.

Program Entrance Requirements Transcript of college record, immunizations, letters of recommendation, RN licensure. Transfer students are accepted. **Standardized tests** *Required:* TOEFL for international students. **Application** *Deadline:* rolling (freshmen), rolling (transfer). *Application fee:* $110.

Advanced Placement Credit by examination available. Credit given for nursing courses completed elsewhere dependent upon specific evaluations.

Expenses (2006–07) *Tuition:* full-time $9750. *International tuition:* $9750 full-time. *Required fees:* full-time $750.

Contact Campus College Chair, Nursing, College of Health and Human Services, University of Phoenix–Oklahoma City Campus, 6501 North Broadway Extension, Suite #100, Oklahoma City, OK 73116-8244. *Telephone:* 405-842-8007.

GRADUATE PROGRAMS

Expenses (2006–07) *Tuition:* full-time $10,608. *International tuition:* $10,608 full-time. *Required fees:* full-time $760.

Contact Campus College Chair, Nursing, College of Health and Human Services, University of Phoenix–Oklahoma City Campus, 6501 North Broadway Extension, Suite #100, Oklahoma City, OK 73116-8244. *Telephone:* 405-842-8007.

MASTER'S DEGREE PROGRAM

Degree MSN

Available Programs Master's.
Concentrations Available Nursing administration.
Site Options Norman, OK.
Study Options Full-time.

Program Entrance Requirements Clinical experience, computer literacy, minimum overall college GPA of 2.5, transcript of college record.

Advanced Placement Credit given for nursing courses completed elsewhere dependent upon specific evaluations.

Degree Requirements 39 total credit hours, thesis or project.

University of Phoenix–Tulsa Campus
College of Health and Human Services
Tulsa, Oklahoma

Founded in 1998

University of Phoenix–Tulsa Campus (continued)

Nursing Student Activities Sigma Theta Tau.

Nursing Student Resources Academic advising; academic or career counseling; assistance for students with disabilities; bookstore; computer lab; library services.

Library Facilities 444 volumes; 666 periodical subscriptions.

University of Tulsa

School of Nursing
Tulsa, Oklahoma

http://www.cba.utulsa.edu/depts/nursing
Founded in 1894

DEGREE • BSN

Nursing Program Faculty 12 (30% with doctorates).

Baccalaureate Enrollment 96
Women 92% **Men** 8% **Minority** 25% **International** 2% **Part-time** 10%

Nursing Student Activities Sigma Theta Tau, Student Nurses' Association.

Nursing Student Resources Academic advising; academic or career counseling; assistance for students with disabilities; bookstore; campus computer network; career placement assistance; computer lab; computer-assisted instruction; daycare for children of students; e-mail services; employment services for current students; externships; housing assistance; interactive nursing skills videos; Internet; learning resource lab; library services; nursing audiovisuals; placement services for program completers; remedial services; resume preparation assistance; skills, simulation, or other laboratory; tutoring.

Library Facilities 1.2 million volumes (4,300 in nursing); 26,228 periodical subscriptions (118 health-care related).

BACCALAUREATE PROGRAMS

Degree BSN

Available Programs Generic Baccalaureate; LPN to RN Baccalaureate; RN Baccalaureate.

Study Options Full-time.

Program Entrance Requirements Minimum overall college GPA of 2.5, transcript of college record, CPR certification, written essay, health exam, immunizations, minimum GPA in nursing prerequisites. Transfer students are accepted. **Standardized tests** *Required:* SAT or ACT, TOEFL for international students. **Application** *Deadline:* rolling (freshmen), rolling (transfer). *Notification:* continuous (freshmen). *Application fee:* $35.

Advanced Placement Credit by examination available. Credit given for nursing courses completed elsewhere dependent upon specific evaluations.

Expenses (2006–07) *Tuition:* full-time $20,658; part-time $741 per course. *International tuition:* $20,658 full-time. *Room and board:* $7052; room only: $3896 per academic year. *Required fees:* full-time $525; part-time $3 per credit.

Financial Aid 90% of baccalaureate students in nursing programs received some form of financial aid in 2005–06. *Gift aid (need-based):* Federal Pell, FSEOG, state, private, college/university gift aid from institutional funds. *Loans:* FFEL (Subsidized and Unsubsidized Stafford PLUS), Perkins. *Work-Study:* Federal Work-Study, part-time campus jobs. *Application deadline (priority):* 4/1.

Contact Dr. Susan Kathleen Gaston, RN, Director, School of Nursing, University of Tulsa, 600 South College Avenue, Tulsa, OK 74104-3189. *Telephone:* 918-631-3116. *Fax:* 918-631-2068. *E-mail:* susan-gaston@utulsa.edu.

OREGON

Linfield College

School of Nursing
McMinnville, Oregon

http://www.linfield.edu/portland
Founded in 1849

DEGREE • BSN

Nursing Program Faculty 45 (42% with doctorates).

Baccalaureate Enrollment 366
Women 85.5% **Men** 14.5% **Minority** 15% **Part-time** 1%

Nursing Student Activities Sigma Theta Tau, Student Nurses' Association, nursing club.

Nursing Student Resources Academic advising; academic or career counseling; bookstore; campus computer network; computer lab; e-mail services; Internet; learning resource lab; library services; nursing audiovisuals; resume preparation assistance; skills, simulation, or other laboratory.

Library Facilities 179,098 volumes (7,201 in health, 1,482 in nursing); 1,268 periodical subscriptions (249 health-care related).

BACCALAUREATE PROGRAMS

Degree BSN

Available Programs Accelerated Baccalaureate for Second Degree; Baccalaureate for Second Degree; Generic Baccalaureate; RN Baccalaureate.

Site Options Portland, OR.

Study Options Full-time.

Program Entrance Requirements Minimum overall college GPA of 2.9, transcript of college record, CPR certification, written essay, health exam, health insurance, immunizations, 1 letter of recommendation, minimum GPA in nursing prerequisites of 2.75, professional liability insurance/malpractice insurance, prerequisite course work. Transfer students are accepted. **Standardized tests** *Required:* SAT or ACT, TOEFL for international students. **Application** *Deadline:* 2/15 (freshmen), 4/15 (transfer). *Early decision:* 11/15. *Notification:* 4/1 (freshmen), 1/15 (early action). *Application fee:* $40.

Advanced Placement Credit given for nursing courses completed elsewhere dependent upon specific evaluations.

Expenses (2006–07) *Tuition:* full-time $23,930; part-time $745 per credit hour. *International tuition:* $23,930 full-time. *Room and board:* room only: $1342 per academic year. *Required fees:* full-time $300; part-time $150 per term.

Financial Aid 94% of baccalaureate students in nursing programs received some form of financial aid in 2005–06. *Gift aid (need-based):* Federal Pell, FSEOG, state, private, college/university gift aid from institutional funds. *Loans:* FFEL (Subsidized and Unsubsidized Stafford PLUS), Perkins, college/university, alternative loans. *Work-Study:* Federal Work-Study, part-time campus jobs. *Application deadline (priority):* 2/1.

Contact Beth A. Woodward, Director, Enrollment Services, School of Nursing, Linfield College, 2255 NW Northrup Street, Portland, OR 97210. *Telephone:* 503-413-8481. *Fax:* 503-413-6283. *E-mail:* bwoodwar@linfield.edu.

CONTINUING EDUCATION PROGRAM

Contact Dr. Beverly Epeneter, Interim Dean, School of Nursing, Linfield College, 2255 NW Northrup Street, Portland, OR 97210. *Telephone:* 503-413-7163. *Fax:* 503-413-6846. *E-mail:* bepenet@linfield.edu.

Oregon Health & Science University

School of Nursing
Portland, Oregon

http://www.ohsu.edu/son
Founded in 1974

DEGREES • BS • MS • MSN/MPH • PHD

Nursing Program Faculty 130 (40% with doctorates).

Baccalaureate Enrollment 637
Minority 12%

Graduate Enrollment 167
Minority 8%

Nursing Student Activities Nursing Honor Society, Sigma Theta Tau, Student Nurses' Association, nursing club.

Nursing Student Resources Academic advising; assistance for students with disabilities; bookstore; campus computer network; computer lab; e-mail services; externships; interactive nursing skills videos; Internet; learning resource lab; library services; nursing audiovisuals; resume preparation assistance; skills, simulation, or other laboratory.

Library Facilities 200,771 volumes (227,344 in health, 7,666 in nursing); 2,110 periodical subscriptions (2,357 health-care related).

BACCALAUREATE PROGRAMS

Degree BS

Available Programs Accelerated Baccalaureate; Generic Baccalaureate; RN Baccalaureate.

Site Options *Distance Learning:* Ashland, OR; Klamath Falls, OR; La Grande, OR.

Study Options Full-time and part-time.

Program Entrance Requirements Minimum overall college GPA of 3.0, transcript of college record, CPR certification, written essay, high school transcript, immunizations, minimum high school GPA of 2.5, minimum GPA in nursing prerequisites of 3.0, prerequisite course work. Transfer students are accepted. **Standardized tests** *Required:* TOEFL for international students. **Application** *Deadline:* 2/1 (transfer). *Application fee:* $125.

Advanced Placement Credit by examination available. Credit given for nursing courses completed elsewhere dependent upon specific evaluations.

Expenses (2006–07) *Tuition, state resident:* full-time $8325; part-time $185 per credit hour. *Tuition, nonresident:* full-time $19,395; part-time $431 per credit hour. *International tuition:* $19,395 full-time. *Required fees:* full-time $4350; part-time $1450 per term.

Financial Aid *Gift aid (need-based):* Federal Pell, FSEOG, state, private, college/university gift aid from institutional funds, Health Profession Scholarships. *Loans:* Federal Nursing Student Loans, Federal Direct (Subsidized and Unsubsidized Stafford PLUS), Perkins, state, college/university, alternative loans. *Work-Study:* Federal Work-Study. *Application deadline:* Continuous.

Contact Admissions Counselor, School of Nursing, Oregon Health & Science University, 3455 SW U.S. Veterans Hospital Road, SN-ADM, Portland, OR 97239-2491. *Telephone:* 503-494-7725. *Fax:* 503-494-6433.

GRADUATE PROGRAMS

Expenses (2006–07) *Tuition, state resident:* full-time $16,740; part-time $372 per credit hour. *Tuition, nonresident:* full-time $16,740; part-time $372 per credit hour. *International tuition:* $16,740 full-time. *Required fees:* full-time $3700; part-time $1250 per term.

Financial Aid 10 fellowships, 42 research assistantships, 8 teaching assistantships were awarded; career-related internships or fieldwork, Federal Work-Study, institutionally sponsored loans, scholarships, and traineeships also available.

Contact Academic Programs Counselor, School of Nursing, Oregon Health & Science University, 3455 SW U.S. Veterans Hospital Road, SN-4N, Portland, OR 97239-2491. *Telephone:* 503-494-7725. *Fax:* 503-494-4350.

MASTER'S DEGREE PROGRAM

Degrees MS; MSN/MPH

Available Programs Accelerated Master's for Non-Nursing College Graduates; Master's; Master's for Non-Nursing College Graduates; Master's for Nurses with Non-Nursing Degrees.

Concentrations Available Health-care administration; nurse anesthesia; nurse-midwifery; nursing administration. *Clinical nurse specialist programs in:* adult health, cardiovascular, community health, family health, gerontology, maternity-newborn, medical-surgical, psychiatric/mental health, public health, women's health. *Nurse practitioner programs in:* adult health, family health, gerontology, pediatric, primary care, psychiatric/mental health, women's health.

Site Options *Distance Learning:* Ashland, OR; Klamath Falls, OR; La Grande, OR.

Study Options Full-time and part-time.

Program Entrance Requirements Clinical experience, computer literacy, minimum overall college GPA of 3.0, transcript of college record, CPR certification, written essay, immunizations, interview, 3 letters of recommendation, physical assessment course, resume, statistics course, GRE General Test. *Application deadline:* For fall admission, 1/15 (priority date). Applications are processed on a rolling basis. *Application fee:* $60.

Advanced Placement Credit given for nursing courses completed elsewhere dependent upon specific evaluations.

Degree Requirements 45 total credit hours, thesis or project.

POST-MASTER'S PROGRAM

Areas of Study Nurse-midwifery; nursing education. *Clinical nurse specialist programs in:* adult health, cardiovascular, family health, gerontology, maternity-newborn, medical-surgical, psychiatric/mental health, women's health. *Nurse practitioner programs in:* adult health, family health, gerontology, pediatric, primary care, psychiatric/mental health, women's health.

DOCTORAL DEGREE PROGRAM

Degree PhD

Available Programs Doctorate; Post-Baccalaureate Doctorate.

Areas of Study Aging, ethics, faculty preparation, family health, gerontology, health policy, health promotion/disease prevention, health-care systems, human health and illness, illness and transition, nursing policy, nursing research, nursing science, women's health.

Site Options *Distance Learning:* Ashland, OR; Klamath Falls, OR; La Grande, OR.

Program Entrance Requirements Clinical experience, minimum overall college GPA of 3.5, interview, 3 letters of recommendation, MSN or equivalent, scholarly papers, statistics course, vita, writing sample, GRE General Test. *Application deadline:* For fall admission, 1/15 (priority date). Applications are processed on a rolling basis. *Application fee:* $60.

Degree Requirements 90 total credit hours, dissertation, oral exam, written exam, residency.

POSTDOCTORAL PROGRAM

Areas of Study Adolescent health, aging, chronic illness, family health, gerontology, health promotion/disease prevention, nursing interventions, nursing research, nursing science, outcomes, self-care, vulnerable population, women's health.

Postdoctoral Program Contact Academic Programs Counselor, School of Nursing, Oregon Health & Science University, 3455 SW U.S. Veterans Hospital Road, SN-4N, Portland, OR 97239-2491. *Telephone:* 503-494-7725. *Fax:* 503-494-4350.

CONTINUING EDUCATION PROGRAM

Contact Paula McNeil, Director of Continuing Education, School of Nursing, Oregon Health & Science University, 3455 SW U.S. Veterans Hospital Road, SN-4N, Portland, OR 97239-2491. *Telephone:* 503-494-6772. *Fax:* 503-494-4350.

University of Portland
School of Nursing
Portland, Oregon

http://www.up.edu

Founded in 1901

DEGREES • BSN • MS

Nursing Program Faculty 73 (7% with doctorates).

Baccalaureate Enrollment 532
Women 91% **Men** 9% **Minority** 8% **International** 2%

Graduate Enrollment 44
Women 91% **Men** 9% **Minority** 9% **International** 2%

Nursing Student Activities Sigma Theta Tau, Student Nurses' Association.

University of Portland (continued)

Nursing Student Resources Academic advising; academic or career counseling; assistance for students with disabilities; bookstore; campus computer network; career placement assistance; computer lab; computer-assisted instruction; e-mail services; employment services for current students; housing assistance; interactive nursing skills videos; Internet; learning resource lab; library services; nursing audiovisuals; remedial services; resume preparation assistance; skills, simulation, or other laboratory; tutoring.

Library Facilities 350,000 volumes (5,090 in health, 1,325 in nursing); 1,400 periodical subscriptions (171 health-care related).

BACCALAUREATE PROGRAMS

Degree BSN

Available Programs Generic Baccalaureate.

Study Options Full-time.

Program Entrance Requirements Minimum overall college GPA of 2.75, transcript of college record, CPR certification, written essay, health exam, health insurance, high school transcript, immunizations, 1 letter of recommendation, minimum high school GPA of 2.5, minimum GPA in nursing prerequisites of 2.75, professional liability insurance/malpractice insurance, prerequisite course work. Transfer students are accepted. **Standardized tests** *Required:* SAT or ACT, TOEFL for international students. **Application** *Deadline:* 6/1 (freshmen), 6/1 (transfer). *Notification:* continuous (freshmen). *Application fee:* $50.

Expenses (2006–07) *Tuition:* full-time $30,208. *International tuition:* $30,208 full-time. *Room and board:* $3935 per academic year. *Required fees:* full-time $2010.

Financial Aid 96% of baccalaureate students in nursing programs received some form of financial aid in 2005–06. *Gift aid (need-based):* Federal Pell, FSEOG, state, private, college/university gift aid from institutional funds. *Loans:* Federal Nursing Student Loans, FFEL (Subsidized and Unsubsidized Stafford PLUS), Perkins, college/university. *Work-Study:* Federal Work-Study, part-time campus jobs. *Application deadline (priority):* 3/1.

Contact Mr. Jason McDonald, Dean of Admissions, School of Nursing, University of Portland, 5000 North Willamette Boulevard, Portland, OR 97203-5798. *Telephone:* 503-943-7147. *E-mail:* mcdonaja@up.edu.

GRADUATE PROGRAMS

Expenses (2006–07) *Tuition:* part-time $728 per credit hour. *Required fees:* part-time $35 per credit.

Financial Aid 85% of graduate students in nursing programs received some form of financial aid in 2005–06. Fellowships, research assistantships, Federal Work-Study and scholarships available. Aid available to part-time students. *Financial aid application deadline:* 3/1.

Contact Miss Stacey Boatright, Nursing Program Counselor, School of Nursing, University of Portland, 5000 North Willamette Boulevard, Portland, OR 97203-5798. *Telephone:* 503-943-7423. *Fax:* 503-943-7729. *E-mail:* boatrigh@up.edu.

MASTER'S DEGREE PROGRAM

Degree MS

Available Programs Master's; Master's for Non-Nursing College Graduates.

Concentrations Available Clinical nurse leader.

Study Options Full-time and part-time.

Program Entrance Requirements Computer literacy, minimum overall college GPA of 3.0, transcript of college record, CPR certification, written essay, immunizations, interview, 2 letters of recommendation, professional liability insurance/malpractice insurance, prerequisite course work, resume, statistics course, GRE General Test. *Application deadline:* Applications are processed on a rolling basis. *Application fee:* $45.

Advanced Placement Credit given for nursing courses completed elsewhere dependent upon specific evaluations.

Degree Requirements 42 total credit hours.

PENNSYLVANIA

Alvernia College
Nursing
Reading, Pennsylvania

http://www.alvernia.edu

Founded in 1958

DEGREE • BSN

Nursing Program Faculty 9 (2% with doctorates).

Baccalaureate Enrollment 161
Women 98% **Men** 2% **Minority** 10% **International** 3% **Part-time** 20%

Nursing Student Activities Nursing Honor Society, Sigma Theta Tau, Student Nurses' Association.

Nursing Student Resources Academic advising; academic or career counseling; bookstore; campus computer network; computer lab; computer-assisted instruction; e-mail services; employment services for current students; externships; interactive nursing skills videos; Internet; learning resource lab; library services; nursing audiovisuals; remedial services; skills, simulation, or other laboratory; tutoring.

Library Facilities 89,399 volumes (2,931 in health, 995 in nursing); 378 periodical subscriptions (89 health-care related).

BACCALAUREATE PROGRAMS

Degree BSN

Available Programs Generic Baccalaureate; LPN to Baccalaureate; LPN to RN Baccalaureate; RN Baccalaureate.

Site Options Reading, PA; Pottsville, PA; Ashland, PA.

Study Options Full-time and part-time.

Program Entrance Requirements Minimum overall college GPA of 2.5, transcript of college record, CPR certification, written essay, health exam, health insurance, high school biology, high school chemistry, 2 years high school math, 2 years high school science, high school transcript, immunizations, 2 letters of recommendation, minimum high school GPA of 2.5, minimum GPA in nursing prerequisites of 2.5. Transfer students are accepted. **Standardized tests** *Required:* SAT or ACT, TOEFL for international students. **Application** *Deadline:* rolling (freshmen), rolling (transfer). *Notification:* continuous (freshmen). *Application fee:* $25.

Advanced Placement Credit by examination available. Credit given for nursing courses completed elsewhere dependent upon specific evaluations.

Financial Aid 75% of baccalaureate students in nursing programs received some form of financial aid in 2005–06. *Gift aid (need-based):* Federal Pell, FSEOG, state, private, college/university gift aid from institutional funds. *Loans:* FFEL (Subsidized and Unsubsidized Stafford PLUS), Perkins, college/university, Health Professions Loans. *Work-Study:* Federal Work-Study, part-time campus jobs. *Application deadline:* Continuous.

Contact Dr. Mary Ellen Symanski, Nursing Department Chair, Nursing, Alvernia College, 400 Saint Bernardine Street, Reading, PA 19607. *Telephone:* 610-796-8460. *Fax:* 610-796-8464. *E-mail:* maryellen.symanski@alvernia.edu.

CONTINUING EDUCATION PROGRAM

Contact Ms. Noreen Kern, Nursing Outreach Coordinator, Nursing, Alvernia College, 400 Saint Bernardine Street, Reading, PA 19607. *Telephone:* 610-796-5611. *Fax:* 610-796-8464. *E-mail:* noreen.kern@alvernia.edu.

Bloomsburg University of Pennsylvania
Department of Nursing
Bloomsburg, Pennsylvania

http://www.bloomu.edu/academic/nur/

Founded in 1839

DEGREES • BSN • MSN • MSN/MBA

Nursing Program Faculty 27 (50% with doctorates).

Baccalaureate Enrollment 300
Women 93% **Men** 7% **Minority** 5% **Part-time** 4%

Graduate Enrollment 50
Women 92% **Men** 8% **Part-time** 92%

Nursing Student Activities Sigma Theta Tau, Student Nurses' Association, nursing club.

Nursing Student Resources Academic advising; academic or career counseling; assistance for students with disabilities; bookstore; campus computer network; career placement assistance; computer lab; computer-assisted instruction; daycare for children of students; e-mail services; employment services for current students; externships; housing assistance; interactive nursing skills videos; Internet; learning resource lab; library services; nursing audiovisuals; paid internships; placement services for program completers; remedial services; resume preparation assistance; skills, simulation, or other laboratory; tutoring; unpaid internships.

Library Facilities 472,982 volumes (6,005 in health, 2,813 in nursing); 1,747 periodical subscriptions (2,783 health-care related).

BACCALAUREATE PROGRAMS

Degree BSN

Available Programs ADN to Baccalaureate; Baccalaureate for Second Degree; Generic Baccalaureate; LPN to RN Baccalaureate; RN Baccalaureate.

Study Options Full-time and part-time.

Program Entrance Requirements Minimum overall college GPA of 2.5, transcript of college record, CPR certification, health exam, health insurance, high school biology, high school chemistry, 2 years high school math, 3 years high school science, high school transcript, immunizations, interview, 3 letters of recommendation, minimum high school GPA of 3.0, minimum high school rank 80%, minimum GPA in nursing prerequisites of 2.5, professional liability insurance/malpractice insurance, prerequisite course work. Transfer students are accepted. **Standardized tests** *Required:* SAT or ACT, TOEFL for international students. **Application** *Deadline:* rolling (freshmen), rolling (transfer). *Early decision:* 11/15. *Notification:* 10/1 (freshmen), 12/1 (out-of-state freshmen), 12/1 (early decision). *Application fee:* $30.

Advanced Placement Credit by examination available. Credit given for nursing courses completed elsewhere dependent upon specific evaluations.

Expenses (2006–07) *Tuition, state resident:* full-time $5038; part-time $210 per credit. *Tuition, nonresident:* full-time $2598; part-time $525 per credit. *International tuition:* $12,598 full-time. *Room and board:* $5616; room only: $3282 per academic year. *Required fees:* full-time $1374; part-time $41 per credit; part-time $66 per term.

Financial Aid 58% of baccalaureate students in nursing programs received some form of financial aid in 2005–06. *Gift aid (need-based):* Federal Pell, FSEOG, state, private, college/university gift aid from institutional funds. *Loans:* FFEL (Subsidized and Unsubsidized Stafford PLUS), Perkins, state, alternative loans. *Work-Study:* Federal Work-Study, part-time campus jobs. *Application deadline (priority):* 3/15.

Contact Dr. M. Christine Alichnie, RN, Chairperson, Department of Nursing/Director, School of Health Sciences, Department of Nursing, Bloomsburg University of Pennsylvania, 400 East Second Street, MCHS 3109, Bloomsburg, PA 17815. *Telephone:* 570-389-4426. *Fax:* 570-389-5008. *E-mail:* calichni@bloomu.edu.

GRADUATE PROGRAMS

Expenses (2006–07) *Tuition, state resident:* full-time $6048; part-time $336 per credit. *Tuition, nonresident:* full-time $9678; part-time $538 per credit. *International tuition:* $9678 full-time. *Required fees:* full-time $1415; part-time $43 per credit; part-time $66 per term.

Financial Aid 29% of graduate students in nursing programs received some form of financial aid in 2005–06. Unspecified assistantships available.

Contact Dr. Michelle Ficca, Coordinator of Graduate Program, Department of Nursing, Bloomsburg University of Pennsylvania, 400 East Second Street, Room 3120, MCHS, Bloomsburg, PA 17815. *Telephone:* 570-389-4615. *Fax:* 570-389-5008. *E-mail:* mficca@bloomu.edu.

MASTER'S DEGREE PROGRAM

Degrees MSN; MSN/MBA

Available Programs Master's; Master's for Nurses with Non-Nursing Degrees; RN to Master's.

Concentrations Available Nursing administration. *Clinical nurse specialist programs in:* adult health, community health, public health, school health. *Nurse practitioner programs in:* adult health.

Study Options Full-time and part-time.

Program Entrance Requirements Clinical experience, computer literacy, minimum overall college GPA of 3.0, transcript of college record, CPR certification, immunizations, interview, 3 letters of recommendation, nursing research course, physical assessment course, professional liability insurance/malpractice insurance, prerequisite course work, resume, statistics course. *Application deadline:* Applications are processed on a rolling basis. *Application fee:* $30.

Advanced Placement Credit by examination available. Credit given for nursing courses completed elsewhere dependent upon specific evaluations.

Degree Requirements 39 total credit hours, comprehensive exam.

POST-MASTER'S PROGRAM

Areas of Study *Clinical nurse specialist programs in:* school health. *Nurse practitioner programs in:* adult health, family health.

California University of Pennsylvania
Department of Nursing
California, Pennsylvania

http://www.cup.edu/eberly/nursing

Founded in 1852

DEGREE • BSN

Nursing Program Faculty 5 (60% with doctorates).

Baccalaureate Enrollment 145
Women 83% **Men** 17% **Minority** 3% **Part-time** 92%

Nursing Student Activities Sigma Theta Tau.

Nursing Student Resources Academic advising; academic or career counseling; assistance for students with disabilities; bookstore; campus computer network; career placement assistance; computer lab; computer-assisted instruction; daycare for children of students; e-mail services; employment services for current students; Internet; library services; nursing audiovisuals; placement services for program completers; remedial services; resume preparation assistance; tutoring.

Library Facilities 437,160 volumes (3,840 in health, 2,010 in nursing); 881 periodical subscriptions (80 health-care related).

BACCALAUREATE PROGRAMS

Degree BSN

Available Programs RN Baccalaureate.

Site Options West Mifflin, PA. *Distance Learning:* Southpointe, PA.

Study Options Full-time and part-time.

Program Entrance Requirements Minimum overall college GPA of 2.0, transcript of college record, CPR certification, health exam, health insurance, immunizations, 2 letters of recommendation, professional liability insurance/malpractice insurance, prerequisite course work, RN licensure. Transfer students are accepted. **Standardized tests** *Required:* SAT, TOEFL for international students. **Application** *Deadline:* 5/1 (freshmen), 5/1 (transfer). *Notification:* continuous (freshmen). *Application fee:* $25.

Advanced Placement Credit by examination available. Credit given for nursing courses completed elsewhere dependent upon specific evaluations.

Financial Aid 80% of baccalaureate students in nursing programs received some form of financial aid in 2005–06.

Contact Ms. Debra Shelapinsky, Chairperson, Department of Nursing, California University of Pennsylvania, 250 University Avenue, Box 60, California, PA 15419-1394. *Telephone:* 724-938-5739. *Fax:* 724-938-1612. *E-mail:* shelapinsky@cup.edu.

Carlow University

School of Nursing
Pittsburgh, Pennsylvania

http://www.carlow.edu/academic/nursing.html

Founded in 1929

DEGREES • BSN • MSN

Nursing Program Faculty 31 (23% with doctorates).

Baccalaureate Enrollment 333
Women 99% **Men** 1% **Minority** 13% **Part-time** 21%

Graduate Enrollment 54
Women 94% **Men** 6% **Minority** 11% **Part-time** 94%

Nursing Student Activities Nursing Honor Society, Sigma Theta Tau, Student Nurses' Association.

Nursing Student Resources Academic advising; academic or career counseling; assistance for students with disabilities; bookstore; campus computer network; career placement assistance; computer lab; computer-assisted instruction; daycare for children of students; e-mail services; employment services for current students; externships; housing assistance; Internet; learning resource lab; library services; nursing audiovisuals; other; paid internships; placement services for program completers; remedial services; resume preparation assistance; skills, simulation, or other laboratory; tutoring; unpaid internships.

Library Facilities 81,532 volumes (14,100 in health, 5,450 in nursing); 382 periodical subscriptions (60 health-care related).

BACCALAUREATE PROGRAMS

Degree BSN

Available Programs Accelerated RN Baccalaureate; Baccalaureate for Second Degree; Generic Baccalaureate.

Site Options Cranberry Township, PA; Greensburg, PA.

Study Options Full-time and part-time.

Program Entrance Requirements Minimum overall college GPA of 3.0, transcript of college record, CPR certification, health exam, health insurance, high school biology, high school chemistry, 2 years high school math, 2 years high school science, high school transcript, immunizations, interview, minimum high school GPA of 3.0, minimum GPA in nursing prerequisites of 2.0, professional liability insurance/malpractice insurance, prerequisite course work. Transfer students are accepted. **Standardized tests** *Required:* SAT or ACT, TOEFL for international students. **Application Deadline:** 4/1 (freshmen), rolling (transfer). *Early decision:* 9/30. *Notification:* continuous (freshmen), 10/30 (early action). *Application fee:* $20.

Advanced Placement Credit by examination available. Credit given for nursing courses completed elsewhere dependent upon specific evaluations.

Expenses (2006–07) *Tuition:* full-time $22,020; part-time $583 per credit. *Room and board:* $7284; room only: $3722 per academic year. *Required fees:* full-time $738; part-time $142 per credit; part-time $369 per term.

Financial Aid 91% of baccalaureate students in nursing programs received some form of financial aid in 2005–06.

Contact Ms. Christine Bell, Associate Provost and Director of Undergraduate Admissions and Enrollment, School of Nursing, Carlow University, Admissions Office, 3333 Fifth Avenue, Pittsburgh, PA 15213. *Telephone:* 412-578-6059. *Fax:* 412-578-6668. *E-mail:* admissions@carlow.edu.

GRADUATE PROGRAMS

Expenses (2006–07) *Tuition:* part-time $626 per credit. *Required fees:* part-time $142 per credit.

Financial Aid 41% of graduate students in nursing programs received some form of financial aid in 2005–06. Career-related internships or fieldwork, Federal Work-Study, scholarships, traineeships, and tuition waivers (partial) available. Aid available to part-time students. *Financial aid application deadline:* 4/1.

Contact Ms. Susan Shutter, Associate Provost and Director of Graduate and Adult Admissions, School of Nursing, Carlow University, 3333 Fifth Avenue, Pittsburgh, PA 15213. *Telephone:* 412-578-8764. *Fax:* 412-578-6321. *E-mail:* gradstudies@carlow.edu.

MASTER'S DEGREE PROGRAM

Degree MSN

Available Programs Accelerated Master's; Master's; RN to Master's.

Concentrations Available Nurse case management; nursing administration; nursing education. *Clinical nurse specialist programs in:* home health care. *Nurse practitioner programs in:* family health.

Site Options Cranberry Township, PA; Greensburg, PA.

Study Options Full-time and part-time.

Program Entrance Requirements Clinical experience, computer literacy, minimum overall college GPA of 3.0, transcript of college record, CPR certification, written essay, immunizations, interview, 3 letters of recommendation, professional liability insurance/malpractice insurance, prerequisite course work, resume, statistics course, GRE General Test. *Application deadline:* For fall admission, 6/15 (priority date); for spring admission, 11/15 (priority date). Applications are processed on a rolling basis. *Application fee:* $20.

Advanced Placement Credit by examination available. Credit given for nursing courses completed elsewhere dependent upon specific evaluations.

Degree Requirements 56 total credit hours, thesis or project, comprehensive exam.

POST-MASTER'S PROGRAM

Areas of Study *Clinical nurse specialist programs in:* home health care. *Nurse practitioner programs in:* family health.

CONTINUING EDUCATION PROGRAM

Contact Ms. Susan Shutter, Associate Provost and Director of Graduate and Adult Admissions, School of Nursing, Carlow University, 3333 Fifth Avenue, Pittsburgh, PA 15213. *Telephone:* 412-578-8764. *Fax:* 412-578-6321. *E-mail:* sshutter@carlow.edu.

Cedar Crest College

Department of Nursing
Allentown, Pennsylvania

http://www.cedarcrest.edu

Founded in 1867

DEGREE • BS

Nursing Student Activities Nursing Honor Society, Sigma Theta Tau, Student Nurses' Association, nursing club.

Nursing Student Resources Academic advising; academic or career counseling; assistance for students with disabilities; bookstore; campus computer network; career placement assistance; computer lab; e-mail services; interactive nursing skills videos; learning resource lab; library services; tutoring.

Library Facilities 140,886 volumes; 1,298 periodical subscriptions.

■ Cedar Crest College offers an undergraduate program in nursing. (Majors in nursing, allied health, and the sciences account for 45 percent of the College's total student enrollment.) The undergraduate nursing program includes clinical experiences at more than a dozen top-rated healthcare facilities within 10 miles of the College, including Pennsylvania's largest teaching hospital. The state-of-the-art Trexler Pavilion for Nursing includes an eight-bed ward for clinical training for nursing students. The program is accredited by the National League for Nursing Accrediting Commission.

BACCALAUREATE PROGRAMS

Degree BS

Available Programs Baccalaureate for Second Degree; Generic Baccalaureate; RN Baccalaureate.

Study Options Full-time and part-time.

Program Entrance Requirements Minimum overall college GPA of 2.5, CPR certification, health exam, health insurance, high school biology, high school chemistry, 3 years high school math, 2 years high school science, high school transcript, immunizations, interview, minimum GPA in nursing prerequisites of 2.5, professional liability insurance/malpractice insurance. Transfer students are accepted. **Standardized tests** *Required:* SAT or ACT, TOEFL for international students. **Application** *Deadline:* rolling (freshmen), rolling (transfer). *Application fee:* $30.

Advanced Placement Credit by examination available. Credit given for nursing courses completed elsewhere dependent upon specific evaluations.

Contact Office of Admissions, Department of Nursing, Cedar Crest College, 100 College Drive, Allentown, PA 18104. *Telephone:* 610-740-3780. *Fax:* 610-606-4647. *E-mail:* cccadmis@cedarcrest.edu.

Clarion University of Pennsylvania
School of Nursing
Oil City, Pennsylvania

Founded in 1867

DEGREES • BSN • MSN

Nursing Program Faculty 19 (21% with doctorates).

Baccalaureate Enrollment 85
Women 93% **Men** 7% **Minority** 4% **Part-time** 88%

Graduate Enrollment 59
Women 97% **Men** 3% **Minority** 3% **Part-time** 97%

Nursing Student Activities Sigma Theta Tau, nursing club.

Nursing Student Resources Academic advising; academic or career counseling; assistance for students with disabilities; bookstore; campus computer network; career placement assistance; computer lab; computer-assisted instruction; daycare for children of students; e-mail services; externships; housing assistance; interactive nursing skills videos; Internet; learning resource lab; library services; nursing audiovisuals; placement services for program completers; remedial services; resume preparation assistance; skills, simulation, or other laboratory; tutoring.

Library Facilities 442,871 volumes (12,000 in health, 6,000 in nursing); 20,264 periodical subscriptions (250 health-care related).

BACCALAUREATE PROGRAMS

Degree BSN

Available Programs ADN to Baccalaureate; RN Baccalaureate.

Site Options *Distance Learning:* Pittsburgh, PA.

Program Entrance Requirements Transfer students are accepted. **Standardized tests** *Required:* SAT or ACT, TOEFL for international students. **Application** *Deadline:* rolling (freshmen), rolling (transfer). *Application fee:* $30.

Financial Aid 60% of baccalaureate students in nursing programs received some form of financial aid in 2004–05.

Contact Mrs. Sally J. Bowser, Acting Director, School of Nursing and Allied Health, School of Nursing, Clarion University of Pennsylvania, 1801 West First Street, Oil City, PA 16301. *Telephone:* 814-676-6591 Ext. 1253. *Fax:* 814-676-0251. *E-mail:* sbowser@clarion.edu.

GRADUATE PROGRAMS

Financial Aid 50% of graduate students in nursing programs received some form of financial aid in 2004–05. 1 research assistantship with full tuition reimbursement available (averaging $4,002 per year) was awarded. *Financial aid application deadline:* 3/1.

Contact Dr. Alice Conway, Coordinator, MSN Family Nurse Practitioner Program, School of Nursing, Clarion University of Pennsylvania, Centennial Hall, Edinboro, PA 16444. *Telephone:* 814-732-2900. *Fax:* 814-732-2536. *E-mail:* aconway@edinboro.edu.

MASTER'S DEGREE PROGRAM

Degree MSN

Available Programs Accelerated RN to Master's; Master's.

Concentrations Available Nursing education. *Nurse practitioner programs in:* family health.

Site Options *Distance Learning:* Edinboro, PA; Pittsburgh, PA; Slippery Rock, PA.

Study Options Full-time and part-time.

Program Entrance Requirements Clinical experience, computer literacy, minimum overall college GPA of 2.7, transcript of college record, CPR certification, written essay, immunizations, interview, 3 letters of recommendation, professional liability insurance/malpractice insurance, statistics course. *Application deadline:* For fall admission, 7/1; for spring admission, 11/1. *Application fee:* $30.

Advanced Placement Credit given for nursing courses completed elsewhere dependent upon specific evaluations.

Degree Requirements 45 total credit hours, thesis or project, comprehensive exam.

POST-MASTER'S PROGRAM

Areas of Study Nursing education. *Nurse practitioner programs in:* family health.

College Misericordia
Department of Nursing
Dallas, Pennsylvania

http://www.misericordia.edu/nursing

Founded in 1924

DEGREES • BSN • MSN

Nursing Program Faculty 35 (10% with doctorates).

Baccalaureate Enrollment 363
Women 80% **Men** 20% **Minority** 3% **Part-time** 65%

Graduate Enrollment 35
Women 95% **Men** 5% **Minority** 1% **Part-time** 100%

Nursing Student Activities Nursing Honor Society, Sigma Theta Tau, Student Nurses' Association, nursing club.

Nursing Student Resources Academic advising; academic or career counseling; assistance for students with disabilities; bookstore; campus computer network; career placement assistance; computer lab; computer-assisted instruction; e-mail services; employment services for current students; externships; housing assistance; interactive nursing skills videos; Internet; learning resource lab; library services; nursing audiovisuals; placement services for program completers; remedial services; resume preparation assistance; skills, simulation, or other laboratory; tutoring.

Library Facilities 75,777 volumes; 995 periodical subscriptions.

BACCALAUREATE PROGRAMS

Degree BSN

Available Programs Accelerated Baccalaureate; Accelerated Baccalaureate for Second Degree; Accelerated RN Baccalaureate; Baccalaureate for Second Degree; Generic Baccalaureate; RN Baccalaureate.

Site Options Nanticoke, PA.

Study Options Full-time and part-time.

Program Entrance Requirements Minimum overall college GPA of 2.5, transcript of college record, health insurance, high school biology, high school chemistry, 1 year of high school math, high school transcript, immunizations, letters of recommendation, minimum high school GPA of 2.0, minimum high school rank, minimum GPA in nursing prerequisites of 2.75. Transfer students are accepted. **Standardized tests** *Required:* SAT or ACT, TOEFL for international students. **Application** *Deadline:* rolling (freshmen), rolling (transfer). *Notification:* continuous (freshmen). *Application fee:* $25.

Advanced Placement Credit by examination available. Credit given for nursing courses completed elsewhere dependent upon specific evaluations.

Expenses (2005–06) *Tuition:* full-time $9350; part-time $425 per credit. *International tuition:* $9350 full-time. *Room and board:* $4070; room only: $2310 per academic year. *Required fees:* full-time $150; part-time $75 per term.

College Misericordia (continued)

Financial Aid 68% of baccalaureate students in nursing programs received some form of financial aid in 2004–05. *Gift aid (need-based):* Federal Pell, FSEOG, state, private, college/university gift aid from institutional funds, Federal Nursing. *Loans:* Federal Nursing Student Loans, FFEL (Subsidized and Unsubsidized Stafford PLUS), Perkins, state. *Work-Study:* Federal Work-Study. *Application deadline (priority):* 3/1.

Contact Glenn Bozinski, Department of Nursing, College Misericordia, 301 Lake Street, Dallas, PA 18612. *Telephone:* 570-674-6434. *E-mail:* gbozinsk@misericordia.edu.

GRADUATE PROGRAMS

Expenses (2005–06) *Tuition:* part-time $500 per credit. *Required fees:* full-time $80; part-time $40 per term.

Financial Aid 60% of graduate students in nursing programs received some form of financial aid in 2004–05. Teaching assistantships, career-related internships or fieldwork, scholarships, traineeships, tuition waivers (partial), and unspecified assistantships available. Aid available to part-time students. *Financial aid application deadline:* 6/30.

Contact Miss Larree Brown, Adult Education Counselor, Graduate Programs, Department of Nursing, College Misericordia, 301 Lake Street, Dallas, PA 18612. *Telephone:* 570-674-6451. *Fax:* 570-674-8902. *E-mail:* lbrown@misericordia.edu.

MASTER'S DEGREE PROGRAM

Degree MSN

Available Programs Accelerated RN to Master's; Master's; RN to Master's.

Concentrations Available Nursing administration; nursing education. *Clinical nurse specialist programs in:* adult health, community health, maternity-newborn, parent-child. *Nurse practitioner programs in:* family health.

Study Options Part-time.

Program Entrance Requirements Clinical experience, computer literacy, minimum overall college GPA of 3.0, transcript of college record, written essay, 3 letters of recommendation, nursing research course, physical assessment course, professional liability insurance/malpractice insurance, statistics course, GRE General Test or MAT. *Application deadline:* For fall admission, 8/7 (priority date); for spring admission, 1/3. Applications are processed on a rolling basis. *Application fee:* $25.

Advanced Placement Credit given for nursing courses completed elsewhere dependent upon specific evaluations.

Degree Requirements 45 total credit hours, thesis or project.

POST-MASTER'S PROGRAM

Areas of Study Nursing education. *Nurse practitioner programs in:* family health.

DeSales University
Department of Nursing and Health
Center Valley, Pennsylvania

http://www.desales.edu

Founded in 1964

DEGREES • BSN • MSN • MSN/MBA

Nursing Program Faculty 23 (26% with doctorates).

Baccalaureate Enrollment 1,858
Women 86% **Men** 14% **Minority** 4% **International** 2% **Part-time** 8%

Graduate Enrollment 100
Women 91% **Men** 9% **Minority** 5% **Part-time** 95%

Nursing Student Activities Nursing Honor Society, Sigma Theta Tau, Student Nurses' Association.

Nursing Student Resources Academic advising; academic or career counseling; bookstore; campus computer network; career placement assistance; computer lab; computer-assisted instruction; e-mail services; employment services for current students; externships; interactive nursing skills videos; Internet; learning resource lab; library services; nursing audiovisuals; paid internships; placement services for program completers; remedial services; resume preparation assistance; skills, simulation, or other laboratory; tutoring; unpaid internships.

Library Facilities 151,999 volumes (1,200 in health); 12,000 periodical subscriptions (100 health-care related).

BACCALAUREATE PROGRAMS

Degree BSN

Available Programs ADN to Baccalaureate; Accelerated Baccalaureate; Accelerated RN Baccalaureate; Generic Baccalaureate; RN Baccalaureate.

Study Options Full-time and part-time.

Program Entrance Requirements High school biology, high school chemistry, high school foreign language, 2 years high school math, 3 years high school science, high school transcript, minimum high school GPA of 2.5, minimum high school rank 33%. Transfer students are accepted. **Standardized tests** *Required:* SAT or ACT, TOEFL for international students. **Application** *Deadline:* 8/1 (freshmen), 8/1 (transfer). *Notification:* continuous (freshmen). *Application fee:* $30.

Advanced Placement Credit by examination available. Credit given for nursing courses completed elsewhere dependent upon specific evaluations.

Expenses (2005–06) *Tuition:* full-time $20,000; part-time $700 per credit hour. *International tuition:* $20,000 full-time. *Required fees:* full-time $700; part-time $350 per term.

Financial Aid 47% of baccalaureate students in nursing programs received some form of financial aid in 2004–05.

Contact Dr. Kerry H. Cheever, Chair, Department of Nursing and Health, DeSales University, 2755 Station Avenue, Center Valley, PA 18034-9568. *Telephone:* 610-282-1100 Ext. 1271. *Fax:* 610-282-2254. *E-mail:* kerry.cheever@desales.edu.

GRADUATE PROGRAMS

Expenses (2005–06) *Tuition:* full-time $15,900; part-time $530 per credit hour. *International tuition:* $15,900 full-time. *Required fees:* full-time $530.

Financial Aid 18% of graduate students in nursing programs received some form of financial aid in 2004–05.

Contact Dr. Carol G. Mest, RN, Director of Graduate Program in Nursing, Department of Nursing and Health, DeSales University, 2755 Station Avenue, Center Valley, PA 18034. *Telephone:* 610-282-1100 Ext. 1271. *Fax:* 610-282-2254. *E-mail:* carol.mest@desales.edu.

MASTER'S DEGREE PROGRAM

Degrees MSN; MSN/MBA

Available Programs Accelerated AD/RN to Master's; Accelerated RN to Master's; Master's; RN to Master's.

Concentrations Available Nursing administration; nursing education. *Clinical nurse specialist programs in:* adult health. *Nurse practitioner programs in:* family health.

Study Options Full-time and part-time.

Program Entrance Requirements Minimum overall college GPA of 3.0, transcript of college record, written essay, interview, 3 letters of recommendation, prerequisite course work, statistics course.

Advanced Placement Credit given for nursing courses completed elsewhere dependent upon specific evaluations.

Degree Requirements 47 total credit hours.

POST-MASTER'S PROGRAM

Areas of Study Nursing education. *Clinical nurse specialist programs in:* adult health. *Nurse practitioner programs in:* family health.

CONTINUING EDUCATION PROGRAM

Contact Dr. Carol G. Mest, RN, Director of Graduate Program in Nursing, Department of Nursing and Health, DeSales University, 2755 Station Avenue, Center Valley, PA 18034. *Telephone:* 610-282-1100 Ext. 1394. *Fax:* 610-282-2254. *E-mail:* carol.mest@desales.edu.

Drexel University
College of Nursing and Health Professions
Philadelphia, Pennsylvania

http://www.drexel.edu

Founded in 1891

DEGREES • BSN • DNP • MSN

Nursing Program Faculty 60 (40% with doctorates).

Baccalaureate Enrollment 998
Women 89% **Men** 11% **Minority** 32% **Part-time** 24%

Graduate Enrollment 505
Women 89% **Men** 11% **Minority** 15% **Part-time** 80%

Nursing Student Activities Nursing Honor Society, Sigma Theta Tau, Student Nurses' Association.

Nursing Student Resources Academic advising; academic or career counseling; assistance for students with disabilities; bookstore; campus computer network; career placement assistance; computer lab; computer-assisted instruction; e-mail services; housing assistance; interactive nursing skills videos; Internet; learning resource lab; library services; nursing audiovisuals; paid internships; placement services for program completers; remedial services; resume preparation assistance; skills, simulation, or other laboratory; tutoring.

Library Facilities 570,335 volumes (51,000 in health, 5,015 in nursing); 8,321 periodical subscriptions (63,000 health-care related).

BACCALAUREATE PROGRAMS
Degree BSN

Available Programs ADN to Baccalaureate; Accelerated Baccalaureate for Second Degree; Generic Baccalaureate; RN Baccalaureate.
Site Options Philadelphia, PA.
Study Options Full-time.
Program Entrance Requirements CPR certification, health insurance, high school biology, high school chemistry, 3 years high school math, 2 years high school science, high school transcript, immunizations. Transfer students are accepted. **Standardized tests** *Required:* SAT or ACT, TOEFL for international students. *Recommended:* SAT. **Application** *Deadline:* 3/1 (freshmen), rolling (transfer). *Notification:* continuous (freshmen). *Application fee:* $50.
Expenses (2006–07) *Tuition:* full-time $26,000. *Room and board:* $11,010; room only: $6555 per academic year. *Required fees:* full-time $1650.
Financial Aid 58% of baccalaureate students in nursing programs received some form of financial aid in 2005–06. *Gift aid (need-based):* Federal Pell, FSEOG, state, private, college/university gift aid from institutional funds, United Negro College Fund. *Loans:* FFEL (Subsidized and Unsubsidized Stafford PLUS), Perkins, college/university. *Work-Study:* Federal Work-Study. *Application deadline:* 3/15.
Contact Ms. Vanessa Thomas, Assistant Director, Office of Enrollment, College of Nursing and Health Professions, Drexel University, 1505 Race Street, Mail Stop 472, Philadelphia, PA 19102-1192. *Telephone:* 215-762-1098. *Fax:* 215-762-6194. *E-mail:* vthomas@drexel.edu.

GRADUATE PROGRAMS
Expenses (2006–07) *Tuition:* part-time $615 per credit.
Financial Aid 27% of graduate students in nursing programs received some form of financial aid in 2005–06. Fellowships, research assistantships, teaching assistantships, career-related internships or fieldwork, Federal Work-Study, institutionally sponsored loans, and tuition waivers (partial) available. Aid available to part-time students. *Financial aid application deadline:* 5/1.
Contact Ms. Maura Wiswall, Program Coordinator, MSN Programs, College of Nursing and Health Professions, Drexel University, 1505 Race Street, Mail Stop 501, Philadelphia, PA 19102-1192. *Telephone:* 215-762-1336. *Fax:* 215-762-1259. *E-mail:* maw86@drexel.edu.

MASTER'S DEGREE PROGRAM
Degree MSN

Available Programs Master's; Master's for Nurses with Non-Nursing Degrees; RN to Master's.

Concentrations Available Nurse anesthesia; nursing administration; nursing education. *Clinical nurse specialist programs in:* women's health. *Nurse practitioner programs in:* acute care, family health, pediatric, psychiatric/mental health, women's health.
Site Options *Distance Learning:* Philadelphia, PA.
Study Options Full-time and part-time.
Program Entrance Requirements Clinical experience, computer literacy, minimum overall college GPA of 3.0, transcript of college record, CPR certification, written essay, immunizations, 2 letters of recommendation, resume. *Application deadline:* Applications are processed on a rolling basis. *Application fee:* $50.
Advanced Placement Credit given for nursing courses completed elsewhere dependent upon specific evaluations.
Degree Requirements 55 total credit hours, thesis or project, comprehensive exam.

POST-MASTER'S PROGRAM
Areas of Study Nurse anesthesia; nursing administration; nursing education. *Nurse practitioner programs in:* acute care, family health, pediatric, psychiatric/mental health, women's health.

DOCTORAL DEGREE PROGRAM
Degree DNP

Available Programs Doctorate; Post-Baccalaureate Doctorate.
Areas of Study Clinical practice, faculty preparation, nursing administration, nursing education, nursing science.
Site Options Philadelphia, PA.
Program Entrance Requirements Clinical experience, minimum overall college GPA of 3.25, interview by faculty committee, 2 letters of recommendation, MSN or equivalent, statistics course, vita, writing sample, GRE General Test. *Application deadline:* Applications are processed on a rolling basis. *Application fee:* $50.
Degree Requirements 48 total credit hours, dissertation, oral exam, written exam, residency.

CONTINUING EDUCATION PROGRAM
Contact Mr. Thomas Harkins, Director of Continuing Nursing Education, College of Nursing and Health Professions, Drexel University, 245 North 15th Street, Mail Stop 1002, Philadelphia, PA 19102-1192. *Telephone:* 215-762-2659. *Fax:* 215-762-8171. *E-mail:* tharkins@drexel.edu.

See full description on page 470.

Duquesne University
School of Nursing
Pittsburgh, Pennsylvania

http://www.nursing.duq.edu

Founded in 1878

DEGREES • BSN • MSN • PHD

Nursing Program Faculty 67 (18% with doctorates).

Baccalaureate Enrollment 398
Women 90% **Men** 10% **Minority** 8% **International** 4%

Graduate Enrollment 225
Women 91% **Men** 9% **Minority** 2% **International** 6% **Part-time** 55%

Nursing Student Activities Nursing Honor Society, Sigma Theta Tau, Student Nurses' Association, nursing club.

Nursing Student Resources Academic advising; academic or career counseling; assistance for students with disabilities; bookstore; campus computer network; career placement assistance; computer lab; computer-assisted instruction; daycare for children of students; e-mail services; employment services for current students; externships; housing assistance; interactive nursing skills videos; Internet; learning resource lab; library services; nursing audiovisuals; paid internships; placement services for program completers; remedial services; resume preparation assistance; skills, simulation, or other laboratory; tutoring; unpaid internships.

Library Facilities 703,981 volumes (27,613 in health, 1,951 in nursing); 20,020 periodical subscriptions (1,779 health-care related).

Duquesne University (continued)

BACCALAUREATE PROGRAMS

Degree BSN

Available Programs Accelerated Baccalaureate for Second Degree; Accelerated RN Baccalaureate; Generic Baccalaureate; International Nurse to Baccalaureate.

Site Options *Distance Learning:* Pittsburgh, PA.

Study Options Full-time and part-time.

Program Entrance Requirements Minimum overall college GPA of 2.5, transcript of college record, written essay, high school biology, high school chemistry, high school foreign language, 2 years high school math, 3 years high school science, high school transcript, 2 letters of recommendation, minimum high school GPA of 3.0, minimum high school rank 40%. Transfer students are accepted. **Standardized tests** *Required:* SAT or ACT. *Recommended:* TOEFL for international students. **Application** *Deadline:* 7/1 (freshmen), 7/1 (transfer). *Early decision:* 11/1, 12/1. *Notification:* continuous (freshmen), 12/15 (out-of-state freshmen), 12/15 (early decision), 1/15 (early action). *Application fee:* $50.

Advanced Placement Credit by examination available. Credit given for nursing courses completed elsewhere dependent upon specific evaluations.

Expenses (2006–07) *Tuition:* full-time $21,571; part-time $718 per credit. *International tuition:* $21,571 full-time. *Room and board:* $8296; room only: $8296 per academic year. *Required fees:* full-time $1810; part-time $71 per credit.

Financial Aid 90% of baccalaureate students in nursing programs received some form of financial aid in 2005–06. *Gift aid (need-based):* Federal Pell, FSEOG, state, private, college/university gift aid from institutional funds, United Negro College Fund. *Loans:* Federal Nursing Student Loans, FFEL (Subsidized and Unsubsidized Stafford PLUS), Perkins, Private Alternative Loans. *Work-Study:* Federal Work-Study. *Application deadline:* 5/1.

Contact Ms. Susan Hardner, RN, Nursing Recruiter, School of Nursing, Duquesne University, 600 Forbes Avenue, Pittsburgh, PA 15282-1760. *Telephone:* 412-396-4945. *Fax:* 412-396-6346. *E-mail:* hardnersue@duq.edu.

GRADUATE PROGRAMS

Expenses (2006–07) *Tuition:* part-time $751 per credit. *International tuition:* $751 full-time. *Room and board:* $4180 per academic year. *Required fees:* part-time $71 per credit.

Financial Aid 50% of graduate students in nursing programs received some form of financial aid in 2005–06. 8 research assistantships (averaging $2,600 per year), 1 teaching assistantship with partial tuition reimbursement available (averaging $2,600 per year) were awarded; institutionally sponsored loans, scholarships, traineeships, tuition waivers (partial), and unspecified assistantships also available.

Contact Ms. Susan Hardner, RN, Nursing Recruiter, School of Nursing, Duquesne University, 600 Forbes Avenue, Pittsburgh, PA 15282-1760. *Telephone:* 412-396-4945. *Fax:* 412-396-6346. *E-mail:* hardnersue@duq.edu.

MASTER'S DEGREE PROGRAM

Degree MSN

Available Programs Master's; RN to Master's.

Concentrations Available Nursing administration; nursing education. *Clinical nurse specialist programs in:* acute care, forensic nursing, psychiatric/mental health. *Nurse practitioner programs in:* family health.

Site Options *Distance Learning:* Pittsburgh, PA.

Study Options Full-time and part-time.

Program Entrance Requirements Clinical experience, computer literacy, minimum overall college GPA of 3.0, transcript of college record, written essay, interview, 2 letters of recommendation, nursing research course, physical assessment course, prerequisite course work, resume, statistics course, MAT, or GRE. *Application deadline:* For fall admission, 5/1; for spring admission, 11/1. *Application fee:* $50.

Advanced Placement Credit given for nursing courses completed elsewhere dependent upon specific evaluations.

Degree Requirements 40 total credit hours, thesis or project.

POST-MASTER'S PROGRAM

Areas of Study Nursing administration; nursing education. *Clinical nurse specialist programs in:* acute care, forensic nursing, psychiatric/mental health. *Nurse practitioner programs in:* family health.

DOCTORAL DEGREE PROGRAM

Degree PhD

Available Programs Doctorate.

Areas of Study Nursing research.

Site Options *Distance Learning:* Pittsburgh, PA.

Program Entrance Requirements Minimum overall college GPA of 3.5, interview by faculty committee, 3 letters of recommendation, MSN or equivalent, scholarly papers, statistics course, vita, writing sample, GRE General Test. *Application deadline:* For fall admission, 5/1; for spring admission, 11/1. *Application fee:* $50.

Degree Requirements 57 total credit hours, dissertation, oral exam, written exam, residency.

CONTINUING EDUCATION PROGRAM

Contact Dr. Shirley P. Smith, Assistant Professor, School of Nursing, Duquesne University, 600 Forbes Avenue, Pittsburgh, PA 15282-1760. *Telephone:* 412-396-6535. *Fax:* 412-396-6346. *E-mail:* smith1@duq.edu.

See full description on page 474.

Eastern University

Program in Nursing
St. Davids, Pennsylvania

http://www.eastern.edu/academics/

Founded in 1952

DEGREE • BSN

Nursing Program Faculty 6 (33% with doctorates).

Baccalaureate Enrollment 97

Women 95% **Men** 5% **Minority** 25% **International** 7%

Nursing Student Activities Sigma Theta Tau.

Nursing Student Resources Academic advising; academic or career counseling; assistance for students with disabilities; bookstore; campus computer network; career placement assistance; computer lab; computer-assisted instruction; e-mail services; employment services for current students; Internet; learning resource lab; library services; nursing audio-visuals; placement services for program completers; remedial services; resume preparation assistance; skills, simulation, or other laboratory; tutoring; unpaid internships.

Library Facilities 143,815 volumes (5,858 in health, 3,000 in nursing); 1,215 periodical subscriptions (821 health-care related).

BACCALAUREATE PROGRAMS

Degree BSN

Available Programs Accelerated RN Baccalaureate; Baccalaureate for Second Degree; International Nurse to Baccalaureate.

Site Options Wynnewood, PA; Phoenixville, PA; Harrisburg, PA.

Study Options Full-time.

Program Entrance Requirements Minimum overall college GPA of 3.0, transcript of college record, CPR certification, written essay, health exam, health insurance, high school chemistry, high school transcript, immunizations, interview, 2 letters of recommendation, minimum GPA in nursing prerequisites of 3.0, professional liability insurance/malpractice insurance, prerequisite course work, RN licensure. Transfer students are accepted. **Standardized tests** *Required:* SAT or ACT, TOEFL for international students. **Application** *Deadline:* rolling (freshmen), rolling (transfer). *Notification:* continuous (freshmen). *Application fee:* $25.

Advanced Placement Credit by examination available. Credit given for nursing courses completed elsewhere dependent upon specific evaluations.

Financial Aid 30% of baccalaureate students in nursing programs received some form of financial aid in 2005–06.

Contact Ms. Kim Skinner, RN-BSN Program Advisor, Program in Nursing, Eastern University, 588 North Gulph Road, King of Prussia, PA 19406. *Telephone:* 800-732-7669. *Fax:* 610-341-1468. *E-mail:* kskinner@eastern.edu.

Contact Ms. Denise Robinson, Program Advisor, Program in Nursing, Eastern University, 1300 Eagle Road, St. Davids, PA 19087. *Telephone:* 484-581-1279. *Fax:* 610-341-1468. *E-mail:* drobinso@eastern.edu.

East Stroudsburg University of Pennsylvania
Department of Nursing
East Stroudsburg, Pennsylvania

http://www3.esu/academics/bshp/nurs/home.asp

Founded in 1893

DEGREE • BS

Nursing Program Faculty 14 (44% with doctorates).

Baccalaureate Enrollment 138
Women 91% **Men** 9%

Nursing Student Activities Nursing Honor Society, Sigma Theta Tau, Student Nurses' Association, nursing club.

Nursing Student Resources Academic advising; academic or career counseling; assistance for students with disabilities; bookstore; campus computer network; career placement assistance; computer lab; computer-assisted instruction; daycare for children of students; e-mail services; employment services for current students; externships; housing assistance; interactive nursing skills videos; Internet; learning resource lab; library services; nursing audiovisuals; other; placement services for program completers; remedial services; resume preparation assistance; skills, simulation, or other laboratory; tutoring; unpaid internships.

Library Facilities 449,107 volumes (16,810 in health, 2,035 in nursing); 1,175 periodical subscriptions (495 health-care related).

BACCALAUREATE PROGRAMS

Degree BS

Available Programs Generic Baccalaureate; LPN to Baccalaureate; RN Baccalaureate.

Study Options Full-time and part-time.

Program Entrance Requirements Minimum overall college GPA of 2.75, transcript of college record, health exam, 2 years high school math, 2 years high school science, high school transcript, minimum high school GPA of 3.0, minimum high school rank 75%, minimum GPA in nursing prerequisites of 2.75. Transfer students are accepted. **Standardized tests** *Required:* SAT or ACT, TOEFL for international students. **Application** *Deadline:* 4/1 (freshmen), 5/1 (transfer). *Notification:* continuous until 5/1 (freshmen). *Application fee:* $35.

Advanced Placement Credit by examination available. Credit given for nursing courses completed elsewhere dependent upon specific evaluations.

Contact Dr. Suzanne Fischer Prestoy, Chairperson and Associate Professor, Department of Nursing, East Stroudsburg University of Pennsylvania, 200 Prospect Street, East Stroudsburg, PA 18301-2999. *Telephone:* 570-422-3474. *Fax:* 570-422-3848. *E-mail:* sprestoy@po-box.esu.edu.

Edinboro University of Pennsylvania
Department of Nursing
Edinboro, Pennsylvania

http://www.edinboro.edu/cwis/nursing/nursing.html

Founded in 1857

DEGREE • BS

Nursing Program Faculty 21 (38% with doctorates).

Baccalaureate Enrollment 297
Women 85% **Men** 15% **Minority** 8% **International** 2% **Part-time** 9%

Nursing Student Activities Sigma Theta Tau, Student Nurses' Association.

Nursing Student Resources Academic advising; academic or career counseling; assistance for students with disabilities; bookstore; campus computer network; career placement assistance; computer lab; computer-assisted instruction; e-mail services; housing assistance; interactive nursing skills videos; Internet; learning resource lab; library services; nursing audiovisuals; remedial services; resume preparation assistance; skills, simulation, or other laboratory; tutoring.

Library Facilities 493,114 volumes; 1,409 periodical subscriptions (105 health-care related).

BACCALAUREATE PROGRAMS

Degree BS

Available Programs ADN to Baccalaureate; Accelerated Baccalaureate for Second Degree; Accelerated RN Baccalaureate; Baccalaureate for Second Degree; Generic Baccalaureate; LPN to Baccalaureate.

Site Options Erie, PA.

Study Options Full-time and part-time.

Program Entrance Requirements Minimum overall college GPA of 2.75, transcript of college record, CPR certification, health exam, high school biology, high school chemistry, 1 year of high school math, 2 years high school science, high school transcript, immunizations, minimum high school rank 40%, minimum GPA in nursing prerequisites of 2.75, professional liability insurance/malpractice insurance, prerequisite course work. Transfer students are accepted. **Standardized tests** *Required:* SAT or ACT, TOEFL for international students. *Required for some:* SAT, ACT. **Application** *Deadline:* 4/1 (freshmen), rolling (transfer). *Notification:* 7/1 (freshmen). *Application fee:* $30.

Advanced Placement Credit by examination available.

Expenses (2006–07) *Tuition, state resident:* full-time $4906; part-time $204 per credit. *Tuition, nonresident:* full-time $7360; part-time $307 per credit. *International tuition:* $7360 full-time. *Room and board:* $5418; room only: $3600 per academic year. *Required fees:* full-time $941; part-time $65 per credit.

Contact Mrs. Patricia Louise Nosel, RN, Chairperson, Department of Nursing, Edinboro University of Pennsylvania, 125 Centennial Hall, Edinboro, PA 16444. *Telephone:* 814-732-1127 Ext. 2900. *Fax:* 814-732-2536. *E-mail:* nosel@edinboro.edu.

Gannon University
Program in Nursing
Erie, Pennsylvania

Founded in 1925

DEGREES • BSN • MSN

Nursing Program Faculty 13 (38% with doctorates).

Baccalaureate Enrollment 220
Women 88% **Men** 12% **Minority** 4% **Part-time** 5%

Graduate Enrollment 81
Women 68% **Men** 32% **Minority** 6% **Part-time** 38%

Nursing Student Activities Nursing Honor Society, Sigma Theta Tau.

Nursing Student Resources Academic advising; academic or career counseling; assistance for students with disabilities; bookstore; campus computer network; career placement assistance; computer lab; computer-assisted instruction; e-mail services; employment services for current students; externships; housing assistance; interactive nursing skills videos; Internet; learning resource lab; library services; nursing audiovisuals; paid internships; placement services for program completers; remedial services; resume preparation assistance; skills, simulation, or other laboratory; tutoring; unpaid internships.

Library Facilities 270,590 volumes (11,604 in health, 1,300 in nursing); 14,301 periodical subscriptions (1,600 health-care related).

BACCALAUREATE PROGRAMS

Degree BSN

Gannon University (continued)

Available Programs ADN to Baccalaureate; Baccalaureate for Second Degree; Generic Baccalaureate; RN Baccalaureate.

Site Options *Distance Learning:* Erie, PA.

Study Options Full-time and part-time.

Program Entrance Requirements Minimum overall college GPA of 2.8, CPR certification, written essay, health exam, health insurance, high school biology, high school chemistry, high school transcript, immunizations, 1 letter of recommendation, minimum high school GPA of 2.5, minimum high school rank 40%. Transfer students are accepted. **Standardized tests** *Required:* SAT or ACT, TOEFL for international students. **Application** *Deadline:* rolling (freshmen), rolling (transfer). *Application fee:* $25.

Advanced Placement Credit by examination available.

Expenses (2006–07) *Tuition:* full-time $20,680; part-time $490 per credit. *International tuition:* $20,680 full-time. *Room and board:* $8400; room only: $4800 per academic year. *Required fees:* full-time $700; part-time $50 per credit; part-time $53 per term.

Financial Aid 70% of baccalaureate students in nursing programs received some form of financial aid in 2005–06. *Gift aid (need-based):* Federal Pell, FSEOG, state, private, college/university gift aid from institutional funds, Federal Nursing. *Loans:* Federal Nursing Student Loans, Federal Direct (Subsidized and Unsubsidized Stafford PLUS), FFEL (Subsidized and Unsubsidized Stafford PLUS), Perkins. *Work-Study:* Federal Work-Study, part-time campus jobs. *Application deadline (priority):* 3/15.

Contact Ms. Patricia Ann Marshall, RN, Undergraduate Program Director, Program in Nursing, Gannon University, 109 University Square, Erie, PA 16541-0001. *Telephone:* 814-871-5470. *Fax:* 814-871-5662. *E-mail:* marshall001@gannon.edu.

GRADUATE PROGRAMS

Expenses (2006–07) *Tuition:* full-time $11,430; part-time $635 per credit. *International tuition:* $11,430 full-time. *Required fees:* full-time $440; part-time $35 per credit.

Financial Aid 90% of graduate students in nursing programs received some form of financial aid in 2005–06. Career-related internships or fieldwork and traineeships available. Aid available to part-time students. *Financial aid application deadline:* 7/1.

Contact Dr. Sharon Thompson, Graduate Program Director, Program in Nursing, Gannon University, 109 University Square, Erie, PA 16541-0001. *Telephone:* 814-871-5345. *Fax:* 814-871-5662. *E-mail:* thompson001@gannon.edu.

MASTER'S DEGREE PROGRAM

Degree MSN

Available Programs Master's; RN to Master's.

Concentrations Available Nurse anesthesia; nursing administration; nursing education. *Clinical nurse specialist programs in:* medical-surgical. *Nurse practitioner programs in:* family health.

Site Options *Distance Learning:* Erie, PA.

Study Options Full-time and part-time.

Program Entrance Requirements Clinical experience, minimum overall college GPA of 3.0, transcript of college record, CPR certification, written essay, interview, 4 letters of recommendation, nursing research course, prerequisite course work, statistics course, GRE General Test, MAT. *Application deadline:* For fall admission, 4/15. *Application fee:* $25.

Advanced Placement Credit given for nursing courses completed elsewhere dependent upon specific evaluations.

Degree Requirements 42 total credit hours, thesis or project.

POST-MASTER'S PROGRAM

Areas of Study Nurse anesthesia; nursing administration; nursing education. *Clinical nurse specialist programs in:* medical-surgical. *Nurse practitioner programs in:* family health.

See full description on page 484.

Gwynedd-Mercy College
School of Nursing
Gwynedd Valley, Pennsylvania

Founded in 1948

DEGREES • BSN • MSN

Nursing Program Faculty 21 (43% with doctorates).

Baccalaureate Enrollment 85
Women 95% **Men** 5% **Minority** 5% **Part-time** 28%

Graduate Enrollment 40
Women 85% **Men** 15% **Minority** 10% **International** 5% **Part-time** 80%

Nursing Student Activities Sigma Theta Tau, Student Nurses' Association.

Nursing Student Resources Academic advising; bookstore; campus computer network; computer lab; computer-assisted instruction; daycare for children of students; e-mail services; interactive nursing skills videos; learning resource lab; library services; nursing audiovisuals; resume preparation assistance; skills, simulation, or other laboratory; tutoring.

Library Facilities 101,552 volumes; 667 periodical subscriptions.

■ Gwynedd-Mercy College's (GMC) School of Nursing is one of the finest nursing schools regionally. The program is one of the few articulated nursing programs in the region, allowing students to progress easily from the A.S.N. to B.S.N. to M.S.N. degrees. The program is clinically oriented, placing students in clinical environments in their freshman year. The program offers personal attention, with a student-teacher ratio of 15:1, and 8:1 in the clinical area. In 2002, the NLNAC informed GMC that the associate degree program was approved for continuing accreditation for eight years, the maximum amount of time that a program can receive.

BACCALAUREATE PROGRAMS

Degree BSN

Available Programs ADN to Baccalaureate; Accelerated RN Baccalaureate; RN Baccalaureate.

Site Options Fort Washington, PA.

Study Options Full-time and part-time.

Program Entrance Requirements Minimum overall college GPA of 2.8, transcript of college record, CPR certification, health exam, health insurance, high school biology, high school chemistry, 2 years high school math, high school transcript, immunizations, letters of recommendation, minimum high school rank 33%, minimum GPA in nursing prerequisites, professional liability insurance/malpractice insurance, RN licensure. Transfer students are accepted. **Standardized tests** *Required:* SAT or ACT. *Recommended:* TOEFL for international students. **Application** *Deadline:* rolling (freshmen), 8/20 (transfer). *Notification:* continuous (freshmen). *Application fee:* $25.

Advanced Placement Credit by examination available. Credit given for nursing courses completed elsewhere dependent upon specific evaluations.

Expenses (2006–07) *Tuition:* full-time $19,720; part-time $470 per credit hour. *International tuition:* $19,720 full-time. *Room and board:* $8100; room only: $4620 per academic year. *Required fees:* full-time $450; part-time $10 per credit; part-time $10 per term.

Financial Aid 90% of baccalaureate students in nursing programs received some form of financial aid in 2005–06.

Contact Ms. JaNell LaRue, Senior Admissions Counselor, School of Nursing, Gwynedd-Mercy College, PO Box 901, Gwynedd Valley, PA 19437. *Telephone:* 215-646-7300 Ext. 425. *Fax:* 215-641-5556 Ext. 528. *E-mail:* larue.jn@gmc.edu.

GRADUATE PROGRAMS

Expenses (2006–07) *Tuition:* part-time $545 per credit hour. *International tuition:* $545 full-time. *Required fees:* full-time $160; part-time $10 per credit.

Financial Aid 60% of graduate students in nursing programs received some form of financial aid in 2005–06. Traineeships and unspecified assistantships available. *Financial aid application deadline:* 8/30.

Contact Dr. Barbara A. Jones, MSN Program Director, School of Nursing, Gwynedd-Mercy College, PO Box 901, 1325 Sumneytown Pike, Gwynedd Valley, PA 19437-0901. *Telephone:* 215-646-7300 Ext. 407. *Fax:* 215-542-5789. *E-mail:* jones.b@gmc.edu.

MASTER'S DEGREE PROGRAM

Degree MSN

Available Programs Master's; RN to Master's.

Concentrations Available *Clinical nurse specialist programs in:* gerontology, oncology, pediatric. *Nurse practitioner programs in:* adult health, pediatric.

Study Options Full-time and part-time.

Program Entrance Requirements Clinical experience, minimum overall college GPA of 3.0, transcript of college record, written essay, immunizations, interview, 2 letters of recommendation, physical assessment course, professional liability insurance/malpractice insurance, statistics course, GRE General Test or MAT. *Application deadline:* For fall admission, 8/1 (priority date); for winter admission, 12/1 (priority date). Applications are processed on a rolling basis. *Application fee:* $25.

Advanced Placement Credit by examination available. Credit given for nursing courses completed elsewhere dependent upon specific evaluations.

Degree Requirements 43 total credit hours.

POST-MASTER'S PROGRAM

Areas of Study *Nurse practitioner programs in:* adult health, pediatric.

Holy Family University
School of Nursing and Allied Health Professions
Philadelphia, Pennsylvania

http://www.holyfamily.edu/school_nursing/index.html

Founded in 1954

DEGREES • BSN • MSN

Nursing Program Faculty 40 (28% with doctorates).

Baccalaureate Enrollment 183
Women 90% **Men** 10% **Minority** 25%

Graduate Enrollment 27
Women 97% **Men** 3% **Part-time** 100%

Nursing Student Activities Sigma Theta Tau, Student Nurses' Association.

Nursing Student Resources Academic advising; academic or career counseling; assistance for students with disabilities; bookstore; campus computer network; career placement assistance; computer lab; computer-assisted instruction; daycare for children of students; e-mail services; interactive nursing skills videos; Internet; learning resource lab; library services; nursing audiovisuals; other; resume preparation assistance; skills, simulation, or other laboratory; tutoring.

Library Facilities 126,780 volumes (8,159 in health, 2,177 in nursing); 742 periodical subscriptions (279 health-care related).

BACCALAUREATE PROGRAMS

Degree BSN

Available Programs ADN to Baccalaureate; Accelerated Baccalaureate; Generic Baccalaureate; International Nurse to Baccalaureate; LPN to Baccalaureate; LPN to RN Baccalaureate; RN Baccalaureate.

Site Options Bensalem, PA; Newtown, PA.

Study Options Full-time and part-time.

Program Entrance Requirements Transcript of college record, health exam, high school biology, high school chemistry, high school foreign language, 3 years high school math, 3 years high school science, high school transcript, immunizations, letters of recommendation, minimum high school GPA of 2.5, minimum high school rank 60%, minimum

GPA in nursing prerequisites of 2.5. Transfer students are accepted. **Standardized tests** *Required:* SAT or ACT, TOEFL for international students. **Application** *Deadline:* rolling (freshmen), rolling (transfer). *Application fee:* $25.

Contact *Telephone:* 215-637-3050. *Fax:* 215-281-1022.

GRADUATE PROGRAMS

Contact *Telephone:* 215-637-7203. *Fax:* 215-637-1478.

MASTER'S DEGREE PROGRAM

Degree MSN

Available Programs Master's.

Concentrations Available Health-care administration; nursing education. *Clinical nurse specialist programs in:* community health.

Site Options Newtown, PA.

Study Options Part-time.

Program Entrance Requirements Transcript of college record, written essay, immunizations, 2 letters of recommendation, nursing research course, professional liability insurance/malpractice insurance, prerequisite course work, resume, statistics course.

Advanced Placement Credit by examination available. Credit given for nursing courses completed elsewhere dependent upon specific evaluations.

Degree Requirements 39 total credit hours, comprehensive exam.

CONTINUING EDUCATION PROGRAM

Contact *Telephone:* 215-637-7700 Ext. 5002. *Fax:* 215-633-0558.

Immaculata University
Department of Nursing
Immaculata, Pennsylvania

http://www.immaculata.edu/nursing/

Founded in 1920

DEGREES • BSN • MSN

Nursing Program Faculty 30 (50% with doctorates).

Baccalaureate Enrollment 620
Women 92% **Men** 8% **Minority** 13% **Part-time** 100%

Graduate Enrollment 32
Women 87% **Men** 13% **Part-time** 100%

Nursing Student Activities Sigma Theta Tau.

Nursing Student Resources Academic or career counseling; bookstore; campus computer network; career placement assistance; e-mail services; Internet; learning resource lab; library services; nursing audiovisuals; resume preparation assistance.

Library Facilities 143,145 volumes; 604 periodical subscriptions (115 health-care related).

BACCALAUREATE PROGRAMS

Degree BSN

Available Programs Accelerated RN Baccalaureate.

Site Options Abington, PA; Lancaster, PA; Christiana, DE.

Program Entrance Requirements Minimum overall college GPA of 2.0, transcript of college record, CPR certification, health exam, interview, prerequisite course work, RN licensure. Transfer students are accepted. **Standardized tests** *Required:* SAT or ACT, TOEFL for international students. *Recommended:* SAT and SAT Subject Tests or ACT. **Application** *Deadline:* 8/15 (freshmen), rolling (transfer). *Notification:* 8/15 (freshmen). *Application fee:* $35.

Expenses (2006–07) *Tuition:* part-time $355 per credit. *Required fees:* full-time $50.

Financial Aid 50% of baccalaureate students in nursing programs received some form of financial aid in 2005–06.

Contact Ms. Tina Floyd, ACCEL Counselors, Department of Nursing, Immaculata University, 1145 King Road, Immaculata, PA 19345. *Telephone:* 610-647-4400 Ext. 3448. *Fax:* 610-251-1668. *E-mail:* accel@immaculata.edu.

Immaculata University (continued)
GRADUATE PROGRAMS

Expenses (2006–07) *Tuition:* part-time $400 per credit.

Financial Aid 25% of graduate students in nursing programs received some form of financial aid in 2005–06.

Contact Dr. Jean McAleer Klein, Coordinator, MSN Program. *Telephone:* 610-644-4400. *E-mail:* jklein@immaculata.edu.

MASTER'S DEGREE PROGRAM

Degree MSN

Available Programs Master's.

Concentrations Available Nursing administration; nursing education.

Study Options Part-time.

Program Entrance Requirements Minimum overall college GPA of 3.0, transcript of college record, interview, 3 letters of recommendation.

Advanced Placement Credit given for nursing courses completed elsewhere dependent upon specific evaluations.

Degree Requirements 36 total credit hours, thesis or project.

Indiana University of Pennsylvania
Department of Nursing and Allied Health
Indiana, Pennsylvania

Founded in 1875

DEGREES • BSN • MSN

Nursing Program Faculty 21 (67% with doctorates).

Baccalaureate Enrollment 435
Women 90% **Men** 10% **Minority** 52%

Graduate Enrollment 53
Women 87% **Men** 13% **International** 4% **Part-time** 62%

Nursing Student Activities Nursing Honor Society, Sigma Theta Tau, nursing club.

Nursing Student Resources Academic advising; academic or career counseling; assistance for students with disabilities; bookstore; campus computer network; career placement assistance; computer lab; computer-assisted instruction; e-mail services; employment services for current students; externships; housing assistance; interactive nursing skills videos; Internet; learning resource lab; library services; nursing audiovisuals; remedial services; resume preparation assistance; skills, simulation, or other laboratory; tutoring.

Library Facilities 852,531 volumes (5,758 in health, 3,395 in nursing); 16,290 periodical subscriptions (225 health-care related).

BACCALAUREATE PROGRAMS

Degree BSN

Available Programs Baccalaureate for Second Degree; Generic Baccalaureate; RN Baccalaureate.

Study Options Full-time and part-time.

Program Entrance Requirements 2 Year (s) high school math, high school transcript, minimum high school rank 20%, prerequisite course work. Transfer students are accepted. **Standardized tests** *Required:* SAT or ACT, TOEFL for international students. **Application** *Deadline:* rolling (freshmen), rolling (transfer). *Notification:* 9/15 (freshmen). *Application fee:* $35.

Advanced Placement Credit by examination available. Credit given for nursing courses completed elsewhere dependent upon specific evaluations.

GRADUATE PROGRAMS

Contact *Telephone:* 724-357-2557. *Fax:* 724-357-3267.

MASTER'S DEGREE PROGRAM

Degree MSN

Available Programs Master's; RN to Master's.

Concentrations Available Nursing administration. *Clinical nurse specialist programs in:* community health.

Site Options Monroeville, PA.

Study Options Full-time and part-time.

Program Entrance Requirements Clinical experience, computer literacy, minimum overall college GPA of 3.0, transcript of college record, written essay, 2 letters of recommendation, nursing research course, professional liability insurance/malpractice insurance, statistics course. *Application deadline:* For fall admission, 7/1 (priority date); for spring admission, 11/1. Applications are processed on a rolling basis. *Application fee:* $30.

Degree Requirements 36 total credit hours, thesis or project.

Kutztown University of Pennsylvania
Department of Nursing
Kutztown, Pennsylvania

http://www.kutztown.edu

Founded in 1866

DEGREE • BSN

Nursing Program Faculty 6 (50% with doctorates).

Baccalaureate Enrollment 122
Women 95% **Men** 5% **Minority** 1% **Part-time** 95%

Nursing Student Activities Sigma Theta Tau.

Nursing Student Resources Academic advising; academic or career counseling; assistance for students with disabilities; bookstore; campus computer network; career placement assistance; computer lab; daycare for children of students; e-mail services; employment services for current students; housing assistance; Internet; library services; nursing audiovisuals; placement services for program completers; remedial services; resume preparation assistance; skills, simulation, or other laboratory; tutoring.

Library Facilities 500,484 volumes (38,000 in health, 15,000 in nursing); 15,600 periodical subscriptions (108 health-care related).

BACCALAUREATE PROGRAMS

Degree BSN

Available Programs RN Baccalaureate.

Site Options *Distance Learning:* Reading, PA; Allentown, PA.

Study Options Full-time and part-time.

Program Entrance Requirements Transcript of college record, CPR certification, health exam, high school transcript, immunizations, minimum GPA in nursing prerequisites of 2.0, professional liability insurance/malpractice insurance, prerequisite course work, RN licensure. Transfer students are accepted. **Standardized tests** *Required:* SAT or ACT, TOEFL for international students. *Required for some:* SAT Subject Tests. **Application** *Deadline:* 3/1 (freshmen), rolling (transfer). *Notification:* 4/15 (freshmen). *Application fee:* $35.

Advanced Placement Credit by examination available. Credit given for nursing courses completed elsewhere dependent upon specific evaluations.

Financial Aid *Gift aid (need-based):* Federal Pell, FSEOG, state, private, college/university gift aid from institutional funds. *Loans:* FFEL (Subsidized and Unsubsidized Stafford PLUS), Perkins. *Work-Study:* Federal Work-Study, part-time campus jobs. *Application deadline (priority):* 2/15.

Contact Prof. Ilene S. Prokup, Chairperson, Department of Nursing, Kutztown University of Pennsylvania, 201 Beekey Education Building, Kutztown, PA 19530. *Telephone:* 610-683-4330. *Fax:* 610-683-4708. *E-mail:* prokup@kutztown.edu.

La Roche College
Department of Nursing and Nursing Management
Pittsburgh, Pennsylvania

http://www.laroche.edu

Founded in 1963

DEGREES • BSN • MSN

Nursing Program Faculty 11 (45% with doctorates).

Baccalaureate Enrollment 46
Women 89% **Men** 11% **International** 17% **Part-time** 74%

Graduate Enrollment 18
Women 83% **Men** 17% **International** 5% **Part-time** 94%

Nursing Student Activities Sigma Theta Tau.

Nursing Student Resources Academic advising; academic or career counseling; assistance for students with disabilities; bookstore; campus computer network; computer lab; e-mail services; externships; Internet; library services; resume preparation assistance; tutoring.

Library Facilities 108,432 volumes; 601 periodical subscriptions (713 health-care related).

BACCALAUREATE PROGRAMS

Degree BSN

Available Programs Accelerated RN Baccalaureate; RN Baccalaureate.
Site Options Pittsburgh, PA.
Study Options Full-time and part-time.
Program Entrance Requirements Minimum overall college GPA of 2.5, transcript of college record, high school transcript, 2 letters of recommendation, professional liability insurance/malpractice insurance, prerequisite course work, RN licensure. Transfer students are accepted.
Standardized tests *Required:* SAT or ACT, TOEFL for international students. **Application** *Deadline:* rolling (freshmen), rolling (transfer). *Notification:* 9/15 (freshmen). *Application fee:* $50.
Advanced Placement Credit by examination available. Credit given for nursing courses completed elsewhere dependent upon specific evaluations.
Expenses (2006–07) *Tuition:* full-time $8810; part-time $528 per credit hour.
Financial Aid 87% of baccalaureate students in nursing programs received some form of financial aid in 2005–06.
Contact Ms. Hope A. Schiffgens, Director, Graduate Studies and Adult Education, Department of Nursing and Nursing Management, La Roche College, Graduate Studies and Adult Education, 9000 Babcock Boulevard, Pittsburgh, PA 15237. *Telephone:* 412-536-1266. *Fax:* 412-536-1283. *E-mail:* hope.schiffgens@laroche.edu.

GRADUATE PROGRAMS

Expenses (2006–07) *Tuition:* full-time $8810; part-time $550 per credit hour.
Contact Ms. Hope A. Schiffgens, Director, Graduate Studies and Adult Education, Department of Nursing and Nursing Management, La Roche College, Graduate Studies and Adult Education, 9000 Babcock Boulevard, Pittsburgh, PA 15237. *Telephone:* 412-536-1262. *Fax:* 412-536-1283. *E-mail:* hope.schiffgens@laroche.edu.

MASTER'S DEGREE PROGRAM

Degree MSN

Available Programs Master's; RN to Master's.
Concentrations Available Nursing administration. *Nurse practitioner programs in:* family health.
Study Options Full-time and part-time.
Program Entrance Requirements Clinical experience, minimum overall college GPA of 3.0, transcript of college record, immunizations, interview, 2 letters of recommendation, professional liability insurance/ malpractice insurance, resume.
Advanced Placement Credit given for nursing courses completed elsewhere dependent upon specific evaluations.
Degree Requirements 41 total credit hours.

CONTINUING EDUCATION PROGRAM

Contact Ms. Hope A. Schiffgens, Director, Graduate Studies and Adult Education, Department of Nursing and Nursing Management, La Roche College, Graduate Studies and Adult Education, 9000 Babcock Boulevard, Pittsburgh, PA 15237. *Telephone:* 412-536-1262. *Fax:* 412-536-1283. *E-mail:* hope.schiffgens@laroche.edu.

La Salle University
School of Nursing and Health Sciences
Philadelphia, Pennsylvania

http://www.lasalle.edu/academ/nursing
Founded in 1863

DEGREES • BSN • MSN • MSN/MBA

Nursing Program Faculty 45 (32% with doctorates).

Nursing Student Activities Sigma Theta Tau, Student Nurses' Association, nursing club.

Nursing Student Resources Academic advising; academic or career counseling; assistance for students with disabilities; bookstore; campus computer network; career placement assistance; computer lab; computer-assisted instruction; e-mail services; employment services for current students; externships; housing assistance; interactive nursing skills videos; Internet; learning resource lab; library services; nursing audiovisuals; placement services for program completers; remedial services; resume preparation assistance; skills, simulation, or other laboratory; tutoring.

Library Facilities 400,000 volumes (8,350 in nursing); 9,250 periodical subscriptions (310 health-care related).

BACCALAUREATE PROGRAMS

Degree BSN

Available Programs Baccalaureate for Second Degree; Generic Baccalaureate; LPN to Baccalaureate; RN Baccalaureate.
Site Options Newtown, PA.
Study Options Full-time and part-time.
Program Entrance Requirements Minimum overall college GPA of 2.75, transcript of college record, CPR certification, written essay, health exam, health insurance, high school biology, high school chemistry, 3 years high school math, 3 years high school science, high school transcript, immunizations, interview, 2 letters of recommendation, minimum high school GPA of 3.0, minimum high school rank 25%, minimum GPA in nursing prerequisites of 2.75, professional liability insurance/malpractice insurance, prerequisite course work. Transfer students are accepted.
Standardized tests *Required:* SAT or ACT, TOEFL for international students. **Application** *Deadline:* 8/15 (transfer). *Early decision:* 11/15. *Notification:* continuous (freshmen), 12/15 (early action). *Application fee:* $35.
Advanced Placement Credit by examination available. Credit given for nursing courses completed elsewhere dependent upon specific evaluations.
Contact *Telephone:* 215-951-1430. *Fax:* 215-951-1896.

GRADUATE PROGRAMS

Contact *Telephone:* 215-951-1413. *Fax:* 215-951-1896.

MASTER'S DEGREE PROGRAM

Degrees MSN; MSN/MBA

Available Programs Master's; RN to Master's.
Concentrations Available Nurse anesthesia; nursing administration. *Clinical nurse specialist programs in:* adult health, public health. *Nurse practitioner programs in:* adult health, family health.
Site Options Newtown, PA.
Study Options Full-time and part-time.
Program Entrance Requirements Clinical experience, minimum overall college GPA of 3.0, transcript of college record, CPR certification, written essay, immunizations, interview, 2 letters of recommendation, nursing research course, physical assessment course, professional liability insurance/malpractice insurance, resume, statistics course.
Advanced Placement Credit given for nursing courses completed elsewhere dependent upon specific evaluations.
Degree Requirements 41 total credit hours.

POST-MASTER'S PROGRAM

Areas of Study Nurse anesthesia; nursing administration; nursing education. *Clinical nurse specialist programs in:* adult health, public health. *Nurse practitioner programs in:* adult health, family health.

La Salle University (continued)
CONTINUING EDUCATION PROGRAM
Contact *Telephone:* 215-951-1432. *Fax:* 215-951-1896.

Mansfield University of Pennsylvania
Robert Packer Department of Health Sciences
Mansfield, Pennsylvania

http://www.mansfield.edu

Founded in 1857

DEGREES • BSN • MSN

Nursing Program Faculty 13 (40% with doctorates).

Baccalaureate Enrollment 190
Women 95% **Men** 5% **Minority** 5% **International** 1% **Part-time** 10%

Graduate Enrollment 38
Women 100% **Minority** 1% **Part-time** 100%

Nursing Student Activities Student Nurses' Association, nursing club.

Nursing Student Resources Academic advising; academic or career counseling; assistance for students with disabilities; bookstore; campus computer network; career placement assistance; computer lab; daycare for children of students; e-mail services; employment services for current students; housing assistance; Internet; learning resource lab; library services; nursing audiovisuals; remedial services; resume preparation assistance; skills, simulation, or other laboratory; tutoring.

Library Facilities 246,141 volumes (12,000 in health, 2,200 in nursing); 2,948 periodical subscriptions (530 health-care related).

BACCALAUREATE PROGRAMS
Degree BSN

Available Programs Generic Baccalaureate; RN Baccalaureate.

Site Options *Distance Learning:* Sayre, PA.

Study Options Full-time and part-time.

Program Entrance Requirements Minimum overall college GPA of 2.7, transcript of college record, CPR certification, health exam, health insurance, high school biology, high school chemistry, 2 years high school math, 2 years high school science, high school transcript, immunizations, minimum high school GPA of 2.7, minimum high school rank 60%, professional liability insurance/malpractice insurance. Transfer students are accepted. **Standardized tests** *Required:* SAT or ACT, TOEFL for international students. **Application** *Deadline:* rolling (freshmen), rolling (transfer). *Notification:* continuous (freshmen). *Application fee:* $25.

Advanced Placement Credit by examination available. Credit given for nursing courses completed elsewhere dependent upon specific evaluations.

Expenses (2006–07) *Tuition, area resident:* full-time $4906; part-time $204 per credit. *Tuition, nonresident:* full-time $12,266; part-time $511 per course. *International tuition:* $12,266 full-time. *Room and board:* $6120; room only: $3824 per academic year. *Required fees:* full-time $1638; part-time $210 per credit.

Financial Aid 90% of baccalaureate students in nursing programs received some form of financial aid in 2005–06.

Contact Admissions Office, Robert Packer Department of Health Sciences, Mansfield University of Pennsylvania, Alumni Hall, Mansfield, PA 16933. *Telephone:* 570-662-4243. *Fax:* 570-662-4121. *E-mail:* admissns@mnsfld.edu.

GRADUATE PROGRAMS
Expenses (2006–07) *Tuition, state resident:* full-time $6048; part-time $336 per credit. *Tuition, nonresident:* full-time $9678; part-time $583 per credit. *International tuition:* $9678 full-time. *Required fees:* full-time $1090; part-time $70 per credit; part-time $420 per term.

Financial Aid 50% of graduate students in nursing programs received some form of financial aid in 2005–06.

Contact Dr. Janeen Bartlett Sheehe, Department Chair and Nursing Program Director, Robert Packer Department of Health Sciences, Mansfield University of Pennsylvania, 212C Elliott Hall, Mansfield, PA 16933. *Telephone:* 570-662-4522. *Fax:* 570-662-4137. *E-mail:* jsheehe@mansfield.edu.

MASTER'S DEGREE PROGRAM
Degree MSN

Available Programs Master's.

Concentrations Available Nursing education.

Study Options Part-time.

Program Entrance Requirements Minimum overall college GPA of 3.0, transcript of college record, 1 letter of recommendation, prerequisite course work.

Degree Requirements 33 total credit hours, thesis or project.

Marywood University
Department of Nursing
Scranton, Pennsylvania

http://www.marywood.edu/uscat/nurs.htm

Founded in 1915

DEGREES • BSN • MSN • MSN/MPH

Nursing Program Faculty 16 (60% with doctorates).

Baccalaureate Enrollment 140
Women 90% **Men** 10% **Minority** 5% **International** 3% **Part-time** 5%

Graduate Enrollment 7
Women 100% **Part-time** 90%

Nursing Student Activities Sigma Theta Tau, Student Nurses' Association.

Nursing Student Resources Academic advising; academic or career counseling; assistance for students with disabilities; bookstore; campus computer network; computer lab; daycare for children of students; e-mail services; employment services for current students; interactive nursing skills videos; Internet; learning resource lab; library services; nursing audiovisuals; skills, simulation, or other laboratory; tutoring.

Library Facilities 219,794 volumes (7,400 in health, 3,006 in nursing); 14,656 periodical subscriptions (750 health-care related).

BACCALAUREATE PROGRAMS
Degree BSN

Available Programs ADN to Baccalaureate; Generic Baccalaureate; International Nurse to Baccalaureate; LPN to Baccalaureate; RN Baccalaureate.

Study Options Full-time and part-time.

Program Entrance Requirements Transcript of college record, high school biology, high school chemistry, 1 year of high school math, high school transcript, 1 letter of recommendation. Transfer students are accepted. **Standardized tests** *Required:* SAT or ACT, TOEFL for international students. **Application** *Deadline:* rolling (freshmen), rolling (transfer). *Notification:* continuous (freshmen). *Application fee:* $30.

Advanced Placement Credit given for nursing courses completed elsewhere dependent upon specific evaluations.

Expenses (2006–07) *Tuition:* full-time $21,840; part-time $600 per credit. *International tuition:* $21,840 full-time. *Room and board:* $9690; room only: $5514 per academic year. *Required fees:* full-time $830; part-time $280 per term.

Financial Aid 90% of baccalaureate students in nursing programs received some form of financial aid in 2005–06.

Contact Dr. Robin Gallagher, Chairperson, Department of Nursing, Marywood University, Center for Natural and Health Science, 2300 Adams Avenue, Scranton, PA 18509. *Telephone:* 570-348-6211 Ext. 2475. *Fax:* 570-961-4761. *E-mail:* gallagher@marywood.edu.

GRADUATE PROGRAMS
Expenses (2006–07) *Tuition:* part-time $672 per credit. *Room and board:* $9690; room only: $5514 per academic year. *Required fees:* full-time $830; part-time $280 per term.

Financial Aid 90% of graduate students in nursing programs received some form of financial aid in 2005–06.

Contact Dr. Robin Gallagher, Chairperson, Department of Nursing, Marywood University, Center for Natural and Health Science, 2300 Adams Avenue, Scranton, PA 18509. *Telephone:* 570-348-6211 Ext. 2475. *Fax:* 570-961-4761. *E-mail:* gallagher@marywood.edu.

MASTER'S DEGREE PROGRAM

Degrees MSN; MSN/MPH

Available Programs Master's.

Concentrations Available Nursing administration.

Study Options Full-time and part-time.

Program Entrance Requirements Clinical experience, minimum overall college GPA of 3.0, transcript of college record, written essay, 2 letters of recommendation, nursing research course, physical assessment course, statistics course.

Degree Requirements 39 total credit hours, thesis or project.

CONTINUING EDUCATION PROGRAM

Contact Dr. Bernadette Russell, Dean, Continuing Education, Department of Nursing, Marywood University, McGowen Center, Room 1039, 2300 Adams Avenue, Scranton, PA 18509. *Telephone:* 570-340-6060. *Fax:* 570-961-4776. *E-mail:* russellb@marywood.edu.

Messiah College
Department of Nursing
Grantham, Pennsylvania

http://www.messiah.edu
Founded in 1909

DEGREE • BSN

Nursing Program Faculty 15 (20% with doctorates).

Baccalaureate Enrollment 215
Women 95% **Men** 5% **Minority** 7% **International** 2% **Part-time** 1%

Nursing Student Activities Nursing Honor Society, Sigma Theta Tau, Student Nurses' Association.

Nursing Student Resources Academic advising; academic or career counseling; assistance for students with disabilities; bookstore; campus computer network; career placement assistance; computer lab; computer-assisted instruction; e-mail services; employment services for current students; interactive nursing skills videos; Internet; learning resource lab; library services; nursing audiovisuals; remedial services; resume preparation assistance; skills, simulation, or other laboratory; tutoring.

Library Facilities 293,357 volumes (7,580 in health, 510 in nursing); 20,219 periodical subscriptions (1,430 health-care related).

BACCALAUREATE PROGRAMS

Degree BSN

Available Programs Generic Baccalaureate.

Study Options Full-time and part-time.

Program Entrance Requirements Minimum overall college GPA of 2.5, transcript of college record, CPR certification, written essay, health exam, health insurance, high school foreign language, 2 years high school math, 2 years high school science, high school transcript, immunizations, 2 letters of recommendation, minimum GPA in nursing prerequisites of 2.5, prerequisite course work. Transfer students are accepted. **Standardized tests** *Required:* TOEFL for international students. *Required for some:* SAT or ACT. **Application** *Deadline:* rolling (freshmen). *Notification:* continuous (freshmen), continuous (early decision). *Application fee:* $30.

Expenses (2006–07) *Tuition:* full-time $22,600; part-time $950 per credit. *International tuition:* $22,600 full-time. *Room and board:* $7060; room only: $3680 per academic year. *Required fees:* full-time $440.

Financial Aid 98% of baccalaureate students in nursing programs received some form of financial aid in 2005–06. *Gift aid (need-based):* Federal Pell, FSEOG, state, private, college/university gift aid from institutional funds. *Loans:* Federal Nursing Student Loans, Federal Direct (Subsidized and Unsubsidized Stafford PLUS), Perkins. *Work-Study:* Federal Work-Study, part-time campus jobs. *Application deadline (priority):* 4/1.

Contact Scott Morrell, Dean of Enrollment Management, Department of Nursing, Messiah College, PO Box 3005, One College Avenue, Grantham, PA 17027. *Telephone:* 800-233-4220. *Fax:* 717-796-5374. *E-mail:* admiss@messiah.edu.

Millersville University of Pennsylvania
Department of Nursing
Millersville, Pennsylvania

http://muweb.millersville.edu/~nursing/
Founded in 1855

DEGREES • BSN • MSN

Nursing Program Faculty 5 (100% with doctorates).

Baccalaureate Enrollment 40
Women 95% **Men** 5% **Minority** 18% **Part-time** 80%

Graduate Enrollment 41
Women 86% **Men** 14% **Minority** 3% **Part-time** 100%

Nursing Student Activities Sigma Theta Tau.

Nursing Student Resources Academic advising; academic or career counseling; assistance for students with disabilities; bookstore; computer lab; e-mail services; interactive nursing skills videos; Internet; library services; nursing audiovisuals.

Library Facilities 515,381 volumes; 10,105 periodical subscriptions (82 health-care related).

BACCALAUREATE PROGRAMS

Degree BSN

Available Programs RN Baccalaureate.

Study Options Full-time and part-time.

Program Entrance Requirements Transcript of college record, CPR certification, health exam, immunizations, professional liability insurance/malpractice insurance, RN licensure. Transfer students are accepted. **Standardized tests** *Required:* SAT or ACT, TOEFL for international students. **Application** *Deadline:* rolling (freshmen), rolling (transfer). *Notification:* continuous (freshmen). *Application fee:* $35.

Expenses (2006–07) *Tuition, state resident:* part-time $630 per course. *Tuition, nonresident:* part-time $1575 per course. *Room and board:* $3114 per academic year. *Required fees:* part-time $186 per term.

Financial Aid 75% of baccalaureate students in nursing programs received some form of financial aid in 2005–06.

Contact Dr. Deborah T. Castellucci, Chairperson, Department of Nursing, Millersville University of Pennsylvania, Caputo Hall, Millersville, PA 17551-0302. *Telephone:* 717-871-5431. *Fax:* 717-871-4877. *E-mail:* Deborah.Castellucci@millersville.edu.

GRADUATE PROGRAMS

Expenses (2006–07) *Tuition, state resident:* part-time $1008 per course. *Tuition, nonresident:* part-time $1614 per course. *Room and board:* $3114 per academic year. *Required fees:* part-time $217 per credit.

Financial Aid 5% of graduate students in nursing programs received some form of financial aid in 2005–06. 1 research assistantship with full tuition reimbursement available (averaging $4,000 per year) was awarded; Federal Work-Study, institutionally sponsored loans, and unspecified assistantships also available. Aid available to part-time students. *Financial aid application deadline:* 3/15.

Contact Dr. Ruth E. Davis, EdD, Graduate Program Coordinator, Department of Nursing, Millersville University of Pennsylvania, Caputo Hall, Room 119, PO Box 1002, Millersville, PA 17551-0302. *Telephone:* 717-871-2183. *Fax:* 717-871-4887. *E-mail:* ruth.davis@millersville.edu.

MASTER'S DEGREE PROGRAM

Degree MSN

Available Programs Master's.

Concentrations Available Nursing education. *Clinical nurse specialist programs in:* family health. *Nurse practitioner programs in:* family health.

Study Options Part-time.

Program Entrance Requirements Clinical experience, minimum overall college GPA of 3.0, transcript of college record, interview, 3 letters of recommendation, nursing research course, physical assessment course, resume, statistics course, GRE. *Application deadline:* For fall admission, 3/1; for spring admission, 10/1. Applications are processed on a rolling basis. *Application fee:* $35.

Millersville University of Pennsylvania (continued)

Advanced Placement Credit given for nursing courses completed elsewhere dependent upon specific evaluations.

Degree Requirements 38 total credit hours, thesis or project.

POST-MASTER'S PROGRAM

Areas of Study *Clinical nurse specialist programs in:* family health. *Nurse practitioner programs in:* family health.

CONTINUING EDUCATION PROGRAM

Contact Ms. Bili Mattes, Director, Professional Training and Education, Department of Nursing, Millersville University of Pennsylvania, Office of Professional Training and Education, PO Box 1002, Millersville, PA 17551-0302. *Telephone:* 717-872-3030. *Fax:* 717-871-2022. *E-mail:* bili. mattes@millersville.edu.

Moravian College
St. Luke's School of Nursing
Bethlehem, Pennsylvania

http://www.moravian.edu/academics/ departments/nursing

Founded in 1742

DEGREE • BS

Nursing Program Faculty 20 (55% with doctorates).

Baccalaureate Enrollment 86
Women 91% **Men** 9% **Minority** 8% **International** 1%

Nursing Student Activities Sigma Theta Tau, Student Nurses' Association.

Nursing Student Resources Academic advising; academic or career counseling; assistance for students with disabilities; bookstore; campus computer network; career placement assistance; computer lab; computer-assisted instruction; e-mail services; employment services for current students; externships; housing assistance; interactive nursing skills videos; Internet; learning resource lab; library services; nursing audiovisuals; paid internships; placement services for program completers; remedial services; resume preparation assistance; skills, simulation, or other laboratory; tutoring.

Library Facilities 260,363 volumes (4,600 in health, 1,900 in nursing); 3,274 periodical subscriptions (275 health-care related).

BACCALAUREATE PROGRAMS

Degree BS

Available Programs Generic Baccalaureate; RN Baccalaureate.

Study Options Full-time.

Program Entrance Requirements CPR certification, written essay, health exam, health insurance, high school foreign language, 3 years high school math, high school transcript, immunizations, interview, professional liability insurance/malpractice insurance. Transfer students are accepted. **Standardized tests** *Required:* SAT or ACT, TOEFL for international students. **Application** *Deadline:* 3/1 (freshmen), 3/1 (transfer). *Early decision:* 2/1. *Notification:* 3/15 (freshmen), 12/15 (out-of-state freshmen), 12/15 (early decision). *Application fee:* $40.

Advanced Placement Credit by examination available. Credit given for nursing courses completed elsewhere dependent upon specific evaluations.

Expenses (2006–07) *Tuition:* full-time $26,300. *International tuition:* $26,300 full-time. *Room and board:* $7485; room only: $4085 per academic year. *Required fees:* full-time $475.

Financial Aid 90% of baccalaureate students in nursing programs received some form of financial aid in 2005–06. *Gift aid (need-based):* Federal Pell, FSEOG, state, private, college/university gift aid from institutional funds. *Loans:* FFEL (Subsidized and Unsubsidized Stafford PLUS), Perkins. *Work-Study:* Federal Work-Study, part-time campus jobs. *Application deadline (priority):* 2/15.

Contact Mr. James P. Mackin, Director of Admissions, St. Luke's School of Nursing, Moravian College, 1200 Main Street, Bethlehem, PA 18018. *Telephone:* 800-441-3191. *E-mail:* mejpm01@moravian.edu.

CONTINUING EDUCATION PROGRAM

Contact Dr. Florence Kimball, Dean, St. Luke's School of Nursing, Moravian College, Continuing and Graduate Studies, 1200 Main Street, Bethlehem, PA 18018. *Telephone:* 610-861-1300. *E-mail:* fkimball@ moravian.edu.

Mount Aloysius College
Department of Nursing
Cresson, Pennsylvania

http://www.mtaloy.edu

Founded in 1939

DEGREE • BSN

Nursing Program Faculty 4 (25% with doctorates).

Baccalaureate Enrollment 76
Women 90% **Men** 10% **Part-time** 91%

Nursing Student Activities Student Nurses' Association.

Nursing Student Resources Academic advising; academic or career counseling; assistance for students with disabilities; bookstore; campus computer network; career placement assistance; computer lab; computer-assisted instruction; daycare for children of students; e-mail services; externships; housing assistance; interactive nursing skills videos; Internet; learning resource lab; library services; nursing audiovisuals; placement services for program completers; remedial services; resume preparation assistance; skills, simulation, or other laboratory; tutoring; unpaid internships.

Library Facilities 91,544 volumes (6,773 in health, 1,121 in nursing); 275 periodical subscriptions (67 health-care related).

BACCALAUREATE PROGRAMS

Degree BSN

Available Programs ADN to Baccalaureate; Accelerated RN Baccalaureate.

Site Options Johnstown, PA; Altoona, PA.

Study Options Full-time and part-time.

Program Entrance Requirements Transcript of college record, CPR certification, health exam, high school transcript, immunizations, RN licensure. Transfer students are accepted. **Standardized tests** *Required:* SAT or ACT, TOEFL for international students. **Application** *Deadline:* rolling (freshmen), rolling (transfer). *Notification:* continuous (freshmen). *Application fee:* $30.

Advanced Placement Credit by examination available. Credit given for nursing courses completed elsewhere dependent upon specific evaluations.

Contact *Telephone:* 814-886-6305. *Fax:* 814-886-6374.

CONTINUING EDUCATION PROGRAM

Contact *Telephone:* 814-886-6361. *Fax:* 814-886-2978.

Neumann College
Program in Nursing and Health Sciences
Aston, Pennsylvania

Founded in 1965

DEGREES • BS • MS

Nursing Program Faculty 26 (24% with doctorates).

Baccalaureate Enrollment 500
Women 93% **Men** 7% **Minority** 15% **International** 2% **Part-time** 22%

Graduate Enrollment 28
Women 91% **Men** 9% **Minority** 12% **Part-time** 4%

Nursing Student Activities Nursing Honor Society, Sigma Theta Tau, Student Nurses' Association.

Nursing Student Resources Academic advising; academic or career counseling; assistance for students with disabilities; bookstore; campus computer network; career placement assistance; computer lab; computer-assisted instruction; daycare for children of students; e-mail services; employment services for current students; externships; interactive nursing skills videos; Internet; learning resource lab; library services; nursing audiovisuals; remedial services; resume preparation assistance; skills, simulation, or other laboratory; tutoring.

Library Facilities 75,000 volumes (3,956 in health, 1,170 in nursing); 400 periodical subscriptions (155 health-care related).

BACCALAUREATE PROGRAMS

Degree BS

Available Programs Baccalaureate for Second Degree; Generic Baccalaureate; International Nurse to Baccalaureate; RN Baccalaureate.

Study Options Full-time and part-time.

Program Entrance Requirements Minimum overall college GPA of 2.5, transcript of college record, CPR certification, health exam, health insurance, high school biology, high school chemistry, high school foreign language, 2 years high school math, 3 years high school science, high school transcript, immunizations, minimum high school GPA of 2.5, minimum GPA in nursing prerequisites of 2.5, prerequisite course work. Transfer students are accepted. **Standardized tests** *Required:* SAT or ACT, TOEFL for international students. **Application** *Deadline:* 4/1 (freshmen), rolling (transfer). *Notification:* continuous (freshmen). *Application fee:* $35.

Advanced Placement Credit by examination available. Credit given for nursing courses completed elsewhere dependent upon specific evaluations.

Expenses (2006–07) *Tuition:* full-time $18,000; part-time $411 per credit hour. *Room and board:* $9100; room only: $6000 per academic year. *Required fees:* full-time $1560; part-time $760 per term.

Financial Aid 95% of baccalaureate students in nursing programs received some form of financial aid in 2005–06. *Gift aid (need-based):* Federal Pell, FSEOG, state, private, college/university gift aid from institutional funds. *Loans:* Federal Nursing Student Loans, Federal Direct (Subsidized and Unsubsidized Stafford PLUS), FFEL (Subsidized and Unsubsidized Stafford PLUS), Perkins. *Work-Study:* Federal Work-Study, part-time campus jobs. *Application deadline:* Continuous.

Contact Miss Brianna Pastor, Admissions Counselor, Program in Nursing and Health Sciences, Neumann College, One Neumann Drive, Aston, PA 19014-1298. *Telephone:* 800-963-8626 Ext. 5531. *Fax:* 610-558-5652. *E-mail:* nursediv@neumann.edu.

GRADUATE PROGRAMS

Expenses (2006–07) *Tuition:* part-time $499 per credit hour.

Financial Aid 50% of graduate students in nursing programs received some form of financial aid in 2005–06. Available to part-time students. *Application deadline:* 3/15.

Contact Mrs. Louise Bank, Admissions Counselor, Program in Nursing and Health Sciences, Neumann College, One Neumann Drive, Aston, PA 19014-1298. *Telephone:* 800-963-8626 Ext. 5613. *Fax:* 610-558-5652. *E-mail:* nursediv@neumann.edu.

MASTER'S DEGREE PROGRAM

Degree MS

Available Programs Master's.

Concentrations Available Nursing education. *Nurse practitioner programs in:* gerontology.

Study Options Full-time and part-time.

Program Entrance Requirements Minimum overall college GPA of 3.0, transcript of college record, CPR certification, immunizations, interview, 2 letters of recommendation, nursing research course, physical assessment course, professional liability insurance/malpractice insurance, statistics course, GRE or MAT. *Application deadline:* Applications are processed on a rolling basis. *Application fee:* $50.

Advanced Placement Credit by examination available. Credit given for nursing courses completed elsewhere dependent upon specific evaluations.

Degree Requirements 45 total credit hours.

POST-MASTER'S PROGRAM

Areas of Study Nursing education. *Nurse practitioner programs in:* gerontology.

Penn State University Park
School of Nursing
State College, University Park, Pennsylvania

http://www.hhdev.psu.edu/nurs
Founded in 1855
DEGREES • BS • MS • MSN/PHD

Nursing Program Faculty 110 (20% with doctorates).

Baccalaureate Enrollment 838
Women 91% **Men** 9% **Minority** 7% **International** 1% **Part-time** 43%

Graduate Enrollment 63
Women 95% **Men** 5% **Minority** 3% **International** 3% **Part-time** 54%

Nursing Student Activities Sigma Theta Tau, Student Nurses' Association.

Nursing Student Resources Academic advising; academic or career counseling; assistance for students with disabilities; bookstore; campus computer network; career placement assistance; computer lab; computer-assisted instruction; daycare for children of students; e-mail services; employment services for current students; externships; housing assistance; interactive nursing skills videos; Internet; learning resource lab; library services; nursing audiovisuals; paid internships; remedial services; resume preparation assistance; skills, simulation, or other laboratory; tutoring.

Library Facilities 5 million volumes (244,000 in health); 68,445 periodical subscriptions (3,500 health-care related).

BACCALAUREATE PROGRAMS

Degree BS

Available Programs ADN to Baccalaureate; Generic Baccalaureate; RN Baccalaureate.

Site Options *Distance Learning:* Altoona, PA; Mont Alto, PA; Worthington-Scranton, PA; Fayette, PA; New Kensington, PA; Harrisburg, PA; Hershey, PA; Shenango Valley, PA.

Study Options Full-time.

Program Entrance Requirements Transcript of college record, 3 years high school math, 3 years high school science, high school transcript. Transfer students are accepted. **Standardized tests** *Required:* SAT or ACT, TOEFL for international students. **Application** *Deadline:* rolling (freshmen), rolling (out-of-state freshmen), rolling (transfer). *Notification:* continuous (freshmen), continuous (out-of-state freshmen). *Application fee:* $50.

Advanced Placement Credit given for nursing courses completed elsewhere dependent upon specific evaluations.

Expenses (2006–07) *Tuition, state resident:* full-time $11,646; part-time $485 per credit hour. *Tuition, nonresident:* full-time $22,194; part-time $925 per credit hour. *Room and board:* $6100; room only: $4200 per academic year. *Required fees:* full-time $518.

Financial Aid 80% of baccalaureate students in nursing programs received some form of financial aid in 2005–06.

Contact Dr. Raymonde Brown, Professor in Charge of Undergraduate Programs, School of Nursing, Penn State University Park, 210 Health and Human Development East, University Park, PA 16802. *Telephone:* 814-863-2235. *Fax:* 814-863-2925. *E-mail:* rab16@psu.edu.

GRADUATE PROGRAMS

Expenses (2006–07) *Tuition, state resident:* full-time $13,972; part-time $582 per credit hour. *Tuition, nonresident:* full-time $24,900; part-time $1038 per credit hour. *Room and board:* $6100; room only: $4200 per academic year. *Required fees:* full-time $518.

Financial Aid 80% of graduate students in nursing programs received some form of financial aid in 2005–06.

Contact Janice Penrod, PhD, Assistant Professor/RN Professor in Charge of Graduate Programs, School of Nursing, Penn State University Park, 210 Health and Human Development East, University Park, PA 16802. *Telephone:* 814-863-2211. *Fax:* 814-865-3779. *E-mail:* jlp198@psu.edu.

MASTER'S DEGREE PROGRAM

Degrees MS; MSN/PhD

Available Programs Master's; RN to Master's.

Penn State University Park (continued)

Concentrations Available Nursing administration. *Clinical nurse specialist programs in:* adult health, community health, gerontology, medical-surgical. *Nurse practitioner programs in:* family health.

Site Options *Distance Learning:* Hershey, PA; Shenango Valley, PA.

Study Options Full-time and part-time.

Program Entrance Requirements Computer literacy, minimum overall college GPA of 3.0, transcript of college record, CPR certification, written essay, immunizations, 2 letters of recommendation, professional liability insurance/malpractice insurance.

Advanced Placement Credit given for nursing courses completed elsewhere dependent upon specific evaluations.

Degree Requirements 34 total credit hours, thesis or project.

POST-MASTER'S PROGRAM

Areas of Study *Nurse practitioner programs in:* family health.

DOCTORAL DEGREE PROGRAM

Degree PhD

Available Programs Doctorate.

Areas of Study Bio-behavioral research, faculty preparation, gerontology, human health and illness, illness and transition, individualized study, nursing research, nursing science.

Site Options *Distance Learning:* Hershey, PA; Shenango Valley, PA.

Program Entrance Requirements Minimum overall college GPA of 3.5, interview, 3 letters of recommendation, MSN or equivalent, writing sample.

Degree Requirements 58 total credit hours, dissertation, oral exam, written exam, residency.

POSTDOCTORAL PROGRAM

Areas of Study Gerontology.

Postdoctoral Program Contact Janice Penrod, PhD, Assistant Professor/RN Professor in Charge of Graduate Programs, School of Nursing, Penn State University Park, 210 Health and Human Development East, University Park, PA 16802. *Telephone:* 814-863-2211. *Fax:* 814-865-3779. *E-mail:* jlp198@psu.edu.

CONTINUING EDUCATION PROGRAM

Contact Ms. Madeline Mattern, Coordinator, Outreach Programs, School of Nursing, Penn State University Park, 204 Health and Human Development East, University Park, PA 16802. *Telephone:* 814-865-8469. *Fax:* 814-865-3779. *E-mail:* mfm107@psu.edu.

Pennsylvania College of Technology

School of Health Sciences
Williamsport, Pennsylvania

Founded in 1965

DEGREE • BSN

Nursing Program Faculty 37 (5% with doctorates).

Baccalaureate Enrollment 12
Women 100% **International** 1% **Part-time** 92%

Nursing Student Activities Student Nurses' Association.

Nursing Student Resources Academic advising; academic or career counseling; assistance for students with disabilities; bookstore; campus computer network; career placement assistance; computer lab; computer-assisted instruction; daycare for children of students; e-mail services; employment services for current students; externships; housing assistance; interactive nursing skills videos; Internet; learning resource lab; library services; nursing audiovisuals; placement services for program completers; remedial services; resume preparation assistance; skills, simulation, or other laboratory; tutoring.

Library Facilities 99,764 volumes; 15,977 periodical subscriptions.

BACCALAUREATE PROGRAMS

Degree BSN

Available Programs RN Baccalaureate.

Site Options *Distance Learning:* Williamsport, PA.

Program Entrance Requirements Transfer students are accepted. **Standardized tests** *Required:* TOEFL for international students. *Required for some:* SAT. **Application** *Deadline:* 7/1 (freshmen), rolling (transfer). *Application fee:* $50.

Contact *Telephone:* 800-367-9222 Ext. 4525.

Robert Morris University

School of Nursing and Allied Health
Moon Township, Pennsylvania

Founded in 1921

DEGREES • BSN • MSN

Nursing Program Faculty 13 (31% with doctorates).

Baccalaureate Enrollment 145
Women 86% **Men** 14% **Minority** 4% **International** 1% **Part-time** 8%

Graduate Enrollment 12
Women 100% **Minority** 8% **Part-time** 100%

Nursing Student Activities Nursing Honor Society, Student Nurses' Association.

Nursing Student Resources Academic advising; academic or career counseling; assistance for students with disabilities; bookstore; campus computer network; career placement assistance; computer lab; computer-assisted instruction; e-mail services; externships; housing assistance; interactive nursing skills videos; Internet; learning resource lab; library services; nursing audiovisuals; placement services for program completers; remedial services; resume preparation assistance; skills, simulation, or other laboratory; tutoring.

Library Facilities 135,806 volumes; 580 periodical subscriptions.

BACCALAUREATE PROGRAMS

Degree BSN

Available Programs Baccalaureate for Second Degree; Generic Baccalaureate; RN Baccalaureate.

Study Options Full-time and part-time.

Program Entrance Requirements Minimum overall college GPA of 2.5, transcript of college record, written essay, health exam, health insurance, high school biology, high school chemistry, 2 years high school math, 2 years high school science, high school transcript, immunizations, 2 letters of recommendation, minimum high school GPA of 3.0, minimum GPA in nursing prerequisites of 2.0, prerequisite course work, RN licensure. Transfer students are accepted. **Standardized tests** *Required:* SAT or ACT, TOEFL for international students. **Application** *Deadline:* 7/1 (freshmen), 7/1 (transfer). *Notification:* continuous (freshmen). *Application fee:* $30.

Expenses (2006–07) *Tuition:* full-time $17,920; part-time $600 per credit hour. *International tuition:* $17,920 full-time. *Room and board:* $8410; room only: $4890 per academic year. *Required fees:* full-time $300.

Financial Aid 80% of baccalaureate students in nursing programs received some form of financial aid in 2005–06. *Gift aid (need-based):* Federal Pell, FSEOG, state, private, college/university gift aid from institutional funds. *Loans:* FFEL (Subsidized and Unsubsidized Stafford PLUS), Perkins, alternative private loans. *Work-Study:* Federal Work-Study, part-time campus jobs. *Application deadline:* Continuous.

Contact Mr. Edward J. Lamm, Assistant Dean, Undergraduate Enrollment, School of Nursing and Allied Health, Robert Morris University, 6001 University Boulevard, Moon Township, PA 15108-1189. *Telephone:* 412-262-8206. *Fax:* 412-397-2425. *E-mail:* lamm@rmu.edu.

GRADUATE PROGRAMS

Expenses (2006–07) *Tuition:* part-time $605 per credit hour. *Room and board:* $8410; room only: $4890 per academic year.

Financial Aid 80% of graduate students in nursing programs received some form of financial aid in 2005–06. Federal Work-Study, institutionally sponsored loans, and unspecified assistantships available. *Financial aid application deadline:* 5/1.

Contact Mr. Barry Bilitski, Assistant Dean, Graduate Enrollment, School of Nursing and Allied Health, Robert Morris University, 6001 University Boulevard, Moon Township, PA 15108-1189. *Telephone:* 412-397-2489. *Fax:* 412-397-2425. *E-mail:* bilitski@rmu.edu.

MASTER'S DEGREE PROGRAM

Degree MSN

Available Programs Master's.

Study Options Part-time.

Program Entrance Requirements Clinical experience, computer literacy, transcript of college record, CPR certification, written essay, 2 letters of recommendation, resume, statistics course. *Application deadline:* For fall admission, 7/1 (priority date); for spring admission, 11/1 (priority date). Applications are processed on a rolling basis. *Application fee:* $35.

Degree Requirements 36 total credit hours.

Saint Francis University
Department of Nursing
Loretto, Pennsylvania

http://www.francis.edu/academic/Undergraduate/Nursing/Nursinghome.shtml

Founded in 1847

DEGREE • BSN

Nursing Program Faculty 6.

Nursing Student Activities Student Nurses' Association, nursing club.

Nursing Student Resources Academic advising; academic or career counseling; assistance for students with disabilities; bookstore; campus computer network; career placement assistance; computer lab; computer-assisted instruction; e-mail services; employment services for current students; externships; interactive nursing skills videos; Internet; learning resource lab; library services; nursing audiovisuals; resume preparation assistance; skills, simulation, or other laboratory; tutoring.

Library Facilities 118,333 volumes (120,000 in nursing); 7,202 periodical subscriptions.

BACCALAUREATE PROGRAMS

Degree BSN

Available Programs Generic Baccalaureate; RN Baccalaureate.

Study Options Full-time and part-time.

Program Entrance Requirements Transcript of college record, high school biology, high school chemistry, 2 years high school math, 2 years high school science, high school transcript, minimum high school GPA of 3.0, minimum high school rank 50%, minimum GPA in nursing prerequisites of 2.0, prerequisite course work. Transfer students are accepted. **Standardized tests** *Required:* SAT or ACT, TOEFL for international students. **Application** *Deadline:* rolling (freshmen), rolling (out-of-state freshmen), rolling (transfer). *Application fee:* $30.

Advanced Placement Credit by examination available. Credit given for nursing courses completed elsewhere dependent upon specific evaluations.

Contact *Telephone:* 814-472-3027. *Fax:* 814-472-3849.

Slippery Rock University of Pennsylvania
Department of Nursing
Slippery Rock, Pennsylvania

http://www.sru.edu/depts/chbs/Nursing/nursing.htm

Founded in 1889

DEGREES • BSN • MSN

Nursing Program Faculty 7 (72% with doctorates).

Baccalaureate Enrollment 254
Women 95% **Men** 5% **Minority** 1% **Part-time** 93%

Graduate Enrollment 65
Women 90% **Men** 10% **Minority** 1% **Part-time** 75%

Nursing Student Activities Sigma Theta Tau, nursing club.

Nursing Student Resources Academic advising; academic or career counseling; assistance for students with disabilities; bookstore; campus computer network; career placement assistance; computer lab; computer-assisted instruction; daycare for children of students; e-mail services; employment services for current students; housing assistance; Internet; library services; nursing audiovisuals; placement services for program completers; resume preparation assistance; tutoring.

Library Facilities 503,376 volumes (7,214 in health, 925 in nursing); 599 periodical subscriptions (1,299 health-care related).

BACCALAUREATE PROGRAMS

Degree BSN

Available Programs ADN to Baccalaureate; RN Baccalaureate.

Study Options Full-time and part-time.

Program Entrance Requirements Minimum overall college GPA of 2.5, transcript of college record, professional liability insurance/malpractice insurance, RN licensure. Transfer students are accepted. **Standardized tests** *Required:* SAT or ACT, TOEFL for international students. **Application Notification:** 9/1 (freshmen). *Application fee:* $25.

Advanced Placement Credit by examination available. Credit given for nursing courses completed elsewhere dependent upon specific evaluations.

Expenses (2006–07) *Tuition, area resident:* full-time $2519; part-time $630 per course. *Tuition, nonresident:* full-time $3779; part-time $643 per course. *Required fees:* full-time $356; part-time $35 per credit.

Financial Aid 45% of baccalaureate students in nursing programs received some form of financial aid in 2005–06. *Gift aid (need-based):* Federal Pell, FSEOG, state, private, college/university gift aid from institutional funds. *Loans:* FFEL (Subsidized and Unsubsidized Stafford PLUS), Perkins. *Work-Study:* Federal Work-Study, part-time campus jobs. *Application deadline (priority):* 5/1.

Contact Dr. Ramona Nelson, Professor and Chair, Department of Nursing, Slippery Rock University of Pennsylvania, 119 Behavioral Science Building, Slippery Rock, PA 16057. *Telephone:* 724-738-2325. *Fax:* 724-738-2509. *E-mail:* ramona.nelson@sru.edu.

GRADUATE PROGRAMS

Financial Aid Teaching assistantships, institutionally sponsored loans, scholarships, traineeships, and unspecified assistantships available.

Contact Dr. Alice Conway, Director and Coordinator, Department of Nursing, Slippery Rock University of Pennsylvania, Edinboro, PA 16444. *Telephone:* 814-732-2285. *E-mail:* aconway@edinboro.edu.

MASTER'S DEGREE PROGRAM

Degree MSN

Available Programs RN to Master's.

Concentrations Available Nursing education. *Nurse practitioner programs in:* family health.

Study Options Full-time and part-time.

Program Entrance Requirements Clinical experience, computer literacy, minimum overall college GPA of 2.75, transcript of college record, CPR certification, written essay, immunizations, interview, 3 letters of recommendation, professional liability insurance/malpractice insurance, statistics course. *Application deadline:* For fall admission, 7/1 (priority date); for spring admission, 11/1 (priority date). Applications are processed on a rolling basis. *Application fee:* $30.

Advanced Placement Credit by examination available. Credit given for nursing courses completed elsewhere dependent upon specific evaluations.

Degree Requirements 45 total credit hours, thesis or project, comprehensive exam.

POST-MASTER'S PROGRAM

Areas of Study Nursing education. *Nurse practitioner programs in:* family health.

Temple University
Department of Nursing
Philadelphia, Pennsylvania

http://www.temple.edu/nursing

Founded in 1884

DEGREES • BSN • MSN

Nursing Program Faculty 37 (50% with doctorates).

Baccalaureate Enrollment 350
Women 85% **Men** 15% **Minority** 49% **Part-time** 62%

Graduate Enrollment 40
Women 95% **Men** 5% **Minority** 16% **Part-time** 100%

Nursing Student Activities Sigma Theta Tau, Student Nurses' Association.

Nursing Student Resources Academic advising; academic or career counseling; assistance for students with disabilities; bookstore; campus computer network; career placement assistance; computer lab; computer-assisted instruction; e-mail services; externships; housing assistance; interactive nursing skills videos; Internet; learning resource lab; library services; nursing audiovisuals; remedial services; resume preparation assistance; skills, simulation, or other laboratory; tutoring.

Library Facilities 3.3 million volumes (60,374 in health, 1,350 in nursing); 20,980 periodical subscriptions (1,350 health-care related).

BACCALAUREATE PROGRAMS
Degree BSN

Available Programs Accelerated Baccalaureate; Accelerated Baccalaureate for Second Degree; Generic Baccalaureate; RN Baccalaureate.

Site Options Ambler, PA; Philadelphia, PA; Bethlehem, PA.

Study Options Full-time and part-time.

Program Entrance Requirements Minimum overall college GPA of 3.0, transcript of college record, CPR certification, written essay, health exam, health insurance, high school biology, high school chemistry, high school foreign language, 3 years high school math, 3 years high school science, high school transcript, immunizations, interview, minimum high school GPA of 2.0, minimum GPA in nursing prerequisites of 3.0, prerequisite course work. Transfer students are accepted. **Standardized tests** *Required:* SAT or ACT, TOEFL for international students. **Application** *Deadline:* 4/1 (freshmen), 6/15 (transfer). *Notification:* continuous (freshmen). *Application fee:* $50.

Advanced Placement Credit given for nursing courses completed elsewhere dependent upon specific evaluations.

Expenses (2006–07) *Tuition, area resident:* part-time $437 per credit. *Tuition, nonresident:* full-time $19,692; part-time $683 per credit. *Required fees:* full-time $500; part-time $200 per term.

Financial Aid 70% of baccalaureate students in nursing programs received some form of financial aid in 2005–06.

Contact Ms. Jeanne Johnson, Director of Student Services, Department of Nursing, Temple University, 3307 North Broad Street, Philadelphia, PA 19140. *Telephone:* 215-707-4688. *Fax:* 215-707-1599. *E-mail:* jjohns13@temple.edu.

GRADUATE PROGRAMS

Expenses (2006–07) *Tuition, area resident:* full-time $9576; part-time $532 per credit hour. *Tuition, state resident:* full-time $9876; part-time $532 per credit hour. *Tuition, nonresident:* full-time $12,294; part-time $683 per credit hour. *Required fees:* full-time $500.

Financial Aid 100% of graduate students in nursing programs received some form of financial aid in 2005–06. Teaching assistantships with full tuition reimbursements available, career-related internships or fieldwork, institutionally sponsored loans, and traineeships available. Aid available to part-time students. *Financial aid application deadline:* 1/15.

Contact Dr. Jane M. Kurz, Director of Graduate Studies, Department of Nursing, Temple University, 3307 North Broad Street, Philadelphia, PA 19140. *Telephone:* 215-707-5017. *Fax:* 215-707-1599. *E-mail:* jkurz@temple.edu.

MASTER'S DEGREE PROGRAM
Degree MSN

Available Programs Master's.

Concentrations Available Nursing education. *Clinical nurse specialist programs in:* maternity-newborn, psychiatric/mental health. *Nurse practitioner programs in:* adult health, family health, pediatric.

Site Options Philadelphia, PA.

Study Options Full-time and part-time.

Program Entrance Requirements Clinical experience, minimum overall college GPA of 3.0, transcript of college record, CPR certification, written essay, immunizations, interview, 2 letters of recommendation, nursing research course, physical assessment course, professional liability insurance/malpractice insurance, statistics course, GRE General Test. *Application deadline:* For fall admission, 8/15 (priority date); for spring admission, 12/15. Applications are processed on a rolling basis. *Application fee:* $50.

Advanced Placement Credit given for nursing courses completed elsewhere dependent upon specific evaluations.

Degree Requirements 36 total credit hours.

POST-MASTER'S PROGRAM

Areas of Study Nursing education. *Clinical nurse specialist programs in:* maternity-newborn, psychiatric/mental health. *Nurse practitioner programs in:* adult health, family health, pediatric.

Thomas Jefferson University
Department of Nursing
Philadelphia, Pennsylvania

http://www.tju.edu

Founded in 1824

DEGREES • BSN • DNP • MSN

Nursing Program Faculty 38 (42% with doctorates).

Baccalaureate Enrollment 350
Women 80% **Men** 20% **Minority** 30% **Part-time** 10%

Graduate Enrollment 198
Women 90% **Men** 10% **Minority** 30% **Part-time** 50%

Nursing Student Activities Nursing Honor Society, Sigma Theta Tau, Student Nurses' Association.

Nursing Student Resources Academic advising; academic or career counseling; assistance for students with disabilities; bookstore; campus computer network; career placement assistance; computer lab; computer-assisted instruction; e-mail services; interactive nursing skills videos; Internet; learning resource lab; library services; nursing audiovisuals; paid internships; placement services for program completers; remedial services; resume preparation assistance; skills, simulation, or other laboratory; tutoring.

Library Facilities 170,000 volumes (146,000 in health, 4,700 in nursing); 2,290 periodical subscriptions (2,100 health-care related).

BACCALAUREATE PROGRAMS
Degree BSN

Available Programs ADN to Baccalaureate; Accelerated Baccalaureate; Accelerated Baccalaureate for Second Degree; Accelerated RN Baccalaureate; Baccalaureate for Second Degree; Generic Baccalaureate; RN Baccalaureate.

Site Options *Distance Learning:* Atlantic City, NJ; Philadelphia, PA.

Study Options Full-time and part-time.

Program Entrance Requirements Minimum overall college GPA of 2.9, transcript of college record, CPR certification, written essay, health exam, health insurance, high school transcript, immunizations, 2 letters of recommendation, prerequisite course work. Transfer students are accepted. **Standardized tests** *Required:* TOEFL for international students. *Recommended:* SAT or ACT. *Required for some:* NET. **Application** *Deadline:* rolling (freshmen), rolling (transfer). *Notification:* continuous (freshmen). *Application fee:* $50.

Advanced Placement Credit by examination available. Credit given for nursing courses completed elsewhere dependent upon specific evaluations.

Expenses (2006–07) *Tuition:* full-time $22,884. *Required fees:* part-time $400 per term.

Financial Aid 70% of baccalaureate students in nursing programs received some form of financial aid in 2005–06. *Gift aid (need-based):* Federal Pell, FSEOG, state, private, college/university gift aid from institutional funds, Scholarships for Disadvantaged Students (SDS). *Loans:* Federal Nursing Student Loans, FFEL (Subsidized and Unsubsidized Stafford PLUS), Perkins, college/university. *Work-Study:* Federal Work-Study. *Application deadline (priority):* 4/1.

Contact Dr. Sandra Krafft, EdD, Associate Dean, Undergraduate Programs, Department of Nursing, Thomas Jefferson University, 130 South Ninth Street, Edison Building, Suite 1230B, Philadelphia, PA 19107. *Telephone:* 215-503-8104. *Fax:* 215-503-0376. *E-mail:* Sandra.Krafft@jefferson.edu.

GRADUATE PROGRAMS

Financial Aid 75% of graduate students in nursing programs received some form of financial aid in 2005–06.

Contact Dr. Beth Ann Swan, Associate Dean, Graduate Program, Department of Nursing, Thomas Jefferson University, 130 South Ninth Street, Suite 1200, Philadelphia, PA 19107. *Telephone:* 215-503-8057. *Fax:* 215-932-1468. *E-mail:* beth.swan@jefferson.edu.

MASTER'S DEGREE PROGRAM

Degree MSN

Available Programs Accelerated Master's; Accelerated RN to Master's; Master's; Master's for Non-Nursing College Graduates; Master's for Nurses with Non-Nursing Degrees; RN to Master's.

Concentrations Available Nurse anesthesia; nursing education; nursing informatics. *Clinical nurse specialist programs in:* acute care, adult health, community health, critical care, home health care, medical-surgical, oncology, pediatric, public health. *Nurse practitioner programs in:* acute care, adult health, family health, neonatal health, oncology, pediatric.

Site Options *Distance Learning:* Philadelphia, PA.

Study Options Full-time and part-time.

Program Entrance Requirements Clinical experience, computer literacy, minimum overall college GPA of 3.0, transcript of college record, CPR certification, written essay, interview, 3 letters of recommendation, nursing research course, physical assessment course, professional liability insurance/malpractice insurance, resume, statistics course.

Advanced Placement Credit given for nursing courses completed elsewhere dependent upon specific evaluations.

Degree Requirements 36 total credit hours.

POST-MASTER'S PROGRAM

Areas of Study Nursing education; nursing informatics. *Nurse practitioner programs in:* acute care, adult health, family health, neonatal health, oncology, pediatric.

DOCTORAL DEGREE PROGRAM

Degree DNP

Available Programs Doctorate.

Areas of Study Advanced practice nursing, clinical practice, individualized study.

Program Entrance Requirements Clinical experience, minimum overall college GPA of 3.2, interview by faculty committee, interview, 3 letters of recommendation, MSN or equivalent, scholarly papers, statistics course, vita, writing sample.

Degree Requirements 36 total credit hours, written exam, residency.

CONTINUING EDUCATION PROGRAM

Contact Dr. Beth Ann Swan, Associate Dean, Graduate Programs, Department of Nursing, Thomas Jefferson University, 130 South Ninth Street, Suite 1200, Philadelphia, PA 19107. *Telephone:* 215-503-8057. *Fax:* 215-503-0376. *E-mail:* beth.swan@jefferson.edu.

See full description on page 534.

University of Pennsylvania
School of Nursing
Philadelphia, Pennsylvania

http://www.nursing.upenn.edu

Founded in 1740

DEGREES • BSN • MSN • MSN/MBA • MSN/MPH • MSN/PHD

Nursing Program Faculty 231 (25% with doctorates).

Baccalaureate Enrollment 507
Women 94% **Men** 6% **Minority** 31% **International** 5% **Part-time** 1%

Graduate Enrollment 448
Women 91% **Men** 9% **Minority** 23% **International** 4% **Part-time** 57%

Nursing Student Activities Nursing Honor Society, Sigma Theta Tau, Student Nurses' Association.

Nursing Student Resources Academic advising; academic or career counseling; assistance for students with disabilities; bookstore; campus computer network; career placement assistance; computer lab; computer-assisted instruction; daycare for children of students; e-mail services; employment services for current students; externships; housing assistance; interactive nursing skills videos; Internet; learning resource lab; library services; nursing audiovisuals; other; paid internships; placement services for program completers; remedial services; resume preparation assistance; skills, simulation, or other laboratory; tutoring; unpaid internships.

Library Facilities 5.9 million volumes; 47,787 periodical subscriptions.

BACCALAUREATE PROGRAMS

Degree BSN

Available Programs ADN to Baccalaureate; Accelerated Baccalaureate; Accelerated Baccalaureate for Second Degree; Accelerated RN Baccalaureate; Baccalaureate for Second Degree; Generic Baccalaureate; RN Baccalaureate.

Study Options Full-time and part-time.

Program Entrance Requirements Minimum overall college GPA of 3.0, transcript of college record, written essay, health exam, health insurance, high school biology, high school chemistry, high school foreign language, 4 years high school math, 4 years high school science, high school transcript, immunizations, interview, 2 letters of recommendation, minimum high school GPA of 3.0, minimum high school rank 10%. Transfer students are accepted. **Standardized tests** *Required:* SAT and SAT Subject Tests or ACT, TOEFL for international students. **Application** *Deadline:* 1/1 (freshmen), 3/15 (transfer). *Early decision:* 11/1. *Notification:* 4/1 (freshmen), 12/15 (out-of-state freshmen), 12/15 (early decision). *Application fee:* $70.

Advanced Placement Credit by examination available. Credit given for nursing courses completed elsewhere dependent upon specific evaluations.

Expenses (2006–07) *Tuition:* full-time $30,598; part-time $3908 per unit. *International tuition:* $30,598 full-time. *Room and board:* $9804; room only: $6022 per academic year. *Required fees:* full-time $3558.

Financial Aid 92% of baccalaureate students in nursing programs received some form of financial aid in 2005–06.

Contact Office of Enrollment Management, School of Nursing, University of Pennsylvania, 420 Guardian Drive, Philadelphia, PA 19104-6096. *Telephone:* 215-898-4271. *Fax:* 215-573-8439. *E-mail:* admissions@nursing.upenn.edu.

GRADUATE PROGRAMS

Expenses (2006–07) *Tuition:* full-time $29,542; part-time $3715 per unit. *International tuition:* $29,542 full-time. *Room and board:* $14,400 per academic year. *Required fees:* full-time $2200.

Financial Aid 89% of graduate students in nursing programs received some form of financial aid in 2005–06. Fellowships, research assistantships, teaching assistantships, career-related internships or fieldwork, Federal Work-Study, and institutionally sponsored loans available. Aid available to part-time students. *Financial aid application deadline:* 12/15.

Contact Office of Enrollment Management, School of Nursing, University of Pennsylvania, 420 Guardian Drive, Philadelphia, PA 19104-6096. *Telephone:* 215-898-4271. *Fax:* 215-573-8439. *E-mail:* admissions@nursing.upenn.edu.

MASTER'S DEGREE PROGRAM

Degrees MSN; MSN/MBA; MSN/MPH; MSN/PhD

Available Programs Accelerated AD/RN to Master's; Accelerated Master's for Non-Nursing College Graduates; Accelerated RN to Master's; Master's.

Concentrations Available Health-care administration; nurse anesthesia; nurse-midwifery; nursing administration; nursing informatics. *Clinical nurse specialist programs in:* acute care, adult health, critical care, family health, gerontology, home health care, maternity-newborn, medical-

University of Pennsylvania (continued)

surgical, oncology, pediatric, perinatal, psychiatric/mental health, women's health. *Nurse practitioner programs in:* acute care, adult health, community health, family health, gerontology, neonatal health, occupational health, oncology, pediatric, primary care, women's health.

Site Options *Distance Learning:* Memphis, TN.

Study Options Full-time and part-time.

Program Entrance Requirements Clinical experience, computer literacy, minimum overall college GPA of 3.0, transcript of college record, CPR certification, written essay, immunizations, interview, 3 letters of recommendation, physical assessment course, prerequisite course work, resume, statistics course, GMAT (MBA/MSN), GRE General Test. *Application deadline:* For fall admission, 2/15 (priority date). Applications are processed on a rolling basis. *Application fee:* $70.

Advanced Placement Credit given for nursing courses completed elsewhere dependent upon specific evaluations.

Degree Requirements 36 total credit hours.

POST-MASTER'S PROGRAM

Areas of Study Health-care administration; nurse anesthesia; nurse-midwifery; nursing administration; nursing education; nursing informatics. *Clinical nurse specialist programs in:* acute care, adult health, critical care, family health, gerontology, home health care, maternity-newborn, medical-surgical, oncology, pediatric, perinatal, psychiatric/mental health, women's health. *Nurse practitioner programs in:* acute care, adult health, community health, family health, gerontology, neonatal health, occupational health, oncology, pediatric, primary care, women's health.

DOCTORAL DEGREE PROGRAM

Degree PhD

Available Programs Doctorate; Post-Baccalaureate Doctorate.

Areas of Study Addiction/substance abuse, aging, bio-behavioral research, biology of health and illness, clinical practice, community health, critical care, ethics, faculty preparation, family health, gerontology, health policy, health promotion/disease prevention, health-care systems, human health and illness, illness and transition, individualized study, information systems, maternity-newborn, neuro-behavior, nursing administration, nursing education, nursing policy, nursing research, nursing science, oncology, urban health, women's health.

Program Entrance Requirements interview by faculty committee, interview, 3 letters of recommendation, MSN or equivalent, statistics course, vita, writing sample, GMAT (MBA/PhD), GRE General Test. *Application deadline:* For fall admission, 2/15 (priority date). Applications are processed on a rolling basis. *Application fee:* $70.

Degree Requirements 39 total credit hours, dissertation, oral exam, written exam, residency.

POSTDOCTORAL PROGRAM

Areas of Study Adolescent health, aging, cancer care, chronic illness, community health, family health, gerontology, health promotion/disease prevention, individualized study, nursing informatics, nursing interventions, nursing research, nursing science, outcomes, self-care, vulnerable population, women's health.

Postdoctoral Program Contact Dr. Linda A. McCauley, Associate Dean for Nursing Research, School of Nursing, University of Pennsylvania, 420 Guardian Drive, Philadelphia, PA 19104-6096. *Telephone:* 215-898-9160. *E-mail:* lmccaule@nursing.upenn.edu.

CONTINUING EDUCATION PROGRAM

Contact Janet L. Tomcavage, Program Management, School of Nursing, University of Pennsylvania, 420 Guardian Drive, Philadelphia, PA 19104-6096. *Telephone:* 215-898-5422. *E-mail:* tomcavag@nursing.upenn.edu.

See full description on page 550.

University of Pittsburgh
School of Nursing
Pittsburgh, Pennsylvania

http://www.nursing.pitt.edu

Founded in 1787

DEGREES • BSN • MSN • PHD

Nursing Program Faculty 103 (63% with doctorates).

Baccalaureate Enrollment 596
Women 88% **Men** 12% **Minority** 8% **International** 2% **Part-time** 17%

Graduate Enrollment 336
Women 84% **Men** 16% **Minority** 8% **International** 2% **Part-time** 50%

Nursing Student Activities Sigma Theta Tau, Student Nurses' Association.

Nursing Student Resources Academic advising; academic or career counseling; assistance for students with disabilities; bookstore; campus computer network; career placement assistance; computer lab; computer-assisted instruction; daycare for children of students; e-mail services; employment services for current students; externships; housing assistance; interactive nursing skills videos; Internet; learning resource lab; library services; nursing audiovisuals; paid internships; placement services for program completers; remedial services; resume preparation assistance; skills, simulation, or other laboratory; tutoring.

Library Facilities 4.6 million volumes; 3,767 periodical subscriptions.

BACCALAUREATE PROGRAMS

Degree BSN

Available Programs ADN to Baccalaureate; Accelerated Baccalaureate for Second Degree; Generic Baccalaureate; RN Baccalaureate.

Site Options *Distance Learning:* Bradford, PA; Johnstown, PA.

Study Options Full-time.

Program Entrance Requirements Minimum overall college GPA of 3.3, transcript of college record, written essay, health exam, health insurance, high school biology, high school chemistry, high school foreign language, 3 years high school math, 3 years high school science, high school transcript, immunizations, 2 letters of recommendation, minimum high school GPA of 3.3, minimum GPA in nursing prerequisites of 2.0. Transfer students are accepted. **Standardized tests** *Required:* SAT or ACT, TOEFL for international students. **Application** *Deadline:* rolling (freshmen), rolling (transfer). *Notification:* continuous (freshmen). *Application fee:* $35.

Advanced Placement Credit by examination available.

Expenses (2006–07) *Tuition, state resident:* full-time $14,308; part-time $596 per credit. *Tuition, nonresident:* full-time $26,290; part-time $1095 per credit. *International tuition:* $26,290 full-time. *Required fees:* full-time $12.

Financial Aid 74% of baccalaureate students in nursing programs received some form of financial aid in 2005–06. *Gift aid (need-based):* Federal Pell, FSEOG, state, private, college/university gift aid from institutional funds. *Loans:* Federal Nursing Student Loans, FFEL (Subsidized and Unsubsidized Stafford PLUS), Perkins, college/university. *Work-Study:* Federal Work-Study. *Application deadline:* 6/1 (priority: 3/1).

Contact Ms. Mary Rodgers Schubert, Associate Director of Recruitment, School of Nursing, University of Pittsburgh, 239 Victoria Building, 3500 Victoria Street, Pittsburgh, PA 15261. *Telephone:* 412-624-1291. *Fax:* 412-624-2409. *E-mail:* mschuber@pitt.edu.

GRADUATE PROGRAMS

Expenses (2006–07) *Tuition, state resident:* full-time $16,384; part-time $671 per credit. *Tuition, nonresident:* full-time $21,280; part-time $872 per credit. *International tuition:* $21,280 full-time. *Required fees:* full-time $644; part-time $322 per term.

Financial Aid 70% of graduate students in nursing programs received some form of financial aid in 2005–06. 21 research assistantships with full and partial tuition reimbursements available (averaging $16,600 per year), 2 teaching assistantships with full and partial tuition reimbursements available (averaging $20,740 per year) were awarded; institutionally sponsored loans, scholarships, traineeships, and unspecified assistantships also available. Aid available to part-time students. *Financial aid application deadline:* 7/1.

Contact Ms. Mary Rodgers Schubert, Associate Director of Recruitment, School of Nursing, University of Pittsburgh, 239 Victoria Building, 3500 Victoria Street, Pittsburgh, PA 15261. *Telephone:* 412-624-1291. *Fax:* 412-624-2409. *E-mail:* mschuber@pitt.edu.

MASTER'S DEGREE PROGRAM

Degree MSN

Available Programs Master's; RN to Master's.

Concentrations Available Nurse anesthesia; nursing administration; nursing education; nursing informatics. *Clinical nurse specialist programs in:* medical-surgical, psychiatric/mental health. *Nurse practitioner programs in:* acute care, adult health, family health, pediatric, psychiatric/mental health.

Site Options *Distance Learning:* Bradford, PA; Johnstown, PA.

Study Options Full-time and part-time.

Program Entrance Requirements Clinical experience, minimum overall college GPA of 3.0, transcript of college record, written essay, immunizations, interview, 3 letters of recommendation, professional liability insurance/malpractice insurance, prerequisite course work, resume, statistics course, GRE or MAT. *Application deadline:* Applications are processed on a rolling basis. *Application fee:* $50.

Advanced Placement Credit by examination available. Credit given for nursing courses completed elsewhere dependent upon specific evaluations.

Degree Requirements 52 total credit hours, comprehensive exam.

POST-MASTER'S PROGRAM

Areas of Study Health-care administration; nursing education; nursing informatics. *Nurse practitioner programs in:* acute care, adult health, pediatric, psychiatric/mental health.

DOCTORAL DEGREE PROGRAM

Degree PhD

Available Programs Doctorate; Post-Baccalaureate Doctorate.

Areas of Study Bio-behavioral research, nursing research, nursing science.

Program Entrance Requirements Minimum overall college GPA of 3.5, interview by faculty committee, interview, 3 letters of recommendation, MSN or equivalent, statistics course, vita, writing sample, GRE. *Application deadline:* Applications are processed on a rolling basis. *Application fee:* $50.

Degree Requirements 64 total credit hours, dissertation, oral exam, written exam, residency.

POSTDOCTORAL PROGRAM

Areas of Study Chronic illness, individualized study, nursing research.

Postdoctoral Program Contact Dr. Judith A. Erlen, PhD Program Coordinator/Associate Director of Center for Research in Chronic Disorders, School of Nursing, University of Pittsburgh, 3500 Victoria Street, Pittsburgh, PA 15261. *Telephone:* 412-624-1905. *Fax:* 412-624-8521. *E-mail:* jae001@pitt.edu.

CONTINUING EDUCATION PROGRAM

Contact Ms. Lisa Bernardo, Director of Continuing Education Program, School of Nursing, University of Pittsburgh, 426 Victoria Building, 3500 Victoria Street, Pittsburgh, PA 15261. *Telephone:* 412-624-7637. *E-mail:* lbe100@pitt.edu.

See full description on page 554.

University of Pittsburgh at Bradford
Department of Nursing
Bradford, Pennsylvania

Founded in 1963

DEGREE • BSN

Nursing Program Faculty 5 (60% with doctorates).

Baccalaureate Enrollment 12
Women 83% **Men** 17%

Nursing Student Activities Nursing club.

Nursing Student Resources Academic advising; academic or career counseling; assistance for students with disabilities; bookstore; campus computer network; career placement assistance; computer lab; computer-assisted instruction; e-mail services; employment services for current students; externships; housing assistance; Internet; learning resource lab;

library services; nursing audiovisuals; remedial services; resume preparation assistance; skills, simulation, or other laboratory; tutoring; unpaid internships.

Library Facilities 95,271 volumes; 343 periodical subscriptions (50 health-care related).

BACCALAUREATE PROGRAMS

Degree BSN

Available Programs RN Baccalaureate.

Study Options Full-time and part-time.

Program Entrance Requirements Transcript of college record, CPR certification, health exam, health insurance, immunizations, minimum GPA in nursing prerequisites of 2.5, professional liability insurance/malpractice insurance, prerequisite course work, RN licensure. Transfer students are accepted. **Standardized tests** *Required:* SAT or ACT, TOEFL for international students. **Application** *Deadline:* rolling (freshmen), rolling (transfer). *Application fee:* $35.

Advanced Placement Credit by examination available. Credit given for nursing courses completed elsewhere dependent upon specific evaluations.

Expenses (2006–07) *Tuition, area resident:* full-time $12,824; part-time $432 per credit. *Tuition, nonresident:* full-time $25,012; part-time $826 per credit. *Room and board:* $6650; room only: $4000 per academic year. *Required fees:* full-time $582.

Financial Aid 85% of baccalaureate students in nursing programs received some form of financial aid in 2005–06. *Gift aid (need-based):* Federal Pell, FSEOG, state, private, college/university gift aid from institutional funds. *Loans:* FFEL (Subsidized and Unsubsidized Stafford PLUS), Perkins. *Work-Study:* Federal Work-Study, part-time campus jobs. *Application deadline (priority):* 3/1.

Contact Department of Nursing Admissions, Department of Nursing, University of Pittsburgh at Bradford, 300 Campus Drive, Bradford, PA 16701. *Telephone:* 800-872-1787.

The University of Scranton
Department of Nursing
Scranton, Pennsylvania

Founded in 1888

DEGREES • BS • MS

Nursing Program Faculty 40 (85% with doctorates).

Baccalaureate Enrollment 245
Women 94% **Men** 6% **Minority** 8% **Part-time** 7%

Graduate Enrollment 105
Women 70% **Men** 30% **Minority** 6% **Part-time** 50%

Nursing Student Activities Nursing Honor Society, Sigma Theta Tau, Student Nurses' Association, nursing club.

Nursing Student Resources Academic advising; academic or career counseling; bookstore; campus computer network; career placement assistance; computer lab; computer-assisted instruction; e-mail services; employment services for current students; interactive nursing skills videos; Internet; learning resource lab; library services; nursing audiovisuals; placement services for program completers; remedial services; resume preparation assistance; skills, simulation, or other laboratory; tutoring.

Library Facilities 481,542 volumes (28,400 in health, 8,484 in nursing); 1,579 periodical subscriptions (106 health-care related).

BACCALAUREATE PROGRAMS

Degree BS

Available Programs ADN to Baccalaureate; Accelerated LPN to Baccalaureate; Baccalaureate for Second Degree; Generic Baccalaureate; LPN to RN Baccalaureate; RN Baccalaureate.

Study Options Full-time and part-time.

Program Entrance Requirements Minimum overall college GPA of 2.5, transcript of college record, written essay, health exam, health insurance, high school biology, high school chemistry, high school foreign language, 3 years high school math, 3 years high school science, high school transcript, immunizations, minimum high school rank 30%. Transfer

The University of Scranton (continued)

students are accepted. **Standardized tests** *Required:* SAT or ACT, TOEFL for international students. **Application** *Deadline:* 3/1 (freshmen), rolling (transfer). *Early decision:* 11/15. *Notification:* continuous until 5/1 (freshmen), 12/15 (early action). *Application fee:* $40.

Advanced Placement Credit by examination available. Credit given for nursing courses completed elsewhere dependent upon specific evaluations.

Expenses (2006–07) *Tuition:* full-time $25,638; part-time $712 per credit. *International tuition:* $25,638 full-time. *Room and board:* $10,216; room only: $6016 per academic year. *Required fees:* full-time $300.

Financial Aid 80% of baccalaureate students in nursing programs received some form of financial aid in 2005–06.

Contact Dr. Patricia Harrington, Chairperson, Department of Nursing, The University of Scranton, McGurrin Hall, Scranton, PA 18510-4595. *Telephone:* 570-941-7673. *Fax:* 570-941-7903. *E-mail:* harringtonp1@scranton.edu.

GRADUATE PROGRAMS

Expenses (2006–07) *Tuition:* full-time $16,416; part-time $684 per credit. *International tuition:* $16,416 full-time. *Room and board:* room only: $4000 per academic year. *Required fees:* full-time $150; part-time $25 per term.

Financial Aid 90% of graduate students in nursing programs received some form of financial aid in 2005–06. 4 teaching assistantships with full and partial tuition reimbursements available (averaging $5,375 per year) were awarded; career-related internships or fieldwork, Federal Work-Study, and unspecified assistantships also available. Aid available to part-time students. *Financial aid application deadline:* 3/1.

Contact Dr. Mary Jane Hanson, Director, Graduate Nursing Program, Department of Nursing, The University of Scranton, McGurrin Hall, Scranton, PA 18510. *Telephone:* 570-941-4060. *Fax:* 570-941-7093. *E-mail:* hansonm2@scranton.edu.

MASTER'S DEGREE PROGRAM

Degree MS

Available Programs Accelerated AD/RN to Master's; Accelerated RN to Master's; Master's; RN to Master's.

Concentrations Available Nurse anesthesia; nursing education. *Clinical nurse specialist programs in:* adult health. *Nurse practitioner programs in:* family health.

Study Options Full-time and part-time.

Program Entrance Requirements Clinical experience, minimum overall college GPA of 3.0, transcript of college record, CPR certification, written essay, immunizations, interview, 3 letters of recommendation, nursing research course, physical assessment course, professional liability insurance/malpractice insurance, prerequisite course work, statistics course. *Application deadline:* For fall admission, 9/1. Applications are processed on a rolling basis. *Application fee:* $50.

Advanced Placement Credit given for nursing courses completed elsewhere dependent upon specific evaluations.

Degree Requirements 46 total credit hours, comprehensive exam.

POST-MASTER'S PROGRAM

Areas of Study Nurse anesthesia; nursing education. *Clinical nurse specialist programs in:* adult health. *Nurse practitioner programs in:* family health.

Villanova University
College of Nursing
Villanova, Pennsylvania

http://www.nursing.villanova.edu/

Founded in 1842

DEGREES • BSN • MSN • PHD

Nursing Program Faculty 77 (45% with doctorates).
Baccalaureate Enrollment 528
Women 96% **Men** 4% **Minority** 24% **International** 4% **Part-time** 3%

Graduate Enrollment 190
Women 88% **Men** 12% **Minority** 12% **International** 8% **Part-time** 78%

Nursing Student Activities Nursing Honor Society, Sigma Theta Tau, Student Nurses' Association, nursing club.

Nursing Student Resources Academic advising; academic or career counseling; assistance for students with disabilities; bookstore; campus computer network; career placement assistance; computer lab; computer-assisted instruction; e-mail services; employment services for current students; externships; housing assistance; interactive nursing skills videos; Internet; learning resource lab; library services; nursing audiovisuals; remedial services; resume preparation assistance; skills, simulation, or other laboratory; tutoring.

Library Facilities 712,000 volumes (22,441 in health, 15,574 in nursing); 12,000 periodical subscriptions (1,900 health-care related).

BACCALAUREATE PROGRAMS

Degree BSN

Available Programs ADN to Baccalaureate; Accelerated Baccalaureate for Second Degree; Baccalaureate for Second Degree; Generic Baccalaureate; International Nurse to Baccalaureate; RN Baccalaureate.

Site Options *Distance Learning:* Villanova, PA.

Study Options Full-time and part-time.

Program Entrance Requirements Transcript of college record, written essay, health exam, health insurance, high school biology, high school chemistry, high school foreign language, 3 years high school math, 3 years high school science, high school transcript, immunizations, minimum high school GPA of 3.0. Transfer students are accepted. **Standardized tests** *Required:* SAT or ACT, TOEFL for international students. **Application** *Deadline:* 1/7 (freshmen), 6/1 (transfer). *Early decision:* 11/1. *Notification:* 4/1 (freshmen), 12/20 (early action). *Application fee:* $70.

Advanced Placement Credit by examination available. Credit given for nursing courses completed elsewhere dependent upon specific evaluations.

Expenses (2006–07) *Tuition:* full-time $33,000; part-time $1375 per credit. *International tuition:* $33,000 full-time. *Room and board:* $9880; room only: $5060 per academic year. *Required fees:* full-time $760; part-time $300 per credit.

Financial Aid 66% of baccalaureate students in nursing programs received some form of financial aid in 2005–06. *Gift aid (need-based):* Federal Pell, FSEOG, state, private, college/university gift aid from institutional funds, endowed and restricted grants. *Loans:* Federal Nursing Student Loans, FFEL (Subsidized and Unsubsidized Stafford PLUS), Perkins, Villanova Loan. *Work-Study:* Federal Work-Study, part-time campus jobs. *Application deadline (priority):* 2/7.

Contact Dr. M. Frances Keen, Assistant Dean and Director, Undergraduate Program, College of Nursing, Villanova University, 800 Lancaster Avenue, Villanova, PA 19085-1690. *Telephone:* 610-519-4926. *Fax:* 610-519-7650. *E-mail:* frances.keen@villanova.edu.

GRADUATE PROGRAMS

Expenses (2006–07) *Tuition:* full-time $10,890; part-time $605 per credit. *International tuition:* $10,890 full-time. *Required fees:* full-time $120; part-time $60 per credit.

Financial Aid 51% of graduate students in nursing programs received some form of financial aid in 2005–06. 4 teaching assistantships with full tuition reimbursements available (averaging $11,750 per year) were awarded; institutionally sponsored loans, scholarships, traineeships, and tuition waivers (full) also available. *Financial aid application deadline:* 3/1.

Contact Dr. Marguerite K. Schlag, Assistant Dean and Director, Graduate Program, College of Nursing, Villanova University, 800 Lancaster Avenue, Villanova, PA 19085-1690. *Telephone:* 610-519-4934. *Fax:* 610-519-7997. *E-mail:* marguerite.schlag@villanova.edu.

MASTER'S DEGREE PROGRAM

Degree MSN

Available Programs Accelerated Master's; Master's.

Concentrations Available Health-care administration; nurse anesthesia; nurse case management; nursing education. *Nurse practitioner programs in:* adult health, gerontology, pediatric.

Site Options *Distance Learning:* Villanova, PA.

Study Options Full-time and part-time.

Program Entrance Requirements Clinical experience, computer literacy, minimum overall college GPA of 3.0, transcript of college record, CPR certification, written essay, immunizations, 3 letters of recommendation, physical assessment course, professional liability insurance/malpractice insurance, prerequisite course work, resume, statistics course, GRE or MAT. *Application deadline:* For fall admission, 7/1 (priority date); for spring admission, 12/1 (priority date). Applications are processed on a rolling basis. *Application fee:* $50.

Advanced Placement Credit given for nursing courses completed elsewhere dependent upon specific evaluations.

Degree Requirements 45 total credit hours, thesis or project.

POST-MASTER'S PROGRAM

Areas of Study Nurse anesthesia; nurse case management; nursing education. *Nurse practitioner programs in:* adult health, gerontology, pediatric.

DOCTORAL DEGREE PROGRAM

Degree PhD

Available Programs Doctorate.

Areas of Study Faculty preparation, nursing education, nursing research.

Site Options *Distance Learning:* Villanova, PA.

Program Entrance Requirements Clinical experience, minimum overall college GPA of 3.5, interview, 3 letters of recommendation, MSN or equivalent, scholarly papers, vita, writing sample, GRE. *Application deadline:* For fall admission, 7/1 (priority date); for spring admission, 12/1 (priority date). Applications are processed on a rolling basis. *Application fee:* $50.

Degree Requirements 51 total credit hours, dissertation, oral exam, written exam.

CONTINUING EDUCATION PROGRAM

Contact Dr. Lynore DeSilets, RN, Assistant Dean and Director, Continuing Education, College of Nursing, Villanova University, 800 Lancaster Avenue, Villanova, PA 19085-1690. *Telephone:* 610-519-4931. *Fax:* 610-519-6780. *E-mail:* lyn.desilets@villanova.edu.

See full description on page 572.

Waynesburg College
Department of Nursing
Waynesburg, Pennsylvania

http://www.waynesburg.edu

Founded in 1849

DEGREES • BSN • DNP • MSN • MSN/MBA

Nursing Program Faculty 48 (38% with doctorates).

Baccalaureate Enrollment 301
Women 87% **Men** 13% **Minority** 3%

Graduate Enrollment 215
Women 96% **Men** 4% **Minority** 1% **Part-time** 100%

Nursing Student Activities Sigma Theta Tau, Student Nurses' Association.

Nursing Student Resources Academic advising; academic or career counseling; assistance for students with disabilities; bookstore; campus computer network; career placement assistance; computer lab; computer-assisted instruction; e-mail services; employment services for current students; externships; Internet; learning resource lab; library services; nursing audiovisuals; paid internships; placement services for program completers; remedial services; resume preparation assistance; skills, simulation, or other laboratory; tutoring.

Library Facilities 100,000 volumes (4,500 in nursing); 1,189 periodical subscriptions (46 health-care related).

BACCALAUREATE PROGRAMS

Degree BSN

Available Programs Accelerated Baccalaureate for Second Degree; Accelerated RN Baccalaureate; Generic Baccalaureate; LPN to Baccalaureate; LPN to RN Baccalaureate.

Site Options Monroeville, PA; Canonsburg, PA; Wexford, PA.

Study Options Full-time.

Program Entrance Requirements Minimum overall college GPA of 3.0, transcript of college record, CPR certification, health exam, high school biology, high school chemistry, 2 years high school math, 2 years high school science, high school transcript, immunizations, minimum high school GPA of 3.0, minimum GPA in nursing prerequisites of 3.0, professional liability insurance/malpractice insurance, prerequisite course work. Transfer students are accepted. **Standardized tests** *Required:* SAT or ACT, TOEFL for international students. **Application** *Deadline:* rolling (freshmen), rolling (transfer). *Notification:* continuous (freshmen). *Application fee:* $20.

Advanced Placement Credit by examination available. Credit given for nursing courses completed elsewhere dependent upon specific evaluations.

Expenses (2006–07) *Tuition:* full-time $15,440. *Room and board:* $6710; room only: $3250 per academic year. *Required fees:* full-time $450.

Financial Aid 90% of baccalaureate students in nursing programs received some form of financial aid in 2005–06. *Gift aid (need-based):* Federal Pell, FSEOG, state, private, college/university gift aid from institutional funds. *Loans:* Federal Nursing Student Loans, FFEL (Subsidized and Unsubsidized Stafford PLUS), Perkins. *Work-Study:* Federal Work-Study. *Application deadline:* Continuous.

Contact Dr. Nancy Mosser, Director and Chair, Department of Nursing, Waynesburg College, 51 West College Street, Waynesburg, PA 15370-1222. *Telephone:* 724-852-3356. *Fax:* 724-852-3220. *E-mail:* nmosser@waynesburg.edu.

GRADUATE PROGRAMS

Expenses (2006–07) *Tuition:* part-time $420 per credit.

Financial Aid 50% of graduate students in nursing programs received some form of financial aid in 2005–06.

Contact Dr. Lynette Jack, Director of Graduate and Professional Studies Program, Department of Nursing, Waynesburg College, 1001 Corporate Drive, Canonsburg, PA 15317. *Telephone:* 724-743-2256. *Fax:* 724-743-4425. *E-mail:* ljack@waynesburg.edu.

MASTER'S DEGREE PROGRAM

Degrees MSN; MSN/MBA

Available Programs Accelerated Master's; Accelerated Master's for Nurses with Non-Nursing Degrees; Accelerated RN to Master's.

Concentrations Available Nursing administration; nursing education.

Site Options Monroeville, PA; Canonsburg, PA; Wexford, PA.

Study Options Part-time.

Program Entrance Requirements Clinical experience, computer literacy, minimum overall college GPA of 3.0, transcript of college record, 2 letters of recommendation, resume.

Degree Requirements 36 total credit hours, thesis or project.

DOCTORAL DEGREE PROGRAM

Degree DNP

Available Programs Doctorate; Post-Baccalaureate Doctorate.

Areas of Study Advanced practice nursing, health-care systems, nursing administration.

Site Options Monroeville, PA.

Program Entrance Requirements Minimum overall college GPA of 3.0, interview by faculty committee, interview, letters of recommendation, MSN or equivalent, statistics course, vita, writing sample.

Degree Requirements 80 total credit hours, oral exam, written exam, residency.

West Chester University of Pennsylvania
Department of Nursing
West Chester, Pennsylvania

http://health-sciences.wcupa.edu/nursing

Founded in 1871

PENNSYLVANIA

West Chester University of Pennsylvania (continued)

DEGREES • BSN • MSN

Nursing Program Faculty 20 (30% with doctorates).

Baccalaureate Enrollment 332
Women 91.9% **Men** 8.1% **Minority** 12% **International** .3% **Part-time** 20.1%

Graduate Enrollment 39
Women 91.3% **Men** 8.7% **Part-time** 84.6%

Nursing Student Activities Nursing Honor Society, Sigma Theta Tau, Student Nurses' Association.

Nursing Student Resources Academic advising; academic or career counseling; assistance for students with disabilities; bookstore; campus computer network; career placement assistance; computer lab; computer-assisted instruction; daycare for children of students; e-mail services; employment services for current students; externships; housing assistance; interactive nursing skills videos; Internet; learning resource lab; library services; nursing audiovisuals; remedial services; resume preparation assistance; skills, simulation, or other laboratory; tutoring.

Library Facilities 752,451 volumes (88 in nursing); 7,755 periodical subscriptions (173 health-care related).

BACCALAUREATE PROGRAMS

Degree BSN

Available Programs Accelerated RN Baccalaureate; Generic Baccalaureate.

Study Options Full-time and part-time.

Program Entrance Requirements Minimum overall college GPA, transcript of college record, written essay, health exam, health insurance, high school biology, high school chemistry, 2 years high school math, 2 years high school science, high school transcript, immunizations, minimum high school GPA, minimum GPA in nursing prerequisites. Transfer students are accepted. **Standardized tests** *Required:* SAT or ACT, TOEFL for international students. **Application** *Deadline:* rolling (freshmen), rolling (transfer). *Notification:* continuous (freshmen). *Application fee:* $35.

Advanced Placement Credit given for nursing courses completed elsewhere dependent upon specific evaluations.

Contact *Telephone:* 610-436-2219. *Fax:* 610-436-3083.

GRADUATE PROGRAMS

Contact *Telephone:* 610-436-2258. *Fax:* 610-436-3083.

MASTER'S DEGREE PROGRAM

Degree MSN

Available Programs Master's.

Concentrations Available *Clinical nurse specialist programs in:* community health.

Study Options Full-time and part-time.

Program Entrance Requirements Clinical experience, minimum overall college GPA of 2.5, transcript of college record, interview, 3 letters of recommendation, physical assessment course, professional liability insurance/malpractice insurance, resume, statistics course, GRE General Test or MAT. *Application deadline:* For fall admission, 4/15 (priority date); for spring admission, 10/15. Applications are processed on a rolling basis. *Application fee:* $35.

Advanced Placement Credit given for nursing courses completed elsewhere dependent upon specific evaluations.

Degree Requirements 39 total credit hours, thesis or project.

Widener University

School of Nursing
Chester, Pennsylvania

http://www.widener.edu
Founded in 1821

DEGREES • BSN • DN SC • MSN

Nursing Program Faculty 56 (38% with doctorates).

Baccalaureate Enrollment 548
Women 90% **Men** 10% **Minority** 34% **International** 1% **Part-time** 10%

Graduate Enrollment 135
Women 92% **Men** 8% **Minority** 23% **Part-time** 76%

Nursing Student Activities Sigma Theta Tau, Student Nurses' Association.

Nursing Student Resources Academic advising; academic or career counseling; assistance for students with disabilities; bookstore; campus computer network; career placement assistance; computer lab; computer-assisted instruction; e-mail services; employment services for current students; housing assistance; interactive nursing skills videos; Internet; learning resource lab; library services; nursing audiovisuals; placement services for program completers; remedial services; resume preparation assistance; skills, simulation, or other laboratory; tutoring.

Library Facilities 223,827 volumes (18,135 in health, 12,162 in nursing); 2,276 periodical subscriptions (254 health-care related).

BACCALAUREATE PROGRAMS

Degree BSN

Available Programs ADN to Baccalaureate; Baccalaureate for Second Degree; Generic Baccalaureate; RN Baccalaureate.

Study Options Full-time and part-time.

Program Entrance Requirements Minimum overall college GPA of 2.75, transcript of college record, health exam, health insurance, high school biology, high school chemistry, high school foreign language, 3 years high school math, 3 years high school science, high school transcript, immunizations, 2 letters of recommendation, minimum high school GPA of 2.85. Transfer students are accepted. **Standardized tests** *Required:* SAT or ACT. **Application** *Deadline:* rolling (freshmen), rolling (out-of-state freshmen), rolling (transfer). *Notification:* continuous (freshmen), continuous (out-of-state freshmen). *Application fee:* $35.

Advanced Placement Credit by examination available. Credit given for nursing courses completed elsewhere dependent upon specific evaluations.

Expenses (2006–07) *Tuition:* full-time $26,350; part-time $595 per credit. *International tuition:* $26,350 full-time. *Room and board:* $8000; room only: $4500 per academic year. *Required fees:* full-time $290.

Financial Aid 90% of baccalaureate students in nursing programs received some form of financial aid in 2005–06. *Gift aid (need-based):* Federal Pell, FSEOG, state, private, college/university gift aid from institutional funds, Federal Nursing. *Loans:* FFEL (Subsidized and Unsubsidized Stafford PLUS), Perkins. *Work-Study:* Federal Work-Study, part-time campus jobs. *Application deadline (priority):* 2/15.

Contact Ms. Cindy Jaskolka, Assistant Dean, Undergraduate Program, School of Nursing, Widener University, One University Place, Chester, PA 19013-5892. *Telephone:* 610-499-4211. *Fax:* 610-499-4216. *E-mail:* amjaskolka@widener.edu.

GRADUATE PROGRAMS

Expenses (2006–07) *Tuition:* full-time $11,700; part-time $650 per credit. *International tuition:* $11,700 full-time. *Required fees:* full-time $150; part-time $75 per term.

Financial Aid 75% of graduate students in nursing programs received some form of financial aid in 2005–06. Career-related internships or fieldwork, Federal Work-Study, and traineeships available. Aid available to part-time students. *Financial aid application deadline:* 4/1.

Contact Dr. Mary B. Walker, Assistant Dean for Graduate Studies, School of Nursing, Widener University, One University Place, Chester, PA 19013-5892. *Telephone:* 610-499-4208. *Fax:* 610-499-4216. *E-mail:* mary.b.walker@widener.edu.

MASTER'S DEGREE PROGRAM

Degree MSN

Available Programs Accelerated Master's; Master's; RN to Master's.

Concentrations Available Nursing education. *Clinical nurse specialist programs in:* adult health, community health, critical care, psychiatric/mental health. *Nurse practitioner programs in:* family health.

Site Options Harrisburg, PA.

Study Options Full-time and part-time.

Program Entrance Requirements Clinical experience, computer literacy, minimum overall college GPA of 3.0, transcript of college record, CPR certification, immunizations, interview, 2 letters of recommendation, nursing research course, physical assessment course, professional liability insurance/malpractice insurance, prerequisite course work, resume, statistics course, GRE General Test. *Application deadline:* For fall admission, 7/1; for winter admission, 3/1; for spring admission, 11/1. Applications are processed on a rolling basis. *Application fee:* $25 ($300 for international students).

Advanced Placement Credit given for nursing courses completed elsewhere dependent upon specific evaluations.

Degree Requirements 40 total credit hours.

POST-MASTER'S PROGRAM

Areas of Study Nursing education. *Clinical nurse specialist programs in:* adult health, community health, critical care, psychiatric/mental health. *Nurse practitioner programs in:* family health.

DOCTORAL DEGREE PROGRAM

Degree DN Sc

Available Programs Doctorate.

Areas of Study Nursing education.

Program Entrance Requirements Minimum overall college GPA of 3.5, interview, 2 letters of recommendation, MSN or equivalent, statistics course, vita, writing sample, GRE General Test. *Application deadline:* For fall admission, 7/1; for winter admission, 3/1; for spring admission, 11/1. Applications are processed on a rolling basis. *Application fee:* $25 ($300 for international students).

Degree Requirements 63 total credit hours, dissertation, written exam.

See full description on page 578.

Wilkes University
Department of Nursing
Wilkes-Barre, Pennsylvania

http://www.wilkes.edu

Founded in 1933

DEGREES • BS • MS

Nursing Program Faculty 17 (40% with doctorates).

Baccalaureate Enrollment 140
Women 85% **Men** 15% **Minority** 5% **Part-time** 39%

Graduate Enrollment 35
Women 84% **Men** 16%

Nursing Student Activities Sigma Theta Tau, Student Nurses' Association, nursing club.

Nursing Student Resources Academic advising; academic or career counseling; assistance for students with disabilities; bookstore; campus computer network; career placement assistance; computer lab; computer-assisted instruction; daycare for children of students; e-mail services; employment services for current students; externships; housing assistance; interactive nursing skills videos; Internet; learning resource lab; library services; nursing audiovisuals; paid internships; placement services for program completers; remedial services; resume preparation assistance; skills, simulation, or other laboratory; tutoring; unpaid internships.

Library Facilities 13,450 volumes in health, 13,000 volumes in nursing; 70 periodical subscriptions health-care related.

BACCALAUREATE PROGRAMS

Degree BS

Available Programs ADN to Baccalaureate; Accelerated Baccalaureate for Second Degree; Accelerated LPN to Baccalaureate; Accelerated RN Baccalaureate; Generic Baccalaureate; LPN to RN Baccalaureate; RN Baccalaureate.

Site Options Scranton, PA; Hazleton, PA.

Study Options Full-time and part-time.

Program Entrance Requirements Minimum overall college GPA of 2.0, transcript of college record, CPR certification, health exam, health insurance, high school biology, high school chemistry, high school foreign language, high school math, high school science, high school transcript, immunizations, minimum high school GPA, professional liability insurance/malpractice insurance, prerequisite course work. Transfer stu-

dents are accepted. **Standardized tests** *Required:* SAT or ACT, TOEFL for international students. **Application** *Deadline:* rolling (freshmen), rolling (transfer). *Notification:* continuous until 8/30 (freshmen). *Application fee:* $40.

Advanced Placement Credit by examination available. Credit given for nursing courses completed elsewhere dependent upon specific evaluations.

Contact *Telephone:* 570-408-4074. *Fax:* 570-408-7807.

GRADUATE PROGRAMS

Contact *Telephone:* 570-408-4076. *Fax:* 570-408-7807.

MASTER'S DEGREE PROGRAM

Degree MS

Available Programs Accelerated AD/RN to Master's; Accelerated RN to Master's; Master's; Master's for Non-Nursing College Graduates; RN to Master's.

Concentrations Available Nursing administration. *Clinical nurse specialist programs in:* gerontology, psychiatric/mental health.

Site Options Scranton, PA.

Study Options Full-time and part-time.

Program Entrance Requirements Clinical experience, minimum overall college GPA of 3.0, transcript of college record, CPR certification, immunizations, interview, 3 letters of recommendation, nursing research course, physical assessment course, professional liability insurance/malpractice insurance, statistics course.

Advanced Placement Credit given for nursing courses completed elsewhere dependent upon specific evaluations.

Degree Requirements 36 total credit hours, thesis or project.

POST-MASTER'S PROGRAM

Areas of Study Nursing administration. *Clinical nurse specialist programs in:* gerontology, psychiatric/mental health.

CONTINUING EDUCATION PROGRAM

Contact *Telephone:* 570-408-4763.

York College of Pennsylvania
Department of Nursing
York, Pennsylvania

http://www.ycp.edu/nursing/index.html

Founded in 1787

DEGREES • BS • MS

Nursing Program Faculty 57 (11% with doctorates).

Baccalaureate Enrollment 579
Women 94% **Men** 6% **Minority** 4% **Part-time** 36%

Graduate Enrollment 61
Women 98% **Men** 2% **Minority** 1% **International** 1% **Part-time** 100%

Nursing Student Activities Sigma Theta Tau, Student Nurses' Association.

Nursing Student Resources Academic advising; academic or career counseling; assistance for students with disabilities; bookstore; campus computer network; career placement assistance; computer lab; computer-assisted instruction; e-mail services; employment services for current students; externships; housing assistance; interactive nursing skills videos; Internet; learning resource lab; library services; nursing audiovisuals; paid internships; placement services for program completers; remedial services; resume preparation assistance; skills, simulation, or other laboratory; tutoring.

Library Facilities 300,000 volumes (6,681 in health, 1,226 in nursing); 1,400 periodical subscriptions (83 health-care related).

BACCALAUREATE PROGRAMS

Degree BS

Available Programs Generic Baccalaureate; LPN to RN Baccalaureate; RN Baccalaureate.

York College of Pennsylvania (continued)

Site Options *Distance Learning:* Harrisburg, PA; Hanover, PA; Chambersburg, PA.

Study Options Full-time and part-time.

Program Entrance Requirements Minimum overall college GPA of 2.8, transcript of college record, CPR certification, written essay, health exam, health insurance, high school biology, high school chemistry, 1 year of high school math, high school science, high school transcript, immunizations, 2 letters of recommendation, minimum high school rank 40%, minimum GPA in nursing prerequisites of 2.8, professional liability insurance/malpractice insurance, prerequisite course work. **Standardized tests** *Required:* SAT or ACT, TOEFL for international students. **Application** *Deadline:* 8/1 (freshmen), rolling (transfer). *Notification:* continuous (freshmen). *Application fee:* $30.

Advanced Placement Credit by examination available. Credit given for nursing courses completed elsewhere dependent upon specific evaluations.

Expenses (2006–07) *Tuition:* full-time $10,160; part-time $318 per credit. *Room and board:* $6950; room only: $3900 per academic year. *Required fees:* full-time $1000; part-time $56 per credit.

Financial Aid 90% of baccalaureate students in nursing programs received some form of financial aid in 2005–06. *Gift aid (need-based):* Federal Pell, FSEOG, state, private, college/university gift aid from institutional funds. *Loans:* Federal Nursing Student Loans, Federal Direct (Subsidized and Unsubsidized Stafford PLUS), FFEL (Subsidized and Unsubsidized Stafford PLUS), Perkins, college/university. *Work-Study:* Federal Work-Study, part-time campus jobs. *Application deadline (priority):* 3/1.

Contact Dr. Jacquelin H. Harrington, RN, Chairperson, Department of Nursing, York College of Pennsylvania, York, PA 17405-7199. *Telephone:* 717-815-1420. *Fax:* 717-849-1651. *E-mail:* jharring@ycp.edu.

GRADUATE PROGRAMS

Expenses (2006–07) *Tuition:* full-time $4293; part-time $477 per credit. *Room and board:* $6950; room only: $3900 per academic year. *Required fees:* full-time $1000; part-time $56 per credit.

Financial Aid 8% of graduate students in nursing programs received some form of financial aid in 2005–06.

Contact Dr. Lynn Warner, RN, Coordinator, Department of Nursing, York College of Pennsylvania, York, PA 17405-7199. *Telephone:* 717-815-1212. *Fax:* 717-849-1651.

MASTER'S DEGREE PROGRAM

Degree MS

Available Programs Master's; RN to Master's.

Concentrations Available Nurse anesthesia; nurse case management; nurse-midwifery; nursing administration; nursing education. *Clinical nurse specialist programs in:* adult health.

Site Options *Distance Learning:* Harrisburg, PA; Hanover, PA; Chambersburg, PA.

Study Options Part-time.

Program Entrance Requirements Clinical experience, computer literacy, minimum overall college GPA of 3.0, transcript of college record, CPR certification, written essay, immunizations, 2 letters of recommendation, nursing research course, physical assessment course, professional liability insurance/malpractice insurance, resume, statistics course.

Advanced Placement Credit given for nursing courses completed elsewhere dependent upon specific evaluations.

Degree Requirements 41 total credit hours, thesis or project.

PUERTO RICO

Inter American University of Puerto Rico, Metropolitan Campus

Carmen Torres de Tiburcio School of Nursing
San Juan, Puerto Rico

http://www.metro.inter.edu/progacad/enfe/ nursing/index.html

Founded in 1960

DEGREE • BSN

Nursing Program Faculty 26 (27% with doctorates).

Baccalaureate Enrollment 312
Women 57% **Men** 43%

Nursing Student Activities Student Nurses' Association.

Nursing Student Resources Academic advising; academic or career counseling; assistance for students with disabilities; bookstore; campus computer network; career placement assistance; computer lab; computer-assisted instruction; daycare for children of students; e-mail services; employment services for current students; externships; interactive nursing skills videos; Internet; learning resource lab; library services; nursing audiovisuals; paid internships; placement services for program completers; remedial services; skills, simulation, or other laboratory; tutoring.

Library Facilities 113,200 volumes (36,000 in health, 21,759 in nursing); 2,771 periodical subscriptions (2,090 health-care related).

BACCALAUREATE PROGRAMS

Degree BSN

Available Programs ADN to Baccalaureate; Accelerated Baccalaureate; Generic Baccalaureate.

Study Options Full-time and part-time.

Program Entrance Requirements Minimum overall college GPA of 2.0, transcript of college record, CPR certification, health exam, health insurance, high school transcript, immunizations, 2 letters of recommendation, minimum high school rank 4%, minimum GPA in nursing prerequisites of 2. Transfer students are accepted. **Standardized tests** *Required for some:* SAT. **Placement:** *Required for some:* SAT. **Application** *Deadline:* 5/15 (freshmen), 5/15 (transfer).

Advanced Placement Credit by examination available. Credit given for nursing courses completed elsewhere dependent upon specific evaluations.

Contact *Telephone:* 787-763-3066. *Fax:* 787-250-1242 Ext. 2159.

Pontifical Catholic University of Puerto Rico

Department of Nursing
Ponce, Puerto Rico

http://www.pucpr.edu/catalogo/espanol/ciencias/ dep_enf.htm

Founded in 1948

DEGREE • BSN

Library Facilities 1,499 volumes in nursing; 58,185 periodical subscriptions.

BACCALAUREATE PROGRAMS

Degree BSN

Available Programs Generic Baccalaureate.

Program Entrance Requirements Minimum overall college GPA of 2.0, CPR certification, health exam, health insurance, immunizations, interview, letters of recommendation, minimum high school GPA of 2.5, prerequisite course work. **Standardized tests** *Required:* SAT. **Application** *Deadline:* 3/15 (freshmen), 3/15 (transfer). *Notification:* continuous (freshmen). *Application fee:* $15.

Contact *Telephone:* 787-841-2000 Ext. 1604.

Universidad Adventista de las Antillas
Department of Nursing
Mayagüez, Puerto Rico

Founded in 1957

DEGREE • BSN

Nursing Program Faculty 9 (22% with doctorates).

Baccalaureate Enrollment 232
Women 78% **Men** 22% **Minority** 100% **International** 4% **Part-time** 9%
Nursing Student Activities Nursing club.

Nursing Student Resources Academic advising; academic or career counseling; campus computer network; computer lab; computer-assisted instruction; e-mail services; employment services for current students; housing assistance; interactive nursing skills videos; Internet; learning resource lab; library services; nursing audiovisuals; remedial services; skills, simulation, or other laboratory; tutoring.

Library Facilities 86,465 volumes (4,360 in health, 3,827 in nursing); 452 periodical subscriptions (70 health-care related).

BACCALAUREATE PROGRAMS

Degree BSN

Available Programs Generic Baccalaureate; RN Baccalaureate.
Study Options Full-time.
Program Entrance Requirements Minimum overall college GPA of 2.3, transcript of college record, health exam, health insurance, high school transcript, immunizations, interview, 2 letters of recommendation, minimum high school GPA of 2.5. Transfer students are accepted. **Standardized tests** *Recommended:* SAT or ACT, PAA. **Application** *Application fee:* $20.
Advanced Placement Credit given for nursing courses completed elsewhere dependent upon specific evaluations.
Contact *Telephone:* 787-834-9595 Ext. 2209. *Fax:* 787-834-9597.

CONTINUING EDUCATION PROGRAM
Contact *Telephone:* 787-834-9595 Ext. 2301. *Fax:* 787-834-9597.

Universidad del Turabo
Nursing Program
Gurabo, Puerto Rico

Founded in 1972

DEGREE • BS

Library Facilities 90,020 volumes; 655 periodical subscriptions.

BACCALAUREATE PROGRAMS

Degree BS

Available Programs Generic Baccalaureate.
Program Entrance Requirements *Placement: Required:* CEEB. **Application** *Deadline:* rolling (freshmen), rolling (transfer). *Notification:* continuous until 8/1 (freshmen). *Application fee:* $15.
Contact Admissions, Nursing Program, Universidad del Turabo, PO Box 3030, Gurabo, PR 00778-3030. *Telephone:* 787-743-7979.

Universidad Metropolitana
Department of Nursing
San Juan, Puerto Rico

http://www.suagm.edu/umet/umet_new_web/ escuelas/ciencias_tecnologia/ciencias_tecnologia. htm
Founded in 1980

DEGREE • BSN

Library Facilities 5,438 volumes in health; 110 periodical subscriptions health-care related.

BACCALAUREATE PROGRAMS

Degree BSN

Program Entrance Requirements Standardized tests *Required:* PAA. **Application** *Deadline:* 7/30 (freshmen), 7/30 (transfer). *Application fee:* $15.
Contact *Telephone:* 787-766-1717 Ext. 6422. *Fax:* 787-769-7663.

University of Puerto Rico at Arecibo
Department of Nursing
Arecibo, Puerto Rico

http://upra.edu/asuntosacademicos/enfermeria/ menu_enfe.htm
Founded in 1967

DEGREE • BSN

Nursing Program Faculty 21.

Library Facilities 65,000 volumes; 3,660 periodical subscriptions.

BACCALAUREATE PROGRAMS

Degree BSN

Available Programs Generic Baccalaureate.
Program Entrance Requirements Standardized tests *Required:* SAT Subject Tests, PAA or SAT, CEEB. *Placement: Required:* SAT Subject Tests. **Application** *Deadline:* 12/8 (freshmen), 2/18 (transfer). *Notification:* 3/18 (freshmen). *Application fee:* $15.
Contact *Telephone:* 787-878-2830. *Fax:* 787-880-4972.

University of Puerto Rico at Humacao
Department of Nursing
Humacao, Puerto Rico

http://cuhwww.upr.clu.edu/~enfe/
Founded in 1962

DEGREE • BS

Nursing Program Faculty 16 (12% with doctorates).
Nursing Student Activities Student Nurses' Association.
Nursing Student Resources Skills, simulation, or other laboratory.
Library Facilities 71,228 volumes; 18,697 periodical subscriptions.

BACCALAUREATE PROGRAMS

Degree BS

Available Programs Generic Baccalaureate.
Study Options Full-time and part-time.

University of Puerto Rico at Humacao (continued)

Program Entrance Requirements Minimum overall college GPA, transcript of college record, health exam, health insurance, high school transcript, immunizations, minimum high school GPA of 2.0, minimum GPA in nursing prerequisites of 2.5. Transfer students are accepted. **Standardized tests** *Required:* CEEB. *Required for some:* SAT or ACT. **Application** *Deadline:* 11/15 (freshmen), 2/15 (transfer). *Notification:* continuous until 4/15 (freshmen). *Application fee:* $20.

Advanced Placement Credit by examination available. Credit given for nursing courses completed elsewhere dependent upon specific evaluations.

Contact *Telephone:* 787-850-9346. *Fax:* 787-850-9411.

University of Puerto Rico, Mayagüez Campus
Department of Nursing
Mayagüez, Puerto Rico

http://www.uprm.edu/enfe/

Founded in 1911

DEGREE • BSN

Nursing Program Faculty 21 (10% with doctorates).

Nursing Student Activities Nursing Honor Society, Sigma Theta Tau, Student Nurses' Association.

Nursing Student Resources Academic advising; academic or career counseling; assistance for students with disabilities; bookstore; campus computer network; career placement assistance; computer lab; computer-assisted instruction; e-mail services; employment services for current students; interactive nursing skills videos; Internet; learning resource lab; library services; nursing audiovisuals; paid internships; placement services for program completers; remedial services; resume preparation assistance; skills, simulation, or other laboratory; tutoring.

Library Facilities 921,392 volumes; 590,716 periodical subscriptions (68 health-care related).

BACCALAUREATE PROGRAMS

Degree BSN

Available Programs Generic Baccalaureate.

Study Options Full-time.

Program Entrance Requirements High school transcript, immunizations. Transfer students are accepted. **Standardized tests** *Required:* SAT, SAT Subject Tests. **Application** *Deadline:* 12/15 (freshmen), 2/15 (transfer). *Notification:* 3/15 (freshmen). *Application fee:* $15.

Advanced Placement Credit by examination available.

Contact *Telephone:* 787-263-3482. *Fax:* 787-832-3875.

CONTINUING EDUCATION PROGRAM

Contact *Telephone:* 787-265-3842. *Fax:* 787-832-3875.

University of Puerto Rico, Medical Sciences Campus
School of Nursing
San Juan, Puerto Rico

Founded in 1950

DEGREES • BSN • MSN

Nursing Program Faculty 37 (25% with doctorates).

Baccalaureate Enrollment 241
Women 85% **Men** 15% **Part-time** 12%

Graduate Enrollment 158
Women 79% **Men** 21% **Part-time** 6%

Nursing Student Activities Sigma Theta Tau, Student Nurses' Association.

Nursing Student Resources Academic advising; academic or career counseling; assistance for students with disabilities; computer lab; computer-assisted instruction; e-mail services; employment services for current students; interactive nursing skills videos; Internet; library services; nursing audiovisuals; skills, simulation, or other laboratory; tutoring.

Library Facilities 46,679 volumes (7,830 in health, 1,143 in nursing); 1,432 periodical subscriptions (1,215 health-care related).

BACCALAUREATE PROGRAMS

Degree BSN

Available Programs ADN to Baccalaureate; Generic Baccalaureate.

Study Options Full-time and part-time.

Program Entrance Requirements Minimum overall college GPA of 2.0, transcript of college record, health exam, immunizations, interview, minimum high school GPA of 2.0, prerequisite course work. Transfer students are accepted. **Application** *Deadline:* 2/18 (transfer). *Application fee:* $20.

Contact *Telephone:* 787-758-2525 Ext. 1984. *Fax:* 787-281-0721.

GRADUATE PROGRAMS

Contact *Telephone:* 787-758-2525 Ext. 3105. *Fax:* 787-281-0721.

MASTER'S DEGREE PROGRAM

Degree MSN

Available Programs Master's.

Concentrations Available Nurse anesthesia; nursing administration; nursing education. *Clinical nurse specialist programs in:* adult health, community health, critical care, gerontology, maternity-newborn, pediatric, psychiatric/mental health.

Site Options Mayaguez, PR.

Study Options Full-time and part-time.

Program Entrance Requirements Clinical experience, minimum overall college GPA of 2.5, transcript of college record, immunizations, interview, resume, statistics course, GRE or EXADEP. *Application deadline:* For fall admission, 3/31 (priority date). *Application fee:* $20.

Degree Requirements 48 total credit hours, thesis or project.

CONTINUING EDUCATION PROGRAM

Contact *Telephone:* 787-758-2525 Ext. 2102. *Fax:* 787-281-0721.

University of the Sacred Heart
Program in Nursing
San Juan, Puerto Rico

Founded in 1935

DEGREES • BSN • MSN

Nursing Student Resources Skills, simulation, or other laboratory.

Library Facilities 1,525 periodical subscriptions.

BACCALAUREATE PROGRAMS

Degree BSN

Available Programs Generic Baccalaureate.

Program Entrance Requirements **Standardized tests** *Required:* PAA, CEEB. **Application** *Deadline:* 6/30 (freshmen), 6/30 (transfer). *Application fee:* $15.

Contact *Telephone:* 787-728-1515. *Fax:* 787-727-1250.

GRADUATE PROGRAMS

Contact *Telephone:* 787-728-1515 Ext. 2427. *Fax:* 787-727-1250.

MASTER'S DEGREE PROGRAM

Degree MSN

Available Programs Master's.

Concentrations Available *Nurse practitioner programs in:* occupational health.

Degree Requirements 37 total credit hours.

RHODE ISLAND

Rhode Island College
Department of Nursing
Providence, Rhode Island

http://www.ric.edu/nursing
Founded in 1854
DEGREE • BS

Nursing Program Faculty 37 (43% with doctorates).

Baccalaureate Enrollment 389
Women 89% **Men** 11% **Minority** 24% **Part-time** 28%

Nursing Student Activities Sigma Theta Tau, Student Nurses' Association, nursing club.

Nursing Student Resources Academic advising; academic or career counseling; assistance for students with disabilities; bookstore; campus computer network; career placement assistance; computer lab; computer-assisted instruction; e-mail services; employment services for current students; housing assistance; interactive nursing skills videos; Internet; learning resource lab; library services; nursing audiovisuals; paid internships; remedial services; resume preparation assistance; skills, simulation, or other laboratory; tutoring.

Library Facilities 664,667 volumes (574 in nursing); 2,251 periodical subscriptions (63 health-care related).

BACCALAUREATE PROGRAMS
Degree BS

Available Programs Baccalaureate for Second Degree; Generic Baccalaureate; RN Baccalaureate.

Site Options Providence, RI.

Study Options Full-time and part-time.

Program Entrance Requirements Minimum overall college GPA of 2.5, CPR certification, health exam, high school biology, high school chemistry, high school foreign language, 4 years high school math, 2 years high school science, high school transcript, immunizations, letters of recommendation, minimum GPA in nursing prerequisites of 2.5, prerequisite course work. Transfer students are accepted. **Standardized tests** *Required:* SAT or ACT, TOEFL for international students. **Application** *Deadline:* 5/1 (freshmen), 5/1 (out-of-state freshmen), 6/1 (transfer). *Notification:* continuous (freshmen), continuous (out-of-state freshmen). *Application fee:* $50.

Advanced Placement Credit given for nursing courses completed elsewhere dependent upon specific evaluations.

Expenses (2005–06) *Tuition, area resident:* full-time $4338; part-time $189 per credit hour. *Tuition, state resident:* full-time $7014; part-time $283 per credit hour. *Tuition, nonresident:* full-time $11,988; part-time $487 per credit hour. *Room and board:* $7060; room only: $3840 per academic year. *Required fees:* full-time $90; part-time $45 per term.

Financial Aid 60% of baccalaureate students in nursing programs received some form of financial aid in 2004–05. *Gift aid (need-based):* Federal Pell, FSEOG, state, private, college/university gift aid from institutional funds. *Loans:* FFEL (Subsidized and Unsubsidized Stafford PLUS), Perkins, state. *Work-Study:* Federal Work-Study. *Application deadline (priority):* 3/1.

Contact Dr. Jane Williams, Chair, Department of Nursing, Rhode Island College, 600 Mount Pleasant Avenue, Providence, RI 02908-1991. *Telephone:* 401-456-8014. *Fax:* 401-456-8206. *E-mail:* jwilliams@ric.edu.

Salve Regina University
Department of Nursing
Newport, Rhode Island

http://www.salve.edu/departments/nur/index.cfm
Founded in 1934

DEGREE • BS

Nursing Program Faculty 23 (39% with doctorates).

Baccalaureate Enrollment 255
Women 96% **Men** 4% **Minority** 5.8% **Part-time** 19%

Nursing Student Activities Student Nurses' Association, nursing club.

Nursing Student Resources Academic advising; academic or career counseling; assistance for students with disabilities; bookstore; campus computer network; career placement assistance; computer lab; computer-assisted instruction; e-mail services; housing assistance; interactive nursing skills videos; Internet; learning resource lab; library services; nursing audiovisuals; paid internships; resume preparation assistance; skills, simulation, or other laboratory; tutoring; unpaid internships.

Library Facilities 139,161 volumes (6,882 in health, 1,081 in nursing); 1,221 periodical subscriptions (76 health-care related).

BACCALAUREATE PROGRAMS
Degree BS

Available Programs Generic Baccalaureate; RN Baccalaureate.

Site Options Warwick, RI; Pawtucket, RI; Providence, RI.

Study Options Full-time and part-time.

Program Entrance Requirements Minimum overall college GPA of 2.7, transcript of college record, CPR certification, written essay, health exam, health insurance, high school biology, high school chemistry, high school foreign language, 4 years high school math, 4 years high school science, high school transcript, immunizations, 2 letters of recommendation, minimum GPA in nursing prerequisites of 2.0, professional liability insurance/malpractice insurance, prerequisite course work. Transfer students are accepted. **Standardized tests** *Required:* SAT or ACT, TOEFL for international students. **Application** *Deadline:* 3/1 (freshmen), rolling (transfer). *Early decision:* 11/1. *Notification:* continuous (freshmen), 12/15 (early action). *Application fee:* $40.

Advanced Placement Credit by examination available. Credit given for nursing courses completed elsewhere dependent upon specific evaluations.

Expenses (2006–07) *Tuition:* full-time $24,975; part-time $833 per credit. *International tuition:* $24,975 full-time. *Room and board:* $9800 per academic year. *Required fees:* full-time $200; part-time $40 per term.

Financial Aid 79% of baccalaureate students in nursing programs received some form of financial aid in 2005–06. *Gift aid (need-based):* Federal Pell, FSEOG, state, private, college/university gift aid from institutional funds. *Loans:* Federal Nursing Student Loans, FFEL (Subsidized and Unsubsidized Stafford PLUS), Perkins, college/university, alternative loans. *Work-Study:* Federal Work-Study, part-time campus jobs. *Application deadline (priority):* 3/1.

Contact Mrs. Laura E. McPhie Oliveira, Vice President for Enrollment Services/Dean of Admissions, Department of Nursing, Salve Regina University, 100 Ochre Point Avenue, Newport, RI 02840-4192. *Telephone:* 888-467-2583. *Fax:* 401-848-2823. *E-mail:* sruadmis@salve.edu.

CONTINUING EDUCATION PROGRAM
Contact Dr. Thomas Sabbagh, Dean/Continuing Education and Graduate Enrollment, Department of Nursing, Salve Regina University, Graduate Studies and Continuing Education Office, Newport, RI 02840-4192. *Telephone:* 800-637-0002. *Fax:* 401-341-2931. *E-mail:* thomas.sabbagh@salve.edu.

University of Rhode Island
College of Nursing
Kingston, Rhode Island

http://www.uri.edu/nursing
Founded in 1892

DEGREES • BS • MS • PHD

Nursing Program Faculty 47 (32% with doctorates).

Baccalaureate Enrollment 404
Women 87% **Men** 13% **Minority** 24% **International** 1% **Part-time** 10%

Graduate Enrollment 110
Women 95% **Men** 5% **Minority** 5% **International** 6% **Part-time** 75%

University of Rhode Island (continued)

Nursing Student Activities Sigma Theta Tau, Student Nurses' Association.

Nursing Student Resources Academic advising; academic or career counseling; assistance for students with disabilities; bookstore; campus computer network; career placement assistance; computer lab; computer-assisted instruction; e-mail services; externships; housing assistance; interactive nursing skills videos; Internet; learning resource lab; library services; nursing audiovisuals; remedial services; resume preparation assistance; skills, simulation, or other laboratory; tutoring.

Library Facilities 1.2 million volumes; 7,926 periodical subscriptions.

BACCALAUREATE PROGRAMS

Degree BS

Available Programs ADN to Baccalaureate; Generic Baccalaureate; RN Baccalaureate.

Site Options Providence, RI.

Study Options Full-time and part-time.

Program Entrance Requirements Minimum overall college GPA of 2.5, transcript of college record, CPR certification, written essay, health exam, health insurance, high school foreign language, 3 years high school math, 2 years high school science, high school transcript, immunizations, 2 letters of recommendation, minimum high school rank 30%, minimum GPA in nursing prerequisites of 2.2. Transfer students are accepted. **Standardized tests** *Required:* SAT or ACT, TOEFL for international students. **Application** *Deadline:* 2/1 (freshmen), 5/1 (transfer). *Early decision:* 12/15. *Notification:* continuous (freshmen), 1/15 (early action). *Application fee:* $50.

Advanced Placement Credit given for nursing courses completed elsewhere dependent upon specific evaluations.

Contact *Telephone:* 401-874-7100.

GRADUATE PROGRAMS

Contact *Telephone:* 401-874-2766. *Fax:* 401-874-2061.

MASTER'S DEGREE PROGRAM

Degree MS

Available Programs Master's; RN to Master's.

Concentrations Available Nurse-midwifery; nursing administration; nursing education. *Clinical nurse specialist programs in:* gerontology, psychiatric/mental health. *Nurse practitioner programs in:* family health.

Site Options Providence, RI.

Study Options Full-time and part-time.

Program Entrance Requirements Clinical experience, minimum overall college GPA of 3.0, transcript of college record, written essay, immunizations, 3 letters of recommendation, nursing research course, professional liability insurance/malpractice insurance, resume, statistics course. *Application deadline:* For fall admission, 4/15. *Application fee:* $35.

Degree Requirements 41 total credit hours, thesis or project, comprehensive exam.

POST-MASTER'S PROGRAM

Areas of Study Nurse-midwifery; nursing administration; nursing education. *Clinical nurse specialist programs in:* gerontology, psychiatric/mental health. *Nurse practitioner programs in:* family health.

DOCTORAL DEGREE PROGRAM

Degree PhD

Available Programs Doctorate.

Areas of Study Nursing research, nursing science.

Program Entrance Requirements Clinical experience, minimum overall college GPA of 3.0, interview by faculty committee, 3 letters of recommendation, MSN or equivalent, scholarly papers, statistics course, vita, writing sample. *Application deadline:* For fall admission, 4/15. *Application fee:* $35.

Degree Requirements 61 total credit hours, dissertation, oral exam, written exam, residency.

SOUTH CAROLINA

Charleston Southern University
Wingo School of Nursing
Charleston, South Carolina

http://www.csuniv.edu

Founded in 1964

DEGREE • BSN

Nursing Program Faculty 11 (20% with doctorates).

Baccalaureate Enrollment 78
Women 90% **Men** 10% **Minority** 25%

Nursing Student Activities Sigma Theta Tau, Student Nurses' Association.

Nursing Student Resources Academic advising; academic or career counseling; assistance for students with disabilities; bookstore; campus computer network; career placement assistance; computer lab; computer-assisted instruction; e-mail services; interactive nursing skills videos; Internet; learning resource lab; library services; nursing audiovisuals; remedial services; resume preparation assistance; skills, simulation, or other laboratory; tutoring.

Library Facilities 192,600 volumes (2,400 in health, 250 in nursing); 1,111 periodical subscriptions (55 health-care related).

BACCALAUREATE PROGRAMS

Degree BSN

Available Programs ADN to Baccalaureate; Generic Baccalaureate; RN Baccalaureate.

Study Options Full-time.

Program Entrance Requirements Minimum overall college GPA of 2.0, transcript of college record, CPR certification, written essay, health exam, health insurance, immunizations, minimum GPA in nursing prerequisites of 2.5, professional liability insurance/malpractice insurance, prerequisite course work. Transfer students are accepted. **Standardized tests** *Required:* SAT or ACT. **Application** *Deadline:* rolling (freshmen), rolling (transfer). *Notification:* continuous (freshmen). *Application fee:* $30.

Advanced Placement Credit given for nursing courses completed elsewhere dependent upon specific evaluations.

Expenses (2006–07) *Tuition:* full-time $16,780; part-time $271 per credit. *Room and board:* $6450 per academic year. *Required fees:* full-time $1000.

Financial Aid 90% of baccalaureate students in nursing programs received some form of financial aid in 2005–06.

Contact Dr. Marian M. Larisey, RN, Dean, Wingo School of Nursing, Charleston Southern University, PO Box 118087, 9200 University Boulevard, Charleston, SC 29423-8087. *Telephone:* 843-863-7075. *Fax:* 843-863-7540. *E-mail:* mlarisey@csuniv.edu.

Clemson University
School of Nursing
Clemson, South Carolina

http://www.hehd.clemson.edu/nursing

Founded in 1889

DEGREES • BS • MS

Nursing Program Faculty 24 (71% with doctorates).

Baccalaureate Enrollment 402
Women 99% **Men** 1% **Minority** 11%

Graduate Enrollment 82
Women 96.3% **Men** 3.7% **Minority** 9.8% **Part-time** 65.9%

Nursing Student Activities Nursing Honor Society, Sigma Theta Tau, Student Nurses' Association.

Nursing Student Resources Academic advising; academic or career counseling; assistance for students with disabilities; bookstore; campus computer network; career placement assistance; computer lab; computer-assisted instruction; e-mail services; employment services for current students; externships; housing assistance; interactive nursing skills videos; Internet; learning resource lab; library services; nursing audiovisuals; other; remedial services; resume preparation assistance; skills, simulation, or other laboratory; tutoring; unpaid internships.

Library Facilities 1.2 million volumes (29,800 in health, 5,548 in nursing); 5,587 periodical subscriptions (877 health-care related).

BACCALAUREATE PROGRAMS

Degree BS

Available Programs Generic Baccalaureate; RN Baccalaureate.
Site Options *Distance Learning:* Greenville, SC.
Study Options Full-time and part-time.
Program Entrance Requirements Minimum overall college GPA of 2.5, transcript of college record, CPR certification, health insurance, high school biology, high school chemistry, 3 years high school math, 3 years high school science, high school transcript, immunizations, minimum high school GPA of 2.5, professional liability insurance/malpractice insurance, prerequisite course work. Transfer students are accepted. **Standardized tests** *Required:* SAT or ACT, TOEFL for international students. **Application** *Deadline:* 5/1 (freshmen), 8/1 (transfer). *Early decision:* 12/1. *Notification:* continuous (freshmen), 2/15 (early action). *Application fee:* $50.
Advanced Placement Credit by examination available. Credit given for nursing courses completed elsewhere dependent upon specific evaluations.
Expenses (2006–07) *Tuition, state resident:* full-time $4700; part-time $386 per credit hour. *Tuition, nonresident:* full-time $9912; part-time $816 per credit hour. *International tuition:* $9912 full-time. *Room and board:* $5780; room only: $3470 per academic year. *Required fees:* full-time $514; part-time $177 per credit; part-time $177 per term.
Financial Aid 90% of baccalaureate students in nursing programs received some form of financial aid in 2005–06. *Gift aid (need-based):* Federal Pell, FSEOG, state, private, college/university gift aid from institutional funds, Federal Nursing. *Loans:* FFEL (Subsidized and Unsubsidized Stafford PLUS), Perkins, state, college/university, private loans. *Work-Study:* Federal Work-Study, part-time campus jobs. *Application deadline (priority):* 4/1.
Contact Mr. Robert S. Barkley, Director of Admissions, School of Nursing, Clemson University, 106 Sikes Hall, Clemson, SC 29634. *Telephone:* 864-656-5463. *Fax:* 864-656-2464. *E-mail:* rbrtbkl@clemson.edu.

GRADUATE PROGRAMS

Expenses (2006–07) *Tuition, state resident:* full-time $4643; part-time $450 per credit hour. *Tuition, nonresident:* full-time $9255; part-time $760 per credit hour. *International tuition:* $9255 full-time. *Room and board:* $5780; room only: $3470 per academic year. *Required fees:* full-time $474; part-time $145 per credit; part-time $237 per term.
Financial Aid 75% of graduate students in nursing programs received some form of financial aid in 2005–06. Fellowships, research assistantships, teaching assistantships, career-related internships or fieldwork and traineeships available.
Contact Ms. Lynne G. McGuirt, Student Services Program Coordinator, School of Nursing, Clemson University, 225 South Pleasantburg Drive, Greenville, SC 29606. *Telephone:* 864-250-8881. *Fax:* 864-250-6711. *E-mail:* lgm@clemson.edu.

MASTER'S DEGREE PROGRAM

Degree MS

Available Programs Master's; RN to Master's.
Concentrations Available Nursing administration; nursing education. *Clinical nurse specialist programs in:* adult health, gerontology, maternity-newborn, parent-child, pediatric. *Nurse practitioner programs in:* adult health, family health, gerontology.
Site Options *Distance Learning:* Greenville, SC.
Study Options Full-time and part-time.

Program Entrance Requirements Clinical experience, computer literacy, minimum overall college GPA of 3.0, transcript of college record, CPR certification, 2 letters of recommendation, nursing research course, physical assessment course, professional liability insurance/malpractice insurance, prerequisite course work, resume, statistics course, GRE General Test. *Application deadline:* For fall admission, 6/1; for spring admission, 12/1. *Application fee:* $50.
Advanced Placement Credit by examination available. Credit given for nursing courses completed elsewhere dependent upon specific evaluations.
Degree Requirements 45 total credit hours, thesis or project, comprehensive exam.

POST-MASTER'S PROGRAM

Areas of Study Nursing administration; nursing education. *Clinical nurse specialist programs in:* adult health, gerontology, maternity-newborn, parent-child, pediatric. *Nurse practitioner programs in:* adult health, family health, gerontology.

CONTINUING EDUCATION PROGRAM

Contact Ms. Olivia Shanahan, Director of Continuing Education, School of Nursing, Clemson University, 430 Edwards Hall, Clemson, SC 29634-0748. *Telephone:* 864-656-3078. *Fax:* 864-656-1877. *E-mail:* olivia@clemson.edu.

Francis Marion University
Department of Nursing
Florence, South Carolina

Founded in 1970
DEGREE • BSN

Library Facilities 396,204 volumes; 1,504 periodical subscriptions.

BACCALAUREATE PROGRAMS
Degree BSN

Available Programs Generic Baccalaureate.
Program Entrance Requirements Standardized tests *Required:* SAT or ACT, TOEFL for international students. **Application** *Deadline:* rolling (freshmen), rolling (transfer). *Notification:* continuous (freshmen). *Application fee:* $30.
Contact Nursing Contact, Department of Nursing, Francis Marion University, PO Box 100547, Florence, SC 29501. *Telephone:* 843-661-1362.

Lander University
School of Nursing
Greenwood, South Carolina

http://www.lander.edu/nursing/
Founded in 1872
DEGREE • BSN

Nursing Program Faculty 15 (13% with doctorates).
Baccalaureate Enrollment 269
Women 91% **Men** 9% **Minority** 20% **Part-time** 18%
Nursing Student Activities Sigma Theta Tau, Student Nurses' Association.
Nursing Student Resources Academic advising; academic or career counseling; assistance for students with disabilities; bookstore; campus computer network; career placement assistance; computer lab; computer-assisted instruction; e-mail services; externships; housing assistance; interactive nursing skills videos; Internet; learning resource lab; library services; nursing audiovisuals; resume preparation assistance; skills, simulation, or other laboratory.
Library Facilities 186,690 volumes (5,743 in health, 5,447 in nursing); 657 periodical subscriptions (53 health-care related).

Lander University (continued)

BACCALAUREATE PROGRAMS

Degree BSN

Available Programs Accelerated Baccalaureate; Accelerated Baccalaureate for Second Degree; Accelerated RN Baccalaureate; Baccalaureate for Second Degree; Generic Baccalaureate; RN Baccalaureate.

Site Options *Distance Learning:* Greenwood, SC.

Study Options Full-time and part-time.

Program Entrance Requirements Minimum overall college GPA of 2.6, transcript of college record, CPR certification, health exam, health insurance, immunizations, professional liability insurance/malpractice insurance, prerequisite course work. Transfer students are accepted. **Standardized tests** *Required:* SAT or ACT, TOEFL for international students. **Application** *Deadline:* 8/1 (freshmen), rolling (transfer). *Notification:* continuous (freshmen). *Application fee:* $35.

Advanced Placement Credit given for nursing courses completed elsewhere dependent upon specific evaluations.

Expenses (2006–07) *Tuition, state resident:* full-time $7152; part-time $298 per credit hour. *Tuition, nonresident:* full-time $13,528; part-time $564 per credit hour. *International tuition:* $13,528 full-time. *Room and board:* $5755; room only: $3543 per academic year. *Required fees:* full-time $1000.

Financial Aid 60% of baccalaureate students in nursing programs received some form of financial aid in 2005–06.

Contact Mr. Jonathan T. Reece, Director of Admissions, School of Nursing, Lander University, 320 Stanley Avenue, Greenwood, SC 29649-2099. *Telephone:* 864-388-8307. *Fax:* 864-388-8125. *E-mail:* jreece@lander.edu.

Medical University of South Carolina

College of Nursing
Charleston, South Carolina

http://www.musc.edu/Nursing

Founded in 1824

DEGREES • BSN • MSN • MSN/PHD

Nursing Program Faculty 94 (32% with doctorates).

Baccalaureate Enrollment 202
Women 90% **Men** 10% **Minority** 13% **International** 1% **Part-time** 15%

Graduate Enrollment 174
Women 91% **Men** 9% **Minority** 9% **Part-time** 58%

Nursing Student Activities Nursing Honor Society, Sigma Theta Tau, Student Nurses' Association.

Nursing Student Resources Academic advising; bookstore; campus computer network; computer lab; computer-assisted instruction; e-mail services; housing assistance; interactive nursing skills videos; Internet; learning resource lab; library services; nursing audiovisuals; resume preparation assistance; skills, simulation, or other laboratory; tutoring.

Library Facilities 225,061 volumes (196,627 in health, 5,824 in nursing); 3,746 periodical subscriptions (5,492 health-care related).

BACCALAUREATE PROGRAMS

Degree BSN

Available Programs ADN to Baccalaureate; Accelerated Baccalaureate; Accelerated RN Baccalaureate; RN Baccalaureate.

Study Options Full-time and part-time.

Program Entrance Requirements Transcript of college record, written essay, 3 letters of recommendation, minimum GPA in nursing prerequisites of 3.0, prerequisite course work. Transfer students are accepted. **Standardized tests** *Required:* TOEFL for international students. **Application** *Deadline:* 2/1 (freshmen), 8/25 (transfer). *Application fee:* $75.

Advanced Placement Credit by examination available. Credit given for nursing courses completed elsewhere dependent upon specific evaluations.

Expenses (2005–06) *Tuition, state resident:* full-time $9060; part-time $410 per credit hour. *Tuition, nonresident:* full-time $24,810; part-time $1148 per credit hour. *International tuition:* $24,810 full-time. *Required fees:* full-time $400; part-time $270 per term.

Financial Aid 82% of baccalaureate students in nursing programs received some form of financial aid in 2004–05.

Contact Ms. Nicole Mullinax, Program Coordinator, College of Nursing, Medical University of South Carolina, PO Box 250160, 99 Jonathan Lucas Street, Charleston, SC 29425. *Telephone:* 843-792-3884. *Fax:* 843-792-9258. *E-mail:* mullinan@musc.edu.

GRADUATE PROGRAMS

Expenses (2005–06) *Tuition, state resident:* full-time $9849; part-time $503 per credit hour. *Tuition, nonresident:* full-time $15,736; part-time $781 per credit hour. *International tuition:* $15,736 full-time. *Required fees:* full-time $1212; part-time $606 per term.

Financial Aid 72% of graduate students in nursing programs received some form of financial aid in 2004–05. Federal Work-Study, scholarships, and traineeships available. Aid available to part-time students. *Financial aid application deadline:* 3/15.

Contact Dr. Mary M. Martin, RN, Assistant Professor, College of Nursing, Medical University of South Carolina, 99 Jonathan Lucas Street, PO Box 250160, Charleston, SC 29425. *Telephone:* 843-792-3084. *Fax:* 843-792-9250. *E-mail:* martinmm@musc.edu.

MASTER'S DEGREE PROGRAM

Degrees MSN; MSN/PhD

Available Programs Accelerated Master's; Accelerated Master's for Nurses with Non-Nursing Degrees; Accelerated RN to Master's; Master's; RN to Master's.

Concentrations Available Nurse-midwifery; nursing administration; nursing education. *Clinical nurse specialist programs in:* adult health, gerontology, parent-child, psychiatric/mental health. *Nurse practitioner programs in:* adult health, family health, gerontology, neonatal health, pediatric, psychiatric/mental health.

Study Options Full-time and part-time.

Program Entrance Requirements Minimum overall college GPA of 3.0, transcript of college record, written essay, interview, 3 letters of recommendation, physical assessment course, prerequisite course work, resume, statistics course, GRE General Test. *Application deadline:* For fall admission, 2/1; for spring admission, 9/15. *Application fee:* $75.

Advanced Placement Credit given for nursing courses completed elsewhere dependent upon specific evaluations.

Degree Requirements 60 total credit hours.

POST-MASTER'S PROGRAM

Areas of Study Nurse-midwifery; nursing administration; nursing education. *Clinical nurse specialist programs in:* adult health, gerontology, parent-child, psychiatric/mental health. *Nurse practitioner programs in:* adult health, family health, gerontology, pediatric, psychiatric/mental health.

DOCTORAL DEGREE PROGRAM

Degree PhD

Available Programs Doctorate; Post-Baccalaureate Doctorate.

Program Entrance Requirements Minimum overall college GPA of 3.5, interview by faculty committee, interview, 3 letters of recommendation, MSN or equivalent, statistics course, vita, writing sample. *Application deadline:* For fall admission, 2/1; for spring admission, 9/15. *Application fee:* $75.

Degree Requirements 62 total credit hours, dissertation, oral exam, written exam.

CONTINUING EDUCATION PROGRAM

Contact Ms. Carol McDougall, Director of Continuing Education, College of Nursing, Medical University of South Carolina, 99 Jonathan Lucas Street, PO Box 260160, Charleston, SC 29425. *Telephone:* 843-792-3682. *Fax:* 843-792-2104. *E-mail:* mcdougac@musc.edu.

South Carolina State University
Department of Nursing
Orangeburg, South Carolina

Founded in 1896
DEGREE • BSN

Library Facilities 1.5 million volumes.

BACCALAUREATE PROGRAMS

Degree BSN

Available Programs Generic Baccalaureate; RN Baccalaureate.

Program Entrance Requirements Minimum overall college GPA of 2.8, immunizations, minimum high school GPA of 2.8. **Standardized tests** *Required:* SAT or ACT, TOEFL for international students. *Recommended:* SAT Subject Tests. **Application** *Deadline:* 7/31 (freshmen), 7/31 (transfer). *Notification:* continuous (freshmen). *Application fee:* $25.
Contact *Telephone:* 803-536-7063. *Fax:* 803-536-8593.

University of South Carolina
College of Nursing
Columbia, South Carolina

http://www.sc.edu/nursing
Founded in 1801

DEGREES • BSN • MSN • MSN/MPH • PHD

Nursing Program Faculty 53 (32% with doctorates).

Baccalaureate Enrollment 808
Women 92% **Men** 8% **Minority** 24% **International** .01% **Part-time** 11%
Graduate Enrollment 132
Women 92% **Men** 8% **Minority** 21% **Part-time** 62%

Nursing Student Activities Sigma Theta Tau, Student Nurses' Association.

Nursing Student Resources Academic advising; academic or career counseling; assistance for students with disabilities; bookstore; campus computer network; career placement assistance; computer lab; computer-assisted instruction; daycare for children of students; e-mail services; housing assistance; interactive nursing skills videos; Internet; learning resource lab; library services; nursing audiovisuals; remedial services; resume preparation assistance; skills, simulation, or other laboratory; tutoring.

Library Facilities 3.6 million volumes (33,888 in health, 3,328 in nursing); 53,610 periodical subscriptions (169 health-care related).

BACCALAUREATE PROGRAMS

Degree BSN

Available Programs Generic Baccalaureate; RN Baccalaureate.
Study Options Full-time and part-time.
Program Entrance Requirements Minimum overall college GPA of 2.75, transcript of college record, high school biology, high school chemistry, high school foreign language, 1.5 years high school math, 1.5 years high school science, high school transcript, immunizations, minimum high school GPA of 3.5, minimum GPA in nursing prerequisites of 2.75. Transfer students are accepted. **Standardized tests** *Required:* SAT or ACT, TOEFL for international students. **Application** *Deadline:* 12/1 (freshmen), 8/1 (transfer). *Notification:* continuous until 10/1 (freshmen). *Application fee:* $50.
Advanced Placement Credit by examination available. Credit given for nursing courses completed elsewhere dependent upon specific evaluations.
Expenses (2006–07) *Tuition, state resident:* full-time $7408; part-time $347 per credit hour. *Tuition, nonresident:* full-time $19,836; part-time $904 per credit hour. *International tuition:* $19,836 full-time. *Room and board:* $6520; room only: $4000 per academic year. *Required fees:* full-time $1954; part-time $89 per credit; part-time $777 per term.
Financial Aid 89% of baccalaureate students in nursing programs received some form of financial aid in 2005–06.

Contact Mrs. Gail S. Vereen, Director of Recruitment and Undergraduate Advisement, College of Nursing, University of South Carolina, 1601 Greene Street, Williams Brice Building, Columbia, SC 29208. *Telephone:* 803-777-2526. *Fax:* 803-777-0616. *E-mail:* gail.vereen@sc.edu.

GRADUATE PROGRAMS

Expenses (2006–07) *Tuition, state resident:* full-time $8288; part-time $411 per credit hour. *Tuition, nonresident:* full-time $17,916; part-time $874 per credit hour. *International tuition:* $17,916 full-time. *Room and board:* $7824; room only: $4824 per academic year. *Required fees:* full-time $2236; part-time $80 per credit; part-time $191 per term.
Financial Aid 64% of graduate students in nursing programs received some form of financial aid in 2005–06. 7 research assistantships with partial tuition reimbursements available (averaging $3,072 per year), 6 teaching assistantships with partial tuition reimbursements available (averaging $3,537 per year) were awarded; scholarships, traineeships, and unspecified assistantships also available. *Financial aid application deadline:* 4/1.
Contact Ms. Cheryl Nelson, Graduate Programs Student Service Coordinator, College of Nursing, University of South Carolina, 1601 Greene Street, Williams Brice Building, Columbia, SC 29208. *Telephone:* 803-777-3754. *Fax:* 803-777-0616. *E-mail:* cheryl.nelson@sc.edu.

MASTER'S DEGREE PROGRAM

Degrees MSN; MSN/MPH
Available Programs Master's.
Concentrations Available Nursing administration; nursing education. *Clinical nurse specialist programs in:* acute care, community health, psychiatric/mental health. *Nurse practitioner programs in:* acute care, adult health, family health, pediatric, psychiatric/mental health, women's health.
Study Options Full-time and part-time.
Program Entrance Requirements Minimum overall college GPA of 2.75, transcript of college record, written essay, immunizations, 2 letters of recommendation, resume, GRE General Test, MAT. *Application deadline:* For fall admission, 7/1; for winter admission, 5/1; for spring admission, 11/15. Applications are processed on a rolling basis. *Application fee:* $40.
Advanced Placement Credit given for nursing courses completed elsewhere dependent upon specific evaluations.
Degree Requirements 45 total credit hours, thesis or project.

POST-MASTER'S PROGRAM

Areas of Study *Nurse practitioner programs in:* acute care, adult health, family health, pediatric, psychiatric/mental health, women's health.

DOCTORAL DEGREE PROGRAM

Degree PhD
Available Programs Doctorate; Post-Baccalaureate Doctorate.
Areas of Study Individualized study, nursing science.
Program Entrance Requirements Minimum overall college GPA of 3.5, interview by faculty committee, 3 letters of recommendation, scholarly papers, vita, writing sample, GRE General Test. *Application deadline:* For fall admission, 7/1; for winter admission, 5/1; for spring admission, 11/15. Applications are processed on a rolling basis. *Application fee:* $40.
Degree Requirements 61 total credit hours, dissertation, written exam, residency.

University of South Carolina Aiken
School of Nursing
Aiken, South Carolina

http://www.usca.edu/nursing/
Founded in 1961
DEGREE • BSN

Nursing Program Faculty 15 (40% with doctorates).
Baccalaureate Enrollment 250
Women 90% **Men** 10% **Minority** 30% **International** 1% **Part-time** 3%
Nursing Student Activities Student Nurses' Association.

University of South Carolina Aiken (continued)

Nursing Student Resources Academic advising; academic or career counseling; assistance for students with disabilities; bookstore; campus computer network; career placement assistance; computer lab; computer-assisted instruction; e-mail services; employment services for current students; housing assistance; interactive nursing skills videos; Internet; learning resource lab; library services; nursing audiovisuals; placement services for program completers; resume preparation assistance; skills, simulation, or other laboratory; tutoring.

Library Facilities 156,750 volumes (200 in health, 100 in nursing); 700 periodical subscriptions (100 health-care related).

BACCALAUREATE PROGRAMS

Degree BSN

Available Programs ADN to Baccalaureate; Generic Baccalaureate.

Study Options Full-time and part-time.

Program Entrance Requirements CPR certification, written essay, health exam, immunizations, 3 letters of recommendation, minimum GPA in nursing prerequisites of 2.75, prerequisite course work. Transfer students are accepted. **Standardized tests** *Required:* SAT or ACT, TOEFL for international students. **Application** *Deadline:* 8/1 (freshmen), 8/1 (out-of-state freshmen), 8/1 (transfer). *Notification:* continuous (freshmen), continuous (out-of-state freshmen). *Application fee:* $35.

Advanced Placement Credit by examination available. Credit given for nursing courses completed elsewhere dependent upon specific evaluations.

Expenses (2006–07) *Tuition, state resident:* full-time $6470; part-time $282 per credit. *Tuition, nonresident:* full-time $1350; part-time $582 per credit. *Room and board:* $5820; room only: $4000 per academic year. *Required fees:* full-time $230; part-time $16 per credit.

Financial Aid 20% of baccalaureate students in nursing programs received some form of financial aid in 2005–06.

Contact Ms. Kathy Simmons, Administrative Assistant, School of Nursing, University of South Carolina Aiken, 471 University Parkway, Aiken, SC 29801. *Telephone:* 803-648-3392. *Fax:* 803-641-3725. *E-mail:* kathers@usca.edu.

CONTINUING EDUCATION PROGRAM

Contact Dr. Julia Ball, RN, Dean, School of Nursing, University of South Carolina Aiken, 471 University Parkway, Aiken, SD 29801. *Telephone:* 803-641-3263 Ext. 3263. *Fax:* 803-641-3725. *E-mail:* juliab@usca.edu.

University of South Carolina Upstate
Mary Black School of Nursing
Spartanburg, South Carolina

http://www.uscs.edu/academics/mbsn/

Founded in 1967

DEGREE • BSN

Nursing Program Faculty 45 (16% with doctorates).

Baccalaureate Enrollment 212
Women 86% **Men** 14% **Minority** 27% **Part-time** 37%

Nursing Student Activities Nursing Honor Society, Sigma Theta Tau, Student Nurses' Association.

Nursing Student Resources Academic advising; academic or career counseling; assistance for students with disabilities; bookstore; campus computer network; computer lab; computer-assisted instruction; daycare for children of students; e-mail services; externships; interactive nursing skills videos; Internet; learning resource lab; library services; nursing audiovisuals; resume preparation assistance; skills, simulation, or other laboratory; tutoring.

Library Facilities 188,572 volumes (214,998 in health, 23,359 in nursing); 31,460 periodical subscriptions.

BACCALAUREATE PROGRAMS

Degree BSN

Available Programs Accelerated RN Baccalaureate; Generic Baccalaureate.

Study Options Full-time.

Program Entrance Requirements Transcript of college record, minimum GPA in nursing prerequisites of 2.5, prerequisite course work. Transfer students are accepted. **Standardized tests** *Required:* SAT or ACT, TOEFL for international students. **Application** *Notification:* continuous (freshmen). *Application fee:* $40.

Advanced Placement Credit by examination available. Credit given for nursing courses completed elsewhere dependent upon specific evaluations.

Contact *Telephone:* 888-551-3858. *Fax:* 864-503-5411.

SOUTH DAKOTA

Augustana College
Department of Nursing
Sioux Falls, South Dakota

http://www.augie.edu

Founded in 1860

DEGREES • BA • MA

Nursing Program Faculty 19 (21% with doctorates).

Baccalaureate Enrollment 254
Women 89% **Men** 11% **Minority** 2% **International** 1% **Part-time** 1%

Graduate Enrollment 16
Women 100% **Part-time** 100%

Nursing Student Activities Sigma Theta Tau, Student Nurses' Association.

Nursing Student Resources Academic advising; academic or career counseling; assistance for students with disabilities; bookstore; campus computer network; career placement assistance; computer lab; computer-assisted instruction; daycare for children of students; e-mail services; employment services for current students; housing assistance; interactive nursing skills videos; Internet; learning resource lab; library services; nursing audiovisuals; remedial services; resume preparation assistance; skills, simulation, or other laboratory; tutoring; unpaid internships.

Library Facilities 279,918 volumes (7,345 in health, 847 in nursing); 595 periodical subscriptions (2,268 health-care related).

BACCALAUREATE PROGRAMS

Degree BA

Available Programs Generic Baccalaureate.

Study Options Full-time.

Program Entrance Requirements Minimum overall college GPA of 2.7, transcript of college record, CPR certification, written essay, health exam, health insurance, high school transcript, immunizations, 2 letters of recommendation, minimum high school GPA of 3.5, minimum GPA in nursing prerequisites of 2.7, prerequisite course work. Transfer students are accepted. **Standardized tests** *Required:* SAT or ACT, TOEFL for international students. **Application** *Deadline:* 8/1 (freshmen), rolling (transfer). *Notification:* continuous (freshmen).

Advanced Placement Credit given for nursing courses completed elsewhere dependent upon specific evaluations.

Expenses (2006–07) *Tuition:* full-time $19,750. *International tuition:* $19,750 full-time. *Room and board:* $5664; room only: $2700 per academic year. *Required fees:* full-time $511.

Financial Aid 100% of baccalaureate students in nursing programs received some form of financial aid in 2005–06. *Gift aid (need-based):* Federal Pell, FSEOG, state, private, college/university gift aid from institutional funds, need-linked special talent scholarships and minority scholarships. *Loans:* Federal Nursing Student Loans, FFEL (Subsidized and Unsubsidized Stafford PLUS), Perkins, college/university, Minnesota SELF Loans, alternative loans. *Work-Study:* Federal Work-Study, part-time campus jobs. *Application deadline (priority):* 3/1.

Contact Mary H. Moline, Secretary, Department of Nursing, Augustana College, 2001 South Summit Avenue, Sioux Falls, SD 57197. *Telephone:* 605-274-4727. *Fax:* 605-274-4723. *E-mail:* mary.moline@augie.edu.

GRADUATE PROGRAMS

Expenses (2006–07) *Tuition:* part-time $350 per credit hour. *International tuition:* $350 full-time.

Contact Dr. Margot Nelson, Professor of Nursing, Department of Nursing, Augustana College, 2001 South Summit Avenue, Sioux Falls, SD 57197. *Telephone:* 605-274-4721. *Fax:* 605-274-4723. *E-mail:* margot.nelson@augie.edu.

MASTER'S DEGREE PROGRAM

Degree MA

Available Programs Master's.

Concentrations Available *Clinical nurse specialist programs in:* community health, public health.

Study Options Part-time.

Program Entrance Requirements Clinical experience, minimum overall college GPA of 3.0, transcript of college record, written essay, immunizations, interview, 3 letters of recommendation, professional liability insurance/malpractice insurance, resume, statistics course.

Advanced Placement Credit given for nursing courses completed elsewhere dependent upon specific evaluations.

Degree Requirements 38 total credit hours, thesis or project.

POST-MASTER'S PROGRAM

Areas of Study *Clinical nurse specialist programs in:* community health, public health.

Mount Marty College
Nursing Program
Yankton, South Dakota

http://www.mtmc.edu

Founded in 1936

DEGREE • BSC PN

Nursing Program Faculty 16 (13% with doctorates).

Baccalaureate Enrollment 106

Women 92% **Men** 8% **Minority** 7% **International** 2% **Part-time** 1%

Nursing Student Activities Student Nurses' Association, nursing club.

Nursing Student Resources Academic advising; academic or career counseling; assistance for students with disabilities; bookstore; campus computer network; career placement assistance; computer lab; computer-assisted instruction; daycare for children of students; e-mail services; employment services for current students; externships; housing assistance; interactive nursing skills videos; Internet; learning resource lab; library services; nursing audiovisuals; paid internships; placement services for program completers; remedial services; resume preparation assistance; skills, simulation, or other laboratory; tutoring.

Library Facilities 76,571 volumes (8,700 in health, 5,300 in nursing); 424 periodical subscriptions (92 health-care related).

BACCALAUREATE PROGRAMS

Degree BSc PN

Available Programs ADN to Baccalaureate; Generic Baccalaureate; International Nurse to Baccalaureate; LPN to Baccalaureate; LPN to RN Baccalaureate; RN Baccalaureate.

Site Options Watertown, SD.

Study Options Full-time and part-time.

Program Entrance Requirements Minimum overall college GPA of 2.7, transcript of college record, CPR certification, health exam, health insurance, high school transcript, immunizations, minimum GPA in nursing prerequisites of 2.0, prerequisite course work. Transfer students are accepted. **Standardized tests** *Required:* SAT or ACT, TOEFL for international students. *Recommended:* ACT. **Application** *Deadline:* rolling (freshmen), rolling (transfer). *Notification:* continuous (freshmen). *Application fee:* $35.

Advanced Placement Credit given for nursing courses completed elsewhere dependent upon specific evaluations.

Contact *Telephone:* 605-668-1594. *Fax:* 605-668-1607.

Presentation College
Department of Nursing
Aberdeen, South Dakota

http://www.presentation.edu

Founded in 1951

DEGREE • BSN

Nursing Program Faculty 21 (14% with doctorates).

Baccalaureate Enrollment 149

Women 96% **Men** 4% **Minority** 4% **Part-time** 28%

Nursing Student Activities Sigma Theta Tau, Student Nurses' Association, nursing club.

Nursing Student Resources Academic advising; academic or career counseling; assistance for students with disabilities; bookstore; campus computer network; career placement assistance; computer lab; computer-assisted instruction; e-mail services; interactive nursing skills videos; Internet; learning resource lab; library services; nursing audiovisuals; placement services for program completers; remedial services; skills, simulation, or other laboratory; tutoring.

Library Facilities 40,000 volumes (378 in health, 353 in nursing); 430 periodical subscriptions (2,172 health-care related).

BACCALAUREATE PROGRAMS

Degree BSN

Available Programs ADN to Baccalaureate; Baccalaureate for Second Degree; Generic Baccalaureate; LPN to Baccalaureate; RN Baccalaureate.

Site Options *Distance Learning:* Wahpeton, ND; Sioux Falls, SD; Fairmont, MN.

Study Options Full-time and part-time.

Program Entrance Requirements Minimum overall college GPA of 2.5, transcript of college record, written essay, high school biology, high school chemistry, 2 years high school math, high school transcript, immunizations, interview, 2 letters of recommendation, minimum high school GPA of 2.0, minimum GPA in nursing prerequisites of 2.5, prerequisite course work. Transfer students are accepted. **Standardized tests** *Required:* SAT or ACT, TOEFL for international students. **Application** *Deadline:* rolling (freshmen), rolling (transfer). *Notification:* continuous (freshmen).

Advanced Placement Credit given for nursing courses completed elsewhere dependent upon specific evaluations.

Contact *Telephone:* 605-229-8492. *Fax:* 605-229-8489.

South Dakota State University
College of Nursing
Brookings, South Dakota

http://www.sdstate.org/Academics/CollegeOfNursing/

Founded in 1881

DEGREES • BS • MS • PHD

Nursing Program Faculty 91 (17% with doctorates).

Baccalaureate Enrollment 445

Women 87% **Men** 13%

Graduate Enrollment 186

Women 87% **Men** 13%

Nursing Student Activities Sigma Theta Tau, Student Nurses' Association, nursing club.

South Dakota State University (continued)

Nursing Student Resources Academic advising; academic or career counseling; assistance for students with disabilities; bookstore; campus computer network; career placement assistance; computer lab; computer-assisted instruction; e-mail services; employment services for current students; externships; interactive nursing skills videos; Internet; learning resource lab; library services; nursing audiovisuals; paid internships; placement services for program completers; remedial services; resume preparation assistance; skills, simulation, or other laboratory; tutoring.

Library Facilities 1 million volumes; 29,255 periodical subscriptions (182 health-care related).

BACCALAUREATE PROGRAMS

Degree BS

Available Programs Accelerated Baccalaureate; Generic Baccalaureate; RN Baccalaureate.

Site Options *Distance Learning:* Rapid City, SD; Sioux Falls, SD.

Study Options Full-time.

Program Entrance Requirements Minimum overall college GPA of 2.7, transcript of college record, CPR certification, health exam, health insurance, immunizations, minimum GPA in nursing prerequisites of 2.5, professional liability insurance/malpractice insurance, prerequisite course work. Transfer students are accepted. **Standardized tests** *Required:* SAT or ACT, TOEFL for international students. **Application** *Deadline:* rolling (freshmen), rolling (transfer). *Application fee:* $20.

Advanced Placement Credit given for nursing courses completed elsewhere dependent upon specific evaluations.

Expenses (2005–06) *Tuition, area resident:* full-time $5047. *Tuition, nonresident:* full-time $7763. *Room and board:* $3912; room only: $2112 per academic year. *Required fees:* full-time $808.

Financial Aid 86% of baccalaureate students in nursing programs received some form of financial aid in 2004–05. *Gift aid (need-based):* Federal Pell, FSEOG, state, private, college/university gift aid from institutional funds, United Negro College Fund, Federal Nursing, agency awards. *Loans:* Federal Nursing Student Loans, FFEL (Subsidized and Unsubsidized Stafford PLUS), Perkins, college/university, alternative loans from private sources. *Work-Study:* Federal Work-Study, part-time campus jobs. *Application deadline (priority):* 3/15.

Contact Dr. Gloria P. Craig, Department Head, Nursing Student Services, College of Nursing, South Dakota State University, Box 2275, Rotunda Lane, NFA 255, Brookings, SD 57007-0098. *Telephone:* 605-688-4106. *Fax:* 605-688-6073. *E-mail:* gloria.craig@sdstate.edu.

GRADUATE PROGRAMS

Expenses (2005–06) *Tuition, state resident:* full-time $2084. *Tuition, nonresident:* full-time $4323. *International tuition:* $4323 full-time. *Room and board:* $2535; room only: $2535 per academic year. *Required fees:* full-time $1464.

Financial Aid 86% of graduate students in nursing programs received some form of financial aid in 2004–05. Fellowships, research assistantships, teaching assistantships, Federal Work-Study available.

Contact Dr. Sandra Bunkers, Department Head, College of Nursing, South Dakota State University, Box 2275, Rotunda Lane, NFA 217, Brookings, SD 57007-0098. *Telephone:* 605-688-4114. *Fax:* 605-688-5827. *E-mail:* sandra.bunkers@sdstate.edu.

MASTER'S DEGREE PROGRAM

Degree MS

Available Programs Master's; RN to Master's.

Concentrations Available Nursing administration; nursing education. *Nurse practitioner programs in:* family health, neonatal health.

Site Options *Distance Learning:* Rapid City, SD; Sioux Falls, SD.

Study Options Full-time and part-time.

Program Entrance Requirements Clinical experience, minimum overall college GPA of 3.0, transcript of college record, CPR certification, written essay, immunizations, 3 letters of recommendation, professional liability insurance/malpractice insurance, statistics course. *Application deadline:* Applications are processed on a rolling basis. *Application fee:* $15.

Advanced Placement Credit given for nursing courses completed elsewhere dependent upon specific evaluations.

Degree Requirements 48 total credit hours, thesis or project, comprehensive exam.

POST-MASTER'S PROGRAM

Areas of Study Nursing education. *Nurse practitioner programs in:* family health.

DOCTORAL DEGREE PROGRAM

Degree PhD

Available Programs Doctorate.

Areas of Study Nursing research.

Site Options *Distance Learning:* Sioux Falls, SD.

Program Entrance Requirements Minimum overall college GPA of 3.3, interview by faculty committee, 6 letters of recommendation, MSN or equivalent, scholarly papers, statistics course, vita, writing sample. *Application deadline:* Applications are processed on a rolling basis. *Application fee:* $15.

Degree Requirements 60 total credit hours, dissertation, oral exam, written exam.

CONTINUING EDUCATION PROGRAM

Contact Dr. Gloria P. Craig, Coordinator, Continuing Nursing Education, College of Nursing, South Dakota State University, Box 2275, Rotunda Lane, NFA 135, Brookings, SD 57007-0098. *Telephone:* 605-688-5745. *Fax:* 605-688-6679. *E-mail:* gloria.craig@sdstate.edu.

TENNESSEE

Aquinas College
Department of Nursing
Nashville, Tennessee

http://www.aquinas-tn.edu/nursing/index.htm

Founded in 1961

DEGREE • BSN

Nursing Student Resources Library services.

Library Facilities 46,549 volumes; 284 periodical subscriptions.

BACCALAUREATE PROGRAMS

Degree BSN

Available Programs RN Baccalaureate.

Program Entrance Requirements Interview, 2 letters of recommendation, RN licensure. **Standardized tests** *Required:* TOEFL for international students. *Required for some:* SAT or ACT. **Application** *Deadline:* rolling (freshmen), rolling (transfer). *Notification:* continuous (freshmen). *Application fee:* $25.

Advanced Placement Credit given for nursing courses completed elsewhere dependent upon specific evaluations.

Contact *Telephone:* 615-222-4038.

Austin Peay State University
School of Nursing
Clarksville, Tennessee

http://www.apsu.edu/nursing01

Founded in 1927

DEGREE • BSN

Nursing Student Activities Nursing Honor Society, Sigma Theta Tau, Student Nurses' Association.

Nursing Student Resources Computer lab; computer-assisted instruction; interactive nursing skills videos; nursing audiovisuals; skills, simulation, or other laboratory.

Library Facilities 400,000 volumes (8,249 in health, 1,111 in nursing); 1,754 periodical subscriptions (146 health-care related).

BACCALAUREATE PROGRAMS

Degree BSN

Available Programs Generic Baccalaureate; RN Baccalaureate.
Study Options Full-time.
Program Entrance Requirements Minimum overall college GPA of 2.8, transcript of college record, CPR certification, health insurance, high school transcript, immunizations, minimum GPA in nursing prerequisites of 2.8. Transfer students are accepted. **Standardized tests** *Required:* TOEFL for international students. *Required for some:* SAT or ACT. **Application** *Deadline:* 8/28 (freshmen), rolling (transfer). *Notification:* continuous (freshmen). *Application fee:* $15.
Contact *Telephone:* 931-221-7710. *Fax:* 931-221-7388.

Baptist College of Health Sciences
Nursing Division
Memphis, Tennessee

Founded in 1994
DEGREE • BSN

Nursing Program Faculty 25.
Baccalaureate Enrollment 63

BACCALAUREATE PROGRAMS

Degree BSN

Available Programs Generic Baccalaureate; LPN to Baccalaureate; RN Baccalaureate.
Study Options Full-time and part-time.
Program Entrance Requirements Minimum overall college GPA of 2.5, CPR certification, health exam, health insurance, 2 years high school math, 2 years high school science, high school transcript, immunizations, 3 letters of recommendation, minimum high school GPA of 2.75. Transfer students are accepted. **Standardized tests** *Required:* ACT, Health Occupations Basic Entrance Test. **Application** *Deadline:* 6/1 (freshmen), 6/1 (transfer). *Application fee:* $25.
Contact *Telephone:* 901-572-2465. *Fax:* 901-572-2461.

Belmont University
School of Nursing
Nashville, Tennessee

http://www.belmont.edu/nursing
Founded in 1951
DEGREES • BSN • MSN

Nursing Program Faculty 43 (21% with doctorates).
Baccalaureate Enrollment 279
Women 90.5% **Men** 9.5% **Minority** 9% **Part-time** 20%
Graduate Enrollment 13
Women 100% **Part-time** 3.3%
Nursing Student Activities Nursing Honor Society, Sigma Theta Tau, Student Nurses' Association.
Nursing Student Resources Academic advising; academic or career counseling; bookstore; campus computer network; career placement assistance; computer lab; computer-assisted instruction; e-mail services; employment services for current students; externships; housing assistance; interactive nursing skills videos; Internet; learning resource lab; library services; nursing audiovisuals; placement services for program completers; remedial services; resume preparation assistance; skills, simulation, or other laboratory; tutoring.
Library Facilities 200,630 volumes (7,552 in health, 43 in nursing); 1,415 periodical subscriptions (262 health-care related).

BACCALAUREATE PROGRAMS

Degree BSN

Available Programs ADN to Baccalaureate; Accelerated Baccalaureate; Accelerated Baccalaureate for Second Degree; Baccalaureate for Second Degree; Generic Baccalaureate; LPN to RN Baccalaureate; RN Baccalaureate.
Site Options *Distance Learning:* Nashville, TN.
Study Options Full-time and part-time.
Program Entrance Requirements Minimum overall college GPA of 2.5, transcript of college record, CPR certification, written essay, health exam, health insurance, high school biology, high school chemistry, 3 years high school math, 3 years high school science, high school transcript, immunizations, 1 letter of recommendation, minimum high school GPA of 2.5, minimum GPA in nursing prerequisites of 3.0. Transfer students are accepted. **Standardized tests** *Required:* SAT or ACT, TOEFL for international students. **Application** *Deadline:* 8/1 (freshmen), 8/1 (transfer). *Notification:* continuous (freshmen). *Application fee:* $35.
Advanced Placement Credit by examination available. Credit given for nursing courses completed elsewhere dependent upon specific evaluations.
Expenses (2006–07) *Tuition:* full-time $8735; part-time $670 per semester. *Room and board:* $3185; room only: $3100 per academic year. *Required fees:* full-time $475; part-time $320 per term.
Financial Aid 75% of baccalaureate students in nursing programs received some form of financial aid in 2005–06.
Contact Mrs. Cathy Hendon, Admissions Coordinator, School of Nursing, Belmont University, 1900 Belmont Boulevard, Nashville, TN 37212-3757. *Telephone:* 615-460-6107. *Fax:* 615-460-6125. *E-mail:* hendonc@mail.belmont.edu.

GRADUATE PROGRAMS

Expenses (2006–07) *Room and board:* $3185; room only: $3100 per academic year. *Required fees:* full-time $230; part-time $115 per term.
Financial Aid 95% of graduate students in nursing programs received some form of financial aid in 2005–06. Scholarships and traineeships available. *Financial aid application deadline:* 3/1.
Contact Dr. Leslie Higgins, Director, Graduate Program, School of Nursing, Belmont University, 1900 Belmont Boulevard, Nashville, TN 37212-3757. *Telephone:* 615-460-6027. *Fax:* 615-460-5644. *E-mail:* higginsl@mail.belmont.edu.

MASTER'S DEGREE PROGRAM

Degree MSN

Available Programs Master's.
Concentrations Available *Nurse practitioner programs in:* family health.
Study Options Full-time and part-time.
Program Entrance Requirements Clinical experience, minimum overall college GPA of 3.0, transcript of college record, CPR certification, written essay, immunizations, interview, 2 letters of recommendation, resume, GRE. *Application deadline:* For fall admission, 5/1 (priority date); for spring admission, 10/15 (priority date). Applications are processed on a rolling basis. *Application fee:* $50.
Degree Requirements 41 total credit hours, comprehensive exam.

POST-MASTER'S PROGRAM

Areas of Study *Nurse practitioner programs in:* family health.

Carson-Newman College
Department of Nursing
Jefferson City, Tennessee

Founded in 1851
DEGREES • BSN • MSN

Nursing Program Faculty 11 (42% with doctorates).
Baccalaureate Enrollment 154
Women 93% **Men** 7% **Minority** 1% **Part-time** 1%
Graduate Enrollment 20
Women 95% **Men** 5% **Minority** 5% **International** 10% **Part-time** 57%
Nursing Student Activities Sigma Theta Tau, Student Nurses' Association, nursing club.

Carson-Newman College (continued)

Nursing Student Resources Academic advising; academic or career counseling; assistance for students with disabilities; bookstore; campus computer network; career placement assistance; computer lab; computer-assisted instruction; e-mail services; employment services for current students; externships; housing assistance; interactive nursing skills videos; Internet; learning resource lab; placement services for program completers; remedial services; resume preparation assistance; skills, simulation, or other laboratory; tutoring; unpaid internships.

Library Facilities 218,371 volumes (1,800 in health); 3,966 periodical subscriptions (180 health-care related).

BACCALAUREATE PROGRAMS

Degree BSN

Available Programs Accelerated Baccalaureate; Generic Baccalaureate; RN Baccalaureate.

Study Options Full-time.

Program Entrance Requirements Minimum overall college GPA of 2.5, transcript of college record, high school transcript, minimum GPA in nursing prerequisites of 2.5, prerequisite course work. Transfer students are accepted. **Standardized tests** *Required:* SAT or ACT, TOEFL for international students. **Application** *Deadline:* 8/1 (freshmen), 8/1 (transfer). *Notification:* continuous (freshmen). *Application fee:* $25.

Advanced Placement Credit given for nursing courses completed elsewhere dependent upon specific evaluations.

Contact *Telephone:* 865-471-3442. *Fax:* 865-471-4574.

GRADUATE PROGRAMS

Contact *Telephone:* 865-471-3429. *Fax:* 865-471-4574.

MASTER'S DEGREE PROGRAM

Degree MSN

Available Programs Master's.

Concentrations Available Nursing education. *Nurse practitioner programs in:* family health.

Study Options Full-time and part-time.

Program Entrance Requirements Minimum overall college GPA of 3.0, transcript of college record, written essay, 3 letters of recommendation. *Application deadline:* For fall admission, 7/15 (priority date). Applications are processed on a rolling basis. *Application fee:* $50.

Advanced Placement Credit given for nursing courses completed elsewhere dependent upon specific evaluations.

Degree Requirements 45 total credit hours, thesis or project, comprehensive exam.

POST-MASTER'S PROGRAM

Areas of Study Nursing education. *Nurse practitioner programs in:* family health.

Cumberland University
Rudy School of Nursing and Health Professions
Lebanon, Tennessee

http://www.cumberland.edu/academics/nursing/ index.html

Founded in 1842

DEGREE • BSN

Nursing Program Faculty 13 (15% with doctorates).

Baccalaureate Enrollment 141
Women 95% **Men** 5% **Minority** 1%

Nursing Student Activities Nursing Honor Society, Student Nurses' Association.

Nursing Student Resources Academic advising; academic or career counseling; assistance for students with disabilities; bookstore; campus computer network; career placement assistance; computer lab; computer-assisted instruction; e-mail services; housing assistance; interactive nursing skills videos; Internet; learning resource lab; library services; nursing audiovisuals; remedial services; resume preparation assistance; skills, simulation, or other laboratory; tutoring.

Library Facilities 50,000 volumes (125 in health, 66 in nursing); 130 periodical subscriptions (25 health-care related).

BACCALAUREATE PROGRAMS

Degree BSN

Available Programs ADN to Baccalaureate; Accelerated Baccalaureate; Accelerated Baccalaureate for Second Degree; Accelerated RN Baccalaureate; Baccalaureate for Second Degree; Generic Baccalaureate; LPN to Baccalaureate; LPN to RN Baccalaureate; RN Baccalaureate.

Study Options Full-time and part-time.

Program Entrance Requirements Minimum overall college GPA of 2.8, CPR certification, health exam, health insurance, immunizations, minimum GPA in nursing prerequisites of 2.8, professional liability insurance/malpractice insurance, prerequisite course work. Transfer students are accepted. **Standardized tests** *Required:* SAT or ACT, TOEFL for international students. *Recommended:* SAT. **Application** *Deadline:* rolling (freshmen), rolling (transfer). *Notification:* continuous (freshmen). *Application fee:* $25.

Advanced Placement Credit given for nursing courses completed elsewhere dependent upon specific evaluations.

Expenses (2006–07) *Tuition:* full-time $14,010; part-time $585 per hour. *International tuition:* $14,010 full-time. *Room and board:* $5300; room only: $2410 per academic year. *Required fees:* full-time $500; part-time $50 per credit; part-time $250 per term.

Financial Aid 95% of baccalaureate students in nursing programs received some form of financial aid in 2005–06.

Contact Dr. Leanne C. Busby, Professor and Dean, Rudy School of Nursing and Health Professions, Cumberland University, One Cumberland Square, Lebanon, TN 37087-3554. *Telephone:* 615-547-1200. *Fax:* 615-444-2569. *E-mail:* lbusby@cumberland.edu.

East Tennessee State University
College of Nursing
Johnson City, Tennessee

http://www.etsu.edu/etsu.con

Founded in 1911

DEGREES • BSN • DSN • MSN

Nursing Program Faculty 58 (41% with doctorates).

Baccalaureate Enrollment 489
Women 84% **Men** 16% **Minority** 6.3% **Part-time** 22%

Graduate Enrollment 110
Women 89% **Men** 11% **Minority** 6.4% **Part-time** 67%

Nursing Student Activities Sigma Theta Tau, Student Nurses' Association.

Nursing Student Resources Academic advising; academic or career counseling; assistance for students with disabilities; bookstore; campus computer network; career placement assistance; computer lab; computer-assisted instruction; daycare for children of students; e-mail services; employment services for current students; externships; housing assistance; interactive nursing skills videos; Internet; learning resource lab; library services; nursing audiovisuals; remedial services; resume preparation assistance; skills, simulation, or other laboratory; tutoring.

Library Facilities 1.1 million volumes; 3,714 periodical subscriptions.

BACCALAUREATE PROGRAMS

Degree BSN

Available Programs ADN to Baccalaureate; Accelerated Baccalaureate for Second Degree; Accelerated RN Baccalaureate; Generic Baccalaureate; LPN to Baccalaureate.

Site Options *Distance Learning:* Sevierville, TN; Morristown, TN; Cleveland, TN.

Study Options Full-time and part-time.

Program Entrance Requirements Minimum overall college GPA of 2.6, transcript of college record, minimum GPA in nursing prerequisites of 2.6, prerequisite course work. Transfer students are accepted. **Standardized tests** *Required:* SAT or ACT, TOEFL for international students. **Application** *Notification:* continuous (freshmen). *Application fee:* $15.
Advanced Placement Credit given for nursing courses completed elsewhere dependent upon specific evaluations.
Financial Aid *Gift aid (need-based):* Federal Pell, FSEOG, state, private, college/university gift aid from institutional funds, Federal Nursing. *Loans:* Federal Nursing Student Loans, FFEL (Subsidized and Unsubsidized Stafford PLUS), Perkins, college/university. *Work-Study:* Federal Work-Study, part-time campus jobs. *Application deadline (priority):* 4/15.
Contact Mr. Scott Vaughn, Advisor, College of Nursing, East Tennessee State University, Office of Student Services, PO Box 70664, Johnson City, TN 37614. *Telephone:* 423-439-4578. *Fax:* 423-439-4522. *E-mail:* admitnur@etsu.edu.

GRADUATE PROGRAMS

Financial Aid 6 research assistantships (averaging $5,500 per year), 4 teaching assistantships (averaging $5,500 per year) were awarded; career-related internships or fieldwork, traineeships, and unspecified assistantships also available.
Contact Ms. Amy Bower, Coordinator, College of Nursing, East Tennessee State University, Office of Student Services, PO Box 70664, Johnson City, TN 37614. *Telephone:* 423-439-4531. *Fax:* 423-439-4522. *E-mail:* bowera@etsu.edu.

MASTER'S DEGREE PROGRAM

Degree MSN
Available Programs Master's; RN to Master's.
Concentrations Available Nursing administration; nursing education. *Nurse practitioner programs in:* adult health, family health, gerontology, psychiatric/mental health.
Study Options Full-time and part-time.
Program Entrance Requirements Minimum overall college GPA of 3.0, transcript of college record, written essay, 3 letters of recommendation, GRE General Test. *Application deadline:* For fall admission, 1/15 (priority date). Applications are processed on a rolling basis. *Application fee:* $25 ($35 for international students).
Advanced Placement Credit given for nursing courses completed elsewhere dependent upon specific evaluations.
Degree Requirements 48 total credit hours, comprehensive exam.

POST-MASTER'S PROGRAM

Areas of Study Health-care administration. *Nurse practitioner programs in:* adult health, family health, gerontology, psychiatric/mental health.

DOCTORAL DEGREE PROGRAM

Degree DSN
Available Programs Doctorate.
Areas of Study Advanced practice nursing, individualized study, nursing administration, nursing education.
Program Entrance Requirements Clinical experience, minimum overall college GPA of 3.0, interview by faculty committee, 3 letters of recommendation, MSN or equivalent, statistics course, vita, writing sample. *Application deadline:* For fall admission, 1/15 (priority date). Applications are processed on a rolling basis. *Application fee:* $25 ($35 for international students).
Degree Requirements 62 total credit hours, dissertation, written exam, residency.

King College
School of Nursing
Bristol, Tennessee

Founded in 1867
DEGREES • BSN • M SC N • MSN/MBA
Nursing Program Faculty 14 (26% with doctorates).

Baccalaureate Enrollment 286
Women 96% **Men** 4% **Minority** 1% **International** 1%
Graduate Enrollment 15
Women 100% **Part-time** 1%
Nursing Student Activities Student Nurses' Association.
Nursing Student Resources Academic advising; academic or career counseling; assistance for students with disabilities; bookstore; campus computer network; career placement assistance; computer lab; computer-assisted instruction; e-mail services; employment services for current students; externships; interactive nursing skills videos; Internet; learning resource lab; library services; nursing audiovisuals; paid internships; remedial services; resume preparation assistance; skills, simulation, or other laboratory; tutoring.
Library Facilities 113,933 volumes (929 in health, 158 in nursing); 468 periodical subscriptions (87 health-care related).

BACCALAUREATE PROGRAMS

Degree BSN
Available Programs Accelerated RN Baccalaureate; Generic Baccalaureate.
Site Options Kingsport, TN.
Study Options Full-time and part-time.
Program Entrance Requirements Minimum overall college GPA of 2.0, transcript of college record, CPR certification, health exam, health insurance, high school biology, high school chemistry, 2 years high school math, 2 years high school science, high school transcript, immunizations, minimum high school GPA of 2.5, minimum high school rank 25%, minimum GPA in nursing prerequisites of 2.5. Transfer students are accepted. **Standardized tests** *Required:* SAT or ACT. *Recommended:* TOEFL for international students. **Application** *Deadline:* rolling (freshmen), rolling (transfer). *Notification:* continuous (freshmen). *Application fee:* $20.
Expenses (2006–07) *Tuition:* full-time $17,290; part-time $575 per credit hour. *Room and board:* $6200; room only: $3100 per academic year. *Required fees:* full-time $1054; part-time $575 per credit.
Financial Aid 90% of baccalaureate students in nursing programs received some form of financial aid in 2005–06. *Gift aid (need-based):* Federal Pell, FSEOG, state, private, college/university gift aid from institutional funds. *Loans:* FFEL (Subsidized and Unsubsidized Stafford PLUS), Perkins, college/university. *Work-Study:* Federal Work-Study, part-time campus jobs. *Application deadline (priority):* 3/1.
Contact Dr. Johanne A. Quinn, Professor and Dean, School of Nursing, King College, 1350 King College Road, Bristol, TN 37620. *Telephone:* 423-652-4748. *Fax:* 423-652-4833. *E-mail:* jaquinn@king.edu.

GRADUATE PROGRAMS

Expenses (2006–07) *Tuition:* full-time $23,000; part-time $500 per credit hour. *Required fees:* full-time $305.
Financial Aid 100% of graduate students in nursing programs received some form of financial aid in 2005–06.
Contact Dr. Johanne A. Quinn, Professor and Dean, School of Nursing, King College, 1350 King College Road, Bristol, TN 37620. *Telephone:* 423-652-4748. *Fax:* 423-652-4833. *E-mail:* jaquinn@king.edu.

MASTER'S DEGREE PROGRAM

Degrees M Sc N; MSN/MBA
Available Programs Master's.
Concentrations Available *Clinical nurse specialist programs in:* acute care, adult health, critical care.
Study Options Full-time and part-time.
Program Entrance Requirements Clinical experience, computer literacy, minimum overall college GPA of 3.0, transcript of college record, CPR certification, written essay, immunizations, 2 letters of recommendation, nursing research course, physical assessment course, resume, statistics course.
Degree Requirements 39 total credit hours, thesis or project.

Lincoln Memorial University
Department of Nursing
Harrogate, Tennessee

*http://www.lmunet.edu/academics/undergrad/
nursing/*

Founded in 1897

DEGREE • BSN

Nursing Program Faculty 7 (57% with doctorates).

Nursing Student Activities Student Nurses' Association.

Nursing Student Resources Academic advising; academic or career counseling; bookstore; campus computer network; career placement assistance; computer lab; e-mail services; externships; interactive nursing skills videos; Internet; learning resource lab; library services; nursing audiovisuals; other; placement services for program completers; skills, simulation, or other laboratory; tutoring.

Library Facilities 174,737 volumes (1,230 in health, 630 in nursing); 20,982 periodical subscriptions (36 health-care related).

BACCALAUREATE PROGRAMS
Degree BSN

Available Programs RN Baccalaureate.

Site Options Knoxville, TN.

Program Entrance Requirements Minimum overall college GPA of 2.25, transcript of college record, CPR certification, immunizations, 3 letters of recommendation, professional liability insurance/malpractice insurance, prerequisite course work, RN licensure. Transfer students are accepted.

Standardized tests *Required:* SAT or ACT, TOEFL for international students. **Application** *Deadline:* rolling (freshmen), rolling (transfer). *Application fee:* $25.

Advanced Placement Credit given for nursing courses completed elsewhere dependent upon specific evaluations.

Contact *Telephone:* 423-869-3611. *Fax:* 423-869-6444.

Middle Tennessee State University
School of Nursing
Murfreesboro, Tennessee

http://www.mtsu.edu/~nursing/

Founded in 1911

DEGREE • BSN

Nursing Student Activities Sigma Theta Tau, Student Nurses' Association.

Library Facilities 748,888 volumes; 4,144 periodical subscriptions.

BACCALAUREATE PROGRAMS
Degree BSN

Available Programs Generic Baccalaureate; RN Baccalaureate.

Program Entrance Requirements Minimum overall college GPA of 2.50, transcript of college record, minimum GPA in nursing prerequisites of 2.50, prerequisite course work. Transfer students are accepted. **Standardized tests** *Required:* SAT or ACT, TOEFL for international students. **Application** *Deadline:* 7/1 (freshmen), 7/1 (transfer). *Notification:* continuous (freshmen). *Application fee:* $25.

Advanced Placement Credit by examination available. Credit given for nursing courses completed elsewhere dependent upon specific evaluations.

Contact *Telephone:* 615-898-2437. *Fax:* 615-898-5441.

CONTINUING EDUCATION PROGRAM
Contact *Telephone:* 615-898-2462. *Fax:* 615-898-3593.

Milligan College
Department of Nursing
Milligan College, Tennessee

Founded in 1866

DEGREE • BSN

Nursing Program Faculty 8 (20% with doctorates).

Baccalaureate Enrollment 55
Women 93% **Men** 7% **Minority** 4% **International** 2%

Nursing Student Activities Nursing Honor Society, Student Nurses' Association.

Nursing Student Resources Academic advising; academic or career counseling; assistance for students with disabilities; bookstore; campus computer network; career placement assistance; computer lab; computer-assisted instruction; e-mail services; employment services for current students; externships; interactive nursing skills videos; Internet; learning resource lab; library services; nursing audiovisuals; paid internships; remedial services; resume preparation assistance; skills, simulation, or other laboratory; tutoring; unpaid internships.

Library Facilities 179,619 volumes (2,430 in health, 184 in nursing); 10,861 periodical subscriptions (340 health-care related).

BACCALAUREATE PROGRAMS
Degree BSN

Available Programs ADN to Baccalaureate; Generic Baccalaureate; International Nurse to Baccalaureate; LPN to Baccalaureate; LPN to RN Baccalaureate; RN Baccalaureate.

Study Options Full-time and part-time.

Program Entrance Requirements Minimum overall college GPA of 2.5, transcript of college record, CPR certification, written essay, health exam, immunizations, minimum GPA in nursing prerequisites of 2.0, professional liability insurance/malpractice insurance, prerequisite course work. Transfer students are accepted. **Standardized tests** *Required:* SAT or ACT, TOEFL for international students. **Application** *Deadline:* 8/1 (freshmen), rolling (transfer). *Notification:* continuous (freshmen). *Application fee:* $30.

Advanced Placement Credit given for nursing courses completed elsewhere dependent upon specific evaluations.

Expenses (2006–07) *Tuition:* full-time $17,800; part-time $490 per credit hour. *International tuition:* $17,800 full-time. *Room and board:* $5030; room only: $2550 per academic year. *Required fees:* full-time $520; part-time $122 per term.

Financial Aid 100% of baccalaureate students in nursing programs received some form of financial aid in 2005–06.

Contact Melinda K. Collins, Area Chair and Director of Nursing, Department of Nursing, Milligan College, Wilson Way, Suite 302, Milligan College, TN 37682. *Telephone:* 423-461-8655.

South College
Department of Nursing
Knoxville, Tennessee

Founded in 1882

DEGREE • BSN

Library Facilities 6,500 volumes; 127 periodical subscriptions.

BACCALAUREATE PROGRAMS
Degree BSN

Available Programs Generic Baccalaureate.

Program Entrance Requirements Immunizations, minimum high school GPA of 2.5. Transfer students are accepted. **Standardized tests** *Required:* TOEFL for international students. **Placement:** *Recommended:* SAT, ACT, or CPT. **Application** *Deadline:* 10/1 (freshmen), rolling (transfer). *Application fee:* $40.

Contact Nursing Contact, Department of Nursing, South College, Knoxville, TN 37909. *Telephone:* 865-251-1800.

Southern Adventist University

School of Nursing
Collegedale, Tennessee

Founded in 1892

DEGREES • BS • MSN • MSN/MBA

Nursing Program Faculty 16 (31% with doctorates).

Baccalaureate Enrollment 65
Women 75% **Men** 25%

Graduate Enrollment 60
Women 84% **Men** 16%

Nursing Student Activities Sigma Theta Tau, nursing club.

Nursing Student Resources Academic advising; academic or career counseling; assistance for students with disabilities; bookstore; campus computer network; computer lab; computer-assisted instruction; e-mail services; employment services for current students; housing assistance; interactive nursing skills videos; Internet; learning resource lab; library services; nursing audiovisuals; remedial services; resume preparation assistance; skills, simulation, or other laboratory; tutoring.

Library Facilities 154,987 volumes (335 in nursing); 21,123 periodical subscriptions (174 health-care related).

BACCALAUREATE PROGRAMS

Degree BS

Available Programs ADN to Baccalaureate.
Site Options Chattanooga, TN.
Study Options Full-time and part-time.
Program Entrance Requirements Minimum overall college GPA of 2.8, transcript of college record, CPR certification, health exam, high school chemistry, high school transcript, immunizations, letters of recommendation, minimum GPA in nursing prerequisites of 2.5, prerequisite course work, RN licensure. Transfer students are accepted. **Standardized tests** *Required:* SAT or ACT, TOEFL for international students. **Application** *Deadline:* rolling (freshmen), rolling (transfer). *Notification:* continuous (freshmen). *Application fee:* $25.
Advanced Placement Credit given for nursing courses completed elsewhere dependent upon specific evaluations.
Expenses (2006–07) *Tuition:* full-time $7248; part-time $604 per credit hour. *Room and board:* $2604 per academic year.
Financial Aid 80% of baccalaureate students in nursing programs received some form of financial aid in 2005–06.
Contact Mrs. Linda Marlowe, Admissions and Progression Coordinator, School of Nursing, Southern Adventist University, PO Box 370, Collegedale, TN 37315-0370. *Telephone:* 423-236-2941. *Fax:* 423-236-1940. *E-mail:* lmarlowe@southern.edu.

GRADUATE PROGRAMS

Expenses (2006–07) *Tuition:* full-time $7506; part-time $417 per hour.
Contact Mrs. Diane Proffitt, Applications Manager, School of Nursing, Southern Adventist University, PO Box 370, Collegedale, TN 37315-0370. *Telephone:* 423-236-2957. *Fax:* 423-236-1940. *E-mail:* dproffit@southern.edu.

MASTER'S DEGREE PROGRAM

Degrees MSN; MSN/MBA

Available Programs Accelerated RN to Master's; Master's.
Concentrations Available Health-care administration; nursing education. *Nurse practitioner programs in:* adult health, family health.
Study Options Full-time and part-time.
Program Entrance Requirements Clinical experience, minimum overall college GPA of 3.0, transcript of college record, CPR certification, written essay, immunizations, interview, 2 letters of recommendation, prerequisite course work, statistics course.
Advanced Placement Credit given for nursing courses completed elsewhere dependent upon specific evaluations.
Degree Requirements 42 total credit hours, thesis or project.

CONTINUING EDUCATION PROGRAM

Contact Mrs. Linda Marlowe, Admissions and Progression Coordinator, School of Nursing, Southern Adventist University, PO Box 370, Collegedale, TN 37315-0370. *Telephone:* 423-236-2941. *Fax:* 423-236-1940. *E-mail:* lmarlowe@southern.edu.

Tennessee State University

School of Nursing
Nashville, Tennessee

http://www.tnstate.edu/nurs
Founded in 1912

DEGREES • BSN • MSN

Nursing Program Faculty 37 (50% with doctorates).

Baccalaureate Enrollment 94
Women 93% **Men** 7% **Minority** 49% **Part-time** 8%

Graduate Enrollment 103
Women 95% **Men** 5% **Minority** 33% **Part-time** 81%

Nursing Student Activities Nursing Honor Society, Sigma Theta Tau, Student Nurses' Association.

Nursing Student Resources Academic advising; academic or career counseling; assistance for students with disabilities; bookstore; campus computer network; computer lab; e-mail services; interactive nursing skills videos; Internet; learning resource lab; library services; nursing audiovisuals; tutoring.

Library Facilities 580,650 volumes (50,000 in health, 25,000 in nursing); 300 periodical subscriptions health-care related.

BACCALAUREATE PROGRAMS

Degree BSN

Available Programs Generic Baccalaureate; LPN to Baccalaureate; RN Baccalaureate.
Site Options *Distance Learning:* Nashville, TN.
Study Options Full-time and part-time.
Program Entrance Requirements Minimum overall college GPA of 2.8, transcript of college record, CPR certification, health exam, health insurance, immunizations, minimum GPA in nursing prerequisites of 2.8, professional liability insurance/malpractice insurance, prerequisite course work. Transfer students are accepted. **Standardized tests** *Required:* SAT or ACT, TOEFL for international students. **Application** *Deadline:* 8/1 (freshmen), 8/1 (transfer). *Notification:* continuous until 8/15 (freshmen). *Application fee:* $15.
Expenses (2006–07) *Tuition, state resident:* full-time $4564; part-time $343 per credit hour. *Tuition, nonresident:* full-time $14,258; part-time $764 per credit hour. *Room and board:* $5960; room only: $3800 per academic year. *Required fees:* full-time $280.
Financial Aid 80% of baccalaureate students in nursing programs received some form of financial aid in 2005–06.
Contact Dr. Barbara W. Buchanan-Covington, RN, Interim BSN Program Director, School of Nursing, Tennessee State University, 3500 John A. Merritt Boulevard, Box 9590, Nashville, TN 37209-1561. *Telephone:* 615-963-7615. *Fax:* 615-963-5593. *E-mail:* bbuchanan@tnstate.edu.

GRADUATE PROGRAMS

Expenses (2006–07) *Tuition, state resident:* full-time $5874; part-time $461 per credit hour. *Tuition, nonresident:* full-time $15,568; part-time $882 per credit hour. *Room and board:* $6320; room only: $4160 per academic year.
Financial Aid 75% of graduate students in nursing programs received some form of financial aid in 2005–06. Research assistantships (averaging $5,500 per year), 2 teaching assistantships (averaging $5,500 per year) were awarded.
Contact Dr. Jane C. Norman, MSN Program Director, School of Nursing, Tennessee State University, 3500 John A. Merritt Boulevard, Box 9590, Nashville, TN 37209-1561. *Telephone:* 615-963-5255. *Fax:* 615-963-7614. *E-mail:* jnorman@tnstate.edu.

Tennessee State University (continued)
MASTER'S DEGREE PROGRAM
Degree MSN

Available Programs RN to Master's.

Concentrations Available Nursing education; nursing informatics. *Clinical nurse specialist programs in:* family health. *Nurse practitioner programs in:* family health.

Site Options Nashville, TN.

Study Options Full-time and part-time.

Program Entrance Requirements Clinical experience, computer literacy, minimum overall college GPA of 3.0, transcript of college record, CPR certification, written essay, immunizations, interview, 3 letters of recommendation, physical assessment course, professional liability insurance/malpractice insurance, resume, statistics course, GRE General Test or MAT. *Application deadline:* Applications are processed on a rolling basis. *Application fee:* $15.

Advanced Placement Credit given for nursing courses completed elsewhere dependent upon specific evaluations.

Degree Requirements 43 total credit hours, comprehensive exam.

POST-MASTER'S PROGRAM
Areas of Study *Clinical nurse specialist programs in:* family health. *Nurse practitioner programs in:* family health.

Tennessee Technological University
School of Nursing
Cookeville, Tennessee

http://www.tntech.edu/www/acad/nursing/

Founded in 1915

DEGREES • BSN • M SC N • MSN

Nursing Program Faculty 17 (18% with doctorates).

Baccalaureate Enrollment 96
Women 94% **Men** 6% **Minority** 4% **Part-time** 2%

Graduate Enrollment 27
Women 93% **Men** 7% **Minority** 7% **Part-time** 85%

Nursing Student Activities Sigma Theta Tau, Student Nurses' Association.

Nursing Student Resources Academic advising; academic or career counseling; assistance for students with disabilities; bookstore; campus computer network; career placement assistance; computer lab; computer-assisted instruction; daycare for children of students; e-mail services; employment services for current students; externships; housing assistance; Internet; learning resource lab; library services; nursing audiovisuals; paid internships; placement services for program completers; remedial services; resume preparation assistance; skills, simulation, or other laboratory; tutoring; unpaid internships.

Library Facilities 640,056 volumes (312,892 in health, 11,893 in nursing); 4,847 periodical subscriptions (96 health-care related).

BACCALAUREATE PROGRAMS
Degree BSN

Available Programs ADN to Baccalaureate; Generic Baccalaureate; RN Baccalaureate.

Study Options Full-time.

Program Entrance Requirements Minimum overall college GPA of 2.5, transcript of college record, CPR certification, health exam, health insurance, high school biology, high school chemistry, high school foreign language, 3 years high school math, 2 years high school science, high school transcript, immunizations, minimum high school GPA of 3.0, minimum GPA in nursing prerequisites of 2.0, professional liability insurance/malpractice insurance, prerequisite course work. Transfer students are accepted. **Standardized tests** *Required:* SAT or ACT, TOEFL for international students. *Recommended:* ACT. **Application** *Deadline:* 8/1 (freshmen), 8/1 (transfer). *Notification:* continuous (freshmen). *Application fee:* $15.

Advanced Placement Credit given for nursing courses completed elsewhere dependent upon specific evaluations.

Expenses (2006–07) *Tuition, state resident:* full-time $2295; part-time $218 per credit hour. *Tuition, nonresident:* full-time $7142; part-time $639 per credit hour. *International tuition:* $7142 full-time. *Room and board:* $5964; room only: $2944 per academic year. *Required fees:* full-time $200; part-time $15 per credit; part-time $45 per term.

Financial Aid 85% of baccalaureate students in nursing programs received some form of financial aid in 2005–06.

Contact Ms. Kristi L. Loftis, Academic Advisor, School of Nursing, Tennessee Technological University, Box 5001, Cookeville, TN 38505-0001. *Telephone:* 931-372-3203. *Fax:* 931-372-6244. *E-mail:* nursing@tntech.edu.

GRADUATE PROGRAMS
Expenses (2006–07) *Tuition, state resident:* part-time $340 per credit hour. *Tuition, nonresident:* part-time $761 per credit hour.

Contact Ms. Kristi L. Loftis, Academic Advisor, School of Nursing, Tennessee Technological University, Box 5001, Cookeville, TN 38505-0001. *Telephone:* 931-372-3203. *Fax:* 931-372-6244. *E-mail:* nursing@tntech.edu.

MASTER'S DEGREE PROGRAM
Degrees M Sc N; MSN

Available Programs Master's; Master's for Nurses with Non-Nursing Degrees.

Concentrations Available Health-care administration; nursing education; nursing informatics. *Nurse practitioner programs in:* family health.

Study Options Full-time and part-time.

Program Entrance Requirements Computer literacy, minimum overall college GPA of 3.0, transcript of college record, CPR certification, immunizations, 3 letters of recommendation, professional liability insurance/malpractice insurance, resume.

Advanced Placement Credit given for nursing courses completed elsewhere dependent upon specific evaluations.

Degree Requirements 46 total credit hours, thesis or project.

Tennessee Wesleyan College
Fort Sanders Nursing Department
Knoxville, Tennessee

http://www.twcnet.edu/academics/nursing

Founded in 1857

DEGREE • BSN

Nursing Program Faculty 15 (20% with doctorates).

Baccalaureate Enrollment 99
Women 86% **Men** 14% **Minority** 2% **Part-time** 9%

Nursing Student Activities Nursing Honor Society, Sigma Theta Tau, Student Nurses' Association.

Nursing Student Resources Academic advising; bookstore; computer lab; Internet; library services; nursing audiovisuals; skills, simulation, or other laboratory.

Library Facilities 156,126 volumes (6,000 in health, 4,000 in nursing); 11,491 periodical subscriptions (175 health-care related).

BACCALAUREATE PROGRAMS
Degree BSN

Available Programs ADN to Baccalaureate; Generic Baccalaureate; RN Baccalaureate.

Site Options Knoxville, TN.

Study Options Full-time and part-time.

Program Entrance Requirements Minimum overall college GPA of 2.7, transcript of college record, CPR certification, written essay, health exam, high school transcript, immunizations, interview, prerequisite course work. Transfer students are accepted. **Standardized tests** *Required:* SAT or ACT. *Recommended:* TOEFL for international students. **Application** *Deadline:* 8/31 (freshmen), 8/31 (transfer). *Notification:* continuous (freshmen). *Application fee:* $25.

Advanced Placement Credit given for nursing courses completed elsewhere dependent upon specific evaluations.

Expenses (2006–07) *Tuition:* full-time $14,000; part-time $638 per credit hour. *Required fees:* full-time $1400; part-time $64 per credit.

Financial Aid 95% of baccalaureate students in nursing programs received some form of financial aid in 2005–06.

Contact Nursing Contact, Fort Sanders Nursing Department, Tennessee Wesleyan College, 9821 Cogdill Road, Suite 2, Knoxville, TN 37932. *Telephone:* 865-777-5100. *Fax:* 865-777-5114.

Union University
School of Nursing
Jackson, Tennessee

http://www.uu.edu/academics/son/

Founded in 1823

DEGREES • BSN • MSN

Nursing Program Faculty 28 (36% with doctorates).

Baccalaureate Enrollment 285
Women 93% **Men** 7% **Minority** 27% **International** 2% **Part-time** 56%

Graduate Enrollment 55
Women 80% **Men** 20% **Minority** 25% **Part-time** 4%

Nursing Student Activities Nursing Honor Society, Sigma Theta Tau, Student Nurses' Association.

Nursing Student Resources Academic advising; academic or career counseling; assistance for students with disabilities; bookstore; campus computer network; career placement assistance; computer lab; computer-assisted instruction; e-mail services; employment services for current students; housing assistance; Internet; learning resource lab; library services; nursing audiovisuals; resume preparation assistance; skills, simulation, or other laboratory; tutoring.

Library Facilities 149,255 volumes (6,005 in nursing); 19,919 periodical subscriptions (1,284 health-care related).

BACCALAUREATE PROGRAMS

Degree BSN

Available Programs Accelerated Baccalaureate for Second Degree; Generic Baccalaureate; LPN to Baccalaureate; RN Baccalaureate.

Site Options Germantown, TN.

Study Options Full-time.

Program Entrance Requirements Minimum overall college GPA of 2.8, transcript of college record, CPR certification, health exam, immunizations, minimum GPA in nursing prerequisites of 2.8, prerequisite course work. Transfer students are accepted. **Standardized tests** *Required:* SAT or ACT, TOEFL for international students. *Recommended:* SAT Subject Tests.

Application *Deadline:* rolling (freshmen), rolling (transfer). *Early decision:* 12/1. *Notification:* continuous until 8/1 (freshmen), 12/15 (early action). *Application fee:* $25.

Advanced Placement Credit by examination available. Credit given for nursing courses completed elsewhere dependent upon specific evaluations.

Expenses (2006–07) *Tuition:* full-time $16,990; part-time $585 per credit hour. *International tuition:* $16,990 full-time. *Required fees:* full-time $2300.

Financial Aid 70% of baccalaureate students in nursing programs received some form of financial aid in 2005–06. *Gift aid (need-based):* Federal Pell, FSEOG, state, private, college/university gift aid from institutional funds. *Loans:* FFEL (Subsidized and Unsubsidized Stafford PLUS), Perkins, college/university, alternative loans. *Work-Study:* Federal Work-Study, part-time campus jobs. *Application deadline (priority):* 3/1.

Contact Ms. Penney Manae Smith, Nursing Admissions Coordinator, School of Nursing, Union University, 1050 Union University Drive, Jackson, TN 38305. *Telephone:* 731-661-5538. *Fax:* 731-661-5504. *E-mail:* psmith@uu.edu.

GRADUATE PROGRAMS

Expenses (2006–07) *Tuition:* full-time $10,200; part-time $340 per credit hour. *International tuition:* $10,200 full-time. *Required fees:* full-time $350.

Financial Aid 90% of graduate students in nursing programs received some form of financial aid in 2005–06. Traineeships available.

Contact Ms. Penney Manae Smith, Nursing Admissions Coordinator, School of Nursing, Union University, 1050 Union University Drive, Jackson, TN 38305. *Telephone:* 731-661-5538. *Fax:* 901-661-5504. *E-mail:* psmith@uu.edu.

MASTER'S DEGREE PROGRAM

Degree MSN

Available Programs Master's.

Concentrations Available Nurse anesthesia; nursing administration; nursing education. *Clinical nurse specialist programs in:* adult health, pediatric. *Nurse practitioner programs in:* family health.

Site Options Germantown, TN.

Study Options Full-time and part-time.

Program Entrance Requirements Minimum overall college GPA of 3.0, transcript of college record, CPR certification, written essay, immunizations, interview, 3 letters of recommendation, professional liability insurance/malpractice insurance, GRE. *Application deadline:* For fall admission, 8/1 (priority date). *Application fee:* $25.

Advanced Placement Credit given for nursing courses completed elsewhere dependent upon specific evaluations.

Degree Requirements 46 total credit hours.

POST-MASTER'S PROGRAM

Areas of Study Nursing administration; nursing education. *Clinical nurse specialist programs in:* adult health, pediatric. *Nurse practitioner programs in:* family health.

CONTINUING EDUCATION PROGRAM

Contact Beckie Kossick, Clinical Simulation Specialist, School of Nursing, Union University, 1050 Union University Drive, Jackson, TN 38305. *Telephone:* 731-661-5152. *Fax:* 731-661-5504. *E-mail:* bkossick@uu.edu.

University of Memphis
Loewenberg School of Nursing
Memphis, Tennessee

http://www.nursing.memphis.edu

Founded in 1912

DEGREES • BSN • MSN

Nursing Program Faculty 65 (22% with doctorates).

Baccalaureate Enrollment 441
Women 91% **Men** 9% **Minority** 23% **Part-time** 15%

Graduate Enrollment 124
Women 92% **Men** 8% **Minority** 30% **Part-time** 75%

Nursing Student Activities Sigma Theta Tau, Student Nurses' Association.

Nursing Student Resources Academic advising; academic or career counseling; assistance for students with disabilities; bookstore; campus computer network; career placement assistance; computer lab; computer-assisted instruction; daycare for children of students; e-mail services; externships; housing assistance; interactive nursing skills videos; Internet; learning resource lab; library services; nursing audiovisuals; paid internships; remedial services; resume preparation assistance; skills, simulation, or other laboratory; tutoring.

Library Facilities 1.3 million volumes (74,513 in health); 9,393 periodical subscriptions (878 health-care related).

BACCALAUREATE PROGRAMS

Degree BSN

Available Programs ADN to Baccalaureate; Accelerated Baccalaureate; Accelerated Baccalaureate for Second Degree; Accelerated RN Baccalaureate; Baccalaureate for Second Degree; Generic Baccalaureate; RN Baccalaureate.

Site Options *Distance Learning:* Jackson, TN.

Study Options Full-time.

University of Memphis (continued)

Program Entrance Requirements Minimum overall college GPA of 2.7, transcript of college record, CPR certification, health exam, high school biology, high school chemistry, high school foreign language, 3 years high school math, 2 years high school science, high school transcript, immunizations, minimum high school GPA of 3.0, minimum GPA in nursing prerequisites of 2.4, prerequisite course work. Transfer students are accepted. **Standardized tests** *Required:* SAT or ACT, TOEFL for international students. **Application** *Deadline:* 7/1 (freshmen), 7/1 (transfer). *Notification:* continuous (freshmen). *Application fee:* $25.

Advanced Placement Credit by examination available. Credit given for nursing courses completed elsewhere dependent upon specific evaluations.

Expenses (2006–07) *Tuition, state resident:* full-time $5300; part-time $247 per credit hour. *Tuition, nonresident:* full-time $15,700; part-time $695 per credit hour. *Room and board:* room only: $3000 per academic year. *Required fees:* full-time $150.

Financial Aid 53% of baccalaureate students in nursing programs received some form of financial aid in 2005–06.

Contact Ms. Sheila Hall, Assistant Dean for Student Affairs, Loewenberg School of Nursing, University of Memphis, 105 Newport Hall, Memphis, TN 38152. *Telephone:* 901-678-2003. *Fax:* 901-678-4906. *E-mail:* shall@memphis.edu.

GRADUATE PROGRAMS

Expenses (2006–07) *Tuition, state resident:* full-time $6400; part-time $349 per credit hour. *Tuition, nonresident:* full-time $16,840; part-time $797 per credit hour.

Contact Dr. Robert Koch, RN, Director of Graduate Program, Loewenberg School of Nursing, University of Memphis, 203 Newport Hall, Memphis, TN 38152. *Telephone:* 901-678-2003. *Fax:* 901-678-4906. *E-mail:* rakoch@memphis.edu.

MASTER'S DEGREE PROGRAM

Degree MSN

Available Programs Accelerated Master's for Nurses with Non-Nursing Degrees; Master's; Master's for Non-Nursing College Graduates; Master's for Nurses with Non-Nursing Degrees.

Concentrations Available Nursing administration; nursing education. *Nurse practitioner programs in:* family health.

Site Options *Distance Learning:* Jackson, TN.

Study Options Full-time and part-time.

Program Entrance Requirements Minimum overall college GPA of 2.8, CPR certification, immunizations, 3 letters of recommendation, professional liability insurance/malpractice insurance.

Advanced Placement Credit given for nursing courses completed elsewhere dependent upon specific evaluations.

Degree Requirements 45 total credit hours, comprehensive exam.

The University of Tennessee
College of Nursing
Knoxville, Tennessee

http://www.nightingale.con.utk.edu

Founded in 1794

DEGREES • BSN • MSN • PHD

Nursing Program Faculty 60 (50% with doctorates).

Baccalaureate Enrollment 242
Women 88% **Men** 12% **Minority** 9.5% **International** 2% **Part-time** 8%

Graduate Enrollment 168
Women 84% **Men** 16% **Minority** 2% **International** 3% **Part-time** 33%

Nursing Student Activities Sigma Theta Tau, Student Nurses' Association.

Nursing Student Resources Academic advising; academic or career counseling; assistance for students with disabilities; bookstore; campus computer network; computer lab; computer-assisted instruction; e-mail services; employment services for current students; externships; interactive nursing skills videos; Internet; learning resource lab; library services; nursing audiovisuals; remedial services; skills, simulation, or other laboratory; tutoring.

Library Facilities 24.4 million volumes (59,214 in health, 3,711 in nursing); 17,628 periodical subscriptions (572 health-care related).

BACCALAUREATE PROGRAMS

Degree BSN

Available Programs Accelerated RN Baccalaureate; Generic Baccalaureate.

Study Options Full-time and part-time.

Program Entrance Requirements Minimum overall college GPA of 2.5, transcript of college record, CPR certification, health exam, health insurance, immunizations, interview, professional liability insurance/malpractice insurance, prerequisite course work. Transfer students are accepted. **Standardized tests** *Required:* SAT or ACT, TOEFL for international students. **Application** *Deadline:* 2/1 (freshmen), 6/1 (transfer). *Early decision:* 11/1. *Notification:* continuous (freshmen), 12/15 (early action). *Application fee:* $30.

Advanced Placement Credit by examination available. Credit given for nursing courses completed elsewhere dependent upon specific evaluations.

Expenses (2006–07) *Tuition, state resident:* full-time $4830; part-time $202 per credit. *Tuition, nonresident:* full-time $16,096; part-time $672 per credit. *International tuition:* $16,096 full-time. *Room and board:* $6054; room only: $3188 per academic year. *Required fees:* full-time $792; part-time $35 per credit.

Financial Aid 50% of baccalaureate students in nursing programs received some form of financial aid in 2005–06.

Contact Director, Student Services, College of Nursing, The University of Tennessee, 1200 Volunteer Boulevard, Knoxville, TN 37996-4180. *Telephone:* 865-974-7606. *Fax:* 865-974-3569. *E-mail:* bbarret@utk.edu.

GRADUATE PROGRAMS

Expenses (2006–07) *Tuition, state resident:* full-time $5574; part-time $310 per credit. *Tuition, nonresident:* full-time $16,840; part-time $672 per credit. *Room and board:* $6054; room only: $3188 per academic year. *Required fees:* full-time $790; part-time $51 per credit.

Financial Aid 75% of graduate students in nursing programs received some form of financial aid in 2005–06. 3 fellowships, 1 research assistantship were awarded; teaching assistantships, Federal Work-Study, institutionally sponsored loans, and unspecified assistantships also available. *Financial aid application deadline:* 2/1.

Contact Dr. Sandra L. McGuire, Chair, Masters Program, College of Nursing, The University of Tennessee, 1200 Volunteer Boulevard, Knoxville, TN 37996-4180. *Telephone:* 865-974-4151. *Fax:* 865-974-3569. *E-mail:* smcguire@utk.edu.

MASTER'S DEGREE PROGRAM

Degree MSN

Available Programs Accelerated Master's for Nurses with Non-Nursing Degrees; Accelerated RN to Master's; Master's; Master's for Non-Nursing College Graduates; Master's for Nurses with Non-Nursing Degrees; RN to Master's.

Concentrations Available Health-care administration; nurse anesthesia; nursing administration. *Clinical nurse specialist programs in:* adult health, gerontology, maternity-newborn, pediatric, perinatal, psychiatric/mental health, women's health. *Nurse practitioner programs in:* adult health, family health, gerontology, neonatal health, pediatric, psychiatric/mental health, women's health.

Study Options Full-time.

Program Entrance Requirements Minimum overall college GPA of 3.0, transcript of college record, CPR certification, written essay, immunizations, 3 letters of recommendation, nursing research course, physical assessment course, professional liability insurance/malpractice insurance, prerequisite course work, statistics course, GRE General Test. *Application deadline:* For fall admission, 2/1 (priority date). Applications are processed on a rolling basis. *Application fee:* $35.

Advanced Placement Credit by examination available. Credit given for nursing courses completed elsewhere dependent upon specific evaluations.

Degree Requirements 41 total credit hours, thesis or project, comprehensive exam.

POST-MASTER'S PROGRAM

Areas of Study   Health-care administration; nurse anesthesia; nursing administration; nursing education. *Clinical nurse specialist programs in:* adult health, gerontology, maternity-newborn, pediatric, perinatal, psychiatric/mental health, women's health. *Nurse practitioner programs in:* adult health, family health, gerontology, neonatal health, pediatric, psychiatric/mental health, women's health.

DOCTORAL DEGREE PROGRAM

Degree   PhD

Available Programs   Doctorate; Post-Baccalaureate Doctorate.

Areas of Study   Bio-behavioral research, biology of health and illness, family health, health policy, health promotion/disease prevention, human health and illness, individualized study, neuro-behavior, nursing administration, nursing education, nursing research, nursing science, women's health.

Program Entrance Requirements   Minimum overall college GPA of 3.0, interview by faculty committee, interview, 3 letters of recommendation, writing sample, GRE General Test. *Application deadline:* For fall admission, 2/1 (priority date). Applications are processed on a rolling basis. *Application fee:* $35.

Degree Requirements   67 total credit hours, dissertation, oral exam, written exam, residency.

CONTINUING EDUCATION PROGRAM

Contact   Dr. Maureen Nalle, Coordinator, Continuing Education, College of Nursing, The University of Tennessee, 1200 Volunteer Boulevard, Knoxville, TN 37996-4180. *Telephone:* 865-974-7598. *Fax:* 865-974-3569. *E-mail:* mnalle@utk.edu.

The University of Tennessee at Chattanooga
School of Nursing
Chattanooga, Tennessee

http://www.utc.edu/~utcnurse/index.btm

Founded in 1886

DEGREES • BSN • MSN

Nursing Program Faculty 25 (65% with doctorates).

Baccalaureate Enrollment 350
Women 85% **Men** 15% **Minority** 12% **Part-time** 5%

Graduate Enrollment 70
Women 60% **Men** 40% **Minority** 20% **Part-time** 30%

Nursing Student Activities Sigma Theta Tau, Student Nurses' Association.

Nursing Student Resources Academic advising; academic or career counseling; assistance for students with disabilities; bookstore; campus computer network; computer lab; e-mail services; interactive nursing skills videos; Internet; learning resource lab; nursing audiovisuals; skills, simulation, or other laboratory.

Library Facilities 491,179 volumes (19,370 in health, 3,100 in nursing); 1,847 periodical subscriptions (200 health-care related).

BACCALAUREATE PROGRAMS

Degree BSN

Available Programs ADN to Baccalaureate; Baccalaureate for Second Degree; Generic Baccalaureate.

Study Options Full-time.

Program Entrance Requirements Minimum overall college GPA of 2.5, transcript of college record, CPR certification, health exam, health insurance, high school foreign language, 3 years high school math, high school transcript, immunizations, 2 letters of recommendation, minimum high school GPA of 2.0, minimum GPA in nursing prerequisites of 2.5, professional liability insurance/malpractice insurance, prerequisite course work. Transfer students are accepted. **Standardized tests** *Required:* SAT or ACT, TOEFL for international students. **Application** *Notification:* continuous (freshmen). *Application fee:* $25.

Advanced Placement   Credit by examination available. Credit given for nursing courses completed elsewhere dependent upon specific evaluations.

Contact   *Telephone:* 423-425-4750. *Fax:* 423-425-4668.

GRADUATE PROGRAMS

Contact   *Telephone:* 423-425-4750. *Fax:* 423-425-4668.

MASTER'S DEGREE PROGRAM

Degree   MSN

Available Programs   Master's.

Concentrations Available   Nurse anesthesia. *Nurse practitioner programs in:* family health.

Site Options   Tupelo, MS.

Study Options   Full-time and part-time.

Program Entrance Requirements   Clinical experience, computer literacy, minimum overall college GPA of 3.0, transcript of college record, CPR certification, written essay, immunizations, interview, 3 letters of recommendation, nursing research course, physical assessment course, resume, statistics course, GRE General Test, MAT. *Application deadline:* For fall admission, 8/1 (priority date); for spring admission, 12/1 (priority date). Applications are processed on a rolling basis. *Application fee:* $25.

Advanced Placement   Credit given for nursing courses completed elsewhere dependent upon specific evaluations.

Degree Requirements   50 total credit hours, thesis or project.

POST-MASTER'S PROGRAM

Areas of Study   Nurse anesthesia. *Nurse practitioner programs in:* family health.

CONTINUING EDUCATION PROGRAM

Contact   *Telephone:* 423-425-4750. *Fax:* 423-425-4668.

The University of Tennessee at Martin
Department of Nursing
Martin, Tennessee

http://www.utm.edu

Founded in 1900

DEGREE • BSN

Nursing Program Faculty 14 (14% with doctorates).

Baccalaureate Enrollment 165
Women 92% **Men** 8% **Minority** 7% **International** 1% **Part-time** 22%

Nursing Student Activities Nursing Honor Society, Sigma Theta Tau, Student Nurses' Association, nursing club.

Nursing Student Resources Academic advising; academic or career counseling; assistance for students with disabilities; bookstore; campus computer network; career placement assistance; computer lab; computer-assisted instruction; daycare for children of students; e-mail services; employment services for current students; housing assistance; interactive nursing skills videos; Internet; learning resource lab; library services; nursing audiovisuals; remedial services; resume preparation assistance; skills, simulation, or other laboratory; tutoring.

Library Facilities 488,807 volumes (3,600 in health, 1,440 in nursing); 2,016 periodical subscriptions (14,700 health-care related).

BACCALAUREATE PROGRAMS

Degree BSN

Available Programs ADN to Baccalaureate; Accelerated RN Baccalaureate; Generic Baccalaureate; LPN to RN Baccalaureate.

Site Options Jackson, TN.

Study Options Full-time.

Program Entrance Requirements Minimum overall college GPA of 2.0, transcript of college record, CPR certification, health exam, health insurance, high school biology, high school chemistry, high school foreign language, 3 years high school math, 2 years high school science, high

The University of Tennessee at Martin (continued)

school transcript, immunizations, interview, minimum high school GPA of 2.8, minimum GPA in nursing prerequisites of 2.0, professional liability insurance/malpractice insurance, prerequisite course work. Transfer students are accepted. **Standardized tests** *Required:* SAT or ACT, TOEFL for international students. **Application** *Deadline:* rolling (freshmen), rolling (transfer). *Notification:* continuous until 8/1 (freshmen). *Application fee:* $30.

Advanced Placement Credit by examination available. Credit given for nursing courses completed elsewhere dependent upon specific evaluations.

Expenses (2006–07) *Tuition, state resident:* full-time $4665; part-time $197 per hour. *Tuition, nonresident:* full-time $14,137; part-time $591 per hour. *International tuition:* $14,137 full-time. *Room and board:* $3000; room only: $2000 per academic year. *Required fees:* full-time $1500; part-time $750 per credit; part-time $750 per term.

Financial Aid 82% of baccalaureate students in nursing programs received some form of financial aid in 2005–06. *Gift aid (need-based):* Federal Pell, FSEOG, state, private, TN minority: Teaching fellowships; TN teachers; Sc. *Loans:* FFEL (Subsidized and Unsubsidized Stafford PLUS), Perkins. *Work-Study:* Federal Work-Study. *Application deadline:* Continuous.

Contact Mrs. Brenda W. Campbell, Program Resource Specialist, Department of Nursing, The University of Tennessee at Martin, Gooch Hall 136J, Martin, TN 38238. *Telephone:* 731-881-7138. *Fax:* 731-881-7939. *E-mail:* brendac@utm.edu.

CONTINUING EDUCATION PROGRAM

Contact Dr. Nancy A. Warren, Professor and Chair, Department of Nursing, The University of Tennessee at Martin, Gooch Hall 136H, Martin, TN 38238. *Telephone:* 731-881-7140. *Fax:* 731-881-7140. *E-mail:* nwarren@utm.edu.

The University of Tennessee Health Science Center
College of Nursing
Memphis, Tennessee

http://www.utmem.edu/nursing

Founded in 1911

DEGREES • BSN • MSN • PHD

Nursing Program Faculty 30 (100% with doctorates).

Baccalaureate Enrollment 65
Women 90% **Men** 10% **Minority** 30%

Graduate Enrollment 164
Women 85% **Men** 15% **Minority** 22%

Nursing Student Activities Sigma Theta Tau, Student Nurses' Association.

Nursing Student Resources Academic advising; academic or career counseling; assistance for students with disabilities; bookstore; campus computer network; computer lab; computer-assisted instruction; e-mail services; housing assistance; Internet; learning resource lab; library services; nursing audiovisuals; paid internships; remedial services; skills, simulation, or other laboratory; tutoring.

Library Facilities 165,200 volumes (194,185 in health, 2,746 in nursing); 1,784 periodical subscriptions (1,852 health-care related).

BACCALAUREATE PROGRAMS

Degree BSN

Available Programs ADN to Baccalaureate; Accelerated Baccalaureate; Accelerated Baccalaureate for Second Degree; Accelerated RN Baccalaureate; Baccalaureate for Second Degree; Generic Baccalaureate; RN Baccalaureate.

Site Options *Distance Learning:* Memphis, TN.
Study Options Full-time and part-time.

Program Entrance Requirements Minimum overall college GPA of 3.0, transcript of college record, CPR certification, written essay, health insurance, high school transcript, immunizations, 3 letters of recommendation, prerequisite course work, RN licensure. Transfer students are accepted. **Application** *Application fee:* $25.

Advanced Placement Credit given for nursing courses completed elsewhere dependent upon specific evaluations.

Expenses (2005–06) *Tuition, state resident:* full-time $6129. *Tuition, nonresident:* full-time $14,355. *Required fees:* full-time $1800.

Financial Aid 52% of baccalaureate students in nursing programs received some form of financial aid in 2004–05.

Contact Mr. Ron Patterson, Assistant Director, Student Affairs, College of Nursing, The University of Tennessee Health Science Center, 877 Madison Avenue, Suite 637, Memphis, TN 38163. *Telephone:* 901-448-1769. *Fax:* 901-448-4121. *E-mail:* rpatte10@utmem.edu.

GRADUATE PROGRAMS

Expenses (2005–06) *Tuition, state resident:* full-time $3853. *Tuition, nonresident:* full-time $9086. *Required fees:* full-time $3500.

Financial Aid 52% of graduate students in nursing programs received some form of financial aid in 2004–05. Fellowships with partial tuition reimbursements available, teaching assistantships, Federal Work-Study, institutionally sponsored loans, scholarships, and traineeships available. Aid available to part-time students. *Financial aid application deadline:* 2/28.

Contact Dr. James Pruett, Assistant Dean, Student Affairs, College of Nursing, The University of Tennessee Health Science Center, 877 Madison Avenue, Suite 637, Memphis, TN 38163. *Telephone:* 901-448-6139. *Fax:* 901-448-4121. *E-mail:* jpruett@utmem.edu.

MASTER'S DEGREE PROGRAM

Degree MSN

Available Programs Master's.

Concentrations Available Nurse anesthesia. *Clinical nurse specialist programs in:* acute care, critical care, psychiatric/mental health. *Nurse practitioner programs in:* acute care, family health, neonatal health, primary care, psychiatric/mental health.

Site Options *Distance Learning:* Memphis, TN.

Study Options Full-time.

Program Entrance Requirements Clinical experience, computer literacy, minimum overall college GPA of 3.0, transcript of college record, CPR certification, written essay, immunizations, interview, 3 letters of recommendation, professional liability insurance/malpractice insurance, prerequisite course work, GRE General Test. *Application deadline:* For fall admission, 2/1; for winter admission, 9/1. *Application fee:* $50.

Degree Requirements 46 total credit hours.

POST-MASTER'S PROGRAM

Areas of Study Nurse anesthesia; nurse-midwifery; nursing administration. *Clinical nurse specialist programs in:* acute care, critical care, psychiatric/mental health, public health. *Nurse practitioner programs in:* acute care, family health, neonatal health, primary care, psychiatric/mental health.

DOCTORAL DEGREE PROGRAM

Degree PhD

Available Programs Doctorate.

Areas of Study Clinical practice, critical care, health promotion/disease prevention, human health and illness, nursing research, nursing science.

Site Options *Distance Learning:* Memphis, TN.

Program Entrance Requirements Clinical experience, minimum overall college GPA of 3.0, interview by faculty committee, 3 letters of recommendation, MSN or equivalent, writing sample. *Application deadline:* For fall admission, 2/1; for winter admission, 9/1. *Application fee:* $50.

Degree Requirements 60 total credit hours, dissertation.

CONTINUING EDUCATION PROGRAM

Contact Dr. Cynthia Russell, Director, Distributive Programs, College of Nursing, The University of Tennessee Health Science Center, 877 Madison Avenue, Suite 645, Memphis, TN 38163. *Telephone:* 901-448-6424. *Fax:* 901-448-4121. *E-mail:* crussell@utmem.edu.

Vanderbilt University
School of Nursing
Nashville, Tennessee

http://www.mc.vanderbilt.edu/nursing/

Founded in 1873

DEGREES • MSN • MSN/MBA • MSN/MDIV • PHD

Nursing Program Faculty 145 (20% with doctorates).

Graduate Enrollment 561
Women 89% **Men** 11% **Minority** 16% **International** 1% **Part-time** 23%
Nursing Student Activities Sigma Theta Tau.

Nursing Student Resources Academic advising; assistance for students with disabilities; bookstore; campus computer network; career placement assistance; computer lab; computer-assisted instruction; daycare for children of students; e-mail services; housing assistance; interactive nursing skills videos; Internet; library services; nursing audiovisuals; remedial services; resume preparation assistance; skills, simulation, or other laboratory.

Library Facilities 1.8 million volumes (201,000 in health); 26,885 periodical subscriptions (3,300 health-care related).

■ Vanderbilt University School of Nursing (VUSN) offers a Master of Science in Nursing (M.S.N.) program with multiple entry options: entry with a non-nursing degree or as a college senior, with an associate degree in nursing, with a diploma in nursing, or with a baccalaureate degree in nursing. VUSN considers the present educational status of each student and incorporates it into an accelerated and highly specialized program that meets individual learning needs. There is even an entry option for students who already have an M.S.N. degree but who want a role change or role expansion. At Vanderbilt, faculty members are committed to the tradition of enhancing the quality of health-care delivery. VUSN's vast selection of nursing specialties allows the School of Nursing to shape the careers of advanced practice nurses today in order to create professional excellence in the health-care leaders of tomorrow.

GRADUATE PROGRAMS

Expenses (2006–07) *Tuition:* full-time $34,827; part-time $893 per credit hour. *Required fees:* full-time $3100.

Financial Aid 94% of graduate students in nursing programs received some form of financial aid in 2005–06. Federal Work-Study, institutionally sponsored loans, and unspecified assistantships available. Aid available to part-time students. *Financial aid application deadline:* 3/15.

Contact Patricia Peerman, Director of Enrollment Management, School of Nursing, Vanderbilt University, 207 Godchaux Hall, Nashville, TN 37240. *Telephone:* 615-322-3800. *Fax:* 615-343-0333. *E-mail:* Paddy.Peerman@vanderbilt.edu.

MASTER'S DEGREE PROGRAM

Degrees MSN; MSN/MBA; MSN/MDIV

Available Programs Accelerated AD/RN to Master's; Accelerated Master's; Accelerated Master's for Non-Nursing College Graduates; Accelerated Master's for Nurses with Non-Nursing Degrees; Accelerated RN to Master's.

Concentrations Available Health-care administration; nurse-midwifery; nursing administration; nursing informatics. *Clinical nurse specialist programs in:* medical-surgical, pediatric, psychiatric/mental health. *Nurse practitioner programs in:* acute care, adult health, family health, gerontology, neonatal health, pediatric, psychiatric/mental health, women's health.

Site Options *Distance Learning:* Nashville, TN.

Study Options Full-time and part-time.

Program Entrance Requirements Computer literacy, minimum overall college GPA of 3.0, transcript of college record, CPR certification, written essay, immunizations, 3 letters of recommendation, physical assessment course, prerequisite course work, statistics course, GRE. *Application deadline:* For fall admission, 12/1 (priority date). Applications are processed on a rolling basis. *Application fee:* $50.

Advanced Placement Credit by examination available. Credit given for nursing courses completed elsewhere dependent upon specific evaluations.

Degree Requirements 39 total credit hours.

POST-MASTER'S PROGRAM

Areas of Study Health-care administration; nurse-midwifery; nursing administration; nursing informatics. *Clinical nurse specialist programs in:* medical-surgical, pediatric, psychiatric/mental health. *Nurse practitioner programs in:* acute care, adult health, family health, gerontology, neonatal health, pediatric, psychiatric/mental health, women's health.

DOCTORAL DEGREE PROGRAM

Degree PhD

Available Programs Doctorate.

Areas of Study Addiction/substance abuse, advanced practice nursing, aging, bio-behavioral research, biology of health and illness, community health, critical care, family health, gerontology, health policy, health promotion/disease prevention, health-care systems, human health and illness, illness and transition, information systems, maternity-newborn, nursing administration, nursing policy, nursing research, nursing science, oncology, women's health.

Program Entrance Requirements Minimum overall college GPA of 3.0, interview by faculty committee, interview, 3 letters of recommendation, MSN or equivalent, statistics course, vita, writing sample, GRE General Test. *Application deadline:* For fall admission, 12/1 (priority date). Applications are processed on a rolling basis. *Application fee:* $50.

Degree Requirements 72 total credit hours, dissertation, oral exam, written exam, residency.

POSTDOCTORAL PROGRAM

Areas of Study Individualized study.

Postdoctoral Program Contact Dr. Melanie Lutenbacher, Director, School of Nursing, Vanderbilt University, 603 Godchaux Hall, Nashville, TN 37240. *Telephone:* 615-343-8977. *Fax:* 615-343-0333. *E-mail:* melanie.lutenbacher@vanderbilt.edu.

CONTINUING EDUCATION PROGRAM

Contact Ms. Ginny Moore, Director of Lifelong Learning, School of Nursing, Vanderbilt University, 461 21st Avenue South, Nashville, TN 37240. *Telephone:* 615-343-8493. *Fax:* 615-322-8816. *E-mail:* ginny.moore@vanderbilt.edu.

See full description on page 570.

TEXAS

Abilene Christian University
Abilene Intercollegiate School of Nursing
Abilene, Texas

See description of programs under
Patty Hanks Shelton School of Nursing
(Abilene, Texas).

Angelo State University
Department of Nursing
San Angelo, Texas

http://www.angelo.edu/dept/nur/
Founded in 1928
DEGREES • BSN • MSN

Nursing Program Faculty 20 (35% with doctorates).
Baccalaureate Enrollment 70
Women 87% **Men** 13% **Minority** 10% **Part-time** 71%
Graduate Enrollment 23
Women 74% **Men** 26% **Minority** 22% **Part-time** 39%
Nursing Student Activities Student Nurses' Association.
Nursing Student Resources Academic advising; academic or career counseling; bookstore; campus computer network; computer lab; computer-assisted instruction; e-mail services; housing assistance; interactive nursing skills videos; Internet; learning resource lab; library services; nursing audiovisuals; skills, simulation, or other laboratory; tutoring.
Library Facilities 50,963 volumes (7,560 in health, 762 in nursing); 22,004 periodical subscriptions (390 health-care related).

BACCALAUREATE PROGRAMS
Degree BSN
Available Programs RN Baccalaureate.
Study Options Full-time and part-time.
Program Entrance Requirements Minimum overall college GPA of 2.5, transcript of college record, CPR certification, immunizations, 3 letters of recommendation. Transfer students are accepted. **Standardized tests** *Required:* SAT or ACT, TOEFL for international students. **Application** *Deadline:* 8/15 (freshmen), 8/15 (transfer). *Notification:* continuous (freshmen). *Application fee:* $25.
Contact *Telephone:* 915-942-2224 Ext. 259. *Fax:* 915-942-2236.

GRADUATE PROGRAMS
Contact *Telephone:* 915-942-2224. *Fax:* 915-942-2236.

MASTER'S DEGREE PROGRAM
Degree MSN
Available Programs Master's.
Concentrations Available Nursing education. *Clinical nurse specialist programs in:* adult health, medical-surgical.
Study Options Full-time and part-time.
Program Entrance Requirements Computer literacy, minimum overall college GPA of 3.0, transcript of college record, 2 letters of recommendation, physical assessment course, statistics course, GRE General Test. *Application deadline:* For fall admission, 7/15 (priority date); for spring admission, 12/8. Applications are processed on a rolling basis. *Application fee:* $25 ($50 for international students).
Advanced Placement Credit given for nursing courses completed elsewhere dependent upon specific evaluations.
Degree Requirements 46 total credit hours, comprehensive exam.

Baylor University
Louise Herrington School of Nursing
Dallas, Texas

http://www.baylor.edu/Nursing
Founded in 1845
DEGREES • BSN • MSN

Nursing Program Faculty 47 (22% with doctorates).
Baccalaureate Enrollment 265
Women 94% **Men** 6% **Minority** 54%
Graduate Enrollment 37
Women 97% **Men** 3% **Minority** 19% **International** 3% **Part-time** 63%
Nursing Student Activities Sigma Theta Tau, Student Nurses' Association.
Nursing Student Resources Academic advising; campus computer network; computer lab; e-mail services; housing assistance; interactive nursing skills videos; Internet; learning resource lab; library services; nursing audiovisuals; skills, simulation, or other laboratory.
Library Facilities 2.3 million volumes (6,000 in health, 5,000 in nursing); 8,429 periodical subscriptions (106 health-care related).

■ Baylor University's Louise Herrington School of Nursing offers B.S.N. and M.S.N. programs in a caring, Christian environment. Low student-teacher ratios allow participatory classroom learning. Clinical instruction is enhanced through access to premier health-care facilities and strong collaboration with health-care providers. Graduates of the B.S.N. program perform well on NCLEX-RN examinations. Graduate programs include family nurse practitioner (FNP) with a missions focus and neonatal nurse practitioner (NNP). Graduates of the FNP and NNP perform well on national certification examinations. Detailed information about programs can be found on the Web at http://www.baylor.edu/Nursing.

BACCALAUREATE PROGRAMS
Degree BSN
Available Programs Generic Baccalaureate.
Study Options Full-time.
Program Entrance Requirements Minimum overall college GPA of 3.0, transcript of college record, CPR certification, written essay, health exam, immunizations, 3 letters of recommendation, minimum GPA in nursing prerequisites of 3.0, prerequisite course work. Transfer students are accepted. **Standardized tests** *Required:* SAT or ACT, TOEFL for international students, ACT essay. **Application** *Deadline:* 2/1 (freshmen), rolling (transfer). *Notification:* 3/15 (freshmen). *Application fee:* $50.
Expenses (2006–07) *Tuition:* full-time $19,050. *Room and board:* $6476; room only: $3346 per academic year. *Required fees:* full-time $2120.
Financial Aid 91% of baccalaureate students in nursing programs received some form of financial aid in 2005–06. *Gift aid (need-based):* Federal Pell, FSEOG, state, private, college/university gift aid from institutional funds. *Loans:* Federal Nursing Student Loans, FFEL (Subsidized and Unsubsidized Stafford PLUS), Perkins, state, college/university. *Work-Study:* Federal Work-Study, part-time campus jobs. *Application deadline (priority):* 3/1.
Contact Miss Tina Sims, Academic Advisor, Louise Herrington School of Nursing, Baylor University, 3700 Worth Street, Dallas, TX 75246. *Telephone:* 214-214-4151. *Fax:* 214-820-3835. *E-mail:* tina_sims@baylor.edu.

GRADUATE PROGRAMS
Expenses (2006–07) *Tuition:* full-time $15,426; part-time $857 per credit hour. *Required fees:* full-time $2140.
Financial Aid 100% of graduate students in nursing programs received some form of financial aid in 2005–06.
Contact Dr. Mary C. Brucker, Director, Graduate Program, Louise Herrington School of Nursing, Baylor University, 3700 Worth Street, Dallas, TX 75246. *Telephone:* 214-820-3361. *Fax:* 214-820-4770. *E-mail:* mary_brucker@baylor.edu.

MASTER'S DEGREE PROGRAM

Degree MSN

Available Programs Master's.

Concentrations Available *Nurse practitioner programs in:* family health, neonatal health.

Site Options *Distance Learning:* Waco, TX.

Study Options Full-time and part-time.

Program Entrance Requirements Clinical experience, minimum overall college GPA of 3.0, transcript of college record, CPR certification, written essay, immunizations, 3 letters of recommendation, prerequisite course work, statistics course, GRE General Test. *Application deadline:* For fall admission, 8/1; for spring admission, 12/1. Applications are processed on a rolling basis. *Application fee:* $25.

Advanced Placement Credit given for nursing courses completed elsewhere dependent upon specific evaluations.

Degree Requirements 45 total credit hours.

POST-MASTER'S PROGRAM

Areas of Study *Nurse practitioner programs in:* family health, neonatal health.

East Texas Baptist University
Department of Nursing
Marshall, Texas

http://www.etbu.edu

Founded in 1912

DEGREE • BSN

Nursing Program Faculty 9 (1% with doctorates).

Baccalaureate Enrollment 48

Women 90% **Men** 10% **Minority** 22%

Nursing Student Activities Student Nurses' Association, nursing club.

Nursing Student Resources Academic advising; academic or career counseling; assistance for students with disabilities; bookstore; campus computer network; career placement assistance; computer lab; computer-assisted instruction; e-mail services; employment services for current students; housing assistance; interactive nursing skills videos; Internet; learning resource lab; library services; nursing audiovisuals; placement services for program completers; remedial services; resume preparation assistance; skills, simulation, or other laboratory; tutoring.

Library Facilities 182,701 volumes (568 in health, 291 in nursing); 15,000 periodical subscriptions (2,100 health-care related).

BACCALAUREATE PROGRAMS

Degree BSN

Available Programs Generic Baccalaureate.

Study Options Full-time.

Program Entrance Requirements Minimum overall college GPA of 2.8, transcript of college record, CPR certification, written essay, health exam, health insurance, immunizations, 2 letters of recommendation, minimum GPA in nursing prerequisites of 2.8, professional liability insurance/malpractice insurance, prerequisite course work. Transfer students are accepted. **Standardized tests** *Required:* SAT or ACT, TOEFL for international students. **Application** *Deadline:* 8/16 (freshmen), 8/16 (out-of-state freshmen), 8/16 (transfer). *Notification:* continuous (freshmen), continuous (out-of-state freshmen). *Application fee:* $25.

Expenses (2006–07) *Tuition:* full-time $12,840; part-time $400 per credit hour. *Room and board:* $3700 per academic year. *Required fees:* full-time $626.

Financial Aid 99% of baccalaureate students in nursing programs received some form of financial aid in 2005–06. *Gift aid (need-based):* Federal Pell, FSEOG, state, private, college/university gift aid from institutional funds. *Loans:* FFEL (Subsidized and Unsubsidized Stafford PLUS), Perkins, state, college/university. *Work-Study:* Federal Work-Study, part-time campus jobs. *Application deadline (priority):* 6/1.

Contact Dr. Carolyn Harvey, Dean, Department of Nursing, East Texas Baptist University, 1209 North Grove Street, Marshall, TX 75670-1498. *Telephone:* 903-923-2210. *Fax:* 903-938-9225. *E-mail:* charvey@etbu.edu.

Hardin-Simmons University
Abilene Intercollegiate School of Nursing
Abilene, Texas

See description of programs under
Patty Hanks Shelton School of Nursing (Abilene, Texas).

Houston Baptist University
College of Nursing
Houston, Texas

Founded in 1960

DEGREE • BSN

Nursing Program Faculty 23 (6% with doctorates).

Baccalaureate Enrollment 60

Women 90% **Men** 10% **Minority** 20% **International** 10%

Nursing Student Activities Nursing Honor Society, Sigma Theta Tau, Student Nurses' Association.

Nursing Student Resources Academic advising; academic or career counseling; assistance for students with disabilities; bookstore; career placement assistance; computer lab; e-mail services; employment services for current students; externships; housing assistance; interactive nursing skills videos; Internet; learning resource lab; library services; nursing audiovisuals; paid internships; placement services for program completers; remedial services; resume preparation assistance; skills, simulation, or other laboratory; tutoring; unpaid internships.

Library Facilities 209,366 volumes (4,276 in health, 1,200 in nursing); 21,000 periodical subscriptions (117 health-care related).

BACCALAUREATE PROGRAMS

Degree BSN

Site Options Houston, TX.

Study Options Full-time.

Program Entrance Requirements Minimum overall college GPA of 2.5, minimum GPA in nursing prerequisites of 2.5. Transfer students are accepted. **Standardized tests** *Required:* SAT or ACT, TOEFL for international students. **Application** *Deadline:* rolling (freshmen), rolling (transfer). *Notification:* continuous (freshmen). *Application fee:* $25.

Advanced Placement Credit by examination available.

Contact *Telephone:* 281-649-3300. *Fax:* 281-649-3340.

Lamar University
Department of Nursing
Beaumont, Texas

http://dept.lamar.edu/nursing/

Founded in 1923

DEGREES • BSN • MSN • MSN/MBA

Nursing Program Faculty 31 (27% with doctorates).

Baccalaureate Enrollment 209

Women 82% **Men** 18% **Minority** 32% **International** 1% **Part-time** 1%

Graduate Enrollment 14

Women 85% **Men** 15% **Minority** 28% **Part-time** 86%

Nursing Student Activities Sigma Theta Tau, Student Nurses' Association.

Nursing Student Resources Academic advising; academic or career counseling; assistance for students with disabilities; bookstore; campus computer network; career placement assistance; computer lab; computer-assisted instruction; daycare for children of students; e-mail services; employment services for current students; housing assistance; interactive

Lamar University (continued)

nursing skills videos; Internet; learning resource lab; library services; nursing audiovisuals; placement services for program completers; remedial services; resume preparation assistance; skills, simulation, or other laboratory; tutoring.

Library Facilities 698,285 volumes (6,825 in health, 1,800 in nursing); 2,900 periodical subscriptions (100 health-care related).

BACCALAUREATE PROGRAMS

Degree BSN

Available Programs ADN to Baccalaureate; Generic Baccalaureate; RN Baccalaureate.

Study Options Full-time.

Program Entrance Requirements Minimum overall college GPA of 2.0, transcript of college record, CPR certification, health exam, immunizations, minimum GPA in nursing prerequisites of 2.0, professional liability insurance/malpractice insurance, prerequisite course work. Transfer students are accepted. **Standardized tests** *Required:* SAT or ACT, TOEFL for international students. *Required for some:* SAT Subject Tests. **Application** *Deadline:* 8/1 (freshmen), 8/1 (transfer). *Notification:* continuous (freshmen).

Advanced Placement Credit given for nursing courses completed elsewhere dependent upon specific evaluations.

Expenses (2006–07) *Tuition, state resident:* full-time $2880; part-time $120 per credit hour. *Tuition, nonresident:* full-time $9480; part-time $395 per credit hour. *International tuition:* $9480 full-time. *Room and board:* $5720; room only: $3990 per academic year. *Required fees:* full-time $1104; part-time $115 per credit.

Financial Aid 80% of baccalaureate students in nursing programs received some form of financial aid in 2005–06. *Gift aid (need-based):* Federal Pell, FSEOG, state, college/university gift aid from institutional funds. *Loans:* FFEL (Subsidized and Unsubsidized Stafford PLUS), Perkins, state, college/university. *Work-Study:* Federal Work-Study, part-time campus jobs. *Application deadline (priority):* 4/1.

Contact Ms. Leah D. East, Advisor, Department of Nursing, Lamar University, PO Box 10081, Beaumont, TX 77710. *Telephone:* 409-880-8868. *Fax:* 409-880-7736. *E-mail:* nursing@lamar.edu.

GRADUATE PROGRAMS

Expenses (2006–07) *Tuition, state resident:* full-time $1872; part-time $272 per credit hour. *Tuition, nonresident:* full-time $4059; part-time $515 per credit hour. *Room and board:* $5888; room only: $3990 per academic year. *Required fees:* full-time $150; part-time $50 per credit.

Financial Aid 35% of graduate students in nursing programs received some form of financial aid in 2005–06.

Contact Dr. Nancy Bume, Director of Graduate Nursing Studies, Department of Nursing, Lamar University, PO Box 10081, Beaumont, TX 77710. *Telephone:* 409-880-7720. *Fax:* 409-880-8698. *E-mail:* nancy.blume@lamar.edu.

MASTER'S DEGREE PROGRAM

Degrees MSN; MSN/MBA

Available Programs Master's.

Concentrations Available Nursing administration; nursing education.

Study Options Full-time and part-time.

Program Entrance Requirements Computer literacy, minimum overall college GPA of 3.0, transcript of college record, immunizations, professional liability insurance/malpractice insurance, prerequisite course work, statistics course.

Advanced Placement Credit given for nursing courses completed elsewhere dependent upon specific evaluations.

Degree Requirements 37 total credit hours, thesis or project, comprehensive exam.

CONTINUING EDUCATION PROGRAM

Contact Dr. Cindy Stinson, RN, Coordinator of Continuing Education, Department of Nursing, Lamar University, PO Box 10081, Beaumont, TX 77710. *Telephone:* 409-880-8833. *Fax:* 409-880-1865. *E-mail:* cynthia.stinson@lamar.edu.

Lubbock Christian University
Department of Nursing
Lubbock, Texas

Founded in 1957

DEGREE • BSN

Nursing Program Faculty 5 (40% with doctorates).

Library Facilities 113,556 volumes; 545 periodical subscriptions.

BACCALAUREATE PROGRAMS

Degree BSN

Available Programs RN Baccalaureate.

Study Options Part-time.

Program Entrance Requirements Minimum overall college GPA of 2.5, transcript of college record, CPR certification, health exam, immunizations, interview, 2 letters of recommendation, minimum high school GPA, minimum GPA in nursing prerequisites of 2.5, professional liability insurance/malpractice insurance, prerequisite course work, RN licensure. Transfer students are accepted. **Standardized tests** *Required:* SAT or ACT, TOEFL for international students. **Application** *Deadline:* 8/1 (freshmen), rolling (transfer). *Notification:* continuous (freshmen). *Application fee:* $25.

McMurry University
Abilene Intercollegiate School of Nursing
Abilene, Texas

See description of programs under
Patty Hanks Shelton School of Nursing (Abilene, Texas).

Midwestern State University
Nursing Program
Wichita Falls, Texas

Founded in 1922

DEGREES • BSN • MN/MHSA • MSN • MSN/MHA

Nursing Program Faculty 22 (4.4% with doctorates).

Baccalaureate Enrollment 271
Women 82% **Men** 18% **Minority** 54% **International** 4% **Part-time** 1%

Graduate Enrollment 65
Women 86% **Men** 14% **Minority** 46% **International** 6% **Part-time** 70%

Nursing Student Activities Nursing Honor Society, Sigma Theta Tau, Student Nurses' Association.

Nursing Student Resources Academic advising; academic or career counseling; assistance for students with disabilities; bookstore; campus computer network; career placement assistance; computer lab; computer-assisted instruction; e-mail services; employment services for current students; externships; housing assistance; interactive nursing skills videos; Internet; learning resource lab; library services; nursing audiovisuals; other; paid internships; placement services for program completers; remedial services; resume preparation assistance; skills, simulation, or other laboratory; tutoring; unpaid internships.

Library Facilities 484,106 volumes (10,000 in health, 5,000 in nursing); 1,582 periodical subscriptions (200 health-care related).

BACCALAUREATE PROGRAMS

Degree BSN

Available Programs ADN to Baccalaureate; Generic Baccalaureate; RN Baccalaureate.

Study Options Full-time and part-time.

Program Entrance Requirements Transcript of college record, CPR certification, health exam, health insurance, high school transcript, immunizations, minimum GPA in nursing prerequisites of 3.0, professional liability insurance/malpractice insurance, prerequisite course work. Transfer students are accepted. **Standardized tests** *Required:* SAT or ACT, TOEFL for international students. **Application** *Deadline:* 8/7 (freshmen), 8/7 (transfer). *Notification:* continuous until 8/31 (freshmen). *Application fee:* $25.

Advanced Placement Credit by examination available. Credit given for nursing courses completed elsewhere dependent upon specific evaluations.

Expenses (2006–07) *Tuition, state resident:* full-time $4715. *Tuition, nonresident:* full-time $5615. *International tuition:* $13,685 full-time. *Room and board:* $5060 per academic year. *Required fees:* full-time $360.

Financial Aid 80% of baccalaureate students in nursing programs received some form of financial aid in 2005–06. *Gift aid (need-based):* Federal Pell, FSEOG, state, private, college/university gift aid from institutional funds. *Loans:* Federal Direct (Subsidized and Unsubsidized Stafford PLUS), FFEL (Subsidized and Unsubsidized Stafford PLUS), Perkins, state, college/university. *Work-Study:* Federal Work-Study, part-time campus jobs. *Application deadline (priority):* 5/1.

Contact Melissa Belle Ford, PhD, Associate Professor and Chair, Wilson School of Nursing, Nursing Program, Midwestern State University, 3410 Taft Boulevard, Bridwell Hall 308B, Wichita Falls, TX 76308. *Telephone:* 940-397-4601. *Fax:* 940-397-4911. *E-mail:* melissa.ford@mwsu.edu.

GRADUATE PROGRAMS

Expenses (2006–07) *Tuition, state resident:* full-time $4715. *Tuition, nonresident:* full-time $5615. *International tuition:* $13,685 full-time. *Room and board:* $5060 per academic year. *Required fees:* full-time $150.

Financial Aid 100% of graduate students in nursing programs received some form of financial aid in 2005–06. Career-related internships or fieldwork, Federal Work-Study, institutionally sponsored loans, scholarships, and unspecified assistantships available. Aid available to part-time students. *Financial aid application deadline:* 5/1.

Contact Melissa Belle Ford, PhD, Associate Professor and Chair, Wilson School of Nursing, Nursing Program, Midwestern State University, 3410 Taft Boulevard, Bridwell Hall 308B, Wichita Falls, TX 76308. *Telephone:* 940-397-4601. *Fax:* 940-397-4911. *E-mail:* melissa.ford@mwsu.edu.

MASTER'S DEGREE PROGRAM

Degrees MN/MHSA; MSN; MSN/MHA

Available Programs Master's; RN to Master's.

Concentrations Available Health-care administration; nursing administration; nursing education. *Nurse practitioner programs in:* family health.

Study Options Full-time and part-time.

Program Entrance Requirements Clinical experience, computer literacy, minimum overall college GPA of 3.0, transcript of college record, CPR certification, immunizations, interview, nursing research course, physical assessment course, professional liability insurance/malpractice insurance, prerequisite course work, statistics course, GRE General Test. *Application deadline:* For fall admission, 7/1; for spring admission, 11/1. Applications are processed on a rolling basis. *Application fee:* $35 ($50 for international students).

Degree Requirements 36 total credit hours, thesis or project.

POST-MASTER'S PROGRAM

Areas of Study Nursing education. *Nurse practitioner programs in:* family health.

CONTINUING EDUCATION PROGRAM

Contact Betty Bowles, Coordinator, Professional Outreach Center, Nursing Program, Midwestern State University, 3410 Taft Boulevard, Wichita Falls, TX 76308. *Telephone:* 940-397-4048. *Fax:* 940-397-4513. *E-mail:* betty.bowles@mwsu.edu.

Patty Hanks Shelton School of Nursing

Patty Hanks Shelton School of Nursing
Abilene, Texas

http://www.aisn.edu/

DEGREES • BSN • MSN

Nursing Program Faculty 17 (33% with doctorates).

Baccalaureate Enrollment 130
Women 90% **Men** 10% **Minority** 15% **International** 4%

Graduate Enrollment 23
Women 75% **Men** 25% **Minority** 10%

Nursing Student Activities Nursing Honor Society, Sigma Theta Tau, Student Nurses' Association.

Nursing Student Resources Academic advising; academic or career counseling; assistance for students with disabilities; bookstore; campus computer network; career placement assistance; computer lab; computer-assisted instruction; e-mail services; employment services for current students; externships; interactive nursing skills videos; Internet; learning resource lab; library services; nursing audiovisuals; remedial services; resume preparation assistance; skills, simulation, or other laboratory; tutoring.

Library Facilities 9,200 volumes in health, 1,300 volumes in nursing; 140 periodical subscriptions health-care related.

BACCALAUREATE PROGRAMS

Degree BSN

Available Programs Generic Baccalaureate; RN Baccalaureate.

Study Options Full-time.

Program Entrance Requirements Minimum overall college GPA of 2.75, transcript of college record, CPR certification, written essay, health exam, health insurance, immunizations, interview, 3 letters of recommendation, minimum GPA in nursing prerequisites of 3.0, professional liability insurance/malpractice insurance, prerequisite course work. Transfer students are accepted.

Advanced Placement Credit by examination available. Credit given for nursing courses completed elsewhere dependent upon specific evaluations.

Expenses (2005–06) *Tuition:* full-time $14,250; part-time $450 per quarter. *Required fees:* full-time $500; part-time $250 per term.

Financial Aid 80% of baccalaureate students in nursing programs received some form of financial aid in 2004–05.

Contact Mr. Brent Wallace, Academic Advisor/Director of Marketing, Patty Hanks Shelton School of Nursing, 2149 Hickory Street, Abilene, TX 79601. *Telephone:* 325-672-2353. *Fax:* 325-671-2386. *E-mail:* bwallace@phssn.edu.

GRADUATE PROGRAMS

Expenses (2005–06) *Tuition:* full-time $5400; part-time $450 per credit hour. *Required fees:* full-time $500.

Financial Aid 50% of graduate students in nursing programs received some form of financial aid in 2004–05.

Contact Dr. Amy Roberts, Director of the Graduate Program, Patty Hanks Shelton School of Nursing, 2149 Hickory Street, Abilene, TX 79601. *Telephone:* 325-671-2361. *Fax:* 325-671-2386. *E-mail:* aroberts@phssn.edu.

MASTER'S DEGREE PROGRAM

Degree MSN

Available Programs Master's.

Concentrations Available Nursing administration; nursing education. *Nurse practitioner programs in:* family health.

Study Options Full-time and part-time.

Program Entrance Requirements Clinical experience, minimum overall college GPA of 3.5, transcript of college record, CPR certification, written essay, immunizations, interview, 3 letters of recommendation, physical assessment course, professional liability insurance/malpractice insurance, resume, statistics course.

Patty Hanks Shelton School of Nursing (continued)

Advanced Placement Credit given for nursing courses completed elsewhere dependent upon specific evaluations.

Degree Requirements 49 total credit hours.

POST-MASTER'S PROGRAM

Areas of Study *Nurse practitioner programs in:* family health.

CONTINUING EDUCATION PROGRAM

Contact Dr. Janet K. Noles, Dean and Associate Professor, Patty Hanks Shelton School of Nursing, 2149 Hickory Street, Abilene, TX 79601. *Telephone:* 325-671-2399. *Fax:* 325-671-2386. *E-mail:* jnoles@phssn.edu.

Prairie View A&M University
College of Nursing
Houston, Texas

http://acad.pvamu.edu/content/nursing/

Founded in 1878

DEGREES • BSN • MSN

Nursing Program Faculty 40.

Nursing Student Activities Nursing Honor Society, Sigma Theta Tau, Student Nurses' Association, nursing club.

Nursing Student Resources Academic advising; bookstore; campus computer network; computer lab; e-mail services; learning resource lab; nursing audiovisuals; skills, simulation, or other laboratory.

Library Facilities 347,477 volumes (109 in nursing); 25,911 periodical subscriptions.

BACCALAUREATE PROGRAMS

Degree BSN

Available Programs Generic Baccalaureate; RN Baccalaureate.

Site Options *Distance Learning:* Huntsville, TX; Woodlands, TX; College Station, TX.

Study Options Full-time and part-time.

Program Entrance Requirements Minimum overall college GPA of 2.5, transcript of college record, CPR certification, health exam, immunizations, minimum GPA in nursing prerequisites of 2.0, professional liability insurance/malpractice insurance, prerequisite course work. Transfer students are accepted. **Standardized tests** *Required:* SAT or ACT, TOEFL for international students. **Application** *Deadline:* 6/1 (freshmen), 6/1 (transfer). *Notification:* continuous (freshmen). *Application fee:* $25.

Advanced Placement Credit given for nursing courses completed elsewhere dependent upon specific evaluations.

Contact *Telephone:* 713-797-7023. *Fax:* 713-797-7013.

GRADUATE PROGRAMS

Contact *Telephone:* 713-797-7003. *Fax:* 713-797-7012.

MASTER'S DEGREE PROGRAM

Degree MSN

Available Programs Master's.

Concentrations Available *Nurse practitioner programs in:* family health.

Study Options Full-time and part-time.

Program Entrance Requirements Clinical experience, minimum overall college GPA of 2.75, transcript of college record, 3 letters of recommendation, physical assessment course, prerequisite course work, resume, statistics course, MAT or GRE. *Application deadline:* For fall admission, 4/1 (priority date); for spring admission, 7/1 (priority date). Applications are processed on a rolling basis. *Application fee:* $50.

Advanced Placement Credit by examination available. Credit given for nursing courses completed elsewhere dependent upon specific evaluations.

Degree Requirements 53 total credit hours.

Southwestern Adventist University
Department of Nursing
Keene, Texas

Founded in 1894

DEGREE • BS

Nursing Program Faculty 12 (25% with doctorates).

Baccalaureate Enrollment 23
Women 83% **Men** 17% **Minority** 56% **International** 17% **Part-time** 25%

Nursing Student Activities Nursing Honor Society, Sigma Theta Tau.

Nursing Student Resources Academic advising; academic or career counseling; assistance for students with disabilities; bookstore; campus computer network; computer lab; computer-assisted instruction; e-mail services; interactive nursing skills videos; Internet; learning resource lab; library services; nursing audiovisuals; remedial services; skills, simulation, or other laboratory; tutoring.

Library Facilities 108,481 volumes (6,575 in nursing); 457 periodical subscriptions (60 health-care related).

BACCALAUREATE PROGRAMS

Degree BS

Available Programs ADN to Baccalaureate; Generic Baccalaureate; LPN to Baccalaureate; RN Baccalaureate.

Study Options Full-time and part-time.

Program Entrance Requirements Transcript of college record, CPR certification, health exam, health insurance, immunizations, 3 letters of recommendation, minimum GPA in nursing prerequisites of 2.75, prerequisite course work. Transfer students are accepted. **Standardized tests** *Required:* SAT or ACT, TOEFL for international students. **Application** *Deadline:* 8/31 (freshmen), 8/31 (transfer). *Notification:* 9/1 (freshmen).

Advanced Placement Credit given for nursing courses completed elsewhere dependent upon specific evaluations.

Expenses (2005–06) *Tuition:* full-time $12,484; part-time $506 per credit hour. *International tuition:* $12,484 full-time. *Room and board:* $3426; room only: $2380 per academic year. *Required fees:* full-time $300.

Financial Aid 60% of baccalaureate students in nursing programs received some form of financial aid in 2004–05.

Contact Dr. Penny Moore, RN, Chair, Baccalaureate Faculty and Curriculum, Department of Nursing, Southwestern Adventist University, Keene, TX 76059. *Telephone:* 817-645-3921 Ext. 519. *Fax:* 817-556-4713. *E-mail:* moorep@swau.edu.

CONTINUING EDUCATION PROGRAM

Contact Dr. Penny Moore, RN, Chair of Nursing Department, Department of Nursing, Southwestern Adventist University, PO Box 567, Keene, TX 76059. *Telephone:* 817-645-3921 Ext. 235. *Fax:* 817-556-4774. *E-mail:* moorep@swau.edu.

Stephen F. Austin State University
Division of Nursing
Nacogdoches, Texas

http://www.fp.sfasu.edu/nursing/

Founded in 1923

DEGREE • BSN

Nursing Program Faculty 19 (16% with doctorates).

Baccalaureate Enrollment 128
Women 96% **Men** 4% **Minority** 1%

Nursing Student Activities Sigma Theta Tau, Student Nurses' Association.

Nursing Student Resources Academic advising; academic or career counseling; bookstore; computer lab; computer-assisted instruction; e-mail services; interactive nursing skills videos; Internet; library services; nursing audiovisuals; skills, simulation, or other laboratory; tutoring.

Library Facilities 722,251 volumes; 1,757 periodical subscriptions.

BACCALAUREATE PROGRAMS

Degree BSN

Available Programs RN Baccalaureate.

Site Options Lufkin, TX.

Study Options Full-time.

Program Entrance Requirements Minimum overall college GPA of 2.75, transcript of college record, CPR certification, health insurance, high school transcript, immunizations, minimum GPA in nursing prerequisites of 2.5, professional liability insurance/malpractice insurance, prerequisite course work. Transfer students are accepted. **Standardized tests** *Required:* SAT or ACT, TOEFL for international students. **Application** *Deadline:* rolling (freshmen). *Notification:* continuous (freshmen). *Application fee:* $35.

Advanced Placement Credit given for nursing courses completed elsewhere dependent upon specific evaluations.

Contact *Telephone:* 936-468-3604. *Fax:* 936-468-1696.

Tarleton State University
Department of Nursing
Stephenville, Texas

http://www.tarleton.edu/~nursing

Founded in 1899

DEGREE • BSN

Nursing Program Faculty 19 (14% with doctorates).

Baccalaureate Enrollment 230
Women 95% **Men** 5% **Minority** 15% **International** 2% **Part-time** 25%

Nursing Student Activities Sigma Theta Tau, Student Nurses' Association.

Nursing Student Resources Academic advising; academic or career counseling; assistance for students with disabilities; bookstore; computer lab; computer-assisted instruction; daycare for children of students; e-mail services; employment services for current students; externships; learning resource lab; library services; nursing audiovisuals; remedial services; resume preparation assistance; skills, simulation, or other laboratory; tutoring; unpaid internships.

Library Facilities 349,979 volumes; 19,844 periodical subscriptions.

BACCALAUREATE PROGRAMS

Degree BSN

Available Programs ADN to Baccalaureate; Generic Baccalaureate; LPN to Baccalaureate.

Site Options *Distance Learning:* Killeen, TX; Brownwood, TX.

Study Options Full-time and part-time.

Program Entrance Requirements Transcript of college record, CPR certification, written essay, health exam, high school transcript, immunizations, 3 letters of recommendation, minimum GPA in nursing prerequisites of 2.75, professional liability insurance/malpractice insurance, prerequisite course work. Transfer students are accepted. **Standardized tests** *Required:* SAT or ACT, TOEFL for international students. **Application** *Deadline:* 8/1 (freshmen), 7/1 (transfer). *Early decision:* 11/30. *Application fee:* $25.

Advanced Placement Credit by examination available. Credit given for nursing courses completed elsewhere dependent upon specific evaluations.

Financial Aid 62% of baccalaureate students in nursing programs received some form of financial aid in 2005–06.

Contact Nursing Contact, Department of Nursing, Tarleton State University, Box T-0500, Stephenville, TX 76402. *Telephone:* 254-968-9139. *Fax:* 254-968-9716. *E-mail:* skinner@tarleton.edu.

CONTINUING EDUCATION PROGRAM

Contact Ms. Dokagari (Dok) Woods, Coordinator of Nursing Professional Development, Department of Nursing, Tarleton State University, Box T-0500, Stephenville, TX 76042. *Telephone:* 325-649-8058. *Fax:* 325-649-8959. *E-mail:* woods@tarleton.edu.

Texas A&M International University
Canseco School of Nursing
Laredo, Texas

Founded in 1969

DEGREES • BSN • MSN

Nursing Program Faculty 18 (20% with doctorates).

Baccalaureate Enrollment 243
Women 70% **Men** 30% **Minority** 98% **International** 1% **Part-time** 25%

Graduate Enrollment 18

Nursing Student Activities Nursing Honor Society, Student Nurses' Association.

Nursing Student Resources Academic advising; academic or career counseling; assistance for students with disabilities; bookstore; campus computer network; career placement assistance; computer lab; computer-assisted instruction; daycare for children of students; e-mail services; employment services for current students; externships; housing assistance; interactive nursing skills videos; Internet; learning resource lab; library services; nursing audiovisuals; paid internships; placement services for program completers; remedial services; resume preparation assistance; skills, simulation, or other laboratory; tutoring.

Library Facilities 237,705 volumes (8,500 in nursing); 5,459 periodical subscriptions (80 health-care related).

BACCALAUREATE PROGRAMS

Degree BSN

Available Programs Generic Baccalaureate; RN Baccalaureate.

Study Options Full-time.

Program Entrance Requirements Minimum overall college GPA of 2.5, transcript of college record, written essay, health exam, immunizations, 2 letters of recommendation, minimum GPA in nursing prerequisites of 2.5, prerequisite course work. Transfer students are accepted. **Standardized tests** *Required:* SAT or ACT, TOEFL for international students. **Application** *Deadline:* 7/1 (freshmen), 7/1 (transfer). *Notification:* 7/15 (freshmen).

Advanced Placement Credit given for nursing courses completed elsewhere dependent upon specific evaluations.

Contact *Telephone:* 956-326-2450. *Fax:* 956-326-2449.

GRADUATE PROGRAMS

Contact *Telephone:* 956-326-2450. *Fax:* 956-326-2449.

MASTER'S DEGREE PROGRAM

Degree MSN

Available Programs Master's; Master's for Nurses with Non-Nursing Degrees.

Concentrations Available *Nurse practitioner programs in:* family health.

Study Options Full-time and part-time.

Program Entrance Requirements Clinical experience, minimum overall college GPA of 3.0, transcript of college record, CPR certification, written essay, immunizations, interview, 2 letters of recommendation.

Advanced Placement Credit given for nursing courses completed elsewhere dependent upon specific evaluations.

Degree Requirements 45 total credit hours.

CONTINUING EDUCATION PROGRAM

Contact *Telephone:* 956-326-2450. *Fax:* 956-326-2449.

Texas A&M University–Corpus Christi
School of Nursing and Health Sciences
Corpus Christi, Texas

http://www.sci.tamucc.edu/nursing/

Founded in 1947

DEGREES • BSN • MSN

Nursing Program Faculty 45 (65% with doctorates).

Baccalaureate Enrollment 211
Women 82% **Men** 18% **Minority** 40% **International** 1% **Part-time** 31%

Graduate Enrollment 191
Women 80% **Men** 20% **Minority** 48% **International** 1% **Part-time** 98%

Nursing Student Activities Nursing Honor Society, Sigma Theta Tau, Student Nurses' Association.

Nursing Student Resources Academic advising; academic or career counseling; assistance for students with disabilities; bookstore; campus computer network; career placement assistance; computer lab; computer-assisted instruction; e-mail services; employment services for current students; housing assistance; interactive nursing skills videos; Internet; learning resource lab; library services; nursing audiovisuals; placement services for program completers; remedial services; resume preparation assistance; skills, simulation, or other laboratory; tutoring.

Library Facilities 731,586 volumes (500 in health, 350 in nursing); 1,901 periodical subscriptions (100 health-care related).

BACCALAUREATE PROGRAMS

Degree BSN

Available Programs ADN to Baccalaureate; Accelerated Baccalaureate for Second Degree; Baccalaureate for Second Degree; Generic Baccalaureate; RN Baccalaureate.

Site Options *Distance Learning:* College Station, TX.

Study Options Full-time and part-time.

Program Entrance Requirements Minimum overall college GPA of 3.0, transcript of college record, CPR certification, immunizations, professional liability insurance/malpractice insurance, prerequisite course work. Transfer students are accepted. **Standardized tests** *Required:* SAT or ACT, TOEFL for international students. **Application** *Deadline:* 7/1 (freshmen). *Application fee:* $20.

Advanced Placement Credit given for nursing courses completed elsewhere dependent upon specific evaluations.

Expenses (2006–07) *Tuition, state resident:* full-time $3544; part-time $123 per credit hour. *Tuition, nonresident:* full-time $11,628; part-time $398 per credit hour. *International tuition:* $11,944 full-time. *Room and board:* $4968; room only: $4560 per academic year. *Required fees:* full-time $1400; part-time $84 per credit; part-time $700 per term.

Financial Aid 70% of baccalaureate students in nursing programs received some form of financial aid in 2005–06.

Contact Dr. Bunny D. Forgione, Associate Dean, School of Nursing and Health Sciences, Texas A&M University–Corpus Christi, 6300 Ocean Drive, Corpus Christi, TX 78412. *Telephone:* 361-825-2740. *Fax:* 361-825-2484. *E-mail:* bunny.forgione@tamucc.edu.

GRADUATE PROGRAMS

Expenses (2006–07) *Tuition, area resident:* full-time $2440; part-time $136 per credit hour. *Tuition, state resident:* full-time $7390; part-time $411 per credit hour. *Tuition, nonresident:* full-time $7390; part-time $411 per credit hour. *International tuition:* $7465 full-time. *Room and board:* $5460; room only: $4660 per academic year. *Required fees:* full-time $972; part-time $359 per term.

Financial Aid 50% of graduate students in nursing programs received some form of financial aid in 2005–06.

Contact Dr. Eve Layman, RN, Graduate Department Chair, School of Nursing and Health Sciences, Texas A&M University–Corpus Christi, 6300 Ocean Drive, CI 372, Corpus Christi, TX 78412. *Telephone:* 361-825-3781. *Fax:* 361-825-5853. *E-mail:* eve.layman@tamucc.edu.

MASTER'S DEGREE PROGRAM

Degree MSN

Available Programs Accelerated AD/RN to Master's; Accelerated Master's for Nurses with Non-Nursing Degrees; Master's.

Concentrations Available Nursing administration. *Clinical nurse specialist programs in:* medical-surgical. *Nurse practitioner programs in:* family health.

Site Options *Distance Learning:* Temple, TX; Laredo, TX.

Study Options Full-time and part-time.

Program Entrance Requirements Minimum overall college GPA of 3.0, transcript of college record, CPR certification, immunizations, nursing research course, professional liability insurance/malpractice insurance, statistics course.

Advanced Placement Credit by examination available. Credit given for nursing courses completed elsewhere dependent upon specific evaluations.

Degree Requirements 45 total credit hours.

POST-MASTER'S PROGRAM

Areas of Study Nursing administration; nursing education. *Clinical nurse specialist programs in:* medical-surgical. *Nurse practitioner programs in:* family health.

CONTINUING EDUCATION PROGRAM

Contact Ms. Petra Martinez, Chair of Continuing Education Committee, School of Nursing and Health Sciences, Texas A&M University–Corpus Christi, 6300 Ocean Drive, ST 316, Corpus Christi, TX 78412. *Telephone:* 361-825-2353. *Fax:* 361-825-3491. *E-mail:* petra.martinez@tamucc.edu.

Texas A&M University–Texarkana
Nursing Department
Texarkana, Texas

Founded in 1971

DEGREE • BSN

Nursing Program Faculty 3 (67% with doctorates).

Baccalaureate Enrollment 21
Women 76% **Men** 24% **Minority** 14% **Part-time** 33%

Nursing Student Activities Nursing club.

Nursing Student Resources Academic advising; academic or career counseling; assistance for students with disabilities; bookstore; campus computer network; career placement assistance; computer lab; computer-assisted instruction; e-mail services; Internet; library services; nursing audiovisuals; resume preparation assistance.

Library Facilities 125,991 volumes (3,735 in health, 2,025 in nursing); 5,709 periodical subscriptions (100 health-care related).

BACCALAUREATE PROGRAMS

Degree BSN

Available Programs ADN to Baccalaureate.

Program Entrance Requirements Transfer students are accepted. **Standardized tests** *Required:* TOEFL for international students. **Application** *Deadline:* rolling (transfer).

Expenses (2006–07) *Tuition, state resident:* full-time $2208. *Tuition, nonresident:* full-time $8808. *International tuition:* $8808 full-time. *Required fees:* full-time $436.

Financial Aid 14% of baccalaureate students in nursing programs received some form of financial aid in 2005–06.

Contact Dean Jo Kahler, EdD, Dean of the College of Health and Behavioral Sciences, Nursing Department, Texas A&M University–Texarkana, 2600 North Robison Road, PO Box 5518, Texarkana, TX 75501. *Telephone:* 903-223-3175. *Fax:* 903-223-3107. *E-mail:* Jo.Kahler@tamut.edu.

Texas Christian University
Harris School of Nursing
Fort Worth, Texas

Founded in 1873

DEGREES • BSN • MSN

Nursing Program Faculty 32 (80% with doctorates).

Baccalaureate Enrollment 500
Women 93.5% **Men** 6.5% **Minority** 18% **International** 2% **Part-time** 1%

Graduate Enrollment 23
Women 95% **Men** 5% **Minority** 17% **Part-time** 43%

Nursing Student Activities Sigma Theta Tau, Student Nurses' Association.

Nursing Student Resources Academic advising; academic or career counseling; assistance for students with disabilities; bookstore; campus computer network; career placement assistance; computer lab; computer-assisted instruction; e-mail services; interactive nursing skills videos; Internet; learning resource lab; library services; nursing audiovisuals; other; resume preparation assistance; skills, simulation, or other laboratory; tutoring.

Library Facilities 1.4 million volumes (16,505 in health, 3,063 in nursing); 32,017 periodical subscriptions (180 health-care related).

BACCALAUREATE PROGRAMS

Degree BSN

Available Programs Accelerated Baccalaureate for Second Degree; Generic Baccalaureate.

Site Options *Distance Learning:* Fort Worth, TX.

Study Options Full-time and part-time.

Program Entrance Requirements Minimum overall college GPA of 2.5, transcript of college record, CPR certification, written essay, 2 years high school math, 4 years high school science, high school transcript, immunizations, minimum high school GPA of 3.0, minimum GPA in nursing prerequisites of 2.5, prerequisite course work. Transfer students are accepted. **Standardized tests** *Required:* SAT or ACT, TOEFL for international students. **Application** *Deadline:* 2/15 (freshmen), 4/15 (transfer). *Early decision:* 11/15. *Notification:* 4/1 (freshmen), 1/1 (early action). *Application fee:* $40.

Advanced Placement Credit by examination available. Credit given for nursing courses completed elsewhere dependent upon specific evaluations.

Expenses (2006–07) *Tuition:* full-time $22,480. *Room and board:* $7520 per academic year. *Required fees:* full-time $440.

Financial Aid 60% of baccalaureate students in nursing programs received some form of financial aid in 2005–06. *Gift aid (need-based):* Federal Pell, FSEOG, state, private, college/university gift aid from institutional funds, United Negro College Fund. *Loans:* Federal Nursing Student Loans, FFEL (Subsidized and Unsubsidized Stafford PLUS), Perkins, state. *Work-Study:* Federal Work-Study, part-time campus jobs. *Application deadline:* 5/1 (priority: 5/1).

Contact Ms. Zoranna Williams, Coordinator of Nursing Recruitment and Retention, Harris School of Nursing, Texas Christian University, 2800 West Bowie, Box 298620, Fort Worth, TX 76129. *Telephone:* 817-257-7650. *Fax:* 817-257-7944. *E-mail:* z.williams@tcu.edu.

GRADUATE PROGRAMS

Expenses (2006–07) *Tuition:* full-time $14,400. *Room and board:* $8780 per academic year. *Required fees:* full-time $100.

Financial Aid 100% of graduate students in nursing programs received some form of financial aid in 2005–06.

Contact Ms. Kathleen M. Baldwin, Director of Graduate Studies, Harris School of Nursing, Texas Christian University, 2800 West Bowie, Box 298620, Fort Worth, TX 76129. *Telephone:* 817-257-7650 Ext. 6748. *Fax:* 817-257-7944. *E-mail:* k.baldwin@tcu.edu.

MASTER'S DEGREE PROGRAM

Degree MSN

Available Programs Master's; RN to Master's.

Concentrations Available Nurse anesthesia; nursing education. *Clinical nurse specialist programs in:* adult health, critical care, medical-surgical.

Site Options *Distance Learning:* Fort Worth, TX.

Study Options Full-time and part-time.

Program Entrance Requirements Clinical experience, computer literacy, minimum overall college GPA of 3.0, transcript of college record, CPR certification, written essay, immunizations, 3 letters of recommendation, professional liability insurance/malpractice insurance, prerequisite course work, resume.

Degree Requirements 38 total credit hours, thesis or project.

CONTINUING EDUCATION PROGRAM

Contact Dr. Linda Curry, Harris School of Nursing, Texas Christian University, Box 298620, Fort Worth, TX 76129. *Telephone:* 817-257-7650 Ext. 7496. *Fax:* 817-257-7944. *E-mail:* l.curry@tcu.edu.

Texas Tech University Health Sciences Center
School of Nursing
Lubbock, Texas

http://www.ttunursing.com

Founded in 1969

DEGREES • BSN • MSN

Nursing Program Faculty 76 (40% with doctorates).

Baccalaureate Enrollment 472
Women 86% **Men** 14% **Minority** 28% **International** 6%

Graduate Enrollment 224
Women 89% **Men** 11% **Minority** 26% **Part-time** 86%

Nursing Student Activities Sigma Theta Tau, Student Nurses' Association.

Nursing Student Resources Academic advising; academic or career counseling; assistance for students with disabilities; bookstore; campus computer network; computer lab; e-mail services; Internet; learning resource lab; library services; nursing audiovisuals; other; skills, simulation, or other laboratory; tutoring.

Library Facilities 303,721 volumes in health, 10,000 volumes in nursing; 12,743 periodical subscriptions health-care related.

BACCALAUREATE PROGRAMS

Degree BSN

Available Programs ADN to Baccalaureate; Accelerated Baccalaureate for Second Degree; Generic Baccalaureate.

Site Options *Distance Learning:* Odessa, TX; Kerrville, TX.

Study Options Full-time.

Program Entrance Requirements Minimum overall college GPA of 2.5, transcript of college record, written essay, immunizations, prerequisite course work.

Advanced Placement Credit given for nursing courses completed elsewhere dependent upon specific evaluations.

Expenses (2006–07) *Tuition, state resident:* full-time $4134; part-time $177 per credit hour. *Tuition, nonresident:* full-time $14,868; part-time $453 per credit hour. *International tuition:* $14,868 full-time. *Room and board:* $8459 per academic year. *Required fees:* full-time $1940.

Financial Aid 72% of baccalaureate students in nursing programs received some form of financial aid in 2005–06.

Contact Dr. Patricia Allen, Associate Dean, Undergraduate Programs, School of Nursing, Texas Tech University Health Sciences Center, 3601 4th Street, MS 6221, Lubbock, TX 79430. *Telephone:* 806-743-2729. *Fax:* 806-743-1648. *E-mail:* patricia.allen@ttuhsc.edu.

GRADUATE PROGRAMS

Expenses (2006–07) *Tuition, state resident:* full-time $4104; part-time $227 per credit hour. *Tuition, nonresident:* full-time $10,848; part-time $503 per credit hour. *International tuition:* $10,848 full-time. *Room and board:* $4080 per academic year. *Required fees:* full-time $1957.

Financial Aid 65% of graduate students in nursing programs received some form of financial aid in 2005–06. Institutionally sponsored loans, scholarships, and traineeships available. Aid available to part-time students. *Financial aid application deadline:* 12/1.

Contact Dr. Barbara Ann Johnston, Associate Dean for Graduate Programs, School of Nursing, Texas Tech University Health Sciences Center, 3601 4th Street, MS6264, Lubbock, TX 79430. *Telephone:* 806-743-3055. *Fax:* 806-743-1622. *E-mail:* barbara.johnston@ttuhsc.edu.

Texas Tech University Health Sciences Center (continued)

MASTER'S DEGREE PROGRAM

Degree MSN

Available Programs Master's; RN to Master's.

Concentrations Available Nursing administration; nursing education. *Nurse practitioner programs in:* acute care, family health, gerontology, pediatric.

Site Options *Distance Learning:* Tyler, TX; Odessa, TX.

Study Options Full-time and part-time.

Program Entrance Requirements Clinical experience, computer literacy, minimum overall college GPA of 3.0, transcript of college record, CPR certification, written essay, immunizations, 3 letters of recommendation, nursing research course, statistics course, GRE General Test or MAT. *Application deadline:* For fall admission, 7/15 (priority date); for spring admission, 11/15 (priority date). Applications are processed on a rolling basis. *Application fee:* $40.

Advanced Placement Credit given for nursing courses completed elsewhere dependent upon specific evaluations.

Degree Requirements 48 total credit hours.

POST-MASTER'S PROGRAM

Areas of Study *Nurse practitioner programs in:* acute care, family health, gerontology, pediatric.

CONTINUING EDUCATION PROGRAM

Contact Ms. Shelley Burson, Director of Continuing Nursing Education, School of Nursing, Texas Tech University Health Sciences Center, 3601 4th Street, Lubbock, TX 79430. *Telephone:* 806-743-2732. *Fax:* 806-743-1198. *E-mail:* shelley.burson@ttuhsc.edu.

Texas Woman's University
College of Nursing
Denton, Texas

Founded in 1901

DEGREES • BS • MS • MSN/MHA • PHD

Nursing Program Faculty 117 (54% with doctorates).

Baccalaureate Enrollment 699
Women 95% **Men** 5% **Minority** 40% **International** 2% **Part-time** 21%

Graduate Enrollment 314
Women 94% **Men** 6% **Minority** 33% **International** 1%

Nursing Student Activities Sigma Theta Tau, Student Nurses' Association.

Nursing Student Resources Academic advising; academic or career counseling; assistance for students with disabilities; bookstore; campus computer network; career placement assistance; computer lab; computer-assisted instruction; e-mail services; employment services for current students; Internet; learning resource lab; library services; nursing audiovisuals; placement services for program completers; remedial services; skills, simulation, or other laboratory.

Library Facilities 572,500 volumes (250,000 in health, 26,463 in nursing); 2,537 periodical subscriptions (2,644 health-care related).

BACCALAUREATE PROGRAMS

Degree BS

Available Programs Baccalaureate for Second Degree; Generic Baccalaureate; RN Baccalaureate.

Site Options Dallas, TX. *Distance Learning:* Houston, TX.

Study Options Full-time and part-time.

Program Entrance Requirements Transcript of college record, CPR certification, high school transcript, immunizations, minimum GPA in nursing prerequisites of 3.0, professional liability insurance/malpractice insurance, prerequisite course work. Transfer students are accepted. **Standardized tests** *Required:* TOEFL for international students. *Required for some:* SAT or ACT. **Application** *Deadline:* 7/1 (freshmen), 7/15 (transfer). *Notification:* continuous until 8/15 (freshmen). *Application fee:* $30.

Advanced Placement Credit given for nursing courses completed elsewhere dependent upon specific evaluations.

Contact *Telephone:* 214-689-6519. *Fax:* 214-689-6539.

GRADUATE PROGRAMS

Contact *Telephone:* 940-898-2418.

MASTER'S DEGREE PROGRAM

Degrees MS; MSN/MHA

Available Programs Master's; RN to Master's.

Concentrations Available Nursing administration. *Clinical nurse specialist programs in:* adult health, community health, pediatric, women's health. *Nurse practitioner programs in:* adult health, family health, pediatric, women's health.

Site Options Dallas, TX. *Distance Learning:* Houston, TX.

Study Options Full-time and part-time.

Program Entrance Requirements Clinical experience, minimum overall college GPA of 3.0, transcript of college record, CPR certification, immunizations, professional liability insurance/malpractice insurance, statistics course, GRE or MAT. *Application deadline:* Applications are processed on a rolling basis. *Application fee:* $30 ($50 for international students).

Advanced Placement Credit given for nursing courses completed elsewhere dependent upon specific evaluations.

Degree Requirements 48 total credit hours, thesis or project.

POST-MASTER'S PROGRAM

Areas of Study *Nurse practitioner programs in:* adult health, family health, pediatric, women's health.

DOCTORAL DEGREE PROGRAM

Degree PhD

Available Programs Doctorate.

Areas of Study Nursing research, nursing science, women's health.

Site Options *Distance Learning:* Houston, TX.

Program Entrance Requirements Minimum overall college GPA of 3.5, 2 letters of recommendation, MSN or equivalent, statistics course, vita, GRE or MAT. *Application deadline:* Applications are processed on a rolling basis. *Application fee:* $30 ($50 for international students).

Degree Requirements 60 total credit hours, dissertation, oral exam, written exam.

University of Mary Hardin-Baylor
College of Nursing
Belton, Texas

Founded in 1845

DEGREE • BSN

Nursing Program Faculty 16 (56% with doctorates).

Baccalaureate Enrollment 213
Women 95% **Men** 5% **Minority** 18% **International** 1% **Part-time** 1%

Nursing Student Activities Sigma Theta Tau, Student Nurses' Association, nursing club.

Nursing Student Resources Academic advising; academic or career counseling; assistance for students with disabilities; bookstore; campus computer network; career placement assistance; computer lab; e-mail services; employment services for current students; housing assistance; Internet; learning resource lab; library services; nursing audiovisuals; placement services for program completers; remedial services; resume preparation assistance; skills, simulation, or other laboratory; tutoring.

Library Facilities 153,120 volumes (7,233 in health, 5,925 in nursing); 1,541 periodical subscriptions (120 health-care related).

BACCALAUREATE PROGRAMS

Degree BSN

Available Programs Baccalaureate for Second Degree; Generic Baccalaureate; RN Baccalaureate.

Study Options Full-time and part-time.

Program Entrance Requirements Minimum overall college GPA of 2.0, transcript of college record, CPR certification, written essay, health exam, health insurance, high school transcript, immunizations, interview, minimum high school rank 50%, minimum GPA in nursing prerequisites of 2.75, professional liability insurance/malpractice insurance, prerequisite course work. Transfer students are accepted. **Standardized tests** *Required:* SAT or ACT. *Recommended:* TOEFL for international students. **Application** *Deadline:* rolling (freshmen), rolling (transfer). *Notification:* continuous (freshmen). *Application fee:* $35.

Advanced Placement Credit given for nursing courses completed elsewhere dependent upon specific evaluations.

Contact *Telephone:* 254-295-4665. *Fax:* 254-295-4141.

CONTINUING EDUCATION PROGRAM

Contact *Telephone:* 254-295-4668. *Fax:* 254-295-4141.

The University of Texas at Arlington
School of Nursing
Arlington, Texas

http://www.uta.edu/nursing

Founded in 1895

DEGREES • BSN • MSN • MSN/MBA • MSN/MHA • MSN/MPH • PHD

Nursing Program Faculty 108 (45% with doctorates).

Baccalaureate Enrollment 546
Women 87.91% **Men** 12.09% **Minority** 55.32% **International** 13% **Part-time** 5.68%

Graduate Enrollment 315
Women 92.69% **Men** 7.31% **Minority** 26.67% **International** 1.27% **Part-time** 87.62%

Nursing Student Activities Nursing Honor Society, Sigma Theta Tau, Student Nurses' Association, nursing club.

Nursing Student Resources Academic advising; assistance for students with disabilities; bookstore; campus computer network; computer lab; e-mail services; externships; interactive nursing skills videos; Internet; learning resource lab; library services; nursing audiovisuals; skills, simulation, or other laboratory.

Library Facilities 1.1 million volumes (35,500 in health, 23,000 in nursing); 16,053 periodical subscriptions (508 health-care related).

BACCALAUREATE PROGRAMS

Degree BSN

Available Programs Generic Baccalaureate; RN Baccalaureate.

Site Options *Distance Learning:* Grayson, TX; Paris, TX; Waco, TX.

Study Options Full-time and part-time.

Program Entrance Requirements Minimum overall college GPA of 2.5, transcript of college record, CPR certification, written essay, immunizations, interview, minimum high school GPA of 2.5, minimum GPA in nursing prerequisites of 2.0, professional liability insurance/malpractice insurance, prerequisite course work. Transfer students are accepted. **Standardized tests** *Required:* SAT or ACT, TOEFL for international students. **Application** *Deadline:* 6/1 (freshmen), rolling (transfer). *Notification:* continuous (freshmen). *Application fee:* $35.

Expenses (2006–07) *Tuition, state resident:* full-time $6868; part-time $240 per credit hour. *Tuition, nonresident:* full-time $13,368; part-time $622 per credit hour. *International tuition:* $14,172 full-time. *Room and board:* $6412; room only: $4112 per academic year. *Required fees:* full-time $1750; part-time $70 per credit; part-time $750 per term.

Financial Aid 40% of baccalaureate students in nursing programs received some form of financial aid in 2005–06. *Gift aid (need-based):* Federal Pell, FSEOG, state, private, college/university gift aid from institutional funds, United Negro College Fund. *Loans:* FFEL (Subsidized and Unsubsidized Stafford PLUS), Perkins, state. *Work-Study:* Federal Work-Study. *Application deadline (priority):* 5/15.

Contact Ms. Jean Ashwill, RN, Director, Undergraduate Student Services, School of Nursing, The University of Texas at Arlington, 411 South Nedderman Drive, Box 19407, Arlington, TX 76019-0407. *Telephone:* 817-272-2776. *Fax:* 817-272-5006. *E-mail:* nursing@uta.edu.

GRADUATE PROGRAMS

Expenses (2006–07) *Tuition, state resident:* full-time $6600; part-time $275 per credit hour. *Tuition, nonresident:* full-time $20,400; part-time $850 per credit hour. *International tuition:* $20,400 full-time. *Room and board:* $6412; room only: $4112 per academic year. *Required fees:* full-time $1920; part-time $80 per credit.

Financial Aid 25% of graduate students in nursing programs received some form of financial aid in 2005–06. 24 fellowships with partial tuition reimbursements available (averaging $3,000 per year), 6 research assistantships (averaging $7,992 per year), 7 teaching assistantships (averaging $10,080 per year) were awarded; career-related internships or fieldwork and traineeships also available. *Financial aid application deadline:* 6/1.

Contact Dr. Susan K. Grove, Associate Dean and Director of Graduate Studies, School of Nursing, The University of Texas at Arlington, 411 South Nedderman Drive, Box 19407, Arlington, TX 76019-0407. *Telephone:* 817-272-7086. *Fax:* 817-272-5006. *E-mail:* grove@uta.edu.

MASTER'S DEGREE PROGRAM

Degrees MSN; MSN/MBA; MSN/MHA; MSN/MPH

Available Programs Master's.

Concentrations Available Health-care administration; nursing administration. *Nurse practitioner programs in:* acute care, adult health, family health, gerontology, pediatric, psychiatric/mental health.

Study Options Full-time and part-time.

Program Entrance Requirements Computer literacy, minimum overall college GPA of 3.0, transcript of college record, CPR certification, written essay, immunizations, 3 letters of recommendation, physical assessment course, statistics course, GRE General Test. *Application deadline:* For fall admission, 6/16. Applications are processed on a rolling basis. *Application fee:* $35 ($50 for international students).

Degree Requirements 48 total credit hours, thesis or project, comprehensive exam.

POST-MASTER'S PROGRAM

Areas of Study Health-care administration. *Nurse practitioner programs in:* acute care, adult health, family health, gerontology, pediatric, psychiatric/mental health.

DOCTORAL DEGREE PROGRAM

Degree PhD

Available Programs Doctorate.

Areas of Study Faculty preparation, nursing education, nursing research.

Program Entrance Requirements Minimum overall college GPA of 3.0, interview, 3 letters of recommendation, MSN or equivalent, statistics course, GRE General Test. *Application deadline:* For fall admission, 6/16. Applications are processed on a rolling basis. *Application fee:* $35 ($50 for international students).

Degree Requirements 58 total credit hours, dissertation, residency.

CONTINUING EDUCATION PROGRAM

Contact Lupita Martinez, Administrative Assistant, School of Nursing, The University of Texas at Arlington, 411 South Nedderman Drive, Box 19407, Arlington, TX 76019-0407. *Telephone:* 817-272-2778. *Fax:* 817-272-5006. *E-mail:* lupita@ua.edu.

The University of Texas at Austin
School of Nursing
Austin, Texas

http://www.utexas.edu/nursing

Founded in 1883

DEGREES • BSN • MSN • MSN/MBA • PHD

Nursing Program Faculty 73 (62% with doctorates).

The University of Texas at Austin (continued)
Baccalaureate Enrollment 701
Women 90.5% **Men** 9.5% **Minority** 33% **International** 1% **Part-time** 13%
Graduate Enrollment 222
Women 88% **Men** 12% **Minority** 27% **International** 9% **Part-time** 24%

Nursing Student Activities Nursing Honor Society, Sigma Theta Tau, Student Nurses' Association, nursing club.

Nursing Student Resources Academic advising; academic or career counseling; assistance for students with disabilities; bookstore; campus computer network; career placement assistance; computer lab; computer-assisted instruction; daycare for children of students; e-mail services; employment services for current students; externships; housing assistance; interactive nursing skills videos; Internet; learning resource lab; library services; nursing audiovisuals; other; paid internships; placement services for program completers; remedial services; resume preparation assistance; skills, simulation, or other laboratory; tutoring; unpaid internships.

Library Facilities 100,000 volumes in health, 80,000 volumes in nursing; 504 periodical subscriptions health-care related.

BACCALAUREATE PROGRAMS

Degree BSN

Available Programs Generic Baccalaureate; RN Baccalaureate.

Study Options Full-time.

Program Entrance Requirements Minimum overall college GPA of 2.5, transcript of college record, CPR certification, written essay, 3 years high school math, 2 years high school science, high school transcript, immunizations, 3 letters of recommendation, minimum GPA in nursing prerequisites of 2.5, professional liability insurance/malpractice insurance, prerequisite course work. Transfer students are accepted. **Standardized tests** *Required:* SAT or ACT, TOEFL for international students. *Required for some:* SAT Subject Tests. **Application** *Deadline:* 2/1 (freshmen), 3/1 (transfer). *Notification:* continuous (freshmen). *Application fee:* $60.

Advanced Placement Credit by examination available. Credit given for nursing courses completed elsewhere dependent upon specific evaluations.

Contact *Telephone:* 512-232-4780. *Fax:* 512-232-4777.

GRADUATE PROGRAMS

Contact *Telephone:* 512-471-7927. *Fax:* 512-232-4777.

MASTER'S DEGREE PROGRAM

Degrees MSN; MSN/MBA

Available Programs Master's; Master's for Non-Nursing College Graduates; Master's for Nurses with Non-Nursing Degrees.

Concentrations Available Nursing administration. *Clinical nurse specialist programs in:* adult health, community health, medical-surgical, public health. *Nurse practitioner programs in:* family health, pediatric.

Study Options Full-time and part-time.

Program Entrance Requirements Clinical experience, minimum overall college GPA of 3.0, transcript of college record, CPR certification, written essay, immunizations, interview, 3 letters of recommendation, physical assessment course, professional liability insurance/malpractice insurance, prerequisite course work, resume, statistics course, GRE General Test. *Application deadline:* For fall admission, 12/1. *Application fee:* $50 ($75 for international students).

Advanced Placement Credit given for nursing courses completed elsewhere dependent upon specific evaluations.

Degree Requirements 48 total credit hours.

POST-MASTER'S PROGRAM

Areas of Study *Nurse practitioner programs in:* family health, pediatric.

DOCTORAL DEGREE PROGRAM

Degree PhD

Available Programs Doctorate.

Areas of Study Aging, community health, faculty preparation, gerontology, health promotion/disease prevention, health-care systems, human health and illness, illness and transition, maternity-newborn, nursing administration, nursing research, women's health.

Program Entrance Requirements Minimum overall college GPA of 3.0, interview, 3 letters of recommendation, MSN or equivalent, statistics course, vita, GRE General Test. *Application deadline:* For fall admission, 12/1. *Application fee:* $50 ($75 for international students).

Degree Requirements 64 total credit hours, dissertation, oral exam, written exam, residency.

POSTDOCTORAL PROGRAM

Areas of Study Women's health.

Postdoctoral Program Contact *Telephone:* 512-232-4751. *Fax:* 512-232-4777.

The University of Texas at Brownsville
Department of Nursing
Brownsville, Texas

http://www.ntmain.utb.edu/shs/nursing_dept.html
Founded in 1973
DEGREES • BSN • MSN

Nursing Program Faculty 25 (12% with doctorates).
Baccalaureate Enrollment 21
Women 90% **Men** 10% **Part-time** 70%
Graduate Enrollment 11
Women 90% **Men** 10% **Part-time** 80%

Nursing Student Resources Academic advising; academic or career counseling; assistance for students with disabilities; bookstore; campus computer network; career placement assistance; computer lab; computer-assisted instruction; daycare for children of students; e-mail services; employment services for current students; housing assistance; interactive nursing skills videos; Internet; learning resource lab; library services; nursing audiovisuals; remedial services; skills, simulation, or other laboratory; tutoring.

Library Facilities 174,660 volumes; 4,447 periodical subscriptions.

BACCALAUREATE PROGRAMS

Degree BSN

Available Programs ADN to Baccalaureate.

Study Options Full-time and part-time.

Program Entrance Requirements Minimum overall college GPA of 2.5, transcript of college record, CPR certification, immunizations, minimum GPA in nursing prerequisites of 2.5, professional liability insurance/malpractice insurance, prerequisite course work, RN licensure. Transfer students are accepted. **Standardized tests** *Recommended:* TOEFL for international students. **Application** *Deadline:* 7/10 (freshmen), 8/1 (transfer).

Advanced Placement Credit by examination available.

Expenses (2006–07) *Tuition, state resident:* full-time $5200.

Contact Dr. Katherine B. Dougherty, Director, RN to BSN Program, Department of Nursing, The University of Texas at Brownsville, 80 Fort Brown, Brownsville, TX 78520. *Telephone:* 956-882-5071. *Fax:* 956-882-5100. *E-mail:* kathy.dougherty@utb.edu.

GRADUATE PROGRAMS

Contact Dr. Eloisa Tamez, Interim Director of Masters Program, Department of Nursing, The University of Texas at Brownsville, 80 Fort Brown, Brownsville, TX 78520. *Telephone:* 956-882-5079. *Fax:* 956-882-5100. *E-mail:* eloisa.tamez@utb.edu.

MASTER'S DEGREE PROGRAM

Degree MSN

Available Programs Master's.

Concentrations Available Nursing administration; nursing education. *Clinical nurse specialist programs in:* public health.

Study Options Full-time and part-time.

Program Entrance Requirements Minimum overall college GPA of 3.0, transcript of college record, immunizations, 2 letters of recommendation, professional liability insurance/malpractice insurance, statistics course.

Degree Requirements 37 total credit hours, thesis or project.

The University of Texas at El Paso
School of Nursing
El Paso, Texas

http://chs.utep.edu/nursing

Founded in 1913

DEGREES • BSN • MSN • PHD

Nursing Program Faculty 55 (33% with doctorates).

Baccalaureate Enrollment 454
Women 80% **Men** 20% **Minority** 81.9% **International** 3% **Part-time** 46.9%

Graduate Enrollment 97
Women 83.5% **Men** 16.5% **Minority** 72% **International** 1% **Part-time** 94.8%

Nursing Student Activities Nursing Honor Society, Sigma Theta Tau, Student Nurses' Association.

Nursing Student Resources Academic advising; academic or career counseling; assistance for students with disabilities; bookstore; campus computer network; career placement assistance; computer lab; computer-assisted instruction; e-mail services; employment services for current students; interactive nursing skills videos; Internet; learning resource lab; library services; nursing audiovisuals; remedial services; skills, simulation, or other laboratory; tutoring.

Library Facilities 961,247 volumes (25,000 in nursing); 3,005 periodical subscriptions.

BACCALAUREATE PROGRAMS

Degree BSN

Available Programs Accelerated Baccalaureate; Generic Baccalaureate; RN Baccalaureate.

Study Options Full-time and part-time.

Program Entrance Requirements Minimum overall college GPA of 2.5, CPR certification, health exam, health insurance, high school biology, high school chemistry, high school math, high school science, high school transcript, immunizations, minimum GPA in nursing prerequisites of 2.5, professional liability insurance/malpractice insurance, prerequisite course work. Transfer students are accepted. **Standardized tests** *Required:* TOEFL for international students. *Required for some:* SAT or ACT, PAA. **Application** *Deadline:* 7/31 (freshmen), 7/31 (transfer).

Advanced Placement Credit by examination available. Credit given for nursing courses completed elsewhere dependent upon specific evaluations.

Expenses (2006–07) *Tuition, state resident:* full-time $3252; part-time $136 per credit hour. *Tuition, nonresident:* full-time $9852; part-time $411 per credit hour. *International tuition:* $9852 full-time. *Room and board:* room only: $5205 per academic year. *Required fees:* full-time $1050; part-time $525 per term.

Financial Aid 74% of baccalaureate students in nursing programs received some form of financial aid in 2005–06.

Contact Ms. Patricia Fowler, Assistant Dean, Undergraduate Education, School of Nursing, The University of Texas at El Paso, 1101 North Campbell Street, El Paso, TX 79902. *Telephone:* 915-747-7267. *Fax:* 915-747-8266. *E-mail:* pfowler@utep.edu.

GRADUATE PROGRAMS

Expenses (2006–07) *Tuition, state resident:* full-time $3123; part-time $174 per credit hour. *Tuition, nonresident:* full-time $8073; part-time $449 per credit hour. *International tuition:* $8073 full-time. *Room and board:* room only: $5205 per academic year. *Required fees:* full-time $1026; part-time $513 per term.

Financial Aid 49% of graduate students in nursing programs received some form of financial aid in 2005–06. Research assistantships with partial tuition reimbursements available (averaging $18,825 per year), teaching assistantships with partial tuition reimbursements available (averaging $18,000 per year) were awarded; fellowships with partial tuition reimbursements available, career-related internships or fieldwork, Federal Work-Study, institutionally sponsored loans, scholarships, and tuition waivers (partial) also available. Aid available to part-time students. *Financial aid application deadline:* 3/15.

Contact Dr. Karen C. Lyon, Assistant Dean, Graduate Education, School of Nursing, The University of Texas at El Paso, 1101 North Campbell Street, El Paso, TX 79902. *Telephone:* 915-747-7279. *Fax:* 915-747-8266. *E-mail:* kclyon@utep.edu.

MASTER'S DEGREE PROGRAM

Degree MSN

Available Programs Master's; RN to Master's.

Concentrations Available Nursing administration; nursing education. *Nurse practitioner programs in:* family health, women's health.

Site Options *Distance Learning:* El Paso, TX.

Study Options Full-time and part-time.

Program Entrance Requirements Clinical experience, minimum overall college GPA of 3.0, transcript of college record, CPR certification, written essay, immunizations, interview, nursing research course, professional liability insurance/malpractice insurance, resume, GRE General Test or MAT. *Application deadline:* For fall admission, 7/1; for spring admission, 11/1. Applications are processed on a rolling basis. *Application fee:* $15 ($65 for international students).

Advanced Placement Credit given for nursing courses completed elsewhere dependent upon specific evaluations.

Degree Requirements 30 total credit hours, thesis or project, comprehensive exam.

POST-MASTER'S PROGRAM

Areas of Study Nursing education. *Nurse practitioner programs in:* family health, women's health.

DOCTORAL DEGREE PROGRAM

Degree PhD

Available Programs Doctorate.

Areas of Study Addiction/substance abuse, biology of health and illness, community health, faculty preparation, health policy, health promotion/disease prevention, health-care systems, human health and illness, illness and transition, nursing research, urban health, women's health.

Site Options *Distance Learning:* Houston, TX.

Program Entrance Requirements interview by faculty committee, interview, letters of recommendation, MSN or equivalent, statistics course, vita. *Application deadline:* For fall admission, 7/1; for spring admission, 11/1. Applications are processed on a rolling basis. *Application fee:* $15 ($65 for international students).

Degree Requirements 60 total credit hours, dissertation.

The University of Texas at Tyler
Program in Nursing
Tyler, Texas

http://www.uttyler.edu/nursing

Founded in 1971

DEGREES • BSN • DNS • MSN • MSN/MBA

Nursing Program Faculty 60 (25% with doctorates).

Baccalaureate Enrollment 563
Women 70% **Men** 30% **Minority** 10% **International** 1% **Part-time** 15%

Graduate Enrollment 175
Women 88% **Men** 12% **Minority** 11% **Part-time** 88%

Nursing Student Activities Nursing Honor Society, Sigma Theta Tau, Student Nurses' Association, nursing club.

Nursing Student Resources Academic advising; academic or career counseling; assistance for students with disabilities; bookstore; campus computer network; career placement assistance; computer lab; computer-assisted instruction; e-mail services; employment services for current students; externships; interactive nursing skills videos; Internet; learning resource lab; library services; nursing audiovisuals; remedial services; resume preparation assistance; skills, simulation, or other laboratory; tutoring.

Library Facilities 486,895 volumes (11,000 in health, 5,500 in nursing); 525 periodical subscriptions (150 health-care related).

The University of Texas at Tyler (continued)

BACCALAUREATE PROGRAMS

Degree BSN

Available Programs ADN to Baccalaureate; Accelerated RN Baccalaureate; Generic Baccalaureate; International Nurse to Baccalaureate; LPN to Baccalaureate; LPN to RN Baccalaureate; RN Baccalaureate.

Site Options *Distance Learning:* Palastine, TX; Longview, TX.

Study Options Full-time and part-time.

Program Entrance Requirements Minimum overall college GPA of 2.75, transcript of college record, CPR certification, health exam, immunizations, minimum GPA in nursing prerequisites of 2.75, professional liability insurance/malpractice insurance, prerequisite course work. Transfer students are accepted. **Standardized tests** *Required:* SAT or ACT, TOEFL for international students. **Application** *Notification:* continuous (freshmen). *Application fee:* $25.

Advanced Placement Credit given for nursing courses completed elsewhere dependent upon specific evaluations.

Expenses (2006–07) *Tuition, state resident:* part-time $50 per credit hour. *Tuition, nonresident:* part-time $325 per credit hour. *International tuition:* $13,640 full-time. *Room and board:* $6030; room only: $4700 per academic year. *Required fees:* full-time $4124; part-time $472 per credit; part-time $2062 per term.

Financial Aid 70% of baccalaureate students in nursing programs received some form of financial aid in 2005–06. *Gift aid (need-based):* Federal Pell, FSEOG, state, private, college/university gift aid from institutional funds, Texas Grant, Teach for Texas Conditional Prog, Institutional Grants (Education Affordability Prog). *Loans:* FFEL (Subsidized and Unsubsidized Stafford PLUS), state. *Work-Study:* Federal Work-Study, part-time campus jobs. *Application deadline (priority):* 4/1.

Contact Ms. Andrea H. Liner, Coordinator, Marketing and Advising, Program in Nursing, The University of Texas at Tyler, 3900 University Boulevard, Tyler, TX 75799. *Telephone:* 903-565-5534. *Fax:* 903-565-5901. *E-mail:* Andrea_Liner@uttyler.edu.

GRADUATE PROGRAMS

Expenses (2006–07) *Tuition, area resident:* part-time $146 per credit hour. *Tuition, state resident:* part-time $421 per credit hour. *Tuition, nonresident:* part-time $421 per credit hour. *Room and board:* $6030; room only: $4700 per academic year.

Financial Aid 60% of graduate students in nursing programs received some form of financial aid in 2005–06. 12 fellowships, 3 research assistantships (averaging $2,200 per year) were awarded; institutionally sponsored loans and AENT grants also available. *Financial aid application deadline:* 8/1.

Contact Ms. Andrea H. Liner, Coordinator, Marketing and Advising, Program in Nursing, The University of Texas at Tyler, 3900 University Boulevard, Tyler, TX 75799. *Telephone:* 903-565-5534. *Fax:* 903-565-5901. *E-mail:* Andrea_Liner@uttyler.edu.

MASTER'S DEGREE PROGRAM

Degrees MSN; MSN/MBA

Available Programs Accelerated AD/RN to Master's; Accelerated RN to Master's; Master's; RN to Master's.

Concentrations Available Nursing administration; nursing education. *Nurse practitioner programs in:* acute care, adult health, family health, gerontology, pediatric, women's health.

Study Options Full-time and part-time.

Program Entrance Requirements Computer literacy, minimum overall college GPA of 3.0, transcript of college record, CPR certification, immunizations, 4 letters of recommendation, nursing research course, professional liability insurance/malpractice insurance, prerequisite course work, resume, statistics course, GRE General Test or MAT, GMAT. *Application deadline:* For fall admission, 3/1 (priority date); for spring admission, 10/1 (priority date). Applications are processed on a rolling basis.

Advanced Placement Credit given for nursing courses completed elsewhere dependent upon specific evaluations.

Degree Requirements 36 total credit hours, thesis or project, comprehensive exam.

POST-MASTER'S PROGRAM

Areas of Study Nursing administration; nursing education. *Nurse practitioner programs in:* acute care, adult health, family health, gerontology, pediatric, women's health.

DOCTORAL DEGREE PROGRAM

Degree DNS

Available Programs Doctorate.

Areas of Study Nursing science.

Program Entrance Requirements Minimum overall college GPA of 3.0, interview by faculty committee, 3 letters of recommendation, MSN or equivalent, scholarly papers, statistics course, vita, writing sample. *Application deadline:* For fall admission, 3/1 (priority date); for spring admission, 10/1 (priority date). Applications are processed on a rolling basis.

Degree Requirements 65 total credit hours, dissertation, written exam.

CONTINUING EDUCATION PROGRAM

Contact Pamela Martin, RN, Assistant Dean of Undergraduate Studies, Program in Nursing, The University of Texas at Tyler, 3900 University Boulevard, Tyler, TX 75799. *Telephone:* 903-566-7320. *Fax:* 903-565-5533. *E-mail:* pmartin@mail.uttyl.edu.

The University of Texas Health Science Center at Houston
School of Nursing
Houston, Texas

http://son.uth.tmc.edu/

Founded in 1972

DEGREES • BSN • DSN • MSN • MSN/MPH

Nursing Program Faculty 76 (72% with doctorates).

Baccalaureate Enrollment 316
Women 85% **Men** 15% **Minority** 53% **International** 4% **Part-time** 14%

Graduate Enrollment 413
Women 71% **Men** 29% **Minority** 33% **International** 3% **Part-time** 46%

Nursing Student Activities Nursing Honor Society, Sigma Theta Tau, Student Nurses' Association.

Nursing Student Resources Academic advising; academic or career counseling; assistance for students with disabilities; bookstore; campus computer network; computer lab; computer-assisted instruction; daycare for children of students; e-mail services; employment services for current students; externships; housing assistance; interactive nursing skills videos; learning resource lab; library services; nursing audiovisuals; remedial services; skills, simulation, or other laboratory; tutoring.

Library Facilities 339,062 volumes; 5,581 periodical subscriptions.

BACCALAUREATE PROGRAMS

Degree BSN

Available Programs ADN to Baccalaureate; Accelerated Baccalaureate for Second Degree; Accelerated RN Baccalaureate; Baccalaureate for Second Degree; Generic Baccalaureate.

Site Options *Distance Learning:* Cypress, TX; Katy, TX.

Study Options Full-time.

Program Entrance Requirements Minimum overall college GPA of 2.75, transcript of college record, CPR certification, written essay, immunizations, minimum GPA in nursing prerequisites of 3.0, prerequisite course work. Transfer students are accepted. **Standardized tests** *Required:* TOEFL for international students. **Application** *Deadline:* 12/31 (transfer). *Application fee:* $30.

Advanced Placement Credit by examination available.

Expenses (2006–07) *Tuition, state resident:* full-time $9573; part-time $124 per credit hour. *Tuition, nonresident:* full-time $13,040; part-time $326 per credit hour. *International tuition:* $13,040 full-time. *Required fees:* full-time $2055; part-time $640 per term.

Financial Aid 95% of baccalaureate students in nursing programs received some form of financial aid in 2005–06.

Contact Mr. William Stewart, Director of Admissions and Recruitment, School of Nursing, The University of Texas Health Science Center at Houston, 6901 Bertner Avenue, Suite 220, Houston, TX 77030. *Telephone:* 800-232-8876. *Fax:* 713-500-2007. *E-mail:* william.stewart@uth.tmc.edu.

GRADUATE PROGRAMS

Expenses (2006–07) *Tuition, state resident:* full-time $3348; part-time $124 per credit hour. *Tuition, nonresident:* full-time $8802; part-time $326 per credit hour. *International tuition:* $8802 full-time. *Required fees:* full-time $1270; part-time $403 per term.

Financial Aid 95% of graduate students in nursing programs received some form of financial aid in 2005–06. Research assistantships with tuition reimbursements available, teaching assistantships with tuition reimbursements available, institutionally sponsored loans, scholarships, traineeships, and tuition waivers (full) available. Aid available to part-time students.

Contact Mr. William Stewart, Director of Admissions and Recruitment, School of Nursing, The University of Texas Health Science Center at Houston, 6901 Bertner Avenue, Suite 220, Houston, TX 77030. *Telephone:* 800-232-8876. *Fax:* 713-500-2007. *E-mail:* william.stewart@uth.tmc.edu.

MASTER'S DEGREE PROGRAM

Degrees MSN; MSN/MPH

Available Programs Accelerated AD/RN to Master's; Master's.

Concentrations Available Nurse anesthesia; nursing administration; nursing education. *Clinical nurse specialist programs in:* acute care, adult health, gerontology, women's health. *Nurse practitioner programs in:* acute care, adult health, family health, gerontology, neonatal health, pediatric, women's health.

Study Options Full-time and part-time.

Program Entrance Requirements Clinical experience, minimum overall college GPA of 3.5, transcript of college record, CPR certification, immunizations, interview, 3 letters of recommendation, prerequisite course work, resume, statistics course, GRE or MAT. *Application deadline:* For fall admission, 5/1 (priority date). Applications are processed on a rolling basis. *Application fee:* $30.

Degree Requirements 49 total credit hours, thesis or project.

POST-MASTER'S PROGRAM

Areas of Study Nursing administration. *Clinical nurse specialist programs in:* acute care, adult health, gerontology, oncology, palliative care, psychiatric/mental health, women's health. *Nurse practitioner programs in:* acute care, adult health, family health, gerontology, neonatal health, oncology, pediatric, psychiatric/mental health, women's health.

DOCTORAL DEGREE PROGRAM

Degree DSN

Available Programs Doctorate.

Areas of Study Addiction/substance abuse, advanced practice nursing, aging, bio-behavioral research, biology of health and illness, clinical practice, community health, critical care, ethics, faculty preparation, family health, gerontology, health policy, health promotion/disease prevention, health-care systems, human health and illness, illness and transition, individualized study, maternity-newborn, neuro-behavior, nurse case management, nursing administration, nursing education, nursing policy, nursing research, nursing science, oncology, urban health, women's health.

Program Entrance Requirements Minimum overall college GPA of 3.5, interview by faculty committee, 3 letters of recommendation, MSN or equivalent, vita, writing sample, GRE. *Application deadline:* For fall admission, 5/1 (priority date). Applications are processed on a rolling basis. *Application fee:* $30.

Degree Requirements 66 total credit hours, dissertation.

CONTINUING EDUCATION PROGRAM

Contact Dr. Vaunette P. Fay, RN, Assistant Dean for e-Learning and Associate Professor of Clinical Nursing, School of Nursing, The University of Texas Health Science Center at Houston, 6901 Bertner Avenue, Suite 846, Houston, TX 77030. *Telephone:* 713-500-2116. *Fax:* 713-500-2026. *E-mail:* vaunette.p.fay@uth.tmc.edu.

The University of Texas Health Science Center at San Antonio
School of Nursing
San Antonio, Texas

http://www.nursing.uthscsa.edu
Founded in 1976

DEGREES • BSN • MSN • MSN/MPH • PHD

Nursing Program Faculty 83 (50% with doctorates).
Baccalaureate Enrollment 675
Women 80% **Men** 20% **Minority** 45% **Part-time** 15%
Graduate Enrollment 150
Women 85% **Men** 15% **Minority** 15% **Part-time** 75%
Nursing Student Activities Nursing Honor Society, Sigma Theta Tau, Student Nurses' Association.

Nursing Student Resources Academic advising; assistance for students with disabilities; bookstore; campus computer network; computer lab; computer-assisted instruction; e-mail services; interactive nursing skills videos; Internet; learning resource lab; library services; nursing audiovisuals; remedial services; skills, simulation, or other laboratory; tutoring.

Library Facilities 192,576 volumes (205,641 in health, 2,056 in nursing); 2,501 periodical subscriptions (250 health-care related).

BACCALAUREATE PROGRAMS

Degree BSN

Available Programs ADN to Baccalaureate; Generic Baccalaureate; LPN to Baccalaureate; LPN to RN Baccalaureate; RN Baccalaureate.

Study Options Full-time and part-time.

Program Entrance Requirements Minimum overall college GPA of 2.0, transcript of college record, CPR certification, health insurance, immunizations, minimum GPA in nursing prerequisites of 2.3, professional liability insurance/malpractice insurance, prerequisite course work. Transfer students are accepted. **Standardized tests** *Required for some:* SAT or ACT, THEA. **Application** *Application fee:* $50.

Advanced Placement Credit by examination available. Credit given for nursing courses completed elsewhere dependent upon specific evaluations.

Contact *Telephone:* 210-567-5810. *Fax:* 210-567-3813.

GRADUATE PROGRAMS

Contact *Telephone:* 210-567-5815.

MASTER'S DEGREE PROGRAM

Degrees MSN; MSN/MPH

Available Programs Master's; RN to Master's.

Concentrations Available Nursing administration; nursing education; nursing informatics. *Clinical nurse specialist programs in:* acute care, critical care, medical-surgical, psychiatric/mental health. *Nurse practitioner programs in:* family health, gerontology, pediatric, psychiatric/mental health.

Study Options Full-time and part-time.

Program Entrance Requirements Clinical experience, computer literacy, minimum overall college GPA of 3.0, transcript of college record, CPR certification, immunizations, 4 letters of recommendation, professional liability insurance/malpractice insurance, prerequisite course work, statistics course, GRE General Test, MAT. *Application deadline:* For fall admission, 4/1; for spring admission, 10/1. *Application fee:* $15.

Advanced Placement Credit given for nursing courses completed elsewhere dependent upon specific evaluations.

Degree Requirements 40 total credit hours, thesis or project.

POST-MASTER'S PROGRAM

Areas of Study *Nurse practitioner programs in:* family health, gerontology, pediatric.

DOCTORAL DEGREE PROGRAM

Degree PhD

Available Programs Doctorate; Post-Baccalaureate Doctorate.

Areas of Study Clinical practice, community health, nursing research.

Site Options *Distance Learning:* Lubbock, TX; Corpus Christi, TX; Edinburg, TX.

Program Entrance Requirements Minimum overall college GPA of 3.0, interview by faculty committee, interview, 4 letters of recommendation, statistics course. *Application deadline:* For fall admission, 4/1; for spring admission, 10/1. *Application fee:* $15.

Degree Requirements 55 total credit hours, dissertation, oral exam, written exam.

The University of Texas Health Science Center at San Antonio (continued)

CONTINUING EDUCATION PROGRAM

Contact *Telephone:* 210-567-5850. *Fax:* 210-567-5909.

The University of Texas Medical Branch

School of Nursing
Galveston, Texas

http://www.son.utmb.edu

Founded in 1891

DEGREES • BSN • MSN • PHD

Nursing Program Faculty 53 (58% with doctorates).

Baccalaureate Enrollment 347
Women 84% **Men** 16% **Minority** 39% **Part-time** 52%

Graduate Enrollment 280
Women 89% **Men** 11% **Minority** 26% **Part-time** 79%

Nursing Student Activities Sigma Theta Tau, Student Nurses' Association.

Nursing Student Resources Academic advising; academic or career counseling; assistance for students with disabilities; bookstore; campus computer network; career placement assistance; computer lab; computer-assisted instruction; e-mail services; employment services for current students; housing assistance; interactive nursing skills videos; Internet; learning resource lab; library services; nursing audiovisuals; resume preparation assistance; skills, simulation, or other laboratory; tutoring.

Library Facilities 248,370 volumes (261,585 in health, 2,921 in nursing); 1,980 periodical subscriptions (25,204 health-care related).

BACCALAUREATE PROGRAMS

Degree BSN

Available Programs Accelerated Baccalaureate for Second Degree; Generic Baccalaureate; RN Baccalaureate.

Study Options Full-time and part-time.

Program Entrance Requirements Minimum overall college GPA of 2.0, transcript of college record, CPR certification, written essay, health exam, immunizations, 3 letters of recommendation, minimum GPA in nursing prerequisites of 2.75, professional liability insurance/malpractice insurance, prerequisite course work. Transfer students are accepted. **Standardized tests** *Required:* TOEFL for international students. **Application** *Application fee:* $25.

Advanced Placement Credit given for nursing courses completed elsewhere dependent upon specific evaluations.

Expenses (2006–07) *Tuition, state resident:* full-time $5760; part-time $120 per credit hour. *Tuition, nonresident:* full-time $18,960; part-time $395 per credit hour. *International tuition:* $18,960 full-time. *Room and board:* $8076; room only: $3876 per academic year. *Required fees:* full-time $3182; part-time $164 per term.

Financial Aid 50% of baccalaureate students in nursing programs received some form of financial aid in 2005–06. *Gift aid (need-based):* Federal Pell, FSEOG, state, private, college/university gift aid from institutional funds. *Loans:* Federal Nursing Student Loans, Federal Direct (Subsidized and Unsubsidized Stafford PLUS), Perkins, state, college/university. *Work-Study:* Federal Work-Study. *Application deadline:* Continuous.

Contact Dr. Margaret Susan Grinslade, Associate Professor and Director of Baccalaureate Programs, School of Nursing, The University of Texas Medical Branch, 301 University Boulevard, 3.526 SON/SAHS Building, Galveston, TX 77555-1029. *Telephone:* 409-772-0396. *Fax:* 409-747-1508. *E-mail:* msgrinsl@utmb.edu.

GRADUATE PROGRAMS

Expenses (2006–07) *Tuition, state resident:* full-time $3900; part-time $130 per credit hour. *Tuition, nonresident:* full-time $4050; part-time $405 per credit hour. *International tuition:* $4050 full-time. *Room and board:* $8076; room only: $3876 per academic year. *Required fees:* full-time $2082; part-time $164 per term.

Financial Aid 25% of graduate students in nursing programs received some form of financial aid in 2005–06.

Contact Dr. Christine A. Boodley, Associate Professor/Interim Masters Program Director, School of Nursing, The University of Texas Medical Branch, 301 University Boulevard, 3.625 SON/SAHS Building, Galveston, TX 77555-1029. *Telephone:* 409-772-0909. *Fax:* 409-772-3770. *E-mail:* cboodley@utmb.edu.

MASTER'S DEGREE PROGRAM

Degree MSN

Available Programs Master's; RN to Master's.

Concentrations Available Nursing administration; nursing education. *Nurse practitioner programs in:* acute care, family health, gerontology, neonatal health, pediatric, women's health.

Site Options Houston, TX.

Study Options Full-time and part-time.

Program Entrance Requirements Clinical experience, computer literacy, minimum overall college GPA of 3.0, transcript of college record, CPR certification, written essay, immunizations, interview, 3 letters of recommendation, statistics course.

Advanced Placement Credit given for nursing courses completed elsewhere dependent upon specific evaluations.

Degree Requirements 48 total credit hours.

POST-MASTER'S PROGRAM

Areas of Study *Nurse practitioner programs in:* acute care, family health, gerontology, neonatal health, pediatric, women's health.

DOCTORAL DEGREE PROGRAM

Degree PhD

Available Programs Doctorate; Post-Baccalaureate Doctorate.

Areas of Study Aging, bio-behavioral research, faculty preparation, gerontology, health promotion/disease prevention, human health and illness, individualized study, maternity-newborn, nursing research, nursing science, women's health.

Program Entrance Requirements Clinical experience, minimum overall college GPA of 3.0, interview by faculty committee, interview, 3 letters of recommendation, MSN or equivalent, statistics course, vita, writing sample.

Degree Requirements 64 total credit hours, dissertation, oral exam, written exam, residency.

CONTINUING EDUCATION PROGRAM

Contact Ms. Phyllis Waters, MSC, Director of Continuing Education, School of Nursing, The University of Texas Medical Branch, 524 Jennie Sealy Hospital, 301 University Boulevard, Galveston, TX 77555-0473. *Telephone:* 409-772-8200. *Fax:* 409-747-1531. *E-mail:* pwaters@utmb.edu.

The University of Texas–Pan American

Department of Nursing
Edinburg, Texas

http://www.panam.edu

Founded in 1927

DEGREES • BSN • MSN

Nursing Program Faculty 23 (35% with doctorates).

Baccalaureate Enrollment 152
Women 79% **Men** 21% **Minority** 91% **Part-time** 3%

Graduate Enrollment 56
Women 80% **Men** 20% **Minority** 77% **International** 4% **Part-time** 95%

Nursing Student Activities Sigma Theta Tau, Student Nurses' Association.

Nursing Student Resources Academic advising; academic or career counseling; assistance for students with disabilities; bookstore; campus computer network; career placement assistance; computer lab; computer-assisted instruction; daycare for children of students; e-mail services;

employment services for current students; housing assistance; interactive nursing skills videos; Internet; learning resource lab; library services; nursing audiovisuals; remedial services; skills, simulation, or other laboratory; tutoring.

Library Facilities 598,008 volumes (230 in health, 200 in nursing); 35,004 periodical subscriptions (300 health-care related).

BACCALAUREATE PROGRAMS

Degree BSN

Available Programs Generic Baccalaureate; RN Baccalaureate.

Study Options Full-time.

Program Entrance Requirements Transcript of college record, CPR certification, health exam, immunizations, minimum GPA in nursing prerequisites of 2.5, professional liability insurance/malpractice insurance, prerequisite course work. Transfer students are accepted. **Standardized tests** *Required:* SAT or ACT, TOEFL for international students. **Application** *Deadline:* 8/11 (freshmen), 8/11 (transfer). *Notification:* continuous (freshmen).

Expenses (2006–07) *Tuition, state resident:* full-time $3464; part-time $1000 per semester. *Tuition, nonresident:* full-time $10,100; part-time $1200 per semester. *International tuition:* $10,100 full-time. *Required fees:* full-time $2500; part-time $200 per credit; part-time $1200 per term.

Financial Aid 90% of baccalaureate students in nursing programs received some form of financial aid in 2005–06.

Contact Dr. Sandy M. Sanchez, BSN Program Coordinator, Department of Nursing, The University of Texas–Pan American, 1201 West University Drive, Edinburg, TX 78541. *Telephone:* 956-381-3491. *Fax:* 956-381-2875. *E-mail:* ssanchez@utpa.edu.

GRADUATE PROGRAMS

Expenses (2006–07) *Tuition, state resident:* full-time $3200; part-time $1200 per semester. *Tuition, nonresident:* full-time $9000; part-time $3000 per semester. *International tuition:* $9000 full-time. *Required fees:* full-time $1000; part-time $50 per credit; part-time $450 per term.

Financial Aid 50% of graduate students in nursing programs received some form of financial aid in 2005–06. Scholarships and traineeships available.

Contact Dr. Jan Maville, EdD, MSN Coordinator, Department of Nursing, The University of Texas–Pan American, 1201 West University Drive, Edinburg, TX 78541. *Telephone:* 956-381-3491. *Fax:* 956-381-2875. *E-mail:* jmaville@utpa.edu.

MASTER'S DEGREE PROGRAM

Degree MSN

Available Programs Master's.

Concentrations Available *Clinical nurse specialist programs in:* adult health. *Nurse practitioner programs in:* family health, pediatric.

Study Options Full-time and part-time.

Program Entrance Requirements Clinical experience, minimum overall college GPA of 3.0, transcript of college record, written essay, immunizations, 3 letters of recommendation, resume, statistics course. *Application deadline:* Applications are processed on a rolling basis. *Application fee:* $35.

Advanced Placement Credit given for nursing courses completed elsewhere dependent upon specific evaluations.

Degree Requirements 48 total credit hours, thesis or project.

POST-MASTER'S PROGRAM

Areas of Study *Nurse practitioner programs in:* family health, pediatric.

University of the Incarnate Word
Program in Nursing
San Antonio, Texas

Founded in 1881

DEGREES • BSN • MSN • MSN/MBA

Nursing Program Faculty 25 (57% with doctorates).

Baccalaureate Enrollment 129

Women 88% **Men** 12% **Minority** 57%

Graduate Enrollment 59

Women 83% **Men** 17% **Minority** 59% **Part-time** 76%

Nursing Student Activities Nursing Honor Society, Sigma Theta Tau, Student Nurses' Association.

Nursing Student Resources Academic advising; academic or career counseling; assistance for students with disabilities; bookstore; campus computer network; career placement assistance; computer lab; computer-assisted instruction; e-mail services; employment services for current students; externships; housing assistance; interactive nursing skills videos; Internet; learning resource lab; library services; nursing audiovisuals; paid internships; placement services for program completers; remedial services; resume preparation assistance; skills, simulation, or other laboratory; tutoring; unpaid internships.

Library Facilities 335,298 volumes (6,000 in health, 6,000 in nursing); 23,551 periodical subscriptions (3,048 health-care related).

BACCALAUREATE PROGRAMS

Degree BSN

Available Programs ADN to Baccalaureate; Generic Baccalaureate.

Study Options Full-time.

Program Entrance Requirements Minimum overall college GPA of 2.5, transcript of college record, CPR certification, health exam, health insurance, immunizations, minimum GPA in nursing prerequisites of 2.5, professional liability insurance/malpractice insurance, prerequisite course work. Transfer students are accepted. **Standardized tests** *Required:* SAT or ACT, TOEFL for international students. **Application** *Deadline:* rolling (freshmen), rolling (transfer). *Application fee:* $20.

Advanced Placement Credit given for nursing courses completed elsewhere dependent upon specific evaluations.

Contact *Telephone:* 210-829-6005.

GRADUATE PROGRAMS

Contact *Telephone:* 210-829-3988. *Fax:* 210-829-3174.

MASTER'S DEGREE PROGRAM

Degrees MSN; MSN/MBA

Available Programs Master's.

Concentrations Available *Clinical nurse specialist programs in:* adult health.

Study Options Full-time and part-time.

Program Entrance Requirements Clinical experience, minimum overall college GPA of 2.5, transcript of college record, immunizations, 3 letters of recommendation, physical assessment course, professional liability insurance/malpractice insurance, statistics course, GRE General Test. *Application deadline:* For fall admission, 8/15 (priority date); for spring admission, 12/31. Applications are processed on a rolling basis. *Application fee:* $20.

Advanced Placement Credit given for nursing courses completed elsewhere dependent upon specific evaluations.

Degree Requirements 36 total credit hours, thesis or project.

West Texas A&M University
Division of Nursing
Canyon, Texas

http://www.wtamu.edu/nursing

Founded in 1909

DEGREES • BSN • MSN

Nursing Program Faculty 30 (13% with doctorates).

Baccalaureate Enrollment 382

Women 88% **Men** 12% **Minority** 22% **International** 1% **Part-time** 26%

Graduate Enrollment 65

Women 85% **Men** 15% **Minority** 17% **Part-time** 75%

Nursing Student Activities Sigma Theta Tau, Student Nurses' Association.

West Texas A&M University (continued)

Nursing Student Resources Academic advising; academic or career counseling; assistance for students with disabilities; bookstore; campus computer network; career placement assistance; computer lab; computer-assisted instruction; daycare for children of students; e-mail services; employment services for current students; housing assistance; interactive nursing skills videos; Internet; learning resource lab; library services; nursing audiovisuals; placement services for program completers; remedial services; resume preparation assistance; skills, simulation, or other laboratory; tutoring.

Library Facilities 1.1 million volumes (16,000 in health, 8,000 in nursing); 5,464 periodical subscriptions (64 health-care related).

BACCALAUREATE PROGRAMS

Degree BSN

Available Programs ADN to Baccalaureate; Generic Baccalaureate; LPN to Baccalaureate.

Study Options Full-time and part-time.

Program Entrance Requirements Minimum overall college GPA of 2.5, transcript of college record, CPR certification, 1 year of high school math, high school transcript, immunizations, minimum GPA in nursing prerequisites of 2.0, prerequisite course work. Transfer students are accepted. **Standardized tests** *Required:* SAT or ACT, TOEFL for international students. **Application** *Deadline:* rolling (freshmen), rolling (transfer). *Notification:* continuous (freshmen). *Application fee:* $25.

Advanced Placement Credit given for nursing courses completed elsewhere dependent upon specific evaluations.

Expenses (2006–07) *Tuition, state resident:* full-time $1600; part-time $50 per credit hour. *Tuition, nonresident:* full-time $10,400; part-time $325 per credit hour. *International tuition:* $10,400 full-time. *Room and board:* $4744; room only: $2310 per academic year.

Financial Aid 63% of baccalaureate students in nursing programs received some form of financial aid in 2005–06.

Contact Ms. Lynda Sue Robinson, Admissions Counselor, Division of Nursing, West Texas A&M University, WTAMU Box 60969, Canyon, TX 79016-0001. *Telephone:* 806-651-2661. *Fax:* 806-651-2632. *E-mail:* lrobinson@mail.wtamu.edu.

GRADUATE PROGRAMS

Expenses (2006–07) *Tuition, state resident:* full-time $1260; part-time $70 per credit hour. *Tuition, nonresident:* full-time $6210; part-time $345 per credit hour. *International tuition:* $6210 full-time. *Room and board:* $4744; room only: $1155 per academic year. *Required fees:* part-time $930 per term.

Financial Aid 30% of graduate students in nursing programs received some form of financial aid in 2005–06. 1 teaching assistantship with partial tuition reimbursement available (averaging $6,750 per year) was awarded; career-related internships or fieldwork, Federal Work-Study, institutionally sponsored loans, scholarships, and tuition waivers (partial) also available. Aid available to part-time students.

Contact Dr. Lisa Davis, Graduate Coordinator, Division of Nursing, West Texas A&M University, WTAMU Box 60969, Canyon, TX 79016-0001. *Telephone:* 806-651-2641. *Fax:* 806-651-2632. *E-mail:* ldavis@mail.wtamu.edu.

MASTER'S DEGREE PROGRAM

Degree MSN

Available Programs Master's; RN to Master's.

Concentrations Available Nursing administration; nursing education. *Nurse practitioner programs in:* family health.

Study Options Full-time and part-time.

Program Entrance Requirements Clinical experience, computer literacy, minimum overall college GPA of 3.0, transcript of college record, CPR certification, immunizations, nursing research course, professional liability insurance/malpractice insurance, prerequisite course work, statistics course, GRE General Test. *Application deadline:* Applications are processed on a rolling basis. *Application fee:* $25 ($75 for international students).

Degree Requirements 39 total credit hours, thesis or project.

POST-MASTER'S PROGRAM

Areas of Study *Nurse practitioner programs in:* family health.

UTAH

Brigham Young University
College of Nursing
Provo, Utah

http://nursing.byu.edu
Founded in 1875
DEGREES • BS • MS

Nursing Program Faculty 49 (45% with doctorates).

Baccalaureate Enrollment 277
Women 92% **Men** 8% **Minority** 7% **International** 3% **Part-time** 11%

Graduate Enrollment 27
Women 75% **Men** 25% **Minority** 6% **International** 2% **Part-time** 1%

Nursing Student Activities Nursing Honor Society, Sigma Theta Tau, Student Nurses' Association.

Nursing Student Resources Academic advising; academic or career counseling; assistance for students with disabilities; bookstore; campus computer network; career placement assistance; computer lab; computer-assisted instruction; e-mail services; employment services for current students; housing assistance; interactive nursing skills videos; Internet; learning resource lab; library services; nursing audiovisuals; other; paid internships; resume preparation assistance; skills, simulation, or other laboratory; tutoring.

Library Facilities 3.5 million volumes (24,471 in health, 3,482 in nursing); 27,161 periodical subscriptions (131 health-care related).

BACCALAUREATE PROGRAMS

Degree BS

Available Programs RN Baccalaureate.

Study Options Full-time and part-time.

Program Entrance Requirements Transcript of college record, CPR certification, written essay, 2 letters of recommendation, minimum GPA in nursing prerequisites of 3.0, prerequisite course work. Transfer students are accepted. **Standardized tests** *Required:* ACT, TOEFL for international students. **Application** *Deadline:* 2/1 (freshmen), 3/1 (transfer). *Notification:* continuous (freshmen). *Application fee:* $30.

Advanced Placement Credit given for nursing courses completed elsewhere dependent upon specific evaluations.

Expenses (2006–07) *Tuition:* full-time $5430; part-time $185 per credit hour. *International tuition:* $5430 full-time. *Room and board:* $3000; room only: $2000 per academic year.

Financial Aid 30% of baccalaureate students in nursing programs received some form of financial aid in 2005–06.

Contact Dr. Mark E. White, Advisement Center Supervisor, College of Nursing, Brigham Young University, 550 SWKT, Provo, UT 84602. *Telephone:* 801-422-7211. *Fax:* 801-422-0536. *E-mail:* mark_white@byu.edu.

GRADUATE PROGRAMS

Expenses (2006–07) *Tuition:* full-time $7290; part-time $255 per credit hour. *International tuition:* $7290 full-time.

Financial Aid 100% of graduate students in nursing programs received some form of financial aid in 2005–06. 2 research assistantships with full and partial tuition reimbursements available (averaging $10,000 per year), 3 teaching assistantships with full and partial tuition reimbursements available (averaging $10,000 per year) were awarded; institutionally sponsored loans, scholarships, tuition waivers (full), and unspecified assistantships also available. Aid available to part-time students. *Financial aid application deadline:* 2/1.

Contact Ms. Denise Gibbons Davis, Research Center and Graduate Program Secretary, College of Nursing, Brigham Young University, 400 SWKT, Provo, UT 84602. *Telephone:* 801-422-4142. *Fax:* 801-422-0536. *E-mail:* denise_gibbons@byu.edu.

MASTER'S DEGREE PROGRAM

Degree MS

Available Programs Master's.

Concentrations Available *Nurse practitioner programs in:* family health.

Study Options Full-time and part-time.

Program Entrance Requirements Clinical experience, minimum overall college GPA of 3.0, transcript of college record, CPR certification, written essay, immunizations, interview, 3 letters of recommendation, prerequisite course work, resume, statistics course, GRE. *Application deadline:* For spring admission, 12/1. Applications are processed on a rolling basis. *Application fee:* $50.

Advanced Placement Credit given for nursing courses completed elsewhere dependent upon specific evaluations.

Degree Requirements 50 total credit hours, thesis or project.

POST-MASTER'S PROGRAM

Areas of Study *Nurse practitioner programs in:* family health.

Southern Utah University
Department of Nursing
Cedar City, Utah

Founded in 1897

DEGREE • BSN

Nursing Program Faculty 11 (9% with doctorates).

Nursing Student Activities Nursing club.

Nursing Student Resources Academic advising; academic or career counseling; assistance for students with disabilities; bookstore; career placement assistance; computer lab; e-mail services; library services.

Library Facilities 180,424 volumes; 6,165 periodical subscriptions.

BACCALAUREATE PROGRAMS

Degree BSN

Available Programs Generic Baccalaureate; LPN to Baccalaureate; RN Baccalaureate.

Study Options Full-time.

Program Entrance Requirements Minimum overall college GPA of 3.0, transcript of college record, high school biology, high school chemistry, 2 years high school math, 2 years high school science, high school transcript, minimum GPA in nursing prerequisites of 3.0, prerequisite course work. Transfer students are accepted. **Standardized tests** *Required:* SAT or ACT, TOEFL for international students. **Application** *Deadline:* 8/1 (freshmen), rolling (transfer). *Notification:* continuous (freshmen). *Application fee:* $35.

Expenses (2006–07) *Tuition, state resident:* full-time $3060. *Tuition, nonresident:* full-time $10,098. *Required fees:* full-time $505.

Contact Vikki Robertson, Department Secretary, Department of Nursing, Southern Utah University, 351 West University Boulevard-GC 005, Cedar City, UT 84720. *Telephone:* 435-586-1906. *E-mail:* robertsonv@suu.edu.

University of Phoenix–Utah Campus
College of Health and Human Services
Salt Lake City, Utah

Founded in 1984

DEGREES • BSN • MSN

Nursing Program Faculty 51 (26% with doctorates).

Baccalaureate Enrollment 88
Women 81.82% **Men** 18.18% **Minority** 3.41%

Graduate Enrollment 23
Women 73.91% **Men** 26.09% **Minority** 25%

Nursing Student Activities Sigma Theta Tau.

Nursing Student Resources Academic advising; academic or career counseling; assistance for students with disabilities; bookstore; computer lab; library services.

Library Facilities 444 volumes; 666 periodical subscriptions.

BACCALAUREATE PROGRAMS

Degree BSN

Available Programs Accelerated Baccalaureate.

Site Options Provo, UT; St. George, UT; Clearfield, UT.

Study Options Full-time.

Program Entrance Requirements Transcript of college record, 1 letter of recommendation, RN licensure. Transfer students are accepted. **Standardized tests** *Required:* TOEFL for international students. **Application** *Deadline:* rolling (freshmen), rolling (transfer). *Application fee:* $110.

Advanced Placement Credit by examination available. Credit given for nursing courses completed elsewhere dependent upon specific evaluations.

Expenses (2006–07) *Tuition:* full-time $10,200. *International tuition:* $10,200 full-time. *Required fees:* full-time $750.

Contact Campus College Chair, Nursing, College of Health and Human Services, University of Phoenix–Utah Campus, 5573 South Green Street, Salt Lake City, UT 84123-4617. *Telephone:* 801-263-1444.

GRADUATE PROGRAMS

Expenses (2006–07) *Tuition:* full-time $9576. *International tuition:* $9576 full-time. *Required fees:* full-time $760.

Contact Campus College Chair, Nursing, College of Health and Human Services, University of Phoenix–Utah Campus, 5573 South Green Street, Salt Lake City, UT 84123-4617. *Telephone:* 801-263-1444.

MASTER'S DEGREE PROGRAM

Degree MSN

Available Programs Master's.

Concentrations Available Nursing administration; nursing education.

Site Options Provo, UT; St. George, UT; Clearfield, UT.

Study Options Full-time.

Program Entrance Requirements Clinical experience, computer literacy, minimum overall college GPA of 2.5, transcript of college record.

Degree Requirements 39 total credit hours, thesis or project.

University of Utah
College of Nursing
Salt Lake City, Utah

http://www.nurs.utah.edu

Founded in 1850

DEGREES • BS • MS • PHD

Nursing Program Faculty 83 (47% with doctorates).

Baccalaureate Enrollment 342
Women 87% **Men** 13% **Minority** 9% **International** 1% **Part-time** 16%

Graduate Enrollment 200
Women 88% **Men** 12% **Minority** 88% **International** 9% **Part-time** 58%

Nursing Student Activities Sigma Theta Tau, Student Nurses' Association.

Nursing Student Resources Academic advising; academic or career counseling; assistance for students with disabilities; bookstore; campus computer network; computer lab; computer-assisted instruction; e-mail services; externships; interactive nursing skills videos; Internet; learning resource lab; library services; nursing audiovisuals; paid internships; resume preparation assistance; skills, simulation, or other laboratory; unpaid internships.

Library Facilities 6.2 million volumes (22,000 in health, 8,000 in nursing); 33,517 periodical subscriptions (2,050 health-care related).

BACCALAUREATE PROGRAMS

Degree BS

Available Programs Generic Baccalaureate; RN Baccalaureate.

Study Options Full-time.

University of Utah (continued)

Program Entrance Requirements Minimum overall college GPA of 2.8, transcript of college record, CPR certification, written essay, health exam, immunizations, 3 letters of recommendation, minimum GPA in nursing prerequisites of 2.8, professional liability insurance/malpractice insurance, prerequisite course work. Transfer students are accepted. **Standardized tests** *Required:* SAT or ACT, TOEFL for international students. *Recommended:* ACT. **Application** *Deadline:* 4/1 (freshmen), 4/1 (transfer). *Application fee:* $35.

Advanced Placement Credit by examination available. Credit given for nursing courses completed elsewhere dependent upon specific evaluations.

Contact *Telephone:* 801-581-3414. *Fax:* 801-581-4642.

GRADUATE PROGRAMS

Contact *Telephone:* 801-581-3414. *Fax:* 801-581-4642.

MASTER'S DEGREE PROGRAM

Degree MS

Concentrations Available Nurse-midwifery; nursing administration; nursing education; nursing informatics. *Clinical nurse specialist programs in:* acute care, adult health, community health, oncology. *Nurse practitioner programs in:* acute care, adult health, family health, gerontology, neonatal health, oncology, pediatric, psychiatric/mental health, women's health.

Study Options Full-time and part-time.

Program Entrance Requirements Computer literacy, minimum overall college GPA of 3.0, transcript of college record, CPR certification, written essay, immunizations, 3 letters of recommendation, professional liability insurance/malpractice insurance, resume, statistics course, GRE General Test. *Application deadline:* For fall admission, 4/1; for spring admission, 11/1. Applications are processed on a rolling basis. *Application fee:* $45 ($65 for international students).

Advanced Placement Credit given for nursing courses completed elsewhere dependent upon specific evaluations.

Degree Requirements 35 total credit hours, thesis or project, comprehensive exam.

POST-MASTER'S PROGRAM

Areas of Study *Clinical nurse specialist programs in:* acute care, adult health, community health, oncology. *Nurse practitioner programs in:* acute care, adult health, family health, gerontology, neonatal health, oncology, pediatric, psychiatric/mental health, women's health.

DOCTORAL DEGREE PROGRAM

Degree PhD

Available Programs Doctorate.

Areas of Study Aging, clinical practice, faculty preparation, gerontology, health promotion/disease prevention, health-care systems, individualized study, information systems, nursing administration, nursing education, nursing policy, nursing research, oncology, women's health.

Program Entrance Requirements Minimum overall college GPA of 3.3, interview by faculty committee, interview, 3 letters of recommendation, MSN or equivalent, vita, writing sample, GRE General Test. *Application deadline:* For fall admission, 4/1; for spring admission, 11/1. Applications are processed on a rolling basis. *Application fee:* $45 ($65 for international students).

Degree Requirements 80 total credit hours, dissertation, oral exam, residency.

POSTDOCTORAL PROGRAM

Areas of Study Gerontology, information systems, nursing informatics, nursing interventions, outcomes.

Postdoctoral Program Contact *Telephone:* 801-585-9609. *Fax:* 801-581-4642.

Utah Valley State College

Department of Nursing
Orem, Utah

http://www.uvsc.edu/nurs/

Founded in 1941

DEGREE • BSN

Nursing Program Faculty 22 (25% with doctorates).

Baccalaureate Enrollment 100
Women 60% **Men** 40% **Part-time** 99%

Nursing Student Activities Student Nurses' Association.

Nursing Student Resources Academic advising; academic or career counseling; assistance for students with disabilities; bookstore; campus computer network; career placement assistance; computer lab; computer-assisted instruction; daycare for children of students; e-mail services; employment services for current students; interactive nursing skills videos; Internet; learning resource lab; library services; nursing audiovisuals; resume preparation assistance; skills, simulation, or other laboratory; tutoring; unpaid internships.

Library Facilities 173,000 volumes (4,640 in health, 361 in nursing); 6,000 periodical subscriptions (200 health-care related).

BACCALAUREATE PROGRAMS

Degree BSN

Available Programs ADN to Baccalaureate.

Study Options Part-time.

Program Entrance Requirements CPR certification, health exam, health insurance, immunizations, minimum GPA in nursing prerequisites of 2.5, prerequisite course work, RN licensure. Transfer students are accepted. **Standardized tests** *Required:* SAT or ACT, TOEFL for international students, or in-house tests. **Application** *Deadline:* 8/15 (freshmen), 8/15 (transfer). *Notification:* continuous (freshmen). *Application fee:* $30.

Advanced Placement Credit by examination available.

Expenses (2006–07) *Tuition, area resident:* full-time $1406; part-time $207 per credit hour. *Tuition, nonresident:* full-time $4921; part-time $721 per credit hour. *International tuition:* $4921 full-time. *Required fees:* full-time $300; part-time $80 per credit.

Financial Aid 10% of baccalaureate students in nursing programs received some form of financial aid in 2005–06. *Gift aid (need-based):* Federal Pell, FSEOG, state, private, college/university gift aid from institutional funds. *Loans:* FFEL (Subsidized and Unsubsidized Stafford PLUS), Perkins, college/university. *Work-Study:* Federal Work-Study. *Application deadline (priority):* 6/1.

Contact Mrs. Lynnae Marsing, Academic Advisor, Department of Nursing, Utah Valley State College, MS 172, 800 West University Parkway, Orem, UT 84058. *Telephone:* 801-863-8199. *Fax:* 801-863-6093. *E-mail:* marsinly@uvsc.edu.

Weber State University

Program in Nursing
Ogden, Utah

Founded in 1889

DEGREE • BSN

Nursing Program Faculty 42 (5% with doctorates).

Baccalaureate Enrollment 250
Women 85% **Men** 15% **Minority** 4% **International** 1% **Part-time** 7%

Nursing Student Activities Sigma Theta Tau, Student Nurses' Association.

Nursing Student Resources Academic advising; academic or career counseling; assistance for students with disabilities; bookstore; campus computer network; career placement assistance; computer lab; computer-assisted instruction; daycare for children of students; e-mail services; employment services for current students; housing assistance; interactive nursing skills videos; Internet; learning resource lab; library services; nursing audiovisuals; placement services for program completers; resume preparation assistance; skills, simulation, or other laboratory; tutoring; unpaid internships.

Library Facilities 734,487 volumes (800 in health, 800 in nursing); 120 periodical subscriptions health-care related.

BACCALAUREATE PROGRAMS

Degree BSN

Available Programs ADN to Baccalaureate.

Site Options *Distance Learning:* South Central, UT; Logan, UT; Central Rotating, UT.

Study Options Full-time and part-time.

Program Entrance Requirements Minimum overall college GPA of 3.0, transcript of college record, CPR certification, written essay, immunizations, minimum GPA in nursing prerequisites of 2.0, prerequisite course work, RN licensure. Transfer students are accepted. **Standardized tests** *Recommended:* TOEFL for international students. *Required for some:* SAT or ACT. **Application** *Deadline:* 8/22 (freshmen), rolling (transfer). *Notification:* continuous (freshmen). *Application fee:* $30.

Advanced Placement Credit by examination available. Credit given for nursing courses completed elsewhere dependent upon specific evaluations.

Expenses (2006–07) *Tuition, state resident:* full-time $2800; part-time $251 per credit. *Tuition, nonresident:* full-time $9776; part-time $880 per credit. *International tuition:* $10,417 full-time. *Required fees:* full-time $642; part-time $83 per credit; part-time $201 per term.

Financial Aid 5% of baccalaureate students in nursing programs received some form of financial aid in 2005–06.

Contact Doug Watson, Academic Admissions Advisor, Program in Nursing, Weber State University, 3907 University Circle, Ogden, UT 84408-3907. *Telephone:* 801-626-6128. *Fax:* 801-626-6382. *E-mail:* dwatson@weber.edu.

Westminster College
School of Nursing and Health Sciences
Salt Lake City, Utah

http://www.westminstercollege.edu

Founded in 1875

DEGREES • BSN • MSN

Nursing Student Activities Sigma Theta Tau, Student Nurses' Association, nursing club.

Nursing Student Resources Academic advising; academic or career counseling; assistance for students with disabilities; bookstore; campus computer network; career placement assistance; computer lab; computer-assisted instruction; e-mail services; employment services for current students; housing assistance; interactive nursing skills videos; Internet; learning resource lab; library services; nursing audiovisuals; placement services for program completers; remedial services; resume preparation assistance; skills, simulation, or other laboratory; tutoring.

Library Facilities 154,069 volumes; 695 periodical subscriptions.

BACCALAUREATE PROGRAMS

Degree BSN

Available Programs Baccalaureate for Second Degree; Generic Baccalaureate; RN Baccalaureate.

Study Options Full-time.

Program Entrance Requirements Transcript of college record, written essay, 3 letters of recommendation, minimum GPA in nursing prerequisites of 2.5, prerequisite course work. Transfer students are accepted. **Standardized tests** *Required:* SAT or ACT, TOEFL for international students. **Application** *Deadline:* rolling (freshmen), rolling (out-of-state freshmen), rolling (transfer). *Notification:* continuous (freshmen), continuous (out-of-state freshmen). *Application fee:* $40.

Contact Department of Nursing, School of Nursing and Health Sciences, Westminster College, 1840 South 1300 East, Salt Lake City, UT 84105. *Telephone:* 801-832-2150. *Fax:* 801-832-3110.

GRADUATE PROGRAMS

Financial Aid Career-related internships or fieldwork and tuition remissions available.

Contact Department of Nursing, School of Nursing and Health Sciences, Westminster College, 1840 South 1300 East, Salt Lake City, UT 84105. *Telephone:* 801-832-2150. *Fax:* 801-832-3110.

MASTER'S DEGREE PROGRAM

Degree MSN

Available Programs Master's.

Concentrations Available Nursing education. *Nurse practitioner programs in:* family health.

Program Entrance Requirements Transcript of college record, written essay, 3 letters of recommendation, resume. *Application deadline:* For fall admission, 8/1 (priority date). Applications are processed on a rolling basis. *Application fee:* $40.

Advanced Placement Credit given for nursing courses completed elsewhere dependent upon specific evaluations.

Degree Requirements 42 total credit hours, thesis or project.

POST-MASTER'S PROGRAM

Areas of Study *Nurse practitioner programs in:* family health.

VERMONT

Norwich University
Division of Nursing
Northfield, Vermont

http://www.norwich.edu/acad/nursing

Founded in 1819

DEGREE • BSN

Nursing Program Faculty 8 (10% with doctorates).

Baccalaureate Enrollment 90
Women 90% **Men** 10% **Minority** 10% **Part-time** 20%

Nursing Student Activities Student Nurses' Association, nursing club.

Nursing Student Resources Academic advising; academic or career counseling; assistance for students with disabilities; bookstore; campus computer network; career placement assistance; computer lab; e-mail services; employment services for current students; externships; housing assistance; interactive nursing skills videos; Internet; learning resource lab; library services; nursing audiovisuals; placement services for program completers; remedial services; resume preparation assistance; skills, simulation, or other laboratory; tutoring; unpaid internships.

Library Facilities 280,000 volumes; 904 periodical subscriptions.

BACCALAUREATE PROGRAMS

Degree BSN

Available Programs ADN to Baccalaureate; Generic Baccalaureate; RN Baccalaureate.

Site Options Rutland, VT.

Study Options Full-time and part-time.

Program Entrance Requirements Minimum overall college GPA of 2.5, transcript of college record, CPR certification, written essay, health exam, health insurance, high school biology, high school chemistry, 2 years high school math, 2 years high school science, high school transcript, immunizations, interview, 2 letters of recommendation, minimum GPA in nursing prerequisites of 2.5. Transfer students are accepted. **Standardized tests** *Required:* SAT or ACT, TOEFL for international students. *Recommended:* SAT Subject Tests. **Application** *Deadline:* rolling (freshmen), rolling (transfer). *Early decision:* 11/15. *Notification:* continuous (freshmen), 12/15 (out-of-state freshmen), 12/15 (early decision). *Application fee:* $35.

Advanced Placement Credit given for nursing courses completed elsewhere dependent upon specific evaluations.

Contact *Telephone:* 802-485-2008. *Fax:* 802-485-2032.

Southern Vermont College
Department of Nursing
Bennington, Vermont

http://www.svc.edu/academics/divisions/nursing.html

Founded in 1926

DEGREE • BSN

Nursing Program Faculty 6.

Library Facilities 26,000 volumes; 250 periodical subscriptions.

BACCALAUREATE PROGRAMS

Degree BSN

Available Programs ADN to Baccalaureate; RN Baccalaureate.

Program Entrance Requirements Standardized tests *Required:* SAT or ACT, TOEFL for international students. **Application** *Deadline:* rolling (freshmen), rolling (transfer). *Notification:* continuous (freshmen). *Application fee:* $30.

Advanced Placement Credit by examination available.

Contact *Telephone:* 802-447-4656. *Fax:* 802-447-4652.

University of Vermont
Department of Nursing
Burlington, Vermont

Founded in 1791

DEGREES • BS • MS

Nursing Program Faculty 34 (41% with doctorates).

Baccalaureate Enrollment 345
Women 92% **Men** 8% **Minority** 3% **Part-time** 5%

Graduate Enrollment 47
Women 100% **Minority** 4% **Part-time** 66%

Nursing Student Activities Nursing Honor Society, Sigma Theta Tau, Student Nurses' Association.

Nursing Student Resources Academic advising; academic or career counseling; assistance for students with disabilities; bookstore; campus computer network; computer lab; computer-assisted instruction; e-mail services; employment services for current students; interactive nursing skills videos; Internet; learning resource lab; library services; nursing audiovisuals; remedial services; resume preparation assistance; skills, simulation, or other laboratory; tutoring.

Library Facilities 2.4 million volumes (1,250 in health, 1,250 in nursing); 20,216 periodical subscriptions (1,492 health-care related).

■ The University of Vermont offers traditional baccalaureate, RN-B.S.-M.S., master's, and post-master's programs in nursing. A Master's Entry Program in nursing is offered for non-nurses who hold a bachelor's degree in another field. The master's program prepares RNs for advanced practice nursing in the areas of community health, primary care (adult or family nurse practitioner), psychiatric–mental health, and clinical systems management. Students completing the master's program are eligible for specialty certification. Nurses with a bachelor's degree in a field other than nursing are eligible to apply to the master's program through a bridge process. Further information can be found on the Web at http://www.uvm.edu/nursing.

BACCALAUREATE PROGRAMS

Degree BS

Available Programs Accelerated RN Baccalaureate; Generic Baccalaureate; RN Baccalaureate.

Study Options Full-time and part-time.

Program Entrance Requirements Minimum overall college GPA of 3.0, transcript of college record, written essay, health insurance, high school biology, high school chemistry, high school foreign language, 3 years high school math, 2 years high school science, high school transcript, immunizations, letters of recommendation, minimum GPA in nursing prerequisites of 2.0. Transfer students are accepted. **Standardized tests** *Required:* SAT or ACT, TOEFL for international students. **Application** *Deadline:* 1/15 (freshmen), 4/1 (transfer). *Early decision:* 11/1. *Notification:* 3/31 (freshmen), 12/15 (early action). *Application fee:* $45.

Advanced Placement Credit by examination available. Credit given for nursing courses completed elsewhere dependent upon specific evaluations.

Expenses (2006–07) *Tuition, state resident:* full-time $9832; part-time $410 per credit hour. *Tuition, nonresident:* full-time $24,816; part-time $1034 per credit hour. *Room and board:* $7642 per academic year. *Required fees:* full-time $1492; part-time $10 per credit.

Financial Aid 87% of baccalaureate students in nursing programs received some form of financial aid in 2005–06.

Contact Ms. Tacy Lincoln, Director of Student Services, Department of Nursing, University of Vermont, Rowell Building, Room 106, Burlington, VT 05405-0068. *Telephone:* 802-656-0968. *E-mail:* tacy.lincoln@uvm.edu.

GRADUATE PROGRAMS

Expenses (2006–07) *Tuition, state resident:* part-time $410 per credit hour. *Tuition, nonresident:* part-time $1034 per credit hour. *Room and board:* $7642 per academic year. *Required fees:* part-time $10 per credit.

Financial Aid 30% of graduate students in nursing programs received some form of financial aid in 2005–06. *Application deadline:* 3/1.

Contact Dr. Gregg Newschwander, Chairman, Department of Nursing, University of Vermont, 216 Rowell Building, 106 Carrigan Drive, Burlington, VT 05405. *Telephone:* 802-656-3051. *Fax:* 802-656-8306. *E-mail:* newsch@uvm.edu.

MASTER'S DEGREE PROGRAM

Degree MS

Available Programs Master's; Master's for Non-Nursing College Graduates; Master's for Nurses with Non-Nursing Degrees; RN to Master's.

Concentrations Available Nursing administration. *Clinical nurse specialist programs in:* community health, psychiatric/mental health, public health. *Nurse practitioner programs in:* adult health, family health, psychiatric/mental health.

Study Options Full-time and part-time.

Program Entrance Requirements Minimum overall college GPA of 3.0, transcript of college record, written essay, 3 letters of recommendation, physical assessment course, statistics course, GRE General Test. *Application deadline:* For fall admission, 4/1 (priority date). Applications are processed on a rolling basis. *Application fee:* $40.

Advanced Placement Credit by examination available. Credit given for nursing courses completed elsewhere dependent upon specific evaluations.

Degree Requirements 57 total credit hours, thesis or project, comprehensive exam.

POST-MASTER'S PROGRAM

Areas of Study *Clinical nurse specialist programs in:* psychiatric/mental health. *Nurse practitioner programs in:* adult health, family health, psychiatric/mental health.

VIRGIN ISLANDS

University of the Virgin Islands
Division of Nursing
Saint Thomas, Virgin Islands

Founded in 1962

DEGREE • BS

Nursing Program Faculty 11 (54% with doctorates).

Baccalaureate Enrollment 51
Women 98.1% **Men** 1.9% **Minority** 88% **International** 17% **Part-time** 9%
Nursing Student Activities Student Nurses' Association.

Nursing Student Resources Academic advising; academic or career counseling; assistance for students with disabilities; bookstore; campus computer network; computer lab; computer-assisted instruction; e-mail services; employment services for current students; externships; housing assistance; interactive nursing skills videos; Internet; learning resource lab; library services; nursing audiovisuals; paid internships; skills, simulation, or other laboratory; tutoring.

Library Facilities 106,361 volumes (95,000 in health, 600 in nursing); 113,623 periodical subscriptions (15 health-care related).

BACCALAUREATE PROGRAMS

Degree BS

Available Programs Generic Baccalaureate; RN Baccalaureate.
Site Options St. Croix, VI.
Study Options Full-time and part-time.

Program Entrance Requirements Minimum overall college GPA of 2.0, CPR certification, health exam, 2 years high school math, high school transcript, immunizations, minimum GPA in nursing prerequisites of 2.0, professional liability insurance/malpractice insurance, prerequisite course work. Transfer students are accepted. **Standardized tests** *Required:* SAT or ACT, TOEFL for international students. **Application** *Deadline:* 4/30 (freshmen), 4/30 (transfer). *Notification:* continuous (freshmen). *Application fee:* $25.

Advanced Placement Credit given for nursing courses completed elsewhere dependent upon specific evaluations.

Expenses (2006–07) *Tuition, state resident:* full-time $3300; part-time $110 per credit. *Tuition, nonresident:* full-time $9900; part-time $330 per credit. *International tuition:* $9900 full-time. *Room and board:* $2675; room only: $1375 per academic year. *Required fees:* full-time $530; part-time $155 per term.

Financial Aid 76% of baccalaureate students in nursing programs received some form of financial aid in 2005–06. *Gift aid (need-based):* Federal Pell, FSEOG, state, college/university gift aid from institutional funds, Federal Nursing. *Loans:* Federal Direct (Subsidized and Unsubsidized Stafford PLUS), Perkins, college/university. *Work-Study:* Federal Work-Study, part-time campus jobs. *Application deadline (priority):* 3/1.

Contact Dr. Gloria B. Callwood, Associate Professor and Chair, Division of Nursing, University of the Virgin Islands, #2 John Brewer's Bay, St. Thomas, VI 00802-9990. *Telephone:* 340-693-1291. *Fax:* 340-693-1285. *E-mail:* gcallwo@uvi.edu.

CONTINUING EDUCATION PROGRAM

Contact Dr. Gloria B. Callwood, Associate Professor and Chair, Division of Nursing, University of the Virgin Islands, #2 John Brewer's Bay, St. Thomas, VI 00802-9990. *Telephone:* 340-693-1291. *Fax:* 340-693-1285. *E-mail:* gcallwo@uvi.edu.

VIRGINIA

Eastern Mennonite University
Department of Nursing
Harrisonburg, Virginia

Founded in 1917
DEGREE • BSN

Nursing Program Faculty 10 (20% with doctorates).
Baccalaureate Enrollment 126
Women 93% **Men** 7% **Minority** 3% **International** 7%
Nursing Student Activities Sigma Theta Tau, Student Nurses' Association.

Nursing Student Resources Academic advising; academic or career counseling; assistance for students with disabilities; bookstore; campus computer network; career placement assistance; computer lab; computer-assisted instruction; e-mail services; employment services for current students; externships; housing assistance; interactive nursing skills videos; Internet; learning resource lab; library services; nursing audiovisuals; placement services for program completers; remedial services; resume preparation assistance; skills, simulation, or other laboratory; tutoring.

Library Facilities 169,785 volumes (1,256 in health, 926 in nursing); 1,033 periodical subscriptions (33 health-care related).

BACCALAUREATE PROGRAMS

Degree BSN

Available Programs ADN to Baccalaureate; Baccalaureate for Second Degree; Generic Baccalaureate; LPN to Baccalaureate.
Site Options Lancaster, PA.
Study Options Full-time and part-time.

Program Entrance Requirements Minimum overall college GPA of 2.6, transcript of college record, CPR certification, written essay, health exam, health insurance, high school chemistry, high school transcript, immunizations, 3 letters of recommendation, minimum high school GPA of 2.0, minimum GPA in nursing prerequisites of 2.6, professional liability insurance/malpractice insurance, prerequisite course work. Transfer students are accepted. **Standardized tests** *Required:* SAT or ACT, TOEFL for international students. **Application** *Deadline:* rolling (freshmen), rolling (out-of-state freshmen), 8/15 (transfer). *Notification:* continuous (freshmen), continuous (out-of-state freshmen). *Application fee:* $25.

Advanced Placement Credit given for nursing courses completed elsewhere dependent upon specific evaluations.

Contact *Telephone:* 800-368-2665. *Fax:* 540-432-4444.

George Mason University
College of Nursing and Health Science
Fairfax, Virginia

http://cnhs.gmu.edu/
Founded in 1957
DEGREES • BSN • MSN • MSN/MBA • PHD

Nursing Program Faculty 39.
Nursing Student Activities Nursing Honor Society, Sigma Theta Tau, Student Nurses' Association.
Nursing Student Resources E-mail services; skills, simulation, or other laboratory.
Library Facilities 1.5 million volumes (16,172 in nursing); 27,708 periodical subscriptions (200 health-care related).

BACCALAUREATE PROGRAMS

Degree BSN

Available Programs Accelerated Baccalaureate for Second Degree; Accelerated LPN to Baccalaureate; Accelerated RN Baccalaureate; Generic Baccalaureate.
Study Options Full-time and part-time.

Program Entrance Requirements Minimum overall college GPA of 3.0, CPR certification, health exam, health insurance, immunizations, minimum GPA in nursing prerequisites, prerequisite course work. Transfer students are accepted. **Standardized tests** *Required:* SAT or ACT, TOEFL for international students. **Application** *Deadline:* 1/15 (freshmen), 3/15 (transfer). *Notification:* 4/1 (freshmen). *Application fee:* $60.

Contact *Telephone:* 703-993-1904. *Fax:* 703-993-3606.

GRADUATE PROGRAMS

Contact *Telephone:* 703-993-1947. *Fax:* 703-993-1949.

MASTER'S DEGREE PROGRAM

Degrees MSN; MSN/MBA
Available Programs Master's; RN to Master's.
Concentrations Available Nursing administration. *Nurse practitioner programs in:* adult health, family health, gerontology, primary care.

George Mason University (continued)
Study Options Full-time and part-time.
Program Entrance Requirements Clinical experience, minimum overall college GPA of 3.0, CPR certification, written essay, immunizations, 3 letters of recommendation, physical assessment course, statistics course. *Application deadline:* For fall admission, 5/1; for spring admission, 11/1.

POST-MASTER'S PROGRAM
Areas of Study Nursing administration; nursing education.

DOCTORAL DEGREE PROGRAM
Degree PhD
Available Programs Doctorate.
Areas of Study Nursing administration.
Program Entrance Requirements Clinical experience, minimum overall college GPA of 3.25, interview, 3 letters of recommendation, MSN or equivalent, statistics course, writing sample, MAT. *Application deadline:* For fall admission, 5/1; for spring admission, 11/1.
Degree Requirements 60 total credit hours, dissertation, oral exam, written exam.

POSTDOCTORAL PROGRAM
Postdoctoral Program Contact *Telephone:* 703-993-1944. *Fax:* 703-993-1942.

CONTINUING EDUCATION PROGRAM
Contact *Telephone:* 703-993-1910. *Fax:* 703-993-3612.

Hampton University
Department of Nursing
Hampton, Virginia

http://www.hamptonu.edu/nursing/Index.htm
Founded in 1868
DEGREES • BS • MS • PHD

Nursing Program Faculty 35 (51% with doctorates).
Baccalaureate Enrollment 388
Women 91% **Men** 9% **Minority** 97% **International** 3% **Part-time** 3%
Graduate Enrollment 72
Women 86% **Men** 14% **Minority** 58% **Part-time** 35%
Nursing Student Activities Nursing Honor Society, Sigma Theta Tau, Student Nurses' Association.
Nursing Student Resources Academic advising; bookstore; computer lab; e-mail services; interactive nursing skills videos; Internet; library services; tutoring.
Library Facilities 336,092 volumes (4,000 in health, 2,000 in nursing); 1,414 periodical subscriptions (500 health-care related).

BACCALAUREATE PROGRAMS
Degree BS
Available Programs ADN to Baccalaureate; Accelerated Baccalaureate; Accelerated RN Baccalaureate; Baccalaureate for Second Degree; Generic Baccalaureate; LPN to Baccalaureate; LPN to RN Baccalaureate; RN Baccalaureate.
Site Options Virginia Beach, VA.
Study Options Full-time and part-time.
Program Entrance Requirements Minimum overall college GPA of 2.3, transcript of college record, CPR certification, written essay, health exam, health insurance, high school biology, high school chemistry, 3 years high school math, 2 years high school science, high school transcript, immunizations, 2 letters of recommendation, minimum high school GPA of 2.0, minimum high school rank 50%, minimum GPA in nursing prerequisites of 2.0, professional liability insurance/malpractice insurance. Transfer students are accepted. **Standardized tests** *Required:* SAT or ACT, TOEFL for international students. **Application** *Deadline:* 3/1 (freshmen). *Notification:* continuous until 7/31 (freshmen). *Application fee:* $25.

Advanced Placement Credit by examination available. Credit given for nursing courses completed elsewhere dependent upon specific evaluations.
Contact *Telephone:* 757-727-5251. *Fax:* 757-727-5423.

GRADUATE PROGRAMS
Contact *Telephone:* 757-727-5251. *Fax:* 757-727-5423.

MASTER'S DEGREE PROGRAM
Degree MS
Available Programs Master's.
Concentrations Available Nursing administration; nursing education. *Clinical nurse specialist programs in:* adult health, community health, psychiatric/mental health. *Nurse practitioner programs in:* family health, gerontology, pediatric, women's health.
Study Options Full-time and part-time.
Program Entrance Requirements Clinical experience, minimum overall college GPA of 2.5, transcript of college record, CPR certification, immunizations, interview, 2 letters of recommendation, nursing research course, physical assessment course, professional liability insurance/malpractice insurance, prerequisite course work, resume, statistics course, GRE General Test. *Application deadline:* For fall admission, 6/1 (priority date); for spring admission, 11/1. Applications are processed on a rolling basis. *Application fee:* $25.
Advanced Placement Credit given for nursing courses completed elsewhere dependent upon specific evaluations.
Degree Requirements 45 total credit hours, thesis or project, comprehensive exam.

POST-MASTER'S PROGRAM
Areas of Study *Nurse practitioner programs in:* family health.

DOCTORAL DEGREE PROGRAM
Degree PhD
Available Programs Doctorate.
Areas of Study Family health.
Program Entrance Requirements Clinical experience, minimum overall college GPA of 3.5, interview, 2 letters of recommendation, MSN or equivalent, scholarly papers, statistics course, vita, writing sample. *Application deadline:* For fall admission, 6/1 (priority date); for spring admission, 11/1. Applications are processed on a rolling basis. *Application fee:* $25.
Degree Requirements 48 total credit hours, dissertation, oral exam, written exam, residency.

James Madison University
Department of Nursing
Harrisonburg, Virginia

http://www.nursing.jmu.edu
Founded in 1908
DEGREES • BSN • MSN

Nursing Program Faculty 22 (36% with doctorates).
Baccalaureate Enrollment 601
Women 96% **Men** 4% **Minority** 6% **Part-time** 1%
Graduate Enrollment 20
Women 90% **Men** 10% **Part-time** 45%
Nursing Student Activities Nursing Honor Society, Sigma Theta Tau, Student Nurses' Association.
Nursing Student Resources Academic advising; academic or career counseling; assistance for students with disabilities; bookstore; campus computer network; career placement assistance; computer lab; computer-assisted instruction; e-mail services; employment services for current students; externships; interactive nursing skills videos; Internet; learning resource lab; library services; nursing audiovisuals; paid internships; remedial services; resume preparation assistance; skills, simulation, or other laboratory; unpaid internships.
Library Facilities 659,136 volumes (67,716 in health, 12,054 in nursing); 15,909 periodical subscriptions (565 health-care related).

BACCALAUREATE PROGRAMS

Degree BSN

Available Programs Accelerated RN Baccalaureate; Generic Baccalaureate.

Site Options Waynesboro, VA; Staunton, VA; Charlottesville, VA.

Study Options Full-time and part-time.

Program Entrance Requirements Minimum overall college GPA of 2.7, transcript of college record, CPR certification, written essay, health exam, health insurance, immunizations, minimum GPA in nursing prerequisites of 2.0, prerequisite course work. Transfer students are accepted. **Standardized tests** *Required:* SAT or ACT, TOEFL for international students. **Application** *Deadline:* 1/15 (freshmen), 3/1 (transfer). *Early decision:* 11/1. *Notification:* 4/1 (freshmen), 1/15 (early action). *Application fee:* $40.

Advanced Placement Credit given for nursing courses completed elsewhere dependent upon specific evaluations.

Expenses (2006–07) *Tuition, state resident:* full-time $6290; part-time $208 per credit. *Tuition, nonresident:* full-time $16,236; part-time $540 per credit. *Room and board:* $3500; room only: $2000 per academic year. *Required fees:* full-time $1100; part-time $36 per credit; part-time $550 per term.

Financial Aid 35% of baccalaureate students in nursing programs received some form of financial aid in 2005–06. *Gift aid (need-based):* Federal Pell, FSEOG, state, private, college/university gift aid from institutional funds. *Loans:* FFEL (Subsidized and Unsubsidized Stafford PLUS), Perkins. *Work-Study:* Federal Work-Study, part-time campus jobs. *Application deadline (priority):* 3/1.

Contact Ms. Stephanie Shifflett, Administrative Office Specialist III, Department of Nursing, James Madison University, 701 Carrier Drive, MSC 4305, Harrisonburg, VA 22807. *Telephone:* 540-568-6314. *Fax:* 540-568-7896. *E-mail:* shiff2sd@jmu.edu.

GRADUATE PROGRAMS

Expenses (2006–07) *Tuition, state resident:* full-time $2376; part-time $264 per credit hour. *Tuition, nonresident:* full-time $6687; part-time $743 per credit hour. *Required fees:* full-time $500; part-time $55 per credit; part-time $250 per term.

Financial Aid 90% of graduate students in nursing programs received some form of financial aid in 2005–06.

Contact Ms. Stephanie Shifflett, Administrative Office Specialist III, Department of Nursing, James Madison University, 701 Carrier Drive, MSC 4305, Harrisonburg, VA 22807. *Telephone:* 540-568-6314. *Fax:* 540-568-7896. *E-mail:* shiff2sd@jmu.edu.

MASTER'S DEGREE PROGRAM

Degree MSN

Available Programs Accelerated AD/RN to Master's; Accelerated RN to Master's; Master's.

Concentrations Available Nursing education. *Nurse practitioner programs in:* adult health, gerontology.

Site Options Waynesboro, VA; Charlottesville, VA.

Study Options Full-time and part-time.

Program Entrance Requirements Clinical experience, computer literacy, minimum overall college GPA of 2.0, transcript of college record, CPR certification, written essay, immunizations, 2 letters of recommendation, physical assessment course, prerequisite course work, resume, statistics course.

Advanced Placement Credit given for nursing courses completed elsewhere dependent upon specific evaluations.

Degree Requirements 47 total credit hours, thesis or project.

POST-MASTER'S PROGRAM

Areas of Study Nursing education. *Nurse practitioner programs in:* adult health, gerontology.

Jefferson College of Health Sciences
Nursing Education Program
Roanoke, Virginia

http://www.jchs.edu

Founded in 1982

DEGREES • BSN • MSN

Nursing Program Faculty 18 (11% with doctorates).

Baccalaureate Enrollment 70
Women 90% **Men** 10% **Minority** 10% **Part-time** 90%

Graduate Enrollment 31
Women 99% **Men** 1% **Minority** 1%

Nursing Student Activities Nursing Honor Society, Student Nurses' Association.

Nursing Student Resources Academic advising; academic or career counseling; assistance for students with disabilities; bookstore; campus computer network; computer lab; computer-assisted instruction; e-mail services; externships; housing assistance; interactive nursing skills videos; Internet; learning resource lab; library services; nursing audiovisuals; skills, simulation, or other laboratory; tutoring.

Library Facilities 10,533 volumes (4,910 in health, 804 in nursing); 376 periodical subscriptions (274 health-care related).

BACCALAUREATE PROGRAMS

Degree BSN

Available Programs ADN to Baccalaureate; Generic Baccalaureate; RN Baccalaureate.

Site Options *Distance Learning:* Roanoke, VA.

Study Options Full-time and part-time.

Program Entrance Requirements Minimum overall college GPA of 2.0, transcript of college record, CPR certification, health exam, health insurance, high school biology, high school chemistry, 2 years high school math, 2 years high school science, high school transcript, immunizations, minimum high school GPA of 2.0, prerequisite course work. Transfer students are accepted. **Standardized tests** *Required:* TOEFL for international students. *Recommended:* SAT. *Required for some:* SAT or ACT, ACT ASSET. **Application** *Deadline:* 7/31 (freshmen). *Early decision:* 10/15. *Notification:* continuous until 7/31 (freshmen), 12/1 (out-of-state freshmen), 12/1 (early decision). *Application fee:* $50.

Advanced Placement Credit by examination available. Credit given for nursing courses completed elsewhere dependent upon specific evaluations.

Expenses (2006–07) *Tuition:* full-time $13,860; part-time $400 per credit hour. *Room and board:* room only: $1800 per academic year.

Financial Aid 97% of baccalaureate students in nursing programs received some form of financial aid in 2005–06. *Gift aid (need-based):* Federal Pell, FSEOG, state, private, college/university gift aid from institutional funds. *Loans:* FFEL (Subsidized and Unsubsidized Stafford PLUS), alternative loans. *Work-Study:* Federal Work-Study. *Application deadline (priority):* 3/1.

Contact Ms. Judith McKeon, Director of Admissions, Nursing Education Program, Jefferson College of Health Sciences, PO Box 13186, Roanoke, VA 24031-3186. *Telephone:* 540-985-9083. *Fax:* 540-224-6703. *E-mail:* jmckeon@jchs.edu.

GRADUATE PROGRAMS

Expenses (2006–07) *Tuition:* part-time $430 per credit hour.

Financial Aid 100% of graduate students in nursing programs received some form of financial aid in 2005–06.

Contact Ms. Judith McKeon, Director of Admissions, Nursing Education Program, Jefferson College of Health Sciences, PO Box 13186, Roanoke, VA 24031-3186. *Telephone:* 540-985-9083. *Fax:* 540-224-6703. *E-mail:* jmckeon@jchs.edu.

MASTER'S DEGREE PROGRAM

Degree MSN

Available Programs Master's; Master's for Nurses with Non-Nursing Degrees.

Jefferson College of Health Sciences (continued)

Concentrations Available Nursing administration; nursing education.

Site Options *Distance Learning:* Roanoke, VA.

Study Options Full-time.

Program Entrance Requirements Clinical experience, computer literacy, transcript of college record, 2 letters of recommendation, nursing research course, resume, statistics course.

Degree Requirements 37 total credit hours, thesis or project.

CONTINUING EDUCATION PROGRAM

Contact Ms. Judy Cusumano, Chair of Department of Arts and Sciences, Nursing Education Program, Jefferson College of Health Sciences, PO Box 13186, Roanoke, VA 24031-3186. *Telephone:* 540-767-6072. *E-mail:* jcusumamo@jchs.edu.

Liberty University
Department of Nursing
Lynchburg, Virginia

http://www.liberty.edu

Founded in 1971

DEGREES • BSN • MSN

Nursing Program Faculty 16 (38% with doctorates).

Baccalaureate Enrollment 236
Women 85% **Men** 15% **Minority** 4% **International** 10% **Part-time** 6%

Graduate Enrollment 24
Women 95% **Men** 5% **Part-time** 60%

Nursing Student Activities Student Nurses' Association.

Nursing Student Resources Academic advising; academic or career counseling; assistance for students with disabilities; bookstore; campus computer network; computer lab; e-mail services; interactive nursing skills videos; Internet; learning resource lab; library services; nursing audiovisuals; resume preparation assistance; skills, simulation, or other laboratory; tutoring.

Library Facilities 199,150 volumes (3,632 in health, 3,000 in nursing); 12,426 periodical subscriptions (46 health-care related).

BACCALAUREATE PROGRAMS

Degree BSN

Available Programs Generic Baccalaureate; RN Baccalaureate.

Study Options Full-time and part-time.

Program Entrance Requirements Minimum overall college GPA of 3.0, transcript of college record, CPR certification, written essay, immunizations, 2 letters of recommendation, minimum GPA in nursing prerequisites of 3.0, professional liability insurance/malpractice insurance, prerequisite course work. Transfer students are accepted. **Standardized tests** *Required:* SAT or ACT, TOEFL for international students. **Application** *Deadline:* 6/30 (freshmen). *Notification:* continuous until 8/15 (freshmen). *Application fee:* $35.

Advanced Placement Credit given for nursing courses completed elsewhere dependent upon specific evaluations.

Expenses (2005–06) *Tuition:* full-time $13,700; part-time $457 per credit hour. *Room and board:* $5400 per academic year. *Required fees:* full-time $850.

Financial Aid 75% of baccalaureate students in nursing programs received some form of financial aid in 2004–05.

Contact Dr. Deanna Britt, Chair, Department of Nursing, Liberty University, 1971 University Boulevard, Lynchburg, VA 24502. *Telephone:* 804-582-2519. *Fax:* 804-582-7035. *E-mail:* dbritt@liberty.edu.

GRADUATE PROGRAMS

Expenses (2005–06) *Tuition:* part-time $339 per credit hour. *Required fees:* part-time $425 per term.

Financial Aid 65% of graduate students in nursing programs received some form of financial aid in 2004–05.

Contact Dr. Hila Spear, Director of Master Program, Department of Nursing, Liberty University, Lynchburg, VA 24502. *Telephone:* 804-582-2519. *E-mail:* hspear@liberty.edu.

MASTER'S DEGREE PROGRAM

Degree MSN

Available Programs Master's.

Concentrations Available *Clinical nurse specialist programs in:* acute care, community health.

Study Options Full-time and part-time.

Program Entrance Requirements Clinical experience, minimum overall college GPA of 3.0, transcript of college record, CPR certification, written essay, immunizations, interview, 3 letters of recommendation, nursing research course, physical assessment course, prerequisite course work, resume, statistics course.

Degree Requirements 36 total credit hours, thesis or project.

Lynchburg College
School of Health Sciences and Human Performance
Lynchburg, Virginia

http://www.lynchburg.edu/schools/NRSG.htm

Founded in 1903

DEGREE • BS

Nursing Program Faculty 13 (23% with doctorates).

Baccalaureate Enrollment 152
Women 85% **Men** 15% **Minority** 10%

Nursing Student Activities Sigma Theta Tau, Student Nurses' Association.

Nursing Student Resources Academic advising; academic or career counseling; assistance for students with disabilities; bookstore; campus computer network; computer lab; computer-assisted instruction; e-mail services; employment services for current students; externships; Internet; learning resource lab; library services; nursing audiovisuals; resume preparation assistance; skills, simulation, or other laboratory; tutoring; unpaid internships.

Library Facilities 225,000 volumes (6,259 in health, 1,881 in nursing); 518 periodical subscriptions (65 health-care related).

BACCALAUREATE PROGRAMS

Degree BS

Available Programs Generic Baccalaureate.

Study Options Full-time and part-time.

Program Entrance Requirements Minimum overall college GPA of 2.0, transcript of college record, CPR certification, written essay, health exam, health insurance, high school biology, high school chemistry, high school foreign language, 3 years high school math, 3 years high school science, high school transcript, immunizations, 1 letter of recommendation, minimum GPA in nursing prerequisites of 2.5, prerequisite course work. Transfer students are accepted. **Standardized tests** *Required:* SAT or ACT, TOEFL for international students. **Application** *Deadline:* rolling (freshmen), rolling (transfer). *Early decision:* 11/15. *Notification:* continuous (freshmen), 12/15 (out-of-state freshmen), 12/15 (early decision). *Application fee:* $30.

Advanced Placement Credit given for nursing courses completed elsewhere dependent upon specific evaluations.

Expenses (2006–07) *Tuition:* full-time $24,960; part-time $350 per credit hour. *International tuition:* $24,960 full-time. *Room and board:* $4450; room only: $1750 per academic year. *Required fees:* full-time $203.

Financial Aid 96% of baccalaureate students in nursing programs received some form of financial aid in 2005–06. *Gift aid (need-based):* Federal Pell, FSEOG, state, college/university gift aid from institutional funds. *Loans:* FFEL (Subsidized and Unsubsidized Stafford PLUS), Perkins. *Work-Study:* Federal Work-Study, part-time campus jobs. *Application deadline (priority):* 3/1.

Contact Linda L. Andrews, Dean, School of Health Sciences and Human Performance, Lynchburg College, McMillan Nursing Building, 1501 Lakeside Drive, Lynchburg, VA 24501-3199. *Telephone:* 434-544-8324. *Fax:* 434-544-8323. *E-mail:* andrews@lynchburg.edu.

Marymount University
School of Health Professions
Arlington, Virginia

http://www.marymount.edu

Founded in 1950

DEGREES • BSN • MSN

Nursing Program Faculty 21 (76% with doctorates).

Baccalaureate Enrollment 297
Women 91% **Men** 9% **Minority** 34% **International** 6% **Part-time** 10%

Graduate Enrollment 40
Women 90% **Men** 10% **Minority** 58% **International** 2% **Part-time** 90%

Nursing Student Activities Sigma Theta Tau, Student Nurses' Association.

Nursing Student Resources Academic advising; academic or career counseling; assistance for students with disabilities; bookstore; campus computer network; career placement assistance; computer lab; computer-assisted instruction; e-mail services; externships; interactive nursing skills videos; Internet; learning resource lab; library services; nursing audiovisuals; paid internships; remedial services; resume preparation assistance; skills, simulation, or other laboratory; tutoring; unpaid internships.

Library Facilities 187,097 volumes (10,000 in health, 1,300 in nursing); 1,048 periodical subscriptions (176 health-care related).

BACCALAUREATE PROGRAMS

Degree BSN

Available Programs ADN to Baccalaureate; Accelerated Baccalaureate; Accelerated Baccalaureate for Second Degree; Accelerated RN Baccalaureate; Baccalaureate for Second Degree; Generic Baccalaureate; RN Baccalaureate.

Site Options *Distance Learning:* Arlington, VA; Reston, VA.

Study Options Full-time and part-time.

Program Entrance Requirements Minimum overall college GPA of 2.0, health exam, health insurance, high school transcript, 2 letters of recommendation, minimum high school GPA of 2.5. Transfer students are accepted. **Standardized tests** *Required:* SAT or ACT, TOEFL for international students. **Application** *Deadline:* rolling (freshmen), rolling (out-of-state freshmen), rolling (transfer). *Notification:* continuous (freshmen), continuous (out-of-state freshmen). *Application fee:* $35.

Advanced Placement Credit by examination available. Credit given for nursing courses completed elsewhere dependent upon specific evaluations.

Expenses (2006–07) *Tuition:* full-time $19,048; part-time $620 per credit hour. *International tuition:* $19,048 full-time. *Room and board:* $8212 per academic year. *Required fees:* full-time $370.

Financial Aid 85% of baccalaureate students in nursing programs received some form of financial aid in 2005–06. *Gift aid (need-based):* Federal Pell, FSEOG, state, private, college/university gift aid from institutional funds. *Loans:* Federal Direct (Subsidized and Unsubsidized Stafford), FFEL, Perkins. *Work-Study:* Federal Work-Study. *Application deadline (priority):* 3/1.

Contact Dr. Sharron Guillett, Chair, School of Health Professions, Marymount University, 2807 North Glebe Road, Arlington, VA 22207-4299. *Telephone:* 703-526-6879. *Fax:* 703-284-3819. *E-mail:* sharron.guillett@marymount.edu.

GRADUATE PROGRAMS

Expenses (2006–07) *Tuition:* part-time $620 per credit hour. *Required fees:* full-time $200.

Financial Aid 46% of graduate students in nursing programs received some form of financial aid in 2005–06. Research assistantships with full tuition reimbursements available, career-related internships or fieldwork and scholarships available. Aid available to part-time students.

Contact Ms. Francesca Reed, Coordinator, Graduate Admissions, School of Health Professions, Marymount University, 2807 North Glebe Road, Arlington, VA 22207-4299. *Telephone:* 703-284-5906. *E-mail:* francesca.reed@marymount.edu.

MASTER'S DEGREE PROGRAM

Degree MSN

Available Programs Master's; RN to Master's.

Concentrations Available Nursing administration; nursing education. *Nurse practitioner programs in:* family health.

Site Options *Distance Learning:* Arlington, VA.

Study Options Full-time and part-time.

Program Entrance Requirements Minimum overall college GPA of 3.0, transcript of college record, CPR certification, immunizations, interview, 2 letters of recommendation, professional liability insurance/malpractice insurance, resume, statistics course, GRE, MAT. *Application deadline:* Applications are processed on a rolling basis. *Application fee:* $35.

Advanced Placement Credit given for nursing courses completed elsewhere dependent upon specific evaluations.

Degree Requirements 40 total credit hours, comprehensive exam.

POST-MASTER'S PROGRAM

Areas of Study Nursing administration; nursing education. *Nurse practitioner programs in:* family health.

Norfolk State University
Department of Nursing
Norfolk, Virginia

http://www.nsu.edu/schools/sciencetech/nursing/

Founded in 1935

DEGREE • BSN

Nursing Program Faculty 20 (13% with doctorates).

Baccalaureate Enrollment 70
Women 94% **Men** 6% **Minority** 90% **International** 9% **Part-time** 45%

Nursing Student Activities Nursing Honor Society, Student Nurses' Association, nursing club.

Nursing Student Resources Academic advising; academic or career counseling; assistance for students with disabilities; bookstore; campus computer network; career placement assistance; computer lab; computer-assisted instruction; daycare for children of students; e-mail services; employment services for current students; externships; housing assistance; interactive nursing skills videos; Internet; learning resource lab; library services; nursing audiovisuals; paid internships; remedial services; resume preparation assistance; skills, simulation, or other laboratory; tutoring.

Library Facilities 378,323 volumes; 88,927 periodical subscriptions.

BACCALAUREATE PROGRAMS

Degree BSN

Available Programs ADN to Baccalaureate; Accelerated Baccalaureate for Second Degree; Accelerated LPN to Baccalaureate; Accelerated RN Baccalaureate; RN Baccalaureate.

Site Options Virginia Beach, VA.

Study Options Full-time and part-time.

Program Entrance Requirements Minimum overall college GPA of 2.5, transcript of college record, CPR certification, health exam, health insurance, high school biology, high school chemistry, 2 years high school math, high school transcript, immunizations, minimum high school GPA of 2.5, minimum GPA in nursing prerequisites of 2.0, professional liability insurance/malpractice insurance, prerequisite course work, RN licensure. Transfer students are accepted. **Standardized tests** *Required:* SAT or ACT, TOEFL for international students. **Application** *Deadline:* 5/31 (freshmen). *Application fee:* $25.

Advanced Placement Credit by examination available. Credit given for nursing courses completed elsewhere dependent upon specific evaluations.

Expenses (2006–07) *Tuition, state resident:* full-time $5556; part-time $226 per credit hour. *Tuition, nonresident:* full-time $15,376; part-time $567 per credit hour. *International tuition:* $15,376 full-time. *Room and board:* $7434; room only: $5000 per academic year. *Required fees:* full-time $256.

Financial Aid 83% of baccalaureate students in nursing programs received some form of financial aid in 2005–06. *Gift aid (need-based):* Federal Pell, FSEOG, state, private, college/university gift aid from institutional funds. *Loans:* Federal Direct (Subsidized and Unsubsidized Stafford), FFEL, Perkins, state, alternative loans. *Work-Study:* Federal Work-Study, part-time campus jobs. *Application deadline:* 5/31.

Norfolk State University (continued)

Contact Dr. Bennie L. Marshall, Department Head, Department of Nursing, Norfolk State University, 700 Park Avenue, Norfolk, VA 23504. *Telephone:* 757-823-9015. *Fax:* 757-823-8241. *E-mail:* blmarshall@nsu.edu.

Old Dominion University
Department of Nursing
Norfolk, Virginia

http://www.odu.edu/nursson

Founded in 1930

DEGREES • BSN • MSN

Nursing Program Faculty 29 (28% with doctorates).

Baccalaureate Enrollment 283
Women 88% **Men** 12% **Minority** 38% **Part-time** 39%

Graduate Enrollment 187
Women 89% **Men** 11% **Minority** 18% **Part-time** 49%

Nursing Student Activities Sigma Theta Tau, Student Nurses' Association.

Nursing Student Resources Academic advising; academic or career counseling; assistance for students with disabilities; bookstore; campus computer network; computer lab; computer-assisted instruction; e-mail services; externships; Internet; learning resource lab; library services; nursing audiovisuals; resume preparation assistance; skills, simulation, or other laboratory; tutoring; unpaid internships.

Library Facilities 968,921 volumes (49,247 in health, 4,758 in nursing); 16,371 periodical subscriptions (1,832 health-care related).

BACCALAUREATE PROGRAMS

Degree BSN

Available Programs Accelerated Baccalaureate; Generic Baccalaureate; RN Baccalaureate.

Site Options *Distance Learning:* Olympia, WA; Yavapai, AZ; Athens, GA.
Study Options Full-time.

Program Entrance Requirements Transcript of college record, minimum GPA in nursing prerequisites of 3.0, prerequisite course work. Transfer students are accepted. **Standardized tests** *Required:* SAT or ACT, TOEFL for international students. **Application** *Deadline:* 3/15 (freshmen), 5/1 (transfer). *Early decision:* 12/1. *Notification:* continuous (freshmen), 1/15 (early action). *Application fee:* $40.

Expenses (2006–07) *Tuition, area resident:* full-time $5430; part-time $181 per credit. *Tuition, state resident:* full-time $6150; part-time $205 per credit. *Tuition, nonresident:* full-time $15,210; part-time $507 per credit. *International tuition:* $15,210 full-time. *Room and board:* $5976; room only: $4740 per academic year. *Required fees:* full-time $158; part-time $30 per credit; part-time $75 per term.

Financial Aid 48% of baccalaureate students in nursing programs received some form of financial aid in 2005–06.

Contact Ms. Phyllis D. Barham, Chief Academic Advisor, Department of Nursing, Old Dominion University, Norfolk, VA 23529-0500. *Telephone:* 757-683-5245. *Fax:* 757-683-5253. *E-mail:* pbarham@odu.edu.

GRADUATE PROGRAMS

Expenses (2006–07) *Tuition, state resident:* full-time $4734; part-time $263 per credit. *Tuition, nonresident:* full-time $11,898; part-time $661 per credit. *International tuition:* $11,898 full-time. *Room and board:* $5976; room only: $4740 per academic year. *Required fees:* full-time $500; part-time $9 per credit; part-time $250 per term.

Financial Aid 41% of graduate students in nursing programs received some form of financial aid in 2005–06.

Contact Dr. Laurel Garzon, Graduate Program Director, Department of Nursing, Old Dominion University, Technology Building, Norfolk, VA 23529-0500. *Telephone:* 757-683-4298. *Fax:* 757-683-5253. *E-mail:* lgarzon@odu.edu.

MASTER'S DEGREE PROGRAM

Degree MSN

Available Programs Master's; RN to Master's.

Concentrations Available Nurse anesthesia; nurse-midwifery; nursing administration; nursing education. *Clinical nurse specialist programs in:* parent-child. *Nurse practitioner programs in:* family health, pediatric, women's health.

Site Options *Distance Learning:* Olympia, WA; Yavapai, AZ; Athens, GA.
Study Options Full-time and part-time.

Program Entrance Requirements Clinical experience, computer literacy, minimum overall college GPA of 3.0, transcript of college record, CPR certification, written essay, immunizations, interview, 3 letters of recommendation, physical assessment course, statistics course.

Advanced Placement Credit given for nursing courses completed elsewhere dependent upon specific evaluations.

Degree Requirements 47 total credit hours, comprehensive exam.

POST-MASTER'S PROGRAM

Areas of Study Nurse anesthesia; nurse-midwifery; nursing administration; nursing education. *Clinical nurse specialist programs in:* parent-child. *Nurse practitioner programs in:* family health, pediatric, women's health.

CONTINUING EDUCATION PROGRAM

Contact Mrs. Kimberly Curry-Lourenco, Lecturer, Department of Nursing, Old Dominion University, 4608 Hampton Boulevard, Norfolk, VA 23529-0500. *Telephone:* 757-683-5261. *Fax:* 757-683-5253. *E-mail:* kcurrylo@odu.edu.

Radford University
School of Nursing
Radford, Virginia

http://www.radford.edu/nurs-web

Founded in 1910

DEGREES • BSN • MSN

Nursing Program Faculty 40 (40% with doctorates).

Baccalaureate Enrollment 143
Women 90% **Men** 10% **Minority** 15% **International** 3%

Graduate Enrollment 44
Women 90% **Men** 10% **Minority** 15% **Part-time** 20%

Nursing Student Activities Nursing Honor Society, Sigma Theta Tau, Student Nurses' Association.

Nursing Student Resources Academic advising; academic or career counseling; assistance for students with disabilities; bookstore; campus computer network; career placement assistance; computer lab; computer-assisted instruction; e-mail services; employment services for current students; externships; housing assistance; interactive nursing skills videos; Internet; learning resource lab; library services; nursing audiovisuals; resume preparation assistance; skills, simulation, or other laboratory; unpaid internships.

Library Facilities 377,110 volumes; 4,801 periodical subscriptions.

BACCALAUREATE PROGRAMS

Degree BSN

Available Programs Generic Baccalaureate; RN Baccalaureate.
Site Options *Distance Learning:* Roanoke, VA.
Study Options Full-time.

Program Entrance Requirements Minimum overall college GPA of 2.5, transcript of college record, CPR certification, written essay, health exam, health insurance, high school biology, immunizations, minimum GPA in nursing prerequisites of 2.5, prerequisite course work. Transfer students are accepted. **Standardized tests** *Required:* SAT or ACT, TOEFL for international students. **Application** *Deadline:* 2/1 (freshmen), 6/1 (transfer). *Notification:* 3/20 (freshmen). *Application fee:* $50.

Advanced Placement Credit given for nursing courses completed elsewhere dependent upon specific evaluations.

Expenses (2005–06) *Room and board:* $6120 per academic year.

Financial Aid 50% of baccalaureate students in nursing programs received some form of financial aid in 2004–05. *Gift aid (need-based):* Federal Pell, FSEOG, state, private, college/university gift aid from institutional funds. *Loans:* Federal Nursing Student Loans, FFEL (Subsidized and Unsubsidized Stafford PLUS), Perkins, state, college/university. *Work-Study:* Federal Work-Study, part-time campus jobs. *Application deadline (priority):* 3/1.

Contact Dr. Marcella Griggs, Director, School of Nursing, Radford University, Box 6964, RU Station, Waldron Hall, Room 305, Radford, VA 24142. *Telephone:* 540-831-7700. *Fax:* 540-831-7716. *E-mail:* nurs-web@ radford.edu.

GRADUATE PROGRAMS

Expenses (2005–06) *Tuition, area resident:* full-time $5710; part-time $238 per credit hour. *Tuition, nonresident:* full-time $10,524; part-time $438 per credit hour.

Financial Aid 90% of graduate students in nursing programs received some form of financial aid in 2004–05. 6 teaching assistantships with tuition reimbursements available (averaging $8,700 per year) were awarded; fellowships with tuition reimbursements available, research assistantships, career-related internships or fieldwork, Federal Work-Study, institutionally sponsored loans, and scholarships also available. *Financial aid application deadline:* 2/1.

Contact Dr. Karolyn Givens, Graduate Program Coordinator, School of Nursing, Radford University, Box 6964, RU Station, Waldron Hall, Radford, VA 24142. *Telephone:* 540-831-7700. *Fax:* 540-831-7716. *E-mail:* nurs-web@ radford.edu.

MASTER'S DEGREE PROGRAM

Degree MSN

Available Programs Accelerated RN to Master's; Master's.

Concentrations Available Nurse-midwifery. *Clinical nurse specialist programs in:* adult health, gerontology. *Nurse practitioner programs in:* family health.

Study Options Full-time and part-time.

Program Entrance Requirements Clinical experience, computer literacy, minimum overall college GPA of 3.0, transcript of college record, CPR certification, written essay, immunizations, interview, 3 letters of recommendation, nursing research course, physical assessment course, professional liability insurance/malpractice insurance, prerequisite course work, resume, statistics course, GMAT, GRE General Test, MAT, or NTE. *Application deadline:* For fall admission, 3/1 (priority date); for spring admission, 10/1. Applications are processed on a rolling basis. *Application fee:* $40.

Advanced Placement Credit given for nursing courses completed elsewhere dependent upon specific evaluations.

Degree Requirements 41 total credit hours, thesis or project, comprehensive exam.

POST-MASTER'S PROGRAM

Areas of Study *Clinical nurse specialist programs in:* gerontology. *Nurse practitioner programs in:* family health.

Shenandoah University
Division of Nursing
Winchester, Virginia

http://www.su.edu/nursing/index.html

Founded in 1875

DEGREES • BSN • MSN

Nursing Program Faculty 44 (30% with doctorates).

Baccalaureate Enrollment 239

Women 97% **Men** 3% **Minority** 10% **International** 3% **Part-time** 15%

Graduate Enrollment 28

Women 97% **Men** 3% **Minority** 10% **Part-time** 25%

Nursing Student Activities Nursing Honor Society, Sigma Theta Tau, Student Nurses' Association.

Nursing Student Resources Academic advising; academic or career counseling; assistance for students with disabilities; bookstore; campus computer network; computer lab; daycare for children of students; e-mail services; interactive nursing skills videos; Internet; learning resource lab; library services; nursing audiovisuals; resume preparation assistance; skills, simulation, or other laboratory; tutoring.

Library Facilities 131,174 volumes (500 in health, 200 in nursing); 19,479 periodical subscriptions (250 health-care related).

BACCALAUREATE PROGRAMS

Degree BSN

Available Programs ADN to Baccalaureate; Accelerated Baccalaureate for Second Degree; Generic Baccalaureate; LPN to Baccalaureate; LPN to RN Baccalaureate; RN Baccalaureate.

Site Options Leesburg, VA.

Study Options Full-time and part-time.

Program Entrance Requirements Minimum overall college GPA of 2.5, transcript of college record, CPR certification, health exam, health insurance, high school biology, high school chemistry, 2 years high school math, high school transcript, immunizations, minimum high school GPA of 2.5, minimum GPA in nursing prerequisites of 2.0, prerequisite course work. Transfer students are accepted. **Standardized tests** *Required:* SAT or ACT, TOEFL for international students. **Application** *Deadline:* rolling (freshmen). *Application fee:* $30.

Advanced Placement Credit by examination available. Credit given for nursing courses completed elsewhere dependent upon specific evaluations.

Expenses (2005–06) *Tuition:* full-time $19,900; part-time $610 per credit hour. *Room and board:* $7550 per academic year. *Required fees:* full-time $775; part-time $575 per term.

Financial Aid 80% of baccalaureate students in nursing programs received some form of financial aid in 2004–05. *Gift aid (need-based):* Federal Pell, FSEOG, state, private, college/university gift aid from institutional funds, Federal Nursing. *Loans:* Federal Nursing Student Loans, Federal Direct (Subsidized and Unsubsidized Stafford PLUS), Perkins, college/university. *Work-Study:* Federal Work-Study, part-time campus jobs. *Application deadline (priority):* 2/15.

Contact Dr. Sheila Sparks Ralph, Director, Division of Nursing, Shenandoah University, 1460 University Drive, Winchester, VA 22601. *Telephone:* 540-678-4381. *Fax:* 540-665-5519. *E-mail:* ssparks@su.edu.

GRADUATE PROGRAMS

Expenses (2005–06) *Tuition:* full-time $21,800; part-time $610 per credit hour. *Room and board:* $7550 per academic year. *Required fees:* full-time $775; part-time $575 per term.

Financial Aid 85% of graduate students in nursing programs received some form of financial aid in 2004–05. 4 fellowships with partial tuition reimbursements available (averaging $1,500 per year), 2 teaching assistantships with partial tuition reimbursements available (averaging $3,474 per year) were awarded; institutionally sponsored loans and scholarships also available. Aid available to part-time students. *Financial aid application deadline:* 3/15.

Contact Dr. Patricia Krauskopf, Coordinator, FNP Graduate Program, Division of Nursing, Shenandoah University, 1775 North Sector Court, Winchester, VA 22601. *Telephone:* 540-665-5512. *Fax:* 540-665-5519. *E-mail:* pkrausko@su.edu.

MASTER'S DEGREE PROGRAM

Degree MSN

Available Programs Master's; RN to Master's.

Concentrations Available Nurse case management; nurse-midwifery. *Clinical nurse specialist programs in:* psychiatric/mental health. *Nurse practitioner programs in:* family health, psychiatric/mental health.

Study Options Full-time and part-time.

Program Entrance Requirements Clinical experience, computer literacy, minimum overall college GPA of 2.8, transcript of college record, CPR certification, immunizations, interview, 3 letters of recommendation, nursing research course, physical assessment course, professional liability insurance/malpractice insurance, prerequisite course work, resume, statistics course, GRE General Test. *Application deadline:* For fall admission, 6/15 (priority date). Applications are processed on a rolling basis. *Application fee:* $30.

Shenandoah University (continued)

Advanced Placement   Credit given for nursing courses completed elsewhere dependent upon specific evaluations.

Degree Requirements   37 total credit hours, thesis or project.

POST-MASTER'S PROGRAM

Areas of Study   Nurse-midwifery. *Nurse practitioner programs in:* family health, psychiatric/mental health.

CONTINUING EDUCATION PROGRAM

Contact   Dr. R.T. Good, Dean, School of Continuing Education, Division of Nursing, Shenandoah University, 1460 University Drive, Winchester, VA 22601. *Telephone:* 540-665-4584. *E-mail:* rtgood@su.edu.

University of Virginia
School of Nursing
Charlottesville, Virginia

http://www.nursing.virginia.edu
Founded in 1819
DEGREES • BSN • MSN • MSN/HSM • MSN/MA • MSN/MBA • MSN/PHD

Nursing Program Faculty 103 (60% with doctorates).
Baccalaureate Enrollment 325
Women 95% **Men** 5% **Minority** 14% **International** 1% **Part-time** 5%
Graduate Enrollment 225
Women 93% **Men** 7% **Minority** 15% **International** 2% **Part-time** 50%
Nursing Student Activities Sigma Theta Tau, Student Nurses' Association, nursing club.
Nursing Student Resources Academic advising; academic or career counseling; assistance for students with disabilities; bookstore; campus computer network; career placement assistance; computer-assisted instruction; e-mail services; housing assistance; interactive nursing skills videos; Internet; learning resource lab; library services; nursing audiovisuals; placement services for program completers; remedial services; resume preparation assistance; skills, simulation, or other laboratory; tutoring.
Library Facilities 5.4 million volumes (180,000 in health); 71,832 periodical subscriptions.

BACCALAUREATE PROGRAMS

Degree BSN

Available Programs ADN to Baccalaureate; Generic Baccalaureate.
Study Options Full-time.
Program Entrance Requirements Transcript of college record, written essay, health insurance, high school biology, 2 years high school math, 1 year of high school science, high school transcript, immunizations, 1 letter of recommendation, minimum GPA in nursing prerequisites of 2.0. Transfer students are accepted. **Standardized tests** *Required:* SAT, TOEFL for international students. *Recommended:* two SAT subject tests (student's choice). **Application** *Deadline:* 1/2 (freshmen), 3/1 (transfer). *Early decision:* 11/1. *Notification:* 4/1 (freshmen), 12/1 (out-of-state freshmen), 12/1 (early decision). *Application fee:* $60.
Expenses (2006–07) *Tuition, state resident:* full-time $7860. *Tuition, nonresident:* full-time $25,960. *International tuition:* $25,960 full-time. *Required fees:* full-time $30; part-time $15 per term.
Financial Aid 30% of baccalaureate students in nursing programs received some form of financial aid in 2005–06. *Gift aid (need-based):* Federal Pell, FSEOG, state, private, college/university gift aid from institutional funds. *Loans:* Federal Nursing Student Loans, Federal Direct (Subsidized and Unsubsidized Stafford PLUS), Perkins, college/university. *Work-Study:* Federal Work-Study. *Application deadline (priority):* 3/1.
Contact   Dr. Theresa J. Carroll, Assistant Dean for Undergraduate Student Services, School of Nursing, University of Virginia, McLeod Hall, PO Box 800782, Charlottesville, VA 22908. *Telephone:* 888-283-8703. *Fax:* 434-924-0528. *E-mail:* nur-osa@virginia.edu.

GRADUATE PROGRAMS

Expenses (2006–07) *Tuition, state resident:* full-time $10,265. *Tuition, nonresident:* full-time $20,265. *International tuition:* $20,265 full-time. *Required fees:* full-time $30; part-time $30 per credit; part-time $30 per term.
Financial Aid 90% of graduate students in nursing programs received some form of financial aid in 2005–06. Fellowships, research assistantships, teaching assistantships, Federal Work-Study and scholarships available. *Financial aid application deadline:* 3/1.
Contact   Mr. Clay D. Hysell, Assistant Dean for Graduate Student Services, School of Nursing, University of Virginia, McLeod Hall, PO Box 800782, Charlottesville, VA 22908. *Telephone:* 888-283-8703. *Fax:* 434-924-0528. *E-mail:* nur-osa@virginia.edu.

MASTER'S DEGREE PROGRAM

Degrees MSN; MSN/HSM; MSN/MA; MSN/MBA; MSN/PhD

Available Programs Accelerated Master's for Non-Nursing College Graduates; Accelerated Master's for Nurses with Non-Nursing Degrees; Master's; Master's for Non-Nursing College Graduates; Master's for Nurses with Non-Nursing Degrees.
Concentrations Available Health-care administration; nursing administration. *Clinical nurse specialist programs in:* acute care, community health, medical-surgical, psychiatric/mental health, public health. *Nurse practitioner programs in:* acute care, family health, gerontology, pediatric, primary care, psychiatric/mental health.
Study Options Full-time and part-time.
Program Entrance Requirements Minimum overall college GPA of 3.0, transcript of college record, written essay, 3 letters of recommendation, physical assessment course, resume, statistics course, GRE General Test, MAT. *Application deadline:* For fall admission, 2/1. Applications are processed on a rolling basis. *Application fee:* $60.
Advanced Placement Credit given for nursing courses completed elsewhere dependent upon specific evaluations.
Degree Requirements 38 total credit hours.

POST-MASTER'S PROGRAM

Areas of Study Health-care administration; nursing administration. *Clinical nurse specialist programs in:* acute care, community health, medical-surgical, psychiatric/mental health, public health. *Nurse practitioner programs in:* acute care, family health, gerontology, pediatric, primary care, psychiatric/mental health.

DOCTORAL DEGREE PROGRAM

Degree PhD

Available Programs Doctorate; Post-Baccalaureate Doctorate.
Areas of Study Advanced practice nursing, aging, community health, critical care, ethics, faculty preparation, family health, gerontology, health policy, health promotion/disease prevention, health-care systems, information systems, maternity-newborn, nursing administration, nursing education, nursing policy, nursing research, nursing science, oncology, women's health.
Program Entrance Requirements Minimum overall college GPA of 3.0, interview by faculty committee, interview, 3 letters of recommendation, statistics course, vita, writing sample, GRE General Test. *Application deadline:* For fall admission, 2/1. Applications are processed on a rolling basis. *Application fee:* $60.
Degree Requirements 51 total credit hours, dissertation, written exam, residency.

POSTDOCTORAL PROGRAM

Areas of Study Aging, cancer care, chronic illness, community health, family health, gerontology, health promotion/disease prevention, nursing interventions, nursing research, nursing science, outcomes, vulnerable population.
Postdoctoral Program Contact Mr. Clay D. Hysell, Assistant Dean for Graduate Student Services, School of Nursing, University of Virginia, McLeod Hall, PO Box 800782, Charlottesville, VA 22908. *Telephone:* 434-924-0141. *Fax:* 434-924-0528. *E-mail:* cdh6n@virginia.edu.

The University of Virginia's College at Wise

Department of Nursing
Wise, Virginia

http://www.wise.virginia.edu/nursing

Founded in 1954

DEGREE • BSN

Nursing Program Faculty 11 (18% with doctorates).

Baccalaureate Enrollment 35
Women 80% **Men** 20% **Minority** 5% **International** 5% **Part-time** 15%

Nursing Student Activities Sigma Theta Tau, Student Nurses' Association.

Nursing Student Resources Academic advising; academic or career counseling; assistance for students with disabilities; bookstore; campus computer network; computer lab; computer-assisted instruction; e-mail services; employment services for current students; externships; housing assistance; interactive nursing skills videos; Internet; learning resource lab; library services; nursing audiovisuals; skills, simulation, or other laboratory; tutoring.

Library Facilities 95,861 volumes (4,654 in health, 2,761 in nursing); 1,029 periodical subscriptions (40 health-care related).

BACCALAUREATE PROGRAMS

Degree BSN

Available Programs Generic Baccalaureate; RN Baccalaureate.

Site Options Abingdon, VA.

Study Options Full-time.

Program Entrance Requirements Minimum overall college GPA of 2.5, transcript of college record, CPR certification, health exam, health insurance, immunizations, 3 letters of recommendation, minimum GPA in nursing prerequisites of 2.5, professional liability insurance/malpractice insurance, prerequisite course work. Transfer students are accepted. **Standardized tests** *Required:* SAT or ACT, TOEFL for international students. **Application** *Deadline:* 8/1 (freshmen), 8/15 (transfer). *Early decision:* 2/1. *Notification:* continuous until 8/20 (freshmen), 2/15 (early action). *Application fee:* $25.

Advanced Placement Credit given for nursing courses completed elsewhere dependent upon specific evaluations.

Expenses (2006–07) *Tuition, state resident:* full-time $3252; part-time $134 per credit hour. *Tuition, nonresident:* full-time $14,238; part-time $587 per credit hour. *Room and board:* $6078; room only: $3230 per academic year. *Required fees:* full-time $2440; part-time $44 per credit.

Financial Aid 90% of baccalaureate students in nursing programs received some form of financial aid in 2005–06. *Gift aid (need-based):* Federal Pell, FSEOG, state, private, college/university gift aid from institutional funds. *Loans:* FFEL (Subsidized and Unsubsidized Stafford PLUS), Perkins, state, college/university. *Work-Study:* Federal Work-Study. *Application deadline (priority):* 4/1.

Contact Dr. Debra Lynn Carter, Chair, Department of Nursing, The University of Virginia's College at Wise, One College Avenue, Wise, VA 24293-4400. *Telephone:* 276-376-1030. *Fax:* 276-376-4589. *E-mail:* dlc4e@uvawise.edu.

Virginia Commonwealth University

School of Nursing
Richmond, Virginia

http://www.nursing.vcu.edu

Founded in 1838

DEGREES • BS • MS • MS/MPH • PHD

Nursing Program Faculty 132 (33% with doctorates).

Baccalaureate Enrollment 613
Women 93% **Men** 7% **Minority** 26% **Part-time** 55%

Graduate Enrollment 269
Women 95% **Men** 5% **Minority** 21% **Part-time** 52%

Nursing Student Activities Sigma Theta Tau, Student Nurses' Association.

Nursing Student Resources Academic advising; academic or career counseling; assistance for students with disabilities; bookstore; campus computer network; career placement assistance; computer lab; computer-assisted instruction; daycare for children of students; e-mail services; employment services for current students; externships; housing assistance; interactive nursing skills videos; Internet; learning resource lab; library services; nursing audiovisuals; paid internships; placement services for program completers; remedial services; resume preparation assistance; skills, simulation, or other laboratory; tutoring.

Library Facilities 1.9 million volumes (360,815 in health, 10,443 in nursing); 18,000 periodical subscriptions (3,618 health-care related).

BACCALAUREATE PROGRAMS

Degree BS

Available Programs ADN to Baccalaureate; Accelerated Baccalaureate for Second Degree; Generic Baccalaureate.

Site Options *Distance Learning:* Portsmouth, VA; Danville, VA.

Study Options Full-time.

Program Entrance Requirements Minimum overall college GPA of 2.5, transcript of college record, CPR certification, written essay, health exam, high school foreign language, 3 years high school math, 2 years high school science, high school transcript, immunizations, 3 letters of recommendation, minimum high school GPA of 3.0, minimum GPA in nursing prerequisites of 2.5, prerequisite course work. Transfer students are accepted. **Standardized tests** *Required:* SAT or ACT. **Application** *Notification:* continuous until 4/1 (freshmen). *Application fee:* $30.

Advanced Placement Credit by examination available. Credit given for nursing courses completed elsewhere dependent upon specific evaluations.

Expenses (2006–07) *Tuition, state resident:* full-time $4227; part-time $176 per credit hour. *Tuition, nonresident:* full-time $15,904; part-time $663 per credit hour. *International tuition:* $15,904 full-time. *Room and board:* $8409; room only: $5209 per academic year. *Required fees:* full-time $1658; part-time $67 per credit; part-time $67 per term.

Financial Aid 70% of baccalaureate students in nursing programs received some form of financial aid in 2005–06.

Contact Ms. Susan L. Lipp, RN, Director of Enrollment and Student Services, School of Nursing, Virginia Commonwealth University, PO Box 980567, Richmond, VA 23298-0567. *Telephone:* 804-828-5171 Ext. 13. *Fax:* 804-828-7743. *E-mail:* slipp@vcu.edu.

GRADUATE PROGRAMS

Expenses (2006–07) *Tuition, state resident:* full-time $6783; part-time $377 per credit hour. *Tuition, nonresident:* full-time $15,904; part-time $884 per credit hour. *International tuition:* $15,904 full-time. *Room and board:* $8781; room only: $5581 per academic year. *Required fees:* full-time $1537; part-time $62 per credit; part-time $62 per term.

Financial Aid 60% of graduate students in nursing programs received some form of financial aid in 2005–06. Fellowships, research assistantships, teaching assistantships, career-related internships or fieldwork and institutionally sponsored loans available.

Contact Ms. Susan L. Lipp, RN, Director of Enrollment and Student Services, School of Nursing, Virginia Commonwealth University, PO Box 980567, Richmond, VA 23298-0567. *Telephone:* 804-828-5171 Ext. 13. *Fax:* 804-828-7743. *E-mail:* slipp@vcu.edu.

MASTER'S DEGREE PROGRAM

Degrees MS; MS/MPH

Available Programs Accelerated Master's for Non-Nursing College Graduates; Accelerated Master's for Nurses with Non-Nursing Degrees; Master's; RN to Master's.

Concentrations Available Nursing administration. *Clinical nurse specialist programs in:* acute care, psychiatric/mental health. *Nurse practitioner programs in:* acute care, adult health, family health, pediatric, primary care, psychiatric/mental health, women's health.

Study Options Full-time and part-time.

Virginia Commonwealth University (continued)

Program Entrance Requirements Computer literacy, minimum overall college GPA of 3.0, transcript of college record, CPR certification, written essay, immunizations, 3 letters of recommendation, prerequisite course work, resume, statistics course, GRE General Test. *Application deadline:* For fall admission, 2/1 (priority date). *Application fee:* $50.

Advanced Placement Credit given for nursing courses completed elsewhere dependent upon specific evaluations.

Degree Requirements 57 total credit hours.

POST-MASTER'S PROGRAM

Areas of Study Nursing administration; nursing education. *Clinical nurse specialist programs in:* acute care, psychiatric/mental health. *Nurse practitioner programs in:* acute care, adult health, family health, pediatric, primary care, psychiatric/mental health, women's health.

DOCTORAL DEGREE PROGRAM

Degree PhD

Available Programs Doctorate; Post-Baccalaureate Doctorate.

Areas of Study Bio-behavioral research.

Program Entrance Requirements Minimum overall college GPA of 3.0, interview by faculty committee, 3 letters of recommendation, MSN or equivalent, statistics course, vita, writing sample, GRE General Test. *Application deadline:* For fall admission, 2/1 (priority date). *Application fee:* $50.

Degree Requirements 63 total credit hours, dissertation, written exam, residency.

See full description on page 574.

WASHINGTON

Eastern Washington University
Intercollegiate College of Nursing/Washington State University
Cheney, Washington

See description of programs under **Intercollegiate College of Nursing/Washington State University (Spokane, Washington).**

Gonzaga University
Department of Nursing
Spokane, Washington

http://www.gonzaga.edu/nursing
Founded in 1887

DEGREES • BSN • MSN

Nursing Program Faculty 24 (50% with doctorates).

Baccalaureate Enrollment 40
Women 86% **Men** 14% **Minority** 7% **Part-time** 50%

Graduate Enrollment 180
Women 94% **Men** 6% **Minority** 94% **International** 7%

Nursing Student Activities Sigma Theta Tau.

Nursing Student Resources Academic advising; assistance for students with disabilities; bookstore; computer lab; Internet; library services.

Library Facilities 305,517 volumes (35,000 in health, 950 in nursing); 32,106 periodical subscriptions (206 health-care related).

BACCALAUREATE PROGRAMS

Degree BSN

Available Programs ADN to Baccalaureate; RN Baccalaureate.

Program Entrance Requirements Transfer students are accepted.
Standardized tests *Required:* SAT or ACT, TOEFL for international students. **Application** *Deadline:* 2/1 (freshmen), 6/1 (transfer). *Early decision:* 11/15. *Notification:* 3/15 (freshmen), 1/15 (early action). *Application fee:* $45.

Contact *Telephone:* 509-323-6643. *Fax:* 509-323-5827.

GRADUATE PROGRAMS

Contact *Telephone:* 509-323-6643. *Fax:* 509-323-5827.

MASTER'S DEGREE PROGRAM

Degree MSN

Available Programs Accelerated RN to Master's; Master's for Nurses with Non-Nursing Degrees; RN to Master's.

Concentrations Available Health-care administration; nurse case management; nursing administration; nursing education. *Clinical nurse specialist programs in:* adult health, critical care, gerontology, medical-surgical, psychiatric/mental health. *Nurse practitioner programs in:* family health, primary care, psychiatric/mental health.

Study Options Full-time and part-time.

Program Entrance Requirements Clinical experience, computer literacy, minimum overall college GPA of 3.0, transcript of college record, written essay, immunizations, 2 letters of recommendation, nursing research course, resume, statistics course, MAT. *Application deadline:* For fall admission, 7/20 (priority date); for spring admission, 11/1. Applications are processed on a rolling basis. *Application fee:* $40.

Advanced Placement Credit given for nursing courses completed elsewhere dependent upon specific evaluations.

Degree Requirements 48 total credit hours, thesis or project.

POST-MASTER'S PROGRAM

Areas of Study Health-care administration; nursing administration; nursing education. *Clinical nurse specialist programs in:* adult health, critical care, gerontology, medical-surgical, psychiatric/mental health. *Nurse practitioner programs in:* family health, primary care, psychiatric/mental health.

CONTINUING EDUCATION PROGRAM

Contact *Telephone:* 509-323-3572. *Fax:* 509-323-5827.

Intercollegiate College of Nursing/Washington State University
Intercollegiate College of Nursing/Washington State University
Spokane, Washington

http://www.nursing.wsu.edu

DEGREES • BSN • MN

Nursing Program Faculty 110 (36% with doctorates).

Baccalaureate Enrollment 739
Women 86% **Men** 14% **Minority** 17% **International** 1% **Part-time** 29%

Graduate Enrollment 187
Women 91% **Men** 9% **Minority** 1% **Part-time** 79%

Nursing Student Activities Sigma Theta Tau, Student Nurses' Association, nursing club.

Nursing Student Resources Academic advising; academic or career counseling; assistance for students with disabilities; bookstore; campus computer network; computer lab; computer-assisted instruction; e-mail services; interactive nursing skills videos; Internet; learning resource lab; library services; nursing audiovisuals; remedial services; resume preparation assistance; skills, simulation, or other laboratory; tutoring; unpaid internships.

Library Facilities 10,000 volumes in health, 10,000 volumes in nursing; 280 periodical subscriptions health-care related.

BACCALAUREATE PROGRAMS

Degree BSN

Available Programs Generic Baccalaureate; RN Baccalaureate.

Site Options *Distance Learning:* Vancouver, WA; Richland, WA; Yakima, WA.

Study Options Full-time and part-time.

Program Entrance Requirements Minimum overall college GPA of 2.5, transcript of college record, CPR certification, immunizations, interview, minimum GPA in nursing prerequisites of 2.5, professional liability insurance/malpractice insurance, prerequisite course work. Transfer students are accepted.

Advanced Placement Credit given for nursing courses completed elsewhere dependent upon specific evaluations.

Expenses (2006–07) *Tuition, area resident:* full-time $5888; part-time $294 per credit. *Tuition, nonresident:* full-time $15,528; part-time $776 per credit. *International tuition:* $15,528 full-time. *Required fees:* full-time $2000.

Contact Ms. Diane Kleweno, Undergraduate Program Coordinator, Intercollegiate College of Nursing/Washington State University, 2917 West Fort George Wright Drive, Spokane, WA 99224-5291. *Telephone:* 509-324-7338. *Fax:* 509-324-7336. *E-mail:* kleweno@wsu.edu.

GRADUATE PROGRAMS

Expenses (2006–07) *Tuition, state resident:* full-time $11,120; part-time $556 per credit. *Tuition, nonresident:* full-time $21,580; part-time $1079 per credit. *International tuition:* $21,580 full-time. *Required fees:* full-time $1000.

Contact Ms. Margaret Ruby, Administrative Assistant for Academic Affairs, Intercollegiate College of Nursing/Washington State University, 2917 West Fort George Wright Drive, Spokane, WA 99224-5291. *Telephone:* 509-324-7334. *Fax:* 509-324-7336. *E-mail:* mruby@wsu.edu.

MASTER'S DEGREE PROGRAM

Degree MN

Available Programs Accelerated Master's for Nurses with Non-Nursing Degrees; Accelerated RN to Master's; Master's.

Concentrations Available Nursing administration; nursing education. *Clinical nurse specialist programs in:* community health. *Nurse practitioner programs in:* family health, psychiatric/mental health.

Site Options *Distance Learning:* Vancouver, WA; Richland, WA; Yakima, WA.

Study Options Full-time and part-time.

Program Entrance Requirements Computer literacy, minimum overall college GPA of 3.0, transcript of college record, CPR certification, written essay, immunizations, 3 letters of recommendation, physical assessment course, prerequisite course work, statistics course.

Advanced Placement Credit given for nursing courses completed elsewhere dependent upon specific evaluations.

Degree Requirements 45 total credit hours, thesis or project.

POST-MASTER'S PROGRAM

Areas of Study *Nurse practitioner programs in:* family health, psychiatric/mental health.

CONTINUING EDUCATION PROGRAM

Contact Ms. Carol Johns, Coordinator of Professional Development, Intercollegiate College of Nursing/Washington State University, 2917 West Fort George Wright Drive, Spokane, WA 99224-5291. *Telephone:* 509-324-7354. *Fax:* 509-324-7341. *E-mail:* cjohns@wsu.edu.

Northwest University
The Mark and Huldah Buntain School of Nursing
Kirkland, Washington

http://www.northwestu.edu/

Founded in 1934

DEGREE • BS

Nursing Program Faculty 17 (17% with doctorates).

Baccalaureate Enrollment 70

Women 93% **Men** 7% **Minority** 11%

Nursing Student Activities Nursing club.

Nursing Student Resources Academic advising; academic or career counseling; assistance for students with disabilities; bookstore; campus computer network; computer lab; computer-assisted instruction; e-mail services; employment services for current students; housing assistance; interactive nursing skills videos; Internet; learning resource lab; library services; nursing audiovisuals; remedial services; resume preparation assistance; skills, simulation, or other laboratory; tutoring; unpaid internships.

Library Facilities 120,226 volumes (1,663 in health, 346 in nursing); 11,454 periodical subscriptions (725 health-care related).

BACCALAUREATE PROGRAMS

Degree BS

Available Programs Generic Baccalaureate.

Study Options Full-time.

Program Entrance Requirements Minimum overall college GPA of 3.0, transcript of college record, CPR certification, written essay, health exam, health insurance, high school transcript, immunizations, 2 letters of recommendation, minimum GPA in nursing prerequisites of 3.0, prerequisite course work. Transfer students are accepted. **Standardized tests** *Required:* SAT or ACT, TOEFL for international students. **Application** *Deadline:* 8/1 (freshmen), 8/1 (transfer). *Notification:* continuous (freshmen). *Application fee:* $30.

Expenses (2006–07) *Tuition:* full-time $17,920; part-time $750 per credit. *Room and board:* $6450 per academic year. *Required fees:* full-time $314.

Financial Aid 99% of baccalaureate students in nursing programs received some form of financial aid in 2005–06. *Gift aid (need-based):* Federal Pell, FSEOG, state, private, college/university gift aid from institutional funds. *Loans:* FFEL (Subsidized and Unsubsidized Stafford PLUS), Perkins, state, alternative loans. *Work-Study:* Federal Work-Study, part-time campus jobs. *Application deadline (priority):* 3/1.

Contact Dr. Carl N. Christensen, Dean, The Mark and Huldah Buntain School of Nursing, Northwest University, 5520 108th Avenue NE, PO Box 579, Kirkland, WA 98083. *Telephone:* 800-669-3781 Ext. 7822. *Fax:* 425-889-7822. *E-mail:* nursing@northwestu.edu.

Pacific Lutheran University
School of Nursing
Tacoma, Washington

http://www.plu.edu/~nurs/

Founded in 1890

DEGREES • BSN • MSN

Nursing Program Faculty 23 (40% with doctorates).

Baccalaureate Enrollment 265

Women 93% **Men** 7% **Minority** 25% **International** 2%

Graduate Enrollment 58

Women 97% **Men** 3% **Minority** 19% **Part-time** 5%

Nursing Student Activities Nursing Honor Society, Sigma Theta Tau, Student Nurses' Association, nursing club.

Nursing Student Resources Academic advising; academic or career counseling; assistance for students with disabilities; bookstore; campus computer network; career placement assistance; computer lab; computer-assisted instruction; e-mail services; employment services for current students; housing assistance; interactive nursing skills videos; Internet; learning resource lab; library services; nursing audiovisuals; paid internships; remedial services; resume preparation assistance; skills, simulation, or other laboratory; tutoring; unpaid internships.

Library Facilities 350,750 volumes (11,300 in health, 5,930 in nursing); 3,433 periodical subscriptions (142 health-care related).

Pacific Lutheran University (continued)

BACCALAUREATE PROGRAMS

Degree BSN

Available Programs ADN to Baccalaureate; Generic Baccalaureate; LPN to Baccalaureate.

Study Options Full-time and part-time.

Program Entrance Requirements Minimum overall college GPA of 3.0, transcript of college record, CPR certification, written essay, health exam, health insurance, 2 years high school math, high school transcript, immunizations, 2 letters of recommendation, minimum GPA in nursing prerequisites of 2.75, professional liability insurance/malpractice insurance, prerequisite course work. Transfer students are accepted. **Standardized tests** *Required:* SAT or ACT, TOEFL for international students. **Application** *Deadline:* rolling (freshmen), rolling (transfer). *Notification:* continuous (freshmen). *Application fee:* $40.

Advanced Placement Credit by examination available. Credit given for nursing courses completed elsewhere dependent upon specific evaluations.

Expenses (2006–07) *Tuition:* full-time $23,450; part-time $731 per credit hour. *International tuition:* $23,450 full-time. *Room and board:* $7140 per academic year. *Required fees:* full-time $418.

Financial Aid 95% of baccalaureate students in nursing programs received some form of financial aid in 2005–06. *Gift aid (need-based):* Federal Pell, FSEOG, state, private, college/university gift aid from institutional funds, Federal Nursing. *Loans:* Federal Nursing Student Loans, FFEL (Subsidized and Unsubsidized Stafford PLUS), Perkins, state, college/university. *Work-Study:* Federal Work-Study, part-time campus jobs. *Application deadline (priority):* 3/1.

Contact Ms. Audrey Cox, Admission, Retention, Recruitment Coordinator, School of Nursing, Pacific Lutheran University, Tacoma, WA 98447-0029. *Telephone:* 253-535-7672. *Fax:* 253-535-7590. *E-mail:* coxae@plu.edu.

GRADUATE PROGRAMS

Expenses (2006–07) *Tuition:* full-time $11,689; part-time $731 per credit hour. *International tuition:* $11,689 full-time.

Financial Aid 100% of graduate students in nursing programs received some form of financial aid in 2005–06. Federal Work-Study, scholarships, and unspecified assistantships available. *Financial aid application deadline:* 3/1.

Contact Ms. Susan Duis, Admissions Coordinator, School of Nursing, Pacific Lutheran University, School of Nursing, Tacoma, WA 98447-0029. *Telephone:* 253-535-8872. *Fax:* 253-535-7590. *E-mail:* duisse@plu.edu.

MASTER'S DEGREE PROGRAM

Degree MSN

Available Programs Accelerated Master's; Master's; Master's for Non-Nursing College Graduates; Master's for Nurses with Non-Nursing Degrees; RN to Master's.

Concentrations Available Health-care administration; nurse case management; nursing administration; nursing education; nursing informatics. *Clinical nurse specialist programs in:* acute care, adult health, medical-surgical. *Nurse practitioner programs in:* family health.

Study Options Full-time and part-time.

Program Entrance Requirements Clinical experience, computer literacy, minimum overall college GPA of 3.0, transcript of college record, CPR certification, written essay, immunizations, interview, 2 letters of recommendation, nursing research course, professional liability insurance/malpractice insurance, prerequisite course work, resume, statistics course, GRE General Test. *Application deadline:* For fall admission, 4/1 (priority date). Applications are processed on a rolling basis. *Application fee:* $35.

Advanced Placement Credit by examination available. Credit given for nursing courses completed elsewhere dependent upon specific evaluations.

Degree Requirements 36 total credit hours, thesis or project.

CONTINUING EDUCATION PROGRAM

Contact Dr. Patsy Maloney, Director, Continuing Nursing Education, School of Nursing, Pacific Lutheran University, Tacoma, WA 98447-0029. *Telephone:* 253-535-7683. *Fax:* 253-535-7590. *E-mail:* malonepl@plu.edu.

Seattle Pacific University
School of Health Sciences
Seattle, Washington

Founded in 1891

DEGREES • BS • MSN

Nursing Program Faculty 27 (37% with doctorates).

Baccalaureate Enrollment 157
Women 90% **Men** 10% **Minority** 21% **International** 5% **Part-time** 37%

Graduate Enrollment 34
Women 97% **Men** 3% **Minority** 9% **Part-time** 41%

Nursing Student Activities Sigma Theta Tau, nursing club.

Nursing Student Resources Academic advising; academic or career counseling; assistance for students with disabilities; bookstore; campus computer network; career placement assistance; computer lab; computer-assisted instruction; e-mail services; employment services for current students; housing assistance; Internet; learning resource lab; library services; nursing audiovisuals; placement services for program completers; remedial services; resume preparation assistance; skills, simulation, or other laboratory; tutoring.

Library Facilities 191,807 volumes (11,316 in health, 1,705 in nursing); 1,230 periodical subscriptions (278 health-care related).

BACCALAUREATE PROGRAMS

Degree BS

Available Programs Generic Baccalaureate; RN Baccalaureate.

Site Options Seattle, WA; Mt. Vernon, WA; Bellingham, WA. *Distance Learning:* Tacoma, WA.

Study Options Full-time.

Program Entrance Requirements Minimum overall college GPA of 2.75, transcript of college record, CPR certification, written essay, health exam, health insurance, immunizations, 1 letter of recommendation, minimum GPA in nursing prerequisites of 2.75, prerequisite course work. Transfer students are accepted. **Standardized tests** *Required:* SAT or ACT, TOEFL for international students. *Recommended:* SAT. **Application** *Deadline:* 2/1 (freshmen), 8/1 (transfer). *Early decision:* 11/15. *Notification:* continuous until 3/1 (freshmen), 1/6 (early action). *Application fee:* $45.

Advanced Placement Credit given for nursing courses completed elsewhere dependent upon specific evaluations.

Expenses (2006–07) *Tuition:* full-time $23,055; part-time $285 per credit. *Room and board:* $7818; room only: $4212 per academic year.

Financial Aid 72% of baccalaureate students in nursing programs received some form of financial aid in 2005–06. *Gift aid (need-based):* Federal Pell, FSEOG, state, private, college/university gift aid from institutional funds. *Loans:* Federal Nursing Student Loans, FFEL (Subsidized and Unsubsidized Stafford PLUS), Perkins, college/university. *Work-Study:* Federal Work-Study, part-time campus jobs. *Application deadline (priority):* 4/1.

Contact Dr. Emily Hitchens, Associate Dean, School of Health Sciences, Seattle Pacific University, Marston Hall, Suite 106, 3307 Third Avenue West, Seattle, WA 98119-1922. *Telephone:* 206-281-2964. *Fax:* 206-281-2767. *E-mail:* hitchens@spu.edu.

GRADUATE PROGRAMS

Expenses (2006–07) *Tuition:* part-time $485 per credit. *Required fees:* full-time $200.

Financial Aid 60% of graduate students in nursing programs received some form of financial aid in 2005–06. 2 teaching assistantships were awarded; career-related internships or fieldwork and traineeships also available.

Contact Mrs. Pam Christensen, Graduate Administrative Assistant, School of Health Sciences, Seattle Pacific University, Marston Hall, 3307 Third Avenue West, Suite 106, Seattle, WA 98119-1922. *Telephone:* 206-281-2616. *Fax:* 206-281-2767. *E-mail:* pjchris@spu.edu.

MASTER'S DEGREE PROGRAM

Degree MSN

Available Programs Master's.

Concentrations Available Nursing administration; nursing education; nursing informatics. *Clinical nurse specialist programs in:* acute care, adult health, cardiovascular, community health, gerontology, maternity-newborn, medical-surgical, oncology, palliative care, pediatric, perinatal, public health, rehabilitation, school health, women's health. *Nurse practitioner programs in:* adult health, family health, gerontology.

Study Options Full-time and part-time.

Program Entrance Requirements Computer literacy, minimum overall college GPA of 3.0, transcript of college record, CPR certification, written essay, interview, 3 letters of recommendation, nursing research course, professional liability insurance/malpractice insurance, prerequisite course work, statistics course, GRE General Test. *Application deadline:* For fall admission, 9/1 (priority date). Applications are processed on a rolling basis. *Application fee:* $50.

Degree Requirements 56 total credit hours, thesis or project, comprehensive exam.

POST-MASTER'S PROGRAM

Areas of Study Nursing education. *Nurse practitioner programs in:* adult health, family health, gerontology.

Seattle University
College of Nursing
Seattle, Washington

http://www.seattleu.edu/nurs

Founded in 1891

DEGREES • BSN • MSN

Nursing Program Faculty 51 (46% with doctorates).

Baccalaureate Enrollment 378
Women 91% **Men** 9% **Minority** 40% **International** 1% **Part-time** 5%

Graduate Enrollment 57
Women 86% **Men** 14% **Minority** 32% **International** 2% **Part-time** 18%

Nursing Student Activities Sigma Theta Tau, Student Nurses' Association.

Nursing Student Resources Academic advising; academic or career counseling; assistance for students with disabilities; bookstore; campus computer network; career placement assistance; computer lab; computer-assisted instruction; e-mail services; housing assistance; interactive nursing skills videos; Internet; learning resource lab; library services; nursing audiovisuals; remedial services; resume preparation assistance; skills, simulation, or other laboratory.

Library Facilities 141,478 volumes (9,534 in health); 2,701 periodical subscriptions (132 health-care related).

BACCALAUREATE PROGRAMS

Degree BSN

Available Programs Baccalaureate for Second Degree; Generic Baccalaureate.

Study Options Full-time and part-time.

Program Entrance Requirements Minimum overall college GPA of 2.75, transcript of college record, written essay, high school chemistry, 3 years high school math, 2 years high school science, high school transcript, 2 letters of recommendation, minimum high school GPA of 2.75, minimum high school rank 50%, minimum GPA in nursing prerequisites of 2.75, prerequisite course work. Transfer students are accepted. **Standardized tests** *Required:* SAT or ACT, TOEFL for international students. **Application** *Deadline:* rolling (freshmen), 8/15 (transfer). *Notification:* continuous (freshmen). *Application fee:* $45.

Advanced Placement Credit given for nursing courses completed elsewhere dependent upon specific evaluations.

Contact *Telephone:* 206-296-2242. *Fax:* 206-296-5544.

GRADUATE PROGRAMS

Contact *Telephone:* 206-296-5666. *Fax:* 206-296-5544.

MASTER'S DEGREE PROGRAM

Degree MSN

Available Programs Accelerated Master's for Nurses with Non-Nursing Degrees; Master's.

Concentrations Available *Clinical nurse specialist programs in:* community health. *Nurse practitioner programs in:* family health, psychiatric/mental health.

Study Options Full-time and part-time.

Program Entrance Requirements Clinical experience, minimum overall college GPA of 3.0, transcript of college record, CPR certification, written essay, immunizations, interview, 2 letters of recommendation, professional liability insurance/malpractice insurance, resume, statistics course, GRE General Test. *Application deadline:* For fall admission, 7/1. *Application fee:* $55.

Advanced Placement Credit given for nursing courses completed elsewhere dependent upon specific evaluations.

Degree Requirements 63 total credit hours, thesis or project.

POST-MASTER'S PROGRAM

Areas of Study *Nurse practitioner programs in:* family health, psychiatric/mental health.

University of Washington
School of Nursing
Seattle, Washington

Founded in 1861

DEGREES • BSN • MN • MN/MPH • PHD

Nursing Program Faculty 166 (64% with doctorates).

Baccalaureate Enrollment 487
Women 92% **Men** 8% **Minority** 24% **International** 1% **Part-time** 54%

Graduate Enrollment 526
Women 91% **Men** 9% **Minority** 14% **International** 6% **Part-time** 60%

Nursing Student Activities Sigma Theta Tau, Student Nurses' Association.

Nursing Student Resources Academic advising; bookstore; campus computer network; computer lab; computer-assisted instruction; e-mail services; employment services for current students; interactive nursing skills videos; Internet; learning resource lab; library services; nursing audiovisuals; skills, simulation, or other laboratory.

Library Facilities 5.8 million volumes (123,098 in health); 50,245 periodical subscriptions (4,000 health-care related).

BACCALAUREATE PROGRAMS

Degree BSN

Available Programs Generic Baccalaureate; RN Baccalaureate.

Site Options Bothell, WA; Tacoma, WA.

Study Options Full-time.

Program Entrance Requirements Minimum overall college GPA of 2.0, transcript of college record, CPR certification, written essay, immunizations, 1 letter of recommendation, minimum GPA in nursing prerequisites of 2.0, prerequisite course work. Transfer students are accepted. **Standardized tests** *Required:* SAT or ACT, TOEFL for international students. **Application** *Deadline:* 1/15 (freshmen), 2/15 (transfer). *Notification:* continuous (freshmen). *Application fee:* $50.

Expenses (2006–07) *Tuition, state resident:* full-time $5985; part-time $199 per quarter hour. *Tuition, nonresident:* full-time $21,285; part-time $710 per quarter hour. *International tuition:* $21,285 full-time. *Room and board:* $8889; room only: $3882 per academic year. *Required fees:* full-time $257.

Financial Aid 44% of baccalaureate students in nursing programs received some form of financial aid in 2005–06.

Contact Ms. Carolyn A. Chow, Director of Admissions and Multicultural Student Affairs, School of Nursing, University of Washington, Health Sciences Building, Box 357260, Seattle, WA 98195. *Telephone:* 206-543-8736. *Fax:* 206-685-1613. *E-mail:* egg@u.washington.edu.

University of Washington (continued)

GRADUATE PROGRAMS

Expenses (2006–07) *Tuition, state resident:* full-time $11,196; part-time $534 per quarter hour. *Tuition, nonresident:* full-time $21,645; part-time $1031 per quarter hour. *International tuition:* $21,645 full-time. *Room and board:* $9777; room only: $4770 per academic year. *Required fees:* full-time $257.

Financial Aid 20% of graduate students in nursing programs received some form of financial aid in 2005–06. Fellowships with full tuition reimbursements available, research assistantships with partial tuition reimbursements available, teaching assistantships with partial tuition reimbursements available, Federal Work-Study, institutionally sponsored loans, scholarships, and traineeships available. *Financial aid application deadline:* 2/28.

Contact Ms. Carolyn A. Chow, Director of Admissions and Multicultural Student Affairs, School of Nursing, University of Washington, Health Sciences Building, Box 357260, Seattle, WA 98195. *Telephone:* 206-543-8736. *Fax:* 206-685-1613. *E-mail:* egg@u.washington.edu.

MASTER'S DEGREE PROGRAM

Degrees MN; MN/MPH

Available Programs Master's; Master's for Non-Nursing College Graduates; Master's for Nurses with Non-Nursing Degrees.

Concentrations Available Nurse-midwifery; nursing education; nursing informatics. *Clinical nurse specialist programs in:* acute care, cardiovascular, community health, critical care, forensic nursing, gerontology, maternity-newborn, medical-surgical, occupational health, oncology, parent-child, pediatric, perinatal, psychiatric/mental health, women's health. *Nurse practitioner programs in:* acute care, adult health, family health, gerontology, neonatal health, pediatric, primary care, psychiatric/mental health, women's health.

Site Options Bothell, WA; Tacoma, WA.

Study Options Full-time and part-time.

Program Entrance Requirements Minimum overall college GPA of 3.0, transcript of college record, CPR certification, written essay, immunizations, 3 letters of recommendation, resume, statistics course, GRE. *Application deadline:* For fall admission, 2/1. *Application fee:* $50.

Degree Requirements 38 total credit hours, thesis or project.

POST-MASTER'S PROGRAM

Areas of Study Nurse-midwifery; nursing education; nursing informatics. *Clinical nurse specialist programs in:* acute care, cardiovascular, community health, critical care, forensic nursing, gerontology, maternity-newborn, medical-surgical, occupational health, oncology, parent-child, pediatric, perinatal, psychiatric/mental health, women's health. *Nurse practitioner programs in:* acute care, adult health, family health, gerontology, neonatal health, pediatric, primary care, psychiatric/mental health, women's health.

DOCTORAL DEGREE PROGRAM

Degree PhD

Available Programs Doctorate for Nurses with Non-Nursing Degrees; Post-Baccalaureate Doctorate.

Areas of Study Individualized study, nursing science.

Program Entrance Requirements Minimum overall college GPA of 3.0, 3 letters of recommendation, scholarly papers, statistics course, vita, writing sample, GRE. *Application deadline:* For fall admission, 2/1. *Application fee:* $50.

Degree Requirements 93 total credit hours, dissertation, oral exam, written exam, residency.

POSTDOCTORAL PROGRAM

Postdoctoral Program Contact Office of Academic Programs, School of Nursing, University of Washington, T-310 Health Sciences Building, Box 357260, Seattle, WA 98195. *Telephone:* 206-543-8736. *Fax:* 206-685-1613. *E-mail:* sonapo@u.washington.edu.

CONTINUING EDUCATION PROGRAM

Contact Dr. Ruth Craven, Associate Dean for Educational Outreach, School of Nursing, University of Washington, Box 357260, Seattle, WA 98195. *Telephone:* 206-616-3549. *Fax:* 206-543-3624. *E-mail:* ruthc@u.washington.edu.

Walla Walla College

School of Nursing
College Place, Washington

http://www.wwc.edu/academics/department/nursing

Founded in 1892

DEGREE • BS

Nursing Program Faculty 17 (17% with doctorates).

Baccalaureate Enrollment 133

Women 83% **Men** 17% **Minority** 14% **International** 1% **Part-time** 1%

Nursing Student Activities Nursing Honor Society, nursing club.

Nursing Student Resources Academic advising; assistance for students with disabilities; bookstore; campus computer network; computer lab; e-mail services; Internet; learning resource lab; library services; nursing audiovisuals; resume preparation assistance; skills, simulation, or other laboratory; tutoring.

Library Facilities 178,450 volumes (10,000 in health, 7,000 in nursing); 1,105 periodical subscriptions (450 health-care related).

BACCALAUREATE PROGRAMS

Degree BS

Available Programs ADN to Baccalaureate; Generic Baccalaureate; LPN to Baccalaureate; RN Baccalaureate.

Site Options Portland, OR.

Study Options Full-time and part-time.

Program Entrance Requirements Minimum overall college GPA of 2.75, transcript of college record, CPR certification, written essay, health exam, health insurance, high school biology, 3 years high school math, 2 years high school science, high school transcript, immunizations, 3 letters of recommendation, minimum high school GPA of 2.75, minimum GPA in nursing prerequisites of 2.75, prerequisite course work. Transfer students are accepted. **Standardized tests** *Required:* SAT, SAT or ACT, TOEFL for international students. **Application** *Deadline:* rolling (freshmen), 9/30 (out-of-state freshmen), rolling (transfer). *Notification:* continuous (freshmen), 9/30 (out-of-state freshmen). *Application fee:* $40.

Advanced Placement Credit given for nursing courses completed elsewhere dependent upon specific evaluations.

Expenses (2006–07) *Tuition:* full-time $19,725; part-time $516 per quarter hour. *International tuition:* $19,725 full-time. *Room and board:* $3993; room only: $2472 per academic year. *Required fees:* full-time $192.

Financial Aid 95% of baccalaureate students in nursing programs received some form of financial aid in 2005–06.

Contact Jan Thurnhofer, RN, Student Program Advisor, School of Nursing, Walla Walla College, 10345 SE Market Street, Portland, OR 97216. *Telephone:* 503-251-6115 Ext. 7304. *Fax:* 503-251-6249. *E-mail:* thurnja@wwc.edu.

Washington State University

Intercollegiate College of Nursing/Washington State University
Pullman, Washington

See description of programs under
Intercollegiate College of Nursing/Washington State University (Spokane, Washington).

Whitworth College
Intercollegiate College of Nursing/Washington State University
Spokane, Washington

See description of programs under **Intercollegiate College of Nursing/Washington State University (Spokane, Washington).**

WEST VIRGINIA

Alderson-Broaddus College
Department of Nursing
Philippi, West Virginia

Founded in 1871

DEGREE • BSN

Nursing Program Faculty 11 (18% with doctorates).

Baccalaureate Enrollment 195
Women 94% **Men** 6% **Minority** 2% **Part-time** 2%

Nursing Student Activities Student Nurses' Association.

Nursing Student Resources Academic advising; academic or career counseling; assistance for students with disabilities; bookstore; campus computer network; career placement assistance; computer lab; computer-assisted instruction; e-mail services; employment services for current students; Internet; learning resource lab; library services; nursing audiovisuals; remedial services; resume preparation assistance; skills, simulation, or other laboratory; tutoring.

Library Facilities 100,000 volumes (6,000 in health); 11,000 periodical subscriptions (172 health-care related).

BACCALAUREATE PROGRAMS

Degree BSN

Available Programs Generic Baccalaureate; LPN to RN Baccalaureate; RN Baccalaureate.

Study Options Full-time.

Program Entrance Requirements Minimum overall college GPA of 2.0, transcript of college record, CPR certification, health exam, high school transcript, immunizations, minimum GPA in nursing prerequisites of 2.0, professional liability insurance/malpractice insurance, prerequisite course work. Transfer students are accepted. **Standardized tests** *Required:* SAT and SAT Subject Tests or ACT, TOEFL for international students. **Application** *Deadline:* rolling (freshmen), rolling (transfer). *Notification:* continuous until 8/31 (freshmen). *Application fee:* $10.

Advanced Placement Credit by examination available. Credit given for nursing courses completed elsewhere dependent upon specific evaluations.

Expenses (2006–07) *Tuition:* full-time $18,890; part-time $630 per credit hour. *Room and board:* $6160 per academic year. *Required fees:* full-time $200.

Financial Aid 98% of baccalaureate students in nursing programs received some form of financial aid in 2005–06.

Contact Dr. Threasia L. Witt, EdD, Chairperson, Department of Nursing, Alderson-Broaddus College, Box 2003, Philippi, WV 26416. *Telephone:* 304-457-6285 Ext. 285. *Fax:* 304-457-6293. *E-mail:* witttl@mail.ab.edu.

Bluefield State College
Program in Nursing
Bluefield, West Virginia

http://www.bluefieldstate.edu

Founded in 1895

DEGREE • BSN

Nursing Program Faculty 3 (30% with doctorates).

Baccalaureate Enrollment 60
Women 95% **Men** 5% **Minority** 1% **Part-time** 2%

Nursing Student Activities Sigma Theta Tau, Student Nurses' Association.

Nursing Student Resources Academic advising; academic or career counseling; assistance for students with disabilities; bookstore; campus computer network; career placement assistance; computer lab; computer-assisted instruction; e-mail services; interactive nursing skills videos; Internet; learning resource lab; library services; nursing audiovisuals; resume preparation assistance; skills, simulation, or other laboratory; tutoring.

Library Facilities 76,391 volumes (5,649 in health, 1,250 in nursing); 2,453 periodical subscriptions (200 health-care related).

BACCALAUREATE PROGRAMS

Degree BSN

Available Programs RN Baccalaureate.

Site Options *Distance Learning:* Beckley, WV.

Study Options Full-time and part-time.

Program Entrance Requirements Minimum overall college GPA of 2.5, transcript of college record, CPR certification, health exam, immunizations, letters of recommendation, minimum GPA in nursing prerequisites, prerequisite course work. Transfer students are accepted. **Standardized tests** *Recommended:* SAT or ACT, TOEFL for international students. **Application** *Deadline:* rolling (freshmen), rolling (transfer). *Notification:* continuous (freshmen).

Expenses (2006–07) *Tuition, area resident:* full-time $5720; part-time $239 per credit hour. *Tuition, state resident:* full-time $3648; part-time $153 per credit hour. *Tuition, nonresident:* full-time $7760; part-time $324 per credit hour. *International tuition:* $7760 full-time. *Required fees:* part-time $1824 per term.

Financial Aid 60% of baccalaureate students in nursing programs received some form of financial aid in 2005–06. *Gift aid (need-based):* Federal Pell, FSEOG, state, private, college/university gift aid from institutional funds. *Loans:* Federal Direct (Subsidized and Unsubsidized Stafford PLUS), Perkins. *Work-Study:* Federal Work-Study, part-time campus jobs. *Application deadline (priority):* 3/1.

Contact Ms. Beth Ann Pritchett, Director, Program in Nursing, Bluefield State College, 219 Rock Street, Bluefield, WV 24701. *Telephone:* 304-327-4139. *Fax:* 304-327-4219. *E-mail:* bpritchett@bluefieldstate.edu.

Fairmont State University
School of Nursing and Allied Health Administration
Fairmont, West Virginia

http://www.fscwv.edu

Founded in 1865

DEGREE • BSN

Nursing Program Faculty 3 (33% with doctorates).

Baccalaureate Enrollment 70
Women 97% **Men** 3% **Part-time** 70%

Nursing Student Activities Student Nurses' Association.

Nursing Student Resources Academic advising; academic or career counseling; assistance for students with disabilities; bookstore; campus computer network; computer lab; computer-assisted instruction; e-mail services; housing assistance; interactive nursing skills videos; Internet;

Fairmont State University (continued)

learning resource lab; library services; nursing audiovisuals; placement services for program completers; remedial services; resume preparation assistance; skills, simulation, or other laboratory; tutoring.

Library Facilities 280,000 volumes (7,000 in health, 1,100 in nursing); 895 periodical subscriptions (50 health-care related).

BACCALAUREATE PROGRAMS

Degree BSN

Available Programs ADN to Baccalaureate; LPN to RN Baccalaureate; RN Baccalaureate.

Study Options Full-time and part-time.

Program Entrance Requirements Minimum overall college GPA of 2.5, transcript of college record, CPR certification, health exam, high school chemistry, immunizations, 1 letter of recommendation, minimum GPA in nursing prerequisites of 3.0, prerequisite course work, RN licensure. Transfer students are accepted. **Standardized tests** *Required:* SAT and SAT Subject Tests or ACT, TOEFL for international students. **Application** *Deadline:* 6/15 (freshmen), 6/15 (transfer).

Advanced Placement Credit by examination available. Credit given for nursing courses completed elsewhere dependent upon specific evaluations.

Expenses (2006–07) *Tuition, state resident:* full-time $4218; part-time $354 per hour. *Tuition, nonresident:* full-time $8808; part-time $736 per hour. *International tuition:* $8808 full-time. *Room and board:* $5674; room only: $2814 per academic year. *Required fees:* full-time $120; part-time $60 per term.

Financial Aid 80% of baccalaureate students in nursing programs received some form of financial aid in 2005–06.

Contact Dr. Mary M. Meighen, Professor, School of Nursing and Allied Health Administration, Fairmont State University, 1201 Locust Avenue, Fairmont, WV 26554. *Telephone:* 304-367-4761. *Fax:* 304-367-4268. *E-mail:* mmeighen@fairmontstate.edu.

CONTINUING EDUCATION PROGRAM

Contact Dr. Mary M. Meighen, Professor, School of Nursing and Allied Health Administration, Fairmont State University, 1201 Locust Avenue, Fairmont, WV 26554. *Telephone:* 304-367-4761. *Fax:* 304-367-4268. *E-mail:* mmeighen@fairmontstate.edu.

Marshall University
College of Health Professions
Huntington, West Virginia

http://www.marshall.edu/conhp

Founded in 1837

DEGREES • BSN • MSN

Nursing Program Faculty 35 (23% with doctorates).
Baccalaureate Enrollment 345
Women 80% **Men** 20% **Minority** 5% **Part-time** 35%
Graduate Enrollment 100
Women 90% **Men** 10% **Part-time** 60%

Nursing Student Activities Sigma Theta Tau, Student Nurses' Association, nursing club.

Nursing Student Resources Academic advising; academic or career counseling; assistance for students with disabilities; bookstore; campus computer network; career placement assistance; computer lab; computer-assisted instruction; daycare for children of students; e-mail services; employment services for current students; externships; housing assistance; interactive nursing skills videos; Internet; learning resource lab; library services; nursing audiovisuals; placement services for program completers; remedial services; resume preparation assistance; skills, simulation, or other laboratory; tutoring.

Library Facilities 1.6 million volumes (20,200 in health, 6,400 in nursing); 22,591 periodical subscriptions (500 health-care related).

BACCALAUREATE PROGRAMS

Degree BSN

Available Programs Accelerated RN Baccalaureate; Generic Baccalaureate.

Site Options *Distance Learning:* South Charleston, WV; Point Pleasant, WV.

Study Options Full-time and part-time.

Program Entrance Requirements Minimum overall college GPA of 2.5, transcript of college record, high school transcript, minimum high school GPA of 2.5. Transfer students are accepted. **Standardized tests** *Required:* SAT or ACT, TOEFL for international students. **Application** *Deadline:* rolling (freshmen), rolling (transfer). *Notification:* continuous (freshmen). *Application fee:* $30.

Advanced Placement Credit given for nursing courses completed elsewhere dependent upon specific evaluations.

Expenses (2006–07) *Tuition, state resident:* full-time $4400; part-time $171 per credit hour. *Tuition, nonresident:* full-time $11,804; part-time $479 per credit hour. *Room and board:* $6000; room only: $4000 per academic year. *Required fees:* full-time $250; part-time $11 per credit; part-time $50 per term.

Financial Aid 52% of baccalaureate students in nursing programs received some form of financial aid in 2005–06. *Gift aid (need-based):* Federal Pell, FSEOG, state, private, college/university gift aid from institutional funds. *Loans:* Federal Direct (Subsidized and Unsubsidized Stafford PLUS), Perkins, state, college/university, alternative loans through outside sources. *Work-Study:* Federal Work-Study, part-time campus jobs. *Application deadline (priority):* 3/1.

Contact Dr. Sandra Marra, Chairman, Nursing, College of Health Professions, Marshall University, One John Marshall Drive, Huntington, WV 25755-9500. *Telephone:* 304-696-2639. *Fax:* 304-696-6739. *E-mail:* Nursing@marshall.edu.

GRADUATE PROGRAMS

Expenses (2006–07) *Tuition, state resident:* full-time $4836; part-time $253 per credit hour. *Tuition, nonresident:* full-time $14,208; part-time $735 per credit hour. *Room and board:* $6000; room only: $4000 per academic year. *Required fees:* full-time $500; part-time $28 per credit; part-time $50 per term.

Financial Aid 51% of graduate students in nursing programs received some form of financial aid in 2005–06.

Contact Dr. Sandra Marra, Chairman, Nursing, College of Health Professions, Marshall University, One John Marshall Drive, Huntington, WV 25755-9500. *Telephone:* 304-696-2639. *Fax:* 304-696-6739. *E-mail:* Nursing@marshall.edu.

MASTER'S DEGREE PROGRAM

Degree MSN

Available Programs Master's.

Concentrations Available Nursing administration; nursing education. *Nurse practitioner programs in:* family health.

Site Options *Distance Learning:* South Charleston, WV; Bluefield, WV; Point Pleasant, WV.

Study Options Full-time and part-time.

Program Entrance Requirements Minimum overall college GPA of 3.0, transcript of college record, nursing research course, resume, statistics course, GRE General Test.

Advanced Placement Credit given for nursing courses completed elsewhere dependent upon specific evaluations.

Degree Requirements 36 total credit hours, thesis or project.

POST-MASTER'S PROGRAM

Areas of Study Nursing administration; nursing education. *Nurse practitioner programs in:* family health.

Mountain State University
Program in Nursing
Beckley, West Virginia

http://www.mountainstate.edu

Founded in 1933

DEGREES • BSN • MSN

Nursing Program Faculty 89 (11% with doctorates).

Baccalaureate Enrollment 388
Women 94% **Men** 6% **Minority** 1% **International** 1% **Part-time** 2%

Graduate Enrollment 120
Women 83% **Men** 17% **Minority** 1% **Part-time** 33%

Nursing Student Activities Nursing Honor Society, Student Nurses' Association.

Nursing Student Resources Academic advising; academic or career counseling; assistance for students with disabilities; bookstore; campus computer network; career placement assistance; computer lab; computer-assisted instruction; e-mail services; employment services for current students; externships; interactive nursing skills videos; Internet; learning resource lab; library services; nursing audiovisuals; placement services for program completers; remedial services; resume preparation assistance; skills, simulation, or other laboratory; tutoring.

Library Facilities 113,361 volumes (10,669 in health, 565 in nursing); 155 periodical subscriptions (1,399 health-care related).

BACCALAUREATE PROGRAMS

Degree BSN

Available Programs ADN to Baccalaureate; Baccalaureate for Second Degree; Generic Baccalaureate; LPN to Baccalaureate; RN Baccalaureate; RPN to Baccalaureate.

Site Options *Distance Learning:* Martinsburg, WV.

Study Options Full-time and part-time.

Program Entrance Requirements Minimum overall college GPA of 2.5, transcript of college record, CPR certification, health exam, health insurance, high school biology, 2 years high school science, high school transcript, immunizations, minimum high school GPA of 2.5. Transfer students are accepted. **Standardized tests** *Recommended:* SAT, ACT, SAT or ACT, SAT Subject Tests. *Required for some:* SAT and SAT Subject Tests or ACT. **Application** *Deadline:* rolling (freshmen), rolling (transfer). *Application fee:* $25.

Advanced Placement Credit by examination available. Credit given for nursing courses completed elsewhere dependent upon specific evaluations.

Expenses (2006–07) *Tuition:* full-time $7320; part-time $30 per credit hour. *International tuition:* $7320 full-time. *Room and board:* $5636; room only: $2810 per academic year. *Required fees:* full-time $1440; part-time $60 per credit.

Financial Aid 83% of baccalaureate students in nursing programs received some form of financial aid in 2005–06.

Contact Dr. Patsy Haslam, Senior Academic Officer, Program in Nursing, Mountain State University, PO Box 9003, Beckley, WV 25802-9003. *Telephone:* 304-929-1327. *Fax:* 304-253-0789. *E-mail:* phaslam@mountainstate.edu.

GRADUATE PROGRAMS

Expenses (2006–07) *Tuition:* full-time $12,395; part-time $335 per credit hour. *International tuition:* $12,395 full-time. *Room and board:* $5636; room only: $2810 per academic year.

Financial Aid 57% of graduate students in nursing programs received some form of financial aid in 2005–06.

Contact Dr. Jessica Sharp, Graduate Program Director, Program in Nursing, Mountain State University, PO Box 9003, Beckley, WV 25802-9003. *Telephone:* 304-929-1425. *E-mail:* jsharp@mountainstate.edu.

MASTER'S DEGREE PROGRAM

Degree MSN

Available Programs Master's.

Concentrations Available Nurse anesthesia; nursing administration; nursing education. *Nurse practitioner programs in:* family health.

Site Options *Distance Learning:* Martinsburg, WV.

Study Options Full-time and part-time.

Program Entrance Requirements Clinical experience, computer literacy, minimum overall college GPA of 3.0, transcript of college record, CPR certification, written essay, immunizations, 3 letters of recommendation, nursing research course, physical assessment course, prerequisite course work, resume, statistics course.

Advanced Placement Credit given for nursing courses completed elsewhere dependent upon specific evaluations.

Degree Requirements 37 total credit hours, thesis or project, comprehensive exam.

POST-MASTER'S PROGRAM

Areas of Study Nurse anesthesia; nursing administration; nursing education. *Nurse practitioner programs in:* family health.

Shepherd University
Department of Nursing Education
Shepherdstown, West Virginia

http://www.shepherd.edu/nurseweb/
Founded in 1871

DEGREE • BSN

Nursing Program Faculty 7 (57% with doctorates).

Baccalaureate Enrollment 99
Women 92% **Men** 8% **Minority** 13%

Nursing Student Activities Nursing Honor Society.

Nursing Student Resources Academic advising; academic or career counseling; assistance for students with disabilities; bookstore; campus computer network; career placement assistance; computer lab; computer-assisted instruction; e-mail services; Internet; learning resource lab; library services; nursing audiovisuals; remedial services; resume preparation assistance; skills, simulation, or other laboratory; tutoring.

Library Facilities 190,586 volumes (3,678 in health, 394 in nursing); 13,376 periodical subscriptions (1,956 health-care related).

BACCALAUREATE PROGRAMS

Degree BSN

Available Programs ADN to Baccalaureate; Generic Baccalaureate; RN Baccalaureate.

Study Options Full-time.

Program Entrance Requirements Minimum overall college GPA of 2.5, transcript of college record, CPR certification, written essay, health exam, immunizations, interview, minimum GPA in nursing prerequisites of 2.0, prerequisite course work. Transfer students are accepted. **Standardized tests** *Required:* SAT or ACT, TOEFL for international students. **Application** *Deadline:* rolling (freshmen), rolling (transfer). *Early decision:* 11/15. *Notification:* continuous until 8/15 (freshmen), 12/15 (early action). *Application fee:* $35.

Advanced Placement Credit by examination available. Credit given for nursing courses completed elsewhere dependent upon specific evaluations.

Expenses (2006–07) *Tuition, state resident:* full-time $4348; part-time $177 per credit hour. *Tuition, nonresident:* full-time $11,464; part-time $473 per credit hour. *International tuition:* $11,464 full-time. *Room and board:* $6456 per academic year. *Required fees:* full-time $220.

Financial Aid 76% of baccalaureate students in nursing programs received some form of financial aid in 2005–06. *Gift aid (need-based):* Federal Pell, FSEOG, state, private, college/university gift aid from institutional funds. *Loans:* Federal Direct (Subsidized and Unsubsidized Stafford PLUS), Perkins. *Work-Study:* Federal Work-Study, part-time campus jobs. *Application deadline (priority):* 3/1.

Contact Dr. Kathleen B. Gaberson, Professor and Chair, Department of Nursing Education, Shepherd University, 301 North King Street, Shepherdstown, WV 25443. *Telephone:* 304-876-5341. *Fax:* 304-876-5169. *E-mail:* kgaberso@shepherd.edu.

CONTINUING EDUCATION PROGRAM

Contact Dr. Kathleen B. Gaberson, Professor and Chair, Department of Nursing Education, Shepherd University, 301 North King Street, Shepherdstown, WV 25443. *Telephone:* 304-876-5341. *Fax:* 304-876-5169. *E-mail:* kgaberso@shepherd.edu.

University of Charleston
Department of Nursing
Charleston, West Virginia

http://www.ucwv.edu/dhs/bsn

Founded in 1888

DEGREE • BSN

Nursing Program Faculty 10 (30% with doctorates).

Baccalaureate Enrollment 103
Women 92% **Men** 8% **Minority** 5% **Part-time** 3%

Nursing Student Activities Sigma Theta Tau, Student Nurses' Association, nursing club.

Nursing Student Resources Academic advising; academic or career counseling; assistance for students with disabilities; bookstore; campus computer network; career placement assistance; computer lab; computer-assisted instruction; e-mail services; employment services for current students; externships; housing assistance; interactive nursing skills videos; Internet; learning resource lab; library services; nursing audiovisuals; paid internships; placement services for program completers; remedial services; resume preparation assistance; skills, simulation, or other laboratory; tutoring; unpaid internships.

Library Facilities 164,457 volumes (3,900 in health, 1,550 in nursing); 14,192 periodical subscriptions (75 health-care related).

BACCALAUREATE PROGRAMS

Degree BSN

Available Programs Generic Baccalaureate.

Study Options Full-time and part-time.

Program Entrance Requirements Minimum overall college GPA of 2.75, transcript of college record, CPR certification, health exam, high school biology, 1 year of high school math, high school transcript, immunizations, minimum high school GPA of 2.75, professional liability insurance/malpractice insurance. Transfer students are accepted. **Standardized tests** *Required:* SAT or ACT, TOEFL for international students. **Application** *Deadline:* rolling (freshmen), rolling (out-of-state freshmen), rolling (transfer). *Notification:* continuous (freshmen). *Application fee:* $25.

Advanced Placement Credit given for nursing courses completed elsewhere dependent upon specific evaluations.

Contact *Telephone:* 304-357-4750 Ext. 4750. *Fax:* 304-357-4781.

West Liberty State College
Department of Health Sciences
West Liberty, West Virginia

http://www.wlsc.edu/nursing/index.htm

Founded in 1837

DEGREE • BSN

Nursing Program Faculty 12 (30% with doctorates).

Baccalaureate Enrollment 100
Women 85% **Men** 15% **Minority** 3% **International** 1% **Part-time** 24%

Nursing Student Activities Student Nurses' Association.

Nursing Student Resources Academic advising; academic or career counseling; assistance for students with disabilities; bookstore; campus computer network; career placement assistance; computer lab; computer-assisted instruction; e-mail services; externships; housing assistance; interactive nursing skills videos; Internet; learning resource lab; library services; nursing audiovisuals; placement services for program completers; remedial services; resume preparation assistance; skills, simulation, or other laboratory; tutoring; unpaid internships.

Library Facilities 194,715 volumes (2,500 in health, 750 in nursing); 485 periodical subscriptions (350 health-care related).

BACCALAUREATE PROGRAMS

Degree BSN

Available Programs Accelerated RN Baccalaureate; Generic Baccalaureate.

Site Options *Distance Learning:* Weirton, WV; Wheeling, WV.

Study Options Full-time and part-time.

Program Entrance Requirements Minimum overall college GPA of 2.8, health exam, minimum high school GPA of 3.0, prerequisite course work. Transfer students are accepted. **Standardized tests** *Required:* SAT or ACT, TOEFL for international students. **Application** *Notification:* continuous (freshmen).

Advanced Placement Credit by examination available. Credit given for nursing courses completed elsewhere dependent upon specific evaluations.

Expenses (2006–07) *Tuition, state resident:* full-time $3946; part-time $159 per credit hour. *Tuition, nonresident:* full-time $9630; part-time $396 per credit hour. *International tuition:* $9630 full-time. *Room and board:* $2867 per academic year.

Financial Aid 80% of baccalaureate students in nursing programs received some form of financial aid in 2005–06.

Contact Dr. Monica Kennison, Nursing Program Director, Department of Health Sciences, West Liberty State College, PO Box 295, CMC #140, West Liberty, WV 26074. *Telephone:* 304-336-8108. *Fax:* 304-336-5104. *E-mail:* mkennison@westliberty.edu.

West Virginia University
School of Nursing
Morgantown, West Virginia

http://www.hsc.wvu.edu/son/

Founded in 1867

DEGREES • BSN • DSN • MSN

Nursing Program Faculty 74 (45% with doctorates).

Baccalaureate Enrollment 550
Women 94% **Men** 6% **Minority** 5% **International** 2% **Part-time** 1%
Graduate Enrollment 101
Women 93% **Men** 7% **Minority** 2% **Part-time** 50%

Nursing Student Activities Nursing Honor Society, Sigma Theta Tau, Student Nurses' Association.

Nursing Student Resources Academic advising; academic or career counseling; assistance for students with disabilities; bookstore; campus computer network; career placement assistance; computer lab; computer-assisted instruction; e-mail services; employment services for current students; externships; housing assistance; interactive nursing skills videos; Internet; learning resource lab; library services; nursing audiovisuals; paid internships; remedial services; resume preparation assistance; skills, simulation, or other laboratory; tutoring.

Library Facilities 1.7 million volumes (211,803 in health, 2,663 in nursing); 9,107 periodical subscriptions (1,662 health-care related).

BACCALAUREATE PROGRAMS

Degree BSN

Available Programs Accelerated Baccalaureate for Second Degree; Generic Baccalaureate; RN Baccalaureate.

Site Options *Distance Learning:* Parkersburg, WV; Glenville, WV; Charleston, WV.

Study Options Full-time and part-time.

Program Entrance Requirements Minimum overall college GPA of 2.8, transcript of college record, CPR certification, written essay, health insurance, high school biology, high school chemistry, 3 years high school math, 2 years high school science, high school transcript, immunizations, interview, minimum high school GPA of 2.5, minimum GPA in nursing prerequisites of 2.8, prerequisite course work. Transfer students are accepted. **Standardized tests** *Required:* SAT or ACT, TOEFL for international students. **Application** *Deadline:* 8/1 (freshmen), 8/1 (transfer). *Application fee:* $25.

Advanced Placement Credit by examination available. Credit given for nursing courses completed elsewhere dependent upon specific evaluations.

Expenses (2006–07) *Tuition, state resident:* full-time $5356; part-time $226 per credit hour. *Tuition, nonresident:* full-time $16,800; part-time $703 per credit hour. *Room and board:* $6400 per academic year.

Financial Aid 70% of baccalaureate students in nursing programs received some form of financial aid in 2005–06. *Gift aid (need-based):* Federal Pell, FSEOG, state, private, college/university gift aid from institutional funds. *Loans:* Federal Direct (Subsidized and Unsubsidized Stafford PLUS), Perkins, college/university. *Work-Study:* Federal Work-Study, part-time campus jobs. *Application deadline:* 3/1.

Contact Dr. Elisabeth N. Shelton, RN, Associate Dean, Undergraduate Academic Affairs, School of Nursing, West Virginia University, PO Box 9600, Morgantown, WV 26506-9600. *Telephone:* 304-293-1386. *Fax:* 304-293-2784. *E-mail:* eshelton@hsc.wvu.edu.

GRADUATE PROGRAMS

Expenses (2006–07) *Tuition, state resident:* full-time $4926; part-time $273 per credit. *Tuition, nonresident:* full-time $14,386; part-time $976 per credit. *International tuition:* $14,386 full-time. *Required fees:* full-time $630; part-time $35 per credit; part-time $315 per term.

Financial Aid 25% of graduate students in nursing programs received some form of financial aid in 2005–06. 1 teaching assistantship was awarded; institutionally sponsored loans, tuition waivers (full and partial), and graduate administrative assistantships also available. *Financial aid application deadline:* 2/1.

Contact Prof. Mary Jane Smith, Associate Dean, Graduate Academic Affairs, School of Nursing, West Virginia University, PO Box 9640, 6417 RCB Health Sciences Center South, Morgantown, WV 26506-9600. *Telephone:* 304-293-4298. *Fax:* 304-293-2784. *E-mail:* mjsmith@hsc.wvu.edu.

MASTER'S DEGREE PROGRAM

Degree MSN

Available Programs Master's; RN to Master's.

Concentrations Available *Nurse practitioner programs in:* family health, neonatal health, pediatric.

Site Options *Distance Learning:* Charleston, WV.

Study Options Full-time and part-time.

Program Entrance Requirements Computer literacy, minimum overall college GPA of 3.0, transcript of college record, CPR certification, written essay, immunizations, 3 letters of recommendation, nursing research course, physical assessment course, resume, statistics course, GRE General Test. *Application deadline:* For fall admission, 6/1. Applications are processed on a rolling basis. *Application fee:* $45.

Advanced Placement Credit by examination available. Credit given for nursing courses completed elsewhere dependent upon specific evaluations.

Degree Requirements 44 total credit hours.

POST-MASTER'S PROGRAM

Areas of Study *Nurse practitioner programs in:* family health, neonatal health, pediatric.

DOCTORAL DEGREE PROGRAM

Degree DSN

Available Programs Doctorate.

Areas of Study Advanced practice nursing, ethics, faculty preparation, family health, health policy, health promotion/disease prevention, health-care systems, human health and illness, illness and transition, nursing education, nursing policy, nursing research, nursing science.

Site Options *Distance Learning:* Charleston, WV.

Program Entrance Requirements Minimum overall college GPA of 3.0, interview by faculty committee, interview, 3 letters of recommendation, MSN or equivalent, scholarly papers, statistics course, vita, writing sample, GRE General Test. *Application deadline:* For fall admission, 6/1. Applications are processed on a rolling basis. *Application fee:* $45.

Degree Requirements 54 total credit hours, dissertation, oral exam, written exam.

West Virginia Wesleyan College
Department of Nursing
Buckhannon, West Virginia

Founded in 1890

DEGREE • BSN

Nursing Program Faculty 6 (50% with doctorates).

Baccalaureate Enrollment 87
Women 91% **Men** 9% **Minority** 4% **International** 1% **Part-time** 30%

Nursing Student Activities Sigma Theta Tau, Student Nurses' Association.

Nursing Student Resources Academic advising; academic or career counseling; assistance for students with disabilities; bookstore; campus computer network; career placement assistance; computer-assisted instruction; e-mail services; employment services for current students; externships; Internet; learning resource lab; library services; nursing audiovisuals; placement services for program completers; remedial services; resume preparation assistance; tutoring.

Library Facilities 91,061 volumes (4,000 in health, 600 in nursing); 2,462 periodical subscriptions (90 health-care related).

BACCALAUREATE PROGRAMS

Degree BSN

Available Programs Generic Baccalaureate; RN Baccalaureate.

Study Options Full-time and part-time.

Program Entrance Requirements Minimum overall college GPA of 2.5, transcript of college record, CPR certification, health exam, health insurance, high school transcript, immunizations, interview, minimum high school GPA of 2.3, minimum GPA in nursing prerequisites of 2.0, prerequisite course work. Transfer students are accepted. **Standardized tests** *Required:* SAT or ACT, TOEFL for international students. *Required for some:* SAT Subject Tests. **Placement:** *Required for some:* SAT or ACT. **Application** *Notification:* continuous (freshmen), continuous (early decision). *Application fee:* $35.

Advanced Placement Credit by examination available. Credit given for nursing courses completed elsewhere dependent upon specific evaluations.

Contact *Telephone:* 304-473-8224. *Fax:* 304-473-8435.

CONTINUING EDUCATION PROGRAM

Contact *Telephone:* 304-473-8224.

Wheeling Jesuit University
Department of Nursing
Wheeling, West Virginia

http://www.wju.edu/academics/nursing/welcome. asp

Founded in 1954

DEGREES • BSN • MSN

Nursing Program Faculty 9 (50% with doctorates).

Library Facilities 144,242 volumes (5,065 in nursing); 456 periodical subscriptions (90 health-care related).

BACCALAUREATE PROGRAMS

Degree BSN

Study Options Full-time and part-time.

Program Entrance Requirements 2 Year (s) high school math, 1 year of high school science, high school transcript, minimum high school rank 50%. Transfer students are accepted. **Standardized tests** *Required:* SAT or ACT, TOEFL for international students. **Application** *Deadline:* rolling (freshmen), rolling (transfer). *Notification:* continuous (freshmen). *Application fee:* $25.

Advanced Placement Credit by examination available. Credit given for nursing courses completed elsewhere dependent upon specific evaluations.

Contact *Telephone:* 304-243-2359. *Fax:* 304-243-2397.

GRADUATE PROGRAMS

Contact *Telephone:* 304-243-2344. *Fax:* 304-243-2608.

Wheeling Jesuit University (continued)

MASTER'S DEGREE PROGRAM

Degree MSN

Available Programs Master's.

Concentrations Available Nursing administration; nursing education. *Nurse practitioner programs in:* family health.

Study Options Full-time and part-time.

Program Entrance Requirements Computer literacy, minimum overall college GPA of 3.0, 3 letters of recommendation, statistics course, GRE General Test. *Application deadline:* For fall admission, 8/1 (priority date); for spring admission, 12/15 (priority date). Applications are processed on a rolling basis. *Application fee:* $25.

Advanced Placement Credit given for nursing courses completed elsewhere dependent upon specific evaluations.

Degree Requirements 42 total credit hours, comprehensive exam.

WISCONSIN

Alverno College
Division of Nursing
Milwaukee, Wisconsin

http://www.alverno.edu

Founded in 1887

DEGREES • BSN • MSN

Nursing Program Faculty 37 (14% with doctorates).

Baccalaureate Enrollment 696
Women 100% **Minority** 28% **Part-time** 21%

Graduate Enrollment 31
Women 94% **Men** 6% **Minority** 13% **Part-time** 42%

Nursing Student Activities Student Nurses' Association.

Nursing Student Resources Academic advising; academic or career counseling; assistance for students with disabilities; bookstore; campus computer network; career placement assistance; computer lab; computer-assisted instruction; daycare for children of students; e-mail services; employment services for current students; externships; housing assistance; interactive nursing skills videos; Internet; learning resource lab; library services; nursing audiovisuals; remedial services; resume preparation assistance; skills, simulation, or other laboratory; tutoring; unpaid internships.

Library Facilities 82,416 volumes; 1,382 periodical subscriptions.

BACCALAUREATE PROGRAMS

Degree BSN

Available Programs ADN to Baccalaureate; Baccalaureate for Second Degree; Generic Baccalaureate; LPN to Baccalaureate; RN Baccalaureate.
Study Options Full-time and part-time.

Program Entrance Requirements Minimum overall college GPA of 2.5, transcript of college record, written essay, high school biology, high school chemistry, 3 years high school math, 2 years high school science, high school transcript, minimum high school GPA of 2.0, prerequisite course work. Transfer students are accepted. **Standardized tests** *Required:* SAT or ACT, TOEFL for international students. **Application** *Deadline:* rolling (freshmen), rolling (transfer). *Notification:* continuous (freshmen). *Application fee:* $20.

Advanced Placement Credit by examination available. Credit given for nursing courses completed elsewhere dependent upon specific evaluations.

Expenses (2006–07) *Tuition:* full-time $16,728; part-time $697 per credit. *International tuition:* $16,728 full-time. *Room and board:* $5954 per academic year. *Required fees:* full-time $175; part-time $175 per term.

Financial Aid 96% of baccalaureate students in nursing programs received some form of financial aid in 2005–06.

Contact Dr. Judeen A. Schulte, Dean, School of Nursing, Division of Nursing, Alverno College, 3400 South 43rd Street, PO Box 343922, Milwaukee, WI 53234-3922. *Telephone:* 414-382-6284. *Fax:* 414-382-6279. *E-mail:* judeen.schulte@alverno.edu.

GRADUATE PROGRAMS

Expenses (2006–07) *Room and board:* $5950 per academic year. *Required fees:* full-time $350.

Financial Aid 65% of graduate students in nursing programs received some form of financial aid in 2005–06.

Contact Ms. Julie L. Millenbruch, MSN Program Director, Division of Nursing, Alverno College, 3400 South 43rd Street, PO Box 343922, Milwaukee, WI 53234-3922. *Telephone:* 414-382-6278. *Fax:* 414-382-6279. *E-mail:* julie.millenbruch@alverno.edu.

MASTER'S DEGREE PROGRAM

Degree MSN

Available Programs Master's.

Concentrations Available Nursing education. *Clinical nurse specialist programs in:* adult health, gerontology, medical-surgical.

Study Options Full-time and part-time.

Program Entrance Requirements Clinical experience, transcript of college record, CPR certification, written essay, immunizations, 3 letters of recommendation, physical assessment course, statistics course.

Advanced Placement Credit given for nursing courses completed elsewhere dependent upon specific evaluations.

Degree Requirements 39 total credit hours, thesis or project.

CONTINUING EDUCATION PROGRAM

Contact Ms. Debra Pass, Director, Institute for Educational Outreach, Division of Nursing, Alverno College, 3400 South 43rd Street, PO Box 343922, Milwaukee, WI 53234-3922. *Telephone:* 414-382-6177. *Fax:* 414-382-6354. *E-mail:* debra.pass@alverno.edu.

Bellin College of Nursing
Nursing Program
Green Bay, Wisconsin

http://www.bcon.edu

Founded in 1909

DEGREES • BSN • MSN

Nursing Program Faculty 19 (16% with doctorates).

Baccalaureate Enrollment 247
Women 91% **Men** 9% **Minority** 4% **Part-time** 14%

Graduate Enrollment 35
Women 97% **Men** 3% **Minority** 2% **Part-time** 94%

Nursing Student Activities Sigma Theta Tau, Student Nurses' Association.

Nursing Student Resources Academic advising; academic or career counseling; assistance for students with disabilities; career placement assistance; computer lab; computer-assisted instruction; e-mail services; interactive nursing skills videos; Internet; learning resource lab; library services; nursing audiovisuals; resume preparation assistance; skills, simulation, or other laboratory; tutoring.

Library Facilities 7,000 volumes (7,000 in health, 4,000 in nursing); 225 periodical subscriptions (190 health-care related).

BACCALAUREATE PROGRAMS

Degree BSN

Available Programs Accelerated Baccalaureate; Accelerated Baccalaureate for Second Degree; Baccalaureate for Second Degree; Generic Baccalaureate.

Study Options Full-time and part-time.

Program Entrance Requirements Minimum overall college GPA of 2.7, transcript of college record, health exam, health insurance, high school biology, high school chemistry, 3 years high school math, 3 years high school science, high school transcript, immunizations, interview, 3 letters of recommendation, minimum high school GPA of 3.25, minimum GPA in nursing prerequisites of 2.7. Transfer students are accepted. **Standardized tests** *Required:* ACT. **Application** *Deadline:* rolling (freshmen), rolling (transfer). *Notification:* continuous (freshmen). *Application fee:* $30.

Advanced Placement Credit by examination available. Credit given for nursing courses completed elsewhere dependent upon specific evaluations.

Expenses (2006–07) *Tuition:* full-time $15,500; part-time $734 per credit. *Required fees:* full-time $339; part-time $234 per credit.

Financial Aid 92% of baccalaureate students in nursing programs received some form of financial aid in 2005–06.

Contact Dr. Penny Croghan, Director of Admission, Nursing Program, Bellin College of Nursing, 725 South Webster Avenue, Green Bay, WI 54301. *Telephone:* 920-433-5803. *Fax:* 920-433-7416. *E-mail:* pcroghan@bcon.edu.

GRADUATE PROGRAMS

Expenses (2006–07) *Tuition:* part-time $535 per credit. *Required fees:* part-time $100 per term.

Financial Aid 63% of graduate students in nursing programs received some form of financial aid in 2005–06.

Contact Dr. Vera Dauffenbach, Interim Director of Graduate Program, Nursing Program, Bellin College of Nursing, 725 South Webster Avenue, PO Box 23400, Green Bay, WI 54305. *Telephone:* 920-433-3409. *Fax:* 920-433-7416. *E-mail:* vkdauffe@bcon.edu.

MASTER'S DEGREE PROGRAM

Degree MSN

Available Programs Master's.

Concentrations Available Nursing administration; nursing education.

Study Options Full-time and part-time.

Program Entrance Requirements Computer literacy, transcript of college record, written essay, interview, 3 letters of recommendation, nursing research course, resume, statistics course.

Advanced Placement Credit given for nursing courses completed elsewhere dependent upon specific evaluations.

Degree Requirements 38 total credit hours, thesis or project.

Cardinal Stritch University

Ruth S. Coleman College of Nursing
Milwaukee, Wisconsin

http://www.stritch.edu/nursing

Founded in 1937

DEGREES • BSN • MSN

Nursing Program Faculty 40 (12% with doctorates).

Baccalaureate Enrollment 50

Graduate Enrollment 25

Nursing Student Activities Student Nurses' Association.

Nursing Student Resources Academic advising; academic or career counseling; bookstore; campus computer network; career placement assistance; computer lab; e-mail services; employment services for current students; interactive nursing skills videos; Internet; learning resource lab; library services; nursing audiovisuals; remedial services; resume preparation assistance; skills, simulation, or other laboratory; tutoring.

Library Facilities 124,897 volumes (119,700 in health, 4,662 in nursing); 667 periodical subscriptions (85 health-care related).

BACCALAUREATE PROGRAMS

Degree BSN

Available Programs Accelerated RN Baccalaureate.

Site Options Milwaukee, WI; Burlington, WI; Kenosha.

Study Options Part-time.

Program Entrance Requirements Minimum overall college GPA of 2.33, transcript of college record, health exam, 2 years high school math, 2 years high school science, high school transcript, minimum high school GPA of 2.33, minimum high school rank 50%, RN licensure. Transfer

students are accepted. **Standardized tests** *Required:* SAT or ACT, TOEFL for international students. *Recommended:* ACT. **Application** *Deadline:* rolling (freshmen), rolling (transfer). *Application fee:* $25.

Advanced Placement Credit by examination available. Credit given for nursing courses completed elsewhere dependent upon specific evaluations.

Expenses (2006–07) *Tuition:* full-time $8800; part-time $615 per credit. *Room and board:* $2795 per academic year. *Required fees:* full-time $200; part-time $150 per term.

Contact Kristy Bueno, BSN Program Contact, Ruth S. Coleman College of Nursing, Cardinal Stritch University, 6801 North Yates Road, Milwaukee, WI 53217-3985. *Telephone:* 414-410-4747. *Fax:* 414-410-4058. *E-mail:* kmbueno@stritch.edu.

GRADUATE PROGRAMS

Expenses (2006–07) *Tuition:* part-time $550 per credit. *Room and board:* $2795 per academic year. *Required fees:* full-time $125.

Contact Ms. Alice Neesley, MSN Program Contact, Ruth S. Coleman College of Nursing, Cardinal Stritch University, 6801 North Yates Road, Milwaukee, WI 53217-3985. *Telephone:* 800-347-8822 Ext. 4427. *Fax:* 414-410-4385. *E-mail:* arneesley@stritch.edu.

MASTER'S DEGREE PROGRAM

Degree MSN

Available Programs Accelerated Master's.

Concentrations Available Nursing education.

Study Options Full-time.

Program Entrance Requirements Computer literacy, minimum overall college GPA of 3.0, transcript of college record, CPR certification, written essay, immunizations, interview, 3 letters of recommendation, nursing research course, resume, statistics course.

Advanced Placement Credit given for nursing courses completed elsewhere dependent upon specific evaluations.

Degree Requirements 36 total credit hours, thesis or project.

Carroll College

Nursing Program
Waukesha, Wisconsin

Founded in 1846

DEGREE • BS

Nursing Student Activities Student Nurses' Association.

Library Facilities 150,000 volumes; 18,000 periodical subscriptions.

BACCALAUREATE PROGRAMS

Degree BS

Available Programs Generic Baccalaureate.

Program Entrance Requirements **Standardized tests** *Required:* SAT or ACT, TOEFL for international students. *Recommended:* ACT. **Application** *Deadline:* rolling (freshmen), rolling (transfer). *Notification:* continuous until 8/20 (freshmen).

Contact Nursing Contact, Nursing Program, Carroll College, 100 North East Avenue, Waukesha, WI 53186. *Telephone:* 262-524-7381.

Columbia College of Nursing/ Mount Mary College Nursing Program

Columbia College of Nursing/Mount Mary College Nursing Program
Milwaukee, Wisconsin

http://www.mtmary.edu/nursing.htm

Founded in 2002

Columbia College of Nursing/Mount Mary College Nursing Program (continued)

DEGREE • BSN

Nursing Program Faculty 20 (7% with doctorates).

Baccalaureate Enrollment 250
Women 95% **Men** 5% **Minority** 15% **Part-time** 20%

Nursing Student Activities Sigma Theta Tau, Student Nurses' Association.

Nursing Student Resources Academic advising; academic or career counseling; bookstore; campus computer network; career placement assistance; computer lab; computer-assisted instruction; daycare for children of students; e-mail services; employment services for current students; interactive nursing skills videos; Internet; learning resource lab; library services; nursing audiovisuals; resume preparation assistance; skills, simulation, or other laboratory; tutoring.

Library Facilities 9,500 volumes in health, 9,000 volumes in nursing; 10 periodical subscriptions health-care related.

■ Columbia College of Nursing has a long history in nursing education dating back to 1901. Since 1913 Mount Mary College has been educating women in liberal studies. Jointly, Columbia College of Nursing and Mount Mary College offer a Bachelor of Science in Nursing degree. Within a liberal arts framework, students integrate nursing instruction with clinical placements, enabling them to meet the challenges of health care today and into the future. The nursing program is approved by the Wisconsin State Board of Nursing and is accredited by the National League for Nursing Accrediting Commission. Students will find more information at the colleges' Web sites (http://www.ccon.edu; http://www.mtmary.edu).

BACCALAUREATE PROGRAMS

Degree BSN

Available Programs ADN to Baccalaureate; Generic Baccalaureate.
Site Options Milwaukee, WI.
Study Options Full-time and part-time.
Program Entrance Requirements Minimum overall college GPA of 2.8, transcript of college record, health exam, health insurance, high school biology, high school chemistry, 2 years high school math, 2 years high school science, high school transcript, minimum high school GPA of 2.5, minimum high school rank 40%, minimum GPA in nursing prerequisites of 2.8, prerequisite course work. Transfer students are accepted.
Advanced Placement Credit by examination available. Credit given for nursing courses completed elsewhere dependent upon specific evaluations.
Expenses (2006–07) *Tuition:* full-time $18,000; part-time $485 per credit. *Room and board:* $4500; room only: $3000 per academic year. *Required fees:* full-time $1000; part-time $50 per credit.
Financial Aid 90% of baccalaureate students in nursing programs received some form of financial aid in 2005–06.
Contact Ms. Ronda Bond, Nursing Recruiter, Columbia College of Nursing/Mount Mary College Nursing Program, 2900 North Menomonee River Parkway, Milwaukee, WI 53222. *Telephone:* 414-256-1219 Ext. 193. *Fax:* 414-256-0180. *E-mail:* bondr@mtmary.edu.

See full description on page 464.

Concordia University Wisconsin
Program in Nursing
Mequon, Wisconsin

http://www.cuw.edu
Founded in 1881

DEGREES • BSN • MSN

Nursing Program Faculty 17 (2% with doctorates).

Baccalaureate Enrollment 210
Women 95% **Men** 5% **Minority** 8% **International** 1%

Graduate Enrollment 217
Women 92% **Men** 8% **Minority** 6% **Part-time** 35%

Nursing Student Activities Nursing Honor Society, Student Nurses' Association.

Nursing Student Resources Academic advising; academic or career counseling; assistance for students with disabilities; bookstore; campus computer network; career placement assistance; computer lab; computer-assisted instruction; e-mail services; employment services for current students; externships; interactive nursing skills videos; Internet; learning resource lab; library services; nursing audiovisuals; paid internships; placement services for program completers; resume preparation assistance; skills, simulation, or other laboratory; tutoring.

Library Facilities 79,341 volumes (3,693 in health, 823 in nursing); 4,440 periodical subscriptions (241 health-care related).

BACCALAUREATE PROGRAMS

Degree BSN

Available Programs ADN to Baccalaureate; LPN to RN Baccalaureate; RN Baccalaureate.
Study Options Full-time.
Program Entrance Requirements Transcript of college record, CPR certification, health exam, health insurance, high school transcript, immunizations, minimum high school GPA of 2.75, minimum GPA in nursing prerequisites of 2.75. Transfer students are accepted. **Standardized tests** *Required:* ACT, TOEFL for international students. **Application** *Deadline:* 8/15 (freshmen). *Notification:* continuous (freshmen). *Application fee:* $35.
Advanced Placement Credit given for nursing courses completed elsewhere dependent upon specific evaluations.
Expenses (2006–07) *Tuition:* full-time $18,050; part-time $752 per credit. *Room and board:* $6860 per academic year. *Required fees:* part-time $752 per credit; part-time $9130 per term.
Financial Aid *Gift aid (need-based):* Federal Pell, FSEOG, state, private, college/university gift aid from institutional funds. *Loans:* Federal Direct (Subsidized and Unsubsidized Stafford PLUS), FFEL (Subsidized and Unsubsidized Stafford PLUS), Perkins, state. *Work-Study:* Federal Work-Study, part-time campus jobs. *Application deadline (priority):* 5/1.
Contact Dr. Grace A. Peterson, Chairperson, Program in Nursing, Concordia University Wisconsin, 12800 North Lake Shore Drive, Mequon, WI 53097. *Telephone:* 262-243-4205 Ext. 4205. *Fax:* 262-243-4466. *E-mail:* grace.peterson@cuw.edu.

GRADUATE PROGRAMS

Expenses (2006–07) *Tuition:* part-time $460 per credit.
Contact Mrs. Teri Kaul, Director, Graduate Nursing, Program in Nursing, Concordia University Wisconsin, 12800 North Lake Shore Drive, Mequon, WI 53097. *Telephone:* 262-243-4538 Ext. 4538. *Fax:* 262-243-4506. *E-mail:* teri.kaul@cuw.edu.

MASTER'S DEGREE PROGRAM

Degree MSN

Available Programs Master's.
Concentrations Available Nursing education. *Nurse practitioner programs in:* family health, gerontology.
Study Options Full-time and part-time.
Program Entrance Requirements Clinical experience, computer literacy, minimum overall college GPA of 3.0, transcript of college record, CPR certification, written essay, immunizations, interview, 2 letters of recommendation, physical assessment course, professional liability insurance/malpractice insurance, resume, statistics course. *Application deadline:* For fall admission, 8/1 (priority date). Applications are processed on a rolling basis. *Application fee:* $35.
Advanced Placement Credit given for nursing courses completed elsewhere dependent upon specific evaluations.
Degree Requirements 44 total credit hours, thesis or project.

Edgewood College
Program in Nursing
Madison, Wisconsin

http://nursing.edgewood.edu

Founded in 1927

DEGREES • BS • MS

Nursing Program Faculty 27 (25% with doctorates).

Baccalaureate Enrollment 201
Women 93% **Men** 7% **Minority** 2% **International** 1% **Part-time** 35%

Graduate Enrollment 51
Women 86% **Men** 14% **Minority** 2% **Part-time** 100%

Nursing Student Activities Sigma Theta Tau, Student Nurses' Association.

Nursing Student Resources Academic advising; academic or career counseling; assistance for students with disabilities; bookstore; campus computer network; career placement assistance; computer lab; computer-assisted instruction; daycare for children of students; e-mail services; employment services for current students; externships; housing assistance; interactive nursing skills videos; Internet; learning resource lab; library services; nursing audiovisuals; paid internships; remedial services; resume preparation assistance; skills, simulation, or other laboratory; tutoring; unpaid internships.

Library Facilities 90,253 volumes (3,000 in health, 935 in nursing); 447 periodical subscriptions (43 health-care related).

BACCALAUREATE PROGRAMS

Degree BS

Available Programs Baccalaureate for Second Degree; Generic Baccalaureate.

Study Options Full-time and part-time.

Program Entrance Requirements Minimum overall college GPA of 2.5, transcript of college record, CPR certification, written essay, health exam, high school biology, high school chemistry, high school foreign language, high school math, high school transcript, immunizations, minimum high school GPA of 2.5, minimum GPA in nursing prerequisites of 2.5, prerequisite course work. Transfer students are accepted. **Standardized tests** *Required:* SAT or ACT, TOEFL for international students. **Application** *Deadline:* rolling (freshmen), rolling (transfer). *Notification:* continuous (freshmen). *Application fee:* $25.

Advanced Placement Credit given for nursing courses completed elsewhere dependent upon specific evaluations.

Expenses (2006–07) *Tuition:* full-time $18,000; part-time $567 per credit. *Room and board:* $5800; room only: $2870 per academic year. *Required fees:* full-time $1134.

Financial Aid 76% of baccalaureate students in nursing programs received some form of financial aid in 2005–06.

Contact Dr. Margaret C. Noreuil, Dean, School of Nursing, Program in Nursing, Edgewood College, 1000 Edgewood College Drive, Madison, WI 53711. *Telephone:* 608-663-2280. *Fax:* 608-663-2863. *E-mail:* mnoreuil@edgewood.edu.

GRADUATE PROGRAMS

Expenses (2006–07) *Tuition:* part-time $588 per credit.

Financial Aid 10% of graduate students in nursing programs received some form of financial aid in 2005–06.

Contact Dr. Margaret C. Noreuil, Dean, School of Nursing, Program in Nursing, Edgewood College, 1000 Edgewood College Drive, Madison, WI 53711. *Telephone:* 608-663-2280. *Fax:* 608-663-2863. *E-mail:* mnoreuil@edgewood.edu.

MASTER'S DEGREE PROGRAM

Degree MS

Available Programs Master's.

Concentrations Available Nursing administration; nursing education.

Study Options Full-time and part-time.

Program Entrance Requirements Clinical experience, computer literacy, minimum overall college GPA of 3.0, transcript of college record, CPR certification, written essay, immunizations, interview, 2 letters of recommendation, nursing research course, prerequisite course work,

statistics course. *Application deadline:* For fall admission, 8/24 (priority date); for spring admission, 1/10 (priority date). Applications are processed on a rolling basis. *Application fee:* $25.

Advanced Placement Credit given for nursing courses completed elsewhere dependent upon specific evaluations.

Degree Requirements 36 total credit hours, thesis or project.

Marian College of Fond du Lac
Nursing Studies Division
Fond du Lac, Wisconsin

http://www.mariancollege.edu

Founded in 1936

DEGREES • BSN • MSN

Baccalaureate Enrollment 221
Women 95% **Men** 5% **Minority** 1% **Part-time** 7%

Graduate Enrollment 39
Women 97% **Men** 3% **Part-time** 15%

Nursing Student Activities Student Nurses' Association.

Nursing Student Resources Academic advising; academic or career counseling; assistance for students with disabilities; bookstore; career placement assistance; computer lab; daycare for children of students; e-mail services; externships; interactive nursing skills videos; Internet; learning resource lab; library services; nursing audiovisuals.

Library Facilities 94,217 volumes (3,000 in health, 2,500 in nursing); 952 periodical subscriptions (91 health-care related).

BACCALAUREATE PROGRAMS

Degree BSN

Available Programs ADN to Baccalaureate; Generic Baccalaureate.

Site Options Appleton, WI; Beaver Dam, WI. *Distance Learning:* Milwaukee, WI.

Study Options Full-time and part-time.

Program Entrance Requirements Transcript of college record, high school biology, high school chemistry, 3 years high school math, high school science, high school transcript, minimum high school GPA of 2.5. Transfer students are accepted. **Standardized tests** *Required:* SAT or ACT, TOEFL for international students. **Application** *Deadline:* rolling (freshmen), rolling (transfer). *Notification:* continuous until 8/15 (freshmen). *Application fee:* $20.

Advanced Placement Credit given for nursing courses completed elsewhere dependent upon specific evaluations.

Contact *Telephone:* 920-923-8732. *Fax:* 920-923-8770.

GRADUATE PROGRAMS

Contact *Telephone:* 920-923-8094. *Fax:* 920-923-8094.

MASTER'S DEGREE PROGRAM

Degree MSN

Available Programs Master's.

Concentrations Available Nursing education. *Nurse practitioner programs in:* adult health.

Site Options *Distance Learning:* Milwaukee, WI.

Study Options Full-time and part-time.

Program Entrance Requirements Clinical experience, minimum overall college GPA of 3.0, transcript of college record, CPR certification, written essay, immunizations, 3 letters of recommendation, nursing research course, professional liability insurance/malpractice insurance, resume, statistics course.

Advanced Placement Credit given for nursing courses completed elsewhere dependent upon specific evaluations.

Degree Requirements 39 total credit hours, thesis or project.

POST-MASTER'S PROGRAM

Areas of Study Nursing education.

Marquette University
College of Nursing
Milwaukee, Wisconsin

http://www.marquette.edu/nursing

Founded in 1881

DEGREES • BSN • MSN • MSN/MBA • PHD

Nursing Program Faculty 43 (65% with doctorates).

Baccalaureate Enrollment 449
Women 95% **Men** 5% **Minority** 12% **Part-time** 6%

Graduate Enrollment 227
Women 94% **Men** 6% **Minority** 4% **International** .8% **Part-time** 51%

Nursing Student Activities Nursing Honor Society, Sigma Theta Tau, Student Nurses' Association.

Nursing Student Resources Academic advising; academic or career counseling; assistance for students with disabilities; bookstore; campus computer network; career placement assistance; computer lab; computer-assisted instruction; daycare for children of students; e-mail services; employment services for current students; externships; housing assistance; interactive nursing skills videos; Internet; learning resource lab; library services; nursing audiovisuals; placement services for program completers; remedial services; resume preparation assistance; skills, simulation, or other laboratory; tutoring.

Library Facilities 1.5 million volumes (58,000 in health, 6,000 in nursing); 23,039 periodical subscriptions (1,200 health-care related).

BACCALAUREATE PROGRAMS

Degree BSN

Available Programs ADN to Baccalaureate; Baccalaureate for Second Degree; Generic Baccalaureate; RN Baccalaureate.

Study Options Full-time and part-time.

Program Entrance Requirements Minimum overall college GPA of 2.5, transcript of college record, written essay, high school biology, high school chemistry, 3 years high school math, high school transcript, minimum high school GPA of 2.5, minimum high school rank 25%. Transfer students are accepted. **Standardized tests** *Required:* SAT or ACT, TOEFL for international students. **Application** *Deadline:* 12/1 (freshmen), 12/1 (transfer). *Notification:* 1/31 (freshmen). *Application fee:* $30.

Advanced Placement Credit given for nursing courses completed elsewhere dependent upon specific evaluations.

Expenses (2006–07) *Tuition:* full-time $24,670; part-time $725 per credit hour. *Room and board:* $8120 per academic year. *Required fees:* full-time $439.

Financial Aid 86% of baccalaureate students in nursing programs received some form of financial aid in 2005–06. *Gift aid (need-based):* Federal Pell, FSEOG, state, private, college/university gift aid from institutional funds. *Loans:* Federal Nursing Student Loans, Federal Direct (Subsidized and Unsubsidized Stafford PLUS), Perkins, state, college/university, alternative loans. *Work-Study:* Federal Work-Study, part-time campus jobs. *Application deadline:* Continuous.

Contact Dr. Janet W. Krejci, RN, Associate Dean for Undergraduate Programs, College of Nursing, Marquette University, Clark Hall, PO Box 1881, Milwaukee, WI 53201-1881. *Telephone:* 414-288-3809. *Fax:* 414-288-1597. *E-mail:* janet.krejci@marquette.edu.

GRADUATE PROGRAMS

Expenses (2006–07) *Tuition:* part-time $750 per credit hour.

Financial Aid 30% of graduate students in nursing programs received some form of financial aid in 2005–06. 6 research assistantships, 1 teaching assistantship were awarded; career-related internships or fieldwork, Federal Work-Study, institutionally sponsored loans, scholarships, and tuition waivers (full and partial) also available. Aid available to part-time students. *Financial aid application deadline:* 2/15.

Contact Dr. Judith Fitzgerald Miller, RN, Associate Dean for Graduate Programs and Research, College of Nursing, Marquette University, Clark Hall, PO Box 1881, Milwaukee, WI 53201-1881. *Telephone:* 414-288-3869. *Fax:* 414-288-1597. *E-mail:* judith.miller@marquette.edu.

MASTER'S DEGREE PROGRAM

Degrees MSN; MSN/MBA

Available Programs Accelerated AD/RN to Master's; Accelerated Master's for Non-Nursing College Graduates; Accelerated RN to Master's; Master's; Master's for Non-Nursing College Graduates; Master's for Nurses with Non-Nursing Degrees; RN to Master's.

Concentrations Available Nurse-midwifery; nursing administration. *Clinical nurse specialist programs in:* adult health, gerontology, pediatric. *Nurse practitioner programs in:* acute care, adult health, gerontology, pediatric.

Study Options Full-time and part-time.

Program Entrance Requirements Minimum overall college GPA of 3.0, transcript of college record, written essay, 3 letters of recommendation, nursing research course, physical assessment course, resume, statistics course, GRE General Test. *Application fee:* $40.

Advanced Placement Credit given for nursing courses completed elsewhere dependent upon specific evaluations.

Degree Requirements 42 total credit hours, comprehensive exam.

POST-MASTER'S PROGRAM

Areas of Study Nurse-midwifery; nursing administration. *Clinical nurse specialist programs in:* adult health, gerontology, pediatric. *Nurse practitioner programs in:* acute care, adult health, gerontology, pediatric.

DOCTORAL DEGREE PROGRAM

Degree PhD

Available Programs Doctorate.

Areas of Study Ethics, faculty preparation, health promotion/disease prevention, health-care systems, human health and illness, illness and transition, nursing administration, nursing education, nursing research, nursing science.

Program Entrance Requirements Minimum overall college GPA of 3.3, interview, 3 letters of recommendation, MSN or equivalent, statistics course, vita, writing sample. *Application fee:* $40.

Degree Requirements 51 total credit hours, dissertation, oral exam, written exam, residency.

CONTINUING EDUCATION PROGRAM

Contact Dr. Lea Acord, Dean, College of Nursing, Marquette University, Clark Hall, PO Box 1881, Milwaukee, WI 53201-1881. *Telephone:* 414-288-3812. *Fax:* 414-288-1597. *E-mail:* lea.acord@marquette.edu.

See full description on page 510.

Milwaukee School of Engineering
School of Nursing
Milwaukee, Wisconsin

http://www.msoe.edu/nursing

Founded in 1903

DEGREE • BSN

Nursing Program Faculty 9 (39% with doctorates).

Baccalaureate Enrollment 110
Women 90% **Men** 10% **Minority** 20%

Nursing Student Activities Student Nurses' Association.

Nursing Student Resources Academic advising; academic or career counseling; assistance for students with disabilities; bookstore; campus computer network; career placement assistance; computer lab; computer-assisted instruction; e-mail services; externships; housing assistance; interactive nursing skills videos; Internet; learning resource lab; library services; nursing audiovisuals; placement services for program completers; remedial services; resume preparation assistance; skills, simulation, or other laboratory; tutoring.

Library Facilities 72,192 volumes (1,956 in health, 1,126 in nursing); 376 periodical subscriptions (116 health-care related).

BACCALAUREATE PROGRAMS

Degree BSN

Available Programs Generic Baccalaureate; RN Baccalaureate.

Study Options Full-time and part-time.

Program Entrance Requirements Minimum overall college GPA of 2.5, transcript of college record, CPR certification, health exam, health insurance, high school biology, high school chemistry, 3 years high school math, 3 years high school science, high school transcript, immunizations, minimum high school GPA of 2.8, professional liability insurance/malpractice insurance. Transfer students are accepted. **Standardized tests** *Required:* SAT or ACT, TOEFL for international students. **Application** *Deadline:* rolling (freshmen), rolling (transfer). *Notification:* continuous (freshmen). *Application fee:* $25.

Advanced Placement Credit by examination available. Credit given for nursing courses completed elsewhere dependent upon specific evaluations.

Contact *Telephone:* 414-277-4516. *Fax:* 414-277-4540.

University of Wisconsin–Eau Claire

College of Nursing and Health Sciences
Eau Claire, Wisconsin

http://www.uwec.edu/Nurs/

Founded in 1916

DEGREES • BSN • MSN

Nursing Program Faculty 40 (43% with doctorates).

Baccalaureate Enrollment 657
Women 92% **Men** 8% **Minority** 4% **International** .5% **Part-time** 17%

Graduate Enrollment 67
Women 97% **Men** 3% **Part-time** 70%

Nursing Student Activities Sigma Theta Tau, Student Nurses' Association.

Nursing Student Resources Academic advising; academic or career counseling; assistance for students with disabilities; bookstore; campus computer network; career placement assistance; computer lab; computer-assisted instruction; daycare for children of students; e-mail services; employment services for current students; housing assistance; interactive nursing skills videos; Internet; learning resource lab; library services; nursing audiovisuals; other; placement services for program completers; remedial services; resume preparation assistance; skills, simulation, or other laboratory; tutoring.

Library Facilities 764,275 volumes (65,000 in nursing); 2,448 periodical subscriptions (4,422 health-care related).

■ The College of Nursing and Health Sciences has an excellent reputation for the high quality of its educational programs and its graduates. The College offers bachelor's and master's degrees in nursing and participates in a statewide Collaborative Nursing Program for registered nurses to earn a B.S.N. Master's-level options include adult or family health specialization and advanced clinical practice, education, or administration role preparation. Baccalaureate-level students receive clinical experiences in acute-care facilities, community health agencies, schools, home-care agencies, and the College of Nursing and Health Sciences clinic. Through distance technology, bachelor's and some master's courses are available at a satellite in Marshfield, Wisconsin.

BACCALAUREATE PROGRAMS

Degree BSN

Available Programs ADN to Baccalaureate; Accelerated Baccalaureate for Second Degree; Generic Baccalaureate; RN Baccalaureate.

Site Options *Distance Learning:* Marshfield, WI.

Study Options Full-time.

Program Entrance Requirements Minimum overall college GPA of 3.0, transcript of college record, CPR certification, written essay, health exam, high school biology, high school chemistry, high school foreign language, 3 years high school math, 3 years high school science, high

school transcript, immunizations, minimum GPA in nursing prerequisites of 2.5, prerequisite course work. Transfer students are accepted. **Standardized tests** *Required:* SAT or ACT, TOEFL for international students. **Application** *Deadline:* rolling (freshmen), 7/1 (transfer). *Notification:* continuous (freshmen). *Application fee:* $35.

Advanced Placement Credit by examination available. Credit given for nursing courses completed elsewhere dependent upon specific evaluations.

Expenses (2006–07) *Tuition, state resident:* full-time $5502; part-time $229 per credit. *Tuition, nonresident:* full-time $12,977; part-time $541 per credit. *Room and board:* $4936; room only: $2640 per academic year.

Financial Aid 70% of baccalaureate students in nursing programs received some form of financial aid in 2005–06.

Contact Dr. Linda Elaine Wendt, Dean, College of Nursing and Health Sciences, University of Wisconsin–Eau Claire, 105 Garfield Avenue, Eau Claire, WI 54701-4004. *Telephone:* 715-836-5287. *Fax:* 715-836-5925. *E-mail:* wendtle@uwec.edu.

GRADUATE PROGRAMS

Expenses (2006–07) *Tuition, state resident:* full-time $6534; part-time $363 per credit. *Tuition, nonresident:* full-time $17,144; part-time $952 per credit. *Room and board:* $4936; room only: $2640 per academic year.

Financial Aid 52% of graduate students in nursing programs received some form of financial aid in 2005–06. 3 teaching assistantships (averaging $3,400 per year) were awarded; Federal Work-Study also available. Aid available to part-time students. *Financial aid application deadline:* 3/1.

Contact Dr. Linda Elaine Wendt, Dean, College of Nursing and Health Sciences, University of Wisconsin–Eau Claire, 105 Garfield Avenue, Eau Claire, WI 54702-4004. *Telephone:* 715-836-5287. *Fax:* 715-836-5925. *E-mail:* wendtle@uwec.edu.

MASTER'S DEGREE PROGRAM

Degree MSN

Available Programs Master's; RN to Master's.

Concentrations Available Nursing administration; nursing education. *Clinical nurse specialist programs in:* adult health, family health. *Nurse practitioner programs in:* adult health, family health.

Site Options *Distance Learning:* Marshfield, WI.

Study Options Full-time and part-time.

Program Entrance Requirements Clinical experience, minimum overall college GPA of 3.0, transcript of college record, CPR certification, written essay, immunizations, 3 letters of recommendation, physical assessment course, professional liability insurance/malpractice insurance, statistics course, GRE General Test. *Application deadline:* For fall admission, 2/1 (priority date). Applications are processed on a rolling basis. *Application fee:* $45.

Advanced Placement Credit given for nursing courses completed elsewhere dependent upon specific evaluations.

Degree Requirements 40 total credit hours.

CONTINUING EDUCATION PROGRAM

Contact Ms. Barbara Enright, Outreach Specialist, College of Nursing and Health Sciences, University of Wisconsin–Eau Claire, Continuing Education Department, Eau Claire, WI 54702-4004. *Telephone:* 715-836-5645. *Fax:* 715-836-5263. *E-mail:* enrighbj@uwec.edu.

University of Wisconsin–Green Bay

BSN–LINC Online RN–BSN Program
Green Bay, Wisconsin

http://www.bsnlinc.wisconsin.edu/

Founded in 1968

DEGREE • BSN

Nursing Program Faculty 6 (50% with doctorates).

Baccalaureate Enrollment 190
Women 90% **Men** 10% **Minority** 8% **Part-time** 80%

University of Wisconsin–Green Bay (continued)

Nursing Student Activities Sigma Theta Tau, Student Nurses' Association.

Nursing Student Resources Academic advising; academic or career counseling; assistance for students with disabilities; bookstore; campus computer network; career placement assistance; computer lab; computer-assisted instruction; e-mail services; employment services for current students; Internet; learning resource lab; library services; nursing audio-visuals; resume preparation assistance; skills, simulation, or other laboratory.

Library Facilities 333,482 volumes (1,000 in health, 675 in nursing); 5,512 periodical subscriptions (100 health-care related).

BACCALAUREATE PROGRAMS

Degree BSN

Available Programs RN Baccalaureate.

Study Options Full-time and part-time.

Program Entrance Requirements Minimum overall college GPA of 2.5, transcript of college record, RN licensure. Transfer students are accepted. **Standardized tests** *Required:* SAT or ACT, TOEFL for international students. **Application** *Notification:* continuous until 8/15 (freshmen). *Application fee:* $35.

Expenses (2006–07) *Tuition, area resident:* part-time $238 per credit. *Tuition, nonresident:* part-time $350 per credit.

Financial Aid 25% of baccalaureate students in nursing programs received some form of financial aid in 2005–06. *Gift aid (need-based):* Federal Pell, FSEOG, state, private, college/university gift aid from institutional funds. *Loans:* FFEL (Subsidized and Unsubsidized Stafford PLUS), Perkins. *Work-Study:* Federal Work-Study, part-time campus jobs. *Application deadline (priority):* 4/15.

Contact Ms. Jennifer Schwahn, Advisor, BSN–LINC Online RN–BSN Program, University of Wisconsin–Green Bay, Professional Program in Nursing, 2420 Nicolet Drive, Green Bay, WI 54311-7001. *Telephone:* 920-465-2934. *Fax:* 920-465-2854. *E-mail:* moyers@uwgb.edu.

University of Wisconsin–Madison
School of Nursing
Madison, Wisconsin

http://www.son.wisc.edu

Founded in 1848

DEGREES • BS • MS • MS/MPH • PHD

Nursing Program Faculty 55 (38% with doctorates).

Baccalaureate Enrollment 365
Women 92% **Men** 8% **Minority** 6% **International** 2% **Part-time** 20%

Graduate Enrollment 176
Women 96% **Men** 4% **Minority** 5% **International** 7% **Part-time** 63%

Nursing Student Activities Nursing Honor Society, Sigma Theta Tau, Student Nurses' Association.

Nursing Student Resources Academic advising; academic or career counseling; assistance for students with disabilities; bookstore; campus computer network; computer lab; computer-assisted instruction; e-mail services; interactive nursing skills videos; Internet; learning resource lab; library services; nursing audiovisuals; resume preparation assistance; skills, simulation, or other laboratory; tutoring.

Library Facilities 334,378 volumes in health, 8,164 volumes in nursing; 1,483 periodical subscriptions health-care related.

BACCALAUREATE PROGRAMS

Degree BS

Available Programs ADN to Baccalaureate; Accelerated RN Baccalaureate; Generic Baccalaureate; RN Baccalaureate.

Site Options *Distance Learning:* LaCrosse, WI.

Study Options Full-time and part-time.

Program Entrance Requirements Minimum overall college GPA of 2.75, transcript of college record, CPR certification, written essay, high school chemistry, high school foreign language, 3 years high school math, 3 years high school science, high school transcript, immunizations,

---

minimum GPA in nursing prerequisites of 2.75, prerequisite course work. Transfer students are accepted. **Standardized tests** *Required:* SAT or ACT, TOEFL for international students. **Application** *Deadline:* 2/1 (freshmen), 2/1 (transfer). *Notification:* continuous (freshmen). *Application fee:* $35.

Advanced Placement Credit by examination available. Credit given for nursing courses completed elsewhere dependent upon specific evaluations.

Expenses (2006–07) *Tuition, state resident:* full-time $6730; part-time $282 per credit. *Tuition, nonresident:* full-time $20,730; part-time $866 per credit.

Financial Aid 33% of baccalaureate students in nursing programs received some form of financial aid in 2005–06. *Gift aid (need-based):* Federal Pell, FSEOG, state, private, college/university gift aid from institutional funds. *Loans:* Federal Nursing Student Loans, FFEL (Subsidized and Unsubsidized Stafford PLUS), Perkins, state, college/university. *Work-Study:* Federal Work-Study. *Application deadline:* Continuous.

Contact Nursing Admissions, School of Nursing, University of Wisconsin–Madison, 600 Highland Avenue, Room K6/146, Madison, WI 53792-2455. *Telephone:* 608-263-5202. *Fax:* 608-263-5296. *E-mail:* ugadmit@son.wisc.edu.

GRADUATE PROGRAMS

Expenses (2006–07) *Tuition, state resident:* full-time $9184; part-time $576 per credit. *Tuition, nonresident:* full-time $24,454; part-time $1530 per credit.

Financial Aid 55% of graduate students in nursing programs received some form of financial aid in 2005–06. 15 fellowships with tuition reimbursements available (averaging $17,000 per year), 12 research assistantships with tuition reimbursements available (averaging $17,000 per year), 8 teaching assistantships with tuition reimbursements available (averaging $11,000 per year) were awarded; career-related internships or fieldwork, Federal Work-Study, institutionally sponsored loans, scholarships, traineeships, and unspecified assistantships also available. Aid available to part-time students. *Financial aid application deadline:* 6/1.

Contact Ms. Marcia Voss, Graduate Program Coordinator, School of Nursing, University of Wisconsin–Madison, 600 Highland Avenue, K6/140, Clinical Science Center, Madison, WI 53792-2455. *Telephone:* 608-263-5258. *Fax:* 608-263-5296. *E-mail:* mlvoss@wisc.edu.

MASTER'S DEGREE PROGRAM

Degrees MS; MS/MPH

Available Programs Accelerated RN to Master's; Master's; Master's for Nurses with Non-Nursing Degrees.

Concentrations Available Nurse case management; nursing education. *Clinical nurse specialist programs in:* adult health, gerontology, medical-surgical, pediatric, perinatal, psychiatric/mental health, women's health. *Nurse practitioner programs in:* acute care, adult health, gerontology, pediatric, psychiatric/mental health, women's health.

Study Options Full-time and part-time.

Program Entrance Requirements Clinical experience, minimum overall college GPA of 3.0, transcript of college record, written essay, immunizations, 3 letters of recommendation, resume, statistics course, GRE General Test. *Application deadline:* For fall admission, 3/1 (priority date); for spring admission, 10/1 (priority date). *Application fee:* $45.

Advanced Placement Credit given for nursing courses completed elsewhere dependent upon specific evaluations.

Degree Requirements 36 total credit hours.

POST-MASTER'S PROGRAM

Areas of Study Nurse case management; nursing education. *Clinical nurse specialist programs in:* adult health, gerontology, medical-surgical, pediatric, perinatal, psychiatric/mental health, women's health. *Nurse practitioner programs in:* acute care, adult health, gerontology, pediatric, psychiatric/mental health, women's health.

DOCTORAL DEGREE PROGRAM

Degree PhD

Available Programs Doctorate; Post-Baccalaureate Doctorate.

Areas of Study Aging, bio-behavioral research, biology of health and illness, community health, faculty preparation, family health, gerontology, health policy, health promotion/disease prevention, human health and illness, information systems, nursing education, nursing research, oncology, women's health.

Program Entrance Requirements Minimum overall college GPA of 3.0, interview, 3 letters of recommendation, scholarly papers, vita, writing sample, GRE General Test. *Application deadline:* For fall admission, 3/1 (priority date); for spring admission, 10/1 (priority date). *Application fee:* $45.

Degree Requirements 60 total credit hours, dissertation, written exam, residency.

POSTDOCTORAL PROGRAM

Areas of Study Adolescent health, aging, cancer care, chronic illness, community health, family health, gerontology, health promotion/disease prevention, individualized study, nursing informatics, nursing interventions, nursing research, vulnerable population, women's health.

Postdoctoral Program Contact Gale Barber, Assistant Dean for Graduate Studies, School of Nursing, University of Wisconsin–Madison, 600 Highland Avenue, Room K6/134, Madison, WI 53792-2455. *Telephone:* 608-263-5172. *Fax:* 608-263-5296. *E-mail:* mgbarber@wisc.edu.

CONTINUING EDUCATION PROGRAM

Contact Ms. Donna Haack, Program Assistant, School of Nursing, University of Wisconsin–Madison, 600 Highland Avenue, H6/158, Clinical Science Center, Madison, WI 53792-2455. *Telephone:* 608-263-5336. *Fax:* 608-263-5332. *E-mail:* dmhaack@wisc.edu.

See full description on page 564.

University of Wisconsin–Milwaukee
College of Nursing
Milwaukee, Wisconsin

http://www.nursing.uwm.edu
Founded in 1956
DEGREES • BSN • MS • MS/MBA • PHD

Nursing Program Faculty 36 (100% with doctorates).
Baccalaureate Enrollment 1,182
Women 89% **Men** 11% **Minority** 18% **International** 1% **Part-time** 27%
Graduate Enrollment 278
Women 68% **Men** 32% **Minority** 16% **International** 2% **Part-time** 69%
Nursing Student Activities Sigma Theta Tau, Student Nurses' Association.

Nursing Student Resources Academic advising; academic or career counseling; campus computer network; computer lab; computer-assisted instruction; e-mail services; interactive nursing skills videos; Internet; learning resource lab; nursing audiovisuals; remedial services; skills, simulation, or other laboratory; tutoring.

Library Facilities 1.4 million volumes (320,089 in health, 178,089 in nursing); 8,240 periodical subscriptions (926 health-care related).

■ The University of Wisconsin–Milwaukee is a Carnegie Foundation–ranked Research Institution. The College of Nursing is nationally recognized for its faculty, programs, and alumni. Students are prepared as nurse leaders at the baccalaureate, master's, and doctoral levels for multiple roles in health care. Faculty members and students are involved in education, research, and service in more than 130 health-care settings. The College supports the Harriet H. Werley Center for Nursing Research and Evaluation, the Center for Cultural Diversity and Health, the Center for Nursing History, and the Nursing Learning Resource Center. The College also has four community nursing centers within its Institute for Urban Health Partnerships, which provides national and international leadership in health promotion and primary health care.

BACCALAUREATE PROGRAMS
Degree BSN
Available Programs Generic Baccalaureate; RN Baccalaureate.
Site Options West Bend, WI; Kenosha, WI.
Study Options Full-time and part-time.
Program Entrance Requirements Minimum overall college GPA of 2.5, transcript of college record, written essay, high school chemistry, high school foreign language, 3 years high school math, 3 years high school science, high school transcript, minimum high school GPA of 2.0, minimum high school rank 50%, minimum GPA in nursing prerequisites of 2.5, prerequisite course work. Transfer students are accepted. **Standardized tests** *Required:* SAT or ACT, TOEFL for international students, ACT for state residents. **Application** *Deadline:* 8/1 (freshmen), 8/1 (transfer). *Notification:* continuous (freshmen). *Application fee:* $35.
Advanced Placement Credit by examination available. Credit given for nursing courses completed elsewhere dependent upon specific evaluations.
Expenses (2006–07) *Tuition, state resident:* full-time $6630; part-time $264 per credit. *Tuition, nonresident:* full-time $16,232; part-time $337 per credit. *International tuition:* $16,232 full-time. *Room and board:* $5556; room only: $3340 per academic year. *Required fees:* full-time $762; part-time $223 per term.
Financial Aid 79% of baccalaureate students in nursing programs received some form of financial aid in 2005–06.
Contact Ms. Donna Wier, Senior Advisor, College of Nursing, University of Wisconsin–Milwaukee, Student Affairs, PO Box 413, Milwaukee, WI 53201. *Telephone:* 414-229-5481. *Fax:* 414-229-5554. *E-mail:* ddw@uwm.edu.

GRADUATE PROGRAMS
Expenses (2006–07) *Tuition, state resident:* full-time $8926; part-time $530 per credit. *Tuition, nonresident:* full-time $23,292; part-time $1428 per credit. *International tuition:* $23,292 full-time. *Room and board:* $6412; room only: $4196 per academic year. *Required fees:* full-time $762; part-time $223 per term.
Financial Aid 87% of graduate students in nursing programs received some form of financial aid in 2005–06. 11 teaching assistantships were awarded; fellowships, research assistantships, career-related internships or fieldwork, Federal Work-Study, and unspecified assistantships also available. Aid available to part-time students. *Financial aid application deadline:* 4/15.
Contact Ms. Carrie Von Bohlen, Advisor, College of Nursing, University of Wisconsin–Milwaukee, Student Affairs, PO Box 413, Milwaukee, WI 53201. *Telephone:* 414-229-5474. *Fax:* 414-229-5554. *E-mail:* cvb@uwm.edu.

MASTER'S DEGREE PROGRAM
Degrees MS; MS/MBA
Available Programs Accelerated Master's for Nurses with Non-Nursing Degrees; Master's; RN to Master's.
Concentrations Available Health-care administration; nursing education. *Clinical nurse specialist programs in:* adult health, community health, parent-child, psychiatric/mental health, women's health. *Nurse practitioner programs in:* family health.
Site Options Kenosha, WI.
Study Options Full-time and part-time.
Program Entrance Requirements Clinical experience, minimum overall college GPA of 2.75, transcript of college record, written essay, interview, 3 letters of recommendation, statistics course, GRE General Test or MAT. *Application deadline:* For fall admission, 1/1 (priority date); for spring admission, 9/1. Applications are processed on a rolling basis. *Application fee:* $45 ($75 for international students).
Advanced Placement Credit given for nursing courses completed elsewhere dependent upon specific evaluations.
Degree Requirements 46 total credit hours, thesis or project.

POST-MASTER'S PROGRAM
Areas of Study *Nurse practitioner programs in:* family health.

DOCTORAL DEGREE PROGRAM
Degree PhD
Available Programs Doctorate; Post-Baccalaureate Doctorate.
Areas of Study Individualized study, nursing research.

University of Wisconsin–Milwaukee (continued)

Program Entrance Requirements Minimum overall college GPA of 3.2, interview, 3 letters of recommendation, MSN or equivalent, scholarly papers, vita, writing sample. *Application deadline:* For fall admission, 1/1 (priority date); for spring admission, 9/1. Applications are processed on a rolling basis. *Application fee:* $45 ($75 for international students).

Degree Requirements 49 total credit hours, dissertation, oral exam, written exam, residency.

CONTINUING EDUCATION PROGRAM

Contact Dr. Elizabeth Fayram, Director, Continuing Education, College of Nursing, University of Wisconsin–Milwaukee, PO Box 413, Milwaukee, WI 53201. *Telephone:* 414-229-5617. *Fax:* 414-229-2596. *E-mail:* fayram@csd.uwm.edu.

See full description on page 566.

University of Wisconsin–Oshkosh
College of Nursing
Oshkosh, Wisconsin

http://www.uwosh.edu/con

Founded in 1871

DEGREES • BSN • MSN

Nursing Program Faculty 71 (25% with doctorates).

Baccalaureate Enrollment 1,031
Women 93% **Men** 7% **Minority** 5% **Part-time** 9%

Graduate Enrollment 75
Women 93% **Men** 7% **Minority** 94% **Part-time** 53%

Nursing Student Activities Sigma Theta Tau, Student Nurses' Association, nursing club.

Nursing Student Resources Academic advising; academic or career counseling; assistance for students with disabilities; bookstore; campus computer network; career placement assistance; computer lab; computer-assisted instruction; daycare for children of students; e-mail services; employment services for current students; externships; interactive nursing skills videos; Internet; learning resource lab; library services; nursing audiovisuals; paid internships; placement services for program completers; resume preparation assistance; skills, simulation, or other laboratory; tutoring; unpaid internships.

Library Facilities 446,774 volumes; 5,219 periodical subscriptions.

BACCALAUREATE PROGRAMS

Degree BSN

Available Programs Accelerated Baccalaureate; Accelerated Baccalaureate for Second Degree; Accelerated RN Baccalaureate; Baccalaureate for Second Degree; Generic Baccalaureate; RN Baccalaureate.

Site Options *Distance Learning:* Wausau, WI; Sheboygan, WI; Manitowoc, WI.

Study Options Full-time and part-time.

Program Entrance Requirements Minimum overall college GPA of 2.75, transcript of college record, CPR certification, written essay, health exam, 3 years high school math, 3 years high school science, immunizations, interview, minimum high school rank 50%, minimum GPA in nursing prerequisites of 2.75, prerequisite course work. Transfer students are accepted. **Standardized tests** *Required:* SAT or ACT, TOEFL for international students, ACT required for state residents. **Application** *Deadline:* rolling (freshmen), rolling (transfer). *Notification:* continuous (freshmen). *Application fee:* $35.

Advanced Placement Credit by examination available. Credit given for nursing courses completed elsewhere dependent upon specific evaluations.

Financial Aid 50% of baccalaureate students in nursing programs received some form of financial aid in 2005–06.

Contact Dr. Suzanne Marnocha, RN, Undergraduate Program Director, College of Nursing, University of Wisconsin–Oshkosh, 800 Algoma Boulevard, Oshkosh, WI 54901-8660. *Telephone:* 920-424-1028. *Fax:* 920-424-0123. *E-mail:* marnocha@uwosh.edu.

GRADUATE PROGRAMS

Financial Aid 40% of graduate students in nursing programs received some form of financial aid in 2005–06. Fellowships, research assistantships with partial tuition reimbursements available, institutionally sponsored loans, scholarships, traineeships, tuition waivers (partial), and unspecified assistantships available. *Financial aid application deadline:* 3/15.

Contact Dr. Roxana Huebscher, RN, Graduate Program Director, College of Nursing, University of Wisconsin–Oshkosh, 800 Algoma Boulevard, Oshkosh, WI 54901-8660. *Telephone:* 920-424-2106. *Fax:* 920-424-0123. *E-mail:* huebsche@uwosh.edu.

MASTER'S DEGREE PROGRAM

Degree MSN

Available Programs Master's.

Concentrations Available Nursing education. *Nurse practitioner programs in:* adult health, family health.

Study Options Full-time and part-time.

Program Entrance Requirements Clinical experience, computer literacy, minimum overall college GPA of 3.0, transcript of college record, CPR certification, written essay, immunizations, interview, 3 letters of recommendation, physical assessment course, statistics course. *Application deadline:* For fall admission, 12/15. *Application fee:* $45.

Degree Requirements 49 total credit hours, thesis or project.

POST-MASTER'S PROGRAM

Areas of Study Nursing education. *Nurse practitioner programs in:* adult health, family health.

CONTINUING EDUCATION PROGRAM

Contact Ms. Billie Gauthier, Director, Continuing Education and Extension, College of Nursing, University of Wisconsin–Oshkosh, 800 Algoma Boulevard, Oshkosh, WI 54901-8660. *Telephone:* 920-424-1129. *Fax:* 920-424-1803. *E-mail:* gauthier@uwosh.edu.

Viterbo University
School of Nursing
La Crosse, Wisconsin

http://www.viterbo.edu

Founded in 1890

DEGREES • BSN • MSN

Nursing Program Faculty 29 (8% with doctorates).

Baccalaureate Enrollment 678
Women 94% **Men** 6% **Minority** 3% **International** 1% **Part-time** 5%

Graduate Enrollment 53
Women 100% **Part-time** 15%

Nursing Student Activities Sigma Theta Tau, Student Nurses' Association.

Nursing Student Resources Academic advising; academic or career counseling; assistance for students with disabilities; bookstore; campus computer network; career placement assistance; computer lab; e-mail services; interactive nursing skills videos; Internet; learning resource lab; library services; nursing audiovisuals; remedial services; resume preparation assistance; skills, simulation, or other laboratory; tutoring.

Library Facilities 92,036 volumes (5,200 in health, 3,398 in nursing); 466 periodical subscriptions (312 health-care related).

BACCALAUREATE PROGRAMS

Degree BSN

Available Programs Generic Baccalaureate; RN Baccalaureate.

Site Options Rochester, MN; Janesville, WI; Madison, WI.

Study Options Full-time and part-time.

Program Entrance Requirements Minimum overall college GPA of 2.5, transcript of college record, CPR certification, health exam, high school chemistry, 1 year of high school math, 2 years high school science, high school transcript, immunizations, minimum high school GPA of 2.0, minimum GPA in nursing prerequisites of 2.5, prerequisite course work.

Transfer students are accepted. **Standardized tests** *Required:* ACT, TOEFL for international students. **Application** *Deadline:* rolling (freshmen), rolling (transfer). *Notification:* continuous until 8/15 (freshmen). *Application fee:* $25.

Advanced Placement Credit given for nursing courses completed elsewhere dependent upon specific evaluations.

Expenses (2006–07) *Tuition:* full-time $17,220; part-time $505 per credit hour. *International tuition:* $17,220 full-time. *Room and board:* $2500 per academic year. *Required fees:* full-time $660.

Financial Aid 88% of baccalaureate students in nursing programs received some form of financial aid in 2005–06.

Contact Dr. Roland Nelson, Director of Admission, School of Nursing, Viterbo University, 900 Viterbo Drive, LaCrosse, WI 54601. *Telephone:* 608-796-3010. *Fax:* 608-796-3050. *E-mail:* adm.buzz@viterbo.edu.

GRADUATE PROGRAMS

Expenses (2006–07) *Tuition:* part-time $525 per credit hour.

Financial Aid 33% of graduate students in nursing programs received some form of financial aid in 2005–06.

Contact Dr. Bonnie Nesbitt, Director, School of Nursing, Viterbo University, 900 Viterbo Drive, LaCrosse, WI 54601. *Telephone:* 608-796-3688. *Fax:* 608-796-3668. *E-mail:* bjnesbitt@viterbo.edu.

MASTER'S DEGREE PROGRAM

Degree MSN

Available Programs Master's.

Concentrations Available Health-care administration; nursing education. *Nurse practitioner programs in:* adult health.

Study Options Full-time and part-time.

Program Entrance Requirements Clinical experience, computer literacy, minimum overall college GPA of 3.0, transcript of college record, CPR certification, written essay, immunizations, interview, 3 letters of recommendation, nursing research course, physical assessment course, resume, statistics course.

Advanced Placement Credit given for nursing courses completed elsewhere dependent upon specific evaluations.

Degree Requirements 37 total credit hours, thesis or project.

POST-MASTER'S PROGRAM

Areas of Study Nursing administration; nursing education. *Nurse practitioner programs in:* adult health.

CONTINUING EDUCATION PROGRAM

Contact Ms. Patricia Wessels, Continuing Education Coordinator, School of Nursing, Viterbo University, 900 Viterbo Drive, La Crosse, WI 54601. *Telephone:* 608-796-3686. *Fax:* 608-796-3668. *E-mail:* pawessels@viterbo.edu.

WYOMING

University of Wyoming
Fay W. Whitney School of Nursing
Laramie, Wyoming

http://www.uwyo.edu/nursing

Founded in 1886

DEGREES • BSN • MS

Nursing Program Faculty 30 (57% with doctorates).

Baccalaureate Enrollment 236
Women 87% **Men** 13% **Minority** 9% **Part-time** 48%

Graduate Enrollment 90
Women 86% **Men** 14% **Minority** 2% **Part-time** 86%

Nursing Student Activities Sigma Theta Tau, Student Nurses' Association.

Nursing Student Resources Academic advising; academic or career counseling; assistance for students with disabilities; bookstore; campus computer network; career placement assistance; computer lab; computer-assisted instruction; e-mail services; employment services for current students; externships; housing assistance; interactive nursing skills videos; Internet; learning resource lab; library services; nursing audiovisuals; paid internships; remedial services; resume preparation assistance; skills, simulation, or other laboratory; tutoring; unpaid internships.

Library Facilities 1.3 million volumes (75,455 in health, 6,082 in nursing); 12,632 periodical subscriptions (1,423 health-care related).

BACCALAUREATE PROGRAMS

Degree BSN

Available Programs ADN to Baccalaureate; Accelerated Baccalaureate for Second Degree; Generic Baccalaureate.

Site Options *Distance Learning:* Laramie, WY.

Study Options Full-time.

Program Entrance Requirements Transcript of college record, CPR certification, written essay, immunizations, 3 letters of recommendation, minimum GPA in nursing prerequisites of 2.5, professional liability insurance/malpractice insurance, prerequisite course work. Transfer students are accepted. **Standardized tests** *Required:* TOEFL for international students. *Required for some:* SAT or ACT. **Application** *Deadline:* 8/10 (freshmen), 8/10 (transfer). *Notification:* continuous (freshmen). *Application fee:* $30.

Advanced Placement Credit given for nursing courses completed elsewhere dependent upon specific evaluations.

Expenses (2006–07) *Tuition, area resident:* part-time $94 per credit hour. *Tuition, nonresident:* part-time $312 per credit hour. *Room and board:* $6836; room only: $2953 per academic year. *Required fees:* part-time $347 per term.

Financial Aid 66% of baccalaureate students in nursing programs received some form of financial aid in 2005–06.

Contact Ms. Claire Hitchcock, Office Associate, Fay W. Whitney School of Nursing, University of Wyoming, Department 3065, 1000 East University Avenue, Laramie, WY 82071. *Telephone:* 307-766-4291. *Fax:* 307-766-4294. *E-mail:* nurs.inq@uwyo.edu.

GRADUATE PROGRAMS

Expenses (2006–07) *Tuition, state resident:* part-time $159 per credit hour. *Tuition, nonresident:* part-time $456 per credit hour. *Required fees:* part-time $347 per term.

Financial Aid 52% of graduate students in nursing programs received some form of financial aid in 2005–06. Research assistantships with full tuition reimbursements available (averaging $10,062 per year), teaching assistantships with full tuition reimbursements available (averaging $10,062 per year) were awarded; career-related internships or fieldwork, institutionally sponsored loans, scholarships, traineeships, and unspecified assistantships also available. Aid available to part-time students. *Financial aid application deadline:* 2/1.

Contact Ms. Claire Hitchcock, Office Associate, Fay W. Whitney School of Nursing, University of Wyoming, Department 3065, 1000 East University Avenue, Laramie, WY 82071. *Telephone:* 307-766-4291. *Fax:* 307-766-4294. *E-mail:* nurs.inq@uwyo.edu.

MASTER'S DEGREE PROGRAM

Degree MS

Available Programs Master's; Master's for Nurses with Non-Nursing Degrees.

Concentrations Available Nursing education. *Nurse practitioner programs in:* family health, psychiatric/mental health.

Site Options *Distance Learning:* Laramie, WY.

Study Options Full-time and part-time.

Program Entrance Requirements Minimum overall college GPA of 3.0, transcript of college record, CPR certification, written essay, immunizations, interview, 3 letters of recommendation, professional liability insurance/malpractice insurance, resume, statistics course, GRE General Test. *Application deadline:* For fall admission, 11/1 (priority date); for spring admission, 2/1 (priority date). *Application fee:* $50.

Advanced Placement Credit given for nursing courses completed elsewhere dependent upon specific evaluations.

Degree Requirements 53 total credit hours, thesis or project.

POST-MASTER'S PROGRAM

Areas of Study Nursing education. *Nurse practitioner programs in:* family health, psychiatric/mental health.

CANADA

ALBERTA

Athabasca University
Centre for Nursing and Health Studies
Athabasca, Alberta

http://www.athabascau.ca/cnhs/

Founded in 1970

DEGREES • BN • MHS

Nursing Program Faculty 42 (28% with doctorates).

Baccalaureate Enrollment 2,502

Graduate Enrollment 962

Nursing Student Resources Academic advising; academic or career counseling; assistance for students with disabilities; computer lab; computer-assisted instruction; e-mail services; interactive nursing skills videos; Internet; library services; nursing audiovisuals; tutoring.

Library Facilities 178,808 volumes; 32,619 periodical subscriptions.

BACCALAUREATE PROGRAMS

Degree BN

Available Programs LPN to Baccalaureate; RN Baccalaureate.

Site Options *Distance Learning:* Calgary, AB.

Study Options Full-time and part-time.

Program Entrance Requirements Minimum overall college GPA of 2.5, transcript of college record, CPR certification, high school chemistry, 3 years high school math, 3 years high school science, immunizations, minimum high school GPA of 2.0, minimum GPA in nursing prerequisites of 2.0, RN licensure. Transfer students are accepted. **Application** *Deadline:* rolling (freshmen), rolling (out-of-state freshmen), rolling (transfer). *Notification:* continuous (freshmen), continuous (out-of-state freshmen). *Application fee:* CAN$60.

Advanced Placement Credit by examination available. Credit given for nursing courses completed elsewhere dependent upon specific evaluations.

Expenses (2006–07) *Tuition, area resident:* part-time CAN$578 per course. *Tuition, state resident:* part-time CAN$661 per course. *Tuition, nonresident:* part-time CAN$884 per course. *International tuition:* CAN$1098 full-time.

Contact Gayle Deren-Purdy, Undergraduate Advisor, Centre for Nursing and Health Studies, Athabasca University, 1 University Drive, Athabasca, AB T9S 3A3. *Telephone:* 800-788-9041 Ext. 6446. *Fax:* 780-675-6468. *E-mail:* gayled@athabascau.ca.

GRADUATE PROGRAMS

Expenses (2006–07) *Tuition, area resident:* part-time CAN$990 per course. *Tuition, state resident:* part-time CAN$1040 per course. *Tuition, nonresident:* part-time CAN$1240 per course. *International tuition:* CAN$1240 full-time.

Contact Donna Dunn, Graduate Advisor, Centre for Nursing and Health Studies, Athabasca University, 1 University Drive, Athabasca, AB T9S 3A3. *Telephone:* 800-788-9041 Ext. 6300. *Fax:* 780-675-6468. *E-mail:* donnad@ athabascau.ca.

MASTER'S DEGREE PROGRAM

Degree MHS

Available Programs Master's; Master's for Nurses with Non-Nursing Degrees.

Concentrations Available Health-care administration. *Nurse practitioner programs in:* community health, primary care.

Study Options Full-time and part-time.

Program Entrance Requirements Clinical experience, computer literacy, minimum overall college GPA of 3.0, transcript of college record, 3 letters of recommendation, resume.

Advanced Placement Credit given for nursing courses completed elsewhere dependent upon specific evaluations.

Degree Requirements 33 total credit hours, thesis or project, comprehensive exam.

University of Alberta
Faculty of Nursing
Edmonton, Alberta

Founded in 1906

DEGREES • BSCN • MN • PHD

Nursing Program Faculty 92 (54% with doctorates).

Baccalaureate Enrollment 1,600
Women 94% **Men** 6% **International** 1% **Part-time** 7%

Graduate Enrollment 266
Women 94% **Men** 6% **International** 3% **Part-time** 61%

Nursing Student Activities Nursing Honor Society, Sigma Theta Tau, Student Nurses' Association.

Nursing Student Resources Academic advising; academic or career counseling; assistance for students with disabilities; bookstore; campus computer network; career placement assistance; computer lab; computer-assisted instruction; daycare for children of students; e-mail services; employment services for current students; housing assistance; interactive nursing skills videos; Internet; learning resource lab; library services; nursing audiovisuals; other; paid internships; remedial services; resume preparation assistance; skills, simulation, or other laboratory; tutoring; unpaid internships.

Library Facilities 9.7 million volumes (115,000 in health, 19,000 in nursing); 2,400 periodical subscriptions health-care related.

BACCALAUREATE PROGRAMS

Degree BScN

Available Programs Baccalaureate for Second Degree; Generic Baccalaureate; LPN to Baccalaureate; RN Baccalaureate; RPN to Baccalaureate.

Site Options Red Deer, AB; Grande Prairie, AB; Fort McMurray, AB.

Study Options Full-time.

Program Entrance Requirements Minimum overall college GPA of 3.0, transcript of college record, CPR certification, health exam, health insurance, high school biology, high school chemistry, 3 years high school math, 3 years high school science, high school transcript, immunizations, minimum high school GPA of 3.5, minimum high school rank 78%. Transfer students are accepted. **Application** *Deadline:* 5/1 (freshmen), 5/1 (transfer). *Notification:* continuous until 9/1 (freshmen). *Application fee:* CAN$100.

Advanced Placement Credit by examination available.

Expenses (2006–07) *Tuition, state resident:* full-time CAN$6000; part-time CAN$151 per credit. *Tuition, nonresident:* full-time CAN$6000; part-time CAN$151 per credit. *International tuition:* CAN$18,000 full-time. *Room and board:* CAN$7080; room only: CAN$3200 per academic year. *Required fees:* full-time CAN$504; part-time CAN$139 per credit; part-time CAN$139 per term.

Financial Aid 50% of baccalaureate students in nursing programs received some form of financial aid in 2005–06. *Loans:* college/university.

Contact Ian Payne, Student Advisor, Faculty of Nursing, University of Alberta, 3-107 Clinical Sciences Building, Edmonton, AB T6G 2G3. *Telephone:* 780-492-9546. *Fax:* 780-492-4844. *E-mail:* ian.payne@ualberta.ca.

GRADUATE PROGRAMS

Expenses (2006–07) *Tuition, state resident:* full-time CAN$3972; part-time CAN$89 per credit. *Tuition, nonresident:* full-time CAN$3972; part-time CAN$89 per credit. *International tuition:* CAN$7563 full-time. *Required fees:* full-time CAN$870.

Financial Aid 47% of graduate students in nursing programs received some form of financial aid in 2005–06. 12 fellowships with partial tuition reimbursements available (averaging $23,868 per year), 27 research assistantships with partial tuition reimbursements available (averaging $6,186 per year), 12 teaching assistantships with partial tuition reimbursements available (averaging $2,365 per year) were awarded; institutionally sponsored loans and scholarships also available.

Contact Barbara Dussault, Director, Graduate Services, Faculty of Nursing, University of Alberta, 3rd Floor, Clinical Sciences Building, Edmonton, AB T6G 2G3. *Telephone:* 780-492-3914. *Fax:* 780-492-2551. *E-mail:* barbara.dussault@ualberta.ca.

MASTER'S DEGREE PROGRAM

Degree MN

Available Programs Master's.

Concentrations Available *Clinical nurse specialist programs in:* acute care, adult health, cardiovascular, community health, critical care, family health, gerontology, maternity-newborn, medical-surgical, oncology, parent-child, pediatric, perinatal, psychiatric/mental health, public health, women's health.

Study Options Full-time and part-time.

Program Entrance Requirements Clinical experience, computer literacy, minimum overall college GPA of 3.0, transcript of college record, CPR certification, 3 letters of recommendation, nursing research course, physical assessment course, resume, statistics course. *Application deadline:* For fall admission, 6/1; for winter admission, 10/1; for spring admission, 2/1. Applications are processed on a rolling basis.

Advanced Placement Credit given for nursing courses completed elsewhere dependent upon specific evaluations.

Degree Requirements 33 total credit hours, thesis or project.

POST-MASTER'S PROGRAM

Areas of Study *Clinical nurse specialist programs in:* acute care, adult health, cardiovascular, community health, critical care, family health, gerontology, maternity-newborn, medical-surgical, oncology, parent-child, pediatric, perinatal, psychiatric/mental health, public health, women's health.

DOCTORAL DEGREE PROGRAM

Degree PhD

Available Programs Doctorate.

Areas of Study Health policy, nursing education, nursing policy, nursing research.

Program Entrance Requirements Clinical experience, minimum overall college GPA of 3.0, 3 letters of recommendation, MSN or equivalent, scholarly papers, statistics course, vita, writing sample. *Application deadline:* For fall admission, 6/1; for winter admission, 10/1; for spring admission, 2/1. Applications are processed on a rolling basis.

Degree Requirements 36 total credit hours, dissertation, oral exam, written exam, residency.

POSTDOCTORAL PROGRAM

Postdoctoral Program Contact Dr. Phyllis Giovannetti, Associate Dean, Graduate Education, Faculty of Nursing, University of Alberta, Clinical Sciences Building, Third Floor, Edmonton, AB T6G 2G3. *Telephone:* 780-492-6764. *Fax:* 780-492-2551. *E-mail:* phyllis.giovannetti@ualberta.ca.

University of Calgary
Faculty of Nursing
Calgary, Alberta

http://www.ucalgary.ca/nu

Founded in 1945

DEGREES • BN • MN • PHD

Nursing Program Faculty 50 (85% with doctorates).

Baccalaureate Enrollment 930
Women 90% **Men** 10% **Minority** 5% **International** 1%

Graduate Enrollment 110
Women 95% **Men** 5% **Minority** 1% **International** 1% **Part-time** 21%

Nursing Student Activities Student Nurses' Association.

Nursing Student Resources Academic advising; academic or career counseling; assistance for students with disabilities; bookstore; campus computer network; career placement assistance; computer lab; computer-assisted instruction; daycare for children of students; e-mail services; externships; housing assistance; interactive nursing skills videos; Internet; learning resource lab; library services; nursing audiovisuals; remedial services; resume preparation assistance; skills, simulation, or other laboratory; tutoring.

Library Facilities 2.4 million volumes; 20,237 periodical subscriptions.

BACCALAUREATE PROGRAMS

Degree BN

Available Programs Accelerated Baccalaureate; Accelerated Baccalaureate for Second Degree; Baccalaureate for Second Degree; Generic Baccalaureate; RN Baccalaureate.

Site Options Medicine Hat, AB. *Distance Learning:* Calgary, AB.

Study Options Full-time.

Program Entrance Requirements Minimum overall college GPA of 3.3, transcript of college record, CPR certification, health exam, high school biology, high school chemistry, 3 years high school math, high school transcript, immunizations, minimum high school rank 78%. Transfer students are accepted. **Standardized tests** *Required for some:* SAT, SAT Subject Tests. **Application** *Deadline:* 4/1 (freshmen). *Notification:* continuous (freshmen). *Application fee:* CAN$130.

Advanced Placement Credit by examination available. Credit given for nursing courses completed elsewhere dependent upon specific evaluations.

Financial Aid *Loans:* college/university. *Application deadline:* 6/15.

Contact Laura Hampson, Student Advisor, Faculty of Nursing, University of Calgary, 2500 University Drive, NW, Calgary, AB T2N 1N4. *Telephone:* 403-220-4636. *Fax:* 403-284-4803. *E-mail:* hampson@ucalgary.ca.

GRADUATE PROGRAMS

Financial Aid 40% of graduate students in nursing programs received some form of financial aid in 2004–05. 8 fellowships (averaging $183,350 per year), 15 teaching assistantships (averaging $103,107 per year) were awarded; institutionally sponsored loans, scholarships, and unspecified assistantships also available. Aid available to part-time students.

Contact Jackie Hendrickx, Administrative Assistant, Graduate Programs, Faculty of Nursing, University of Calgary, Faculty of Nursing, 2500 University Drive, NW, Calgary, AB T2N 1N4. *Telephone:* 403-220-6241. *Fax:* 403-284-4803. *E-mail:* nursgrad@ucalgary.ca.

MASTER'S DEGREE PROGRAM

Degree MN

Available Programs Master's; RN to Master's.

Concentrations Available *Clinical nurse specialist programs in:* acute care, adult health, cardiovascular, community health, critical care, family health, gerontology, maternity-newborn, medical-surgical, parent-child, pediatric, perinatal, psychiatric/mental health, public health, rehabilitation, women's health. *Nurse practitioner programs in:* acute care, adult health, neonatal health.

Study Options Full-time and part-time.

University of Calgary (continued)

Program Entrance Requirements Clinical experience, computer literacy, minimum overall college GPA of 3.0, transcript of college record, CPR certification, written essay, 3 letters of recommendation, nursing research course, statistics course. *Application deadline:* For fall admission, 2/1. *Application fee:* $100 ($130 for international students).

Advanced Placement Credit given for nursing courses completed elsewhere dependent upon specific evaluations.

Degree Requirements 30 total credit hours, thesis or project, comprehensive exam.

POST-MASTER'S PROGRAM

Areas of Study *Nurse practitioner programs in:* acute care, adult health, neonatal health.

DOCTORAL DEGREE PROGRAM

Degree PhD

Available Programs Doctorate; Doctorate for Nurses with Non-Nursing Degrees.

Areas of Study Advanced practice nursing, aging, clinical practice, community health, critical care, ethics, family health, gerontology, health promotion/disease prevention, health-care systems, human health and illness, illness and transition, individualized study, maternity-newborn, neuro-behavior, nursing research, women's health.

Site Options *Distance Learning:* Calgary, AB.

Program Entrance Requirements Clinical experience, minimum overall college GPA of 3.0, 3 letters of recommendation, MSN or equivalent, scholarly papers, statistics course, vita, writing sample. *Application deadline:* For fall admission, 2/1. *Application fee:* $100 ($130 for international students).

Degree Requirements Dissertation, oral exam, written exam.

University of Lethbridge
School of Health Sciences
Lethbridge, Alberta

http://home.uleth.ca/hlsc/

Founded in 1967

DEGREES • BN • M SC

Nursing Program Faculty 30 (20% with doctorates).

Baccalaureate Enrollment 228
Women 91% **Men** 9% **Part-time** 3%

Graduate Enrollment 3
Women 67% **Men** 33%

Nursing Student Activities Nursing club.

Nursing Student Resources Academic advising; academic or career counseling; assistance for students with disabilities; bookstore; campus computer network; computer lab; e-mail services; employment services for current students; housing assistance; interactive nursing skills videos; Internet; learning resource lab; library services; nursing audiovisuals; remedial services; resume preparation assistance; skills, simulation, or other laboratory; tutoring; unpaid internships.

Library Facilities 560,427 volumes (14,743 in health, 2,554 in nursing); 1,300 periodical subscriptions (11,168 health-care related).

BACCALAUREATE PROGRAMS

Degree BN

Available Programs Generic Baccalaureate; RN Baccalaureate.

Site Options Lethbridge, AB.

Study Options Full-time.

Program Entrance Requirements CPR certification, high school biology, high school chemistry, 3 years high school math, 3 years high school science, high school transcript, immunizations, minimum high school rank 70%. Transfer students are accepted. **Application** *Deadline:* 6/1 (freshmen), 6/1 (transfer). *Early decision:* 4/1. *Notification:* continuous (freshmen), 4/22 (out-of-state freshmen), 4/22 (early decision). *Application fee:* CAN$60.

Advanced Placement Credit given for nursing courses completed elsewhere dependent upon specific evaluations.

Contact *Telephone:* 403-329-2649. *Fax:* 403-329-2668.

GRADUATE PROGRAMS

Contact *Telephone:* 403-329-2649. *Fax:* 403-329-2668.

MASTER'S DEGREE PROGRAM

Degree M Sc

Available Programs Master's.

Study Options Full-time and part-time.

Program Entrance Requirements Clinical experience, minimum overall college GPA of 3.0, transcript of college record, CPR certification, immunizations, interview.

Advanced Placement Credit given for nursing courses completed elsewhere dependent upon specific evaluations.

Degree Requirements Thesis or project, comprehensive exam.

BRITISH COLUMBIA

British Columbia Institute of Technology
School of Health Sciences
Burnaby, British Columbia

http://www.health.bcit.ca/nursing/

Founded in 1964

DEGREE • BSCN

Nursing Program Faculty 44.

Nursing Student Activities Student Nurses' Association.

Nursing Student Resources Academic advising; academic or career counseling; assistance for students with disabilities; bookstore; campus computer network; computer lab; computer-assisted instruction; housing assistance; interactive nursing skills videos; Internet; learning resource lab; library services; nursing audiovisuals; skills, simulation, or other laboratory; tutoring; unpaid internships.

Library Facilities 169,404 volumes (100 in health, 50 in nursing); 1,080 periodical subscriptions (100 health-care related).

BACCALAUREATE PROGRAMS

Degree BScN

Available Programs Generic Baccalaureate; RPN to Baccalaureate.

Study Options Full-time.

Program Entrance Requirements CPR certification, written essay, high school biology, high school chemistry, high school math, immunizations, interview, 1 letter of recommendation, prerequisite course work.

Application *Application fee:* CAN$60.

Contact *Telephone:* 604-432-8884. *Fax:* 604-436-9590.

CONTINUING EDUCATION PROGRAM

Contact *Telephone:* 604-451-7100.

Kwantlen University College
Faculty of Community and Health Sciences
Surrey, British Columbia

Founded in 1981

DEGREE • BSN

Nursing Program Faculty 60 (13% with doctorates).

Baccalaureate Enrollment 320
Women 90% **Men** 10% **Part-time** 13%

Nursing Student Activities Student Nurses' Association.

Nursing Student Resources Academic advising; academic or career counseling; assistance for students with disabilities; bookstore; campus computer network; career placement assistance; computer lab; computer-assisted instruction; e-mail services; employment services for current students; interactive nursing skills videos; Internet; learning resource lab; library services; nursing audiovisuals; remedial services; resume preparation assistance; skills, simulation, or other laboratory.

BACCALAUREATE PROGRAMS

Degree BSN

Available Programs Generic Baccalaureate; RN Baccalaureate.
Study Options Full-time.

Program Entrance Requirements CPR certification, health insurance, high school biology, high school chemistry, high school math, 2 years high school science, high school transcript, immunizations. Transfer students are accepted. **Application** *Deadline:* 6/30 (freshmen), 5/30 (out-of-state freshmen), 6/30 (transfer). *Early decision:* 2/28. *Notification:* continuous until 6/30 (freshmen), 5/30 (out-of-state freshmen), 3/31 (out-of-state freshmen), 3/31 (early decision). *Application fee:* CAN$40.

Advanced Placement Credit given for nursing courses completed elsewhere dependent upon specific evaluations.

Contact Ms. Barbara Maxwell, Admissions Assistant, Faculty of Community and Health Sciences, Kwantlen University College, 12666 72nd Avenue, Surrey, BC V3W 2M8. *Telephone:* 604-599-2317. *E-mail:* kim.jans@kwantlen.ca.

Malaspina University-College
Department of Nursing
Nanaimo, British Columbia

http://www.mala.bc.ca/www/discover/health/index.htm

Founded in 1969

DEGREE • BSCN

Nursing Program Faculty 42 (2% with doctorates).

Baccalaureate Enrollment 224
Women 98% **Men** 2% **Minority** 5.5%

Nursing Student Activities Student Nurses' Association.

Nursing Student Resources Academic advising; academic or career counseling; assistance for students with disabilities; bookstore; campus computer network; computer lab; computer-assisted instruction; daycare for children of students; e-mail services; employment services for current students; housing assistance; interactive nursing skills videos; Internet; learning resource lab; library services; nursing audiovisuals; paid internships; remedial services; resume preparation assistance; skills, simulation, or other laboratory; unpaid internships.

Library Facilities 9,475 volumes in health, 1,299 volumes in nursing; 800 periodical subscriptions health-care related.

BACCALAUREATE PROGRAMS

Degree BScN

Available Programs Generic Baccalaureate; LPN to Baccalaureate; RN Baccalaureate.
Study Options Full-time.

Program Entrance Requirements CPR certification, written essay, health exam, health insurance, high school biology, high school chemistry, 11 years high school math, high school transcript, immunizations, minimum GPA in nursing prerequisites of 3.0, prerequisite course work, RN licensure. Transfer students are accepted. **Application** *Application fee:* CAN$30.

Advanced Placement Credit given for nursing courses completed elsewhere dependent upon specific evaluations.

Expenses (2006–07) *Tuition, area resident:* full-time CAN$4855. *Room and board:* CAN$1700; room only: CAN$1400 per academic year. *Required fees:* full-time CAN$30.

Financial Aid 65% of baccalaureate students in nursing programs received some form of financial aid in 2005–06.

Contact Mrs. Madelene J. Heffel Ponting, RN, Chair of Bachelor of Science in Nursing Programs, Department of Nursing, Malaspina University-College, 900 Fifth Street, Nanaimo, BC V9R 5S5. *Telephone:* 250-740-6260. *Fax:* 250-740-6468. *E-mail:* heffelpom@mala.bc.ca.

Thompson Rivers University
School of Nursing
Kamloops, British Columbia

http://www.cariboo.bc.ca/nursing/index.html

Founded in 1970

DEGREE • BSN

Nursing Program Faculty 56.

Library Facilities 273,900 volumes (7,326 in health, 2,275 in nursing); 13,709 periodical subscriptions (89 health-care related).

BACCALAUREATE PROGRAMS

Degree BSN

Study Options Full-time and part-time.

Program Entrance Requirements Minimum overall college GPA of 2.7, transcript of college record, CPR certification, health exam, high school biology, high school chemistry, high school foreign language, high school math, high school science, high school transcript, immunizations, interview, 2 letters of recommendation, minimum high school GPA of 2.3, minimum GPA in nursing prerequisites of 2.3. Transfer students are accepted. **Application** *Deadline:* 3/1 (freshmen), 3/1 (transfer). *Notification:* continuous until 3/1 (freshmen). *Application fee:* CAN$25.

Advanced Placement Credit given for nursing courses completed elsewhere dependent upon specific evaluations.

Contact *Telephone:* 250-828-5435. *Fax:* 250-828-5450.

CONTINUING EDUCATION PROGRAM

Contact *Telephone:* 250-828-5210. *Fax:* 250-371-5510.

Trinity Western University
Department of Nursing
Langley, British Columbia

Founded in 1962

DEGREE • BSCN

Nursing Program Faculty 9 (33% with doctorates).

Baccalaureate Enrollment 151
Women 93.4% **Men** 6.6% **Minority** 11.9% **International** 12.6%

Nursing Student Activities Student Nurses' Association.

Nursing Student Resources Academic advising; academic or career counseling; assistance for students with disabilities; bookstore; campus computer network; computer lab; computer-assisted instruction; e-mail services; employment services for current students; housing assistance; interactive nursing skills videos; Internet; learning resource lab; library services; nursing audiovisuals; resume preparation assistance; skills, simulation, or other laboratory.

Library Facilities 190,565 volumes (2,500 in health, 800 in nursing); 11,000 periodical subscriptions (369 health-care related).

BACCALAUREATE PROGRAMS

Degree BScN

Available Programs Generic Baccalaureate.
Study Options Full-time.

Program Entrance Requirements Minimum overall college GPA of 2.0, CPR certification, health exam, health insurance, high school biology, high school chemistry, 1 year of high school math, 2 years high school science, high school transcript, immunizations, 2 letters of recommendation, minimum high school GPA of 2.7, minimum GPA in nursing

Trinity Western University (continued)
prerequisites of 2.3. Transfer students are accepted. **Standardized tests** *Required for some:* SAT or ACT. **Application** *Deadline:* 6/15 (freshmen), 6/15 (transfer). *Notification:* continuous (freshmen). *Application fee:* $40.

Advanced Placement Credit given for nursing courses completed elsewhere dependent upon specific evaluations.

Financial Aid 50% of baccalaureate students in nursing programs received some form of financial aid in 2005–06. *Gift aid (need-based):* private, college/university gift aid from institutional funds. *Loans:* FFEL (Subsidized and Unsubsidized Stafford PLUS), federal and provincial loans. *Application deadline (priority):* 2/28.

Contact Ms. Barbara Pesut, Director of Nursing, Department of Nursing, Trinity Western University, 7600 Glover Road, Langley, BC V2Y 1Y1. *Telephone:* 604-888-7511 Ext. 3283. *Fax:* 604-513-2018. *E-mail:* pesut@ twu.ca.

The University of British Columbia
School of Nursing
Vancouver, British Columbia

http://www.nursing.ubc.ca
Founded in 1915
DEGREES • BSN • MSN • PHD

Nursing Program Faculty 51 (60% with doctorates).

Baccalaureate Enrollment 600

Graduate Enrollment 300

Nursing Student Activities Nursing Honor Society, Sigma Theta Tau, Student Nurses' Association.

Nursing Student Resources Academic advising; academic or career counseling; assistance for students with disabilities; bookstore; campus computer network; career placement assistance; computer lab; computer-assisted instruction; daycare for children of students; e-mail services; employment services for current students; housing assistance; interactive nursing skills videos; Internet; learning resource lab; library services; nursing audiovisuals; skills, simulation, or other laboratory.

Library Facilities 5.1 million volumes; 51,553 periodical subscriptions.

BACCALAUREATE PROGRAMS
Degree BSN

Available Programs Accelerated Baccalaureate for Second Degree; RN Baccalaureate.

Study Options Full-time.

Program Entrance Requirements Minimum overall college GPA of 3.6, transcript of college record, CPR certification, written essay, health exam, health insurance, high school transcript, immunizations, interview, professional liability insurance/malpractice insurance, prerequisite course work. **Standardized tests** *Required for some:* SAT and SAT Subject Tests or ACT. **Application** *Deadline:* 2/28 (freshmen), 2/28 (transfer). *Notification:* continuous until 8/31 (freshmen). *Application fee:* CAN$100.

Expenses (2006–07) *Tuition, area resident:* full-time CAN$3339. *International tuition:* CAN$10,282 full-time. *Room and board:* CAN$10,282 per academic year.

Financial Aid *Gift aid (need-based):* private, college/university gift aid from institutional funds, provincial scholarships/grants, Federal Canada Study Grants. *Loans:* FFEL (Subsidized and Unsubsidized Stafford PLUS), college/university, Canadian Student Loans, Provincial Student Loans. *Work-Study:* part-time campus jobs. *Application deadline:* 9/15 (priority: 4/15).

Contact Nursing Programs, School of Nursing, The University of British Columbia, T201-2211 Wesbrook Mall, Vancouver, BC V6T 2B5. *Telephone:* 604-822-7420. *Fax:* 604-822-7466. *E-mail:* information@nursing.ubc.ca.

GRADUATE PROGRAMS
Expenses (2006–07) *International tuition:* CAN$14,062 full-time. *Required fees:* full-time CAN$3861.

Financial Aid 10% of graduate students in nursing programs received some form of financial aid in 2005–06. 4 fellowships (averaging $8,000 per year), 14 research assistantships (averaging $800 per year), 3 teaching assistantships were awarded.

Contact Dr. Carol Jillings, MSN Advisor, School of Nursing, The University of British Columbia, T201-2211 Wesbrook Mall, Vancouver, BC V6T 2B5. *Telephone:* 604-822-7479. *Fax:* 604-822-7466. *E-mail:* jillings@ nursing.ubc.ca.

MASTER'S DEGREE PROGRAM
Degree MSN

Available Programs Master's.

Concentrations Available Nursing administration; nursing education. *Clinical nurse specialist programs in:* adult health, community health, family health, psychiatric/mental health, public health. *Nurse practitioner programs in:* family health, primary care.

Site Options *Distance Learning:* Kamloops, BC.

Study Options Full-time and part-time.

Program Entrance Requirements Computer literacy, minimum overall college GPA of 3.3, transcript of college record, 3 letters of recommendation, resume, GRE. *Application deadline:* For fall admission, 1/31; for spring admission, 6/30. *Application fee:* $90 ($150 for international students).

Advanced Placement Credit given for nursing courses completed elsewhere dependent upon specific evaluations.

Degree Requirements 33 total credit hours, thesis or project.

DOCTORAL DEGREE PROGRAM
Degree PhD

Available Programs Doctorate.

Areas of Study Advanced practice nursing, aging, clinical practice, community health, ethics, faculty preparation, family health, gerontology, health policy, health promotion/disease prevention, health-care systems, individualized study, maternity-newborn, nursing administration, nursing education, nursing research, nursing science, oncology, women's health.

Program Entrance Requirements interview, 3 letters of recommendation, MSN or equivalent, statistics course, vita, writing sample, GRE. *Application deadline:* For fall admission, 1/31; for spring admission, 6/30. *Application fee:* $90 ($150 for international students).

Degree Requirements 18 total credit hours, dissertation, oral exam, written exam, residency.

POSTDOCTORAL PROGRAM
Areas of Study Health promotion/disease prevention, individualized study, nursing research, nursing science, vulnerable population.

Postdoctoral Program Contact Dr. Pamela Ratner, PhD Advisor, School of Nursing, The University of British Columbia, T201-2211 Wesbrook Mall, Vancouver, BC V6T 2B5. *Telephone:* 604-822-7427. *Fax:* 604-822-7869. *E-mail:* pam.ratner@ubc.ca.

The University of British Columbia–Okanagan
School of Nursing
Kelowna, British Columbia

Founded in 2005
DEGREE • BSN

Nursing Program Faculty 40 (20% with doctorates).

Baccalaureate Enrollment 292
Women 90% **Men** 10%

Nursing Student Resources Academic advising; academic or career counseling; assistance for students with disabilities; bookstore; campus computer network; computer lab; computer-assisted instruction; daycare for children of students; e-mail services; Internet; learning resource lab; library services; nursing audiovisuals; resume preparation assistance; skills, simulation, or other laboratory.

BACCALAUREATE PROGRAMS

Degree BSN

Available Programs Generic Baccalaureate; LPN to RN Baccalaureate; RN Baccalaureate.

Study Options Full-time and part-time.

Program Entrance Requirements Minimum overall college GPA, transcript of college record, CPR certification, health exam, health insurance, high school biology, high school chemistry, high school math, 2 years high school science, high school transcript, immunizations, minimum high school GPA, minimum high school rank 67%, minimum GPA in nursing prerequisites. Transfer students are accepted.

Contact *Telephone:* 250-762-5445 Ext. 7951. *Fax:* 250-470-6085.

University of Northern British Columbia
Nursing Programme
Prince George, British Columbia

http://www.unbc.ca/nursing/

Founded in 1994

DEGREE • BSN

Nursing Program Faculty 12 (18% with doctorates).

Nursing Student Activities Student Nurses' Association.

Nursing Student Resources Academic or career counseling; computer lab; e-mail services; Internet; learning resource lab; library services; skills, simulation, or other laboratory.

Library Facilities 617,236 volumes (4,000 in health, 2,000 in nursing); 7,854 periodical subscriptions (300 health-care related).

BACCALAUREATE PROGRAMS

Degree BSN

Available Programs Generic Baccalaureate.

Site Options Prince George, BC.

Study Options Full-time and part-time.

Program Entrance Requirements Minimum overall college GPA of 2.33, transcript of college record, CPR certification, health exam, high school biology, high school chemistry, 1 year of high school math, 4 years high school science, high school transcript, immunizations, minimum high school GPA of 2.3, minimum high school rank 65%, minimum GPA in nursing prerequisites of 2.0, professional liability insurance/malpractice insurance. Transfer students are accepted. **Application** *Deadline:* 3/1 (freshmen), 3/1 (transfer). *Application fee:* CAN$25.

Advanced Placement Credit given for nursing courses completed elsewhere dependent upon specific evaluations.

Contact *Telephone:* 250-960-6309. *Fax:* 250-960-5744.

University of Victoria
School of Nursing
Victoria, British Columbia

http://web.uvic.ca/nurs/

Founded in 1963

DEGREES • BSN • MN • PHD

Nursing Program Faculty 21 (95% with doctorates).

Baccalaureate Enrollment 1,100

Women 95% **Men** 5% **Part-time** 50%

Nursing Student Activities Student Nurses' Association.

Nursing Student Resources Academic advising; assistance for students with disabilities; bookstore; campus computer network; computer lab; e-mail services; employment services for current students; interactive nursing skills videos; Internet; library services; nursing audiovisuals; remedial services; resume preparation assistance; unpaid internships.

Library Facilities 1.8 million volumes; 14,000 periodical subscriptions.

BACCALAUREATE PROGRAMS

Degree BSN

Site Options Vancouver, BC.

Program Entrance Requirements Minimum overall college GPA of 3.5, transcript of college record, CPR certification, high school transcript, immunizations, prerequisite course work. Transfer students are accepted. **Application** *Deadline:* 4/30 (freshmen), 4/30 (transfer). *Early decision:* 2/28. *Notification:* continuous (freshmen), 5/1 (early action). *Application fee:* CAN$100.

Contact *Telephone:* 250-721-7961. *Fax:* 250-721-6231.

GRADUATE PROGRAMS

Contact *Telephone:* 250-721-7961. *Fax:* 250-721-6231.

MASTER'S DEGREE PROGRAM

Degree MN

Available Programs Master's.

Site Options Victoria.

Study Options Full-time and part-time.

Program Entrance Requirements Clinical experience, transcript of college record, letters of recommendation.

Advanced Placement Credit given for nursing courses completed elsewhere dependent upon specific evaluations.

Degree Requirements 18 total credit hours, thesis or project.

DOCTORAL DEGREE PROGRAM

Degree PhD

Program Entrance Requirements Clinical experience, MSN or equivalent.

Degree Requirements Dissertation.

MANITOBA

Brandon University
School of Health Studies
Brandon, Manitoba

http://www.brandonu.ca/academic/health studies

Founded in 1899

DEGREE • BN

Nursing Program Faculty 16.

Baccalaureate Enrollment 44

Women 100% **Minority** 6% **Part-time** 2%

Nursing Student Activities Student Nurses' Association.

Nursing Student Resources Academic advising; academic or career counseling; assistance for students with disabilities; bookstore; campus computer network; career placement assistance; computer lab; e-mail services; employment services for current students; housing assistance; interactive nursing skills videos; Internet; library services; resume preparation assistance; skills, simulation, or other laboratory; tutoring.

Library Facilities 238,816 volumes; 1,699 periodical subscriptions.

BACCALAUREATE PROGRAMS

Degree BN

Available Programs Baccalaureate for Second Degree; Generic Baccalaureate; LPN to Baccalaureate; RN Baccalaureate.

Study Options Full-time and part-time.

Program Entrance Requirements Minimum overall college GPA of 2.0, CPR certification, immunizations, minimum GPA in nursing prerequisites of 2.0, prerequisite course work. Transfer students are accepted. **Application** *Deadline:* rolling (freshmen), rolling (transfer). *Notification:* continuous until 9/30 (freshmen). *Application fee:* CAN$60.

Brandon University (continued)

Advanced Placement Credit given for nursing courses completed elsewhere dependent upon specific evaluations.

Contact *Telephone:* 204-571-8567. *Fax:* 204-571-8568.

University of Manitoba
Faculty of Nursing
Winnipeg, Manitoba

http://www.umanitoba.ca/faculties/nursing/

Founded in 1877

DEGREES • BN • MN • PHD

Nursing Program Faculty 54 (51% with doctorates).

Baccalaureate Enrollment 1,170
Women 89% **Men** 11% **Part-time** 39%

Graduate Enrollment 91
Women 91% **Men** 9% **Part-time** 68%

Nursing Student Activities Nursing Honor Society, Sigma Theta Tau, Student Nurses' Association.

Nursing Student Resources Academic advising; academic or career counseling; assistance for students with disabilities; bookstore; campus computer network; computer lab; daycare for children of students; e-mail services; employment services for current students; housing assistance; interactive nursing skills videos; Internet; learning resource lab; library services; skills, simulation, or other laboratory; unpaid internships.

Library Facilities 1.6 million volumes (137,100 in health, 5,000 in nursing); 12,800 periodical subscriptions (2,208 health-care related).

BACCALAUREATE PROGRAMS
Degree BN

Available Programs Baccalaureate for Second Degree; Generic Baccalaureate; RN Baccalaureate.

Site Options Norway House, MB.

Study Options Full-time and part-time.

Program Entrance Requirements Minimum overall college GPA of 2.5, transcript of college record, CPR certification, high school chemistry, high school math, high school science, high school transcript, immunizations, minimum high school GPA of 2.5, prerequisite course work. Transfer students are accepted. **Application** *Deadline:* 7/1 (freshmen), 7/1 (transfer). *Notification:* continuous (freshmen). *Application fee:* CAN$35.

Advanced Placement Credit given for nursing courses completed elsewhere dependent upon specific evaluations.

Expenses (2006–07) *Tuition, area resident:* full-time CAN$3400.

Financial Aid *Gift aid (need-based):* state, private, college/university gift aid from institutional funds. *Loans:* Federal Direct (Subsidized and Unsubsidized Stafford PLUS), FFEL (Subsidized and Unsubsidized Stafford PLUS), Perkins, state, college/university, TERI Loans. *Work-Study:* part-time campus jobs. *Application deadline (priority):* 6/30.

Contact Dr. Christine Ateah, Associate Dean, Undergraduate Program, Faculty of Nursing, University of Manitoba, 277 Helen Glass Centre for Nursing, Winnipeg, MB R3T 2N2. *Telephone:* 204-474-6220. *Fax:* 204-474-7682. *E-mail:* christine_ateah@umanitoba.ca.

GRADUATE PROGRAMS
Contact Dr. Pamela Hawranik, Associate Dean, Graduate Programs, Faculty of Nursing, University of Manitoba, 281-89 Curry Place, Winnipeg, MB R3T 2N2. *Telephone:* 204-474-9317. *Fax:* 204-474-7682. *E-mail:* nursing_grad@umanitoba.ca.

MASTER'S DEGREE PROGRAM
Degree MN

Available Programs Master's.

Concentrations Available Nursing administration. *Clinical nurse specialist programs in:* acute care, gerontology, perinatal. *Nurse practitioner programs in:* primary care.

Study Options Full-time and part-time.

Program Entrance Requirements Clinical experience, minimum overall college GPA of 3.0, transcript of college record, written essay, 3 letters of recommendation, nursing research course, resume, statistics course. *Application deadline:* For fall admission, 3/1. *Application fee:* CAN$50.

Advanced Placement Credit given for nursing courses completed elsewhere dependent upon specific evaluations.

Degree Requirements 27 total credit hours, thesis or project, comprehensive exam.

DOCTORAL DEGREE PROGRAM
Degree PhD

Available Programs Doctorate.

Areas of Study Oncology.

Program Entrance Requirements Clinical experience, letters of recommendation, MSN or equivalent. *Application deadline:* For fall admission, 3/1. *Application fee:* CAN$50.

Degree Requirements 21 total credit hours, dissertation.

CONTINUING EDUCATION PROGRAM
Contact Dr. Dean Care, Dean, Faculty of Nursing, University of Manitoba, 293 Helen Glass Centre for Nursing, Winnipeg, MB R3T 2N2. *Telephone:* 204-474-9201. *Fax:* 204-474-7500. *E-mail:* dean_care@umanitoba.ca.

NEW BRUNSWICK

Université de Moncton
School of Nursing
Moncton, New Brunswick

Founded in 1963

DEGREES • BSCN • M SC N

Nursing Program Faculty 24 (25% with doctorates).

Baccalaureate Enrollment 570
Women 90% **Men** 10% **International** 1%

Graduate Enrollment 8

Nursing Student Activities Student Nurses' Association.

Nursing Student Resources Academic or career counseling; assistance for students with disabilities; bookstore; campus computer network; career placement assistance; computer lab; computer-assisted instruction; daycare for children of students; e-mail services; externships; housing assistance; Internet; library services; nursing audiovisuals; placement services for program completers; resume preparation assistance; unpaid internships.

Library Facilities 789,046 volumes; 2,059 periodical subscriptions.

BACCALAUREATE PROGRAMS
Degree BScN

Available Programs RN Baccalaureate.

Site Options Moncton, NB; Edmundston, NB; Bathurst, NB.

Study Options Full-time and part-time.

Program Entrance Requirements Transcript of college record, CPR certification, high school biology, high school chemistry, 12 years high school math, high school science, high school transcript, immunizations, minimum high school rank 65%. Transfer students are accepted. **Application** *Deadline:* 6/1 (freshmen), 2/1 (out-of-state freshmen), 6/1 (transfer). *Notification:* continuous until 9/1 (freshmen), continuous until 8/15 (out-of-state freshmen). *Application fee:* $30.

Advanced Placement Credit given for nursing courses completed elsewhere dependent upon specific evaluations.

Contact *Telephone:* 506-858-4443. *Fax:* 506-858-4544.

GRADUATE PROGRAMS
Contact *Telephone:* 506-858-4443. *Fax:* 506-858-4544.

MASTER'S DEGREE PROGRAM

Degree M Sc N

Available Programs Master's; RN to Master's.

Concentrations Available Health-care administration; nurse case management; nursing administration; nursing education. *Clinical nurse specialist programs in:* community health, family health, home health care, occupational health, pediatric, psychiatric/mental health, public health, school health. *Nurse practitioner programs in:* adult health, community health, family health, oncology, primary care.

Site Options Moncton, NB.

Study Options Full-time and part-time.

Program Entrance Requirements Minimum overall college GPA of 3.0, transcript of college record, CPR certification, written essay, 2 letters of recommendation, resume, statistics course.

Advanced Placement Credit given for nursing courses completed elsewhere dependent upon specific evaluations.

Degree Requirements 45 total credit hours, thesis or project.

CONTINUING EDUCATION PROGRAM

Contact *Telephone:* 506-858-4121.

University of New Brunswick Fredericton

Faculty of Nursing
Fredericton, New Brunswick

http://www.unbf.ca/nursing/

Founded in 1785

DEGREES • BN • MN

Nursing Program Faculty 68 (8% with doctorates).

Baccalaureate Enrollment 585
Women 95% **Men** 5%

Graduate Enrollment 54
Women 99% **Men** 1% **Part-time** 82%

Nursing Student Activities Student Nurses' Association, nursing club.

Nursing Student Resources Academic advising; academic or career counseling; assistance for students with disabilities; bookstore; campus computer network; computer lab; computer-assisted instruction; daycare for children of students; e-mail services; interactive nursing skills videos; Internet; learning resource lab; library services; nursing audiovisuals; resume preparation assistance; skills, simulation, or other laboratory; tutoring.

Library Facilities 1.1 million volumes (12,547 in health, 1,910 in nursing); 4,817 periodical subscriptions (250 health-care related).

BACCALAUREATE PROGRAMS

Degree BN

Available Programs Generic Baccalaureate.

Site Options *Distance Learning:* Moncton, NB; Bathurst, NB.

Study Options Full-time.

Program Entrance Requirements Transcript of college record, CPR certification, written essay, health exam, high school biology, high school chemistry, high school math, high school transcript, immunizations, interview, minimum high school rank 70%, minimum GPA in nursing prerequisites, prerequisite course work. Transfer students are accepted.

Standardized tests *Required for some:* SAT. **Application** *Deadline:* 3/31 (freshmen), 3/31 (transfer). *Notification:* continuous until 8/31 (freshmen). *Application fee:* CAN$45.

Advanced Placement Credit given for nursing courses completed elsewhere dependent upon specific evaluations.

Expenses (2006–07) *Tuition:* full-time CAN$5246. *Room and board:* CAN$6951 per academic year.

Financial Aid 73% of baccalaureate students in nursing programs received some form of financial aid in 2005–06. *Gift aid (need-based):* private, college/university gift aid from institutional funds. *Loans:* Federal Direct (Subsidized and Unsubsidized Stafford PLUS), college/university, federal/provincial loans. *Work-Study:* part-time campus jobs. *Application deadline:* 5/15 (priority: 2/15).

Contact Mr. Lee Heenan, Administrative Assistant, Faculty of Nursing, University of New Brunswick Fredericton, PO Box 4400, Fredericton, NB E3B 5A3. *Telephone:* 506-458-7670. *Fax:* 506-447-3374. *E-mail:* lheenan@unb.ca.

GRADUATE PROGRAMS

Expenses (2006–07) *Tuition:* full-time CAN$5322; part-time CAN$1300 per term. *International tuition:* CAN$10,620 full-time. *Room and board:* CAN$6951 per academic year. *Required fees:* full-time CAN$1365; part-time CAN$596 per term.

Financial Aid 95% of graduate students in nursing programs received some form of financial aid in 2005–06.

Contact Mr. Francis Perry, Graduate Assistant, Faculty of Nursing, University of New Brunswick Fredericton, PO Box 4400, Fredericton, NB E3B 5A3. *Telephone:* 506-451-6844. *Fax:* 506-447-3374. *E-mail:* fperry@unb.ca.

MASTER'S DEGREE PROGRAM

Degree MN

Available Programs Master's.

Concentrations Available Nurse case management; nursing administration; nursing education; nursing informatics. *Clinical nurse specialist programs in:* acute care, adult health, cardiovascular, community health, critical care, family health, gerontology, maternity-newborn, medical-surgical, oncology, parent-child, pediatric, psychiatric/mental health, public health, school health, women's health. *Nurse practitioner programs in:* acute care, adult health, community health, family health, gerontology, neonatal health, pediatric, primary care, psychiatric/mental health, women's health.

Study Options Full-time and part-time.

Program Entrance Requirements Clinical experience, computer literacy, minimum overall college GPA of 3.3, transcript of college record, written essay, 3 letters of recommendation, nursing research course, physical assessment course, prerequisite course work, statistics course.

Advanced Placement Credit given for nursing courses completed elsewhere dependent upon specific evaluations.

Degree Requirements 27 total credit hours, thesis or project.

CONTINUING EDUCATION PROGRAM

Contact Nursing Contact, Faculty of Nursing, University of New Brunswick Fredericton, PO Box 4400, Fredericton, NB E3B 5A3. *Telephone:* 506-453-4642. *Fax:* 506-447-3057. *E-mail:* nursing@unb.ca.

NEWFOUNDLAND AND LABRADOR

Memorial University of Newfoundland

School of Nursing
St. John's, Newfoundland and Labrador

http://www.nurs.mun.ca

Founded in 1925

DEGREES • BN • M SC

Nursing Program Faculty 42 (30% with doctorates).

Baccalaureate Enrollment 642
Women 92% **Men** 8% **International** 2% **Part-time** 50%

Memorial University of Newfoundland (continued)
Graduate Enrollment 100
Women 91% **Men** 9% **International** 1% **Part-time** 82%
Nursing Student Activities Student Nurses' Association.

Nursing Student Resources Academic advising; academic or career counseling; assistance for students with disabilities; bookstore; campus computer network; computer lab; computer-assisted instruction; daycare for children of students; e-mail services; employment services for current students; externships; interactive nursing skills videos; Internet; learning resource lab; library services; nursing audiovisuals; remedial services; skills, simulation, or other laboratory; tutoring.

Library Facilities 1.7 million volumes (40,000 in health, 5,000 in nursing); 17,170 periodical subscriptions (3,800 health-care related).

BACCALAUREATE PROGRAMS
Degree BN

Available Programs Accelerated Baccalaureate for Second Degree; Generic Baccalaureate; RN Baccalaureate.
Study Options Full-time.

Program Entrance Requirements CPR certification, written essay, health exam, health insurance, high school biology, high school chemistry, high school math, high school science, high school transcript, immunizations, 2 letters of recommendation, minimum high school GPA. Transfer students are accepted. **Application** *Deadline:* rolling (freshmen), 3/1 (out-of-state freshmen), 3/1 (transfer). *Application fee:* CAN$40.

Advanced Placement Credit given for nursing courses completed elsewhere dependent upon specific evaluations.

Expenses (2006–07) *Tuition, area resident:* full-time CAN$2805; part-time CAN$85 per credit hour. *International tuition:* CAN$9669 full-time. *Room and board:* CAN$3315; room only: CAN$1804 per academic year. *Required fees:* full-time CAN$165; part-time CAN$20 per term.

Financial Aid 10% of baccalaureate students in nursing programs received some form of financial aid in 2005–06. *Loans:* college/university. *Application deadline:* Continuous.

Contact Ms. June Ellis, Consortium Coordinator, School of Nursing, Memorial University of Newfoundland, St. John's, NF A1B 3R6. *Telephone:* 709-737-6871. *Fax:* 709-737-3890. *E-mail:* junee@mun.ca or nursing@mun.ca.

GRADUATE PROGRAMS
Expenses (2006–07) *Tuition, state resident:* full-time CAN$2000; part-time CAN$733 per semester. *Tuition, nonresident:* full-time CAN$2000; part-time CAN$733 per semester. *International tuition:* CAN$2600 full-time. *Room and board:* CAN$3829; room only: CAN$2318 per academic year. *Required fees:* full-time CAN$140; part-time CAN$80 per term.

Financial Aid 25% of graduate students in nursing programs received some form of financial aid in 2005–06. Fellowships, research assistantships, teaching assistantships available. *Financial aid application deadline:* 12/31.

Contact Dr. Donna Moralejo, Acting Associate Director, Graduate Program and Research, School of Nursing, Memorial University of Newfoundland, 300 Prince Philip Parkway, St. John's, NF A1B 3V6. *Telephone:* 709-777-6679. *Fax:* 709-777-7037. *E-mail:* lenac@mun.ca or nursing@mun.ca.

MASTER'S DEGREE PROGRAM
Degree M Sc

Available Programs Master's.
Concentrations Available *Clinical nurse specialist programs in:* adult health, community health, pediatric, psychiatric/mental health. *Nurse practitioner programs in:* acute care, psychiatric/mental health.
Study Options Full-time and part-time.

Program Entrance Requirements Clinical experience, minimum overall college GPA of 3.0, transcript of college record, CPR certification, written essay, 3 letters of recommendation, nursing research course, professional liability insurance/malpractice insurance, resume, statistics course. *Application deadline:* For fall admission, 2/15 (priority date). Applications are processed on a rolling basis. *Application fee:* CAN$40.

Advanced Placement Credit given for nursing courses completed elsewhere dependent upon specific evaluations.

Degree Requirements 34 total credit hours, thesis or project.

NOVA SCOTIA

Dalhousie University
School of Nursing
Halifax, Nova Scotia

http://www.dal.ca/nursing
Founded in 1818
DEGREES • BSCN • MN • MN/MHSA • PHD
Nursing Program Faculty 57 (32% with doctorates).

Baccalaureate Enrollment 543
Women 90% **Men** 10% **Minority** 2% **Part-time** 2%
Graduate Enrollment 109
Women 96% **Men** 4% **Minority** 3% **Part-time** 71%
Nursing Student Activities Nursing Honor Society, Sigma Theta Tau, Student Nurses' Association.

Nursing Student Resources Academic advising; academic or career counseling; assistance for students with disabilities; bookstore; campus computer network; computer lab; computer-assisted instruction; daycare for children of students; e-mail services; employment services for current students; externships; housing assistance; interactive nursing skills videos; Internet; learning resource lab; library services; nursing audiovisuals; resume preparation assistance; skills, simulation, or other laboratory; tutoring.

Library Facilities 1.7 million volumes; 8,306 periodical subscriptions.

BACCALAUREATE PROGRAMS
Degree BScN

Available Programs Accelerated Baccalaureate; Accelerated Baccalaureate for Second Degree; Baccalaureate for Second Degree; Generic Baccalaureate; RN Baccalaureate.
Site Options Yarmouth, NS.
Study Options Full-time.

Program Entrance Requirements Minimum overall college GPA of 2.5, transcript of college record, high school biology, high school chemistry, 3 years high school math, high school transcript, immunizations, minimum high school rank 70%, minimum GPA in nursing prerequisites of 2.5, prerequisite course work. Transfer students are accepted. **Standardized tests** *Required:* SAT. **Application** *Deadline:* 6/1 (freshmen), 6/1 (transfer). *Early decision:* 3/15. *Notification:* continuous (freshmen). *Application fee:* CAN$45.

Advanced Placement Credit given for nursing courses completed elsewhere dependent upon specific evaluations.

Financial Aid *Gift aid (need-based):* private, college/university gift aid from institutional funds, Vermont Grants, Rhode Island grants. *Loans:* FFEL (Subsidized and Unsubsidized Stafford PLUS), Canadian Loans; Private Bank Loans. *Application deadline:* Continuous.

Contact Prof. Lucille Wittstock, Associate Director, Undergraduate Student Affairs, School of Nursing, Dalhousie University, 5869 University Avenue, Halifax, NS B3H 3J5. *Telephone:* 902-494-2004. *Fax:* 902-494-3487. *E-mail:* lucille.wittstock@dal.ca.

GRADUATE PROGRAMS
Financial Aid 21% of graduate students in nursing programs received some form of financial aid in 2005–06. Fellowships, research assistantships, teaching assistantships available.

Contact Dr. Ruth Martin-Misener, Associate Director, Graduate Programs, School of Nursing, Dalhousie University, 5869 University Avenue, Halifax, NS B3H 3J5. *Telephone:* 902-494-2250. *Fax:* 902-494-3487. *E-mail:* ruth.martin-misener@dal.ca.

MASTER'S DEGREE PROGRAM
Degrees MN; MN/MHSA
Available Programs Master's.
Concentrations Available *Clinical nurse specialist programs in:* adult health, community health, family health, maternity-newborn, parent-child, pediatric, psychiatric/mental health, public health. *Nurse practitioner programs in:* acute care, adult health, gerontology, neonatal health, oncology.

Study Options Full-time and part-time.

Program Entrance Requirements Clinical experience, minimum overall college GPA of 3.0, transcript of college record, immunizations, interview, 3 letters of recommendation, nursing research course, prerequisite course work, statistics course, GRE General Test. *Application deadline:* For fall admission, 4/1 (priority date); for winter admission, 10/31. Applications are processed on a rolling basis. *Application fee:* $60.

Degree Requirements 36 total credit hours, thesis or project.

POST-MASTER'S PROGRAM

Areas of Study *Nurse practitioner programs in:* acute care, adult health, gerontology, neonatal health, oncology.

DOCTORAL DEGREE PROGRAM

Degree PhD

Available Programs Doctorate.

Areas of Study Advanced practice nursing, aging, community health, family health, health policy, health promotion/disease prevention, human health and illness, illness and transition, maternity-newborn, nursing policy, nursing research, nursing science, oncology, women's health.

Program Entrance Requirements Clinical experience, minimum overall college GPA of 3.3, interview, 3 letters of recommendation, MSN or equivalent, vita, writing sample. *Application deadline:* For fall admission, 4/1 (priority date); for winter admission, 10/31. Applications are processed on a rolling basis. *Application fee:* $60.

Degree Requirements 27 total credit hours, dissertation, oral exam, written exam, residency.

St. Francis Xavier University
Department of Nursing
Antigonish, Nova Scotia

http://www.stfx.ca

Founded in 1853

DEGREE • BSCN

Nursing Program Faculty 67 (10% with doctorates).

Baccalaureate Enrollment 1,067
Women 90% **Men** 10% **Minority** 5% **International** 1% **Part-time** 40%

Nursing Student Activities Student Nurses' Association, nursing club.

Nursing Student Resources Academic advising; academic or career counseling; assistance for students with disabilities; bookstore; campus computer network; career placement assistance; computer lab; computer-assisted instruction; daycare for children of students; e-mail services; employment services for current students; externships; housing assistance; interactive nursing skills videos; Internet; learning resource lab; library services; nursing audiovisuals; other; paid internships; placement services for program completers; remedial services; resume preparation assistance; skills, simulation, or other laboratory; tutoring; unpaid internships.

Library Facilities 632,575 volumes (4,000 in health, 4,000 in nursing); 3,282 periodical subscriptions (1,015 health-care related).

BACCALAUREATE PROGRAMS

Degree BScN

Available Programs Accelerated Baccalaureate; Accelerated Baccalaureate for Second Degree; Accelerated LPN to Baccalaureate; Generic Baccalaureate; RN Baccalaureate.

Site Options Sydney, NS.

Study Options Full-time.

Program Entrance Requirements Transcript of college record, CPR certification, health exam, high school biology, high school chemistry, 2 years high school math, 2 years high school science, high school transcript, immunizations, minimum high school GPA, prerequisite course work. Transfer students are accepted. **Standardized tests** *Recommended:* SAT or ACT, SAT Subject Tests. *Required for some:* SAT or ACT. **Application** *Deadline:* rolling (freshmen), rolling (transfer). *Notification:* continuous until 8/15 (freshmen). *Application fee:* CAN$40.

Advanced Placement Credit given for nursing courses completed elsewhere dependent upon specific evaluations.

Contact *Telephone:* 902-867-5386. *Fax:* 902-867-2329.

CONTINUING EDUCATION PROGRAM

Contact *Telephone:* 902-867-5186. *Fax:* 902-867-5154.

ONTARIO

Brock University
Department of Nursing
St. Catharines, Ontario

http://www.brocku.ca/nursing/

Founded in 1964

DEGREE • BSCN

Nursing Student Resources Computer-assisted instruction.

Library Facilities 1.6 million volumes; 856,587 periodical subscriptions.

BACCALAUREATE PROGRAMS

Degree BScN

Available Programs Generic Baccalaureate; RN Baccalaureate.

Study Options Full-time and part-time.

Program Entrance Requirements Application *Deadline:* 4/1 (freshmen), 4/1 (transfer). *Notification:* continuous (freshmen). *Application fee:* CAN$115.

Contact *Telephone:* 905-688-5550 Ext. 4781.

Lakehead University
School of Nursing
Thunder Bay, Ontario

http://www.lakeheadu.ca

Founded in 1965

DEGREE • BSN

Nursing Program Faculty 11 (27% with doctorates).

Baccalaureate Enrollment 450

Nursing Student Activities Nursing club.

Nursing Student Resources Academic advising; academic or career counseling; assistance for students with disabilities; bookstore; campus computer network; computer lab; daycare for children of students; e-mail services; interactive nursing skills videos; library services; nursing audiovisuals; skills, simulation, or other laboratory; tutoring.

Library Facilities 780,974 volumes; 10,300 periodical subscriptions.

BACCALAUREATE PROGRAMS

Degree BSN

Available Programs Generic Baccalaureate; RN Baccalaureate.

Study Options Full-time and part-time.

Program Entrance Requirements Transcript of college record, CPR certification, health insurance, high school biology, high school chemistry, 4 years high school math, high school transcript, immunizations. Transfer students are accepted. **Standardized tests** *Required:* SAT or ACT. **Application** *Deadline:* 9/19 (freshmen), 9/19 (transfer). *Application fee:* CAN$105.

Advanced Placement Credit given for nursing courses completed elsewhere dependent upon specific evaluations.

Contact *Telephone:* 807-343-8115. *Fax:* 807-343-8246.

Laurentian University
School of Nursing
Sudbury, Ontario

Founded in 1960

DEGREE • BSCN

Nursing Program Faculty 20 (20% with doctorates).
Nursing Student Resources Internet.
Library Facilities 696,838 volumes.

BACCALAUREATE PROGRAMS

Degree BScN

Study Options Full-time and part-time.
Program Entrance Requirements CPR certification, health exam, high school biology, high school chemistry, high school transcript, immunizations, prerequisite course work. Transfer students are accepted. **Application** *Deadline:* 2/1 (freshmen), rolling (transfer). *Application fee:* CAN$55.
Advanced Placement Credit given for nursing courses completed elsewhere dependent upon specific evaluations.
Contact *Telephone:* 705-675-1151 Ext. 3808. *Fax:* 705-675-4861.

CONTINUING EDUCATION PROGRAM

Contact *Telephone:* 705-675-1151 Ext. 3808. *Fax:* 705-675-4861.

McMaster University
School of Nursing
Hamilton, Ontario

http://www.fhs.mcmaster.ca/nursing
Founded in 1887

DEGREES • BSCN • M SC • MSN/PHD

Nursing Program Faculty 53 (47% with doctorates).
Baccalaureate Enrollment 548
Women 90% **Men** 10% **Part-time** 20%
Nursing Student Activities Student Nurses' Association.
Nursing Student Resources Academic advising; academic or career counseling; assistance for students with disabilities; bookstore; campus computer network; career placement assistance; computer lab; daycare for children of students; e-mail services; employment services for current students; housing assistance; Internet; learning resource lab; library services; nursing audiovisuals; placement services for program completers; remedial services; resume preparation assistance; skills, simulation, or other laboratory; tutoring.
Library Facilities 1.7 million volumes (150,446 in health); 11,976 periodical subscriptions (89,267 health-care related).

BACCALAUREATE PROGRAMS

Degree BScN

Available Programs Baccalaureate for Second Degree; Generic Baccalaureate; RN Baccalaureate.
Site Options Kitchener, ON.
Study Options Full-time and part-time.
Program Entrance Requirements CPR certification, health exam, high school biology, high school chemistry, 4 years high school math, 4 years high school science, high school transcript, immunizations, minimum high school GPA of 3.0, minimum high school rank 75%. Transfer students are accepted. **Application** *Deadline:* 7/15 (freshmen), 5/1 (out-of-state freshmen), 7/15 (transfer). *Early decision:* 3/1. *Notification:* continuous until 9/1 (freshmen), 6/12 (early action). *Application fee:* CAN$95.
Advanced Placement Credit by examination available. Credit given for nursing courses completed elsewhere dependent upon specific evaluations.
Contact *Telephone:* 905-525-9140 Ext. 22232. *Fax:* 905-528-4727.

GRADUATE PROGRAMS

Contact *Telephone:* 905-525-9140 Ext. 22982. *Fax:* 905-546-1129.

MASTER'S DEGREE PROGRAM

Degrees M Sc; MSN/PhD
Available Programs Master's.
Concentrations Available *Clinical nurse specialist programs in:* perinatal. *Nurse practitioner programs in:* neonatal health.
Study Options Full-time and part-time.
Program Entrance Requirements Transcript of college record, written essay, 2 letters of recommendation.
Advanced Placement Credit given for nursing courses completed elsewhere dependent upon specific evaluations.
Degree Requirements Thesis or project.

DOCTORAL DEGREE PROGRAM

Degree PhD
Available Programs Doctorate.
Program Entrance Requirements 2 letters of recommendation, MSN or equivalent, vita.
Degree Requirements Dissertation, oral exam.

Nipissing University
Nursing Department
North Bay, Ontario

Founded in 1992

DEGREE • BSCN

Nursing Program Faculty 11 (3% with doctorates).
Baccalaureate Enrollment 145
Women 98% **Men** 2% **Minority** 2% **International** 1% **Part-time** 10%
Nursing Student Activities Student Nurses' Association.
Nursing Student Resources Academic advising; academic or career counseling; assistance for students with disabilities; bookstore; campus computer network; career placement assistance; computer lab; computer-assisted instruction; daycare for children of students; e-mail services; employment services for current students; housing assistance; interactive nursing skills videos; Internet; learning resource lab; library services; nursing audiovisuals; placement services for program completers; remedial services; resume preparation assistance; skills, simulation, or other laboratory; tutoring; unpaid internships.
Library Facilities 180,397 volumes (2,800 in health, 1,820 in nursing); 5,680 periodical subscriptions (2,430 health-care related).

BACCALAUREATE PROGRAMS

Degree BScN

Available Programs Generic Baccalaureate.
Study Options Full-time.
Program Entrance Requirements Minimum overall college GPA of 3.0, transcript of college record, high school biology, high school chemistry, high school transcript, immunizations, minimum high school rank 70%. Transfer students are accepted. **Application** *Deadline:* 6/1 (freshmen), 6/1 (transfer). *Notification:* continuous until 6/1 (freshmen). *Application fee:* CAN$40.
Financial Aid 44% of baccalaureate students in nursing programs received some form of financial aid in 2004–05.
Contact Admissions Office. *Telephone:* 705-474-3450 Ext. 4521.

Queen's University at Kingston
School of Nursing
Kingston, Ontario

http://meds.queensu.ca/nursing
Founded in 1841

DEGREES • BNSC • M SC

Nursing Program Faculty 20 (80% with doctorates).

Baccalaureate Enrollment 400
Women 95% **Men** 5%

Graduate Enrollment 25
Women 95% **Men** 5%

Nursing Student Activities Student Nurses' Association.

Nursing Student Resources Academic advising; academic or career counseling; assistance for students with disabilities; bookstore; campus computer network; career placement assistance; computer lab; computer-assisted instruction; daycare for children of students; e-mail services; employment services for current students; housing assistance; interactive nursing skills videos; Internet; learning resource lab; library services; nursing audiovisuals; resume preparation assistance; skills, simulation, or other laboratory; tutoring; unpaid internships.

Library Facilities 3.5 million volumes (5,209 in health, 3,652 in nursing); 16,109 periodical subscriptions (1,054 health-care related).

BACCALAUREATE PROGRAMS

Degree BNSc

Available Programs Accelerated Baccalaureate; Generic Baccalaureate; RN Baccalaureate.

Study Options Full-time.

Program Entrance Requirements CPR certification, high school biology, high school chemistry, high school math, high school science, high school transcript, immunizations, minimum high school GPA, minimum high school rank. Transfer students are accepted. **Standardized tests** *Required:* SAT or ACT. **Application** *Deadline:* 2/16 (freshmen), 5/15 (transfer). *Notification:* continuous until 5/28 (freshmen). *Application fee:* CAN$165.

Financial Aid 41% of baccalaureate students in nursing programs received some form of financial aid in 2005–06. *Gift aid (need-based):* state, private, college/university gift aid from institutional funds. *Loans:* FFEL (Subsidized and Unsubsidized Stafford PLUS), college/university, federal aid provincial loans, alternative loans. *Work-Study:* part-time campus jobs. *Application deadline (priority):* 7/1.

Contact Prof. Susan Laschinger, Chair, Admissions Committee, School of Nursing, Queen's University at Kingston, Cataraqui Building, 92 Barrie Street, Kingston, ON K7L 3N6. *Telephone:* 613-533-6000 Ext. 74743. *Fax:* 613-533-6770. *E-mail:* lasching@post.queensu.ca.

GRADUATE PROGRAMS

Financial Aid 100% of graduate students in nursing programs received some form of financial aid in 2005–06. 25 fellowships (averaging $6,636 per year), 4 research assistantships, 9 teaching assistantships (averaging $2,592 per year) were awarded; institutionally sponsored loans and scholarships also available. *Financial aid application deadline:* 2/1.

Contact Dr. Marianne Lamb, Graduate Coordinator, School of Nursing, Queen's University at Kingston, Cataraqui Building, 92 Barrie Street, Kingston, ON K7L 3N6. *Telephone:* 613-533-6000 Ext. 74764. *Fax:* 613-533-6770. *E-mail:* marianne.lamb@queensu.ca.

MASTER'S DEGREE PROGRAM

Degree M Sc

Available Programs Master's.

Study Options Full-time.

Program Entrance Requirements Transcript of college record, 2 letters of recommendation, nursing research course, prerequisite course work, statistics course. *Application deadline:* For winter admission, 2/1 (priority date). Applications are processed on a rolling basis. *Application fee:* CAN$70.

Degree Requirements Thesis or project.

Ryerson University
Program in Nursing
Toronto, Ontario

http://www.ryerson.ca/nursing
Founded in 1948

DEGREES • BSCN • MN

Nursing Program Faculty 80 (19% with doctorates).

Baccalaureate Enrollment 1,881
Women 92% **Men** 8% **Part-time** 38%

Nursing Student Activities Sigma Theta Tau, Student Nurses' Association, nursing club.

Nursing Student Resources Academic advising; academic or career counseling; assistance for students with disabilities; bookstore; campus computer network; career placement assistance; computer lab; computer-assisted instruction; daycare for children of students; e-mail services; employment services for current students; housing assistance; interactive nursing skills videos; Internet; learning resource lab; library services; nursing audiovisuals; remedial services; resume preparation assistance; skills, simulation, or other laboratory; tutoring.

Library Facilities 606,603 volumes (70,000 in health, 7,000 in nursing); 25,675 periodical subscriptions (5,000 health-care related).

BACCALAUREATE PROGRAMS

Degree BScN

Available Programs Generic Baccalaureate; International Nurse to Baccalaureate; RN Baccalaureate; RPN to Baccalaureate.

Study Options Full-time.

Program Entrance Requirements Transcript of college record, CPR certification, health exam, health insurance, high school biology, high school chemistry, high school math, high school transcript, immunizations, minimum high school rank 75%. **Application** *Deadline:* 3/1 (freshmen). *Notification:* continuous (freshmen). *Application fee:* CAN$95.

Advanced Placement Credit given for nursing courses completed elsewhere dependent upon specific evaluations.

Expenses (2006–07) *Required fees:* full-time CAN$27; part-time CAN$19 per credit; part-time CAN$19 per term.

Financial Aid 45% of baccalaureate students in nursing programs received some form of financial aid in 2005–06. *Gift aid (need-based):* college/university gift aid from institutional funds. *Loans:* Federal Direct (Subsidized and Unsubsidized Stafford). *Application deadline:* 1/15.

Contact Richard Perras, Student Affairs Coordinator, Program in Nursing, Ryerson University, 350 Victoria Street, Room POD-474, Toronto, ON M5B 2K3. *Telephone:* 416-979-5000 Ext. 6318. *Fax:* 416-979-5332. *E-mail:* rperras@ryerson.ca.

GRADUATE PROGRAMS

Expenses (2006–07) *Tuition, state resident:* full-time CAN$5376; part-time CAN$896 per course. *Tuition, nonresident:* full-time CAN$5376; part-time CAN$896 per course. *Required fees:* full-time CAN$906; part-time CAN$279 per credit.

Financial Aid 67% of graduate students in nursing programs received some form of financial aid in 2005–06.

Contact Mr. Gerry Warner, Program Administrator, Program in Nursing, Ryerson University, 350 Victoria Street, Toronto, ON M5B 2K3. *Telephone:* 416-979-5000 Ext. 7852. *Fax:* 416-979-5332. *E-mail:* g2warner@ryerson.ca.

MASTER'S DEGREE PROGRAM

Degree MN

Available Programs Master's.

Concentrations Available *Clinical nurse specialist programs in:* adult health, community health, family health, public health.

Study Options Full-time and part-time.

Program Entrance Requirements Minimum overall college GPA of 3.33, transcript of college record, CPR certification, written essay, immunizations, letters of recommendation, nursing research course, resume.

Advanced Placement Credit given for nursing courses completed elsewhere dependent upon specific evaluations.

Degree Requirements 10 total credit hours, thesis or project.

CONTINUING EDUCATION PROGRAM

Contact Paula Mastrilli, Program Manager, Program in Nursing, Ryerson University, 350 Victoria Street, Room POD-476A, Toronto, ON M5B 2K3. *Telephone:* 416-979-5178. *Fax:* 416-979-5277. *E-mail:* pmastril@ryerson.ca.

Trent University
Nursing Program
Peterborough, Ontario

http://www.trentu.ca/nursing/

Founded in 1963

DEGREE • BSCN

Nursing Program Faculty 42 (14% with doctorates).

Baccalaureate Enrollment 438

Nursing Student Activities Student Nurses' Association.

Nursing Student Resources Academic advising; academic or career counseling; assistance for students with disabilities; bookstore; campus computer network; computer lab; computer-assisted instruction; e-mail services; employment services for current students; housing assistance; interactive nursing skills videos; Internet; learning resource lab; library services; nursing audiovisuals; remedial services; resume preparation assistance; skills, simulation, or other laboratory; tutoring.

Library Facilities 606,422 volumes (6,393 in health, 1,281 in nursing); 9,388 periodical subscriptions (360 health-care related).

BACCALAUREATE PROGRAMS

Degree BScN

Available Programs Accelerated Baccalaureate; RN Baccalaureate.

Site Options Peterborough, ON.

Study Options Full-time.

Program Entrance Requirements CPR certification, health exam, high school biology, high school chemistry, 4 years high school math, 4 years high school science, high school transcript, immunizations, minimum high school rank 70%. Transfer students are accepted. **Standardized tests** *Required for some:* SAT or ACT. **Application** *Deadline:* 6/1 (freshmen), 6/1 (transfer). *Application fee:* CAN$95.

Expenses (2006–07) *Tuition, area resident:* full-time CAN$5600. *Room and board:* CAN$7200 per academic year.

Contact Ms. Carol Weafer-Lloyd, Liaison and Admissions Officer, Nursing Program, Trent University, Trent/Fleming Nursing Program, 1600 Westbank Drive, Peterborough, ON K9J 7B8. *Telephone:* 705-748-1011 Ext. 7809. *Fax:* 705-748-1088. *E-mail:* nursing@trentu.ca.

University of Ottawa
School of Nursing
Ottawa, Ontario

http://www.health.uottawa.ca/sn/

Founded in 1848

DEGREES • BSCN • M SC N • PHD

Nursing Program Faculty 150 (18% with doctorates).

Baccalaureate Enrollment 1,324
Women 94% **Men** 6% **Part-time** 21%

Graduate Enrollment 78
Women 95% **Men** 5% **Part-time** 79%

Nursing Student Activities Sigma Theta Tau, Student Nurses' Association.

Nursing Student Resources Academic advising; academic or career counseling; assistance for students with disabilities; bookstore; campus computer network; computer lab; e-mail services; employment services for current students; housing assistance; learning resource lab; library services; nursing audiovisuals; remedial services; skills, simulation, or other laboratory; tutoring.

Library Facilities 2.6 million volumes (54,000 in health, 7,000 in nursing); 9,183 periodical subscriptions (1,050 health-care related).

BACCALAUREATE PROGRAMS

Degree BScN

Available Programs Generic Baccalaureate; International Nurse to Baccalaureate; RN Baccalaureate; RPN to Baccalaureate.

Site Options *Distance Learning:* Pembroke, ON; Kingston, PQ; Montreal, QC.

Study Options Full-time.

Program Entrance Requirements Transcript of college record, CPR certification, high school biology, high school chemistry, high school math, high school transcript, immunizations. Transfer students are accepted. **Application** *Deadline:* 6/1 (freshmen). *Notification:* continuous until 8/30 (freshmen). *Application fee:* CAN$165.

Advanced Placement Credit given for nursing courses completed elsewhere dependent upon specific evaluations.

Financial Aid *Gift aid (need-based):* state, private, college/university gift aid from institutional funds. *Loans:* provincial and federal loans. *Work-Study:* Federal Work-Study, part-time campus jobs. *Application deadline:* 1/31.

Contact Ms. Suzanne Biagé, Academic Advisor, School of Nursing, University of Ottawa, 451 Smyth Road, Ottawa, ON K1H 8M5. *Telephone:* 613-562-5800 Ext. 5404. *Fax:* 613-562-5470. *E-mail:* sbiage@uottawa.ca.

GRADUATE PROGRAMS

Financial Aid Fellowships, research assistantships, teaching assistantships, career-related internships or fieldwork, Federal Work-Study, scholarships, traineeships, tuition waivers (full and partial), and unspecified assistantships available.

Contact Dr. Pierrrette Guimond, Assistant Director of Graduate Program, School of Nursing, University of Ottawa, 451 Smyth Road, Ottawa, ON K1H 8M5. *Telephone:* 613-562-5800 Ext. 8422. *Fax:* 613-562-5473. *E-mail:* pguimond@uottawa.ca.

MASTER'S DEGREE PROGRAM

Degree M Sc N

Available Programs Master's.

Concentrations Available *Clinical nurse specialist programs in:* acute care, community health. *Nurse practitioner programs in:* primary care.

Program Entrance Requirements Clinical experience, minimum overall college GPA of 3.0, transcript of college record, written essay, immunizations, 3 letters of recommendation, nursing research course, physical assessment course, prerequisite course work, statistics course. *Application deadline:* For fall admission, 8/1 (priority date); for winter admission, 11/15 (priority date); for spring admission, 4/1 (priority date). *Application fee:* $75.

Advanced Placement Credit given for nursing courses completed elsewhere dependent upon specific evaluations.

Degree Requirements 24 total credit hours, thesis or project.

DOCTORAL DEGREE PROGRAM

Degree PhD

Available Programs Doctorate; Doctorate for Nurses with Non-Nursing Degrees.

Areas of Study Health promotion/disease prevention, health-care systems, nursing policy, nursing research, nursing science.

Program Entrance Requirements Minimum overall college GPA of 3.5, 3 letters of recommendation, MSN or equivalent, statistics course, vita, writing sample. *Application deadline:* For fall admission, 8/1 (priority date); for winter admission, 11/15 (priority date); for spring admission, 4/1 (priority date). *Application fee:* $75.

Degree Requirements 18 total credit hours, dissertation, oral exam, written exam, residency.

POSTDOCTORAL PROGRAM

Areas of Study Community health, nursing interventions.

Postdoctoral Program Contact Dr. Nancy Edwards, CIHR/CHSRF Chair/Professor, School of Nursing, University of Ottawa, 451 Smyth Road, Ottawa, ON K1H 8M5. *Telephone:* 613-562-5800 Ext. 8040. *E-mail:* nedwards@uottawa.ca.

University of Toronto
Faculty of Nursing
Toronto, Ontario

http://www.nursing.utoronto.ca/

Founded in 1827

DEGREES • BSCN • MN • PHD

Nursing Program Faculty 45 (58% with doctorates).

Baccalaureate Enrollment 300

Graduate Enrollment 360
Part-time 45%

Nursing Student Activities Sigma Theta Tau, Student Nurses' Association, nursing club.

Nursing Student Resources Academic advising; academic or career counseling; assistance for students with disabilities; bookstore; campus computer network; career placement assistance; computer lab; computer-assisted instruction; e-mail services; employment services for current students; externships; housing assistance; interactive nursing skills videos; Internet; learning resource lab; library services; nursing audiovisuals; resume preparation assistance; skills, simulation, or other laboratory; unpaid internships.

Library Facilities 10.3 million volumes; 53,547 periodical subscriptions.

BACCALAUREATE PROGRAMS

Degree BScN

Available Programs Accelerated RN Baccalaureate.

Study Options Full-time.

Program Entrance Requirements Application *Deadline:* 3/1 (freshmen), 7/1 (transfer). *Notification:* continuous (freshmen). *Application fee:* CAN$43.

Financial Aid 60% of baccalaureate students in nursing programs received some form of financial aid in 2005–06. *Loans:* . *Work-Study:* Federal Work-Study.

Contact Office of Student Affairs, Faculty of Nursing, University of Toronto, 155 College Street, Suite 132, Toronto, ON M5T 1P8. *Telephone:* 416-978-2863. *Fax:* 416-978-8222. *E-mail:* inquiry.nursing@utoronto.ca.

GRADUATE PROGRAMS

Financial Aid 14% of graduate students in nursing programs received some form of financial aid in 2005–06.

Contact Office of Student Affairs, Faculty of Nursing, University of Toronto, 155 College Street, Suite 132, Toronto, ON M5T 1P8. *Telephone:* 416-978-2863. *Fax:* 416-978-8222. *E-mail:* inquiry.nursing@utoronto.ca.

MASTER'S DEGREE PROGRAM

Degree MN

Available Programs Master's.

Concentrations Available Nursing administration. *Clinical nurse specialist programs in:* adult health, community health, critical care, pediatric, psychiatric/mental health, women's health. *Nurse practitioner programs in:* acute care, adult health, family health, pediatric, primary care.

Study Options Full-time and part-time.

Program Entrance Requirements Clinical experience, minimum overall college GPA of 3.0, transcript of college record, written essay, 2 letters of recommendation, prerequisite course work, resume, statistics course.

Advanced Placement Credit given for nursing courses completed elsewhere dependent upon specific evaluations.

Degree Requirements 9 total credit hours, thesis or project.

POST-MASTER'S PROGRAM

Areas of Study *Nurse practitioner programs in:* acute care.

DOCTORAL DEGREE PROGRAM

Degree PhD

Available Programs Doctorate.

Areas of Study Community health, family health, human health and illness, nursing administration, nursing science, women's health.

Program Entrance Requirements Minimum overall college GPA of 3.3, 2 letters of recommendation, MSN or equivalent, scholarly papers, vita, writing sample.

Degree Requirements Dissertation, oral exam.

POSTDOCTORAL PROGRAM

Postdoctoral Program Contact Graduate Department, Faculty of Nursing, University of Toronto, 50 St. George Street, Toronto, ON M5S 3H4. *Telephone:* 416-978-8069.

The University of Western Ontario
School of Nursing
London, Ontario

Founded in 1878

DEGREES • BSCN • M SC N • PHD

Nursing Program Faculty 76 (5% with doctorates).

Baccalaureate Enrollment 812
Women 96% **Men** 4% **Part-time** 2%

Graduate Enrollment 54
Women 89% **Men** 11% **Part-time** 28%

Nursing Student Activities Nursing Honor Society, Sigma Theta Tau, Student Nurses' Association.

Nursing Student Resources Academic advising; academic or career counseling; assistance for students with disabilities; bookstore; campus computer network; computer lab; computer-assisted instruction; daycare for children of students; e-mail services; employment services for current students; housing assistance; interactive nursing skills videos; Internet; learning resource lab; library services; nursing audiovisuals; resume preparation assistance; unpaid internships.

Library Facilities 3.1 million volumes (357,263 in health, 40 in nursing); 38,517 periodical subscriptions (250 health-care related).

BACCALAUREATE PROGRAMS

Degree BScN

Available Programs Accelerated Baccalaureate; Accelerated Baccalaureate for Second Degree; Generic Baccalaureate; RN Baccalaureate.

Study Options Full-time.

Program Entrance Requirements CPR certification, high school biology, high school chemistry, 4 years high school math, high school science, high school transcript, immunizations, minimum high school rank 80%. Transfer students are accepted. **Standardized tests** *Required for some:* SAT. **Application** *Deadline:* 6/1 (freshmen), 5/15 (out-of-state freshmen), 6/1 (transfer). *Application fee:* CAN$100.

Advanced Placement Credit given for nursing courses completed elsewhere dependent upon specific evaluations.

Expenses (2006–07) *Room and board:* $9016; room only: $5286 per academic year. *Required fees:* full-time $5252; part-time $997 per credit.

Financial Aid 30% of baccalaureate students in nursing programs received some form of financial aid in 2005–06. *Gift aid (need-based):* private, college/university gift aid from institutional funds. *Loans:* . *Work-Study:* part-time campus jobs. *Application deadline:* Continuous.

Contact Ms. Denice Litzan, Academic Counselor, School of Nursing, The University of Western Ontario, London, ON N6A 5C1. *Telephone:* 519-661-2111 Ext. 86564. *Fax:* 519-850-2514. *E-mail:* dlitzan@uwo.ca.

GRADUATE PROGRAMS

Expenses (2006–07) *Tuition:* full-time CAN$7380; part-time CAN$1098 per term. *International tuition:* CAN$18,264 full-time. *Required fees:* part-time CAN$1098 per term.

Financial Aid 25% of graduate students in nursing programs received some form of financial aid in 2005–06. 5 research assistantships (averaging $7,500 per year), 10 teaching assistantships (averaging $8,900 per year) were awarded. *Financial aid application deadline:* 4/1.

Contact Ms. Lori Johnson, Graduate Affairs Assistant, School of Nursing, The University of Western Ontario, Health Sciences Addition, London, ON N6A 5C1. *Telephone:* 519-661-3409. *Fax:* 519-661-3928. *E-mail:* ljohns24@uwo.ca.

MASTER'S DEGREE PROGRAM

Degree M Sc N

Available Programs Master's.

Concentrations Available Health-care administration; nursing administration; nursing education. *Clinical nurse specialist programs in:* acute care, adult health, community health, psychiatric/mental health, public health, women's health. *Nurse practitioner programs in:* community health.

Study Options Full-time and part-time.

The University of Western Ontario (continued)

Program Entrance Requirements Minimum overall college GPA of 3.5, transcript of college record, written essay, interview, 2 letters of recommendation, nursing research course, prerequisite course work, resume, statistics course. *Application deadline:* For fall admission, 2/1. *Application fee:* $50.

Advanced Placement Credit given for nursing courses completed elsewhere dependent upon specific evaluations.

Degree Requirements 7 total credit hours, thesis or project.

DOCTORAL DEGREE PROGRAM

Degree PhD

Available Programs Doctorate.

Areas of Study Addiction/substance abuse, advanced practice nursing, aging, clinical practice, community health, faculty preparation, health policy, health promotion/disease prevention, health-care systems, human health and illness, individualized study, nurse case management, nursing administration, nursing education, nursing research, nursing science, women's health.

Program Entrance Requirements Clinical experience, minimum overall college GPA of 3.5, interview by faculty committee, interview, 2 letters of recommendation, MSN or equivalent, scholarly papers, statistics course, vita, writing sample. *Application deadline:* For fall admission, 2/1. *Application fee:* $50.

Degree Requirements 4 total credit hours, dissertation, written exam.

POSTDOCTORAL PROGRAM

Areas of Study Addiction/substance abuse, community health, health promotion/disease prevention, vulnerable population, women's health.

Postdoctoral Program Contact Dr. Dolly Goldenberg, Chair, Graduate Programs, School of Nursing, The University of Western Ontario, Health Sciences Addition, London, ON N6A 5C1. *Telephone:* 519-661-2111 Ext. 86573. *E-mail:* dgoldenb@uwo.ca.

University of Windsor

School of Nursing
Windsor, Ontario

http://www.uwindsor.ca/nursing

Founded in 1857

DEGREES • BSCN • M SC

Nursing Program Faculty 21 (65% with doctorates).

Baccalaureate Enrollment 584
Women 89% **Men** 11% **Part-time** 10%

Graduate Enrollment 34
Women 97% **Men** 3% **Part-time** 91%

Nursing Student Activities Nursing Honor Society, Student Nurses' Association, nursing club.

Nursing Student Resources Academic advising; academic or career counseling; assistance for students with disabilities; bookstore; campus computer network; computer lab; computer-assisted instruction; daycare for children of students; e-mail services; employment services for current students; externships; housing assistance; interactive nursing skills videos; Internet; learning resource lab; library services; nursing audiovisuals; remedial services; resume preparation assistance; skills, simulation, or other laboratory; tutoring; unpaid internships.

Library Facilities 2.8 million volumes (41,874 in health); 25,458 periodical subscriptions (521 health-care related).

BACCALAUREATE PROGRAMS

Degree BScN

Available Programs Generic Baccalaureate; RN Baccalaureate.
Study Options Full-time and part-time.
Program Entrance Requirements CPR certification, health exam, health insurance, high school biology, high school chemistry, high school math, 4 years high school science, high school transcript, immunizations, minimum high school rank 72%. Transfer students are accepted. **Stan-**

dardized tests *Required for some:* SAT. **Application** *Deadline:* rolling (freshmen), 7/1 (out-of-state freshmen), rolling (transfer). *Notification:* continuous until 8/30 (freshmen). *Application fee:* CAN$60.

Advanced Placement Credit given for nursing courses completed elsewhere dependent upon specific evaluations.

Contact *Telephone:* 519-253-3000 Ext. 2258. *Fax:* 519-973-7084.

GRADUATE PROGRAMS

Contact *Telephone:* 519-253-3000 Ext. 2268. *Fax:* 519-973-7084.

MASTER'S DEGREE PROGRAM

Degree M Sc

Available Programs Master's.
Study Options Full-time and part-time.
Program Entrance Requirements Transcript of college record, written essay, interview, 3 letters of recommendation, nursing research course, physical assessment course, statistics course.

Advanced Placement Credit given for nursing courses completed elsewhere dependent upon specific evaluations.

Degree Requirements 10 total credit hours, thesis or project.

CONTINUING EDUCATION PROGRAM

Contact *Telephone:* 519-253-3000. *Fax:* 519-971-3608.

York University

School of Nursing, Atkinson Faculty of Liberal and Professional Studies
Toronto, Ontario

Founded in 1959

DEGREE • BSCN

Nursing Program Faculty 19 (79% with doctorates).

Baccalaureate Enrollment 850
Women 96% **Men** 4% **Minority** 30% **International** 1% **Part-time** 15%

Nursing Student Resources Academic advising; academic or career counseling; assistance for students with disabilities; bookstore; campus computer network; career placement assistance; computer lab; computer-assisted instruction; daycare for children of students; e-mail services; employment services for current students; housing assistance; interactive nursing skills videos; Internet; learning resource lab; library services; nursing audiovisuals; skills, simulation, or other laboratory; unpaid internships.

Library Facilities 6.1 million volumes; 540,000 periodical subscriptions.

BACCALAUREATE PROGRAMS

Degree BScN

Available Programs Generic Baccalaureate; RN Baccalaureate.
Site Options King City, ON; Barrie, ON; Oshawa, ON.
Study Options Full-time and part-time.
Program Entrance Requirements CPR certification, written essay, health exam, high school biology, high school chemistry, high school math, high school science, high school transcript, immunizations, 1 letter of recommendation, minimum high school GPA, minimum GPA in nursing prerequisites. Transfer students are accepted. **Standardized tests** *Required:* SAT or ACT. **Application** *Deadline:* 2/1 (freshmen), 2/1 (transfer). *Early decision:* 2/1. *Notification:* 6/1 (early action). *Application fee:* CAN$90.

Advanced Placement Credit by examination available. Credit given for nursing courses completed elsewhere dependent upon specific evaluations.

Contact *Telephone:* 416-736-5271 Ext. 66351. *Fax:* 416-736-5714.

CONTINUING EDUCATION PROGRAM

Contact *Telephone:* 416-736-5271. *Fax:* 416-736-5714.

PRINCE EDWARD ISLAND

University of Prince Edward Island
School of Nursing
Charlottetown, Prince Edward Island

Founded in 1834
DEGREE • BSCN

Nursing Program Faculty 10 (2% with doctorates).

Baccalaureate Enrollment 211
Women 97% **Men** 3% **International** 1%

Nursing Student Activities Nursing Honor Society, Student Nurses' Association, nursing club.

Nursing Student Resources Academic advising; academic or career counseling; assistance for students with disabilities; bookstore; campus computer network; career placement assistance; computer lab; computer-assisted instruction; daycare for children of students; e-mail services; employment services for current students; housing assistance; interactive nursing skills videos; Internet; learning resource lab; library services; nursing audiovisuals; placement services for program completers; remedial services; resume preparation assistance; skills, simulation, or other laboratory; tutoring.

Library Facilities 359,403 volumes; 17,232 periodical subscriptions.

BACCALAUREATE PROGRAMS

Degree BScN

Available Programs Generic Baccalaureate.

Study Options Full-time and part-time.

Program Entrance Requirements Transcript of college record, CPR certification, high school chemistry, high school math, high school science, high school transcript, immunizations, minimum high school GPA of 3.0, minimum high school rank 75%, minimum GPA in nursing prerequisites of 3.0, prerequisite course work. Transfer students are accepted. **Application** *Deadline:* 8/1 (freshmen), 8/1 (out-of-state freshmen), 8/1 (transfer). *Notification:* continuous until 8/31 (freshmen), continuous until 8/31 (out-of-state freshmen). *Application fee:* CAN$50.

Advanced Placement Credit given for nursing courses completed elsewhere dependent upon specific evaluations.

Contact *Telephone:* 902-566-0733. *Fax:* 902-566-0777.

QUEBEC

McGill University
School of Nursing
Montréal, Quebec

http://www.nursing.mcgill.ca
Founded in 1821
DEGREES • BSCN • M SC • PHD

Nursing Program Faculty 16 (56% with doctorates).

Baccalaureate Enrollment 193
Women 94% **Men** 6% **Minority** 3% **International** 2% **Part-time** 23%

Graduate Enrollment 96
Women 93% **Men** 7% **International** 2% **Part-time** 5%

Nursing Student Activities Student Nurses' Association.

Nursing Student Resources Academic advising; academic or career counseling; assistance for students with disabilities; bookstore; campus computer network; career placement assistance; computer lab; e-mail services; Internet; learning resource lab; library services; nursing audiovisuals; skills, simulation, or other laboratory; tutoring; unpaid internships.

Library Facilities 4.2 million volumes (250,000 in health); 49,433 periodical subscriptions (1,500 health-care related).

BACCALAUREATE PROGRAMS

Degree BScN

Available Programs Generic Baccalaureate; RN Baccalaureate.
Study Options Full-time.

Program Entrance Requirements Minimum overall college GPA of 3.0, transcript of college record, high school chemistry, 4 years high school math, 4 years high school science, high school transcript, minimum high school GPA of 3.3, minimum high school rank 25%. Transfer students are accepted. **Standardized tests** *Required for some:* SAT and SAT Subject Tests or ACT. **Application** *Deadline:* 1/15 (freshmen), 1/15 (transfer). *Notification:* continuous until 1/15 (freshmen). *Application fee:* CAN$80.

Financial Aid 19% of baccalaureate students in nursing programs received some form of financial aid in 2004–05. *Loans:* FFEL (Subsidized and Unsubsidized Stafford PLUS), college/university, alternative loans. *Application deadline (priority):* 6/1.

Contact Ms. Celine Arseneault, Student Affairs Coordinator, Undergraduate Programs, School of Nursing, McGill University, Wilson Hall Building, Room 203, 3506 University Street, Montreal, QC H3A 2A7. *Telephone:* 514-398-3784. *Fax:* 514-398-8455. *E-mail:* celine.arseneault@mcgill.ca.

GRADUATE PROGRAMS

Financial Aid Institutionally sponsored loans and scholarships available.

Contact Ms. Anna Santandrea, Students Affairs Coordinator, Graduate and Post-Doctoral Studies, School of Nursing, McGill University, 3506 University Street, Montreal, QC H3A 2A7. *Telephone:* 514-398-4151. *Fax:* 514-398-8455. *E-mail:* anna.santandrea@mcgill.ca.

MASTER'S DEGREE PROGRAM

Degree M Sc

Available Programs Master's; Master's for Non-Nursing College Graduates.

Concentrations Available *Clinical nurse specialist programs in:* acute care, adult health, cardiovascular, community health, critical care, family health, gerontology, home health care, maternity-newborn, medical-surgical, oncology, parent-child, pediatric, perinatal, psychiatric/mental health, public health, rehabilitation, women's health. *Nurse practitioner programs in:* neonatal health.

Study Options Full-time.

Program Entrance Requirements Clinical experience, minimum overall college GPA of 3.0, transcript of college record, CPR certification, written essay, immunizations, interview, 3 letters of recommendation, resume, statistics course, GRE General Test. *Application deadline:* For fall admission, 3/1 (priority date). Applications are processed on a rolling basis. *Application fee:* CAN$60.

Degree Requirements 53 total credit hours, thesis or project.

DOCTORAL DEGREE PROGRAM

Degree PhD

Available Programs Doctorate; Post-Baccalaureate Doctorate.

Areas of Study Family health, health-care systems, human health and illness, nursing administration, nursing research, oncology.

Program Entrance Requirements Minimum overall college GPA of 3.3, interview, 2 letters of recommendation, MSN or equivalent, statistics course, vita, writing sample, GRE General Test. *Application deadline:* For fall admission, 3/1 (priority date). Applications are processed on a rolling basis. *Application fee:* CAN$60.

Degree Requirements Dissertation, oral exam, written exam, residency.

POSTDOCTORAL PROGRAM

Areas of Study Cancer care, chronic illness.

Postdoctoral Program Contact Dr. C. Celeste Johnston, Associate Director, Research, School of Nursing, McGill University, 3506 University Street, Montreal, QC H3A 2A7. *Telephone:* 514-398-4157. *Fax:* 514-398-8455. *E-mail:* celeste.johnston@mcgill.ca.

Université de Montréal

Faculty of Nursing
Montréal, Quebec

http://www.scinf.umontreal.ca

Founded in 1920

DEGREES • BSCN • M SC • PHD

Nursing Program Faculty 35 (80% with doctorates).

Nursing Student Activities Student Nurses' Association.

Library Facilities 4 million volumes (32,536 in health, 32,536 in nursing); 18,330 periodical subscriptions (1,319 health-care related).

BACCALAUREATE PROGRAMS

Degree BScN

Study Options Full-time and part-time.

Program Entrance Requirements Transfer students are accepted. **Application** *Deadline:* 3/1 (freshmen), 3/1 (transfer). *Notification:* 5/15 (freshmen). *Application fee:* CAN$50.

Contact *Telephone:* 514-343-6439. *Fax:* 514-343-2306.

GRADUATE PROGRAMS

Contact *Telephone:* 514-343-6111 Ext. 7098. *Fax:* 514-343-2306.

MASTER'S DEGREE PROGRAM

Degree M Sc

Study Options Full-time and part-time.

Program Entrance Requirements Transcript of college record, nursing research course, statistics course. *Application deadline:* For fall and spring admission, 2/1 (priority date); for winter admission, 11/1 (priority date). Applications are processed on a rolling basis. *Application fee:* $30.

Degree Requirements 45 total credit hours.

DOCTORAL DEGREE PROGRAM

Degree PhD

Program Entrance Requirements MSN or equivalent. *Application deadline:* For fall and spring admission, 2/1 (priority date); for winter admission, 11/1 (priority date). Applications are processed on a rolling basis. *Application fee:* $30.

Degree Requirements 90 total credit hours, dissertation.

Université de Sherbrooke

Department of Nursing
Sherbrooke, Quebec

http://www.usherbrooke.ca/scinf/

Founded in 1954

DEGREES • BSCN • M SC • PHD

Nursing Program Faculty 17 (76% with doctorates).

Baccalaureate Enrollment 482
Women 90% **Men** 10% **Minority** .5% **Part-time** 30%

Graduate Enrollment 61
Women 95% **Men** 5% **Part-time** 50%

Nursing Student Activities Student Nurses' Association.

Nursing Student Resources Academic advising; academic or career counseling; assistance for students with disabilities; bookstore; computer lab; computer-assisted instruction; e-mail services; externships; housing assistance; Internet; learning resource lab; library services; nursing audio-visuals; tutoring.

Library Facilities 1.2 million volumes (40,000 in health, 4,000 in nursing); 5,937 periodical subscriptions (3,000 health-care related).

BACCALAUREATE PROGRAMS

Degree BScN

Available Programs RN Baccalaureate.

Site Options Longueuil, QC.

Study Options Full-time and part-time.

Program Entrance Requirements Transcript of college record, high school chemistry, 4 years high school math, immunizations, professional liability insurance/malpractice insurance, RN licensure. Transfer students are accepted. **Application** *Deadline:* 3/1 (freshmen). *Notification:* continuous until 5/15 (freshmen). *Application fee:* CAN$70.

Advanced Placement Credit given for nursing courses completed elsewhere dependent upon specific evaluations.

Expenses (2005–06) *Room and board:* room only: CAN$1800 per academic year.

Financial Aid *Gift aid (need-based):* state, private, college/university gift aid from institutional funds. *Loans:* state, college/university. *Work-Study:* part-time campus jobs. *Application deadline:* 3/31.

Contact Mr. Luc Mathieu, Director, Department of Nursing, Université de Sherbrooke, 3001, 12e Avenue Nord, Sherbrooke, QC J1H 5N4. *Telephone:* 819-563-5355. *Fax:* 819-820-6816. *E-mail:* luc.mathieu@usherbrooke.ca.

GRADUATE PROGRAMS

Expenses (2005–06) *Room and board:* room only: CAN$1800 per academic year.

Contact Dr. Frances Gallagher, Coordinator, Department of Nursing, Université de Sherbrooke, 3001, 12e Avenue Nord, Sherbrooke, QC J1H 5N4. *Telephone:* 819-564-5354. *Fax:* 819-820-6816. *E-mail:* frances.gallagher@usherbrooke.ca.

MASTER'S DEGREE PROGRAM

Degree M Sc

Available Programs Master's.

Concentrations Available *Clinical nurse specialist programs in:* acute care, community health, family health, gerontology.

Site Options Longueuil, QC.

Study Options Full-time and part-time.

Program Entrance Requirements Transcript of college record, interview, 3 letters of recommendation, nursing research course, professional liability insurance/malpractice insurance, resume.

Degree Requirements 45 total credit hours, thesis or project.

DOCTORAL DEGREE PROGRAM

Degree PhD

Available Programs Doctorate.

Areas of Study Advanced practice nursing, aging, biology of health and illness, clinical practice, community health, critical care, family health, gerontology, health promotion/disease prevention, human health and illness, illness and transition, information systems, maternity-newborn, neuro-behavior, nurse case management, nursing administration, nursing education, nursing policy, nursing research, nursing science, oncology, women's health.

Site Options Longueuil, QC.

Program Entrance Requirements Clinical experience, interview, 3 letters of recommendation, MSN or equivalent, statistics course, vita, writing sample.

Degree Requirements 90 total credit hours, dissertation, oral exam, written exam.

POSTDOCTORAL PROGRAM

Postdoctoral Program Contact Dr. Luc Mathieu, Director, Department of Nursing, Université de Sherbrooke, 3001, 12e Avenue Nord, School of Nursing, Sherbrooke, QC J1H 5N4. *Telephone:* 819-564-5355. *Fax:* 819-820-6816. *E-mail:* luc.mathieu@usherbrooke.ca.

Université du Québec à Chicoutimi

Program in Nursing
Chicoutimi, Quebec

Founded in 1969

DEGREES • BNSC • MSN

Nursing Program Faculty 8 (25% with doctorates).

Baccalaureate Enrollment 600
Women 90% **Men** 10% **Minority** 5% **Part-time** 75%

Graduate Enrollment 30
Women 90% **Men** 10% **Minority** 1% **Part-time** 100%

Nursing Student Activities Student Nurses' Association.

Nursing Student Resources Academic advising; academic or career counseling; assistance for students with disabilities; bookstore; campus computer network; computer lab; computer-assisted instruction; e-mail services; employment services for current students; externships; housing assistance; interactive nursing skills videos; Internet; learning resource lab; library services; nursing audiovisuals; resume preparation assistance; skills, simulation, or other laboratory; tutoring; unpaid internships.

Library Facilities 689,214 volumes; 5,092 periodical subscriptions.

BACCALAUREATE PROGRAMS

Degree BNSc

Available Programs Accelerated RN Baccalaureate; RN Baccalaureate.

Site Options Alma, PQ. *Distance Learning:* Sept-Iles, PQ; St. Felicien, PQ.

Study Options Full-time and part-time.

Program Entrance Requirements Health exam, high school chemistry, immunizations, interview. Transfer students are accepted. **Application** *Deadline:* 3/1 (freshmen). *Notification:* 5/15 (freshmen).

Advanced Placement Credit given for nursing courses completed elsewhere dependent upon specific evaluations.

Financial Aid *Gift aid (need-based):* private, college/university gift aid from institutional funds. *Loans:* college/university. *Work-Study:* part-time campus jobs.

Contact Mme. Anna Gauthier, Secretere, Program in Nursing, Université du Québec à Chicoutimi, 555 Boulevard de l'Universite, Chicoutimi, QC G7H 2B1. *Telephone:* 418-545-5011 Ext. 5315. *Fax:* 418-545-5012. *E-mail:* anna_gauthier@uqac.ca.

GRADUATE PROGRAMS

Financial Aid 2% of graduate students in nursing programs received some form of financial aid in 2004–05.

Contact Francoise Courville, Director of Master's Degree Program, Program in Nursing, Université du Québec à Chicoutimi, 555 Boulevard de l'Université, Chicoutimi, QC G7H 2B1. *Telephone:* 418-545-5011 Ext. 2374. *Fax:* 418-545-5012. *E-mail:* francoise_courville@uqac.ca.

MASTER'S DEGREE PROGRAM

Degree MSN

Available Programs Accelerated RN to Master's; RN to Master's.

Concentrations Available *Clinical nurse specialist programs in:* acute care, adult health, cardiovascular, community health, critical care, family health, gerontology, home health care, maternity-newborn, medical-surgical, occupational health, oncology, parent-child, pediatric, perinatal, psychiatric/mental health, public health, rehabilitation, school health, women's health.

Site Options Alma, PQ. *Distance Learning:* St. Felicien, PQ.

Study Options Part-time.

Program Entrance Requirements Clinical experience, minimum overall college GPA of 3.0, transcript of college record, written essay, interview, 3 letters of recommendation, nursing research course, professional liability insurance/malpractice insurance, statistics course.

Advanced Placement Credit given for nursing courses completed elsewhere dependent upon specific evaluations.

Degree Requirements 45 total credit hours, thesis or project.

Université du Québec à Rimouski
Program in Nursing
Rimouski, Quebec

http://www.uquebec.ca/mscinf/

Founded in 1973

DEGREES • BSCN • M SC N

Nursing Program Faculty 8 (38% with doctorates).

Baccalaureate Enrollment 750
Women 90% **Men** 10% **Part-time** 74%

Graduate Enrollment 13
Women 93% **Men** 7% **Part-time** 100%

Nursing Student Activities Student Nurses' Association.

Nursing Student Resources Academic advising; academic or career counseling; assistance for students with disabilities; bookstore; campus computer network; career placement assistance; computer lab; daycare for children of students; e-mail services; employment services for current students; housing assistance; Internet; learning resource lab; library services; nursing audiovisuals; other; placement services for program completers; resume preparation assistance; skills, simulation, or other laboratory; tutoring.

Library Facilities 263,142 volumes (5,200 in health, 1,100 in nursing); 3,951 periodical subscriptions (1,300 health-care related).

BACCALAUREATE PROGRAMS

Degree BScN

Available Programs RN Baccalaureate.

Site Options Levis, QC.

Study Options Full-time and part-time.

Program Entrance Requirements Transcript of college record, professional liability insurance/malpractice insurance, prerequisite course work. Transfer students are accepted. **Application** *Deadline:* 3/1 (freshmen). *Notification:* 5/15 (freshmen).

Advanced Placement Credit by examination available.

Contact *Telephone:* 418-723-1986 Ext. 1730. *Fax:* 418-724-1849.

GRADUATE PROGRAMS

Contact *Telephone:* 418-723-1986 Ext. 1874. *Fax:* 418-724-1849.

MASTER'S DEGREE PROGRAM

Degree M Sc N

Available Programs Master's.

Concentrations Available *Clinical nurse specialist programs in:* community health, critical care, gerontology, psychiatric/mental health.

Study Options Full-time and part-time.

Program Entrance Requirements Clinical experience, transcript of college record, interview, 3 letters of recommendation, nursing research course, prerequisite course work, statistics course.

Advanced Placement Credit given for nursing courses completed elsewhere dependent upon specific evaluations.

Degree Requirements 45 total credit hours, thesis or project.

CONTINUING EDUCATION PROGRAM

Contact *Telephone:* 418-723-1986 Ext. 1818. *Fax:* 418-724-1525.

Université du Québec à Trois-Rivières
Program in Nursing
Trois-Rivières, Quebec

Founded in 1969

DEGREES • BSN • MSN

Library Facilities 464,338 volumes.

BACCALAUREATE PROGRAMS

Degree BSN

Program Entrance Requirements Transfer students are accepted. **Application** *Deadline:* 3/1 (freshmen). *Notification:* 6/1 (freshmen). *Application fee:* CAN$30.

Contact *Telephone:* 819-376-5011 Ext. 3471. *Fax:* 819-376-5218.

Université du Québec à Trois-Rivières (continued)

GRADUATE PROGRAMS

Contact *Telephone:* 819-376-5011 Ext. 3464.

MASTER'S DEGREE PROGRAM

Degree MSN

Université du Québec en Abitibi-Témiscamingue
Département des sciences sociales et de la santé
Rouyn-Noranda, Quebec

http://www.uqat.uquebec.ca/gestac/prg/7855.asp

Founded in 1983

DEGREE • BN

Nursing Program Faculty 12.

Baccalaureate Enrollment 78
Women 95% **Men** 5% **Part-time** 64%

Nursing Student Resources Academic advising; assistance for students with disabilities; bookstore; campus computer network; computer lab; computer-assisted instruction; housing assistance; Internet; library services; resume preparation assistance; skills, simulation, or other laboratory.

Library Facilities 135,882 volumes (3,239 in health, 715 in nursing); 302 periodical subscriptions (17 health-care related).

BACCALAUREATE PROGRAMS

Degree BN

Program Entrance Requirements Transfer students are accepted. **Application** *Deadline:* rolling (freshmen). *Notification:* 5/15 (freshmen). *Application fee:* CAN$30.

Contact *Telephone:* 819-762-0971 Ext. 2370. *Fax:* 819-797-4727.

Université du Québec en Outaouais
Département des Sciences Infirmières
Gatineau, Quebec

Founded in 1981

DEGREES • BSCN • M SC N

Nursing Program Faculty 10 (60% with doctorates).

Baccalaureate Enrollment 450
Women 90% **Men** 10% **Minority** 20% **International** 1% **Part-time** 90%

Graduate Enrollment 30
Women 97% **Men** 3% **Minority** 3% **Part-time** 97%

Nursing Student Activities Student Nurses' Association.

Nursing Student Resources Academic advising; academic or career counseling; bookstore; campus computer network; computer lab; daycare for children of students; e-mail services; employment services for current students; externships; housing assistance; Internet; learning resource lab; library services; nursing audiovisuals; placement services for program completers; skills, simulation, or other laboratory.

Library Facilities 230,910 volumes; 12,351 periodical subscriptions.

BACCALAUREATE PROGRAMS

Degree BScN

Available Programs ADN to Baccalaureate; Generic Baccalaureate; RN Baccalaureate.
Site Options St-Jerome, PQ; Laval, PQ; Mont-Laurier, PQ.
Study Options Full-time.

Program Entrance Requirements CPR certification, high school chemistry, immunizations, interview, RN licensure. Transfer students are accepted. **Application** *Deadline:* 3/1 (freshmen), 3/1 (out-of-state freshmen). *Notification:* 5/15 (freshmen). *Application fee:* CAN$30.
Advanced Placement Credit by examination available. Credit given for nursing courses completed elsewhere dependent upon specific evaluations.

Contact *Telephone:* 819-595-3900 Ext. 2345. *Fax:* 819-595-3801.

GRADUATE PROGRAMS

Contact *Telephone:* 819-595-3900 Ext. 2344. *Fax:* 819-595-3801.

MASTER'S DEGREE PROGRAM

Degree M Sc N

Available Programs Master's.
Concentrations Available *Clinical nurse specialist programs in:* community health, critical care, psychiatric/mental health, rehabilitation.
Study Options Full-time and part-time.
Program Entrance Requirements Computer literacy, 3 letters of recommendation, nursing research course, resume, statistics course.
Advanced Placement Credit given for nursing courses completed elsewhere dependent upon specific evaluations.
Degree Requirements 45 total credit hours, thesis or project.

Université Laval
Faculty of Nursing
Québec, Quebec

http://www.fsi.ulaval.ca

Founded in 1852

DEGREES • BSCN • MSN • PHD

Nursing Program Faculty 25 (64% with doctorates).
Library Facilities 3 million volumes (118,994 in health, 3,781 in nursing); 13,928 periodical subscriptions (624 health-care related).

BACCALAUREATE PROGRAMS

Degree BScN

Program Entrance Requirements Transfer students are accepted. **Application** *Deadline:* 3/1 (freshmen), 3/1 (out-of-state freshmen), 5/1 (transfer). *Notification:* 5/15 (freshmen). *Application fee:* CAN$30.
Contact *Telephone:* 418-656-2131 Ext. 3388. *Fax:* 418-656-7747.

GRADUATE PROGRAMS

Contact *Telephone:* 418-656-3356. *Fax:* 418-656-7304.

MASTER'S DEGREE PROGRAM

Degree MSN

Concentrations Available *Nurse practitioner programs in:* community health.
Program Entrance Requirements Clinical experience, 3 letters of recommendation, nursing research course, resume, statistics course, French exam. *Application deadline:* For fall admission, 2/1 (priority date); for winter admission, 11/1 (priority date); for spring admission, 4/1 (priority date). Applications are processed on a rolling basis. *Application fee:* $30.
Degree Requirements 48 total credit hours.

DOCTORAL DEGREE PROGRAM

Degree PhD

Areas of Study Community health.

CONTINUING EDUCATION PROGRAM

Contact *Telephone:* 418-656-2131 Ext. 2633. *Fax:* 418-656-7747.

SASKATCHEWAN

University of Saskatchewan
College of Nursing
Saskatoon, Saskatchewan

http://www.usask.ca/nursing/
Founded in 1907
DEGREES • BSN • MN

Nursing Program Faculty 130 (20% with doctorates).

Baccalaureate Enrollment 1,200
Women 93% **Men** 7% **Minority** 5% **Part-time** 17%

Graduate Enrollment 50
Women 94% **Men** 6% **Minority** 2% **Part-time** 62%

Nursing Student Activities Student Nurses' Association.

Nursing Student Resources Academic advising; academic or career counseling; assistance for students with disabilities; bookstore; campus computer network; computer lab; computer-assisted instruction; daycare for children of students; e-mail services; employment services for current students; interactive nursing skills videos; Internet; learning resource lab; library services; nursing audiovisuals; other; remedial services; resume preparation assistance; skills, simulation, or other laboratory; tutoring.

Library Facilities 1.8 million volumes (120,000 in health, 7,000 in nursing); 16,900 periodical subscriptions (1,000 health-care related).

BACCALAUREATE PROGRAMS

Degree BSN

Available Programs Accelerated Baccalaureate; Accelerated RN Baccalaureate; Baccalaureate for Second Degree; Generic Baccalaureate; RN Baccalaureate; RPN to Baccalaureate.

Site Options Regina, SK; Prince Albert, SK. *Distance Learning:* Saskatoon, SK.

Study Options Full-time and part-time.

Program Entrance Requirements Transcript of college record, high school biology, high school chemistry, 4 years high school math, 4 years high school science, high school transcript, minimum high school GPA of 2.0. Transfer students are accepted. **Application** *Deadline:* 5/1 (freshmen), 5/1 (transfer). *Notification:* continuous (freshmen). *Application fee:* CAN$75.

Advanced Placement Credit given for nursing courses completed elsewhere dependent upon specific evaluations.

Financial Aid 80% of baccalaureate students in nursing programs received some form of financial aid in 2005–06. *Gift aid (need-based):* private, college/university gift aid from institutional funds. *Loans:* FFEL (Subsidized and Unsubsidized Stafford PLUS), college/university, Canadian Student Loans, Provincial Loans. *Application deadline:* 3/15 (priority: 2/15).

Contact Ms. Shelley Bueckert, Admissions and Records Secretary, College of Nursing, University of Saskatchewan, 107 Wiggins Road, Saskatoon, SK S7N 5E5. *Telephone:* 306-966-6231. *Fax:* 306-966-6621. *E-mail:* shelley.bueckert@usask.ca.

GRADUATE PROGRAMS

Expenses (2006–07) *Tuition, state resident:* full-time CAN$3000; part-time CAN$500 per unit. *Tuition, nonresident:* full-time CAN$3000; part-time CAN$500 per unit. *International tuition:* CAN$3000 full-time. *Required fees:* full-time CAN$420; part-time CAN$95 per credit.

Financial Aid 30% of graduate students in nursing programs received some form of financial aid in 2005–06. Fellowships, research assistantships, teaching assistantships available. *Financial aid application deadline:* 1/31.

Contact Dr. Lynnette Stamler, Chairperson, Graduate Program, College of Nursing, University of Saskatchewan, 107 Wiggins Road, Saskatoon, SK S7N 5E5. *Telephone:* 306-966-1477. *Fax:* 306-966-6703. *E-mail:* lynnette.stamler@usask.ca.

MASTER'S DEGREE PROGRAM

Degree MN

Available Programs Master's.

Concentrations Available Nursing education. *Nurse practitioner programs in:* primary care.

Site Options *Distance Learning:* Saskatoon, SK.

Study Options Full-time and part-time.

Program Entrance Requirements Minimum overall college GPA of 2.5, transcript of college record, 3 letters of recommendation, nursing research course, statistics course. *Application deadline:* For fall admission, 7/1 (priority date). Applications are processed on a rolling basis. *Application fee:* $50.

Advanced Placement Credit given for nursing courses completed elsewhere dependent upon specific evaluations.

Degree Requirements 24 total credit hours, thesis or project.

DOCTORAL DEGREE PROGRAM

Site Options *Distance Learning:* Saskatoon, SK.

CONTINUING EDUCATION PROGRAM

Contact Ms. Kyla Avis, Coordinator, College of Nursing, University of Saskatchewan, Continuing Nursing Education, Box 60000, RPO, Saskatoon, SK S7N 4J8. *Telephone:* 306-966-6261. *Fax:* 306-966-7673. *E-mail:* kyla.avis@usask.ca.

CLOSE-UPS OF NURSING PROGRAMS

Baker University
School of Nursing
Baldwin City, Kansas

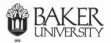

THE UNIVERSITY

Baker University was established in 1858 as the first four-year college in the state of Kansas. With 147 years of tradition, Baker embodies an unusual blend of innovation, tradition, quality, and community. Affiliated with the United Methodist Church, the University is dedicated to excellence in liberal and professional education, to the integration of learning with faith and values, and to the personal development of each community member.

The University attracts the serious student who expects to encounter challenge in the classroom but also enjoys participating in a multitude of extracurricular activities—sports, forensics, radio, the newspaper, theater, music, and departmental and special interest organizations.

THE SCHOOL OF NURSING

The Baker University School of Nursing was established in the Pozez Education Center at Stormont-Vail Health*Care* in Topeka, Kansas, to provide much-needed nursing education for the students in Baker's service region. The School of Nursing offers an academic program leading to a baccalaureate degree. The generic baccalaureate degree program in nursing comprises four full-time semesters of upper-division study after completion of general education requirements. A baccalaureate degree completion program for registered nurses is composed of one year of full-time study or part-time study over several semesters. Students may enter the nursing program during the fall or spring semester.

The mission of Baker University School of Nursing is to prepare nurses for professional practice as providers of general health care for individuals, families, and communities within the global environment. As an institution related to the United Methodist Church, the School embodies the belief that the integration of faith and values into the curriculum promotes the intellectual growth and personal development of each individual. The nurse will have the ability to communicate; think critically; perform clinical skills competently; participate in lifelong education; assume the roles of care provider, manager, and member of a profession; and make ethical decisions based on a sound value system and broad knowledge base.

While course demands are rigorous, the goals of nursing education at Baker are accomplished in a climate of collaboration and cooperation among faculty members and students—a hallmark of the Baker experience. Classes are small and friendly. The teacher-student ratio is approximately 1:9. Baker takes a holistic approach to nursing, teaching the art and science of nursing to those who want to make a critical difference in a profession that is more important today than ever before.

Baker University is accredited by the Higher Learning Commission of the North Central Association of Colleges and Schools and the Kansas State Board of Education. The School of Nursing program is accredited by the Commission on Collegiate Nursing Education and approved by the Kansas State Board of Nursing.

PROGRAMS OF STUDY

Baker University offers two degree tracks in nursing education. Both lead to a Bachelor of Science in Nursing (B.S.N.) degree. One program is for students who have not practiced in the nursing profession. They have attended college for two years either at Baker's College of Arts and Sciences in Baldwin City or elsewhere and are accepted for their final two years of study into Baker's School of Nursing.

The other program is for registered nurses who wish to complete a baccalaureate degree in nursing. This program offers courses at convenient times and addresses topics in a way that is most meaningful to nurses in practice.

ACADEMIC FACILITIES

The Pozez Education Center at Stormont-Vail Health*Care* in Topeka, Kansas, provides both administrative offices and excellent educational facilities for the School of Nursing. Large modern classrooms, fully equipped clinical laboratories, and individual study areas provide functional and appealing space. A computer lab is accessible to students for both word processing and interactive tutorial programs in nursing. The Stauffer Health Science Library, located on the ground level of the Pozez Education Center, provides a strong learning resource for both students and faculty members.

LOCATION

The main campus of Baker University and home of the College of Arts and Sciences is in Baldwin City, Kansas, a beautiful small community of tree-lined streets and rich tradition that is about 40 miles southwest of Kansas City and 40 miles southeast of Topeka. The historic campus is only a few blocks south of the old Santa Fe Trail, now followed by U.S. Highway 56. It is easily accessible from north or south by U.S. 59 and from east or west by U.S. 56.

The School of Nursing is located in the Pozez Education Center of Stormont-Vail Health*Care* in Topeka. This modern facility provides administrative offices, classrooms, laboratories, and a library.

STUDENT SERVICES

Baker University offers many services to meet individual student needs. These include orientation, career counseling and placement, personal counseling, tutoring, and other academic support services. Academic support resources available to students in the School of Nursing include academic advising, tutoring, counseling, orientation, and testing. In addition, nursing students are encouraged to use, at no cost, the Mabee Health and Fitness Center.

Each student is assigned a faculty adviser upon entering the nursing program. The adviser provides the student with assistance in academic program planning and matters pertaining to academic work and can also provide assistance with study habits and personal adjustment problems.

THE NURSING STUDENT GROUP

There are approximately 142 students enrolled in the under-graduate nursing program. Approximately 90 percent are women and 8 percent are members of minority groups. Virtually all graduates find employment within three months of graduation, and most secure jobs while they are still in school.

COSTS

Tuition for the 2006–07 academic year for full-time students (12–18 credit hours) at Baker University School of Nursing was $11,400 per year. Part-time students paid $380 per credit hour. The cost for fees and books was approximately $600 per semester for full-time students. Uniforms, supplies, and a background check are additional expenses for first-semester students. There are also specific costs associated with graduation for fourth-semester students.

FINANCIAL AID

Baker University is committed to helping students and parents find resources to finance their university experience. Approximately 95 percent of Baker's undergraduate students receive some form of financial assistance. Financial need is met through a combination of scholarships, grants, and loans. By completing the Free Application for Federal Student Aid (FAFSA), a student is considered for all federal, state, and institutional funds administered by Baker.

APPLYING

Students may be admitted to the nursing program after two years of study in Baker's College of Arts and Sciences or after successful completion of program requirements at other universities.

The Student Affairs Committee selects students from applicants who best meet requirements. All program prerequisites must be completed with a grade of C or higher, with an overall prerequisite cumulative GPA of at least 2.7. Each individual is considered for admission based on the following factors: academic history, prerequisite cumulative GPA, math and science prerequisite GPA, number of prerequisite courses completed, other degrees conferred, and interview with faculty. Applicants who do not meet all School of Nursing admission requirements may be reviewed for further consideration by the Student Affairs Committee upon request by the applicant.

For further information about applying to the College of Arts and Sciences, applicants should refer to *Peterson's Guide to Four-Year Colleges,* or applicants should go online to http://www.bakeru.edu/index.php.

The School of Nursing admits students in both the fall and spring semesters. Baker College of Arts and Sciences students receive priority admission to the nursing school. Interested applicants should Janet Creager, Student Affairs Specialist, 785-354-5850 or 888-866-4242 (toll-free).

CORRESPONDENCE AND INFORMATION:

Baker University
School of Nursing
Stormont-Vail Health*Care* Campus
1500 Southwest 10th Street
Topeka, Kansas 66604-1351
Phone: 785-354-5850
      800-866-4242 (toll-free)

Janet Creager
Student Affairs Specialist
School of Nursing
Phone: 785-354-5850
      888-866-4242 (toll-free)
E-mail: janet.creager@bakeru.edu

Daniel McKinney
Director of Admissions
Phone: 785-594-8458
      800-873-4282 (toll-free)
E-mail: daniel.mckinney@bakeru.edu

Jeanne Mott
Director of Financial Aid
Phone: 785-594-4595
      800-873-4282 (toll-free)
E-mail: jeanne.mott@bakeru.edu

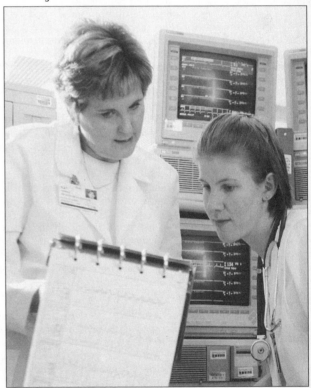

After learning basic skills during the beginning five weeks of the first semester in the nursing program, students begin clinical experiences in a variety of settings.

Blessing-Rieman College of Nursing

Quincy, Illinois

THE COLLEGE

Blessing-Rieman College of Nursing (B-RCN) prides itself on personal attention tailored to each student's needs and the high-quality nursing education it has offered for more than 100 years. Blessing Hospital School of Nursing, one of the first nursing schools in the state of Illinois, was founded in 1891 to train nurses for area health-care needs. Today, it is a small private college offering a Bachelor of Science in Nursing (B.S.N.) degree conferred jointly with a partner college, either Culver-Stockton College in Canton, Missouri, or Quincy University in Quincy, Illinois. This flexibility offers students many options not available from other programs while providing a high-quality college education and excellent nursing education at a regional medical center.

Culver-Stockton College (C-SC) is an independent, private college with a scenic campus overlooking the Mississippi River in Canton, Missouri. The College offers music, theater, intercollegiate and intramural sports, student government, residence and dining halls, numerous clubs and organizations, and Greek life. Quincy University (QU) is an independent private institution rooted in the Catholic tradition. Cultural, social, and recreational opportunities include intercollegiate sports, a new fitness center with an indoor pool, fine arts, student government, radio and TV studios, and housing options.

Blessing-Rieman is accredited by the National League for Nursing Accrediting Commission (NLNAC), the Commission on Collegiate Nursing Education, and the Higher Learning Commission (HLC) of the North Central Association of Colleges and Schools (NCACS). Students participate in the Student Nurse Organization and can act as representatives on College committees. The College offers apartments for upper-level students, a state-of-the-art child-care facility, a fitness center, and meal discounts at the hospital cafeteria.

To learn more about a career in nursing, the College offers Nursing in Action, a half-day program designed to show students the advantages and opportunities of a versatile career in nursing. Nurse Shadow visits are also offered, which involves following a staff nurse in the hospital during a normal morning or afternoon. To receive more information on these programs or to schedule a campus tour, students should contact the Admissions Office.

PROGRAM OF STUDY

Nursing courses are designed to help students acquire the knowledge, skills, and values needed to become professional nurses fully equipped to handle today's practice. Graduates are also prepared for leadership positions or further education in specialty fields. The joint Bachelor of Science in Nursing degree program for new college students is typically four years of study. Students are nursing majors all four years, and nursing classes begin in the freshman year. All freshman classes are provided on the partner campus, and students are required to live on campus. During the sophomore year, students come together for nursing classes on the Blessing-Rieman campus but continue to live on the partner campus. Nursing clinical experiences begin in the sophomore year at Blessing Hospital and other area health-care agencies. In the junior and senior years, students have usually completed most general education courses on the partner campus and may choose to live on the Blessing campus while focusing more on nursing courses and clinicals. Junior-level nursing instruction includes medical-surgical, psychiatric, obstetrical, and pediatric course work and clinicals. Senior nursing courses include community health, acute-care nursing, professionalism, leadership, and research. Blessing-Rieman has separate tracks for LPNs and RNs and an Advanced Placement track for those who already have a degree and wish to complete their B.S.N. degree.

The joint-degree program with Culver-Stockton requires 124 semester hours, including English, speech, physical education, and religion core courses; computer science, fine arts, social science, and humanities general education courses; natural science, mathematics, psychology, and philosophy support courses; and 61 hours of nursing courses.

The joint-degree program with Quincy University requires 126 semester hours, including English, social sciences, humanities, fine arts, theology, and physical education general education courses; computer science and statistics tool courses; natural science and speech support courses; and 61 hours of nursing courses.

AFFILIATIONS WITH HEALTH-CARE FACILITIES

Blessing-Rieman is located on the campus of Blessing Hospital, a fully accredited major medical facility serving the surrounding 100-mile radius. Blessing Hospital has state-of-the-art cancer and heart centers. Students have direct access to clinical areas of the hospital, with College instructors and hospital staff members providing guidance. Nearby clinics, health departments, nursing homes, and other health agencies offer additional clinical experiences.

ACADEMIC FACILITIES

Blessing-Rieman has computer-networked, air-conditioned classrooms and offices. A student lounge and locker room are adjacent to the classrooms. The Blessing Health Professions Library provides an extensive collection of books, journals, and audiovisual teaching materials as well as study areas and a computer lab open to students that provides software, Internet access, online research databases, and other resources. Students on the C-SC and QU campuses also have access to computers and libraries equipped with extensive resources.

Hands-on training in the College Skills Lab is provided prior to clinical experience. After demonstration by the Lab Coordinator, students use actual clinical equipment in a simulated hospital setting to practice nursing skills and clinical decision making. Skills Lab practice allows students to approach actual clinical experiences with confidence.

LOCATION

Blessing-Rieman College of Nursing is located in Quincy, Illinois, a city of around 45,000 people, on the bluff overlooking the Mississippi River in west-central Illinois. The city is known for its history, architecture, arts, and quality of life. The Adams County seat, Quincy has an Amtrak station, regional airport, TV and radio stations, convention center, numerous hotels and restaurants, shopping malls, theaters, and a symphony orchestra, and it is the site of fairs, festivals, and cultural events.

STUDENT SERVICES

One of the greatest benefits of the joint programs in nursing is that throughout their four-year concurrent enrollment, students enjoy all of the services and activities of Blessing-Rieman and the partnering institution as well as those of Blessing Hospital, whose state-of-the-art child-care center and fitness center are available for students.

THE NURSING STUDENT GROUP

Most students receive some form of financial aid. Many students choose to hold part-time jobs, including some who work in the College as Student Assistants. Enrollment is approximately 250 students. Five to 10 percent of the students are men, and about 5 percent are members of minority groups. Of the graduates who seek employment, 100 percent have a position before graduation.

COSTS

According to the College's partnership agreements, tuition and fees for the first two years are set by the partner institutions, and the last two years are set by B-RCN. Approximate tuition for the Culver-Stockton program is $14,250, and the Quincy University program is about $17,800. B-RCN tuition is $9115 for the junior and senior years. Students should check with the Admissions Office for current rates.

FINANCIAL AID

Significant scholarships and financial aid (federal, local, state, and private) are available at each institution, whether need-based and/or for academic achievement. Students should contact the admissions office for further information.

APPLYING

Qualifications for acceptance as a nursing major include a minimum 3.0 high school GPA, graduation in the upper half of the class, and a composite ACT score of at least 22 or an SAT combined score of at least 920. High school courses must include 4 units of English; at least 2 units of science, including biology and chemistry; 3 units of social science; and 2 units of math, including 1 unit of algebra. Nontraditional students should contact the admissions office for requirements.

CORRESPONDENCE AND INFORMATION:

Blessing-Rieman College of Nursing
Broadway at 11th
Quincy, Illinois 62305-7005
Phone: 217-228-5520
       800-877-9140 Ext. 6949 (toll-free)
E-mail: admissions@brcn.edu
Web site: http://www.brcn.edu

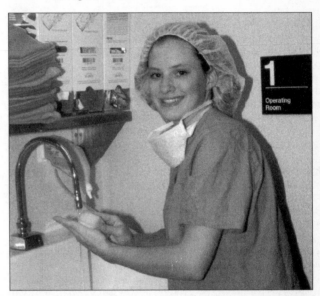

Nursing clinical experiences take place at Blessing Hospital and at other area health-care agencies.

Boston College
William F. Connell School of Nursing
Chestnut Hill, Massachusetts

THE COLLEGE
Boston College is a coeducational university with more than 9,000 undergraduate students and 4,700 graduate students who represent every state and more than ninety-nine countries. Founded in 1863, it is one of the oldest Jesuit-affiliated universities in the country and one of the largest private universities in the nation.

The reputation of the university, securely established after more than a century of proven excellence, continues to gain stature. In recent years, surveys undertaken by periodicals such as *Barron's* and *U.S. News & World Report* have consistently ranked Boston College among the top colleges and universities in the nation and as one of the best values in higher education.

THE SCHOOL OF NURSING
Founded in 1947, the Boston College William F. Connell School of Nursing is one of the largest Jesuit schools of nursing. The baccalaureate and master's programs are accredited by the Commission on Collegiate Nursing Education. Currently, the School of Nursing offers baccalaureate, master's, master's entry (for students with an undergraduate degree in a field other than nursing), RN-to-M.S., M.S./M.B.A., M.S./M.A., Ph.D., and continuing education programs. Graduates of the programs are highly successful in clinical, academic, administrative, and research careers in nursing. They are widely respected and sought after for regional, national, and international positions.

The School of Nursing has 47 full-time faculty members teaching and advising in both the undergraduate and graduate programs. They are highly qualified, clinically and academically, and many are certified for advanced clinical practice. More than 90 percent of the tenured and tenure-track faculty members hold an earned doctorate in nursing or in related fields and are actively engaged in research. The faculty is widely published and includes nursing scholars who are recognized as experts and leaders in their fields both nationally and internationally.

PROGRAMS OF STUDY
The baccalaureate program is a full-time, four-year program of study. The thirty-eight-course curriculum that is required for graduation consists of university core requirements; electives; nursing courses, which include simulated and audiovisual laboratory activities on campus; and clinical learning activities in a vast variety of health-care settings. The curriculum is designed to develop students' diagnostic, therapeutic, and ethical reasoning in nursing practice. The graduate is prepared as a generalist able to care for individuals and groups at each developmental level and in various health-care settings. Options are available for baccalaureate students to begin master's-level courses during their undergraduate nursing program.

Undergraduate nursing students may enroll for one semester during their junior or senior year in any number of study-abroad programs sponsored by Boston College or by other U.S. colleges and universities.

The main objective of the master's program is to prepare nurses for advanced practice roles, including clinical nurse specialist, nurse anesthetist, and nurse practitioner. There are nine areas of specialization: adult health, community health, family health, gerontological health, pediatric health, nurse anesthesia, palliative care, and psychiatric-mental health. An Additional Specialty Certificate is available for those with an M.S. in nursing who desire expertise in an additional specialty area. Two dual-degree programs are offered: M.S. in nursing/ M.B.A. and M.S. in nursing/M.A. in pastoral ministry. In addition, individuals with a non-nursing baccalaureate may apply to the M.S. Entry into Nursing Program. The focus in the specialty areas is on human responses to actual or potential health problems. The approach to clients is multifaceted and includes the development of advanced competencies in clinical judgment. Numerous community agencies in and around Boston are used for the clinical practicum of the program. Full-time students can complete the program in one to two years, and part-time students may take up to five years.

The Ph.D. program in nursing was the first doctoral program in nursing to be offered at a Jesuit university. Each student is mentored by a faculty member with expertise in the student's area of interest. Core areas of doctoral study are concepts of nursing science, methods of theory development, and qualitative and quantitative research methods needed to extend nursing knowledge. The full-time plan allows the student to take 10 credits of course work per semester for the first two years of study before entering the dissertation phase of the program. The part-time plan allows the student to take 6 to 7 credits of course work per semester for the first three years of study before entering the dissertation phase of the program. Various learning opportunities are available through interdisciplinary colloquia at the university and health-care agencies and clinical research practica with faculty mentors.

ACADEMIC FACILITIES
A member of the Association of Research Libraries, Boston College's libraries offer a wealth of resources and services to support faculty and student research activities. The book collection consists of more than 2 million volumes, and the nursing holdings have been characterized by nursing leaders as one of the finest collections in the world. A special reference librarian serves as a liaison for all School of Nursing needs. Other nursing resource facilities include the Kennedy Resource Center, the Nursing Simulation Laboratory, and a computer lab, all housed within the School of Nursing. The university also offers a wide range of services, such as technical support, audiovisual and computing facilities, and academic and research centers.

LOCATION
Boston College is located in a beautiful suburban setting just minutes from downtown Boston. Boston is a city that offers an outstanding combination of history, culture, and vitality, and it is home to a number of the world's most renowned health-care institutions. Students and faculty members enjoy the unique advantages of metropolitan Boston in addition to the beauty and tranquility of the suburban campus. The scenic grounds and stately Gothic architecture of the 200-acre campus provide an atmosphere conducive to both study and socializing.

STUDENT SERVICES
Health, counseling, and career planning services are available to all graduate and undergraduate students, including programs for African-American, Hispanic, Asian, and Native American students as well as for international students. A wide variety of recreational and cultural facilities and on- and off-campus housing options are available to students.

THE NURSING STUDENT GROUP

Students at Boston College reflect a diversity of interests and backgrounds. The student body is drawn from every race, religion, and economic background as well as from every state in the Union and numerous countries. Currently, the School of Nursing has approximately 330 undergraduate students, 140 master's students, and 45 doctoral students. The students' ages range from 18 to 50, and many are employed and/or married with children.

COSTS

For 2006–07, undergraduate tuition was $33,000. Freshman room rates were $6620, board was approximately $4100, and health, recreation, and activity fees averaged $875. Books, supplies, and personal expenses were estimated at $1650.

For 2006–07, graduate tuition was $922 per credit hour. Charges for books, fees, supplies, housing, and transportation are additional.

FINANCIAL AID

Boston College offers a variety of scholarships, grants, loans, and employment to assist students in financing their education. The majority of undergraduate students receive some form of financial aid. Financial aid awards are made by the Financial Aid Office to freshmen and transfer students on the basis of academic promise and demonstrated financial need. Notice of such awards made to incoming freshmen and transfer students usually accompanies notification of the students' acceptance by the university. Opportunities include work-study and job referral positions and undergraduate research fellowships.

Graduate students may apply for financial assistance from both the university Financial Aid Office and the School of Nursing. Opportunities include federal traineeships, tuition remission scholarships, university fellowships, and teaching and research assistantships. The university also has competitive minority fellowships for doctoral students.

APPLYING

For the undergraduate program, the type of college-preparatory program viewed as the best foundation for college work usually includes at least 4 units of English, a foreign language, math, social science, and a laboratory science. Students applying to the School of Nursing are required to complete at least 1 unit of chemistry. All applicants must complete the SAT and two Subject Tests of the applicant's choice. In place of the SAT, applicants may take the ACT, including the writing exam. Qualifying Advanced Placement scores or successful completion of college courses prior to freshman enrollment may help students to place out of core requirements.

Students applying to the undergraduate program are required to submit the Common Application, the Boston College Supplemental Application for Admission, and the nonrefundable application fee of $70 by January 2. It is the candidate's responsibility to ensure that all credentials are sent to and received by the Office of Undergraduate Admissions. Candidates are notified of action taken on their applications between April 1 and 15. Candidates accepted for admission are required to forward an acceptance fee by May 1.

Applicants to the master's program should submit GRE scores, three references, and a personal goal statement. A minimum GPA of 3.0, a transcript from an accredited baccalaureate nursing program, and previous course work in statistics are required. Application deadlines are as follows: for full-time and part-time study for May or September admission, March 15; and for January admission, October 15. November 1 is the deadline for applicants with non-nursing baccalaureate or higher degrees to apply to the Master's Entry into Nursing Program. Applications to the nurse anesthesia program are due September 15 for January enrollment.

Applicants to the doctoral program should submit GRE scores; three references; a career goals statement; evidence of scholarship, including a writing sample; a curriculum vitae; transcripts from an accredited M.S. program in nursing; and previous course work in statistics. An interview is required. The deadline is January 31 of the year of admission. The application fee for each graduate program is $40 and is nonrefundable. International students must also provide TOEFL scores.

CORRESPONDENCE AND INFORMATION

For the undergraduate program:
Director of Undergraduate Admissions
Boston College
Devlin Hall, Room 208
Chestnut Hill, Massachusetts 02467-3812
Phone: 617-552-3100

Associate Dean, Undergraduate Program
William F. Connell School of Nursing
Boston College
Chestnut Hill, Massachusetts 02467-3812
Phone: 617-552-4925

For the graduate programs:
Associate Dean, Graduate Programs
William F. Connell School of Nursing
Boston College
Chestnut Hill, Massachusetts 02467-3812
Phone: 617-552-4928
Web site: http://bc.edu/nursing

The College of New Rochelle
School of Nursing
New Rochelle, New York

THE COLLEGE

One of the oldest in Westchester County, The College of New Rochelle was founded in 1904 by Mother Irene Gill, OSU, as the first Catholic college for women in New York State. The College, now independent, established the Graduate School in 1969, the School of New Resources (for adult learners) in 1972, and the School of Nursing in 1976. The School of Arts and Sciences (the seminal unit) continues the tradition of enrolling only women; the other three schools admit both women and men. The College of New Rochelle is chartered by the New York State Board of Regents and is accredited by the Middle States Association of Colleges and Schools.

There are nineteen major buildings, including Leland Castle, a National Historic Site and the first home of the College; the 180,000-volume Mother Irene Gill Library, currently undergoing a multimillion dollar renovation; a chapel; four large residence halls; a Student Service Center; two science buildings; and the Mooney Center, formerly known as the College Center.

Although there have been fundamental changes in the expression of the College's Mission since the late 1960s, The College of New Rochelle has remained faithful to its mission and has responded flexibly to the higher learning needs of the community it serves. From this tradition, the College derives its dedication to the education of women and men in the liberal arts and in professional studies. Building on its original commitment to women, the College also reaches out to those who have not previously had access to higher education. It places particular emphasis on the concept of lifelong learning.

The College is committed to a respect and concern for each individual. It seeks to challenge students to achieve the full development of their individual talents and a greater understanding of themselves. It encourages the examination of values through the creative and responsible use of reason. The College strives to articulate its academic tradition and religious heritage in ways that are consonant with the best contemporary understandings of both. It provides opportunities for spiritual growth in a context of freedom and ecumenism.

Finally, with justice as its guiding principle, the College tries to respond to the needs of society through its education programs and service activities and through fostering the concept of education for service.

THE SCHOOL OF NURSING

In May 1975, the Board of Trustees of The College of New Rochelle approved a proposal to establish a School of Nursing. The curriculum, leading to a Bachelor of Science in Nursing degree, was approved by the New York State Education Department in spring 1976. In fall 1976, the first freshmen were admitted to the program, and in 1980, the first class graduated.

PROGRAMS OF STUDY

The School of Nursing offers undergraduate programs that are open to women and men: an undergraduate program leading to a Bachelor of Science in Nursing (B.S.N.); two programs, an RN-B.S.N. and an RN-M.S., are offered to registered nurses; and a Second Degree B.S.N. Program is offered for persons holding degrees in other fields. Second degree students are those students who hold undergraduate degrees from four-year colleges or universities in an area of study other than nursing. Five semesters of clinical nursing courses are required after completing all prerequisite courses. Students may begin studies in the fall, spring, or summer semesters and may include prerequisite courses in their individualized plan of study. Opportunities for acceleration in the program are also available.

In 1983, a Master's Program in Nursing was established in the School of Nursing, funded for a three-year period by a half-million-dollar federal grant from the Division of Nursing of the Department of Health and Human Services. The Master of Science degree program offered by the School of Nursing is designed to prepare graduates for the roles of advanced-practice nursing (clinical nurse specialist in holistic nursing, family nurse practitioner, nurse educator, and nursing and health-care management). Post-master's certificate programs are offered for all advanced-practice tracks. The programs are designed to accommodate the needs of part-time or full-time students, with theoretical courses offered in the late afternoon or evenings.

The philosophy of the Master's Program is grounded in a holistic framework that recognizes caring/healing as the foundation for preparing a nurse professional at an advanced level of practice. Consistent wit the philosophy of The College of New Rochelle, the Master's Program in Nursing provides small classes and individualized advisement and program planning.

ACADEMIC FACILITIES

The Learning Center for Nursing (LCN) is a multiresource facility for the School. It is composed of five specialized areas. The Nursing Laboratory is designed for the teaching and reinforcement of basic and advanced nursing skills development. Simulating a hospital setting, client-care units are equipped with variable-height beds, overbed tables, bedside cabinets, and medication areas. Each unit has wall-mounted otoscopes, ophthalmoscopes, and blood pressure cuffs. In addition, to facilitate learning in the primary care clinical practice settings, there are client areas equipped with examination tables. There are several mannequins, models, and simulators that facilitate learning and allow for realistic practice of a wide array of skills. Registered nurses serve as preceptors to students for individualized instruction and mentoring. There is also a computer interactive video system that supports students' skill development.

The Media Laboratory offers a variety of audiovisual resources for self-guided study. Audiovisual equipment includes color television/VCR centers and slide projectors for a media library containing more than 470 videotapes and more than fifty-five slide sets. This area is also equipped with viewing carrels and a 25-inch color television/VCR for group or classroom use.

The Computer Center is the third area where students learn, practice, and apply a variety of computer skills. This area contains multimedia personal computers, IBM or IBM-compatible personal computers, printers, and interactive video systems. The College of New Rochelle School of Nursing has served as a Fuld Institute for Technology in Nursing Education (FITNE) Interactive Demonstration Center for computer-interactive video system technology. A CD-ROM version of the Cumulative Index to Nursing and Allied Health Literature (CINAHL), an easy-to-search index, provides coverage of articles included in more than 550 nursing journals and primary publications. A variety of software is available, including RNCAT (a computerized adaptive testing program simulating NCLEX-

RN), computer-assistive instruction software, and popular business applications (word processing, database management, spreadsheet, and graphics).

The fourth area is the Group Instruction Room, which is designed to facilitate independent and small-group study and support research activity. It houses a small library of current textbooks on clinical skills and issues, including a section referenced by the computer-based health-care consulting system.

The Electronic Classroom is equipped with personal computers for both students and faculty members. State-of-the-art computers, printers, a projection boxlight, and scanner are housed here. The goal of the Electronic Classroom is to facilitate group learning through technology using Internet and instructional software.

LOCATION
The School of Nursing is located on the principal campus of The College of New Rochelle, which is situated on 20 beautiful acres in the southeastern corner of Westchester County, New York, 1 mile west of Long Island Sound and 16 miles north of mid-Manhattan. It is easily accessible by commuter trains and school-sponsored buses. The area contains numerous parks and recreational areas; the Long Island Sound, with its many beaches, is within walking distance; and New York City is a half hour away.

STUDENT SERVICES
The Mentor Connection Program provides professional and leadership development opportunities for undergraduate and graduate students. Mentors consist of alumni, faculty members, administrators, peers, and professional nurses. The mentor-protégé relationship is a developmental process that empowers and nurtures the participants over time. Mutual growth, learning, and sharing occur in an atmosphere of affirmation, collegiality, respect, and support.

THE NURSING STUDENT GROUP
There are 657 students in the programs of the School of Nursing. Of those, 112 are in the graduate program, 211 are in the RN-B.S.N. Completion Program, 241 are in the basic undergraduate program, and 93 are in the second degree program. Ninety-five percent of the students are women, and 60 percent are part-time.

COSTS
Tuition and other changes are set at the minimum for financially responsible operations and are below actual costs. Gifts and grants received through the generosity of alumni, friends, corporations, and foundations play a significant part in reducing this difference. Undergraduate tuition for full-time students (12–16 credits) is $10,730. Part-time charges are $722 per credit. Nonmatriculated students also pay $722 per credit. The charge to audit a course is one half the usual tuition per credit hour.

Students enrolled in the RN-B.S.N. Second Degree Programs are billed at the per-credit rates listed above.

Graduate tuition is $650 per credit as of the 2007–08 academic year.

FINANCIAL AID
The Financial Aid Program of The College of New Rochelle fulfills several objectives. The College firmly believes that by providing financial assistance to needy and deserving students of diverse economic and social backgrounds and by rewarding academic achievement, it may best promote and maintain the educational goals that are central to the mission of the institution. The ability to furnish a financial aid package to students who might otherwise be unable to obtain a high-quality education clearly benefits and enriches the College community.

The Office of Financial Aid is dedicated to the service of students. The financial aid staff is trained to provide individual and group counseling to students about their financial responsibilities and available aid programs.

APPLYING
Admission to the B.S.N. program is open to high school graduates, transfer students from two- or four-year colleges or universities, registered nurses who are graduates of diploma or associate degree programs, and college graduates with non-nursing degrees. To be considered for admission, applicants must have taken 16 academic units in secondary school that include three science courses, including a laboratory chemistry and a laboratory biology, and three courses in mathematics (algebra I and II and geometry). A written statement of the candidate's academic and personal qualities should be prepared by the principal or guidance counselor and submitted with the transcript. Applicants are encouraged to submit other information in support of their credentials. SAT or ACT scores are also required. There is a $20 nonrefundable application fee. In cases of economic hardship, a fee waiver may be requested. Admission requirements for the RN-B.S.N. option include current professional registered nurse licensure and an employer recommendation.

Residents of New York State who do not qualify for regular admission and who come from low-income backgrounds may be considered for the College's Community Leadership Program.

Admission to the graduate program is selective. Criteria for admission include graduation from an accredited baccalaureate nursing program or a nursing program deemed comparable by the World Education Services with a minimum GPA of 3.0; an application, including an essay describing goals for graduate study in nursing; a resume; a personal interview (distance permitting); two letters of recommendation, preferably from a nursing administrator and a faculty member; completion of a basic statistics course (course may be taken concurrently with graduate study); current malpractice insurance; current New York State RN licensure; completion of health requirements; completion of a physical assessment course for clinical majors; one year of clinical experience for the family nurse practitioner track and holistic clinical nurse specialist track; and a nonrefundable $30 application fee. Applicants who do not meet the 3.0 GPA requirement for admission may submit a written request to the Graduate Nursing Admissions Committee for a review of their application portfolio.

CORRESPONDENCE AND INFORMATION:
The College of New Rochelle
29 Castle Place
New Rochelle, New York 10805-2339

Phone: 914-654-5436
E-mail: mdonius@cnr.edu
Web site: http://www.cnr.edu

Columbia College of Nursing
Mount Mary College
Nursing Program
Milwaukee, Wisconsin

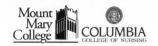

THE COLLEGES

In 1901, Columbia College of Nursing (CCON) began as part of the Knowlton Hospital and Training School. In 1909, the Columbia Hospital Corporation took over Knowlton Hospital and changed the name to the Columbia Hospital School of Nursing. In 1919, both hospital and school moved to their current location on Milwaukee's east side. In 1956, an addition to the original 1919 building was completed, and it serves, in part, as the present-day Columbia College of Nursing building. By 1983, college-based nursing course work was replacing diploma nursing education. CCON joined with a liberal arts college in order to confer an intercollegiate degree. In 2002, CCON and Mount Mary College entered into a partnership to confer the Bachelor of Science in Nursing degree.

Mount Mary College, an urban Catholic college for women sponsored by the School Sisters of Notre Dame, is located on the northwest side of Milwaukee. Mount Mary's roots are deep in the history of Wisconsin. St. Mary's Institute was founded in Prairie du Chien in 1872. In 1913, it extended its educational program to the postsecondary level and was chartered as St. Mary's College, a four-year Catholic college for women, the first in the state to grant degrees. Its academic standards were accepted by the North Central Association of Colleges in 1926. The institution changed its name to Mount Mary College when it moved to its present location in 1929.

The Mount Mary College campus is home to freshman and sophomore nursing students as well as other Mount Mary students. The student residence, Caroline Hall, provides sports and recreational facilities, a student lounge, and the Marian Art Gallery. Notre Dame Hall is the location of administrative offices, classrooms, laboratories, art and music studios, the Walter and Olive Stiemke Memorial Hall and Conference Center, Macintosh computer laboratories, and two chapels. The Gerhardinger Center opened in 2004, providing state-of-the-art science and nursing laboratories, an electronic lecture hall, a cyber café, and student study areas. Dining facilities, the bookstore, the post office, and the Advising and Career Development Center are found in Bergstrom Hall. In fall 2006, the new Bloechl Recreation Center opened; it houses a full-size collegiate gym, practice courts, locker rooms, fitness center, and dance/yoga classroom.

Minutes away, on Milwaukee's east side, the Columbia College of Nursing campus is home to junior and senior nursing students. In addition to comprehensive, state-of-the-art academic facilities, the campus includes the Columbia Residence Hall, the Campus Center, bookstore, fitness center, laundry room, kitchenette, and recreational facilities.

THE INTERCOLLEGIATE NURSING PROGRAM

In summer 2002, Mount Mary College and the Columbia College of Nursing established a joint Bachelor of Science in Nursing (B.S.N.) degree program. The combination of Columbia's history of excellence with Mount Mary's highly respected liberal arts education offers a program of high-quality preparation for a career in nursing. Within the liberal arts framework, students integrate the most up-to-date nursing instruction with challenging clinical placements. The nursing program is approved by the Wisconsin State Board of Nursing and is accredited by the National League for Nursing Accrediting Commission. Mount Mary College is approved by the State of Wisconsin to confer degrees and by the

Wisconsin State Department of Public Instruction for teachers' certificates. Both colleges are fully accredited by the Higher Learning Commission.

PROGRAMS OF STUDY

Columbia College of Nursing and Mount Mary College offer a unique intercollegiate program leading to a Bachelor of Science in Nursing degree. A completion program leading to a Bachelor of Science in Nursing degree is also available for students who are registered nurses and have an associate degree or diploma in nursing.

AFFILIATIONS WITH HEALTH-CARE FACILITIES

Affiliations between Columbia College of Nursing and Southeastern Wisconsin community clinical sites further guarantee that students, while experiencing the latest advances in nursing education, also remain on the cutting edge of today's changing health-care environment.

ACADEMIC FACILITIES

On the Mount Mary campus, the Patrick and Beatrice Haggerty Library collection includes more than 110,000 volumes and 500 subscription periodical titles, along with a significant collection of audiovisual materials. Several offices are located in the lower level of Haggerty Library, including the Teacher Education Center, the Academic Resource Center, the Development Office, and Computer Services, which includes three computer labs. Mount Mary College recently constructed the Gerhardinger Center. This $7-million, 33,000-square-foot, three-story science, technology, and campus center is a state-of-the-art facility that includes science, nursing, and occupational therapy labs; classrooms; a cyber café; meeting rooms; a theater/conference area; and student social areas.

The Columbia College of Nursing campus houses newly renovated classrooms with state-of-the-art projection technology and Internet access. The College's Ellen A. Bacon Library hosts a collection of 9,200 professional books, journals, and bound volumes. The Helene Fuld Learning Resource Center affords students 24-hour access to computers, printers, and scanners.

LOCATION

Columbia College of Nursing, located on Milwaukee's east side, is surrounded by residential neighborhoods near Lake Michigan and the University of Wisconsin–Milwaukee. The College is served by most of the city's major bus routes and is near a diverse assortment of shops, restaurants, and entertainment and recreational facilities.

Located on 80 acres on Milwaukee's northwest side, Mount Mary provides a park-like campus featuring stately stone buildings, gorgeous green lawns, and beautiful wooded areas in a residential area of Milwaukee.

STUDENT SERVICES

To broaden their cultural awareness, Columbia College of Nursing and Mount Mary encourage their students to take advantage of a variety of study-abroad opportunities. Accordingly, Mount Mary College sponsors trips to Rome, Peru, Guatemala, England, Ireland, Nicaragua, France, and China. In addition to these study-abroad programs, the College maintains affiliate relationships with numerous international colleges and universities, including the American College, Dublin, Ireland; the American Intercontinental University, London and Dubai; Nanzan College, Japan; Universidad Católica de Santa Maria (UCSM), Arequipa, Peru; and

Notre Dame College, Kyoto, Japan. Mount Mary is a part of a consortium directed by the Wisconsin Association of Independent Colleges and Universities that enables member institutions to share study-abroad opportunities.

Mount Mary College sponsors many social activities, including performances by musicians and comedians, dances, and picnics. These events are sponsored by the Mount Mary Programming and Activities Council (MMPAC), Student Government, Residence Hall Association, and other groups on campus. Other events include films, concerts, and lectures. Through participation in clubs/organizations, students have opportunities to develop leadership skills, collaborate with other clubs/organizations, network, and explore areas of interest. Special and professional interests are served by affiliates of national societies. Physical fitness and an interest in athletics are fostered through various activities, fitness programs, health and dance courses, and intramural and intercollegiate athletics. Mount Mary College is a provisional member of NCAA Division III. The Blue Angels compete in basketball, soccer, softball, tennis, and volleyball.

Academic and professional student services are available to all students. Services include tutoring and assistance with tests through the Academic Resource Center; advising, resume writing, and career planning through the Advising and Career Development Center; and personal counseling through the Counseling Center.

COSTS
For the 2006–07 academic year, full-time undergraduate tuition was $17,938 per year, and $485 per credit for part-time undergraduates. There was a $1000 per year nursing program fee for full-time undergraduates, and, for part-time undergraduates, the nursing fee was $50 per credit. Various other fees also apply. Room and board costs averaged $5990.

FINANCIAL AID
The Financial Aid Office at Mount Mary College develops a financial package on an individual basis for each qualified student. More than 90 percent of full-time Columbia/Mount Mary students receive some form of financial assistance. Students filing for financial aid should complete the Free Application for Federal Student Aid (FAFSA). Additional information on numerous merit-based scholarships, grants, and work-study opportunities is available for incoming first-year as well as transfer students. Students should contact the Admission Office for more information.

APPLYING
Candidates for admission are considered on the basis of academic preparation, scholarship, and evidence of the ability to do college work and benefit from it. Fifteen secondary school units are required for students entering directly from high school into the nursing program. The 15 units must consist of 2 in biology; 2 in chemistry; 2 in algebra; 3 in English; 4 in history, language, or social science; and 2 electives. Each applicant is reviewed individually. International students must take the Test of English as a Foreign Language (TOEFL). Early acceptance is available at Mount Mary College and advanced placement is honored. Mount Mary has a rolling admission policy. An admission decision is sent as soon as all required materials have been received and reviewed by the Admission Office. After notification of acceptance, students wishing to enroll need to submit the $200 tuition deposit. Student make application for acceptance by Columbia College of Nursing to the nursing major upon completion of required college course work and demonstration of the required college grade point average. Neither Columbia College of Nursing nor Mount Mary discriminate against any individual for reasons of race, color, religion, age, disability, or national or ethnic origin. The nursing program is open to both men and women.

CORRESPONDENCE AND INFORMATION
Admission Office
Mount Mary College
2900 North Menomonee River Parkway
Milwaukee, Wisconsin 53222-4597

Phone: 414-256-1219
    800-321-6265 (toll-free)
Web site: http://www.mtmary.edu

Columbia College of Nursing
2121 East Newport
Milwaukee, Wisconsin 53211
Web site: http://www.ccon.edu

THE FACULTY OF COLUMBIA COLLEGE OF NURSING, INC.
Ann Aschenbrenner, Assistant Professor; M.S.N., Marquette, 2001. Adult nurse practitioner.

Virginia Bastian, Clinical Assistant Professor; M.S., Wisconsin–Milwaukee, 1996; Nurse Practitioner. Child and adolescent health.

Renee Bender. Assistant Professor; M.S.N., Marian, 2005. Nursing education.

Nancy Boehm. Instructor; B.S.N., Wisconsin–Madison. Adult health nursing.

Susan Cole, Assistant Professor; M.S, Marquette, 1991. Medical surgical nursing.

Ann Cook, Professor; Ph.D., Wisconsin–Milwaukee, 1995. Community and medical-surgical nursing.

Katherine Dimmock, Professor and Dean; Ed.D., Northern Illinois, 1985; J.D., Indiana–Purdue at Indianapolis, 1998; M.S.N., Indiana University, 1980.

Hope Fox, Assistant Professor; M.S.N., Vanderbilt, 2000; M.B.A., Wisconsin-Milwaukee, 2004; Acute Care Nurse Practitioner. Nephrology.

Dorothy Hagemeier, Assistant Professor; M.S.N., Marquette, 1974. Medical-surgical nursing.

Mark Hirschmann, Professor; Ph.D., Purdue, 1986. Psychiatric and mental health nursing, community nursing.

Debra Johnson, Associate Professor; M.S.N., Wisconsin–Madison, 1977. Pediatrics.

Annika Joy, Assistant Professor; M.S., Minnesota, 2004. Medical and surgical nursing.

Judy Kopka, Assistant Professor; M.S.N., Cardinal Stritch, 2002. Health promotion and mental health.

Tammy Kasprovich, Clinical Instructor; B.S.N., Carroll College; M.S.N. candidate, Cardinal Stritch. Emergency medicine.

Sandra Pasch, Assistant Professor; M.S., Rochester, 1981; M.A., Medical College of Wisconsin, 1999. Psychiatric and mental health nursing; bioethics.

Mary Ross, Clinical Assistant Professor; M.S., Ohio State, 1992; Medical-surgical nursing.

Shawneen Schmitt, Clinical Assistant Professor; M.S.N. candidate, Phoenix. Parish nurse and certified wound, ostomy, and continence nurse specialist.

Kimberly Schuster, Clinical Assistant Professor; M.S.N., Northern Illinois, 1985. Medical-surgical nursing, oncology.

Gladys Simandl, Professor; Ph.D., Wisconsin–Milwaukee, 1990. Community nursing.

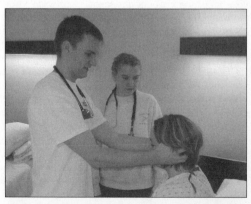

Clinical experiences are an integral part of the Columbia College of Nursing/Mount Mary College nursing program.

Columbia University
School of Nursing
New York, New York

THE UNIVERSITY

By royal charter of King George III of England, Columbia University was founded in 1754 as King's College. It is the oldest institution of higher learning in New York State and the fifth oldest in the nation. A private, nonsectarian institution, Columbia University has, since its inception, addressed the issues of the moment, making important contributions to American life through teaching and research. It is organized into fifteen schools and is associated with more than seventy research and public service institutions and twenty-two scholarly journals. One of its most notable affiliations is with the research-oriented New York–Presbyterian Medical Center. The New York–Presbyterian Hospital, together with the Health Science Division of Columbia University, which includes the Schools of Medicine, Dental and Oral Surgery, Nursing, and Public Health and programs in physical therapy, nutrition, and occupational therapy, constitute the Columbia University Medical Center. Total enrollment is close to 2,500 at the Health Science Campus and nearly 17,500 at the Morningside Campus.

THE SCHOOL OF NURSING

Founded in 1892 as the Presbyterian Hospital School of Nursing, the School first offered the baccalaureate degree when it joined Columbia University. In 1956, it became the first nursing program in the country to award a master's degree in a clinical nursing specialty. Today, the primary focus of the School is to educate advanced practice nurses: nurse practitioners, nurse midwives, and nurse anesthetists. This is done through the academic program at the graduate and advanced certificate levels. The School also offers two doctoral programs. The Doctor of Nursing Science (D.N.Sc.) is a research-intensive program that prepares nurse scholars to independently conduct research in outcomes and health policy. The Doctor of Nursing Practice (Dr.N.P.) prepares nurse clinicians with the knowledge and skills necessary for fully accountable practice with patients across sites and over time.

The curriculum is focused on preparing professional nurses who think critically, exercise technical competence, and make socially significant contributions to society through theory-based practice. The faculty members endeavor to provide knowledge, to stimulate learning, to define issues, and to serve as resource persons, clinicians, administrators, leaders, and innovators in nursing. A major strength of the School is that the faculty members maintain clinical practices in their advanced roles and incorporate students into these settings. One of these practices, Columbia Advanced Practice Nurse Associates (CAPNA), has gained national exposure as an innovative model of primary-care delivery by advanced practice nurses who are on the primary provider panels of several major managed-care organizations.

In addition to these programs, the School contains four academic centers: the Center for AIDS Research, the Center for Health Policy and Health Services Research, the Center for Evidence-Based Practice, and the World Health Organization Collaborating Center for International Nursing Development in Advanced Practice. Columbia was the first nursing school to be awarded this designation, which makes the School an active participant in international exchange and collaborative research in advanced practice and health services research. It also facilitates the development of international study opportunities for its students.

PROGRAMS OF STUDY

The School of Nursing offers four levels of educational programs. The Entry to Practice (ETP) Program is an accelerated combined-degree program (B.S./M.S.) for non-nurse baccalaureate-prepared graduates, designed to prepare the student for a career as an advanced practice nurse. Academic studies are closely integrated with clinical experience. The prelicensure phase of the program consists of 60 credits, which are completed through full-time study. Upon completion, the student is eligible to take the professional nurse licensure examination in any state. In the specialty phase (postlicensure), the student follows the curriculum for a clinical specialty, which is described later in this section. Part-time study is available during the specialty phase.

The Graduate Program, leading to the M.S. degree, affords baccalaureate-prepared nurses the opportunity to increase their knowledge in advanced nursing practice. The School currently offers eleven graduate majors that include anesthesia, acute-care, neonatal, psychiatric–mental health nursing, midwifery, oncology, the primary-care specialties (adult, family, geriatric, and pediatric), and women's health. The credit requirements range from 45 to 59 and are allocated among core, major, and elective courses. Cross-site curricula are available in selected programs. Joint degrees are available with the Schools of Public Health and Business Administration.

The Advanced Certificate Program allows RNs with a master's degree in nursing to pursue an advanced practice program as a nurse practitioner. The credit requirements range from 23 to 36 credits.

The Doctor of Nursing Science Program is designed to prepare clinical nurse scholars to examine, shape, and refine the health-care delivery system. The program consists of 90 credits beyond the baccalaureate degree. Of these, 45 credits are credits earned at the master's level in a clinical specialist/nurse practitioner program.

The Doctor of Nursing Practice Program prepares nurses with the knowledge, skills, and attributes necessary for fully accountable practice with patients across sites and over time. The Dr.N.P. is the natural evolution and needed expansion of existing clinical degrees in nursing, the basic B.S. and the site-specific M.S. Currently, it is a 40-credit program designed for post-master's nurse practitioners.

AFFILIATIONS WITH HEALTH-CARE FACILITIES

The center of clinical activity at Columbia University Medical Center is the New York Presbyterian Medical Center, which includes a number of world-renowned facilities. Among the most notable are the Neurological Institute, the Eye Institute, Children's Hospital of New York, Sloane Hospital for Women, the Center for Geriatrics and Gerontology, the Organ Transplant Center, and the Center for Health Promotion and Disease Prevention. In addition, approximately 150 other sites in the tristate area are available for clinical education.

ACADEMIC FACILITIES

The Augustus C. Long Library is the fourth-largest academic medical library in the country and is part of the Columbia

University Library system, which encompasses approximately forty libraries and more than 4 million volumes. The Long Library houses more than 400,000 volumes and receives more than 4,500 journals, most of which can be accessed through online computer search programs. The Media and Computer Center contains more than 3,000 audiovisual and computer-assisted instruction programs, including slides, videodiscs, tapes, and a wide variety of personal computer applications. Other services include microfilming, interlibrary loans, study and conference facilities, and photocopying services. The Special Collections Section houses several thousand rare works including the Florence Nightingale Collection, which is featured at exhibitions along with rare holdings of Freud and Webster.

The School of Nursing building houses two Technology Learning Centers (TLC). The TLCs include a mock hospital unit containing several patient units and an ambulatory-care area for practicing primary-care skills; it is used by graduate and undergraduate students for skills development, including physical assessment and state-of-the-art monitoring technology. There are also two informatics laboratories available to School of Nursing students.

LOCATION

The School of Nursing is part of the Columbia University Medical Center, a 20-acre campus overlooking the Hudson River on Manhattan's Upper West Side. Students can avail themselves of the recreational, cultural, and educational events and entertainment that have made New York City famous.

STUDENT SERVICES

The Office of Student Administrative Services is the hub of all student projects, programs, and services, and it coordinates activities with many other departments. Among the organizations and services provided are housing, dining, health, athletic facilities, a Wellness Program, counseling and advisement, parking, shuttle bus, financial aid, a bookstore, orientation, student records, the Office of Multicultural Affairs, Disability Services, and the International Student Office.

THE NURSING STUDENT GROUP

About 600 students are enrolled each year in the School of Nursing, and they represent a diverse group of nursing professionals. They come from all over the country, but most are from the tristate area.

COSTS

During the 2006–07 academic year, tuition for undergraduates was $991 per credit. For graduate students, tuition ranged from $991 to $1258 per credit. Average housing costs at the Medical Center ranged from $4000 to $6000. Other expenses, including health fees, books, personal expenses, transportation, and uniforms, were estimated at $5000.

FINANCIAL AID

The goal of the School of Nursing financial aid program is to provide as many students as possible with sufficient resources to meet their needs and to distribute funds to eligible students in a fair and equitable manner. Financial aid is met through a combination of scholarships, grants, work, and loans. Students should be able to meet all expenses for the academic year through a combination of these resources.

APPLYING

Columbia University School of Nursing has two semesters: one begins in September (fall semester) and the other in May (summer semester). The School has rolling admissions for most master's specialties. All clinical sequences begin in the fall semester.

Admission is based on past academic and professional performance. Admission requirements include an application form with a fee; a typed, double-spaced, one-page personal statement describing professional goals and aspirations; three competed recommendation forms; official transcripts from all postsecondary schools; official GRE scores; a copy of an RN license and current registration; and an undergraduate course in statistics and in physical assessment.

CORRESPONDENCE AND INFORMATION

Columbia University School of Nursing
Office of Admissions
630 West 168th Street Box 6
New York, New York 10032

Phone: 800-899-8895
Fax: 212-305-3680
E-mail: nursing@columbia.edu
Web site: http://www.nursing.hs.columbia.edu

Dominican University of California
School of Arts and Sciences
San Rafael, California

THE UNIVERSITY

Dominican University of California is a coeducational, independent, liberal arts university of Dominican heritage offering more than thirty bachelor's and master's degrees. Dominican has a commitment to interdisciplinary study in the humanities, a global perspective, and the involvement of students in their own intellectual, spiritual, ethical, and social development. The University was founded in 1890 by the Dominican Sisters of San Rafael. It was the first Catholic college in the state of California to offer the baccalaureate degree to women. Today, Dominican derives no direct financial support from the church or the state.

THE SCHOOL

The School of Arts and Sciences strives to support the idea that nursing is a dynamic and interpersonal process based on the premise of individual worth and human dignity and to teach that the goal of nursing is to help individuals, families, and groups achieve and maintain self-care in coping with actual and potential health problems. Nursing is a human service provided when clients' self-care capabilities are inadequate to promote, maintain, and restore health. The Department of Nursing faculty members bring deep understanding and rich backgrounds of both clinical and teaching experience to the program. All full-time faculty members have master's degrees, and the majority have doctorates or are currently engaged in doctoral work.

PROGRAMS OF STUDY

Dominican University offers a Bachelor of Science in Nursing (B.S.N.) for women and men wishing to enter the field of professional nursing. Students complete one and a half years of prerequisite courses before beginning the clinical nursing major in the sophomore year. Clinical experiences in the sophomore, junior, and senior years take place at a variety of Bay Area hospitals. Throughout the four-year program, lecture classes are held on the Dominican campus. Upon satisfactory completion of the nursing curriculum, students are granted the Bachelor of Science in Nursing degree, are eligible to take the State Board Examination for licensure as a registered nurse (RN), and can obtain a California Public Health Nursing Certificate. Advanced placement is available for transfer students from other nursing programs, registered nurses, and licensed vocational nurses who wish to obtain a bachelor's degree in nursing. A 30-unit option is also available for licensed vocational nurses. Dominican also offers two Master of Science in Nursing (M.S.N.) programs that prepare nurses for advanced practice as clinical nurse specialists in integrated health practices or geriatrics and nurse education. The nursing program is accredited by the California Board of Registered Nursing and the National League for Nursing Accrediting Commission.

AFFILIATIONS WITH HEALTH-CARE FACILITIES

The Department of Nursing is affiliated with a number of health-care agencies and institutions in the Bay Area, offering students clinical learning opportunities with diverse populations in a wide variety of settings. Agencies include Marin General Hospital; Marin County Health Department; St. Francis Medical Center, San Francisco; and Kaiser Permanente in San Rafael, among others.

ACADEMIC FACILITIES

The Archbishop Alemany Library houses more than 100,000 volumes in open stacks, 3,200 reels of microfilm, 775 videocassettes, 225 audiocassettes and CDs, subscriptions to more than 370 periodicals in print, and another 19,000 periodical titles in full-text online. About 4,000 online journals are health and nursing related, with more than 100 print periodicals related to nursing and occupational therapy. Reference services, including access to a variety of computerized database and indexes, and multimedia facilities are provided to assist students with their studies and assignments. Nursing students have access to CINAHL, MEDLINE, ProQuest Nursing Journals, PsycINFO, and other online health-related information resources. The library also houses the campus computer center.

The E. L. Wiegand Nursing Laboratory offers students the opportunity to acquire nursing skills in a simulated clinical setting on campus. Computer-assisted instruction and a number of other audiovisual programs are available for student use in this lab.

In fall 2006 a new nursing simulation lab opened after a generous grant from the Texas-based RGK Foundation. The state-of-the-art lab will provide Dominican nursing students with clinical experiences in a risk-free virtual-reality environment. This simulation lab, with two programmable mannequins, will put Dominican in the forefront of nursing education today by providing students with the real-world clinical experience they need to transition quickly into the role of an independently functioning caregiver. The lab also will be available to community health practitioners.

LOCATION

The University is located on 80 wooded acres in a peaceful residential neighborhood in San Rafael, just 15 minutes north of San Francisco and less than a half hour's drive from Pacific Ocean beaches. Students at the University enjoy the intimacy of a small university while benefiting from easy access to the resources of Marin County and the broader San Francisco Bay Area. Marin offers hills for hiking, redwood forests, and ocean shoreline for walking, and, in general, an unsurpassed lifestyle. In addition, students are only a short distance from San Francisco, which offers world-renowned opera, symphonies, ballet, museums, and championship athletic teams. Dominican is also less than an hour's drive from California's wine country and Silicon Valley.

STUDENT SERVICES

The University offers many services that support the University's educational mission and the personal, social, physical, spiritual, and professional development of students. Services provided include career services, athletics (NAIA Division II men's and women's basketball, soccer, and golf and women's volleyball, tennis, and softball and men's lacrosse), recreational sports, on-campus housing, campus ministry, the campus health center, counseling services, and student government (ASDU). There are also many student-formed groups and clubs to choose from on campus. The School of Arts and Sciences has an active chapter of the California Nurses Students' Association and a nursing honor society.

THE NURSING STUDENT GROUP

There are approximately 388 students enrolled in the undergraduate nursing programs; of these, 90 percent are women, 54 percent are members of minority groups, and 2 percent are international. There are currently 17 M.S.N. students.

COSTS

The 2006–07 tuition costs for full-time students (12–17 units) were $27,770. Part-time students paid $1160 per unit. Room and board cost approximately $10,080. The registration fee was $250 per semester, and there was an additional nursing major fee of $400 per semester when taking clinicals. Mandatory health insurance was approximately $1500 per year for those without coverage. Additional expenses for the nursing program included uniforms, books, supplies, a physical examination, annual tuberculosis screening and immunization, and transportation between the University and affiliated clinical agencies.

FINANCIAL AID

The University manages an extensive financial assistance program to ensure that a highly qualified and diverse population is able to matriculate and continue to graduation. The assistance programs take two major forms: scholarships and need-based financial aid. In addition to administering federal and state aid programs, Dominican also awards a number of scholarships and grants annually from income provided by annual gifts and endowed funds as well as from its own general funds. The Financial Aid Office matches the intentions of the donor to the academic and other qualifications of students with need.

APPLYING

Applicants who are qualified for admission to Dominican are admitted as prenursing majors. After students have completed the fourteen prerequisite courses with at least a 3.0 GPA, they are accepted into the nursing courses as nursing majors. Transfer students are considered for placement in sophomore clinical classes in the fall or spring semesters once they have completed a minimum four-semester wait period and if the following minimal admission criteria are fulfilled: completion of elementary algebra, completion of all prerequisite courses (inorganic and organic chemistry; human anatomy and physiology; microbiology; statistics; nutrition; introduction to psychology, lifespan development, sociology, or anthropology; public speaking; and English), and maintenance of an overall GPA of at least 3.0. Advanced placement students can be admitted for either the spring or fall semesters.

CORRESPONDENCE AND INFORMATION:

Office of Admissions
Dominican University of California
50 Acacia Avenue
San Rafael, California 94901-2298

Phone: 415-485-3204
      888-323-6763 (toll-free)
E-mail: enroll@dominican.edu
Web site: http://www.dominican.edu

Dominican University of California
School of Arts and Sciences
Department of Nursing
Phone: 415-485-3295
E-mail: nursing@dominican.edu

THE FACULTY

Nicole Barnett, Assistant Professor; Ed.D., RN.
Kathleen Beebe, Assistant Professor; Ph.D., RN.
Christina Campbell, Assistant Professor; Ed.D., RN.
Olivia Catolico, Associate Professor; Ph.D., RN.
Debbie Daunt, Assistant Professor; M.S.N., RN.
Margaret Fink, Assistant Professor; M.S.N., RN.
Linda Gabriel-Marin, Assistant Professor; M.S.N., RN.
Barbara Ganley, Assistant Professor; Ph.D., RN.
Mary Ann Haeuser, Assistant Professor; M.S.N.
Adrina Lemos, Assistant Professor; M.S.N., RN.
Luanne Linnard-Palmer, Department Chair; Ed.D., RN.
Ingrid Sheets, Assistant Professor; M.S., RN.

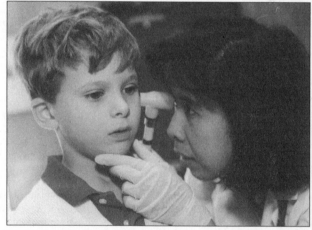

The School of Arts and Sciences at Dominican University of California offers its students a wide variety of clinical experiences.

Drexel University
College of Nursing and Health Professions
Philadelphia, Pennsylvania

THE UNIVERSITY

On July 1, 2002, Drexel University's Board of Trustees unanimously voted to merge the academic programs of Drexel and MCP Hahnemann Universities. With the addition of the nation's largest private medical school, an outstanding college of nursing and health professions, and one of only two schools of public health in Pennsylvania, Drexel University now comprises thirteen colleges and schools. This combination of expertise in advanced technology and cooperative education and academic programs in medicine and health-related fields means that students are offered an exceptional set of skills with which to succeed in today's ever-changing world.

THE COLLEGE OF NURSING AND HEALTH PROFESSIONS

Drexel has a 130-year legacy of educating nurses. Hospital-based nursing programs began in 1864 at what was then the Female Medical College of Pennsylvania and in 1890 at the Hahnemann Hospital Training School for Nurses. With the consolidation of Medical College of Pennsylvania and Hahnemann University in 1993, Hahnemann's undergraduate and graduate nursing programs and Medical College of Pennsylvania's nurse anesthesia program were combined into the College of Nursing and Health Professions (CNHP).

Since the merger of MCP Hahnemann with Drexel University, this tradition of health sciences education has taken another step forward. Undergraduate and graduate programs in health professions, nursing, public health, medicine, and biomedical graduate studies stand alongside Drexel's established and renowned programs.

PROGRAMS OF STUDY

Drexel's College of Nursing and Health Professions offers a variety of educational programs that prepare nurses and future nurses for exciting opportunities. Several undergraduate programs are offered. The Bachelor of Science in Nursing (B.S.N.) Co-op program is a full-time, five-year program that leads to the B.S.N. The program is one of only two in the country that offers three paid, six-month cooperative education experiences in the field of nursing in addition to traditional clinical experiences. The Accelerated B.S.N./M.S.N. program allows students to complete both the Bachelor of Science in Nursing and the Master of Science in Nursing degrees in five years. The Accelerated Career Entry (ACE) program is an eleven-month, intensive, full-time B.S.N. program for students who already have bachelor's or graduate degrees in another field. The R.N./B.S.N Completion program, available online or in class, is a B.S.N. completion program for nurses from associate and diploma nursing programs. The R.N./B.S.N./M.S.N. program is an accelerated program designed for graduates of associate degree and diploma nursing programs who are committed to earning the Master of Science in Nursing degree.

The M.S.N. programs prepare nurse practitioners in a variety of specialty areas, such as urban family health care, acute care, psychiatric–mental health care, and women's health. (Women's health is offered in collaboration with Planned Parenthood Federation of America.) Online M.S.N. programs in nursing education, nursing leadership and management, and clinical trials research are also offered. An exciting option is the online M.S.N. in Innovation and Entrepreneurship in Advanced Nursing Practice Program—the first such M.S.N. degree in the nation. It is designed for creative individuals who seek to build, construct, or design products or projects that will advance nursing practice, education, and administration. In response to health-care-system needs, innovative M.S.N. tracks are always in continuous development.

The M.S.N. in nurse anesthesia is a nationally recognized program that prepares nurses to practice as anesthetists. The R.N./M.S.N. program is for nurses who hold a B.A. or B.S. in an area other than nursing. An M.S.N. Completion program is offered for graduates of certificate nurse practitioner or nurse anesthesia programs. Certificate programs are offered for individuals who have earned an M.S.N. and seek further preparation to qualify for state or national certification. Currently, there are certificate programs in nursing education, nursing leadership and management, and clinical trials research.

In fall 2005, Drexel began the first clinical research Doctor of Nursing Practice (Dr.N.P.) program in the country. Rather than a D.N.P., Drexel's Dr.N.P. is a hybrid program combining the professional practice doctorate and the academic research doctorate. It is similar to a Ph.D. because it requires a clinical dissertation. Students can choose from the program's four tracks: Practitioner, Educator, Clinical Scientist, or Clinical Executive. Drexel's aim for this new practice doctoral degree is to develop clinical scholars who can make a major impact on nursing practice, as well as contribute to nursing science knowledge development.

The B.S.N. and M.S.N. programs are accredited by the National League for Nursing Accrediting Commission and the Commission on Collegiate Nursing Education (CCNE). The nurse anesthesia M.S.N. program is accredited by the Council on Accreditation of the Nurse Anesthesia Educational Programs.

ACADEMIC FACILITIES

The Clinical Resource Learning Center (CRLC) provides a simulated environment in which students can safely learn and practice clinical skills. Students practice head-to-toe assessments, invasive as well as noninvasive procedures, and interpersonal skills. Students also have an opportunity learn how to manage real-life emergencies and clinical situations with SIM-MAN®, a simulated patient that can mimic patient signs and symptoms. The CRLC consists of a physical assessment lab, media center and media classroom, nursing therapeutics lab, and two rehabilitation sciences labs. In addition, a hallmark of the nursing programs at Drexel is the intensive application of patient care and information technologies, including personal digital assistants (PDA's) and other evolving information management platforms.

The Drexel University CNHP has strong relationships with the vast array of premier health systems and hospitals located in the Philadelphia metropolitan area, and students have access to these for clinical experiences and for co-operative employment.

LOCATION

Drexel University's Center City Hahnemann Campus is spread over more than a city block and includes classrooms, research areas, student lounge and activity areas, and an array of educational and student-life resources. Students have the use of the Student Life Center, which includes a Nautilus-equipped fitness center, and there are lounges throughout the campus that offer video games and television as well as comfortable space to eat and socialize. Intramural sports teams are also available at the Center City campus.

The 636-bed Hahnemann University Hospital is located on the campus. In 2002, Drexel University merged with MCP Hahnemann University, and the Center City location name reflects its history as one of Philadelphia's progressive medical institutions. At the Center City Hahnemann Campus, the College of Nursing and Health Profession's Nursing Co-op Program provides eighteen months of co-op education designed to expose students to various career options.

STUDENT SERVICES
Many services are offered to students. These include Academic Enrichment Services (ACT 101), the Center for Student Academic Resources, the Office of International Student Services, the Office of Multicultural Programs and Special Projects, Residential Life and Off-Campus Housing, Student Counseling Center, and Student Disability Services as well as student organizations and government and many activities for students. There is a Health Sciences Campus Bookstore and a chapter of the Student Nurses' Association of Pennsylvania.

THE NURSING STUDENT GROUP
There are more than 1,200 undergraduates and 900 graduate students in the nursing and health professions programs. Most undergraduates attend on a full-time basis, while most graduate students attend part-time.

COSTS
Tuition for the 2006 academic year was $26,000 per year for the B.S.N. Co-op program and $440 per credit for the RN-B.S.N. program. The ACE program tuition was $30,000.

FINANCIAL AID
Drexel University offers a full program of financial aid in the form of low-interest educational loans, alumni endorsement scholarships, grants, and campus work-study opportunities. Additional financial aid and work programs are available to students who qualify.

APPLYING
Drexel University offers programs for applicants with both nursing and non-nursing backgrounds. Admissions requirements vary by program. Students should visit http://www.drexel.edu.em to apply.

CORRESPONDENCE AND INFORMATION
Office of Health Sciences Admissions
Drexel University
3141 Chestnut Street
Philadelphia, Pennsylvania 19104
Phone: 800-2DREXEL (toll-free)
E-mail: enroll@drexel.edu
Web site: http://www.drexel.edu/em

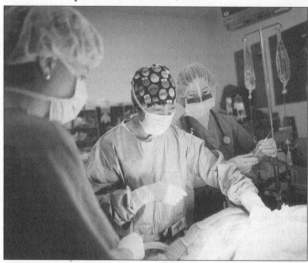

The M.S.N. in nurse anesthesia is a nationally recognized program that prepares nurses to practice as anesthetists.

Duke University
School of Nursing
Durham, North Carolina

THE UNIVERSITY

Since its founding in 1839 as the Union Institute, and later as Trinity College before incorporating in 1924, the basic principles of Duke University have remained constant. Through changing generations of students, the objective has been to encourage individuals to achieve, to the extent of their capacities, an understanding and appreciation of the world in which they live, their relationship to it, their opportunities, and their responsibilities. Today, Duke University has 12,000 students, of whom 5,250 (400 part-time) are enrolled in the graduate and professional programs, representing nearly every state and many countries.

The School of Medicine, School of Nursing, and Duke Hospital and Health Network are the core institutions of the Duke University Medical Center and Health System, which ranks among the outstanding health-care providers of the world. The opening of Duke Hospital North in 1980 made Duke Hospital, with 1,048 beds, one of the most modern patient-care facilities available anywhere. The mission of the Health System is to be a leader in world health care. This involves maintaining superiority in its four primary functions: excellent patient care, dedication to educational programs, national and international distinction in the quality of research, and service to the region.

THE SCHOOL OF NURSING

Since the founding of the School in 1930, Duke has prepared outstanding clinicians, educators, and researchers and is continuing this tradition. Drawing on the intellectual and clinical resources of both Duke University Medical Center and Duke University, the School offers an Accelerated Bachelor of Science in Nursing degree (for second degree students) and a Master of Science in Nursing degree program that balances education, practice, and research.

Faculty members work closely with students to challenge and nurture them; students not only practice with state-of-the-art science and technology in a great medical center but also have opportunities to work in rural and underserved areas.

PROGRAMS OF STUDY

The School of Nursing offers a 58-credit-hour, full-time, Accelerated Bachelor of Science in Nursing (B.S.N.) degree program in a sixteen-month, intensive format. In addition, a flexible, 39- to 59-credit program leading to the Master of Science in Nursing (M.S.N.) degree is offered. There are also two joint-degree programs: in conjunction with the Fuqua School of Business, a joint M.S.N./M.B.A. degree, and, in conjunction with the Divinity School, a joint M.S.N./Master of Church Ministries degree. The School of Nursing also offers a collaborative arrangement with Meredith College in Raleigh, North Carolina, that facilitates completion of the M.S.N. degree in nursing and health-care leadership or clinical research management at the Duke School of Nursing and the M.B.A. at Meredith College. The School of Nursing also offers a post-master's certificate to students who have already earned an M.S.N. The purpose of the Master of Science in Nursing program is to prepare professional nurses for advanced practice in a clinical specialty, administration, or education. Graduates are prepared as clinical nurse specialists in gerontology, oncology, critical care, pediatrics, or neonatal care; as adult nurse practitioners (with specialization in primary care, acute care, cardiovascular care, or oncology/HIV); as gerontological nurse practitioners, family nurse practitioners, neonatal nurse practitioners, pediatric acute/chronic care nurse practitioners, pediatric nurse practitioners, or combined neonatal-pediatric nurse practitioners with an emphasis on rural health care; as nursing health-care leadership administrators and managers and clinical research managers; as nurse anesthetists; as advanced practice nurses prepared to serve faith communities; and as nurse educators. The clinical research management program, the nursing and health-care leadership program, the nursing education program, the nursing informatics program, and selected nurse practitioner core courses are available online to distance education students. The family nurse practitioner, adult nurse practitioner, and gerontological nurse practitioner programs are also available online. The integration of education, practice, and research is basic to the entire curriculum as well as to the activities of each student, and the program is designed to provide maximum flexibility for full-time or part-time study.

The School of Nursing also offers a Ph.D. in nursing. The Ph.D. program in nursing prepares nurse scientists to conduct nursing research in the broad area of trajectories of chronic illness and care systems. Graduates assume roles primarily in academic and research settings. The approach is to admit a small number of highly qualified applicants so every student can work closely with one or more faculty members in a series of mentored experiences supported by formal course work, to ensure socialization to the role of research scientist, ensure significant knowledge and skill acquisition for launching a successful program of independent post-doctorate research, and prepare for an entry-level role in an academic setting. The program requires a minimum of 54 credit hours of graduate course work (post-M.S.N.) prior to a dissertation. Students work on active research projects, and it is expected that most students graduate with a record of publication. Course work is structured with a substantial core (36 credits) of nursing science and research methods to be taken in the School of Nursing. This core is expanded with elected statistics, research methods, and minor area courses (18 credits) to be taken mainly outside of nursing in other Duke University departments. In addition to course work and a dissertation, the Ph.D. program in nursing includes two program-long structured activities that include mentored research and teaching experiences and development of the student's scholarly portfolio. Each student takes a comprehensive exam at the end of the second year or at the beginning of the third year of residence. The final requirement is the presentation of a dissertation. Students are expected to complete the program in four to five years. For more information and further details, students should inquire by e-mail at nursephd@notes.duke.edu.

AFFILIATIONS WITH HEALTH-CARE FACILITIES

As one of the leading national and international academic health systems, Duke University Health System has assembled and integrated a comprehensive range of health-care resources providing the very best in patient care, health education, and clinical research. The clinical faculty members of the Duke University School of Nursing number more than 100 and represent all specialties. Clinical faculty members actively participate in nursing education and practice nursing in hospitals and ambulatory settings. Cooperative teaching and clinical facilities, including health departments, retirement centers, and private practices in both urban and rural settings, are available to students mostly within the state of North Carolina. Occasionally, placements are arranged out-of-state or in other countries to accommodate the student's needs.

Nationally recognized centers with which the School of Nursing is affiliated include the Duke Heart Center, the Center for Aging and Human Development, the Comprehensive Cancer Center, the Comprehensive Sickle Cell Center, Alzheimer's Disease Research Center, Duke Hypertension Center, Duke–VA Center for Cerebrovascular Research, Cystic Fibrosis/Chest Center and Clinic, Sleep Disorders Center, the Eye Center, and the Geriatric Research, Education, and Clinical Center.

ACADEMIC FACILITIES

The goal of the Duke Nursing Research Center is to facilitate the conduct of clinical research by the students and faculty and nursing staff members. The center provides support for research through assistance with literature searches, development of research designs, the Institutional Review Board and/or the protection of human subjects consultation, data collection and data management, grant proposal development, and editorial review.

The Duke School of Nursing is a national leader in online education; all of the School's courses are enriched by the use of technology. There is a student computer laboratory containing fifteen computer workstations, and a computing orientation seminar enables students to take full advantage of technology. The School also supports a new Center for Instruction Technology and Distance Learning, the purpose of which is to provide technical support for online education and classroom technology.

The Medical Center Library, located in the Seeley G. Mudd Communications Center and Library Building, provides services and collections necessary to support educational, research, and clinical activities. The library has sizable holdings of nursing books and journals, including 300,000 bound volumes in health, 6,000 bound volumes in nursing, 2,375 health-care-related periodical titles, and 1,000 electronic journals, including thirty-five in nursing.

LOCATION
Durham, a city of 223,000, is about 250 miles south of Washington, D.C. Durham and nearby Raleigh and Chapel Hill constitute the three points of the Research Triangle, one of the nation's foremost centers of research-oriented industries and government, research, and regulatory agencies.

STUDENT SERVICES
The University has many resources and activities to offer students. These include the Graduate and Professional Student Council, the Women's Center, the Mary Lou Williams Center for Black Culture, and the International House as well as the full programs of the Office of Cultural Affairs, the Duke University Campus Ministry, the Duke University Union, the Office of Student Activities, and recreational clubs.

THE NURSING STUDENT GROUP
Approximately 115 students are enrolled in the accelerated B.S.N. degree program, 347 students are enrolled in the M.S.N. and post-master's certificate programs, and 5 students are enrolled in the Ph.D. program. About 13 percent are men, and 13 percent are members of minority groups.

COSTS
Tuition in 2006–07 was $785 per credit hour for graduate nursing courses and $619 per credit hour for undergraduate nursing courses.

FINANCIAL AID
Merit and need-based scholarships, traineeships, and federal/state loan programs are generally available. Approximately 80 percent of School of Nursing students receive some form of financial aid.

APPLYING
Admission requirements for the Accelerated B.S.N. program include a bachelor's degree from an accredited college or university, a minimum 3.0 GPA on a 4.0 scale, three letters of recommendation, 1000 or greater on the GRE (scores not more than five years old), and completion of all required prerequisites. Admission requirements for the graduate program include a bachelor's degree with an upper-division nursing major from an NLNAC- or CCNE-accredited program, a preferred undergraduate scholastic average of 3.0 or better on a 4.0 scale, an introductory course in descriptive and inferential statistics, 1000 or greater on the GRE (scores not more than five years old), and licensure as a registered nurse in North Carolina. An interview is requested; if distance prohibits this, a telephone interview may be arranged. Exceptions to any of the above qualifications are considered on an individual basis.

Duke University does not discriminate on the basis of race, color, national and ethnic origin, handicap, sexual orientation or preference, gender, or age in the administration of educational policies, admission policies, financial aid, employment, or any other University program or activity. It admits qualified students to all the rights, privileges, programs, and activities generally accorded or made available to students.

CORRESPONDENCE AND INFORMATION
Office of Admissions and Student Services
Duke University School of Nursing
Box 3322 Medical Center
Durham, North Carolina 27710

Phone: 919-684-4248
   877-415-3853 (toll-free)
Fax: 919-668-4693
E-mail: SONAdmissions@mc.duke.edu
Web site: http://www.nursing.duke.edu

THE FACULTY
Ruth Anderson, Associate Professor; Ph.D., Texas at Austin, 1987; RN.
Donald Bailey, Assistant Professor; Ph.D., North Carolina at Chapel Hill, 2002; RN.
Julie V. Barroso, Assistant Professor; Ph.D., Texas at Austin; RN, ANP, CS.
Jane Blood-Siegfried, Assistant Professor; D.N.S., UCLA, 1995; RN, PNP.
Margaret Bowers, Assistant Clinical Professor; M.S.N., Duke, 1990; RN, FNP.
Wanda Bradshaw, Assistant Clinical Professor; M.S.N., Duke, 1996; RN, PNP, NNP.
Debra Brandon, Assistant Professor; Ph.D., North Carolina at Chapel Hill, 2000; RN.

Mary T. Champagne, Associate Professor; Ph.D., Texas at Austin; 1981; RN.
Elizabeth Clipp, Ph.D., Professor and Associate Dean of Research Affairs; Cornell, 1984; RN.
Janice Collins-McNeil, Assistant Research Professor; Ph.D., Tennessee Health Science Center, 2005.
Kirsten Corazzini, Assistant Professor; Ph.D., Massachusetts Boston, 2000.
Linda Davis, Professor; Ph.D., Maryland, 1984; RN.
Susan Denman, Assistant Professor; Ph.D., North Carolina at Chapel Hill, 1996; RN, FNP.
Wendy Demark-Wahnefried, Professor; Ph.D., Syracuse, 1988; RD, LDN.
Sharron Docherty, Assistant Professor; Ph.D., North Carolina at Chapel Hill, 1999; RN.
Anthony T. Dren, Consulting Professor; Ph.D., Michigan, 1966.
Pamela Edwards, Associate Consulting Professor; M.S.N., Ed.D., North Carolina State, 1989; RN, BC.
Catherine Gilliss, Dean and Vice Chancellor for Nursing Affairs for Duke University Health System; D.N.Sc., Duke, 1971; RN.
Linda K. Goodwin, Assistant Professor; Ph.D., Kansas, 1992; RN.
Helen Gordon, Assistant Clinical Professor; M.S., Utah, 1978; RN, CNM.
Judith C. Hays, Associate Professor and Chair of the Accelerated B.S.N. Program; Ph.D., Yale, 1991; RN.
Sharon Hawks, Assistant Professor; M.S.N., North Carolina at Greensboro, 1993; RN, CRNA.
Cristina Hendrix, Assistant Professor; Ph.D., LSU, 2001; RN.
Elizabeth Hill, Assistant Professor; D.N.Sc., Catholic University, 1993; RN.
Diane Holdtich-Davis, Professor; Ph.D., Connecticut, 1985; RN, FAAN.
Constance Johnson, Assistant Professor; Ph.D., Texas Health Science Center at Houston, 2003; RN.
Lawrence Landerman, Associate Research Professor; Ph.D., Duke, 1979.
Holly Lieder, Assistant Clinical Professor; M.S.N., Duke, 2000; RN, CPNP.
Kelly Lochmuller, Instructor; M.S.N., Pittsburgh, 2003; RN, CRNA.
Marcia S. Lorimer, Assistant Clinical Professor; M.S.N., Virginia, 1988; RN, PNP.
Michelle Martin, Assistant Professor; Ph.D., Case Western Reserve, 2001; RN.
Eleanor S. McConnell, Assistant Research Professor; Ph.D., North Carolina at Chapel Hill, 1995; RN.
Mary Miller-Bell, Adjunct Associate Professor; Pharm.D., North Carolina at Chapel Hill, 1998.
Brenda M. Nevidjon, Associate Clinical Professor and Chair of the M.S.N. Program; M.S.N., North Carolina at Chapel Hill, 1978; RN.
Judith K. Payne, Assistant Professor; Ph.D., Iowa, 1998; RN, AOCN, CS.
Katherine Pereira, Assistant Clinical Professor; M.S.N., Duke, 2002; RN.
Beth Phillips, Assistant Clinical Professor; M.S.N., Duke, 1993; RN.
Dorothy Powell, Clinical Professor; Ed.D., William and Mary, 1983; RN, FAAN.
Marva M. Price, Assistant Professor; Dr.P.H., North Carolina at Chapel Hill, 1994; RN, FNP; FAAN.
Carla Rapp, Assistant Professor; Ph.D., Iowa, 1999; RN, CRRN.
Susan Schneider, Assistant Professor; Ph.D., Case Western Reserve, 1998; RN.
Nancy Short, Assistant Professor; M.B.A., Dr.P.H., North Carolina at Chapel Hill, 2003; RN.
Steven Talbert, Assistant Professor; Ph.D., Kentucky, 2002; RN.
Joshua M. Thorpe, Assistant Research Professor; Ph.D., North Carolina at Chapel Hill, 2005.
J. Frank Titch, Assistant Clinical Professor; M.S.N.A., Virginia Commonwealth, 1994; RN, CRNA.
Kathryn Trotter, Assistant Clinical Professor; M.S.N., Kentucky, 1988; RN, CNM, FNP.
Barbara S. Turner, Professor, Associate Dean, Director of Nursing Research, and Division Chief; D.N.Sc., California, San Francisco, 1984; RN; FAAN.
George H. Turner III, Assistant Clinical Professor; M.A., Webster, 1978; RPh.
Kathleen M. Turner, Assistant Clinical Professor and Associate Director of the Accelerated B.S.N. Program; M.S.N., Duke, 1993; RN.
Queen Utley-Smith, Assistant Professor; Ed.D., North Carolina State, 1999; RN.

Duquesne University
School of Nursing
Pittsburgh, Pennsylvania

THE UNIVERSITY

Duquesne University, located in Pittsburgh, Pennsylvania, America's renaissance city, is a private coeducational Catholic university with ten schools and an enrollment of more than 10,000 students. Currently, the University is experiencing a period of unprecedented growth, and nearly 100 nations and every state are represented in Duquesne's student body.

With a long tradition of scholarship and community service, Duquesne is among the top Catholic universities in the United States and has a well-deserved reputation for providing an education for the mind, heart, and spirit. The University offers a wide variety of activities and volunteer opportunities that complement the curriculum and provide a broad, well-balanced, and fully integrated education.

THE SCHOOL OF NURSING

Founded in 1937, the School of Nursing at Duquesne was the first nursing school in Pennsylvania to offer a baccalaureate program in nursing, and it was among the first in the nation to offer an online doctoral program in nursing. Continuing that tradition of innovation, Duquesne's School of Nursing offers a wide variety of online and traditional degree and certificate programs. A leader in nursing education for generations, the School of Nursing at Duquesne maintains the highest standards of clinical competency, academic achievement, and dedication to helping others.

Community service integrated with an unmatched educational experience is the hallmark of a nursing education at Duquesne. This commitment to service holds true for the faculty and staff, as well. Members of the School of Nursing's award-winning faculty have been widely recognized for their volunteer work as well as their clinical expertise, research accomplishments, and teaching skills.

Faculty members operate a number of Nurse-Managed Wellness Centers in underserved communities, where nurses and other health-care providers promote health and wellness and monitor chronic medical conditions. The clinics offer students an invaluable clinical learning experience and an ongoing opportunity for community service.

Duquesne's Center for International Nursing offers students a transcultural perspective on health care. Through student/faculty exchange programs, collaborative international research projects, and hands-on training in other countries, the Center provides a range of educational, research, and nursing leadership opportunities for students and faculty members. The Center for International Nursing is designed to meet curricular requirements as well as individual student needs at the undergraduate, graduate, and postgraduate levels.

The Center for Health Care Diversity addresses health-care equity and diversity issues in minority populations through community-focused research, nursing education programs, health policy development, and community service.

PROGRAMS OF STUDY

The School of Nursing offers baccalaureate, master's, and doctoral degrees as well as a variety of professional certificates. School of Nursing students may enroll part-time or full-time. The undergraduate program of the School of Nursing leads to the degree of Bachelor of Science in Nursing (B.S.N.). At the undergraduate level, Duquesne offers a four-year B.S.N., the

RN-B.S.N./M.S.N., and the Second Degree B.S.N. The B.S.N. program is designed to educate nurse generalists and usually requires four years of full-time study. The curriculum (130 credits) provides students with a strong foundation in the natural, biological, and behavioral sciences, most of which are taken during the first two years of study. Students receive an introduction to the nursing profession at the freshman level and begin clinical experience with clients and families during the sophomore year. The junior and senior years are devoted almost exclusively to clinical experience. Undergraduate minors for nursing students are available in business, psychology, sociology, Spanish, and communication. In addition, the School offers a unique undergraduate focus area in music therapy as well as a business certificate for nursing students.

Pittsburgh is home to a number of world-class medical centers that provide Duquesne nursing students with state-of-the-art clinical experience. Duquesne faculty members teach all professional courses as well as guide and direct the clinical learning experiences.

The Second Degree B.S.N. program allows the non-nurse with a baccalaureate degree to achieve a Bachelor of Science in Nursing degree in twelve months. After all requirements for the B.S.N. degree have been completed, students are eligible to take the state board examination for nursing licensure. The program begins in August and includes three semesters of intensive course work using traditional classroom instruction, creative Web-enhanced seminars for nonclinical courses, and more than 1,000 hours of clinical practice in leading health-care settings.

The RN-B.S.N./M.S.N. program, for registered nurses pursuing B.S.N. and M.S.N. degrees, is offered entirely online. Through transfer credits and CLEP testing, this program permits a registered nurse to apply previous learning experience toward the requirements of a B.S.N. degree. After completing the required core curriculum and nursing prerequisites, the B.S.N. program can be completed online and part-time in five semesters. In this program, a B.S.N. is awarded after the completion of 31–32 nursing credits, 19–20 of which are master's-level credits. Students who have earned a 3.0 QPA in the B.S.N. course work have the option of earning an M.S.N. degree at Duquesne in one of six specialties (see below). The Miller Analogies Test (MAT), a required admission test for the M.S.N. program, is waived for students with a 3.0 GPA who have met all graduate admissions criteria.

The M.S.N. program, which is offered entirely online, is based on the belief that specialization in nursing is acquired at the graduate level. This program is designed to meet the current and future needs of nurses who are likely to hold leadership positions. It educates nurses to plan, initiate, effect, and evaluate change; ensure high-quality patient care; and enhance the profession. Working nurses may continue their employment while undertaking this course of study through part-time enrollment, or course work may be undertaken on a full-time basis for most programs.

Six areas of specialization exist in the M.S.N. program: nursing education (39 credits), nursing administration (37 credits), family nurse practitioner (46 credits), forensic nursing (36 credits), acute-care clinical nurse specialist (41 credits), and psychiatric–mental health clinical nurse specialist (37 credits).

Post-master's certificates offered online give professional nurses the opportunity to learn skills and acquire information that may not have been offered in graduate programs. Course work in these nondegree programs is designed to prepare nurses for certification through applicable professional organizations. Duquesne offers the following post-master's certificates: acute-care clinical nurse specialist (28 credits), nursing administration (15 credits), nursing education (12 credits), family nurse practitioner (33 credits), forensic nursing (17 credits), psychiatric–mental health clinical nurse specialist (21 credits), and transcultural/international nursing (12 credits).

The online Doctor of Philosophy (Ph.D.) degree (57 credits) prepares nurses for a lifetime of intellectual inquiry and creative scholarship. This online program permits students to earn a doctoral degree in nursing using state-of-the-art distance education technology. Online courses are asynchronous, meaning that students can complete their work anytime and anywhere via the Internet. Mandatory fieldwork can be conducted near the student's home. Ph.D. students are required to be on campus for one week each spring during the completion of their required course work (a period that varies from two to four years). During that week, students meet with faculty advisers, attend lectures by visiting professors, participate in seminars for required courses, complete examinations, and participate in program evaluation.

ACADEMIC FACILITIES
Duquesne University's Gumberg Library houses extensive collections of digital research databases and electronic journals, books, and reference works that are accessible from remote locations. The library's facilities include CD-ROM collections as well as numerous computers and multimedia learning tools. The School of Nursing has technologically advanced facilities, which include sophisticated educational tools and a realistic practice setting for learning clinical skills and procedures.

LOCATION
Duquesne's campus provides a comfortable and secure academic and social atmosphere that is just minutes from downtown Pittsburgh. The scenic, hilltop campus is readily accessible to the city's business, cultural, entertainment, and shopping districts while still offering students the privacy and peaceful atmosphere of a self-contained 47-acre campus. Home to emerging technologies as well as established corporations and rated as one of the nation's most livable cities, Pittsburgh combines the best features of urban life with the charm, pace, and personality of small-town living.

STUDENT SERVICES
Duquesne University offers a variety of services that help students achieve their academic and professional goals and grow socially, spiritually, and personally. Support services include student Health Service, the Office of Freshman Development and Special Student Services, Career Services Center, Comprehensive Student Advisement, University Counseling Center, Learning Skills Center, and Campus Ministry. In addition, the Office of International Programs assists students and scholars from other countries who are pursuing undergraduate and graduate studies at Duquesne.

THE NURSING STUDENT GROUP
The School of Nursing currently has an enrollment of more than 400 B.S.N. students, of whom 5 percent are enrolled part-time. Ten percent are members of minority groups, and 10 percent are men. Of the nearly 150 M.S.N. students, 95 percent are part-time. The Ph.D. program has more than 50 students. Duquesne's nursing students come from around the United States and the world. In addition to challenging clinical and classroom learning, Duquesne's nursing students are involved in a full range of campus activities, including student government, fraternities, sororities, and social and professional organizations (Alpha Tau Delta, Chi Eta Phi, Male Association of Nursing, Nurses Christian Fellowship, Sigma Theta Tau International Honor Society, and the Student Nurses Association of Pennsylvania). Nursing students have excelled in a number of competitive sports, including football, baseball, crew, volleyball, soccer, lacrosse, cross-country, swimming, and diving.

COSTS
For the 2006–07 academic year, undergraduate full-time students (12–18 credits) paid $23,381 per year for tuition and fees. Undergraduate room and board per semester were $4148 (double room). Undergraduate tuition and fees were $789 per credit for part-time students. Graduate tuition and fees (part-time or full-time) were $822 per credit. Other estimated undergraduate nursing school expenses each semester included books and supplies, $500; student liability insurance, $25; and uniforms, $150.

FINANCIAL AID
Tuition at Duquesne is among the lowest among private national universities, and competitive financial aid packages make a Duquesne education more affordable. Financial aid includes scholarships, grants, loans, and part-time employment awarded to help students meet the costs of education. Awards, both merit-based and need-based, come through a variety of sources, including programs administered by the federal and state government, private organizations, and the University. Duquesne is constantly developing resources for funding scholarships and providing financial assistance, and the School of Nursing maintains numerous listings of nursing funding sources for undergraduate and graduate nursing education, including federal, state, and private organizations and local hospital discounts. Students must apply for any awards by May 1 of each year.

APPLYING
Students with above-average high school records whose first college of choice is Duquesne may apply for early decision admission. Early decision applications must be submitted on or before November 1 of the student's senior year for consideration for the following fall semester. Early decision acceptance notifications are made by December 15, after which time students have two weeks to submit the required deposit. Admission requirements for the undergraduate and graduate programs are specific for each degree option. Transfer and international applicants must fulfill all undergraduate or graduate admission requirements. A personal or telephone interview with a School of Nursing representative is highly recommended and may be required, depending on the program of study. Interested applicants should contact the School of Nursing or visit http://www.nursing.duq.edu for detailed information.

CORRESPONDENCE AND INFORMATION
Duquesne University School of Nursing
600 Forbes Avenue
Pittsburgh, Pennsylvania 15282-1760
Phone: 412-396-6550 (general information)
       412-396-4945 (program inquiries)
Fax: 412-396-6346
E-mail: nursing@duq.edu
Web site: http://www.nursing.duq.edu

D'Youville College
Department of Nursing
Buffalo, New York

THE COLLEGE

D'Youville College is a private, coeducational liberal arts and professional college offering students a high-quality education in more than thirty undergraduate and graduate degree programs. Founded in 1908 by the Grey Nuns as the first college for women in western New York to offer baccalaureate degrees to women, it was named for their founder, Saint Marguerite D'Youville. The current enrollment is 2,500 men and women. Students' learning is facilitated by the low 14:1 student-faculty ratio. The College is committed to helping its students grow not only academically but also in the social and personal areas of their college experience.

THE DEPARTMENT OF NURSING

D'Youville College has been educating and preparing professional nurses for careers since 1942; the first Bachelor of Science in Nursing (B.S.N.) class graduated in 1946. In 1957, the RN to B.S.N. degree program was initiated, offering a specialized curriculum for the working professional nurse. All programs offered by the nursing department are fully accredited by the Commission on Collegiate Nursing Education (CCNE) and approved by the New York State Education Department.

The nursing faculty members are committed, dedicated educators who pride themselves on providing individual attention. Faculty members, the majority of whom are prepared at the doctoral level, represent diverse backgrounds, both clinically and educationally, providing numerous specialty areas for the students to draw upon.

PROGRAMS OF STUDY

D'Youville College has been growing and attracting students from all over the world since 1908, playing a leadership role in the areas of professional health training. D'Youville offers a four-year Bachelor of Science in Nursing degree program, and students who are interested in pursuing careers in nursing also have the option of completing a dual-degree, five-year sequence to graduate with both a baccalaureate and a master's degree. It is a direct-entry program in which accepted students do not have to reapply or requalify for upper-division courses. The B.S.N. degree program combines a liberal arts foundation with professional nursing course work. Students begin their clinical experiences at area hospitals and health facilities in their sophomore year. Areas of clinical experience include geriatrics, pediatrics, OB/maternity, and medical/surgical nursing. To hone their clinical and research skills, students participate in internships during the summer of their junior year. The two-year RN to B.S.N. degree program includes an RN to B.S.N./M.S. option and an RN to B.S.N./M.S. in community health nursing option, in which RNs complete an additional year of study and graduate with both degrees. Convenient class scheduling provides working nursing professionals with the opportunity to study full-time by attending only two days a week. This alternative scheduling allows students to continue working in their professions while earning their degrees. In 2005, a new nursing flextrack program became available for students who want a B.S.N. but have a bachelor's degree in another major.

At the graduate level, nursing programs include the Master of Science (M.S.) in community health nursing, with concentrations in holistic nursing, hospice and palliative-care nursing, nursing management, and nursing education; the M.S. in

nursing, with choice of clinical focus; and the Master of Science in family nurse practitioner studies as well as a post-master's certificate in family nurse practitioner studies.

AFFILIATIONS WITH HEALTH-CARE FACILITIES

Specific facilities with which D'Youville has affiliations include Catholic Health System, which encompasses Mercy Hospital of Buffalo and Kenmore Mercy Hospital; Erie County Medical Center; WNY's Level I Trauma and Burn Center; Buffalo Psychiatric Center; Kaleida Health Care System, which comprises Women and Children's Hospital of Buffalo, Buffalo General Hospital, Millard Fillmore Hospital, and the Visiting Nurses Association of Western New York; BryLin Hospital; and the world-renowned Roswell Park Cancer Institute.

ACADEMIC FACILITIES

D'Youville's modern Library Resource Center, which was completed in 1999, contains 154,000 volumes, including microtext and software and subscriptions to 870 periodicals and newspapers. The multimillion-dollar Health Science Building houses laboratories, including those for anatomy, organic chemistry, quantitative analysis, and computer science. It also houses classrooms, faculty offices, and development centers, including one for career development. In addition, an academic center opened in 2001.

LOCATION

D'Youville is situated on Buffalo's residential west side. The College is within minutes of many social attractions, including the downtown shopping center, the Kleinhans Music Hall, the Albright-Knox Art Gallery, two museums, and several theaters that offer stage productions. Seasonal changes in the area offer a variety of recreational opportunities. Buffalo is only 90 miles from Toronto and 25 minutes from Niagara Falls.

STUDENT SERVICES

The College offers a full range of student services. The D'Youville Freshman Experience (DFX) is designed to help make the students' first year exciting, fun, and challenging. At orientation, students are assigned a College mentor and register for the FOCUS Freshmen Seminar. There are also activities and leadership opportunities (D'Youville Leads) as well as a peer mentor program coordinated through the Leadership Development Institute. The College also has a Career Services Center, the Learning Center, the Multicultural Affairs Office, and the Personal Counseling Center. A new apartment residence opened in January 2005.

THE NURSING STUDENT GROUP

D'Youville has both traditional and nontraditional students from a variety of ethnic backgrounds in the nursing program, enhancing the educational and social experiences. Nursing organizations on campus include the National Student Nurse Association (NSNA), which is open to all nursing students. Students who excel academically may be invited to join the Society of Nursing, Sigma Theta Tau International.

COSTS

For 2004–05, tuition was $7345 per semester, and room and board cost $3670 per semester. A general College fee is required and is based on credit hours taken. Graduate tuition for

2004–05 was $520 per credit hour. Students in the B.S.N./M.S. programs pay undergraduate tuition.

FINANCIAL AID

All students enrolled in the RN degree-completion program are offered a 50 percent tuition reduction. Ninety percent of D'Youville freshmen receive financial aid. This includes nearly $2 million in grants and scholarships. Grants include Federal Pell Grants and Federal Supplemental Educational Opportunity Grants, the New York State Tuition Assistance Program, and the Aid for Part-Time Study Program. The Federal Work-Study Program, federally insured loans, and flexible payment plans are also available. All applicants are reviewed for academic scholarships at the time of acceptance. D'Youville's new Instant Scholarship Program offers scholarships with total values up to $45,900 for undergraduate and dual-degree programs.

APPLYING

D'Youville admits students on a rolling admission basis; therefore, applications are reviewed as they are received by the Admissions Office. Undergraduate applicants must submit a completed application along with a $25 processing fee; official high school transcripts or, for transfer students, official transcripts from colleges previously attended; SAT or ACT scores; and letters of recommendation.

Applicants to the master's program must present a baccalaureate degree in nursing from an accredited college or university program; a valid New York state or provincial license to practice nursing; evidence of an undergraduate course in statistics and an undergraduate course in computer science or its equivalent; and evidence of capability to succeed in a graduate program, as shown by an overall undergraduate GPA of at least 3.0 (based on a 4.0 system); an overall undergraduate GPA of at least 2.7, with a 3.0 or better in the upper half of undergraduate work; an overall undergraduate GPA of at least 2.7, with a 3.0 or better in the major field; or a baccalaureate degree in nursing plus a master's degree in another field from an accredited college or university with an overall GPA of at least 3.5. Candidates for the post-master's certificate program in family nurse practitioner studies must have a master's degree in nursing.

CORRESPONDENCE AND INFORMATION

Department of Nursing
D'Youville College
320 Porter Avenue
Buffalo, New York 14201-9985

Phone: 716-829-7613
Fax: 716-829-8159
E-mail: admissions@dyc.edu
Web site: http://www.dyc.edu

THE FACULTY

Patricia Bahn, M.S., RN. Adult health/nursing administration, holistic health/oncology.

Joan Cookfair, Ed.D., RN. Publications and practice center on community health nursing specialty.

Carol Gutt, Ed.D., RN. Child health/curriculum/wellness.

Dorothy Hoehne, Ph.D., RN. Maternal child nursing/teaching higher education, instructional communications, research and evaluation.

Janet Ihlenfeld, Ph.D., RN. Social support and job satisfaction, pediatric/neonatal critical care, children in the community.

Verna Kieffer, D.N.S., RN. Community wellness, adult health, gerontology, quality-of-life and quality-of-care issues.

Edith Malizia, Ed.D., RN. Adult health, education administration.

Pamela Miller, M.S., RN, WHNP.

Karen Piotrowski, M.S., RN. Labor, childbirth.

Bernadette Pursel, M.S. Community health nursing.

Connie Jozwiak Shields, Ph.D., RN, ANP. Adult primary-care nursing.

Judith Stanley, M.S.N., RN. Hospital patient advocacy and education, supervision and administration of home infusion therapy, complementary and alternative healing modalities (biofeedback, hypnosis, imagery).

Paul Violanti, M.S., RN, PNP, FNP. International medical missions and refugees.

Dawn Williams, M.S., RN. Adult health, medical surgery.

Emory University
Nell Hodgson Woodruff School of Nursing
Atlanta, Georgia

THE UNIVERSITY
Emory University, founded by the Methodist Church in 1836, has approximately 12,000 students and 2,500 faculty members who represent all regions of the United States and about ninety other nations. Emory has nine major academic divisions, numerous centers for advanced study, and a host of prestigious affiliated institutions. The University has a two-year and four-year undergraduate college, a graduate school of arts and sciences, and professional schools of medicine, theology, law, nursing, public health, and business.

THE SCHOOL OF NURSING
The Nell Hodgson Woodruff School of Nursing was founded in 1905 as the Training School for Nurses at Wesley Memorial Hospital in Atlanta. In 1922, the hospital and school of nursing were moved to the Emory University campus and functioned as a diploma school with a three-year hospital program. In 1944, the school became an integral part of Emory University, offering the Bachelor of Science in Nursing degree. The diploma program was offered concurrently until its discontinuation in 1949. The School of Nursing was named the Nell Hodgson Woodruff School of Nursing in 1968 in honor of Mrs. Woodruff, who supported the School of Nursing throughout her lifetime. The School offers undergraduate, graduate, and doctoral nursing education to nearly 300 students.

PROGRAMS OF STUDY
The Bachelor of Science in Nursing (B.S.N.) degree provides a strong academic foundation that focuses on connecting the theoretical basis of nursing with the development of critical-thinking and decision-making skills. The first two years of general education course work (including prerequisites) may be taken at any accredited college or university. Specific physical science, humanities, social science, and elective courses that total 60 semester hours are required for admission to the B.S.N. program at Emory. During the second year of prerequisite course work, students apply for admission to the School of Nursing. Qualified students are then admitted for the remaining two years of professional study. The four-semester, 60-semester-hour nursing program combines clinical and in-class experiences. The goals of the School of Nursing are to advance nursing knowledge, produce nurse leaders, and design new models of care.

Students who hold a bachelor's degree in another area but are interested in becoming nurses are eligible for the second degree B.S.N. program. Students enroll into the B.S.N. program and complete their nursing studies in four semesters of full-time course work. Emory University also has a B.S.N./M.S.N. Segue Option for non-nurses interested in becoming nurse practitioners or certified nurse midwives. Students must have a bachelor's degree in an area other than nursing to be eligible. This program provides a seamless course of study through admission into the B.S.N. program followed by direct entry into the M.S.N. program after receiving RN licensure.

The degree programs at Emory University School of Nursing combine the advantages of outstanding facilities, a well-crafted curriculum, high-quality instruction, a prestigious and far-reaching reputation, and courses that are relevant to today's evolving practice environment. A wealth of clinical venues are available in the Atlanta metropolitan area, and clinical experiences are precisely geared to students' career focuses. Emory offers B.S.N., M.S.N., RN-M.S.N., Bridge, M.S.N./M.P.H., post-master's, and Ph.D. programs.

Programs of study leading to the Master of Science in Nursing (M.S.N.) include the following specialties: acute care nurse prac-

titioner, adult nurse practitioner, adult oncology nurse practitioner, emergency nurse practitioner, family nurse-midwife, family nurse practitioner, gerontological nurse practitioner, international health (M.S.N./M.P.H. only), leadership and administration in health care, public-health nursing leadership, nurse-midwifery, pediatrics, pediatric nurse practitioner-acute care, pediatric nurse practitioner-primary care, women's health nurse practitioner, women's health care (Title X), and women's health/adult health nurse practitioner. Length of the specialty programs ranges from three (one calendar year) to five consecutive semesters of full-time study. Part-time study is available. Students are eligible to sit for certification as nurse practitioners or certified nurse midwives.

The RN-M.S.N. bridge program provides an opportunity for associate degree or diploma-prepared nurses to obtain the Master of Science in Nursing. Students in the RN-M.S.N. program complete 24 semester hours of bridge course work prior to beginning the specialty curriculum of choice. In addition, a dual Master of Science in Nursing/Master of Public Health (M.S.N./M.P.H.) is available, and post-master's options are available in all graduate specialty areas except the Emergency Nurse Practitioner Program.

The Ph.D. in nursing offers flexible specialization options and is a four-year, full-time program. Students accepted to the program receive an annual stipend plus financial support to cover tuition for a maximum of four years.

AFFILIATIONS WITH HEALTH-CARE FACILITIES
The Nell Hodgson Woodruff School of Nursing maintains close ties with the Centers for Disease Control and Prevention (CDC), and the American Cancer Society. The School of Nursing at Emory is also the home of the Lillian Carter Center for International Nursing. Students at Emory have access to more than 200 diverse clinical learning sites.

ACADEMIC FACILITIES
In January 2001, the School of Nursing opened a state-of-the-art facility for nursing study and research. The building unites scholarship and teaching under one roof. The School of Nursing is part of the Robert W. Woodruff Health Sciences Center, a major provider of patient care and a national leader in clinical and research programs. Emory University is a close collaborator with the Carter Center, a nonprofit, nonpartisan public policy institute founded by former President Jimmy Carter and his wife Rosalynn.

LOCATION
Emory University is located 6 miles northeast of downtown Atlanta. Emory is positioned along Clifton Road, which is also the home of the U.S. Centers for Disease Control and Prevention and the American Cancer Society. With top-tier entertainment, cultural attractions, sports, and shopping, Atlanta has something for everyone.

STUDENT SERVICES
Nursing students at Emory enjoy a vibrant campus life. Opportunities for involvement on campus and within the nursing school are abundant. Emory students also have the opportunity to participate in student nursing organizations on the local, state, and national levels.

THE NURSING STUDENT GROUP
During the 2006–07 academic year, the School of Nursing enrolled 213 undergraduate students, 177 graduate students, and 17 doctoral students from across the nation and around the world.

COSTS

In 2006–07, full-time undergraduate tuition was $14,400 per semester. The student activity fee was $71 per semester or $5 per semester hour. The student athletic fee was $132 per semester or $40 for the summer semester.

Full-time graduate tuition was $14,400 per semester or $1200 per semester hour for part-time students (fewer than 12 semester hours). The student activity fee was $71 per semester or $5 per semester hour. The student athletic fee was $102 per semester or $40 for the summer semester.

FINANCIAL AID

Emory University and Nell Hodgson Woodruff School of Nursing are committed to providing a generous package of financial assistance to all who qualify. Currently, 96 percent of undergraduate nursing students and 95 percent of graduate nursing students receive financial assistance.

Students who apply for financial assistance at Emory University are considered for a combination of scholarships, grants, and low-interest loans. Merit-based scholarships are available at both the undergraduate and graduate levels.

APPLYING

All applicants to the School of Nursing are considered on an individual basis. Applications and supporting credentials should be submitted by January 15 for priority admission and scholarships; however, applications are reviewed as long as class space is available. The School of Nursing selects those applicants who are best qualified academically and have a strong desire of commitment to the field of nursing. After all application materials are received, the Admissions Committee reviews the applicant's credentials and makes the decision to accept or deny admission. Final acceptance is contingent upon satisfactory completion of prerequisite course work.

CORRESPONDENCE AND INFORMATION

Office of Admission
Emory University School of Nursing
1520 Clifton Road
Atlanta, Georgia 30322
Phone: 404-727-7980
　　　　800-222-3879 (toll-free)
Fax: 404-727-8509
E-mail: admit@nursing.emory.edu
Web site: http://www.nursing.emory.edu

THE FACULTY

Corrine Abraham, Associate; M.N., Emory, 1985. Adult and elder health.

Kelly Brewer, Associate; M.S.N., Arkansas, 1992. Adult and elder health.

Holly L. Brown, Associate; M.S.N., Pennsylvania, 1989. Adult and elder health.

Ann Connor, Clinical Assistant Professor; M.S.N., Alabama, 1980. Family and community nursing.

Jo Ann Dalton, Professor and Chair, Adult and Elder Health; Ed.D., North Carolina State, 1984.

Madge M. Donnellan, Clinical Associate Professor; Ph.D., Tennessee, 1988. Family and community nursing.

Elizabeth Downes, Clinical Assistant Professor; M.S.N., Tennessee, 1986. Family and community nursing.

Sandra B. Dunbar, Professor and Coordinator of the Doctoral Program; D.S.N., Alabama at Birmingham, 1982. Adaptation to the stresses of acute and chronic cardiovascular illness.

Sara Edwards, Instructor; M.S.N./M.P.H., Emory, 1994. Family and community nursing.

Sarah B. Freeman, Clinical Professor; Ph.D., Georgia State, 1989. Family and community nursing.

Mary L. Garvin-Surpris, Instructor; M.S., New Rochelle, 1993. Adult and elder health.

Maggie P. Gilead, Associate Professor; Ph.D., Emory, 1981. Adult and elder health.

Judy Gretz, Instructor; M.S., Texas Woman's, 1977. Family and community nursing.

Jill Hamilton, Assistant Professor; Ph.D., North Carolina at Chapel Hill, 2001.

Kenneth Hepburn, Associate Dean for Research; Ph.D., Washington, 1968.

Leslie Holmes, Instructor; M.S.N., Medical University of South Carolina, 1993. Family and community nursing.

Barbara Kaplan, Instructor; M.S.N., Emory, 1992. Family and community nursing.

Maureen A. Kelley, Clinical Associate Professor and Chair, Family and Community Nursing; Ph.D., Medical College of Georgia, 1993. Midwifery.

Joyce L. King, Clinical Assistant Professor; Ph.D., Emory, 1995. Family and community nursing.

Sally T. Lehr, Clinical Assistant Professor; Ph.D., Georgia State, 2001. Adult and elder health.

Marsha Lewis, Associate Dean for Education; Ph.D., Minnesota, 1992.

Maureen O. Lobb, Clinical Assistant Professor; Ph.D., Georgia State, 1992. Family and community nursing.

Kathy Markowski, Instructor; M.S.N., DePaul, 1980. Adult and elder health.

Jane E. Mashburn, Clinical Associate Professor and Director, M.S.N. Program; M.N., Emory, 1978. Midwifery, Family and community nursing.

Kathryn Matthews, Instructor; M.S.N., Pennsylvania, 1976. Family and community nursing.

Marcia K. McDonnell-Holstad, Assistant Professor; D.S.N., Alabama, 1996. Family and community nursing.

Joyce P. Murray, Professor; Ed.D., Georgia, 1989. Adult and elder health.

Lynda P. Nauright, Professor; Ed.D., Georgia, 1975. Adult and elder health.

Michael W. Neville, Clinical Associate Professor; Pharm.D., Georgia, 1992. Adult and elder health.

Helen S. O'Shea, Professor Emerita; Ph.D., Georgia State, 1980. Adult health.

Kathy Parker, Professor; Ph.D., Georgia State, 1990. Family and community nursing.

Quyen Phan, Instructor; M.S.N., Emory, 2004. Adult and elder health.

Marcene L. Powell, Professor; D.S.W., Utah, 1981. Family and community nursing.

Barbara D. Reeves, Clinical Assistant Professor; M.S.N., Vanderbilt, 1979. Family and community nursing.

Bethany D. Robertson, Instructor; M.S.N., Emory, 1992. Family and community nursing.

Martha F. Rogers, Clinical Professor; M.D., Medical College of Georgia, 1976. Family and community nursing.

Deborah A. Ryan, Clinical Associate Professor and Director, B.S.N. Program; M.S.N., Marquette, 1981. Family and community nursing.

Marla E. Salmon, Professor, Dean, and Director of LCCIN; Sc.D., Johns Hopkins, 1977. Health workforce and health services.

Lynn Sibley, Associate Professor; Ph.D., Colorado, 1993. Family and community nursing.

Linda Smith, Instructor; M.N., South Carolina, 1980; M.Div., Emory, 2004. Adult and elder health.

Linda Spencer, Clinical Associate Professor; Ph.D., Georgia State, 1988. Family and community nursing.

Ora Strickland, Professor; Ph.D., North Carolina at Greensboro, 1977. Family and community nursing.

Darla R. Ura, Clinical Associate Professor; M.A., Ball State, 1974. Adult and elder health.

Jeannie Weston, Instructor; M.S., Maryland, 1982. Family and community nursing.

Lynette Wright, Clinical Associate Professor; M.N., Emory, 1974. Distance learning strategies.

Erin M. York, Associate; M.S., Georgia State, 1995. Family and community nursing.

Weihua Zhang, Clinical Assistant Professor; Ph.D., Georgia State, 2004. Adult and elder health.

Excelsior College
Nursing Program
Albany, New York

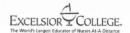
EXCELSIOR COLLEGE.
The World's Largest Educator of Nurses At-A-Distance

THE COLLEGE

Excelsior College, formerly Regents College, was founded in 1971 to make college degrees more accessible to busy, working adults. Most Excelsior College students are returning to college to complete an education begun elsewhere. Because it has no residency requirement, the College accepts a broad array of prior college-level credit in transfer, including credit earned in classroom and distance courses from Excelsior College and other accredited colleges and universities; proficiency examinations such as Excelsior College Examinations and CLEP; and corporate and military training recognized for the award of college-level credit by the American Council on Education (ACE), Center for Adult Learning and Educational Credentials. A recognized leader in distance education, Excelsior College offers degree programs in nursing, health sciences, business, liberal arts, and technology, and certificates in health science specialties. With more than 115,000 graduates, the College's associate, baccalaureate, and master's degree programs and certificate programs are accessible worldwide. This enables students to work at their own pace while maintaining a full-time work schedule and family and civic responsibilities.

Since 1977, Excelsior College has been accredited by the Commission on Higher Education of the Middle States Association of Colleges and Schools, 3624 Market Street, Philadelphia, Pennsylvania 19104, 215-662-5606. The Commission on Higher Education is an institutional accrediting agency recognized by the U.S. Secretary of Education and the Council for Higher Education Accreditation (CHEA). All the College's academic programs, including its undergraduate and graduate programs in nursing, are registered (i.e., approved) by the New York State Education Department. The associate, baccalaureate, and master's degree programs in nursing are accredited by the National League for Nursing Accrediting Commission (NLNAC), 61 Broadway, New York, New York 10006, 800-669-1656. The NLNAC is a specialized accrediting agency recognized by the U.S. Secretary of Education. The Excelsior College School of Nursing is one of only seven schools of nursing in the nation and the only one in New York State to be designated an NLN Center of Excellence for 2005–08 by the National League for Nursing in recognition of the College's sustained efforts to create environments that promote student learning and professional development.

Excelsior College Examinations are recognized by the American Council on Education (ACE), Center for Adult Learning and Educational Credentials, for the award of college-level credit. Excelsior College Examinations in nursing are the only nursing examinations approved by ACE. This school is a nonprofit corporation authorized by the State of Oregon to offer and confer the academic degrees described herein, following a determination that state academic standards will be satisfied under OAR 583-030. Inquiries concerning the standards or school compliance may be directed to the Oregon Office of Educational Policy and Planning, 255 Capitol Street, NE, Suite 126, Salem, Oregon 97310-1338.

THE NURSING PROGRAM

The Excelsior College School of Nursing, honored as one of only seven NLN Centers of Excellence in the nation, is the largest distance educator of nurses in the world. The Nursing Program began offering the first nontraditional distance nursing programs in the United States in 1975. Today, it has more than 35,000 graduates among its several programs. Representing the largest assessment-based undergraduate nursing program in the nation, Excelsior College's programs have served as models for the development of other nontraditional programs. Faculty members are selected for their expertise in curriculum development and program evaluation. They represent leaders in nursing education.

At the undergraduate level, Excelsior College offers nursing degree programs leading to an Associate in Science, an Associate in Applied Science, and a Bachelor of Science degree in nursing (completion program for RNs). All offered at a distance, its undergraduate programs have been specifically designed to meet the educational needs of qualified individuals with significant background and/or experience in clinically oriented health-care disciplines. The requirements for the associate degree programs may be met by completing a series of examinations that measure a student's knowledge of nursing theory and a student's clinical competency. Excelsior College performance (clinical) examinations are administered through a national network of Regional Performance Assessment Centers (RPAC).

The nursing component of the bachelor's degree program comprises 30 transfer credits (validated by successful completion of the NCLEX-RN), Excelsior college courses, and Excelsior college examinations. Students may also transfer in most, if not all, of their general education credits, or finish with Excelsior college courses and Excelsior college examinations.

At the graduate level, delivered online, Excelsior offers a Master of Science degree in nursing with specializations in clinical systems management and nursing education, and an RN-M.S. in nursing program.

The School of Health Sciences offers a Bachelor of Science in health sciences with concentrations in management, health education, gerontology, and end-of-life-care, as well as online Nursing Management, End-of-Life Care, and Health-Care Informatics Certificate programs.

PROGRAMS OF STUDY

The purpose of the Excelsior College associate degree nursing program is to provide an alternative educational approach to earning an associate degree in nursing. The student's qualifications as a learned individual and a competent member of the nursing profession are documented through an objective assessment program in general education and nursing. The program is designed to promote a sense of social responsibility and personal fulfillment by emphasizing the need for students to evaluate their own learning and potential achievements in terms of professional relevance and personal goals, proficiency in the practice of nursing, and a foundation for lifelong learning. The associate degree program is divided into two components: general education (31 semester hours) and nursing (36 semester hours). The general education component is very flexible so that adult students can build the degree to meet their interests and needs. It includes requirements in anatomy, physiology, microbiology, lifespan developmental psychology, sociology, and English composition. Students can meet these requirements through classroom or distance courses from Excelsior College and other regionally accredited colleges or through proficiency examinations. The nursing component comprises seven Excelsior College theory examinations and one performance examination.

The purpose of the bachelor's degree in nursing program is to offer an alternative educational approach to earning a baccalaureate degree in nursing. The student's qualifications as a learned individual and competent member of the nursing profession are documented through an objective assessment program of general and professional education designed to promote an awareness of the human experience and an appreciation for the contributions of people from diverse cultures through the study of liberal arts and sciences; a sense of social responsibility and personal fulfillment by emphasizing the need for individuals to evaluate their own potential and learning achievements in terms of professional relevance and personal goals; proficiency in the practice of professional nursing by providing assessment of baccalaureate-level competencies in the liberal arts and sciences and in nursing; and a foundation for graduate specialization.

The bachelor's degree program is divided into two components: general education (61 semester hours) and nursing (60 semester hours). The general education component is very flexible so that adult students may build the degree to meet their interests and needs. It includes requirements in anatomy, physiology, microbiology, psychology, sociology, statistics, and English composition. Students can meet these requirements through classroom or distance courses from Excelsior College and other accredited colleges or through proficiency examinations. The nursing component comprises three Excelsior College theory examinations and four performance examinations. Students are granted 30 semester hours of nursing credit for prior learning validated by successful completion of the NCLEX-RN.

To test the clinical competencies of its nursing students, Excelsior College pioneered the creation of rigorous performance examinations. The program is self-paced, and students can take performance examinations at any of four RPACs located in California, Georgia, New York, and Wisconsin.

College courses in nursing and nursing theory examinations may not be accepted for credit if they were completed more than five years prior to enrollment.

Excelsior College's certificate programs (through the School of Health Sciences) offer instruction that helps busy health-care professionals to enhance their knowledge in specific areas and take their careers to the next level. The online Nursing Management Certificate program provides the formal management preparation necessary to excel in a demanding management role. From budgeting and finance to human resources and ethics, the program's five credit-bearing courses give students a complete framework of knowledge about the field. The total program is 15 credits for students who do not already have a bachelor's degree. Those who already have a bachelor's degree may substitute two 4-credit graduate-level courses to earn 17 credits. The 12-credit End-of-Life Care Certificate equips current and aspiring palliative care nurses with the skills to provide more effective high-quality care. Online courses cover topics from therapeutic communications through coping strategies for patients and families. A Health-Care Informatics Certificate program is available as a 17-hour curriculum, 6 of which may be applied toward the online master's degree program.

The purpose of the online Master of Science (M.S.) in nursing degree program is to offer a high-quality educational program in clinical systems management or to prepare students for a career in nursing education. It is also available as the RN-M.S. degree program for registered nurses, who must complete requirements for both the bachelor's and master's program segments. Engaging in the study of foundational material for advanced nursing roles, master's-level students in the program earn a total of 38 or 39 graduate-level credits (for clinical systems management and nursing education specializations, respectively) through online course work and an interactive capstone experience.

ACADEMIC FACILITIES

As a distance education program, Excelsior College promotes students' success with a variety of guided learning services to students, such as study guides, learning modules, online workshops, performance examination workshops, teleconferences, comprehensive online library services, an online bookstore, and computer conference groups facilitated at the College's Electronic Peer Network (EPN), a "virtual student union." Academic advisers and nurse faculty members are available to provide services to students by telephone, fax, computer, and mail.

LOCATION

Because its programs are provided at a distance, the College allows students to pursue their degrees wherever they are. The administrative offices are located in Albany, the capital of New York State. Each year the College holds a formal commencement ceremony

to recognize all who have completed a degree that year. Proud of their accomplishment, many students travel great distances to participate in commencement festivities.

THE NURSING STUDENT GROUP

The 1,500 adult students enrolled in the Bachelor of Science in nursing program represent diverse backgrounds in terms of age, ethnicity, nationality, and professional experience. Most are registered nurses. Of the more than 16,000 students enrolled in the associate degree program, most are licensed practical/vocational nurses (LPNs/LVNs). The average student has ten years of health-care experience. Graduates of the College are employed in various health-care settings and are accepted into most graduate programs.

COSTS

Undergraduate tuition for Excelsior College distance courses is $275 per credit hour. Excelsior College charges an $895 (associate degree programs) or $995 (baccalaureate degree programs) fee at enrollment, which covers initial evaluation of a student's existing academic records and academic advisement and program planning services for one year; a $450 (associate) or $515 (baccalaureate) annual fee for each year after the first, which covers the ongoing evaluation of academic records submitted by a student and academic and program planning services for an additional twelve months; and a $490 (associate) or $495 (baccalaureate) fee for a final evaluation and verification of all academic records prior to program completion and graduation. Different fees and fee structures apply to military students, certificate and graduate programs, and to students who choose to budget their Excelsior College enrollment expenses via the College's FACTS Payment Plan. Detailed fee schedules are available in hard copy and on the College's Web site. Additional costs depend on the amount of credit students need to earn and what credit sources they choose. Proficiency examinations are the least expensive mode of earning credit. Students should also figure in costs for books and other learning materials, travel, postage, online resources, and miscellaneous charges and supplies.

FINANCIAL AID

Some financial aid is available, particularly the College's President's Scholarships and aid connected with Veterans Affairs benefits. The College participates in a variety of alternative loan programs. Students seeking financial aid should contact the Excelsior College Financial Aid Office before enrolling.

APPLYING

Students must apply for admission to the Excelsior College School of Nursing and, once accepted, enroll in Excelsior College. The Excelsior College nursing degree programs are specifically designed to serve individuals with significant background or experience in clinically oriented health-care disciplines. Therefore, undergraduate admission to the program is open to registered nurses, licensed practical/vocational nurses, paramedics, military service corpsmen, individuals who hold a degree in a clinically oriented health-care field in which they have had the opportunity to provide direct patient care (i.e., physicians, respiratory therapists, respiratory care practitioners, and physicians' assistants), or individuals who have completed, in the last five years, 50 percent or more of the clinical nursing courses in a program leading to RN licensure. Exceptions may be made for individuals who do not meet these qualifications but who can document significant clinical background. Specific admission requirements regarding the RN-M.S. and M.S. programs are detailed in the nursing catalog.

CORRESPONDENCE AND INFORMATION

Admissions Office
Excelsior College
7 Columbia Circle
Albany, New York 12203-5159

Phone: 888-647-2388 (press 2-7) (toll-free)
Fax: 518-464-8777
E-mail: admissions@excelsior.edu
Web site: http://nursing8.excelsior.edu

Fairleigh Dickinson University
Henry P. Becton School of Nursing and Allied Health
Teaneck-Hackensack, New Jersey

THE UNIVERSITY
Founded in 1942, Fairleigh Dickinson University (FDU) is an independent nonsectarian institution of higher education offering high-quality, career-oriented undergraduate and graduate programs. Fairleigh Dickinson is one of New Jersey's leading institutions of private higher education, with nearly 100 career-oriented programs at the undergraduate and graduate levels. Beginning in spring 2007, the University is scheduled to launch its third doctoral-level program: a Doctor of Nursing Practice (D.N.P.), offered through the Henry P. Becton School of Nursing and Allied Health.

The University has two campuses in northern New Jersey—the Metropolitan Campus in Teaneck and the College at Florham in Madison—and the Wroxton College campus in Oxfordshire, England. The nursing program is offered at the Metropolitan Campus; however, nursing students may take non-nursing classes at either the College at Florham or the Metropolitan Campus. Clinical site experiences are prearranged at a wide variety of health-care agencies.

THE SCHOOL OF NURSING
Established in 1952, Fairleigh Dickinson's nursing program focuses on preparing individuals who will enhance society and the health-care environment. It does so through course work that prepares graduates to function within a global health-care system. This philosophy reflects the educational tradition that has been the hallmark of the University, long recognized for its career-oriented studies enriched by a liberal arts tradition.

The faculty of the School of Nursing and Allied Health is committed to the belief that a basis of scientific knowledge is essential for professional nursing practice. The program views the professional nurse as an independent and interdependent practitioner who functions as a client advocate, change agent, innovator, planner, leader, and consumer of research. Nursing education at FDU encourages students to understand cultural differences and the relationship between human beings and their environment. The School approaches nursing as a collaborative learning process. Courses reflect a strong commitment to the development of critical thinking, ethical decision making, and cultural competence.

PROGRAMS OF STUDY
As of spring 2007, Fairleigh Dickinson is one of only two schools in New Jersey to offer a clinical doctoral degree in nursing. The Doctor of Nursing Practice is designed to prepare fully accountable professionals who are clinically expert as providers and educators.

The undergraduate program offers three specific study tracks leading to the Bachelor of Science in Nursing (B.S.N.) degree: basic four-year studies, a choice of accelerated one-year (full-time) or two-year (part-time, evening) studies for individuals who hold a non-nursing baccalaureate degree, and a B.S.N. to M.S.N. program for RNs from diploma or associate degree nursing programs. The basic four-year B.S.N. program is offered during the daytime, although many of the required and elective liberal arts courses for the degree are also available during the evening. The Accelerated B.S.N. program is an intensive, concentrated course of study designed to enable participants to complete their degrees in as little as one year. Nursing courses for full-time, one-year students are offered during the daytime and evening, starting in mid-May, five days per week; nursing courses for part-time, two-year students are offered during the evening, starting in September, four evenings per week.

Students who are interested in the RN to B.S.N. to M.S.N. program can enroll at any time during the academic year and take classes on a part-time or full-time basis. Two graduate nursing

courses are offered in the RN to B.S.N. curriculum as an incentive for students who are pursuing the M.S.N. degree.

The Master of Science in Nursing (M.S.N.) program offers studies in the following areas of specialization: adult nurse practitioner, adult nursing practitioner with educator or administrator tracks, clinical nurse leadering, forensic nursing, psychiatric/mental health, nursing educator, and nursing information systems. The School also offers a bridge program to the M.S.N. for RNs with non-nursing Bachelor of Science (B.S.) degrees.

The M.S.N. program consists of 28 to 40 credits, which full-time students can complete in two academic years, including the intervening summer. Graduates of the program are eligible to take the national certification exams of the American Academy of Nurse Practitioners (AANP) and the American Nurses Credentialing Center (ANCC) to become certified nurse practitioners. Nationally certified graduates may also obtain licensure from the New Jersey Board for Prescriptive Practice.

Individuals holding an M.S.N. degree may pursue a post-M.S.N. graduate certificate in the following areas: adult nurse practitioner, family nurse practitioner, forensic nursing, nursing education, nursing administration, or nursing information systems.

A variety of allied health programs are offered by the School: Associate in Science in radiography, which is a collaborative program with Valley Hospital, and Bachelor of Science programs in allied health (diagnostic medical sonography, nuclear medicine, respiratory care, or vascular technology), clinical laboratory science (cytotechnology or medical laboratory science), and medical technology. The School also offers studies leading to a doctorate in physical therapy. Both the B.S. in clinical laboratory science and doctorate in physical therapy are collaborative programs with the University of Medicine and Dentistry of New Jersey/SHRP.

AFFILIATIONS WITH HEALTH-CARE FACILITIES
The School of Nursing and Allied Health has built a strong network of participating clinical agencies to provide excellent and diverse clinical experiences for nursing students. These agencies include American Red Cross; Atlantic Health System; Barnert Hospital; Bergen Regional Medical Center; Charter Care One at Paramus; Children's Specialized Hospital; Chilton Memorial Hospital; Christian Health Care Center; Eastern Christian Children's Retreat; Englewood Hospital and Medical Center; Englewood Hospital Home Health Service and Hospice; Essex County Hospital Center; Essex Valley Visiting Nurse Association; Hackensack University Medical Center and Home Health Agency of Hackensack University Medical Center; Holy Name Hospital; Holy Name Home Care, Hospice and Adult Day Away; Hospice of New Jersey; Loving Care Pediatric Home Care; Morristown Memorial Hospital; New Jersey Veterans Memorial Home at Paramus; Overlook Hospital; Palisades Medical Center; Pascack Valley Hospital; Passaic Valley Hospice; Passaic Valley Hospice/Visiting Health Services of New Jersey; Robert Wood Johnson University Hospital; St. Clare's Hospital; St. Joseph's Home for the Elderly, Little Sisters of the Poor; St. Joseph's Regional Medical Center; St. Joseph's Wayne Hospital; St. Mary's Hospital; St. Vincent's Nursing Home; Summit Oaks Hospital; Teaneck Nursing and Rehabilitation Center; University of Medicine and Dentistry of New Jersey; the Valley Hospital; Valley Home Care, Inc.; VA New Jersey Health Care System; Van Dyk at Park Place; the Wanaque Center; Wellington Health Care Center; and Youth Consultation Services.

ACADEMIC FACILITIES
The Metropolitan Campus has nearly sixty buildings situated on 88 acres. In addition to the computer and laboratory facilities available at any major institution of higher education, FDU pro-

vides state-of-the-art equipment specifically for nursing students. The School of Nursing and Allied Health maintains modern facilities located in Dickinson Hall on the Metropolitan Campus. In its four specialized laboratories, students are taught patient care and a wide variety of nursing skills by the faculty members. The nursing laboratories are well equipped with realistic "hospital environments" as well as a separate clinical lab for learning with the simulated mannequin SimMan. The skills labs have interactive computer programs that enable students to practice and develop their skills independently using the technology frequently found in clinical settings.

LOCATION
The Metropolitan Campus is situated along the east and west banks of the Hackensack River, about 10 minutes from New York City. The campus is directly accessible from Route 4 and is 6 miles west of the George Washington Bridge. Easy access to New York City enables students and faculty members to take advantage of the city's financial, cultural, and international activities. The College at Florham is located at the outskirts of Morristown on Route 124, 35 miles from New York City. It is convenient to both the railroad and New Jersey bus transit. The Florham campus is 166 acres of beautifully landscaped property. Originally an estate, its Georgian-style buildings have been adapted to the University's needs.

STUDENT SERVICES
The University community is a total learning environment shared by students and faculty and staff members. To this end, strong support services are provided to enhance both the classroom and extracurricular experiences. Academic and career advisement and library and computer services are complemented by personal counseling, social and cultural activities, and programs that promote cross-cultural understanding. Lectures, seminars, concerts, performances, and special events are frequently offered on both campuses. Each year, the Fairleigh Dickinson University Student Nurses Association sponsors a variety of professional and social activities. Fairleigh Dickinson is home to the Epsilon Rho chapter of Sigma Theta Tau, the international nursing honor society.

THE NURSING STUDENT GROUP
Approximately 300 students are enrolled at the School. Five percent of students in the traditional baccalaureate program are men, and more than 50 percent are members of minority groups.

COSTS
For the 2006–07 academic year, undergraduate full-time tuition (12 to 18 credits per semester) was $24,072 at the Metropolitan Campus in Teaneck. All full-time undergraduates also paid an inclusive charge of $1868 for fees. The individual undergraduate per-credit rate was $772. Graduate nursing tuition was $839 per credit plus an additional technology fee of $274 for part-time students or $572 for full-time students. Nursing students also pay for nursing lab fees, books, and uniforms. Although costs varied by residence hall and meal plan, average annual room and board costs in 2006–07 were $9574 at the Metropolitan Campus.

FINANCIAL AID
Each year, the University awards more than $27 million from federal, state, and University sources in financial aid to students. In addition to its excellent need-based financial aid awards, the University also recognizes outstanding academic performance through its annually renewable Col. Fairleigh S. Dickinson Scholarships, which are worth up to $18,000 per year. For information on merit- and need-based financial aid, students should contact the Office of Financial Aid on the Metropolitan Campus at 201-692-2368.

APPLYING
For admission into the basic 128-credit, four-year track leading to the B.S.N. degree, applicants should be graduates of an accredited secondary school, with a record indicating the potential to succeed in college. Applicants should have completed the following high school studies: 4 units of English, 2 units of history, 1 unit of chemistry with lab, 1 unit of biology with lab, and 2 units of college-preparatory mathematics. In addition, 2 units of foreign language and 1 unit of physics are recommended. A minimum of 16 high school academic units is required for admission. A minimum score of 1000 on the SAT (math and critical reading) is necessary for admission. November, December, or January test scores are preferred. An interview with the nursing faculty is recommended.

Applicants to the 62-credit accelerated track leading to the B.S.N. degree should have earned a baccalaureate degree from a regionally accredited college or university, with a cumulative GPA of 3.0 or higher (based on a 4.0 scale). The following prerequisites, completed at a college level, are also required for enrollment: human anatomy and physiology (8 credits, with lab), chemistry (4 credits, with lab), microbiology (4 credits, with lab), economics (3 credits), bioethics (3 credits), and statistics (3 credits). An interview with the nursing faculty is also required.

To be considered for the M.S.N. program, applicants should be graduates of a National League for Nursing (NLN)–accredited B.S.N. program, with an undergraduate cumulative GPA of 3.0 or higher. Proof of registered nurse licensure, two essays showing evidence of suitability for graduate study in nursing, and proficiency in spoken and written English also are required. Undergraduate prerequisites include courses in health assessment, statistics, and nursing research. A personal interview may be necessary on request from the faculty.

Applicants to the post-M.S.N. program should hold an M.S.N. from an accredited college or university and be eligible for licensure in New Jersey. A personal interview may be requested.

Students who are interested in transferring to FDU's School of Nursing and Allied Health from regionally accredited institutions may be admitted with advanced standing upon presentation of official transcripts to the Office of University Admissions and an interview with a School of Nursing and Allied Health faculty member. To transfer, a student must have a cumulative GPA of at least 3.0 (based on a 4.0 scale) and grades of C or higher for liberal arts and sciences courses (a stronger emphasis is placed on science grades). Students transferring from accredited baccalaureate degree nursing programs may be awarded credit for nursing courses with grades of C+ or higher that are comparable to FDU's courses. A student interview and catalog descriptions and syllabi of previous courses are used to determine comparability.

CORRESPONDENCE AND INFORMATION
Dr. Minerva Guttman
Director, School of Nursing and Allied Health
Fairleigh Dickinson University
1000 River Road, H-DH4-02
Teaneck, New Jersey 07666

Phone: 201-692-2888 (Nursing and Allied Health)
       800-338-8803 (University Admissions, toll-free)

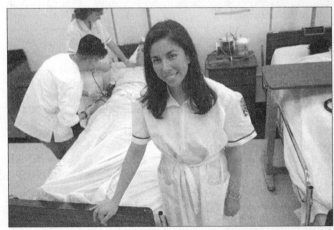

The School of Nursing and Allied Health provides excellent and diverse clinical experiences for nursing students.

Gannon University
Villa Maria School of Nursing
Erie, Pennsylvania

THE UNIVERSITY

A Catholic, diocesan, student-centered university, Gannon University is dedicated to holistic education in the Judeo-Christian tradition. The University faculty and staff members are committed to excellence and continuous improvement in teaching, learning, scholarship, research, and service.

Gannon University is a coeducational institution with 3,800 students, providing a caring environment that fosters inclusiveness and cultural diversity. Gannon's outstanding values-based education combines liberal arts with professional specializations to prepare students for leadership roles in their careers, society, and church. A range of campus organizations and activities encourages academic interests, community service, and moral and spiritual growth. Gannon also offers students a broad program of intramural and intercollegiate athletics.

Gannon offers associate, bachelor's, master's, doctoral, and preprofessional degrees in more than seventy academic majors in sciences, health sciences, engineering, humanities, business, and education.

THE SCHOOL OF NURSING

The Villa Maria School of Nursing offers baccalaureate and master's degree programs. Gannon's community-based nursing curriculum maintains a balanced study of natural and social sciences and the humanities within the context of professional education, fosters creative thinking and effective communication, and promotes caring, respect, and concern for individuals, communities, and society. All programs hold preliminary accreditation by the Commission on Collegiate Nursing Education (CCNE). Gannon's nursing faculty members have graduate preparation in their clinical areas of specializations and are skilled clinical practitioners.

All of Gannon's Villa Maria School of Nursing graduates are employed at various health-care facilities across the nation. Nursing students have the opportunity to participate in clinical experiences at more than forty local hospitals, clinics, and community agencies. For the past two years, 100 percent of nursing graduates have passed the licensure examination on their first attempt.

The purpose of the professional nursing program is to prepare students for life as well as for the practice of professional nursing. The community-based baccalaureate program provides competencies, knowledge, values, and roles that prepare professional nurses to provide high-quality care to diverse populations, in and across all environments.

The Villa Maria School of Nursing is able to accommodate an entering baccalaureate class of 60 each year.

PROGRAMS OF STUDY

In the baccalaureate program, the professional nurse's role is integrated into each clinical nursing course. The Villa Maria School of Nursing prepares high-quality graduates. Freshman students begin the investigation into the profession of nursing with seminar courses. Clinical course work begins in the sophomore year.

The Villa Maria School of Nursing offers a certification program for school nurses, in cooperation with the School of Education. The certification, which is available to registered nurses with an earned B.S.N. and a current registered nurse license in the commonwealth of Pennsylvania, consists of 17 credits: 3 credits in education, 5 credits in nursing, 3 credits in sociology, and 6 credits in math.

Options for registered nurses are available, including RN to B.S.N. and RN to M.S.N., offering an articulation path to the B.S.N. or the M.S.N. degree. Students follow a course of study that includes challenge exams, transfer credits, and validation of prior learning via student-created portfolios. The options focus on nonduplication of previously learned nursing knowledge.

Gannon also offers a graduate program in nursing. The Master of Science in Nursing (M.S.N.) program integrates nursing education, research, and practice and is designed so that the professional nurse can respond to the challenge of unresolved problems in nursing and in health-care systems. Students may choose the Master of Science in Nursing degree program with options in nursing administration, medical-surgical nursing, family nurse practitioner, or nurse anesthesia. Each graduate student is expected to conduct research and prepare a research thesis or project. The program may be completed by enrolling full-time or part-time, with the exception of the nurse anesthesia option, which can be completed only by enrolling full-time.

ACADEMIC FACILITIES

The Nash Library currently has more than 260,000 bound volumes. The library subscribes to more than 850 periodicals, with additional online access to more than 10,000 journals in full text. The library contains the Cyber Café, with personal computers, laptop ports, and cappuccino and juice machines; lounges; study rooms; typing rooms; a TV studio; the latest audiovisual and tape equipment; and a multimedia studio. New library services that have been recently added include electronic reserves and wireless connections and ITH laptops that are available for use within the building. In addition, students may use the facilities and resources of the Erie County Law Library and the Erie County Library. For specialized research projects, an efficient interlibrary loan service is available.

The Zurn Science Center has laboratories for research in biology, anatomy, physics, chemistry, and engineering. The building also houses three computer laboratories, including an IBM PC lab. The A. J. Palumbo Academic Center houses Gannon's Villa Maria School of Nursing and features modern nursing arts labs and classrooms so that students can apply theory to practice. Additional features of the A. J. Palumbo Academic Center include state-of-the-art multimedia tiered classrooms with video teleconferencing capabilities for distance learning opportunities, additional computer labs, and student study lounges. Other University facilities include a radio station, a theater, the Career Development and Employment Services Center, and the Waldron Campus Center.

All academic buildings at Gannon are wireless.

LOCATION

Erie is Pennsylvania's fourth-largest city and is located in the northwest corner of the state on the shores of Lake Erie. It is approximately 120 miles north of Pittsburgh, Pennsylvania; 90 miles east of Cleveland, Ohio; and 90 miles west of Buffalo, New York. The campus is within 5 miles of Interstates 79 and 90 and 5 miles from Erie International Airport. Erie is also serviced by rail and bus transportation.

STUDENT SERVICES

Gannon prides itself on meeting the personal and professional needs of all students. The Career Development and Employment Services Center for Experiential Education helps students in all stages of career preparation, from determining interests and aptitudes to writing a resume and conducting a job search. Counseling Services also provides support for students' personal concerns. Gannon students can visit the academic advising center in addition to the math and writing centers for additional help on assignments.

THE NURSING STUDENT GROUP

There are currently 206 students in the Bachelor of Science in Nursing program and 59 students in the Master of Science in Nursing program. One hundred percent of the B.S.N. graduates are employed in their field, and more than 90 percent of the M.S.N. graduates are employed in the nursing profession.

COSTS

In 2006–07, full-time undergraduate tuition was $9750 per semester, or $19,500 per academic year ($20,680 for engineering and health sciences, which includes the nursing program). Tuition for part-time students was $605–$640 per credit hour. Room and board costs were approximately $3895 per semester. The total cost for the academic year at Gannon, including books and supplies, was between $19,996 and $21,856 for commuting students and $27,786 and $29,648 for resident students, depending on the program of study.

FINANCIAL AID

In order to bring a Gannon education to qualified students who could not otherwise afford it, the University offers an integrated financial aid program of scholarships, grants, loans, and employment. An application for financial aid should be filed with the application for admission. The filing has no effect on the decision of the Admissions Committee. Gannon's financial aid program is open to all full-time students attending classes during the period from August to May. All students seeking aid should file the admission and financial aid applications no later than March 1.

Nursing students wishing to pursue a career in the Army may participate in Gannon's Army ROTC program through the Partnership in Nursing Education (PNE) program. PNE students receive officer training in addition to their required course work and have the opportunity to apply for ROTC scholarships.

APPLYING

To obtain admission into the B.S.N. program, students must have completed work equal to a standard high school curriculum with a minimum of 16 units, including 4 units of English, 3 units of social studies, 2 units of mathematics (one of which is algebra), and 2 units of science with a related laboratory or the equivalent. Additional requirements include a minimum GPA of 2.5 (transfer students must have at least a 2.8 GPA); a combined SAT score of 1010 or higher (out of 1600 for math and critical reading), with a mathematics score of at least 510; and a rank in the top 40 percent of the high school class. All applicants are required to submit scores on either the SAT or ACT, an up-to-date transcript of the high school record showing rank in class (plus a college transcript for transfer applicants), a completed application form, and a nonrefundable $25 application fee.

Requirements for students applying to graduate programs include an introductory statistics course and a research course with a grade of at least a B in both courses, competitive scores on the GRE, three letters of recommendation, RN licensure, and an interview.

CORRESPONDENCE AND INFORMATION

Director of Admissions
Gannon University
109 University Square
Erie, Pennsylvania 16541
Phone: 814-871-7240
       800-GANNON-U (toll-free)
Fax: 814-871-5803
E-mail: admissions@gannon.edu
Web site: http://www.gannon.edu

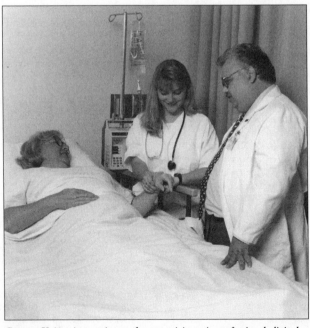

Gannon University nursing students participate in professional clinical rotations offering a variety of specialty areas with patients of different age groups and health conditions.

Georgetown University
School of Nursing and Health Studies
Washington, D.C.

THE UNIVERSITY

Georgetown University was founded in 1789 and is the oldest Catholic, Jesuit institution of higher learning in the United States. Washington, D.C., the nation's capital, is one of the most important cities in the world. Health policy and medical economics decisions are debated daily in many arenas, and decisions are made that shape the delivery of health care in this country and abroad. Cultural and social opportunities are limitless.

The diversity of the student population at Georgetown provides a stimulating environment for student life and study. All fifty states and more than 100 countries are represented by the 12,000 men and women currently enrolled in undergraduate, graduate, and professional programs.

THE SCHOOL OF NURSING AND HEALTH STUDIES

The School, founded in 1903, is conveniently located on the Main Campus next to the Georgetown University Medical Center. The Concentrated Care Center, Georgetown University Hospital, Pasquerilla Healthcare Center, Perinatal Center, and Lombardi Cancer Research Center provide access to an abundant patient population, while their proximity to the John Vinton Dahlgren Medical Library yields an ideal coordination of academic, clinical, and research facilities. This physical and functional relationship among research, nursing, medical, and academic facilities creates an integrated, comprehensive educational environment unavailable at many other universities.

PROGRAMS OF STUDY

The School of Nursing and Health Studies offers baccalaureate and master's degrees in nursing as well as non-nursing degrees. All nursing programs have been accredited by the National League for Nursing Accrediting Commission. There are four undergraduate majors offered in the School: the traditional Bachelor of Science in Nursing (B.S.N.) degree program and Bachelor of Science (B.S.) degrees in health-care management and policy, human science, and international health. An accelerated second-degree B.S.N. program for students with a bachelor's degree in a non-nursing field and a traditional transfer option into the B.S.N. and the three B.S. programs are also offered. The nursing and health studies components are a balance between a strong theoretical base and clinical skills. Students study the curative and restorative aspects of health care, as well as health maintenance and health education. Clinical practice culminates in the senior practicum. This practicum is designed to ease the transition of the individual from the role of student to that of graduate health-care professional. Students are permitted to choose an area of concentration based on the various clinical settings available to the School. In keeping with the University's commitment to international work and study, students have opportunities for intercultural clinical experience; to date, these have included work in Appalachia, Guatemala, England, Ireland, and Australia.

The Master of Science degree programs lead to advanced nursing practice in six specialty areas: nurse education, nurse midwifery, acute-care nurse practitioner, acute and critical-care clinical nurse specialist, family nurse practitioner, and nurse anesthesia. The Master of Science in health systems administration is taught in conjunction with the School of Business and does not require a B.S.N. All bachelor's degrees are welcome. Post-master's options are available in all programs except nurse anesthesia.

AFFILIATIONS WITH HEALTH-CARE FACILITIES

In addition to the Georgetown University Hospital, the School is affiliated with many of the Washington-area health institutions. Some of these include Bethesda Naval Medical Center, National Children's Hospital, U.S. Department of Human Services, Walter Reed Hospital, and Hospice of the District of Columbia, to name only a few.

ACADEMIC FACILITIES

The School's classrooms, faculty, and administration are located in St. Mary's Hall. Students also have classes and laboratories on the main campus and in the medical school. The Medical Center's exciting research, innovative techniques, and sophisticated instrumentation provide an exemplary background for student clinical practice. A special clinical emphasis in home health care is included. There are varied educational resources at Georgetown's three campus libraries: the Lauinger Library, the Riggs Bioethics Library, and the Dahlgren Medical Library.

A simulation center contains five hospital-bed units, storage cabinets for teaching models, and equipment for teaching physical assessment. The center also includes a new METI Human Patient Simulator, which is used by faculty members and students, both undergraduate and graduate, in various courses.

LOCATION

The University is located in historic Georgetown. Students come to the University recognizing the special opportunities, the wealth of experience, and the insights and exposure that life in Washington will provide. Located less than 2 miles from the White House and 3 miles from the Capitol, the University is set high on a bluff overlooking picturesque Georgetown and the Potomac River. The Lauinger Library provides a panoramic view of Washington's skyline, including the Washington Monument, the Lincoln and Jefferson memorials, and the John F. Kennedy Center for the Performing Arts. More than 240 other libraries, museums, and research facilities in the city are open to Georgetown students, including the world-famous Library of Congress, National Archives, Smithsonian Institution, Folger Shakespeare Library, and National Gallery of Art. Most international embassies and federal government agencies have library facilities with staff members who are willing to help students.

STUDENT SERVICES

The Leavey Center serves as a hub of activity for social and academic campus life. The building includes three distinct components: a Conference Center, Guest House, and Student Activities Building. The Leavey Center also contains a 450-seat cafeteria, fast-food shops, a bookstore, the Faculty Club, and Hoya's. At Georgetown, athletic activity and physical well-being are integral to the happiness and health of its students, and Yates Field House provides every means necessary to achieve this goal. It is a four-level, 142,300-square-foot structure with facilities for tennis, squash, basketball, racquetball, badminton, handball, swimming, volleyball, weightlifting, and track.

THE NURSING STUDENT GROUP

Approximately 450 undergraduate students are currently enrolled in the nursing and health studies programs. The master's program has approximately 185 students enrolled both full- and part-time.

COSTS

Undergraduate tuition for the 2005–06 academic year was $31,656. Room and board were $10,739 per academic year. Full-time graduate program tuition was $29,448 per academic year. Part-time graduate program tuition was $1227 per credit hour. University housing includes apartments, dormitories, town houses, and college houses. Accommodations are also available in apartments and houses in the Georgetown area surrounding the University. Both the University and the public transportation system provide excellent facilities to meet students' needs.

FINANCIAL AID

Georgetown's financial aid is need-based. In cases of economic need, the University makes every effort to provide financial aid in the form of scholarships, grants, loans, and jobs to enable students to come to Georgetown. The amount of financial assistance given varies with the demonstrated financial need of the applicant. Qualified applicants may be admitted to the U.S. Army or Naval ROTC, which supports a unit on the Georgetown campus. An Air Force unit is available at a neighboring institution. Full-tuition scholarship assistance and subsistence allowances are available.

APPLYING

The School welcomes applications from men and women, without distinction on the basis of race, sex, or religious beliefs. Transfer students and candidates with degrees in fields other than nursing are encouraged to apply. All candidates are required to take the SAT or the ACT. Candidates are also strongly encouraged to take three SAT Subject Tests.

Graduate school admission requirements include a baccalaureate degree, a minimum undergraduate GPA of 3.0 on a 4.0 scale, RN licensure, three letters of reference, Graduate Record Examinations scores or the Miller Analogies Test scores, completion of an introductory course in statistical methods, and one year's experience as an RN. Those applying for the health systems administration program must have a bachelor's degree, but a nursing major is not required. For a more detailed description of the application process, students should contact the admissions office.

CORRESPONDENCE AND INFORMATION

Office of Undergraduate Admissions
White Gravenor, 101
Georgetown University
37th and O Street, NW
Washington, D.C. 20057

Phone: 202-687-3600

Office of Graduate Admissions
Intercultural Center, 302
Georgetown University
37th and O Street, NW
Washington, D.C. 20057

Phone: 202-687-5568

School of Nursing and Health Studies
3700 Reservoir Road, NW
Washington, D.C. 20007

Phone: 202-687-8439 (undergraduate programs)
       202-687-2781 (graduate programs)
Fax: 202-687-3703

Office of Student Financial Services
G-19 Healy Hall, Box 571252
Washington, D.C. 20057

Phone: 202-687-4547
Fax: 202-687-6542

THE ADMINISTRATION

Better R. Keltner, Dean; Ph.D.; RN, FAAN.
Michael Relf, Chair, Department of Professional Nursing; Ph.D.; RN.

Goshen College
Department of Nursing
Goshen, Indiana

THE COLLEGE

Goshen College is a four-year liberal arts college owned by and operated as a ministry of the Mennonite Church. Founded in 1894, the College is nationally recognized for its excellent academic program and Christian ideals. The College stresses academic excellence, international education, and personal and spiritual growth. There is a diverse student body of about 1,000 students from thirty-seven states and Puerto Rico, Canada, and thirty other countries. A majority of the classes have 25 or fewer students. The College motto is "Culture for Service."

The College is fully accredited by the North Central Association of Colleges and Schools.

THE DEPARTMENT OF NURSING

The Department of Nursing was founded in 1950. Programs offered are the generic baccalaureate and an accelerated RN baccalaureate.

Goshen College is home to the oldest private baccalaureate nursing program in Indiana. The nursing program recently received ten years of accreditation by the Commission on Collegiate Nursing Education. Clinical experiences in the nursing major include a wide range of hospital and community experiences. The B.S.N. completion option for RNs allows the student to work while pursuing further education, with classes conducted in the evening hours and individually arranged clinical experiences.

Goshen College's nursing program is highly respected in this country and abroad. Its graduates are known by their ethical standards, personal integrity, Christian commitment, caring attitude, and clinical knowledge. Goshen College is primarily a teaching institution. The faculty members are highly committed to teaching and maintaining up-to-date clinical practice through faculty practice arrangements.

There are approximately 95 students enrolled in the two educational tracks. Students enjoy small class sizes in clinical courses, one-on-one student-faculty relationships, and interactive learning experiences. Students are encouraged to foster personal wellness in a variety of ways, including active participation in sports, music, drama, campus clubs, service, and commitment to a liberal arts education.

The Department's mission statement holds that within the community of faith and learning at Goshen College, the nursing program nurtures students in the process of becoming informed, articulate, sensitive, and responsible professional nurses. Graduates are prepared to engage in lifelong learning and in right relationships with recipients of care and the dynamic environmental system to promote health, healing, and wholeness.

PROGRAMS OF STUDY

The Department is committed to a high-quality program with an emphasis in liberal arts and the discipline of nursing. The nursing program has a basic and a B.S.N. completion track. The program outcomes are the same for students enrolled in either track. Both programs confer the Bachelor of Science in Nursing (B.S.N.) degree.

Graduation requirements for the generic baccalaureate track are completion of 120 credit hours accepted by Goshen College, successful completion of all nursing courses, a cumulative grade point average of 2.5 or higher in college course work, and demonstration of competency. Of the required 120 credit hours, 41 are in supporting courses and 46 are in nursing courses. Nursing students complete the same general education course requirements as students in other majors.

A typical plan of study for this track involves taking chemistry and the physics of life, human anatomy and physiology, general psychology, principles of sociology, and general education the first year. Second-year courses are microbiology, human nutrition, developmental psychology, marriage and family, theories and practice of nursing, nursing skills and physical assessment, and general education. Human pathophysiology, abnormal psychology, pharmacology and drug administration, nursing care of the adult, gerontological nursing, bioethics, nursing care of the expanding family, and nursing care of the child are typical third-year courses. In the fourth year, courses in nursing research, psychiatric/mental health nursing, nursing care in the home, community health nursing, acute-care nursing, leadership in nursing, senior seminar in nursing, and general education are usually taken.

The core requirements in international/intercultural education provide students with an opportunity to learn about the values and assumptions of their own and other cultures. Most students choose to meet this requirement by participating in the unique Study-Service Term (SST). SST requirements may be met by spending fourteen weeks in a developing nation. Groups of about 20 students are led by a Goshen College professor. Students live with host families and study the language and culture of the host country. The SST requirement may also be met by taking 12 hours of SST alternate courses on campus, which must include one in language

The RN to B.S.N. Completion Program allows registered nurses to complete a B.S.N. degree program in about eighteen months. The track is designed to affirm personal and professional strengths. The program is offered in collaboration with the Division of Adult and External Studies (DAES). Each group of RNs progresses through the courses as a cohort group. Classes meet one night a week for 4 hours and vary in length from two to ten weeks. Clinical experiences for specified courses are arranged at other times during the week. There are thirteen courses that provide 40 credit hours, of which 28 are upper-level nursing credits and 12 are general education credits.

ACADEMIC FACILITIES

The campus library has 123,000 volumes (2,023 in health and nursing) and 672 periodical subscriptions (fifty-five health-related). In addition, the library offers individualized reference service, computerized database searching, and computerized catalog capabilities. The College is home to the Mennonite Historical Library and the archives of the Mennonite Church.

Departmental resources include a computer lab, nursing audiovisuals, interactive nursing skills videos, CD-ROM resources, and a learning resource lab.

Computing resources include two large computer labs on campus to which students have access 22 hours a day. Student rooms within residence halls are wired for campus computer network access. Computing Services provides an expanding array of network services and technical support to the campus. Thirteen campus classrooms are wired for computer-generated multimedia presentations.

LOCATION

This residential college is located in Goshen, Indiana, a town of about 24,000 people. Goshen is 120 miles east of Chicago and approximately 40 miles from South Bend airport.

STUDENT SERVICES

Student services and resources include a health clinic, child-care facilities, personal and career counseling, an institutionally sponsored work-study program, job placement, a campus safety program, and special assistance for disabled students.

The College's cabin and meditation garden are available for quiet reflection and contemplation. The Recreation-Fitness Center includes three basketball courts, a swimming pool, a jogging track, racquetball courts, a weight room, classrooms, and an athletic training room.

COSTS

In 2006–07, tuition was $20,300, room was $3600, and board was $3100. Books and supplies cost approximately $800 and personal expenses, approximately $1100.

FINANCIAL AID

Institutionally sponsored need-based and non-need-based grants and scholarships, institutionally sponsored long-term loans, the Federal Work-Study Program, Federal Supplemental Educational Opportunity Grants, Federal Direct Student Loans, Federal Perkins Loans, and Federal Nursing Student Loans are available sources of financial aid. In 2004–05, 98 percent of undergraduate nursing students received some form of financial aid. Specialized scholarships are available for nursing students who demonstrate leadership abilities, high scholastic standing, financial need, and/or the desire to work in a mission/service setting. All the nursing students who applied for financial aid during the 2004–05 academic year received it.

APPLYING

Students seeking admission to the nursing program must first be admitted to Goshen College. Admission to the nursing major is a separate process that is usually initiated during the second semester of the first year. Admission criteria include essential abilities necessary to learn the professional nurse role and a cumulative GPA of 2.5 or higher.

CORRESPONDENCE AND INFORMATION

Goshen College
Admissions Department
1700 South Main
Goshen, Indiana 46526

Phone: 800-348-7422 (toll-free)
Fax: 219-535-7609
E-mail: admissions@goshen.edu
Web site: http://www.goshen.edu

THE FACULTY

Vicky S. Kirkton, Director of Nursing and Associate Professor of Nursing; M.S., Ball State, 1983.

Fern L. Brunner, Associate Professor of Nursing; M.S.N., Indiana–Purdue at Indianapolis, 1990.

Evelyn J. Driver, Associate Professor of Nursing; Ph.D., Virginia, 1997.

Mervin R. Helmuth, Associate Professor of Nursing; M.N., Florida, 1970.

Joyce Bedsworth Hoffman, Associate Professor of Nursing; M.S., M.A., Wichita State, 1988.

Dawn Hoover, Assistant Professor of Nursing; M.S., Indiana Wesleyan, 2001.

Nancy Liechty Loewen, Associate Professor of Nursing; M.S., Georgetown, 1988.

Brenda S. Srof, Associate Professor of Nursing; M.S.N., Oral Roberts, 1986; Ph.D. candidate.

Gail Weybright, Associate Professor of Nursing; M.S.N., Valparaiso, 1999.

Grand Canyon University
College of Nursing
Phoenix, Arizona

THE UNIVERSITY

Grand Canyon University (GCU) is Arizona's only private, Christian university. Grand Canyon University prepares learners to become global citizens, critical thinkers, effective communicators, and responsible leaders by providing an academically challenging, values-based curriculum. GCU is often referred to as "The University with a Heart" because personal, individual commitment is at the core of each instructor's approach to the student-teacher relationship. In addition, students and faculty and staff members share the essential belief that service is more important than self and the greatest blessing in life is to be able to give. At Grand Canyon University, students of diverse backgrounds and faiths, of every race and ethnicity, and from every socioeconomic situation find a sense of community, a demanding academic curriculum, and countless opportunities for community leadership and service both on and off campus.

THE COLLEGE OF NURSING

More than two decades after the College of Nursing was founded, the College continues to educate students of diverse backgrounds through rigorous academic and clinical preparation within an environment of Christian values and with a commitment to the enhancement of health and wellness in society. The College's high-quality undergraduate and graduate degree programs meet each student's career and academic needs, and the spiritual dimension that is fundamental to caring for one's self and others is integrated into every nursing course. The faculty members are experienced, caring professionals who are dedicated to service and the mission of the University.

The College of Nursing is accredited by the Commission on Collegiate Nursing Education.

PROGRAMS OF STUDY

The College of Nursing offers a wide range of professional nurse education programs that are anchored in strong Judeo-Christian values and ethical principles. Two of the three undergraduate nursing degree programs are prelicensure programs: a traditional Bachelor of Science in Nursing (B.S.N.) program aimed at new students interested in becoming RNs and an accelerated baccalaureate-level professional registered nurse program tailored for students with an existing baccalaureate degree in another subject or at least 90 credit hours of college course work. The third is an RN to B.S.N. program for registered nurses who have completed an associate degree or diploma program in professional nursing. Building on the baccalaureate degree, the College offers the Master of Science degree (M.S.) in nursing with four tracks: clinical nurse specialist (M.S.-CNS) (also with optional nursing education focus), family nurse practitioner (M.S.-FNP), nursing education (M.S.-NEd), and nursing leadership in the health-care system (M.S.-NL). Faculty-student ratios in both the undergraduate and graduate nursing programs are limited to 1:10 in the clinical setting, though they are often lower than this (1:6 in the FNP concentration). The College also offers three post-master's certificates: family nurse practitioner, adult clinical nurse specialist, and nursing education.

Students in the traditional B.S.N. program enter as freshmen to begin the prerequisites for the nursing major. The program's focus on leading, critical thinking, teaching, and meeting spiritual needs fosters quality development in each student.

Approximately 30 students are admitted to the major each fall and spring and begin clinical practice in groups of 10 or fewer in the very first semester. During the last two years of study, students spend up to 18 hours per week in an assigned clinical practice area learning to apply theory in direct patient care situations. Students learn to assess the individual, the family, and communities; utilize functional health patterns within a variety of clinical settings; formulate nursing diagnoses; plan and evaluate nursing interventions; and function as professionals within the health-care team. Prelicensure students complete a practicum in nursing as their last course in the curriculum. This course is designed to assist students in role transition and in gaining confidence in their practice. Development of a resume and interview skills are also part of senior studies. As a result of rigorous training and hard work, GCU nursing graduates have an exceptional record of success on the NCLEX-RN, the RN licensure examination, and are highly recruited by health-care facilities.

The accelerated/fast track B.S.N. track allows students who have fulfilled all prerequisites to complete a degree in approximately eighteen months. It encompasses all of the components of the traditional B.S.N. track in a contracted period. This track begins in August of each year and ends in February, eighteen months later. The number of nursing courses and clinical hours are the same as those for the traditional track.

The RN to B.S.N. program responds to the needs of registered nurses and equips them with relevant knowledge and skills. Participants focus on one area of study at a time through the block instruction format. Classes meet one night a week. The fifty-seven-week program requires the completion of 128 credits (45 hours upper-division) that are earned through a combination of nursing core requirements, transfer credits, and earned life-learning credits. Work experiences are applied to meet clinical requirements—there is no clinical testing.

The graduate nursing programs prepare experienced nurses for advanced professional nursing roles. The graduate core provides content essential to all advanced professional nurses, while the specialty areas expand and extend this knowledge and offer the opportunity for students to develop skills in evidence-based practice. The program is offered on a part-time schedule to allow nurses to continue working as they pursue their graduate degrees. The design of the College's Web-enhanced courses enables students to experience a rich and dynamic classroom environment along with the flexibility of the Internet. Class sizes are kept small to allow students to work closely with their peers and faculty members.

The FNP concentration prepares the advanced professional nurse for advanced practice as a primary-care provider. Family nurse practitioners make independent critical judgments in all levels of prevention, including health promotion, health screening, illness prevention, and restoration and rehabilitation for individuals, families, communities, and populations. The FNP performs comprehensive health assessments, diagnoses, and prescribes pharmacologic and non-pharmacologic treatments to manage acute and chronic health problems to achieve cost-effective outcomes in a culturally sensitive context.

The nursing leadership track prepares the advanced professional nurse for distinction in a leadership role for today's rapidly changing health-care delivery systems. This track is designed to apply both the cognitive and behavioral skill sets necessary to be an effective leader. The entire curriculum of the M.S.-NL program explores values, content knowledge, and skills required to understand and apply effective leadership requirements in the health-care environment.

The M.S.-CNS concentration prepares the advanced professional nurse as an advanced practice nurse. Clinical nurse specialists address health-care needs in the three CNS spheres of influence: the patient/client, nurses and nursing practice, and systems and organizations. The dimensions of the CNS role include clinical judgment, clinical inquiry, facilitator of learning, collaboration, systems thinking, advocacy/moral agency, caring practices, and response to diversity. This track may also be pursued with a nursing education focus.

The nurse educator track prepares advanced professional nurses in the nursing role specialty of nursing education and addresses the expanding educational needs of the nursing profession. The nurse educator may practice in a variety of settings. Nurses who pursue this track are prepared to practice in acute- or chronic-care settings as staff-educators and to plan, implement, and evaluate continuing education programs. The advanced-professional nurse educator is also qualified to assume a faculty position in a traditional college of nursing or in a nontraditional program that relies on online technology as a teaching medium.

ACADEMIC FACILITIES

Grand Canyon University consists of thirty-six buildings on a 90-acre campus. The campus features the Fleming Library, which houses a collection of more than 166,000 volumes, 700 periodicals, newspapers, microfilm, and audiovisual materials. Library holdings are expanded by CD-ROM databases, computerized database searches, and interlibrary loans. Computers housed in the library have Internet access to assist students.

The College of Nursing houses a fully equipped clinical skills lab. The lab consists of a simulated hospital room and three exam rooms, all appropriately equipped to enable students to practice and hone their clinical skills.

There are two computer labs on campus that offer Internet access and a host of applications for use outside of the classroom. Each student has an individual login, which includes secured space on a server to store personal files. In addition to the lab computers, wireless access is available for students with laptops.

LOCATION

Grand Canyon University is located just minutes from Phoenix, Arizona's state capital and sixth-largest city in the United States. Phoenix is the nerve center of the Southwest, one of the fastest-growing regions in the nation. Grand Canyon University students flourish in the school's southwestern environment. Surrounded by rugged mountains, lush valleys, and the arid beauty of the Sonoran Desert, Grand Canyon students feel a part of the larger human experience.

THE NURSING STUDENT GROUP

A maximum of 30 students are admitted to the B.S.N. program each semester. Although there are more women, there has been an increase in the ratio of men. The population is quite diverse and includes students from Africa, China, and Japan.

COSTS

In 2006–07, undergraduate tuition and fees were $6000 per semester for in-state students (12 to 18 hours) and $6000 per semester for out-of-state students. Room and board cost $7130. Graduate nursing students paid $475 per credit hour.

FINANCIAL AID

Scholarships are available based on a student's previous academic work and need, and various loan and payment-option programs are available. Financial aid processing and advising are available through the University's Office of Financial Aid.

APPLYING

Application and admission to Grand Canyon University are required for consideration for admission into the College of Nursing bachelor's degree programs. To apply to the University, students must submit an application, official high school transcripts, and SAT or ACT scores. Acceptance into the College of Nursing is then determined by the College of Nursing faculty and availability of clinical spaces. Applicants to the accelerated B.S.N. track are required to have completed a baccalaureate degree or have senior standing (at least 90 credits) and have a strong academic record (3.0 GPA). Applicants for the RN to B.S.N. track must be licensed RNs in the State of Arizona and be employed as RNs and have a minimum of two years (60 semester hours) of credit from a regionally accredited college or university with a minimum cumulative GPA of 2.8. The transfer work must contain at least 6 hours of college-level English. Applicants should also possess professional training and life experiences for which equivalent college credit can be awarded.

Requirements for the graduate nursing programs are a bachelor's degree in nursing from NLNAC/CCNE accredited program; a valid unrestricted unencumbered U.S. RN license with no history of discipline in state of practice; a cumulative grade point average of 3.0 or above (on a 4.0 scale); undergraduate courses in statistics, research, health assessment (FNP, CNS, NEd), and pathophysiology (FNP, CNS, NEd); an essay of 250 words or less describing the applicant's desire to obtain a master's degree and why a Web-enhanced course of study has been chosen; two letters of reference (one for GCU graduates); admission to Grand Canyon University and College of Nursing; official transcripts from all colleges or universities attended; and a resume that details education, work experience, and pertinent clinical experience.

CORRESPONDENCE AND INFORMATION:

Office of Admission
Grand Canyon University
3300 West Camelback Road
Phoenix, Arizona 85017

Phone: 800-800-9776 (toll-free)
E-mail: admissionsground@gcu.edu
Web site: http://www.gcu.net

Hawai'i Pacific University
School of Nursing
Kaneohe, Hawaii

THE UNIVERSITY

Hawai'i Pacific University (HPU) is an independent, coeducational, career-oriented, comprehensive university with a foundation in the liberal arts. Undergraduate and graduate degrees are offered in more than fifty different areas. Hawai'i Pacific prides itself on maintaining small class size and individual attention to students.

Students at HPU come from every state in the union and more than 100 countries around the world. The diversity of the student body stimulates learning about other cultures firsthand, both in and out of the classroom. There is no majority population at HPU. Students are encouraged to examine the values, customs, traditions, and principles of others to gain a clearer understanding of their own perspectives. HPU students develop friendships with students from throughout the United States and the world and make important connections for success in the global community of the twenty-first century.

THE SCHOOL OF NURSING

The School of Nursing began with 36 students in the fall of 1982 as a program designed to facilitate the completion of the baccalaureate degree by registered nurses. In September 1984, the program was expanded to accommodate the educational needs of licensed practical nurses. In the fall of 1987, 24 students were accepted into a newly developed four-year program. The qualities of humanism, caring, and collaboration provide a foundation to the comprehensive study of the art and science of nursing. Students learn in a flexible, multicultural environment and receive high-quality instruction in classrooms consisting of 24 to 32 students and clinical groups consisting of 8 to 10 students.

The School of Nursing at Hawai'i Pacific University has grown into the largest nursing program in the state of Hawaii, with more than 1,300 students in the baccalaureate and master's programs. Despite its size, the faculty members strive to provide individual attention to students.

The education and expertise gained by HPU nursing students allow them to gain experience in the physical, mental, emotional, and spiritual care of clients from varied age groups and multiple ethnic backgrounds.

PROGRAMS OF STUDY

The baccalaureate nursing program offers four pathways toward a Bachelor of Science in Nursing degree: a Basic Pathway for the beginning or transfer student with fewer than 45 college credits, an LPN to B.S.N. Pathway for U.S. licensed practical nurses, an RN to B.S.N. Pathway for licensed registered nurses from associate degree or diploma programs, and an International Nurse Pathway for persons who have graduated from a nursing program in another country and are not licensed in the United States.

HPU's graduate nursing program brings together theory and community-based practice in an M.S.N. program that offers the registered nurse the opportunity to advance as either a community clinical nurse specialist (CNS) or family nurse practitioner (FNP). Students interested in gaining a solid foundation in current business and management practice may pursue a joint M.S.N./M.B.A. degree. An RN to M.S.N. Pathway allows registered nurses without baccalaureate degrees in nursing to make the transition into the M.S.N. program.

Students entering the RN to M.S.N. Pathway are granted provisional admission status until all prerequisites are completed.

A post-master's certificate as a family nurse practitioner is also possible for nurses with master's degrees seeking to expand their practice. A certificate program in nursing education can be taken as part of the CNS concentration or as a stand-alone certificate.

The goal of the School of Nursing at Hawai'i Pacific University is to prepare a liberally educated professional nurse. The professional nurse has the following attributes: he or she synthesizes knowledge from the humanities, the arts, and the natural, behavioral, and nursing sciences to provide competent nursing services within a multicultural society; incorporates the caring ethic as the foundation of nursing practice; develops a commitment to altruistic service valued by society, is sensitive to the diverse needs of vulnerable groups, and has active involvement in health-care delivery policy; and promotes the integration of body, mind, and spirit through utilizing the nursing process, diagnostic and ethical reasoning, and critical thinking to assist the client in achieving mutually determined health goals. The professional nurse also practices autonomously along the continuum of novice to expert through collaboration and consultation as a member of a multidisciplinary health-care team; applies beginning leadership and management knowledge and skills to nursing practice; participates in the research process, evaluates findings for applicability and utilization in nursing practice, and contributes to the body of nursing practice; and continues to pursue knowledge and expertise commensurate with the evolving professional scope of practice.

AFFILIATIONS WITH HEALTH-CARE FACILITIES

The School of Nursing chooses facilities that give students the best experience possible. Within these facilities, the choice of clinical units is made based upon the learning needs of the students. The majority of clinical faculty members are currently actively employed in the clinical specialties and/or facilities where they teach.

ACADEMIC FACILITIES

All nursing lecture and science laboratory classes are held on the suburban and residential windward Hawai'i Loa campus where life revolves around the Amos N. Starr and Juliette Montague Cooke Academic Center (AC). The AC houses faculty and staff offices, classrooms and nursing laboratories, an art gallery, and the Atherton Learning Resources Center, which includes a library with extensive collections in the areas of Asian studies, marine science, and nursing. The Educational Technology Center provides access to both Macintosh and IBM computers and includes a collection of automated audio, video, and interactive nursing learning resources.

LOCATION

With three campuses linked by shuttle, Hawai'i Pacific combines the excitement of an urban downtown campus with the serenity of the windward side of the island. The main campus is located in downtown Honolulu, the financial center of the Pacific, and is home to the business, communication, international studies, professional studies, and liberal arts programs. The Hawai'i Loa residential campus is 8 miles away in Kane'ohe at the base of the

Ko'olau Mountains; it is the site of the School of Nursing, the marine science program, and a variety of other course offerings. The third campus, Oceanic Institute, is an aquaculture research facility located on a 56-acre site, providing a global center for research and education in marine environmental and life sciences. The University also offers classes at six military locations on Oahu.

STUDENT SERVICES
The University has many services to meet student needs, including a professional staff of advisers who are available throughout the year to assist undergraduate students in advising and counseling matters. Other services include career placement programs; a cooperative education program; international student advising; various student organizations, including the Student Nurses' Association; and numerous honor societies, including Sigma Theta Tau International Nursing Honor Society. A director of student life and a residence life staff are actively involved in all aspects of student life.

HPU competes in NCAA Division II intercollegiate sports. Men's athletic programs include baseball, basketball, cross-country, and tennis. Women's athletics include cross-country, softball, tennis, and volleyball.

The Housing Office at HPU offers many services and options for students. On-campus residence halls with cafeteria service are available on the windward Hawai'i Loa campus, while off-campus apartments are available in the Waikiki area, near the downtown campus, for those seeking more independent living arrangements.

THE NURSING STUDENT GROUP
The students in the School of Nursing are representative of the global community in terms of age, ethnicity, citizenship, gender, and professional experience. Students may attend either full- or part-time, with a substantial number of students choosing to accelerate the completion of their degree by studying during summer sessions. Various nursing courses are offered during summer sessions.

COSTS
Tuition for the 2006–07 academic year was $12,232 for freshmen and sophomores and $17,400 for juniors and seniors. Part-time student tuition was $240 per unit for 1 to 7 credits and $510 per unit for 8 to 11 credits for freshmen and sophomores. For part-time juniors and seniors, the tuition was $725 per unit for 1 to 11 credits. Residence hall room and board were $9840, and off-campus apartments rented between $2900 and $3300 per semester. (There was an additional $500 refundable security deposit required for residence halls and off-campus apartments.)

FINANCIAL AID
The University provides financial aid for qualified students through institutional, state, and federal aid programs. Approxi-mately 40 percent of the University's students receive financial aid. Among the forms of aid available are Federal Perkins Loans, Federal Stafford Student Loans, Guaranteed Parental Loans, Federal Pell Grants, and Federal Supplemental Educational Opportunity Grants. To apply for aid, students must submit the Free Application for Federal Student Aid (FAFSA). The FAFSA may be submitted at any time, but the priority deadline is March 1. Several local health-care agencies award low-interest loans to student nurses, which are forgiven for various lengths of service following successful completion of the NCLEX-RN examination.

APPLYING
Candidates are notified of admission decisions on a rolling basis, usually within two weeks of receipt of application materials. Early entrance and deferred entrance are available. HPU accepts the Common Application form.

CORRESPONDENCE AND INFORMATION
Office of Admissions
Hawai'i Pacific University
1164 Bishop Street, Suite 200
Honolulu, Hawaii 96813
Phone: 808-544-0238
　　　　866-CALL-HPU (toll-free)
Fax: 808-544-1136
E-mail: admissions@hpu.edu
Web site: http://www.hpu.edu/Petersons

THE FACULTY
Dale Allison, Professor; Ph.D., Pennsylvania; APRN-Rx, RNC, FAAN.

Margaret Anderson, Associate Professor; Ed.D, M.S.N., San Francisco; RN, APRN.

Patricia Burrell, Associate Professor and Assistant Dean of Nursing for Students; Ph.D., Utah; RN, APRN, BC.

ReNel Davis, Associate Professor; Ph.D., Colorado; RN.

Hobie Etta Feagai, Assistant Professor and Nursing Chair of Faculty and Learning Resources; M.S.N., Tennessee, Knoxville; RN, FNP, APRN.

Janice Haley, Assistant Professor; Ph.D., Hawaii; APRN, CRNP, FNP.

Judith Holland, Assistant Professor and RN-B.S.N. Coordinator; Ph.D., Denver; RN.

Patricia Lange-Otsuka, Associate Professor and Associate Dean of Nursing for Administration; Ed.D., Nova Southeastern; RN, APRN, BC.

Michelle Marineau, Assistant Professor; Ph.D., Hawaii; RN, FNP, APRN.

Catherine Ryan, Assistant Professor; D.N.P., Case Western Reserve; RN, APRN, CNM.

Illinois State University
Mennonite College of Nursing
Normal, Illinois

THE UNIVERSITY

Illinois State University was founded in 1857 and was the first public university in the state of Illinois. The mission of the University is to expand the horizons of knowledge and culture among students, colleagues, and the general public through teaching and research. As a multidimensional, residential university, it has one of the largest undergraduate programs in Illinois, with six colleges and forty-one academic departments that offer more than ninety-five major/minor options. The Graduate School coordinates forty master's, specialist, and doctoral programs. Illinois State University is highly committed to a student-centered focus as evidenced by approximately 90 percent of undergraduate credit hours being taught by faculty members.

Illinois State University has thirteen residence halls with lifestyle options. A floor of one of these residence halls is reserved for Mennonite College of Nursing students.

THE COLLEGE OF NURSING

Mennonite College of Nursing at Illinois State University began as a private, diploma program in 1918. Mennonite made the transition to an upper-division baccalaureate program in 1982 and began a graduate program in 1995. On July 1, 1999, the nursing college merged with Illinois State University and moved from the private to the public sector, making Mennonite the sixth college and first professional college at Illinois State University. The nursing program is located on the campus quad in a building remodeled with state-of-the-art facilities. The mission is to educate students to serve the citizens of Illinois and the global community, with a particular responsibility to address the nursing and health-care needs of urban and rural populations, especially the vulnerable and underserved. There is a dynamic community of learning in which reflective thinking and ethical decision making are valued. The College is committed to being purposeful, open, just, caring, disciplined, and celebratory. Students work closely with faculty members of Mennonite College of Nursing, who actively engage in research, write for publication, give professional presentations, and participate in clinical practice. Graduates possess outcome abilities of caring, critical thinking, communication, and professional practice. Mennonite College of Nursing is accredited by the Commission on Collegiate Nursing Education.

Current research activities of the faculty include the areas of aging, HIV prevention among women at high-risk, evidence-based practice, research ethics, quality outcomes in long-term care, exercise adherence, informatics, and increasing the attractiveness of long-term care as a career choice.

PROGRAMS OF STUDY

In the Prelicensure/Bachelor of Science in Nursing Program, students complete the University's General Education program or the Illinois Transferable General Education Core Curriculum, including required courses and additional requirements. To be admitted to the nursing major, completion of 56 semester hours is required. The nursing major requires completion of 65 semester hours in nursing courses. These requirements make up the 121 semester hours required for graduation.

The faculty of the nursing college provides a curriculum that responds to both the nursing needs of society and the learning needs of students. Students have frequent contact with faculty members on an individual and group basis. The nursing curriculum is four semesters of full-time study. Each semester provides for the practice of skills and application of knowledge through a variety of classroom and laboratory experiences.

Nursing students actively participate in the University-wide Honors Program and the Transcultural Program, which allows students the opportunity to examine nursing care in a location culturally different from central Illinois. In the past, students have had experiences in Texas, Kentucky, Montana, and England.

The Registered Nurse/Bachelor of Science in Nursing (RN/B.S.N.) Completion Program at Mennonite College of Nursing offers full-time, three-semester plans and part-time plans. All RN/B.S.N. courses are offered online. Proficiency examinations and portfolio processes are available in select courses.

Thirty-three nursing hours are granted for prior lower-division courses upon successful completion of all general education requirements. Sixty-four nursing hours are required, of which 33 may be earned as escrow credit for prior learning. Requirements for the B.S.N. include a minimum of 120 hours, a 30-hour residency, a cumulative grade point average (GPA) of at least 2.0 on a 4.0 scale, and a grade of C or better in all required courses. Fifty-six General Education hours are required for graduation. Additional University graduation requirements include a 3-hour global studies course and a University writing examination.

The Master of Science in Nursing (M.S.N.) Program offers two sequences, Family Nurse Practitioner (FNP) and Nursing Systems Administration (NSA), and two certificates, Nurse Educator Certificate (NEC) and Post-Master's Family Nurse Practitioner Certificate. The FNP sequence offers a 44-hour option or a 48-hour option with a thesis. The NSA sequence offers a 30-hour option or a 34-hour option with a thesis. The NSA specialty courses are offered online. NEC course work prepares graduates to function in the areas of nursing education and nursing service/clinical practice. Candidates for the certificate must complete a total of 15 credits. The Post-Master's FNP Certificate requires a minimum of 26 credits at Mennonite College of Nursing.

A collaborative doctoral in nursing with a focal area in aging has been developed with the University of Iowa with the support of a three-year Advanced Education Nursing Grant from the Health Resources and Services Administration. Students take courses at both institutions, with the degree being awarded by the University of Iowa until program approval has been completed at Illinois State University, tentatively scheduled for 2008.

AFFILIATIONS WITH HEALTH-CARE FACILITIES

Mennonite College of Nursing has a clinical network of approximately sixty off-campus agencies, such as hospitals, nursing homes, public health departments, and community centers. Student experiences are extended to include surrounding communities in which specialty health services are provided to various clients. This type of clinical rotation allows students to have a complex, diverse orientation to multiple health-care approaches.

ACADEMIC FACILITIES

Milner Library at Illinois State University has more than 1.58 million cataloged books, magazines, and journals; 400,000 government publications; 2 million microforms; 440,000 maps; and 35,000 audio recordings. In addition, there is state-of-the-art technology in classrooms, including computer, video, and Internet resources. A distance education classroom/computer lab and futuristic clinical laboratories are available in Edwards Hall, which houses Mennonite College of Nursing.

LOCATION

Illinois State University is located in the community of Bloomington–Normal with a population of approximately 150,000. Bloomington–Normal is located in central Illinois, 137 miles southwest of Chicago and 164 miles northeast of St. Louis, and is one of the fastest-growing communities in Illinois. The University is near three major interstate highways and the railway between St. Louis and Chicago. The local airport offers a wide range of flights on a daily basis.

THE NURSING STUDENT GROUP

Xi Pi, a chapter of nursing's honor society, Sigma Theta Tau International, is located at Mennonite College of Nursing. Students are eligible for application to the honor society and the Student Nursing Association (SNA). An additional opportunity for involvement is the Peer Support Program, in which outstanding students are selected to support incoming students.

All graduate students belong to the campuswide Graduate Student Association. In addition, students can become involved in the Mennonite Graduate Student Organization, which is one of 250 registered student organizations at Illinois State University.

COSTS

For students enrolled for fall 2006, tuition per credit hour was assessed at $205. General fees were $52.45 per semester hour.

Graduate study costs were $185 per credit hour, with a fee assessment of $52.45 per semester hour.

FINANCIAL AID

The Financial Aid Office at Illinois State University administers from federal, state, institutional, and private sources to ensure that eligible students have access to an education. Prospective students should visit the Web site at http://fao.ilstu.edu for further financial aid information.

Mennonite College of Nursing awards scholarships in conjunction with the Financial Aid Office and the Illinois State University Foundation. Scholarship information and application forms may be found at http://www.mcn.ilstu.edu by selecting "Prospective Students."

Graduate students may apply for graduate assistantships that include tuition waivers. Traineeships may be available for full-time nurse practitioner students.

APPLYING

For the Prelicensure/Bachelor of Science in Nursing Sequence, a total of 56 semester college hours is required to be considered for admission. Students must receive a C or better in designated required courses. Admission is competitive and the number of students admitted may vary from year to year depending on program capacity. Students may be admitted to the program following completion of their sophomore year in college. Class cohorts begin in the fall semester only. Applications received prior to January 15 for admission consideration the following fall receive preferential admission review. Academic preferences and early admission criteria are available upon request.

For the Registered Nurse/Bachelor of Science in Nursing Program, an applicant must be a graduate of a state-approved diploma school of nursing or an associate-degree nursing program, be licensed as a registered nurse in the state of Illinois, have completed specific required courses with a C or better, and submit one recommendation form. Applicants are considered for admission for fall semester only.

For the Master of Science in Nursing Program, an applicant must hold a B.S.N. from an accredited program, have a minimum GPA of 3.0 for the last 60 semester hours of undergraduate course work, satisfactorily complete a graduate-level statistics course (300 level or higher), submit official scores from the Graduate Record Examinations (GRE) General Test, be licensed as a registered nurse in the state of Illinois, and submit a resume, three letters of reference, and an essay discussing professional and educational goals. GRE scores are not required for those applicants with a GPA of 3.4 or higher for the last 60 hours of undergraduate course work.

All applicants to the Nurse Educator Certificate Program must show evidence of current enrollment in an accredited master's degree nursing program or evidence of graduation from an accredited master's degree nursing program, complete a Nurse Educator Certificate application form, submit one reference from a person qualified to assess the applicant's potential to succeed as a nurse educator, and must meet general admission requirements as designated for Mennonite College of Nursing's Master of Science in Nursing Program.

For the Family Nurse Practitioner Post-Master's Certificate Program, course work is determined for each student after an assessment of the applicant's prior graduate nursing education to determine equivalency to the master's degree core and support courses.

For admission to the collaborative doctoral program, applications must be submitted to both the University of Iowa and Mennonite College of Nursing at Illinois State University. Students should contact the College or visit the College Web site for the latest information regarding the application process.

CORRESPONDENCE AND INFORMATION:

Illinois State University
Mennonite College of Nursing
Campus Box 5810
Normal, Illinois 61790-5810

Phone: 309-438-7400
Web site: http://www.mcn.ilstu.edu

PROGRAM HEADS

Sara L. Campbell, D.N.S., RN, CNAA, BC; Associate Dean.
  (e-mail: slcampb2@ilstu.edu)
Pamela Lindsey, D.N.Sc., RN; Undergraduate Program Director.
  (e-mail: pllinds@ilstu.edu)
Brenda Recchia Jeffers, Ph.D., RN; Graduate Program Director.
  (e-mail: brjeffe@ilstu.edu)

Indiana University
School of Nursing
Indianapolis, Bloomington, and Columbus, Indiana

THE UNIVERSITY

Founded in 1820, Indiana University (IU) has grown from its modest beginnings into one of the oldest and largest universities in the Midwest and one of the nation's finest educational institutions. Offering 838 degree programs at eight campuses around the state, IU attracts students from every state in the United States and around the world. IU's residential campus at Bloomington and its urban center in Indianapolis form the core of the University, bringing a high-quality education within the reach of any student. IU is accredited by the North Central Association of Colleges and Schools.

THE SCHOOL OF NURSING

Since its inception as the Indiana University Training School for Nurses in 1914, the Indiana University School of Nursing (IUSON) has become one of the largest multipurpose schools of nursing in the United States. Ranked fifteenth nationally (*U.S. News & World Report,* 2003), IUSON offers the following academic degrees, ranging from the baccalaureate to the doctoral levels: the Bachelor of Science in Nursing (B.S.N.), the Master of Science in Nursing (M.S.N.), and the Ph.D. in nursing science.

The School's B.S.N. and M.S.N. programs are accredited by the National League for Nursing Accrediting Commission (NLNAC). The B.S.N. and M.S.N. programs are also accredited by the Commission on Collegiate Nursing Education (CCNE), the B.S.N. program is accredited by the Indiana State Board of Nursing, and the School's continuing education department is accredited by the American Nurses Credentialing Center's Commission on Accreditation. IUSON is an agency member of the NLN, AACN, and CIC.

PROGRAMS OF STUDY

The B.S.N. degree program provides a comprehensive academic foundation in the sciences and humanities that is essential for preparing students for a generalist practice role. The baccalaureate program appeals to students wishing to combine general education with professional course work and also serves as a foundation for graduate study. (It is recommended that those interested in graduate studies enter nursing education at the B.S.N. level.) The program takes a minimum of four years of full-time study to complete. The program emphasizes health promotion, maintenance, and prevention as well as managing individuals and families coping with acute and chronic illnesses. Indiana University–Purdue University offers the B.S.N. degree to both traditional and second-degree students, as well as the RN to B.S.N. program. Indiana University–Purdue University at Columbus offers the LPN to A.S.N. mobility option and the RN to B.S.N. mobility option. Indiana University Bloomington offers the B.S.N. degree.

The goal of the M.S.N. degree program is to prepare graduates for leadership roles in advanced nursing practice, clinical specialization, and nursing administration. Majors are offered in twelve areas: adult health clinical nurse specialist studies, adult psychiatric/mental health nursing, child/adolescent psychiatric/mental health nursing, community health nursing, nursing administration, pediatric nurse practitioner studies, pediatric clinical nurse specialist studies, adult nurse practitioner studies, neonatal nurse practitioner studies, family nurse practitioner studies, acute-care nurse practitioner studies, and women's health nurse practitioner studies. A graduate certificate in nursing informatics is also available. Post-master's options are available in all clinical areas and in nursing administration and teaching in

nursing education. Students select a major area of study when they apply for admission. Students may elect to follow a full- or part-time course of study. All degree requirements must be met within six years of initial enrollment.

The Ph.D. in Nursing Science program builds on baccalaureate nursing education and focuses on the discovery and creation of nursing knowledge through evidence-based inquiry. The primary goal of the program is the preparation of scholars, researchers, and future nursing faculty members. The Ph.D. in Nursing Science program has two focus areas: clinical nursing and health systems. The 90-credit curriculum includes concentrations in theory, research, and statistics; nursing science and research; an external or internal cognate minor; and a dissertation. The Ph.D. program is post-B.S.N. or post-master's.

Nurses wishing to pursue additional academic education at IUSON can also take advantage of several "mobility options." The LPN to A.S.N. mobility program enables students to apply previous nursing education toward earning an Associate of Science in Nursing degree. Graduates are eligible to take the registered nurse licensure examination. The associate/diploma RN to B.S.N. mobility option facilitates the application of previous course work toward the Bachelor of Science in Nursing degree. Nursing knowledge is substantiated through "bridging courses" rather than through testing. The associate/diploma RN to M.S.N. mobility program offers a unique opportunity for those individuals who have accumulated advanced nursing knowledge and skill through additional experiences. The RN to M.S.N. educational mobility option is available to qualified registered nurses who do not hold a baccalaureate degree in nursing but who have earned academic credit in addition to their initial registered nurse program. Included are those whose highest academic credential is the diploma in nursing or the A.S.N. degree. Specific mobility courses are offered on the Indianapolis, Bloomington, and Columbus campuses and through distance education, including the Internet.

AFFILIATIONS WITH HEALTH-CARE FACILITIES

The Indiana University Medical Center (IUMC), which is located on the Indiana University–Purdue University Indianapolis (IUPUI) campus, includes the Schools of Nursing, Medicine, Social Work, Health and Rehabilitation Services, and Dentistry. IUMC's extensive diagnostic clinics and five teaching hospitals are Indiana's primary referral hospitals and its chief centers for clinical instruction in the health professions. The School's commitment to practice is also reflected in the number of its innovative programs and ongoing cutting-edge research. The Maternity Outreach Mobilization (MOM) project provides prenatal care to needy women in Indianapolis. The Institute of Action Research for Community Health, which is dedicated to working with cities across the state to improve community health, has been designated a World Health Organization (WHO) Collaborating Center in Healthy Cities. The Mary Margaret Walther Program for Cancer Care Research Center, which is located on the IUPUI campus, is a leader in oncology care research.

ACADEMIC FACILITIES

Library facilities for student use are extensive. IUPUI facilities include the University Library, the School of Law Library, the School of Dentistry Library, the Medical Science Library, Herron School of Art Library, and a School of Nursing reference library. The Medical Science Library houses the largest and most complete health science library in Indiana. The multimillion-dollar University Library employs state-of-the-art electronic information systems technology.

LOCATION
The B.S.N., M.S.N., and Ph.D. nursing programs are offered on the IUPUI campus; Columbus Center offers the LPN to A.S.N. mobility option, RN to B.S.N. mobility option, and selected general education courses for the B.S.N.; and the B.S.N. degree may be obtained at IU Bloomington. Graduate programs are offered through the campus of IUPUI in Indianapolis. Selected baccalaureate- and core master's-level nursing courses are offered over the Internet.

STUDENT SERVICES
The mission of the Center for Academic Affairs is to ensure the integrity of the School of Nursing's academic programs and to assist learners to meet their educational goals by effectively using resources to serve and support students, faculty and staff members, and external communities.

THE NURSING STUDENT GROUP
The headquarters of the Honor Society of Nursing, Sigma Theta Tau International, is located on the Indianapolis campus, where it was founded in 1922. All prenursing and nursing undergraduates are eligible for membership in the National Student Nurses Association and the Indiana Chapter of the Student Nurses Association. Chi Eta Phi Sorority is a service organization that is open to all qualified undergraduate nursing students.

COSTS
Tuition and fees vary by campus. Indiana residents pay $197.46 per credit hour for undergraduate courses and $272.80 per credit hour for graduate courses. Nonresidents pay approximately $558.86 per credit hour for undergraduate courses and $825.05 per credit hour for graduate courses. Students are also responsible for student technology fees, student activity fees, clinical and laboratory fees, and other fees.

FINANCIAL AID
Financial aid, including scholarships, grants, and loans, is provided by the federal government, the state of Indiana, Indiana University, IUSON, and individual donors. Prenursing undergraduate students should contact the Office of Scholarships and Financial Aid at the campus they wish to attend for information. Students admitted to graduate programs should visit the School's Web site for information about scholarships.

APPLYING
Students who are interested in the B.S.N. degree program must be accepted to the Indianapolis or Bloomington campus and begin studies with required prerequisite general education course work as prenursing students. Students who meet all application requirements are eligible to apply competitively for admission to the B.S.N. program.

Requirements for unconditional admission to the M.S.N. program are as follows: a B.S.N. from an accredited program or its equivalent, a minimum 3.0 GPA on a 4.0 scale, a 200- to 250-word personal essay outlining career goals and aspirations, a current Indiana registered nurse license (international applicants must submit evidence of passing the Council of Graduates of Foreign Nursing Schools (CGFNS) qualifying examination and must receive licensure in Indiana prior to enrollment), a TOEFL score of 550 or above for those whose native language is not English, completion of a 3-credit statistics course within the last seven years with a grade of at least B–, verification of ability to use computer technologies, and verification of physical assessment skills. Requirements for admission into the RN to M.S.N. mobility option are the same, except the student does not need to have completed a B.S.N. degree prior to applying. Students who meet the above requirements but whose highest credential in nursing is an A.S.N. degree or diploma are eligible for admission.

The criteria for consideration for admission to the Ph.D. program are a baccalaureate degree with a major in nursing from an accredited program or its equivalent, a baccalaureate cumulative GPA of 3.0 or higher on a 4.0 scale (for those holding a master's degree, a graduate GPA of 3.5 or higher is required), completion of a 3-credit graduate-level statistics course with a grade of B or higher within three years before the date of proposed enrollment, ability to secure current registered nurse licensure in Indiana, scores of 600 or better on all sections of the GRE, scores of 600 or better on the TOEFL for students whose first language is not English (a written test of English is also required), a two- to three-page essay, evidence of the capacity for original scholarship and research in nursing, three references, and an interview. Applicants to the Ph.D. program must also have a research mentor, who must be a nursing faculty member with full IU graduate school status.

CORRESPONDENCE AND INFORMATION
Center for Academic Affairs
Indiana University School of Nursing
1111 Middle Drive, NU 122
Indianapolis, Indiana 46202

Phone: 317-274-2806
Fax: 317-274-2996
E-mail: nursing@iupui.edu
Web site: http://nursing.iupui.edu

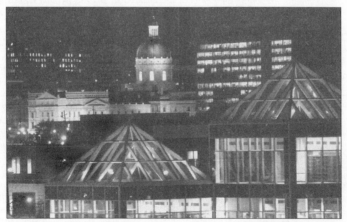

In the foreground is the IUPUI Medical Library. In the background is downtown Indianapolis.

The Johns Hopkins University
School of Nursing
Baltimore, Maryland

THE UNIVERSITY

Since its founding in 1876, Johns Hopkins University has been in the forefront of higher education. Originally established as an institution oriented toward graduate study and research, it is often called America's first true university. Today, Johns Hopkins' commitment to academic excellence continues in its eight academic divisions: Nursing, Medicine, Public Health, Arts and Science, Engineering, Continuing Studies, Advanced International Studies, and the Peabody Conservatory of Music. With a full-time enrollment of approximately 7,000 students, it is the smallest of the top-ranked universities in the United States and, by its own choice, remains small.

THE SCHOOL OF NURSING

The School of Nursing was established in 1983 by Johns Hopkins University. It is known worldwide for innovation and excellence in teaching, research, and patient care.

By choosing to attend Johns Hopkins University School of Nursing, students become leaders in the nursing profession. A Hopkins education provides a solid foundation on which to base a lifelong career in the ever-growing field of nursing. Hopkins students enjoy the advantages of an education at an institution with a worldwide reputation and an outstanding network of alumni who are willing to serve as guides and mentors. Students at the School of Nursing are given the opportunity to participate in designing an educational program tailored to their individual needs. A rigorous academic curriculum, which includes a strong scientific orientation, gives students the background to understand the health-care decisions they will make as professionals. Students learn in an atmosphere where excellence is expected, valued, and reinforced.

The School of Nursing emphasizes undergraduate research. Its graduates are prepared for professional practice through an educational process that emphasizes clinical excellence, critical thinking, and intellectual curiosity.

PROGRAMS OF STUDY

Johns Hopkins University School of Nursing prepares students for professional nursing practice through an educational process that combines a strong academic curriculum with intensive clinical experience. The program is built on the University's commitment to research, teaching, patient service, educational innovation, and excellence in clinical practice. The School's mission is to prepare its students academically and technologically for challenges of the future and to graduate professional nurses who can participate in all aspects of modern health care.

The School of Nursing offers an NLNAC-accredited upper-division baccalaureate program leading to a Bachelor of Science degree with a major in nursing. College graduates with a degree in any major other than nursing are eligible to apply to either the 13½-month accelerated program, which begins annually in June, or to the two-year traditional program, which begins in September.

The Johns Hopkins University School of Nursing is proud to offer the only Peace Corps Fellows Program in nursing. Returned Peace Corps Volunteers are eligible to participate in the Peace Corps Fellows program while enrolled in the school. This provides a unique opportunity for clinical education in community health nursing through the Community Outreach Program while meeting the human needs of low-income, underserved, and homeless families through preventive health services.

The School of Nursing also offers a Direct Entry to Combined B.S./M.S.N. option. In addition, an NLNAC-accredited master's program leading to the Master of Science in Nursing (M.S.N.) degree is offered. The goal of the master's program is to prepare nurse experts in advanced practice and/or management for leadership in professional nursing practice and patient-centered health-care delivery. Master's study and research opportunities are available in selected clinical areas, health policy, and management of nursing and health-care services. The program broadens the perspective of students by requiring them to take innovative interdisciplinary approaches to the resolution of health-care problems. Graduates are prepared to work throughout the health-care system in both the public and private sectors, including community-based primary care, acute care, subacute care, specialty care, and integrated systems of managed care.

Students planning a career path that focuses on nursing care for a specific population of patients may choose from several advanced practice nursing options. These include nurse practitioner in adult, family, pediatric primary care, or adult acute/critical care; health-systems management; clinical nurse specialist; or a combination of both management and clinical nurse specialist as a dual degree. A master's specialty in health systems focuses on emergency preparedness and disaster response and prepares nurses for pivotal leadership roles during disaster and mass casualty incidents. The clinical nurse specialist role allows students to select a focus, such as forensic, geriatric, oncology, or public health nursing. Nurses with master's degrees in nursing are eligible to apply to the post-master's nurse practitioner option, which also includes an adult, family, or pediatric focus, as well as the accelerated adult acute-/critical-care nurse practitioner or the post-master's emergency preparedness/disaster response. Other options include a joint M.S.N./M.P.H. degree program with the Bloomberg School of Public Health in public health nursing or a nurse practitioner role with a public health focus and a joint M.S.N./M.B.A. and the Hopkins Business of Nursing certificate program for midlevel career nurses, which are both offered in conjunction with the School of Professional Studies in Business and Education.

The Ph.D. program prepares nurse scholars to conduct original research that advances the theoretical foundation of nursing practice and health-care delivery. The School offers Ph.D. students the combination of a strong nursing science base, a broad range of faculty expertise, and unmatched opportunities for creative interdisciplinary collaboration.

AFFILIATIONS WITH HEALTH-CARE FACILITIES

The Johns Hopkins Medical Institutions (JHMI) campus is part of a world-renowned academic health center that includes the Schools of Nursing, Medicine, and Public Health; the Johns Hopkins Hospital; and the William H. Welch Medical Library.

The Johns Hopkins Health System includes, in addition to Johns Hopkins Hospital, three other hospital campuses, one of which houses the National Institute on Aging Gerontology Center and the National Institute on Drug Abuse Addiction Research Center.

ACADEMIC FACILITIES

The William H. Welch Medical Library provides the Johns Hopkins Medical Institutions and its affiliates with information services that advance research, teaching, and patient care. The Welch Library Gateway menu leads library users to remote and local online databases, including the JHMI Online Catalog and complete MEDLINE; a dynamic array of other databases, including WelchWeb and JHMI InfoNet; and a growing number of databases and full-text journals offered by the Milton S. Eisenhower Library. The Nursing Information Resource Center is managed by the Welch Library and maintains a core collection of books to support student course work.

The Center for Nursing Research provides support services to the School of Nursing faculty members and students, such as consultation on research design and conduct, including data management and analysis; information on funding sources and grant application processes; advice on career development and continuing education and research; and other resources.

The Nursing Research Laboratory is dedicated to research projects in nursing that incorporate basic biological science methods. The Research Laboratory consists of a dark room, microscopy facilities, tissue culture facilities, a core equipment area, an electrophysiologic lab, a vivarium, a cold room, a utility area, and bench space for research.

Three nursing practice labs are available to provide the student with an opportunity to gain experience and confidence in performing a wide variety of nursing technologies. Patient care stations in the laboratories, designed to closely approximate inpatient areas and stocked with necessary supplies, are available for students to practice both basic and advanced nursing technologies.

LOCATION

The School of Nursing is located on the campus of the Johns Hopkins Medical Institutions, including the School of Medicine, the Bloomberg School of Public Health, and the Johns Hopkins Hospital. Located 10 minutes away is the Homewood Campus of Johns Hopkins University, which is accessible to students via a free shuttle service.

STUDENT SERVICES

There are more than seventy student organizations within the University, including fraternities and sororities and social, religious, and cultural groups. Each class within the School of Nursing has a government board and a president. There is also the Student Government Association (SGA), which includes all divisions of the entire University. Each class has two representatives to the SGA, and anyone may attend the meetings.

THE NURSING STUDENT GROUP

The School of Nursing attracts a national and international student body of just over 700 students, including undergraduate and graduate students.

COSTS

For the 2005–06 academic year, baccalaureate tuition was $23,784, and master's tuition was $25,440. For the M.S.N./M.P.H. and the Ph.D. programs, tuition was $42,567 and $30,960, respectively.

FINANCIAL AID

Johns Hopkins University School of Nursing attempts to provide financial assistance to all eligible accepted students. The School of Nursing assists those students who qualify for need-based aid. Such assistance is usually in the form of loans, grants, scholarships, and work-study programs. While most of the financial aid received by students is based on financial need, many students also benefit from awards based on academic merit and achievement.

APPLYING

The School seeks individuals who will bring to the student body the qualities of scholarship, motivation, and commitment.

A complete baccalaureate and master's application consists of an application form and a nonrefundable $75 application fee. Doctoral applicants pay an application fee of $100.

Applicants to the baccalaureate program are required to have three recommendations, official college transcripts, an official high school transcript (unless the applicant has already completed a college degree), and SAT I or ACT scores, if they are not more than five years old and the student does not already hold a bachelor's degree. A grade point average above 3.0 (on a 4.0 scale) is recommended. Personal interviews may be requested.

Applicants to the master's program are required to have graduated from a baccalaureate or master's degree program in nursing with a GPA above 3.0 (on a 4.0 scale), a current Maryland state nursing license, competitive scores on the Graduate Record Examinations (GRE), academic and professional references, and official transcripts from all previous schools attended. Personal interviews may be requested. Students interested in a Ph.D. program should contact the Office of Admissions and Student Services for individual counseling regarding entrance requirements.

International students whose native language is not English must submit official test score reports of the Test of English as a Foreign Language (TOEFL). In order to be considered for admission, nonpermanent residents must establish their ability to finance their education in the United States. International students must submit official records of all university-level course work. To be considered for transfer toward a degree, any courses listed on an international transcript must be submitted by the student to the World Education Service (WES). International RN students may have their transcripts evaluated by the Commission on Graduates of Foreign Nursing Schools (CGFNS). Students should contact the Office of Admissions and Student Services for additional information regarding WES and CGFNS.

CORRESPONDENCE AND INFORMATION

Office of Admissions and Student Services, Suite 113
School of Nursing
The Johns Hopkins University
525 North Wolfe Street
Baltimore, Maryland 21205-2110

Phone: 410-955-7548
Fax: 410-614-7086
E-mail: jhuson@son.jhmi.edu
Web site: http://www.son.jhmi.edu

THE DEANS

Martha N. Hill, Dean, Professor, and Director of Center for Nursing Research; Ph.D., RN, FAAN.

Anne E. Belcher, Senior Associate Dean for Academic Affairs; Ph.D., RN, FAAN.

Jerilyn Allen, Associate Dean for Research; Sc.D., RN, FAAN.

Sandra Angell, Associate Dean for Student Affairs; M.L.A., RN.

Claire Bogdanski, Associate Dean for Finance and Administration; M.B.A., CPA.

Kennesaw State University
WellStar School of Nursing
Kennesaw, Georgia

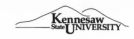

THE UNIVERSITY

Kennesaw State University (KSU) is a public university in the University System of Georgia, located in northwest greater metropolitan Atlanta. Chartered in 1963, KSU serves as a rich resource for the region's educational, economic, social, and cultural advancement, offering baccalaureate and professional master's degrees to its more than 18,000 students in the arts, humanities, sciences, and professional fields of business, social services, and nursing. Although KSU was originally a commuter school, the campus now provides on-campus apartment housing for students in recently completed building complexes.

KSU offers a high-quality teaching/learning environment that sustains instructional excellence, serves a diverse student body, and promotes high levels of student achievement. It educates the whole person through a supportive campus climate, necessary services, and leadership development opportunities and promotes cultural, ethnic, racial, and gender diversity by practices and programs that embody the ideals of an open, democratic, and global society.

THE SCHOOL OF NURSING

Nursing at KSU began as an associate degree program in 1968. The Baccalaureate Degree Nursing Program was added in 1985 and included a generic baccalaureate degree option and an RN-B.S.N. completion program. In 2003, an accelerated track for degreed students was added. In 1995, the associate degree program was discontinued and an M.S.N. program, to prepare primary-care nurse practitioners, accepted its first class. Both programs were merged into WellStar School of Nursing in 2001. All the baccalaureate nursing programs and the M.S.N. program are accredited by the Commission on Collegiate Nursing Education.

PROGRAMS OF STUDY

KSU offers baccalaureate and master's degree programs in nursing. The baccalaureate nursing program offers a generic B.S.N. program, an accelerated program for students with degrees in other fields, and an online B.S.N. completion option for registered nurses. The curriculum includes courses in the humanities and the biological and social sciences as well as the theoretical and clinical practice background necessary for the practice of professional nursing. Generic students are admitted twice annually to maintain smaller classes.

The B.S.N. accelerated track for degreed applicants is an intensive accelerated program for students who hold degrees in other disciplines from an accredited institution. The sixteen-month-program provides an excellent career migration for those with B.A.'s or B.S.'s from a variety of fields, particularly psychology, biology, the social sciences, and the humanities. The curriculum includes both theoretical and clinical nursing classes. Accelerated program students are admitted each semester as full-time students, with fall admissions being assigned to the satellite campus at Georgia Highlands College in Rome, Georgia. Only the B.S.N. accelerated track is offered at the KSU satellite campus in Rome, Georgia, at the Georgia Highlands College campus.

The B.S.N. completion option for registered nurses is based on the statewide articulation plan formulated by nursing programs in the state of Georgia. Upon completion of a bridge course, registered nurse students receive credit for 24 semester hours of sophomore- and junior-level nursing courses and may enter the senior-level courses. This program admits students once a year in the spring semester and includes online, Web-based courses to provide flexible options for the working nurse. Emphasis at the senior level is on community and family nursing, career development, and professional growth. Clinicals are individually tailored to meet students' needs.

There are two M.S.N. programs. WellStar Primary-Care Nurse Practitioner Program prepares experienced registered nurses as primary-care nurse practitioners who are eligible for national certification as family or adult nurse practitioners. The M.S.N. in Advanced Care Management and Leadership Program is designed to provide experienced registered nurses with advanced preparation in clinical management and leadership with the option of preparing for certification as a CNS. Additional tracks are planned in this program for fall 2006. Students should contact the School of Nursing office for further information. Both programs are designed for working professional nurses, with all classes scheduled on alternate weekends. Students are admitted to both graduate programs once a year in the fall.

AFFILIATIONS WITH HEALTH-CARE FACILITIES

WellStar School of Nursing has affiliations with more than sixty health and community agencies in the metropolitan Atlanta area and northwest Georgia. Two of the major reasons cited by students for choosing KSU are location and access to experience in both the major acute-care facilities in Atlanta and a tremendous diversity of other community-based health and social agencies.

The primary-care nurse practitioner program collaborates with more than 150 nurse practitioners, physicians, and physician assistants in a variety of primary-care settings. These professionals serve as clinical preceptors for the nurse practitioner students.

ACADEMIC FACILITIES

WellStar School of Nursing is located on the main campus of KSU. Modern classrooms, faculty offices, conference rooms, study areas, a learning resource center, a campus health center, and computer facilities are all located in the same building. A new Health Sciences Building has been approved by the Georgia Board of Regents, and construction should begin within the year. The KSU library is housed in a 100,000-square-foot building and is networked with online computer databases and document retrieval facilities. Students have access to library resources, e-mail, and the Internet both on campus and from home computers. WellStar School of Nursing has a goal of increasing the use of technology in the classroom and has invested in many computer learning resources that are available to students.

LOCATION

Nestled in the hills just 20 miles north of downtown Atlanta, KSU is easily accessible to its more than 18,000 students. The 182-acre campus is memorable for its beautiful grounds, oak-lined streets, manicured lawns, and colorful flower beds. The University offers a diverse array of cultural enrichment opportunities for the community, including concerts, recitals, art exhibitions, plays, and lectures. It has NCAA national baseball, basketball, and softball championships. Its proximity to

Atlanta offers a vast field of cultural and recreational opportunities, from theater productions and major art exhibits to professional football, basketball, baseball, and soccer.

STUDENT SERVICES

KSU encourages student involvement through more than forty campus activities, social fraternities and sororities, student government, student publications, and intramural and leisure programs. Support services include career planning and placement, personal counseling, financial aid, an Advisement Center, a Wellness Center, and a special Lifelong Learning Center that caters to the nontraditional-age student. There are a limited child-care facility, a well-equipped gym, a campus health center, and a Student Development Center, which concentrates support services for minority, international, and special needs students.

THE NURSING STUDENT GROUP

KSU is a nontraditional, commuter university serving a diverse student body. There are more than 400 students enrolled in the undergraduate and graduate nursing programs. Generic students tend to be slightly older than traditional college-age students, with an average age of 27 years and a range of 20 to 54 years. RN-B.S.N. students average 35 years of age, with a range of 25 to 47 years. Approximately 10 percent of the students are male, and approximately 30 percent have a previous degree in another field. KSU has a growing population of international and historically underrepresented students.

Students in the master's program are professional nurses with a minimum of three years of experience. They work in a variety of settings scattered over the geographic region of northwest Georgia and the metropolitan Atlanta area.

COSTS

Tuition for full-time undergraduate students who are Georgia residents is approximately $1268 per semester (based on a two-semester year). Graduate student tuition is slightly higher. Nonresident fees for out-of-state students are an estimated $5474 per semester including parking and other fees. On-campus housing is available. Special nursing expenses include an initial $150 to $200 required for the purchase of uniforms, a suitable watch, a stethoscope, and other supplies; a $305 testing fee is charged initially upon admission to the program; a $35 lab fee is charged for each required clinical nursing course per semester; and malpractice insurance coverage fees are charged every semester.

FINANCIAL AID

The University financial assistance program provides need-based, scholastic, and athletic scholarships. The Office of Student Financial Aid processes need-based scholarships and grants, government-guaranteed loans, and work-study programs. Co-op programs and Army and Air Force ROTC also help defray costs. In addition, KSU participates in the HOPE program for superior students. Nursing students are also eligible for Service Cancellable Loans and various targeted scholarships.

APPLYING

All B.S.N. applicants must have full admittance to the University, which requires an official transcript from high school and SAT I or ACT scores and/or official transcripts from each university attended, along with a $20 application fee.

Applications are taken for acceptance into the fall, spring, or summer generic B.S.N. class. For admission, prospective students must be fully admitted to KSU and have completed all Regent's testing requirements and College Preparatory Curriculum (CPC) deficiencies. Student must complete seven of the twelve prerequisite courses to be considered for admission and five of the seven must be math or natural science courses. Courses with a lab component are considered as one prerequisite. Applicants must have at least a 2.7 cumulative grade point average (GPA) and a minimum grade of C in each required science and math course. In addition, applicants who repeat two different natural science courses or repeat the same natural science course twice because of grades below C within the past 5 years will not be considered for admission to the program. To be considered for admission, applicants must not have more than two withdrawals per course from any prerequisite nursing courses on their academic transcripts. Admission is based on a combination of grades in prerequisite courses, total number of prerequisite courses completed, and total number of college credits completed. Applicants must meet published application deadlines. Decisions regarding admission into the nursing sequence and progression in the program is made by a nursing admissions committee. All applicants must complete a pre-entrance admission exam (limited to two attempts) as designated by the School of Nursing. Cost for the exam is incurred by the student. Finalists for admission are notified and must attend a mandatory interview session as the final step in the admissions process. Applicants previously enrolled in a nursing program and not eligible to return to their former program are not eligible for admission to the KSU School of Nursing. All applicants must be aware that the Georgia Board of Nursing has the right to refuse to grant a registered nurse license to any individual regardless of educational credentials under circumstances of falsification of application for licensure or conviction of a felony or crime of moral turpitude or other moral and legal violations specified by the Board of Nursing.

The B.S.N. accelerated track for degreed applicants is highly competitive. Students are admitted every semester to the accelerated program, including summer. Accelerated students in the Rome, Georgia, satellite campus at Georgia Highlands College are admitted in the fall. Because of the program's accelerated pace, it is most advantageous for the student to discuss goals, timeline, and outside commitments with the nursing admissions coordinator to determine if the program is right for the student and to review specific admission requirements to the accelerated program, which are the same as the requirements for the generic nursing program. Students applying to this track must have completed or complete a bachelor's degree in another field prior to being admitted.

Registered nurses are admitted during the fall semester to begin the one-year completion program in the spring. Students must complete fifteen prerequisite courses with a minimum grade point average of 2.7 and include a letter of reference for consideration.

Applications to the M.S.N. WellStar Primary-Care Nurse Practitioner Program must have a baccalaureate degree in nursing from an accredited institution, with a GPA of at least 3.0; a minimum of three years' full-time professional experience within the last five years involving direct patient care, documented in a professional resume; a current RN license in the state of Georgia; an acceptable score on the GRE; a statement of personal goals for the program; an undergraduate physical-assessment course; an undergraduate research course; and full admission into KSU.

CORRESPONDENCE AND INFORMATION

Fran Paul, Undergraduate Advising Coordinator
or
Timothy St. Marie, Graduate Advising Coordinator
WellStar School of Nursing
Kennesaw State University
1000 Chastain Road, #1601
Kennesaw, Georgia 30144-5519
Phone: 770-499-3211
      770-423-6061
Fax: 770-423-6870
Web site: http://www.kennesaw.edu/chhs/schoolofnursing/

Kent State University
College of Nursing
Kent, Ohio

THE UNIVERSITY

Founded in 1910, Kent State University is today ranked among the Doctoral/Research Universities–Extensive by the Carnegie Foundation and is one of the largest public universities in Ohio. The eight-campus system throughout northeastern Ohio enrolls nearly 34,000 students. The Kent campus offers baccalaureate, master's, and doctoral study in the Colleges of Arts and Science, Business Administration, Communication and Information, Education, Fine and Professional Arts, and Nursing and the School of Technology. At the seven regional campuses, associate degrees in technical, business, and health fields are offered as well as lower-division baccalaureate study.

The University's primary concern is the student. It has a commitment to providing the academic atmosphere and curricular and extracurricular activities that stimulate curiosity, broaden perspective, enrich awareness, deepen understanding, establish disciplined habits of thought, prepare for a vocation, and help realize potential as an individual and as a responsible and informed citizen.

THE COLLEGE OF NURSING

The Kent State University College of Nursing, established in 1967, offers the most comprehensive program of study in nursing in Ohio, ranks in the 98th percentile in size in the nation, and enjoys a reputation for excellent academic performance, clinical knowledge, and leadership ability of its students and graduates. The associate degree in nursing (ADN) program is accredited by the National League for Nursing Accrediting Commission. The B.S.N. and M.S.N. programs are accredited by the Commission on Collegiate Nursing Education (CCNE).

Since its founding, nursing at Kent State University has enjoyed continued growth, and today it is the largest college of nursing in Ohio. The mission of Kent State University College of Nursing reflects a commitment to furthering nursing knowledge, to excellence in instruction, and to preparing graduates who are able to address changing societal needs. There exists an academic atmosphere that fosters intellectual curiosity, develops professional and personal values, and facilitates the acquisition, interpretation, utilization, and expansion of nursing knowledge for the discipline and for professional practice.

Kent's faculty, skilled in the scholarship of teaching, discovery, application, and integration, fosters the intellectual life of the University. The College of Nursing's faculty members, who number more than 85, are active, creative contributors to the advancement of nursing knowledge and to the improvement of health-care delivery through teaching, research, and service activities at the local, regional, national, and international levels. The nursing faculty is composed of scholars, researchers, and those with strong clinical skills.

PROGRAMS OF STUDY

The College of Nursing offers associate, baccalaureate, master's, and Ph.D. degree programs in nursing. The baccalaureate degree program accommodates generic as well as second-degree, licensed practical nurse, and registered nurse students. In addition, there is an accelerated option for second-degree students. B.S.N. students who qualify may apply to the M.S.N. program and begin taking graduate-level courses in their junior year under the B.S.N.-to-M.S.N. Bridge Option. The master's

degree nursing program offers clinical concentrations in nursing of adults, family, gerontology, psychiatric–mental health nursing, women's health and pediatrics, as well as functional concentrations in nurse practitioner clinical specialization and administration. Post-master's nurse practitioner certificate programs are also available in acute, family, gerontology, and primary care as well as women's health, pediatrics, and psychiatric–mental health nursing. A Web-based certificate program in nursing education is also offered. In addition, dual-degree M.S.N./M.P.A. and M.S.N./M.B.A. options are available. There is also a Ph.D. in nursing program.

An associate degree in nursing program is offered at four regional campuses (Ashtabula, East Liverpool, Geauga, and Tuscarawas). The associate degree program prepares practitioners to assume responsibility for the provision of technical nursing care.

The baccalaureate nursing program is an undergraduate program leading to the Bachelor of Science in Nursing degree. The curriculum includes courses in the humanities and biological and social sciences as well as theoretical knowledge and clinical practice in the discipline of nursing. Both generic students and nontraditional students (second-degree, RNs, and LPNs) are admitted to the program. Currently, nearly 1,500 students are enrolled in the baccalaureate program. The baccalaureate program is available at four of the regional campuses. An accelerated program is available for students who hold a degree in another field.

The master's program is an accelerated graduate program leading to a Master of Science in Nursing degree. The purpose of this program is to prepare specialists for leadership and advanced practice roles in professional nursing. Enrollment in the master's program is more than 225, with approximately 85 percent of these students pursuing graduate study on a part-time basis.

The purpose of the Doctor of Philosophy (Ph.D.) degree program is to develop scholars in nursing who are informed about the many dimensions of scholarship, with balance, and synthesis among research, practice, and teaching. This program is conducted in collaboration with the University of Akron College of Nursing and rests on the belief that strength can be achieved through strong linkages among faculty members and students and among the diverse units of both universities. The program consists of five components: nursing knowledge; research methods, designs, and statistics; cognates; health-care and nursing policy; and the dissertation. Full- and part-time students are accommodated in this program.

A program of continuing nursing education is also offered. The College of Nursing is an Ohio Nurses Association–approved provider of continuing education and awards continuing education units (CEUs) for program offerings.

AFFILIATIONS WITH HEALTH-CARE FACILITIES

The College of Nursing has established affiliations with more than seventy-five health agencies throughout northeastern Ohio for clinical learning experiences. These range from large urban medical centers, including The Cleveland Clinic Foundation and University Hospitals of Cleveland, to small rural hospitals and clinics as well as a variety of long-term and community health-care agencies.

ACADEMIC FACILITIES

The College of Nursing is located in Henderson Hall, a building designed specifically to house the nursing programs. It contains classrooms, faculty offices, conference rooms, study areas, nursing multipurpose and computer laboratories, a learning resource center, a nursing research center, and a 250-seat auditorium. In addition, the excellent services and resources of the entire Kent State University are available. The twelve-story open-stack library is a member of the Association of Research Libraries and holds more than 1.5 million volumes, including an extensive collection of nursing and medical references. The basic science complex of Northeastern Ohio Universities College of Medicine is located 6 miles from the Kent campus and is an integral part of Kent State.

LOCATION

Located in Kent, Ohio (population approximately 30,000), the Kent campus is situated on a beautiful 2,264-acre tree-covered area. Close by are the metropolitan areas of Cleveland (35 miles), Akron (15 miles), Canton (35 miles), and Youngstown (35 miles). The seven regional campuses are located in communities 35–80 miles from the Kent campus. The most populous of Ohio's four quadrants, northeastern Ohio is an area rich with cultural and recreational activities. Among these are Kent's Porthouse Theatre and Blossom Music Center, summer home of the Cleveland Orchestra.

STUDENT SERVICES

A comprehensive array of student services is available through the College of Nursing Office of Student Affairs and the University's Michael Schwartz Student Service Center. In addition to academic services, health services, counseling and guidance, career planning and placement, financial aid, residential service, recreation, and student activities programming are provided. More than 200 undergraduate and graduate student organizations on campus welcome members from throughout the University. Students can also participate in a variety of intercollegiate sports.

THE NURSING STUDENT GROUP

Kent serves a talented, culturally rich student body from Ohio and around the world, including historically underrepresented and nontraditional students. Students in nursing reflect a microcosm of the University student body.

Students for Professional Nursing (SPN) provides opportunities for development of leadership skills, promoting health-care activities on campus, and facilitating socialization into the professional role. In addition, a chapter of the Ohio Nursing Students Association (ONSA) at Kent is active. Graduate students can take an active role in the University Graduate Student Senate and the Graduate Nurse Student Organization (GNSO).

COSTS

Kent State's tuition is set by the Board of Trustees. For current tuition information, students should visit the Bursar's Office's Web site at http://www.kent.edu/bursar.

FINANCIAL AID

Kent State University has developed a financial aid program to assist students who lack the necessary funds for a college education. This program consists of scholarships, loans, grants-in-aid, and part-time employment. Registered nurses may find additional financial assistance through the clinical agencies with whom they are employed. Federal traineeships, graduate assistantships, scholarships, and special awards, such as the Ohio Board of Regents Scholars program, are additional sources of financial assistance for graduate students.

APPLYING

Applicants to the B.S.N. program need to submit a completed Kent State University application; a high school transcript; ACT or SAT scores (for students under 21 years of age); an official transcript from each college, university, or school attended; and a $30 application fee.

Students completing prenursing requirements with a GPA of 2.5 or higher and a 2.5 average or higher in the first-year science courses are eligible to make application to the nursing sequence, which begins in the second year of the program. Registered nurses and persons holding a non-nursing degree are admitted directly to the College of Nursing.

Applicants to the master's program must have current Ohio licensure as a registered nurse, have a baccalaureate degree from an accredited program, achieve a grade point average of at least 3.0 on a 4.0 scale from the undergraduate program, and have completed an elementary course in research methodology. In addition to an application form, $30 application fee, and official transcripts, prospective students are asked to submit three letters of reference and an essay not exceeding 300 words describing previous education and experience, future professional goals, and reasons for seeking graduate nursing education. A satisfactory score on the Graduate Record Examinations is required for applicants with a GPA below 3.0. A preadmission interview is recommended.

Admission to the Joint Ph.D. in Nursing Program (JPDN) is determined by a review committee of JPDN faculty members. Each applicant must provide evidence of successful completion of a master's degree in nursing at an accredited program with a minimum grade point average of 3.0 on a 4.0 scale; evidence of current licensure or eligibility for licensure by the Ohio Board of Nursing; official reports of scores on the Graduate Record Examinations; a clear and succinct statement of the applicant's clearly defined career goals; a sample of written work that indicates logic and writing skills (an essay, term paper, thesis, published article, or professional report); and three letters of reference from professionals or professors who can adequately evaluate the applicant and the applicant's previous work and potential for success. Applicants must also complete a personal interview with a graduate faculty member to assess research interests and motivation for successful completion of doctoral study. Accepted applicants must register for courses within two years of acceptance into the JPDN.

CORRESPONDENCE AND INFORMATION

Office of Student Services
College of Nursing
216 Henderson Hall
Kent State University
P.O. Box 5190
Kent, Ohio 44242-0001

Phone: 330-672-7911
Fax: 330-672-2061
Web site: http://www.kent.edu/nursing

Loma Linda University

School of Nursing

Loma Linda, California

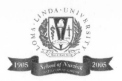

THE UNIVERSITY

Loma Linda University (LLU) is a Seventh-day Adventist educational health sciences institution located in southern California. Offering more than fifty-five programs to more than 3,000 students, Loma Linda University consists of eight schools: the Schools of Allied Health Professions, Dentistry, Medicine, Nursing, Pharmacy, Public Health, and Science and Technology and the Faculty of Graduate Studies.

The University is dedicated to promoting physical, intellectual, social, and spiritual growth in its faculty members and students. The University's mission, "To continue the healing and teaching ministry of Jesus Christ, to make man whole," describes the essence of what it stands for.

THE SCHOOL OF NURSING

The School of Nursing, which was established in 1905, has California Board of Registered Nursing approval and is accredited by the Commission on Collegiate Nursing Education until 2009.

The faculty members in the School of Nursing are known for their commitment to mentoring students and providing a rich learning environment. The School believes that one-on-one interaction between faculty members and students is the essence of study. Thus, its programs are orchestrated to consider individual needs and professional goals. Along with their focus on teaching, many of the faculty members maintain individual research programs with ongoing externally funded projects that provide opportunities for student involvement. They demonstrate both Christian values and competence in their scholarship and professions.

PROGRAMS OF STUDY

Loma Linda University School of Nursing offers students many choices in pursuing their nursing education. Three degree programs are offered through the School: the Bachelor of Science (B.S.), the Master of Science (M.S.), and the Doctor of Philosophy in nursing (Ph.D.).

The following tracks are offered in the undergraduate department of the School of Nursing: basic B.S. program; B.A./B.S. to B.S. track, for those with a baccalaureate degree in another area; accelerated M.S. track, for those with a baccalaureate degree in another area; LVN to B.S. track, for LVNs with a license in California; RN to B.S. track, for RNs with a license in California; and RN to B.S./M.S. track, for RNs with a license in California and a minimum of three years' experience.

The B.S. degree prepares students for professional nursing practice in acute and community settings. It may be completed in eight quarters after the initial year of prerequisites. Students may sit for boards after completing approximately five to six quarters in this program and receiving the A.S. degree.

The M.S. degree program is designed to engage students in scientific inquiry and to apply their discoveries in a variety of clinical, teaching, and administrative settings. Graduate students may select a focus in advanced practice nursing as a nurse practitioner (NP) or clinical nurse specialist (CNS), in nursing administration or nurse educator studies, or in a combined-degree program. Post-master's certificate programs are also available through the graduate program in nursing. Upon completion of the M.S. degree, graduates are eligible for appropriately related certification by the American Nurses Association and by the California Board of Registered Nursing.

The Ph.D. degree in nursing is designed to prepare nurse scholars for leadership in education, health-care administration, clinical practice, and research. It is expected that a doctorally prepared nurse scientist will be committed to the generation of knowledge that is critical to development of nursing science and practice.

ACADEMIC FACILITIES

The academic resources and the clinical facilities of the University constitute a rich environment for the nursing student, both in classroom instruction and in clinical experience. The University Medical Center and other hospitals and community agencies are used for student clinical experience.

LOCATION

Loma Linda University is centrally located in beautiful, sunny southern California. It is approximately 60 miles east of Los Angeles and is located in an enviable geographic location, offering the best of both urban and rural settings. Students can snow ski at Big Bear, enjoy outdoor recreation in the desert, go surfing at the beach, or experience the arts of Los Angeles.

STUDENT SERVICES

The University offers students a variety of services, including access to the Drayson Center, the University's 100,000-square-foot, state-of-the-art fitness/wellness facility. There is also a Student Association that represents the unified efforts of the student body to bring together, in purpose and activities, students from all programs and schools on the campus. Loma Linda University is also very involved in local as well as international outreach activities. International students receive guidance and assistance from the Office of International Student Services. Loma Linda University is committed to whole-person student development.

THE NURSING STUDENT GROUP

The School's primary responsibility is the education of students, who come from diverse ethnic and cultural backgrounds, enabling them to acquire the foundation of knowledge, skills, values, attitudes, and behaviors appropriate for their chosen academic or health-care ministry. A personal Christian faith that permeates the lives of the students is encouraged. Loma Linda University School of Nursing has a low student-faculty ratio, which ensures that nursing students receive personal attention from their professors. Graduates from the School are in high demand and are employed in large medical centers, community health centers, primary-care facilities, and small community hospitals.

COSTS

Tuition for the 2006–07 school year was $485 per credit unit for undergraduate students and $525 per credit unit for graduate students. Tuition and fees may vary according to degree level and program.

In addition to on-campus dormitories, there are a number of apartments within walking distance of the University. The Office of Student Affairs maintains information on local housing on its Web site at http://www.llu.edu/llu/housing.

FINANCIAL AID

Loma Linda University offers financial aid programs for eligible students with documented needs. A financial aid adviser is dedicated to assisting students with financial aid planning and debt-management counseling. In addition to tuition, a student should budget for room and board for a nine-month period if on-campus residence is desired. Books, uniforms, and other supplies must also be considered. Students who think they will be in need of financial assistance should apply early. Information is available from the LLU Student Financial Aid Office at http://www.llu.edu/ssweb/finaid.

APPLYING

For the undergraduate program, new students are accepted for the fall, winter, and spring quarters. Applications can be found on the University's Web site at http://nursing.llu.edu. Students must have completed the nursing prerequisites and have maintained a cumulative college GPA of 3.0 or better, schedule a personal interview with the admissions director, and take a nurse entrance exam.

For the M.S. program, students must have a B.S. degree in nursing and an undergraduate GPA of at least 3.0 and participate in an interview; the GRE is not required but is recommended. A current California RN license is required for enrollment in clinical nursing courses. Nursing experience in the area of the desired clinical option is preferred before beginning graduate study.

For the Ph.D. program, students must possess a master's degree in nursing with a minimum 3.5 GPA at that level, have taken the GRE within the last five years and received satisfactory scores, participate in a personal interview, and show evidence of scholarly work.

CORRESPONDENCE AND INFORMATION

For the bachelor's degree:
Office of Admissions
School of Nursing
Loma Linda University
Loma Linda, California 92350
Phone: 909-558-4923
        800-422-4558 (toll-free)
E-mail: nursing@llu.edu
Web site: http://nursing.llu.edu

For the graduate degrees:
Office of Admissions
Graduate School
Loma Linda University
Loma Linda, California 92350
Phone: 909-558-4529
        800-422-4558 (toll-free)
E-mail: nursing@llu.edu
Web site: http://nursing.llu.edu

Long Island University, Brooklyn Campus
School of Nursing
Brooklyn, New York

THE UNIVERSITY AND THE CAMPUS

Celebrating nearly eighty years of access to the American dream through excellence in higher education, Long Island University is the nation's seventh-largest private university. The University offers 563 undergraduate, graduate, and doctoral-level degree programs and certificates. Nearly 700 full-time faculty members educate more than 31,000 students on six metropolitan-area campuses in Brooklyn, Brookville (C.W. Post), Southampton, Brentwood, Rockland, and Westchester, and at six overseas sites. The Arnold & Marie Schwartz College of Pharmacy and Health Sciences prepares students for successful careers in pharmacy and health care. The accomplishments of more than 116,000 living alumni testify to the success of the University's mission—to provide the highest level of education to people from all walks of life.

With more than 11,000 students and 250 certificate and undergraduate and graduate degree programs in the arts and media, the natural sciences, business, social policy, urban education, the health professions, and pharmacy, the Brooklyn Campus is distinguished by dynamic curricula reflecting the great urban community it serves. Students enjoy the benefits of living and learning in a multicultural environment that promotes growth and a progressive exchange of knowledge and ideas.

THE SCHOOL OF NURSING

The School of Nursing is exceptionally well positioned to fill the need for nursing professionals in the growing areas of health promotion; home care of the acutely, long-term, and chronically ill; and community health. The School offers the B.S. in nursing and an RN/B.S. Connection Program as well as the M.S. for adult nurse practitioners, family nurse practitioners, and geriatric nurse practitioners; the M.S. in Nursing: Executive Program for Nursing and Health Care Management, an advanced certificate for adult nurse practitioners, family nurse practitioners, and geriatric nurse practitioners; a B.S./M.S. Accelerated Program in Nursing/Executive Program for Nursing and Health Care Management; a post-master's certification in nursing education; and a B.S./M.S. Accelerated Program for Nursing/Adult Nurse Practitioners. Graduates of the bachelor's program are eligible to take the examination for licensure of registered professional nurses in New York State. Registered professional nurses who have earned a diploma or associate degree at other institutions may apply credits toward completion of the Bachelor of Science degree through the RN/B.S. Connection Program.

PROGRAMS OF STUDY

The program leading to the B.S. in nursing is accredited by the Commission on Collegiate Nursing Education (CCNE). It is designed to prepare students who are beginning nursing studies to develop the competencies essential for professional nursing practice, sit for the state licensure examination for registered nurses, and build a foundation for graduate study. The program's proximity to Manhattan creates the opportunity for clinical experiences in some of the world's most prestigious hospitals and health-care agencies. Candidates must successfully complete 128 credits, including 4 credits in noncore freshman courses; 36 credits in the humanities, social sciences, and sciences and mathematics; 62 credits in nursing requirements; 7 credits in distribution; and 19 credits in ancillary requirements. Graduates are able to incorporate knowledge synthesized from the nursing, humanities, psychosocial, and biophysical curriculum into all aspects of professional nursing practice; use critical thinking, communication, and therapeutic intervention skills; embody the characteristics of humanism and caring in the practice of nursing; facilitate adaptive responses of individuals and families within the community in the promotion, maintenance, and restoration of health; and assume leadership roles in structured and unstructured health-care settings. The program is also available to registered nurses seeking the baccalaureate degree through the RN/B.S. Connection Program. Registered nurses admitted into the program may receive up to 64 transfer credits, including required core curriculum, prerequisite, and distribution credits. Transferred credits may also include up to 31 credits in nursing courses for work previously completed. Flexible course schedules are available for the working professional.

The M.S. for adult nurse practitioners, M.S. for family nurse practitioners, and M.S. for geriatric nurse practitioners are designed to prepare advanced practice nurses in primary-care roles for adult and family populations. Clinical expertise is stressed, resulting in the graduate's ability to assess, diagnose, monitor, coordinate, and manage the health care of their clients in both primary- and acute-care settings; perform and interpret physical examinations and laboratory tests; select and prescribe appropriate drug therapy for common acute and chronic child and adult disorders; and articulate the role of the nurse practitioner as a collaborative member of the health team. Candidates for the degree must successfully complete 43 credits of theory, equivalent to 495 hours, and clinical laboratory work of 600 hours for the adult and geriatric programs and 49 credits and 900 clinical hours for the family nurse practitioner program.

An advanced certificate for adult nurse practitioners is also available to nurses who have earned a master's degree in nursing and are seeking clinical expertise in the advanced practice role for the care of adult clients. Candidates must successfully complete 35 credits of theory, equivalent to 360 hours, in addition to clinical laboratory work of 600 hours for the adult and geriatric programs and 41 credits and 900 clinical hours for the family nurse practitioner program.

The M.S. in Nursing: Executive Program for Nursing and Health Care Management provides a unique opportunity to educate the nurse executive with needed skills for today's complex health-care environment. The program combines both nursing and business courses, fulfilling the growing need for executive nurses who are responsible for multimillion-dollar budgets, cost-benefit analyses, reduction of overtime expenses, and staff. Graduates are prepared to assume leadership positions in hospitals, nursing homes, community health centers, HMOs, home-care agencies, consulting firms, and entrepreneurial ventures. Candidates must successfully complete 43 credits, including two semesters of internship experience in management of a nursing or health-care organization. The graduate programs are accredited by the Commission on Collegiate Nursing Education.

A post-master's certificate in nursing education is available for registered nurses with a master's degree in nursing who wish to prepare themselves for teaching in schools of nursing and clinical education positions. It is a 12-credit program with additional hours in mentored teaching experience.

AFFILIATIONS WITH HEALTH-CARE FACILITIES

Due to the campus's proximity to Manhattan, students often have the opportunity to learn through clinical experiences and after graduation obtain jobs in some of the top hospitals and health-care facilities in the world. The School's affiliates encompass a wide range of clinical health-care settings, including acute-care and community agencies and prestigious hospitals, such as

Beth Israel Medical Center, Montefiore Medical Center, New York Methodist Hospital, Maimonides Medical Center, and St. Luke's–Roosevelt Hospital Center.

ACADEMIC FACILITIES
The campus has invested more than $40 million to construct and renovate buildings and academic facilities. The William Zeckendorf Health Sciences Center houses state-of-the-art classrooms and labs for students in nursing, pharmacy, and the health professions. Ten academic computing laboratories offer user-friendly environments to work on homework assignments, research, and class projects. Dorm rooms are wired for computers and Internet access. The Salena Library Learning Center provides access to more than 2.8 million library volumes University-wide as well as its own substantial collection of books, periodicals, microfilms, and recordings.

LOCATION
The 11-acre Brooklyn Campus is located in the heart of downtown Brooklyn, only minutes from Manhattan. Some of Brooklyn's richest cultural and historic attractions are within walking distance, including the Brooklyn Academy of Music, known for its innovative drama, music, and dance productions; the Brooklyn Heights Promenade, featuring world-famous panoramic views of the Manhattan skyline; the Brooklyn Bridge; and the Statue of Liberty. The campus is surrounded by neighborhoods the New York City Landmarks Preservation Commission recognizes as historic districts. Close to the campus are the Brooklyn Museum, Prospect Park, and the Brooklyn Botanic Garden.

STUDENT SERVICES
On any given day, students can participate in more than sixty on-campus clubs and organizations. Nursing students can also join the Nursing Association. The campus Frosh Center offers incoming students a support network that includes academic advising, financial aid service, counseling, tutoring, and computer-assisted instruction.

THE NURSING STUDENT GROUP
The undergraduate student body pursuing the B.S. in nursing is composed of students just beginning their nursing studies and practicing registered nurses who seek the baccalaureate degree. Upon completion of all requirements, these students are eligible to take the state licensure examination for registered professional nurses. The graduate student body pursuing the M.S. in nursing is composed of students preparing to become advanced practice nurses in primary-care roles. RN/B.S. students are normally registered nurses who already hold registered nurse licensure and are interested in earning the B.S. in nursing. Candidates for the M.S. in Nursing: Executive Program for Nursing and Health Care Management are nursing professionals interested in pursuing careers as nurse executives and administrators. The advanced certificate for adult nurse practitioners is available to nurses who have earned a master's degree and are seeking clinical expertise in the advanced practice role for the care of adult clients.

COSTS
Brooklyn Campus undergraduate tuition rates for 2006–07 were $729 per credit. Graduate tuition was $790 per credit. These rates do not include University fees of approximately $550 for student activities and specific programs or miscellaneous costs such as books, supplies, and personal expenses. On-campus room and board charges averaged $3140 per semester.

FINANCIAL AID
Ninety-three percent of undergraduate students attending the Brooklyn Campus receive financial aid to help meet college expenses. Parental contributions, government aid programs, Long Island University Scholarships, student earnings, loans, and scholarships from outside sources are all considered by the financial aid office when formulating a student's aid package. Full, partial, and transfer academic scholarships, Dean's Awards, and activity awards are available if the student qualifies. Complete details about all of these options are included in the Brooklyn Campus financial aid information publication, which is available through the admissions office. TAP and Pell grants are also available to those who qualify.

APPLYING
Before beginning the professional phase of the B.S. in nursing program, students must satisfy all proficiency requirements, complete all prerequisite courses, obtain a grade of 70 or above on the HESI A2 tests, and have a minimum grade point average (GPA) of 2.75. In addition, a personal interview may be required. Prior to entry into the first nursing course, students are responsible for obtaining certification in cardiopulmonary resuscitation (CPR).

An application for admission; an official high school transcript, evidence of graduation from high school, or GED scores; SAT or ACT test results; and a $30 application fee must be submitted to be considered for undergraduate admission. Transfer applicants must submit a completed transfer application form, an official transcript from all colleges previously attended, a $30 application fee, and financial aid records from all colleges previously attended.

To qualify for admission into the RN/B.S. Connection Program, registered nurses must possess a current RN license, be a graduate from an accredited nursing program, demonstrate evidence of clinical competency, and have at least a 2.75 cumulative grade point average from previous academic studies.

Acceptance requirements for the M.S. for nurse practitioners include a B.S. degree from a CCNE- or NLNAC-accredited school of nursing, with a minimum 3.0 GPA in the nursing major and at least a 2.75 overall GPA; a New York State RN license; two years of recent clinical experience or the equivalent; three professional references; and a personal interview. Research, statistics, and health-assessment courses or certificate are also a prerequisite but may be completed during the first year of graduate work. Registered nurses with non-nursing baccalaureate degrees may be able to qualify for entrance to the graduate program by validation of knowledge through required tests.

Acceptance requirements for the advanced certificate program include an M.S. from a CCNE- or NLNAC-accredited school of nursing with a minimum 3.0 GPA, a New York State RN license, two years of recent clinical experience or equivalent, three professional references, and a personal interview.

Acceptance requirements for the M.S. in Nursing: Executive Program for Nursing and Health Care Management include a B.S. degree from an NLNAC-accredited school of nursing, with a minimum 3.0 GPA in the nursing major and at least a 2.75 overall GPA; a New York State RN license; two years of recent clinical experience or the equivalent; three professional references; a personal interview; and research and statistics prerequisites, which may be completed during the first year of graduate work.

CORRESPONDENCE AND INFORMATION:
Kristin Cohen, Dean of Admissions
Office of Admissions
Long Island University, Brooklyn Campus
1 University Plaza
Brooklyn, New York 11201-5372

Phone: 718-488-1011
Fax: 718-797-2399
E-mail: alan.chaves@liu.edu
Web site: http://www.liu.edu

Dawn F. Kilts, Dean
School of Nursing, Room 401
Zeckendorf Health Sciences Center
Long Island University, Brooklyn Campus
1 University Plaza
Brooklyn, New York 11201-5372

Phone: 718-488-1059
Fax: 718-780-4019
E-mail: dawn.kilts@liu.edu

Luther College
Department of Nursing
Decorah, Iowa

THE COLLEGE

Luther College, founded in 1861, is a four-year, residential liberal arts college of the Evangelical Lutheran Church in America. The College, which was founded by Norwegian immigrants, is an academic community of faith and learning where students of promise from all beliefs and backgrounds have the freedom to learn, to express themselves, to perform, to compete, and to grow. The College, located in Decorah, Iowa, is home to 2,550 students from thirty-six states and twenty-six countries around the world. Thirty-seven percent of the students are from the state of Iowa; 89 percent come from the four-state area of Iowa, Minnesota, Wisconsin, and Illinois. Each year, approximately 70 international students (3 percent of the student body) choose to study at Luther. The College offers more than sixty majors and preprofessional programs leading to the Bachelor of Arts degree.

THE DEPARTMENT OF NURSING

The goals of Luther's nursing program are to prepare nurses to function autonomously and interdependently with individuals, families, groups, and communities to promote, maintain, and restore optimal health in a variety of health-care settings. The nursing major, therefore, offers an integrated program of liberal arts and fourteen professional nursing courses. The program gives students a broad approach to nursing, providing a base for graduate study or immediate entry into the nursing profession. Following graduation with a Bachelor of Arts in nursing, Luther nursing students may write the National Council Licensure Examination for Registered Nurses (NCLEX-RN).

PROGRAMS OF STUDY

It is Luther's mission to produce well-rounded and capable students. In the context of a Christian, liberal arts institution, student nurses explore the sciences and the humanities in addition to their nursing courses. The first year provides a foundation in the liberal arts. An introductory course in nursing gives the student an overview of the nursing profession. Faculty members advise each student about career opportunities in nursing.

Students entering the nursing program should have a solid background in English, math, biology, and chemistry.

Clinical nursing courses begin in the fall of the sophomore year. Nursing courses at this level emphasize health assessment throughout the life span in a variety of settings. These learning experiences develop new communication and interpersonal skills.

Third-year students engage in a concentrated study of nursing concepts through caring for children and adults with physical and emotional problems. The sites for the clinical experiences include Rochester Methodist Hospital and St. Mary's Hospital, affiliates of the Mayo Medical Center, and the Federal Medical Center as well as a variety of community-based health-care agencies in Rochester, Minnesota.

The senior year provides final preparation for entry into the practice of professional nursing. Courses focus on promoting health and preventing illness in childbearing families and in community groups. One feature of the senior year is the assignment of an expectant mother to each nursing student. The student follows the mother through the pregnancy and is present at birth. Following graduation, an NCLEX review course is available to all nursing students.

AFFILIATIONS WITH HEALTH-CARE FACILITIES

Luther College conducts its clinical nursing experiences during the junior year at Mayo Medical Center facilities in Rochester, Minnesota, as well as a variety of community-based facilities. These affiliations afford students the opportunity for exposure to the most recent technical and personal strategies for effective nursing care. Additional clinical experiences occur with Winneshiek County Memorial Hospital, the Oneota Riverview Care Facility, the Winneshiek County Public Health Nursing Service, Minowa Cancer Detection, and a variety of community-based programs in Northeast Iowa.

ACADEMIC FACILITIES

The 1,000-acre campus includes the Preus Library, housing 350,000 volumes, 1,100 periodicals, and the College art collection. The library offers five online indexes and ten commercial online services and provides access to more than 480 other libraries. Modern, well-equipped laboratories in the Valders Hall of Science are supplemented by several other science-teaching facilities on campus, including a planetarium, a greenhouse, an herbarium, a live-animal center, a human anatomy laboratory, a natural history museum, and a psychology sleep laboratory. The science facilities also include an extensive field study area and two electron microscopes. Within easy walking distance of the campus, the field study area offers an ideal setting for studies in aquatic biology, ecology, and field biology. Five ponds, two reestablished prairies, marshes, wooded areas, and agricultural lands are available for classwork and independent study. The College has a fiber-based campus network connecting a variety of PC and Macintosh computers (in several environments) to shared computing resources and to the Internet. More than 400 microcomputers and terminals are available for student use throughout the campus.

LOCATION

The College is located in Decorah, a city of 8,500 people in the scenic bluff country of northeast Iowa. The Upper Iowa River, which runs through the campus, is one of twenty-seven rivers throughout the country designated as a National Scenic and Recreational River. Rich in Scandinavian heritage, Decorah is a popular recreation area, providing opportunities for canoeing, fishing, hunting, cross-country skiing, camping, hiking, cycling, and spelunking. Three airports are located within a 75-mile radius of Decorah: in Rochester, Minnesota; Waterloo, Iowa; and La Crosse, Wisconsin.

STUDENT SERVICES

Luther provides numerous student services in a setting that includes programming seven days a week. The Regents Center for recreation, the Centennial Union, and the Center for Faith and Life serve as hubs of student life activities. Students are involved in the governance of the College through involvement on college committees and student government organizations. Luther fields nineteen athletic teams and provides more than forty intramural activities. In addition, students from every academic department participate in the broad-based music program.

THE NURSING STUDENT GROUP

The Luther College nursing program enrolls approximately 100 students, with 30 students graduating annually. Since the program was established in 1978, the retention rate of nursing students from sophomore to senior year has typically been 90 percent. Nursing students generally have an average of more than 25 on the ACT and are challenged in a very rigorous program that prepares them well for the profession or for graduate study. Nursing students must achieve a Luther College grade point average of at least 2.5.

COSTS

For 2006–07, the comprehensive fee was $30,670, which includes tuition, general fees, facilities fees, room, board, subscriptions to student publications, and admission to College-supported concerts, lectures, and other events. A room telephone, cable TV, computer access from residence hall rooms, and a health-service program were also included. Private music lessons were $225 per semester. It is estimated that an additional $3000 was adequate for books, clothing, entertainment, and other personal expenses.

FINANCIAL AID

More than 97 percent of all Luther students receive some financial aid in the form of grants, such as the Federal Pell Grant, scholarships from Luther and other sources, loans, and jobs on campus. Luther awards Regent and Presidential scholarships to applicants demonstrating superior academic achievement. The amount of aid given is determined by the College's analysis of the Free Application for Federal Student Aid. The priority deadline for a financial aid application is March 1 each year. Students receive notification of their aid awards after their acceptance for admission. All nursing students benefit from the Bernice Fischer Cross and Bert S. Cross Perpetual Endowment for the Luther College Mayo Nursing Program and Health Sciences Program. This endowment is used for equal-share assistance for the Luther College nursing students enrolled in the curriculum provided in the Mayo Medical Center in Rochester, Minnesota. This is not a need-based scholarship.

APPLYING

An application, SAT or ACT scores, an educator's reference, a transcript of previous academic work, and a $25 application fee are required for admission. On-campus interviews are recommended but not required. Admission is selective. An applicant must be a graduate of an accredited high school and have completed at least 4 units of English, 3 units of mathematics, 3 units of social science, and 2 units of natural science. It is strongly recommended that the applicant have at least two years of a foreign language.

CORRESPONDENCE AND INFORMATION

Admissions Office
Luther College
Decorah, Iowa 52101
Phone: 563-387-1287
           800-458-8437 (toll-free)
Fax: 563-387-2159
E-mail: admissions@luther.edu
Web site: http://www.luther.edu/~nursing

THE FULL-TIME FACULTY

Donna Kubesh, Department Head; Ph.D.; RN.
Corine Carlson, M.S.; RN.
Penny Leake, Ph.D.; RN.
Jayme Nelson, M.S.; RN.
Mary Overvold-Ronningen, M.S.; RN.

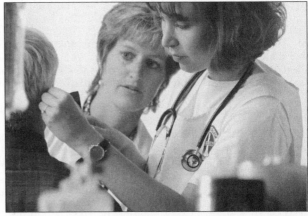

Luther College nursing students gain significant clinical experience in facilities associated with the Mayo Medical Center.

Marquette University
College of Nursing
Milwaukee, Wisconsin

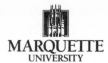

MARQUETTE
UNIVERSITY

THE UNIVERSITY
Established in 1881, Marquette University (MU) is recognized for its rigorous core curriculum and professional preparation in the Jesuit tradition. An enrollment of 11,000 includes students from all fifty states and eighty countries. Colleges and Schools of the University include Arts and Sciences, Business Administration, Communication, Dental, Education, Engineering, Health Sciences, Law, Nursing, and Professional Studies. The location in the heart of Milwaukee affords students opportunities to apply learning in partnership with the dynamic urban community. The Marquette experience is personally transformational as it prepares graduates to transform society for the better.

THE COLLEGE OF NURSING
Marquette's College of Nursing has its roots in 1899 as St. Joseph's Hospital School of Nursing and established its baccalaureate program as Marquette University College of Nursing in 1936 and master's program in 1938. Established in 2003, the Ph.D. program has an emphasis on preparing teacher-scholars, with a focus on developing the body of knowledge related to vulnerable populations. The College focuses on excellence in clinical teaching and health care of the vulnerable, those at risk for adverse health outcomes. The graduate program is ranked among the top 20 percent in the nation.

PROGRAMS OF STUDY
The four-year Bachelor of Science in Nursing (B.S.N.) degree program provides a strong academic foundation in nursing, natural and social science, and humanities. Preparation for a professional nursing role is emphasized through the development of clinical, cognitive, and leadership skills and personal and professional values. Students are admitted directly as freshmen into the College of Nursing, which assures placement in clinical nursing courses. Nursing courses begin on the first day of enrollment. Clinical skills, introduced in the second year through clinical laboratory experiences, are developed through seven clinical rotations in health-care agencies in the junior and senior years. A low student-teacher ratio (8:1) affords personal attention in all clinical rotations, including adult care, maternity, mental health, pediatric, and community health and a synthesis course in a setting of the student's choice.

The 128-credit B.S.N. program includes courses in the humanities, physical-biological sciences, and social-behavioral sciences as well as electives and courses in the nursing major. A University Core of Common Studies is foundational for all majors at Marquette University. Lower-division nursing courses are Dimensions of Professional Nursing, Health Assessment, Foundations of Nursing Practice, Pathophysiology 1 and 2, and Pharmacotherapeutics. Upper-division courses include Nursing Research, Care of Adults*, Childbearing Family Nursing*, Mental Health Nursing*, Primary Health Care Concepts, Gerontological Nursing, Family Centered Nursing of Children*, Nursing of Communities*, Care of Acutely Ill Adults*, Nursing Synthesis*, and Nursing Leadership. The asterisk (*) denotes clinical practice courses.

Additional options for student in the B.S.N. program include a nursing/psychology double major, B.S.N./premedicine studies, B.S.N./pre–Doctor of Physical Therapy program, and minors in Spanish for health professionals and family studies. ROTC programs are offered with the Army, Air Force, and Navy. Study-abroad options are also available in sixteen countries. Students may elect an internship at the Les Aspin Center for Government in Washington, D.C., in the area of health policy. The Advanced Nurse Scholar (ANS) program offers select freshmen entry into the nurse practitioner/clinical nurse specialist, health-care systems leadership, nurse midwifery, or clinical nurse leader M.S.N. programs.

The RN to B.S.N. program is available for ADN and diploma RNs. Prior course work is evaluated, and students may be awarded credits through credit transfer and a validation process.

Marquette University College of Nursing offers the Master of Science in Nursing (M.S.N.) degree and post-master's certificates that prepare graduates for advanced practice roles or leadership roles within health-care systems. Individuals may enter through four pathways: post-B.S.N.; Direct Entry (DE), a combined RN and M.S.N. for those with non-nursing bachelor's degrees; RN to B.S.N. to M.S.N.; and ADN-prepared nurses with bachelor's degrees in other disciplines. Graduates are academically eligible to seek formal professional certification as nurse practitioners, clinical nurse specialists, nurse midwives, or nurse administrators. Seven specialty options are available: health-care systems leadership, clinical nurse leadership, and advanced practice programs in nurse midwifery, children, adults, older adults, and acute care. Full-time students complete the 33–45 credit programs in four semesters.

A 51-credit post-M.S.N./Ph.D. program to prepare teachers/scholars focuses on knowledge generation related to vulnerable populations.

AFFILIATIONS WITH HEALTH-CARE FACILITIES
The College is affiliated with more than eighty health-care agencies in Wisconsin and the surrounding states. These agencies include hospitals, clinics, home care facilities, public health departments, schools, parishes, long-term-care facilities, hospice, and clinics. Many of these agencies offer excellent student employment opportunities as well as financial aid and loan forgiveness programs once students graduate from the program.

ACADEMIC FACILITIES
Marquette is located on an 80-acre campus with excellent facilities. State-of-the-art libraries support student and faculty needs through their collections, services, and connections to worldwide resources. The Instructional Media Center provides a broad range of media support to faculty members and students. Information Technology Services offer voice and data communications and computer-based services to students all around campus, with Internet access from the residence hall rooms. The College of Nursing has many technology-enhanced classrooms and a well-equipped Simulation Technology and Learning Resource Center (STLRC), including SIM-MAN and many advanced simulation technology models for student learning. The STLRC provides computer access, media resources, and practice labs supplied with state-of-the-art models and equipment necessary to develop a solid foundation for clinical practice. Students participate in simulation exercises that are videotaped for maximal learning before entering into complex health-care systems.

LOCATION
The College is located in a metropolitan area on the shore of Lake Michigan with a population of more than 1 million people. The city of Milwaukee is known as the city of festivals and for the friendliness of its residents (the Germans call it *gemütlichkeit*). Students can enrich their lives with theater, music, art, major-league sports, and world-class dining.

STUDENT SERVICES
Students take advantage of a wide range of student services including individual advising with faculty members, student health services, a writing center, free tutoring services, a counseling center, 160 student organizations, and the University ministry with a

staff dedicated to students' needs. Student development includes leadership and service opportunities. Marquette students, administrators, and faculty and staff members provide more than 100,000 hours of service per year. The University Task Force on Diversity attends to recruitment and the needs of a diverse group of students and faculty members and addresses multicultural appreciation.

THE NURSING STUDENT GROUP
Currently, more than 440 undergraduates are enrolled from throughout the U.S. Approximately 10 percent are students of color and about 10 percent are men. Nurses from Kenya, the Republic of Georgia, and other countries, attending Marquette for special programs, join them in some classes. In the past five years, nursing students have earned local, regional, national, and University student leadership awards and have competed in varsity soccer, basketball, tennis, and track and cross-country as well as club sports.

There are 209 graduate students enrolled in the College of Nursing. Approximately 20 percent are full-time students and most are employed while attending classes. Graduates from the M.S.N. programs are employed in various leadership positions that currently include hospital presidents, chief nursing officers of health-care systems, academic leaders, partners in group practices, nursing faculty members, clinical nurse specialists, nurse midwives, and nurse practitioners.

COSTS
The annual tuition for the undergraduate nursing program in 2006–07 was $24,670, and the cost for the graduate program was $750 per credit.

FINANCIAL AID
More than 90 percent of undergraduate students receive financial aid, including scholarships, grants, and low-interest loans. The rising demand for nurses has increased support for nursing education from federal and state sources as well as from health-care organizations. Applicants should complete the FAFSA (Free Application for Federal Student Aid) and work with the University's financial aid counselors to optimize support. Graduate student aid includes federal traineeships, teaching assistantships, research assistantships, Marquette University Tuition Scholarships, health-care agency tuition programs, and other option-specific dedicated scholarships.

APPLYING
Requirements for the prelicensure B.S.N. program include high school academic record; one year of algebra, geometry, biology, and chemistry; and ACT or SAT scores. Interested students are encouraged to visit in person or on the Web at http://www.marquette.edu/nursing. For detailed information, students should contact University Admissions toll-free at 800-222-6544.

Routes to admission to the M.S.N. program vary depending upon the student's background. Students with the following backgrounds are encouraged to apply for the M.S.N. program: those who have a B.S.N., those who are RNs who want to complete the accelerated B.S.N./M.S.N., or those associate degree nurses who have completed a degree in another discipline other than nursing. Admission requirements include the completed Marquette University Graduate School application (available online at http://www.grad.mu.edu), three completed reference forms, an up-to-date resume, a brief goal statement, GRE scores (only if the undergraduate GPA is equal to or less than 3.2), and an undergraduate GPA of 3.0 or better.

Direct Entry students are to have completed the following: bachelor's degree with a GPA of 3.0 or better; 5–6 credits in anatomy and physiology; 5–6 credits of another science, such as chemistry, biology, or microbiology; 3 credits of social science; and 3 credits of statistics.

The application deadline for the Direct Entry program is early January. Financial aid applications are due by February 15 for the following fall semester. DE students begin as a cohort in the last week in May and complete the pre-M.S.N. course work and an

initial 9 graduate credits in fifteen months. At the completion of the pre-M.S.N. phase, they are eligible to take the professional licensing exam leading to licensure in the state of Wisconsin and, if successful, proceed into their desired graduate option.

Application requirements for the Ph.D. program include the MU Graduate School Application, a Master of Science in Nursing with a GPA of 3.0 or better, GRE scores (verbal, quantitative, and writing), three letters of recommendation, a goal statement, a curriculum vita, a writing sample and a personal interview.

CORRESPONDENCE AND INFORMATION
College of Nursing
Marquette University
P.O. Box 1881
Milwaukee, Wisconsin 53201

Phone: 414-288-3803
E-mail: judith.miller@marquette.edu (graduate)
janet.krejci@marquette.edu (undergraduate)
Web site: http://www.marquette.edu/nursing

THE FACULTY
Lea Acord, Ph.D; RN. Dean and Educational Administration Professor.

Cheryl Anderson, M.S.N., M.A.; RN, CCRN. Health-care ethics.

Ruth Ann Belknap, Ph.D.; APRN, BC. Family violence in Hispanic women.

Kathleen Bobay Ph.D.; RN, CS, FNP. Health-care systems, measuring clinical nursing expertise.

Marilyn Bratt, Ph.D.; RN. Nurse residency programs.

Margaret Bull, Ph.D.; RN, FAAN. Continuity of care, community elder care.

Diane Dressler, M.S.N.; RN, CCRN, CCTC. Critical care, heart transplant, heart failure.

Richard J. Fehring, D.N.Sc.; RN, CNFPP, CNFPE. Natural family planning, adult health.

Marilyn Frenn, Ph.D.; RN. Health promotion, adolescent health.

Mary Beth Gosline, Ph.D.; RN, CS. Elder care, emergency care, education.

Kristin Haglund, M.S.N., Ph.D.; RN, FNP, PNP. Pediatric primary care, adolescent sexual behavior.

Lisa Hanson, D.N.Sc.; RN, CNM. Women's health, nurse midwifery care.

Kathryn Harrod, D.N.Sc.; RN, CNM. Caring behaviors in labor.

Kerry Kosmoski-Goepfert, Ph.D.; RN. Critical care, health-care systems.

Judith Kowatsch, M.S.N.; RN-C. Maternal-child care.

Janet Wessel Krejci, Ph.D.; RN, CNAA. Systems, health-care leadership development.

Carolyn Laabs, M.S.N.; APRN-BC, FNP-C. Primary care, health-care ethics.

Mary Ann Lough, Ph.D.; RN. Community delivery systems, chronically ill elders.

Ruth McShane, Ph.D.; RN. Family caregiving, chronic illness.

Judith Fitzgerald Miller, Ph.D.; RN, FAAN. Hope, chronic illness, self-management.

Maureen O'Brien, Ph.D.; RN. Technology-dependent children.

Linda Sauer, M.S.N.; RN. Mental health, dementia.

Doris Schoneman, Ph.D.; RN, CS. Community health interventions and outcomes.

Marge Sebern, Ph.D.; RN. Adults, informal caregivers, home health care.

Christine Shaw, Ph.D.; RN, BC, FNP, ANP. Primary care of underserved.

Leona VandeVusse, Ph.D.; RN, CNM. Primary care of women, birth stories.

Marianne Weiss, D.N.Sc.; RN. Preterm labor, postpartum follow-up, outcomes.

Sarah A. Wilson, Ph.D.; RN. Community health and culture, dying and hospice.

Jill Winters, Ph.D.; RN. Critical care, music therapy, outcome measures, telehealth.

Medical College of Georgia
School of Nursing
Augusta, Georgia

THE COLLEGE

The Medical College of Georgia (MCG), Georgia's health sciences university, is located at Georgia's eastern border on the Savannah River and is the state's primary institution to educate health-care professionals. It is the third-largest of the thirty-four colleges and universities in the University System of Georgia, with approximately 2,500 students, interns, residents, and fellows. It is the largest single employer in the city of Augusta, with more than 5,000 faculty and staff members.

THE SCHOOL OF NURSING

In response to the wartime need for additional nurses, the University System of Georgia voted August 11, 1943, to offer courses in nursing education. This participation in the U.S. Cadet Nurse Corps paved the way for establishing a department of nursing at the University of Georgia the following fall. The program moved from Athens, Georgia, to Augusta in 1956 and became a part of the Medical College of Georgia. The first B.S.N. degrees were awarded in 1958. The School of Nursing, with a strong commitment to research, authorized a graduate program in nursing in 1966. The first Master of Science in Nursing degrees were conferred in 1969, and the first Ph.D. in nursing degrees were conferred in 1990.

In 1974, to meet Georgia's growing need for baccalaureate-prepared nurses, a free-standing, self-contained satellite campus was opened in Athens, Georgia. This campus, for more than thirty years, has consistently prepared one third of the graduates of the baccalaureate program each year. To assist faculty research, an essential component in graduate education, the Center for Nursing Research was established in 1987. In 1995, the Nursing Anesthesia Program was started. In 1996, an RN to B.S.N. program by distance learning was started in cooperation with Gordon College, located in Barnesville, Georgia. In 1999, a Family Nurse Practitioner program by distance learning was started in cooperation with Columbus State University, located in Columbus, Georgia. In 2000, an Adult Acute Care Clinical Nurse Specialist and a CRNA Completion program were approved for immediate implementation. In 2005, a Doctorate of Nursing program (DLP) was approved and implemented, and in 2006 a Clinical Nurse Leader program (CNL) was approved and implemented. In 2006, the School of Nursing and School of Allied Health Sciences moved into a state-of-the-art health sciences building, equipped with the latest technology available in patient care.

The School of Nursing is accredited by the National League for Nursing Accrediting Commission, the Commission on Colleges of the Southern Association of Colleges and Schools, and the Commission of Collegiate Nursing Education (CCNE) and is approved by the Georgia Board of Nursing. The School is a member of the agency of the National League for Nursing Baccalaureate and Higher Degree Program.

PROGRAMS OF STUDY

Degrees offered are the Bachelor of Science in Nursing (B.S.N.), Master of Science in Nursing (M.S.N.) (clinical nurse leader, clinical nurse specialist, nurse practitioner, and nurse anesthesia), Doctor of Philosophy (Ph.D.) in nursing, and Doctor of Nursing Practice (D.N.P.). The baccalaureate program has a community-based curriculum that incorporates a wide variety of clinical experiences in inpatient, outpatient, and community settings. As part of the baccalaureate program, a B.S.N. completion program for registered nurses is offered online.

The Master of Science in Nursing program offers specialties in adult and community health nursing, clinical nurse leader (new), family nurse practitioner studies, and nursing anesthesia.

The Ph.D. program specialty is health care across the life span. The D.N.P. is one of only ten such programs in the nation providing advanced practice education for nurse clinicians.

AFFILIATIONS WITH HEALTH-CARE FACILITIES

MCG's campus includes MCG Hospital, the Children's Medical Center, and more than eighty specialty clinics. The MCG Medical Center complex forms the core of MCG Health System's facilities and includes a 478-bed hospital, an Ambulatory Care Center with more than eighty outpatient clinics in one convenient setting, a Specialized Care Center housing a thirteen-county regional trauma center, and a 154-bed Children's Medical Center. The facility is a leading referral center for Georgia and the region. To meet the clinical learning needs of students and the baccalaureate program, more than 275 contracts exist between the School of Nursing and a variety of health-care agencies throughout Georgia and South Carolina.

ACADEMIC FACILITIES

The five-school campus of almost 90 acres includes forty-seven buildings, with construction of new buildings plus expansion and renovation of present buildings continuing the growth trend of the institution.

The University operates community outreach clinics in twenty-eight counties. Telemedicine sites are located throughout the state. The institution also has a satellite campus in Athens, Georgia, and delivers distance learning to students in Albany, Atlanta, Barnesville, Columbus, Morrow, and Valdosta. The University houses a large multimedia library that participates in the state library system, GALILEO, with MERLIN. GALILEO provides access to more than fifty databases and services pertinent to undergraduate studies. The library also offers an extensive public computing area with Macintosh and IBM-compatible microcomputers, terminals with access to MERLIN and GALILEO, and programs for word processing, spreadsheets, graphics, and other services. In addition, students have access to computers within their respective schools.

LOCATION

Augusta, the second-largest city in Georgia, is located on the south bank of the Savannah River, midway between the Great Smokey Mountains and the Atlantic Ocean. It is a growing and thriving city with a metropolitan-area population of around 200,000, and was recently ranked as the second most favorable place to live in Georgia. The area is known for its balmy climate, with an annual mean temperature of 64 degrees.

Founded in 1836 by General James Oglethorpe, Augusta is Georgia's second-oldest city. Augusta was Georgia's capital in 1778 and from 1785 to 1795. The city offers a wide array of cultural and recreational activities. Augusta has an impressive riverwalk, the site of many activities such as the Augusta Invitation Regatta, a national collegiate rowing event. The city also is a short drive from Lake Thurmond Reservoir, the site of such outdoor activities as waterskiing, swimming, boating, and camping. Augusta is world-renowned as the home of the Masters Golf Tournament.

Augusta has many associations dedicated to the performing and visual arts, including the Augusta Opera Association, the Augusta Ballet, the Augusta Players, the Augusta Children's Theatre, the Augusta Symphony, and the Augusta Art Association. The Medical College of Georgia, Augusta State University, and Paine College often bring prestigious films, speakers, and special events to the city.

Augusta offers exceptional shopping and features a downtown art and antiques district. The area's hundreds of restaurants range from fine to casual dining, featuring everything from ethnic specialties to burgers.

Augusta is within an easy 3-hour drive to Atlanta, the University of Georgia, the Atlantic Ocean, and the mountains.

Augusta is a leading health-care center of the Southeast and has a rapidly developing and diversified industrial base. The area's nine hospitals serve the Southeast and beyond.

STUDENT SERVICES

MCG's Student Health Services provides primary care for MCG students' medical, dental, and psychological needs. The Minority Academic Advisement Program ensures the recruitment and retention of minority students in schools through the University System of Georgia. The School of Nursing houses the Learning Resources Center and Simulation Center, where students train to manage emergencies in a safe, controlled, and replicable environment and learn psychomotor skills needed to practice nursing. Students also have access to computers, audiovisual materials, nursing journals, and classroom materials.

THE NURSING STUDENT GROUP

Student life at the Medical College of Georgia offers many learning experiences in a variety of settings. The School of Nursing has approximately 350 undergraduate students and 150 graduate students. Many student organizations are available to enhance the student's career, including the Georgia Association of Nursing Students (GANS); the IMHOTEP-Leadership Honor Society; MCG Student Government Association; Sigma Theta Tau, Beta Omicron Chapter; and Phi Chi Beta of Chi Eta Phi

Sorority. The Augusta and Athens chapters of GANS are active on local, state, and national levels. Several students have held national offices.

COSTS

Full-time undergraduate tuition for 2006–07 was $2250 for in-state students and $7965 for out-of-state students per semester. Part-time tuition costs were $160 per credit hour for in-state students and $637 per credit hour for out-of-state students. On-campus housing costs ranged from $1278 to $1750; off-campus room and board expenses ranged from $9000 to $13,000. Books, uniforms, and equipment fees were approximately $400 to $800 per academic year.

FINANCIAL AID

For a copy of the *Student Financial Aid Bulletin*, students should contact the Financial Aid Office (706-721-4901) or refer to the Web site (http://www.mcg.edu/students/finaid/). A limited number of part-time employment opportunities are available through the MCG Personnel Office.

APPLYING

Admission to the Medical College of Georgia School of Nursing is based on high school graduation or its equivalent; scores on the SAT or ACT; cumulative GPA, with some preference given for outstanding grades in courses supporting nursing; completion of all prerequisite course work; and references.

CORRESPONDENCE AND INFORMATION

Office of Academic Admissions
AA-170 Kelly Building
Medical College of Georgia
Augusta, Georgia 30912

Phone: 706-721-2725
      800-519-3388 (toll-free)
Fax: 706-721-0186
E-mail: underadm@mail.mcg.edu
      gradadm@mail.mcg.edu
Web site: http://www.mcg.edu/son

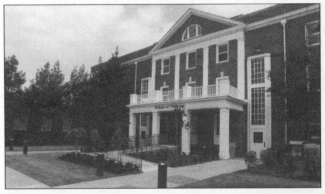

The School of Nursing was founded in 1943 and serves as the University System of Georgia's flagship nursing school, meeting the challenges of an evolving health-care system.

MGH Institute of Health Professions
Graduate Program in Nursing
Boston, Massachusetts

THE SCHOOL

The MGH Institute of Health Professions, founded in 1977, is an innovative graduate school affiliated with the internationally known Massachusetts General Hospital (MGH). The Institute offers programs in nursing, communication sciences and disorders, physical therapy, clinical investigation, and medical imaging. A faculty of more than 80 members, half of whom are practicing clinicians, teaches more than 750 students. The Institute is accredited by the New England Association of Schools and Colleges. The Graduate Program in Nursing is approved by the Board of Registration in Nursing of the Commonwealth of Massachusetts and is accredited by the National League for Nursing Accrediting Commission.

Located in Boston, the Institute was formed to meet the need for master clinicians—leaders in the health-care professions with an education formed by theory and simultaneous practice and based upon a thorough understanding of specialized clinical practice, planning and management of clinical services, and research. The Institute offers an impressive student-faculty ratio of 7:1, enabling students to receive personalized attention from faculty members. The setting also promotes small-group interactions that advance the health professions through interdisciplinary models of education, research, and practice. For more information, prospective students should consult the Institute's Web site, listed in this In-Depth Description.

THE NURSING PROGRAM

With internationally recognized faculty members who are researchers, clinicians, and mentors to students, the Graduate Program in Nursing is designed to prepare advanced practice nurses to assume leadership roles in the health-care system of the future. This includes engaging diverse individuals, families, groups, and communities in pursuit of healing and wholeness, by providing excellence and innovation in education, scholarship, and service.

The program is based on the philosophy that nursing is caring for the body, mind, and spirit of persons in relation to their environment at every level of human connection: individuals, families, groups, and communities. From this framework, nursing addresses promotion, maintenance, and restoration of health while underscoring the political, economic, and social forces that have impacted a person. These forces create a diverse environment within which nursing seeks to maximize health at every level of human existence.

The Graduate Program in Nursing is the largest program at the MGH Institute of Health Professions and has more than 200 students. The Master of Science in Nursing (M.S.N.) degree program accepts both college graduates and nurses with bachelor's degrees in nursing and other fields. A nondegree Certificate of Advanced Study (CAS) is available for RNs holding a master's degree in nursing. Registered nurses with an associate degree in nursing or diploma in nursing are also eligible for admission provided they have completed specific prerequisite general education requirements. Upon graduation, all students are eligible to take nurse practitioner certification and clinical nurse specialist examinations in their selected specialty or specialties.

PROGRAMS OF STUDY

The Graduate Program in Nursing offers the following programs of study, which are designed to be congruent with the individual student's prior preparation and professional goals: Master of Science in Nursing degree for college graduates (entry-level program); Master of Science in Nursing degree for registered nurses with an associate degree in nursing, a diploma in nursing, or a bachelor's degree in nursing or other discipline (RN-to-M.S. program); and Certificates of Advanced Study in primary care, psychiatric–mental health, and acute care for registered nurses holding a Master of Science degree in nursing (CAS program).

There are also certificate programs for non-degree students. The HIV/AIDS care certificate is a 9-credit program. Health-care educators can earn the 9-credit Teaching and Learning Certificate or take the

15-credit option for a Certificate of Advanced Studies. These programs are offered on a distance-learning platform.

A new, fourteen-month entry-level Fast Track B.S.N. is planned to be offered summer 2008

The current Master's entry-level program requires three years of full-time study (no summers) and consists of generalist and advanced practice courses. Upon successful completion of the generalist courses (at the end of the fall semester, year two), entry-level students are eligible to apply for and take the examination for registered nurse licensure (NCLEX-RN®). The Massachusetts Board of Registration in Nursing administers this examination. All entry-level students must achieve RN licensure prior to entering the final (third) year of their program. RN and CAS students may complete the program on a full- or part-time basis, with courses offered in the daytime, evenings, and during the summer. Total credits depend on the specialties selected.

All programs offer opportunities to develop specializations in a variety of areas. Current specialties include acute-care and primary-care specialties in family, pediatrics, and general adult. Dual primary-care specialties are available in adult/women's health, adult/gerontology, adult/HIV/AIDS, and adult/psychiatric–mental health. Upon graduation, all students are eligible to sit for one or more nurse practitioner certification examinations within selected clinical specialties. Prospective students should see the Institute's online catalog by visiting the Web site for additional information and curriculum plans.

The Graduate Program in Nursing has an outstanding faculty, with strong academic preparation and clinical expertise, reflecting diverse backgrounds and geographical origins. Faculty members practice in a variety of health-care settings and maintain active programs of clinical research in areas such as maternal-infant health, aging, women's health, HIV/AIDS, spirituality and health, and cultural diversity. Through their practice, research, and scholarship, faculty members provide excellent role models for student learning and professional practice.

Institute students have a high pass rate in both the RN licensure (NCLEX-RN) and Advanced Practice Certification exams. Over the past few years, 94–100 percent of first-time takers have passed the NCLEX-RN. All entry-level nursing students have successfully passed the exam prior to entering their third year of study. Advanced Practice Certification pass rates and scores are consistently above national averages.

AFFILIATIONS WITH HEALTH-CARE FACILITIES

The MGH Institute of Health Professions is affiliated with Massachusetts General Hospital and Partners HealthCare System. Established in 1994, Partners was created by the affiliation of Massachusetts General Hospital and Brigham and Women's Hospital. The Partners system also includes area community health centers and hospitals, the Institute, and many private primary-care practices throughout New England. Partners provides primary and specialty care and serves as a referral center for patients throughout the region and around the world. Its clinical facilities are an extraordinary resource for the education of health-care professionals. Affiliations also exist with a large number of clinical sites in the Boston area and nationwide. Students work with and are precepted by highly experienced clinicians in a wide variety of settings: community health centers, homeless shelters, outpatient clinics, elderly housing, private practices, health maintenance organizations, nurse-managed clinics, school-based clinics, and various acute-care settings, among others.

With more than 400 contractual agreements throughout the greater New England area, clinical learning offers the setting whereby theory is joined with practice to increase students' confidence in their skills, clinical judgment, and ability to make a valuable contribution to improving health care within society. In addition, many students find part-time work in these institutions during their course of study. Entry-level students often work full-time during the summer, first as patient care assistants and then as RNs during the second summer. This provides an opportunity to gain additional nursing experience prior to graduation.

ACADEMIC FACILITIES
Clinical and research opportunities are provided at MGH and in more than 500 other major health-care centers and community settings in the greater Boston area. Through MGH's Treadwell Library, which contains major basic science, medical, and nursing collections, students may access online computer databases and an extensive reference and periodical collection. The Institute's Ruth Sleeper Learning Center provides computers and modern technology for interactive learning.

LOCATION
Located in the historic Charlestown Navy Yard, overlooking Boston's famed waterfront, the Institute offers students a stimulating environment. There are numerous opportunities for extracurricular activities, including theaters, museums, concerts, and professional sports events. Boston has an excellent public transportation system and is located in proximity to rivers, lakes, mountains, and parks.

STUDENT SERVICES
The Office of Student Affairs offers a wide variety of student services, including student activities and programming. The office also advises student government, provides financial support for the National Student Nurses Association and student conferences, and oversees accommodations for students with disabilities.

THE NURSING STUDENT GROUP
Institute students come from a wide variety of disciplines and educational backgrounds. Entry-level students vary from new liberal arts or basic science graduates to students with a master's or Ph.D. degree and strong experience in another field. RN students also have diverse backgrounds and bring their unique nursing experience to share. The wide age range and diverse backgrounds enhance learning opportunities for all. Exposure to different ideas is provided, and the development of the skills and ability for critical thinking and collaboration are strengthened.

COSTS
Tuition for the 2006–07 academic year was $800 per credit hour, with the number of credits dependent on individual program requirements. A general student fee is assessed each semester for lab and clinical expenses, technical support, and student services. Books and supplies cost about $1500 per year.

FINANCIAL AID
Financial assistance is supplemental to the student's financial resources. Whenever possible, financial need is met through a combination of sources that may include federal loans, scholarships, graduate assistantships, and federal traineeships.

APPLYING
Entry-level students are graduates of baccalaureate programs in fields other than nursing and must complete prerequisite course work in anatomy, physiology, chemistry, microbiology, nutrition, and statistics before matriculation. Applicants may complete those prerequisites, with the exception of statistics, at the Institute in "Science Summer," the summer preceding matriculation. RN program students must hold a bachelor's degree in nursing, an associate degree in nursing, or a diploma in nursing. Prerequisites include a statistics course and a current RN license. Associate degree and diploma students are required to successfully complete additional general education prerequisites. All applicants must take the Graduate Record Examinations (GRE) unless they qualify for a waiver as explained in the Institute's application instructions. Advanced Practice Certificate applicants are not required to take the GRE. Prospective students should see the Institute's online catalog by visiting the Web site for admission application requirements and available nurse practitioner specialty areas.

CORRESPONDENCE AND INFORMATION
Office of Student Affairs
MGH Institute of Health Professions
P.O. Box 6357
Boston, Massachusetts 02114-0016

Phone: 617-726-3140
Fax: 617-726-8010
E-mail: admissions@mghihp.edu
Web site: http://www.mghihp.edu

THE FACULTY
Linda Andrist, Associate Professor; Ph.D., Brandeis; RN,C; WHNP. Women's health research.

Deborah Bradford, Clinical Instructor; M.S.N., Boston College; RN, ANP.

Cheryl Cahill, Amelia Peabody Professor in Nursing Research; Ph.D., Michigan; RN.

Jeanne Cartier, Assistant Professor: Ph.D., Massachusetts Lowell; APRN,BC.

Margery Chisholm, Professor and Director; Ed.D., Boston University; RN, CS, ABPP.

Steve Coffey, Clinical Instructor; M.S.N., Syracuse; RN,C; ARNP.

Inge Corless, FAAN Professor; Ph.D., Brown; RN. HIV/AIDS and palliative-care research.

Deborah D'Avolio, Assistant Professor; Ph.D., Boston College; RN, ANP; Hartford Fellow. Geriatric health care and domestic violence research.

Elizabeth Friedlander, Clinical Assistant Professor; Ph.D., Capella; RNC, ANP.

Janice Goodman, Assistant Professor; Ph.D., Boston College; APRN,BC; IBCLC.

Alex Hoyt, Instructor; M.S.N., MGH Institute of Health Professions; RNC, FNP.

Veronica Kane, Clinical Assistant Professor; Ph.D., Capella; RNC, PNP.

Ursula Kelly, Assistant Professor; Ph.D., Boston College; APRN. Domestic violence in Latina women.

Elissa Ladd, Clinical Instructor; Ph.D., Massachusetts Boston; APRN, ANP/FNP.

Ellen Long-Middleton, Assistant Professor; Ph.D., Boston College; RNC, FNP.

Ruth Palan Lopez, Assistant Clinical Professor; Ph.D., Boston College; APRN,BC. Gerontology research.

Patricia Lussier-Duynstee, Assistant Professor; Ph.D., Massachusetts Lowell; RN. Community health.

Talli McCormick, Clinical Assistant Professor; M.S.N., MGH Institute of Health Professions; RNC, GNP. Gerontology research.

Diane Feeney Mahoney, Jacques Mohr Professor of Geriatric Nursing and Director of Gerontechnology; Ph.D., Brandeis; ARNP,BC. Gerontology and technology.

Janice Bell Meisenhelder, Associate Professor; D.N.Sc., Boston University; RN. Spirituality research.

Jacqueline Sue Myers, Assistant Professor; Ph.D., George Mason; RN, PNP.

Patrice Nicholas, Professor; M.P.H., Harvard; D.N.Sc., Boston University; RNC, ANP; Fulbright Fellow.

Joanne O'Sullivan, Assistant Professor; M.S.N., Ph.D., Boston College; RN, FNP. Adolescent research.

Alexandra Paul-Simon, Assistant Professor; Ph.D., Boston College; RN.

Patricia Reidy, Assistant Clinical Professor; M.S., Massachusetts Lowell; APRN; FNP,BC.

Deborah Rosenbloom-Brunton, Clinical Instructor; M.S.N., MGH Institute of Health Professions; APRN,BC.

Pamela Senesac, Assistant Professor and Associate Director of Academic Programs; Ph.D., Boston College; RN.

Katherine Simmonds, Clinical Instructor; M.S.N., MGH Institute of Health Professions; M.P.H., Harvard; RNC, WHNP.

Kathleen Solomon, Clinical Assistant Professor; M.S.N., Massachusetts Lowell; RNC, FNP.

Sharon Sullivan, Clinical Instructor; M.S., Boston University; RN.

Nancy Terres, Assistant Professor; Ph.D., Tufts; RN. Pediatric research.

Carmela Townsend, Clinical Instructor and Academic Coordinator of Clinical Education; M.S./M.B.A., Northeastern; RN.

John Twomey, Associate Professor; Ph.D., Virginia; RNC, PNP. Ethics.

John Twomey, Associate Professor; Ph.D., Virginia; RNC, PNP. Pediatric research.

Maria Winne, Clinical Instructor; M.S., Massachusetts Boston; RN.

Karen Anne Wolf, Clinical Associate Professor and Associate Director of Administration and Development; Ph.D., Brandeis; RNC, ANP. Nursing historical research and community health promotion.

Mount Carmel College of Nursing

Columbus, Ohio

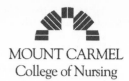

MOUNT CARMEL
College of Nursing

THE COLLEGE

Mount Carmel College of Nursing (MCCN) is a private, specialized institution of higher education offering a Bachelor of Science in Nursing degree, a Second Degree Accelerated Program, an RN to B.S.N. program, a Master of Science program in adult health and nursing education, a Post-Master's Certificate in Nursing Education, a Dietetic Internship Program, and programs through its Division of Continuing Education. The College's baccalaureate degree in nursing includes both the prelicensure program and a curriculum option called the RN to B.S.N. Completion Program for registered nurses seeking a baccalaureate degree.

The College is accredited by the North Central Association of Colleges and Schools, and the nursing program is accredited by the National League for Nursing Accrediting Commission.

Mount Carmel College of Nursing is a subsidiary of Mount Carmel Health and is proud to offer one of the largest undergraduate nursing programs among all Ohio private colleges with nursing programs. The learning is enhanced by experiences and opportunities made possible by the College's inclusion in Mount Carmel Health System, an integrated delivery system. Mount Carmel includes three acute-care hospitals, community outreach programs, hospice, home health, and ambulatory-care centers.

Founded in 1903 by the Congregation of the Sisters of the Holy Cross, Mount Carmel offered a diploma program until 1993. In 1990, Mount Carmel College of Nursing was established. MCCN offers small classes, one-on-one instruction, and the opportunity to form lifelong friendships. A variety of cocurricular activities exists to enrich the college experience.

Mount Carmel College of Nursing is committed to respect for all persons, holistic development of individuals, and encouragement of social responsibility.

PROGRAMS OF STUDY

MCCN offers a comprehensive approach to health-care education. The Prelicensure Program leads to a Bachelor of Science in Nursing degree. This traditional four-year program is designed for students without previous nursing experience. The first two years of study focus on completing general education requirements, which provide the foundation for the nursing program. Nursing studies begin in the sophomore year, when the curriculum combines hands-on clinical experiences with classroom theory. Nursing course work emphasizes clinical practice in a variety of acute-care hospitals and community-based centers. In addition to regular classes, the nursing and humanity seminars encourage students to explore personal health-related interests and provide them with rich cultural experiences.

The Advanced Placement Program allows students to transfer in all non-nursing courses from their first two years of study at other institutions of higher learning. When degree requirements (prerequisite courses completed) are met, a nursing degree can be obtained in five semesters. All transfer students must complete a twelve-week summer advanced-placement tract at the College prior to the fall semester start.

The RN to B.S.N. Completion Program is designed for registered nurses who want to earn a Bachelor of Science in Nursing degree. The registered nurse can complete degree requirements in four semesters of full-time study. Classes are scheduled one full day per week, so that RNs may work full-time if necessary. Class sizes are small and designed to meet the individual needs of the student. The program offers flexibility for the nurse seeking his or her level of expertise within the confines of course objectives.

The new thirteen-month Second Degree Accelerated Program allows students who have already earned at least a bachelor's degree in any other major to pursue a career in nursing. Applications are now being accepted for the January 2008 class.

The Master of Science degree programs in adult health and nursing education are designed for career-minded baccalaureate-prepared registered nurses who want to take their calling to a higher level. With a master's degree from Mount Carmel, students can increase professional responsibility, teach patients, educate future nurses and health-care workers, and become eligible for Certified Nurse Specialist (CNS) credentials.

Offered on both a full- and part-time basis, the master's programs offer flexibility for the nurse seeking his or her level of expertise. Class sizes are small and designed to meet the individual needs of the student. Other advantages to Mount Carmel's program are that students attend classes only one day a week, there are no GRE requirements for admission, undergraduate work and nursing licensure count toward requirements, and there is flexible scheduling of classes.

Offered online or on-site, the Post-Master's Certificate in Nursing Education program prepares licensed registered nurses who already have a master's degree in nursing for another level of practice—the role of qualified educator in an academic or a health-care setting.

AFFILIATIONS WITH HEALTH-CARE FACILITIES

Clinical learning experiences are offered at several hospitals, including those within the Mount Carmel network and at Children's Hospital in Columbus. Other clinical opportunities are conducted in conjunction with numerous community health agencies within central Ohio. Clinical sites may include Mount Carmel West Hospital, Mount Carmel East Hospital, Mount Carmel St. Ann's Hospital, Children's Hospital, neighboring elementary schools, Maryhaven Drug and Substance Abuse Center, and community-based agencies. The clinical areas of study offer students an excellent and well-rounded opportunity to experience all elements of nursing care in a variety of environments.

ACADEMIC FACILITIES

As part of a large health-care delivery system, students at MCCN have access to a full professional library. The library provides a full range of reference, bibliographic, and interlibrary loan services.

Students also have access to an on-site Learning Resource Center, which is designed specifically to support studies. The center includes a fully equipped computer lab for student use and a multimedia area that houses state-of-the-art instructional technology.

LOCATION

Mount Carmel College of Nursing is located on the near West Side of Columbus, Ohio, on the hospital campus of Mount Carmel West. With well over a million residents in its metropolitan area, Columbus is a diverse city. Mount Carmel is located just minutes from the exciting downtown area, which is conveniently located near shopping theaters, sporting events, and parks.

Columbus has all the benefits of a large city without losing the feeling of small-town warmth and spontaneity.

STUDENT SERVICES

MCCN has a full range of services to meet students' needs. There are a Student Union, complete with a kitchen, vending machines, and numerous sitting and reading areas; a gymnasium and exercise room; and Mount Carmel intramural sports, which include organized basketball, volleyball, and softball teams. A student nursing organization, SNAM, is an excellent resource for students to establish friendships while providing community service and enhancing their skills in the field of nursing.

For students wishing to live on campus, MCCN maintains a full-service dormitory within the College for easy access to classes and the faculty. In addition, students, both commuter and resident, have access to three on-campus dining options: the hospital cafeteria, Wendy's, and Tim Hortons.

For those who are interested in spectator sports, the Ohio State University and other nearby colleges and universities have regularly scheduled sporting events. Sports fans can enjoy games hosted by the Columbus Clippers, a Triple-A farm baseball team of the New York Yankees; the Columbus Blue Jackets, a professional ice-hockey team; and the Columbus Crew, a professional soccer team.

In addition, Columbus offers an outstanding symphony orchestra, a jazz orchestra, numerous music clubs of all genres, both opera and ballet companies, and world-class shopping and entertainment facilities, including Easton Town Center and Polaris Fashion Place.

THE NURSING STUDENT GROUP

More than 70 faculty members teach 650 students in the College's nursing programs. Faculty and staff members are committed to fostering personal and academic growth—an approach that transcends into such areas as graduation and retention rates, which are among the highest in the state and far surpass national averages. For those who need help academically, "Success in College" courses are available to promote academic improvement and development.

Mount Carmel's cultural environment is one that embraces diversity. The highly successful "Learning Trail Program" assists students of various cultural backgrounds by nurturing academic, personal, and professional growth through one-on-one consultation. Minority student retention and graduation rates far exceed national averages.

Diversity extends beyond the richness that people of different backgrounds bring to the campus. Outreach programs have enabled students to visit many places, including a Native American reservation, an Appalachian mining town, and Europe.

Job placement services are available both during college and upon graduation. As an undergraduate, many opportunities exist within Mount Carmel, including those in hospitals, hospice, and home care. While there are no guarantees, these positions often lead to the first employment opportunity after graduation. In addition, senior students find assistance with referrals, job placement, resume writing, and job-seeking skills.

COSTS
Fees range from approximately $6230 for the first year to $17,275 during the fourth year. Housing costs associated with living in the dormitory are $964 per semester for double occupancy.

FINANCIAL AID
Numerous financial aid options are available to students. Financial aid is awarded based on demonstrated financial need, scholastic achievement, and other considerations in the form of loans, employment opportunities, scholarships, and grants. Students may find assistance through the College's own financial aid programs and through federal programs. Representatives from the MCCN financial aid department can assist students in exploring various options.

APPLYING
Applicants with college credit must meet MCCN general admission requirements and must have earned a college GPA of 2.75 or higher. ACT or SAT scores need not be submitted if at least 30 hours of college credit have been successfully completed. Applicants should submit official transcripts from all colleges and universities attended. Transfer students must also submit an official high school transcript.

The following criteria are used for admission to the bachelor's program: a high school diploma (or GED certificate) with a minimum cumulative GPA of 2.75 is required; a GPA of at least 3.0 is preferred. The applicant may submit evidence of a college GPA of 2.75 or higher in lieu of the high school GPA. High school course requirements are English, four courses; college-preparatory math, two courses (three recommended); laboratory science, two courses (biology and chemistry); social science, two courses; foreign language, two courses (sign language is an option); and visual or performing arts, one course (two recommended). If any of the above courses are not passed in high school, the applicant is required to take these classes at the college level and earn a minimum grade of C (+/-). The courses must be completed prior to the applicant attending Mount Carmel College of Nursing. (All applicants must submit a transcript from high school.) All applicants must provide ACT or SAT scores, except applicants who have been out of high school more than five years or have at least 30 college/university credits. An essay is also required. To schedule a visit and tour or for information about all programs within MCCN, students should contact the College.

Admission to the master's program is determined on the following criteria: a baccalaureate degree in nursing from an accredited program/accreditation by either NLNAC or CCNE, a current unrestricted Ohio RN license, a minimum cumulative GPA of 3.0 (on a 4.0 scale) in a baccalaureate nursing program, and a minimum score of 550 on the TOEFL for international students whose native language is not English. Admission materials to be submitted include official transcripts from all previous academic work; a current resume; a statement of career goals, objectives, and plans for graduate study; and letters of recommendation from professional associates.

CORRESPONDENCE AND INFORMATION
Office of Admission
Mount Carmel College of Nursing
127 South Davis Avenue
Columbus, Ohio 43222

Phone: 614-234-4CON
        800-556-6942 (toll-free)
Web site: http://www.mccn.edu

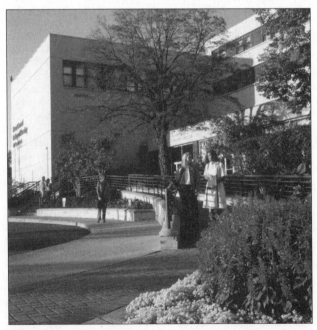

Individualized attention, small classes, and highly experienced and caring faculty members foster excellence in education at Mount Carmel College of Nursing.

Mount Saint Mary College
Division of Nursing
Newburgh, New York

THE COLLEGE

Mount Saint Mary College is a private, four-year liberal arts college for men and women with an enrollment of 2,600 students. With a favorable student-faculty ratio of 16:1, the Mount provides a warm and personal atmosphere. Mount Saint Mary College is a young, vibrant, growing school where group commitment is made to the individual student.

Since opening its doors in 1960, the College's basic goals have been the pursuit and dissemination of knowledge and the development of the capacity to discern and use it. The Mount maintains a firm belief in the value of a liberal arts education and a commitment to the Judeo-Christian traditions upon which is was founded. It retains the spirit of the intellectual, cultural, ethical, spiritual, and social philosophies of its founders.

The College's mission is to form a vital academic community characterized by the attitude that learning is a lifelong process. This process involves the ongoing acquisition of knowledge, skills, and experience and a continuing selection of values and a commitment to a value system.

THE DIVISION OF NURSING

Mount Saint Mary College's nursing program prepares students to practice as highly skilled professionals capable of meeting the demands of a rapidly evolving health-care system. Students who graduate from the Mount have a strong theoretical basis enhanced by development of clinical skills. This is achieved through nursing course work, clinical experiences, and a liberal arts background. Students apply what they learn in class directly to real-life experiences in their clinical experiences and cooperative education placements.

Intimate with today's ever-racing, ever-changing atmosphere, the faculty emphasizes a critical-thinking, problem-solving approach to nursing care. Students are prepared to work in multicultural health-care settings, where they utilize creative solutions to make independent patient care decisions. Students collaborate with other members of a health-care team to provide the best possible care.

PROGRAMS OF STUDY

The Bachelor of Science degree program in nursing prepares graduates for diverse careers in nursing and for graduate study. The program integrates professional nursing courses with a liberal arts education that emphasizes evidence-based practice, professional values, development of a strong knowledge base, skill competence, an appreciation of human and cultural diversity, and the development of leadership skills.

There are 120 credits required for the degree. In addition to the liberal arts core requirements and nursing courses, nursing students take multiple courses in biology and chemistry. The nursing program is accredited by the Commission on Collegiate Nursing Education.

The baccalaureate program offers several options for undergraduate study, including the traditional track (fall and spring semesters), evening accelerated track, and the RN Fast Track. Upon completion of all program requirements, graduates take the NCLEX for licensure as registered nurses.

Graduates are employed worldwide in hospitals, long-term-care facilities, community agencies, management, research, academia, government, private corporations, and professional organizations. Alumni have earned master's and doctoral degrees as well as certifications in many nursing specialty areas.

AFFILIATIONS WITH HEALTH-CARE FACILITIES

Mount Saint Mary College's nursing students begin working in health-care settings the second semester of the sophomore year and continue throughout their senior year. Students are assigned to a variety of hospitals and community agencies for clinical experiences. Assignments vary from semester to semester but typically include St. Luke's hospital in Newburgh, New York; St. Francis and Vassar Brothers hospitals in Poughkeepsie, New York; Cornwall Hospital in Cornwall, New York; Orange Medical Center in Goshen and Middletown, New York; Westchester Medical Center in Valhalla, New York; Danbury Hospital in Danbury, Connecticut; and VA Medical Centers as well as area health departments, community health centers, schools, homes, nursing homes, and senior citizens centers.

ACADEMIC FACILITIES

The fully computerized Curtin Memorial Library provides a state-of-the-art Integrated Online Library System that provides access to the library's holdings and an automated check-out system. Students are able to use the system from the library, the Academic Computer Center, and their dorm rooms. Students have access to online search services. These search services provide access to periodical databases with journal article citations and some full-text articles. The library has online access to First Search and the Expanded Academic Index. The library has several periodical databases on CD-ROM.

The library collection has more than 120,000 volumes, more than 1,100 periodical subscriptions, and an extensive video collection. The College coordinates an interlibrary loan program with public and private libraries throughout the Hudson Valley region.

The newly renovated Nursing Learning Resource Center (LRC) is open to nursing students to gain practical experience in nursing techniques. Hospital equipment and patient simulators are available to aid in the acquisition of nursing skills. The LRC also includes ten computer workstations with state-of-the-art interactive software to enhance learning.

Students have access to the campus network, online library resources, e-mail, and the Internet from residence halls and many other campus facilities via the Wireless Academic Network. The Academic Computer Center contains six separate computer facilities using the latest PC technology, including multimedia capabilities. Teaching facilities include modern classrooms equipped with television monitors, two 20-station PC classrooms, a state-of-the-art multimedia production center, faculty technology center, and the availability of laptops with LCD projection screens for computer presentations outside the laboratories.

LOCATION

Mount Saint Mary College's campus sits on the banks of the scenic Hudson River in a residential section of Newburgh, New York, approximately halfway between Albany and New York City. The campus is served by Stewart International Airport. The nearby Catskill Mountains offer recreational opportunities all year long, including ski trips and hikes.

STUDENT SERVICES

The Mount offers students more than classes, tests, and term papers. Students are encouraged to take advantage of the 30 clubs and organizations on campus. The Student Government Association is the legislative body for student life.

All undergraduate nursing majors belong to the Nursing Student Union (NSU) from the time they enter the College. NSU is an integral part of nursing students' experiences since its inception in the 1960s. This group offers students the opportunity to develop leadership skills by participating in college governance, networking, and community service activities. The organization is governed by students with the assistance of a nursing faculty adviser who is selected by the students. Students elect their own officers, administer their own budget, and determine their own agenda. All activities required for NSU events are planned and carried out by the students, including the invitation of speakers, printing invitations, and other program activities. Students also participate in health fairs and organize study groups for freshmen nursing students. Students may also get involved with the National Student Nurses Association and the international chapter of Sigma Theta Tau, the honor society for nursing. The experience of working together as a team and coordinating important events offers the students invaluable experience as they prepare for careers as professional nurses. Ninety percent of all nursing graduates are employed in the nursing field or enrolled in graduate school within six months of graduation.

THE NURSING STUDENT GROUP

The nursing program provides an opportunity for close interaction between faculty and students. All undergraduate nursing students belong to the Nursing Student Union from the time they enter as nursing majors until they graduate. The feasibility of establishing a chapter of the National Student Nurses Association is being explored, and it would provide numerous membership benefits beyond the College. Selected senior nursing students are invited to join the College's chapter of Sigma Theta Tau International, the honor society for nursing. A nursing student listserv keeps students and faculty members connected in a meaningful way.

COSTS

For the 2006–07 academic year, undergraduate tuition was $17,730. Graduate program tuition for the academic year was $660 per credit.

FINANCIAL AID

Mount Saint Mary College's financial aid program provides assistance in the form of federal, state, and campus-based scholarships, and grants, loans, and part-time employment for students who demonstrate academic potential but whose resources are insufficient to meet the costs of higher education. High-achieving students may also benefit from awards based solely on previous academic performance. Using March 15 as a priority date, students apply for financial aid by completing the admissions process and filing the Free Application for Federal Student Aid (FAFSA).

APPLYING

Students who wish to apply to the Mount's undergraduate nursing program should submit a completed application form and a $35 application fee to the Admissions Office. Students should also make arrangements for their high school transcript and SAT scores to be forwarded to the same office. Letters of recommendation, while not required, are strongly advised. Mount Saint Mary College operates on a rolling admissions

policy. Once a student's file is complete, he or she is usually notified of the admissions decision within two to four weeks.

The graduate nursing division requires applicants to submit an application at least six weeks before the desired entry date. Applicants must submit a completed application form and fee; official transcripts from all institutions attended, undergraduate and graduate; a photocopy of New York State RN license/registration and malpractice insurance identification; official GRE or MAT scores; three letters of recommendation; a personal statement of interest; qualifications; career goals; official TOEFL score (if applicable); and a completed health form. Upon receipt of all documents, the applicant is notified and instructed to arrange an interview with the Program Coordinator.

CORRESPONDENCE AND INFORMATION

Director of Admissions
Mount Saint Mary College
330 Powell Avenue
Newburgh, New York 12550
Phone: 845-569-3248
          888-YES-MSMC (toll-free)
E-mail: mtstmary@msmc.edu
Web site: http://www.msmc.edu

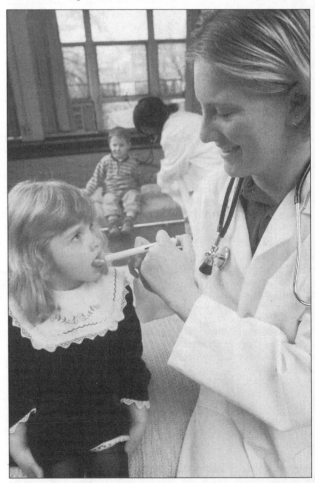

Students are assigned to a variety of hospitals and community agencies for clinical experiences.

New York University
College of Nursing
New York, New York

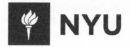

THE UNIVERSITY

New York University (NYU), one of the largest private university in the country, was founded in 1831. NYU draws top students from every state and from 140 countries. The University attracts a world-famous faculty and distinguished student body.

The University includes fourteen schools and colleges. In NYU's College of Nursing, students have all the advantages and resources found only at a major research university, yet they are also part of a small college community that shares a commitment to the health and welfare of humanity. Exchanging ideas with scholars in health, education, and the arts assists nursing students' growth as professionals and people.

THE COLLEGE OF NURSING

Excellence has placed New York University's College of Nursing among the nation's top nursing programs. The intellectual energies of the faculty and students, the quality of the academic resources, and the rich interaction with a vibrant city provide a learning experience that is unique in its rigor and diversity. All programs—baccalaureate, master's, and doctoral—provide a dynamic balance between nursing theory and practice. These programs prepare graduates for leadership roles in direct care, administration, research, or teaching. They reflect the latest advances in knowledge and technology as well as today's modern health-care environment. When students graduate, in addition to a wealth of knowledge and skills, they take with them the ability to think analytically—the hallmark of a successful nursing career.

All of the College of Nursing's full-time, tenure-track faculty members are doctorate prepared. Full-time clinical faculty members are all master's or doctorate prepared expert practitioners. Part-time faculty members hold at least a master's degree in their clinical specialty area.

NYU's College of Nursing alumni are in positions of leadership throughout the world, where they practice in diverse clinical, academic, and administrative settings. Many are making their mark through nursing science research. Others have forged new roles as entrepreneurs in private practice or as consultants to health insurers, pharmaceutical companies, and international health organizations.

PROGRAMS OF STUDY

The NYU College of Nursing offers B.S., M.S., post-master's certificate, and Ph.D. programs. Bachelor of Science programs include a traditional, four-year program that includes a special sequence of courses for registered nurses; a college-graduates program, which may be completed in a regular track or fifteen-month accelerated track; and dual-degree B.S./M.S. programs. Master of Science programs are offered in midwifery, nursing administration, nursing education, and nursing informatics. Master of Science programs in advanced practice nursing are offered in adult acute care, adult primary care, adult primary care/geriatric, geriatrics, holistic nursing, home health nursing, mental health, palliative care, pediatrics, and pediatrics/children with special needs. A joint degree program (M.S. in nursing administration/M.S. in management) is offered with the NYU Wagner Graduate School of Public Service. Post-master's certificate programs are offered in midwifery, nursing administration, nursing education, and nursing informatics. Post-master's certificate programs in advanced practice nursing are available in adult acute care, adult primary care, adult primary care/geriatric, children with special needs, geriatrics, holistic nursing, home health nursing, mental health, and palliative care. A Doctor of Philosophy program in research and theory development is also available. In addition to these programs, the College offers a sequence of courses in substance abuse disorders and a master's completion sequence for certificate-prepared nurse practitioners and certified nurse midwives.

The B.S. program in nursing prepares students to manage the full scope of nursing care responsibilities in today's complex health-care environment. The nursing science curricula emphasize a humanistic approach that examines the social, emotional, and environmental context in which wellness and illness occur. Students examine the growth and development of the family structure, patterns that characterize different age groups, human behavior in health and illness, and the effects of chronic illness. In the classroom, students learn nursing theories, nursing process, and relevant knowledge. Students apply these theories in practice through laboratory and clinical study. Students gain experience in all clinical areas, including maternal-child health, adult medical-surgical nursing, community/psychiatric nursing, geriatric nursing, and nursing leadership. Students work with all ages and cultures in a range of settings.

The M.S. programs in advanced education in nursing science prepare students for leadership roles in management, nursing education, informatics, and advanced nursing practice. They are unique programs that subscribe to a philosophy and vision of nursing reflecting a commitment to human values and the advancement of nursing as a profession. The programs emphasize critical thinking, the development and use of a theoretical base for advanced practice, the application of evidence-based practice to further nursing practice knowledge, and the promotion of a professional identity. The 45- to 48-point curricula include a core in nursing theory, clinical advanced practice core, an area of concentration, and related cognates and electives. Graduates of the clinical programs are eligible to sit for ANCC and other certification examinations as nurse practitioners and/or clinical nurse specialists or are eligible for American College of Nurse-Midwives certification and licensure as professional midwives in New York State. All advanced practice nursing programs are registered by the state of New York as nurse practitioner programs. The post-M.S. advanced certificate programs require 12 to 30 points.

The Ph.D. program in research and theory development in nursing science educates scholars in the critical and creative study of human beings and their environment and prepares leaders to examine issues in nursing and health care. The required course work of approximately 52 points is taken in the College of Nursing and other University departments on a full- or part-time basis. The curriculum is designed to provide a solid research foundation in quantitative and qualitative methods, which generates nursing knowledge and furthers theory development and substantive practice within the discipline.

AFFILIATIONS WITH HEALTH-CARE FACILITIES

The College of Nursing offers clinical and practicum experience at many of the nation's foremost hospitals, including NYU Medical Center, Bellevue Hospital Center, Mt. Sinai Medical Center, St. Vincent's Hospital, Beth Israel Medical Center, and more than fifty other acute-care hospitals. Students also gain significant experience in community settings, including the Visiting Nurse Service, and other ambulatory and home-care settings.

ACADEMIC FACILITIES

NYU's Bobst Library is one of the largest open-stack research libraries in the world. Bobst is one of eight NYU libraries, including the Frederick L. Ehrman Medical Library, to which nursing students have access. The College of Nursing's Nursing Arts Laboratories enable students to practice their nursing skills in a simulated hospital setting.

LOCATION

NYU is located in historic Greenwich Village, traditionally a community of artists and intellectuals. NYU's campus is within minutes of off-Broadway theaters, Little Italy, Chinatown, and renowned museums. As an international center of finance, culture, and communications, New York City offers unmatched educational, internship, and social opportunities.

STUDENT SERVICES

The University offers students a variety of services and resources, including the Student Resource Center; the Center for Multicultural Education and Programs; the Student Health Center; the Wasserman Center for Career Development; the Coles Sports and Recreation Center; Information Technology Services; and the Henry and Lucy Moses Center for Students with Disabilities.

THE NURSING STUDENT GROUP

The student body represents most of the fifty states and many other countries. This diversification affords opportunities for rich and lasting relationships. The average student is a mature, self-directed individual who assumes both professional and academic responsibilities, often in addition to family commitments.

COSTS

Tuition and fees for 2006–07 were $31,534 (plus nonrefundable registration and service fees of $1886) for full-time undergraduates. Graduate students paid $1063 per point (plus nonrefundable registration and service fees of $611).

FINANCIAL AID

Financial aid at NYU comes from many sources. In order to meet an applicant's financial need, the University may offer a package of aid that includes scholarships or grants, loans, or work-study programs. NYU requires the submission of the Free Application for Federal Student Aid (FAFSA).

The College of Nursing offers a competitive financial aid program. Scholarships for full-time and part-time study are available. For master's and doctoral candidates, a number of fellowships and assistantships are available. Information on financial aid may be obtained from the NYU Office of Financial Aid at http://www.nyu.edu/financial.aid.

APPLYING

As baccalaureate program requirements differ for the traditional, RN, college-graduate, and dual-degree B.S./M.S. programs, interested students should contact the College of Nursing Office of Student Affairs and Admissions for specific requirements (http://www.nyu.edu/info/nursingprogram; 212-998-5317). For admission to the M.S. program, a candidate must have a baccalaureate nursing degree from an accredited nursing program. A minimum overall GPA of 3.0, RN licensure, two professional letters of reference, and a goal statement are required. TOEFL scores are required for students whose native language is not English. Students who have not met the prerequisites of basic statistics and nursing research may take them while in the program. Applicants with an associate degree in nursing and a bachelor's degree in another field may apply to the M.S. program.

Admission requirements for the post-master's advanced certificate programs are a master's degree in nursing with a minimum 3.0 GPA. For admission to the Ph.D. program, the applicant must be a nurse with baccalaureate and master's degrees acceptable to NYU, with at least one degree in nursing. A minimum grade point average of 3.0 on a scale of 4.0 and GRE scores of at least 1000 are required. In addition, the applicant must submit a resume, demonstration of professional performance/contribution to the nursing profession, two professional reference letters, a three- to five-page goal statement, copies of GRE scores, and transcripts of college-level work.

CORRESPONDENCE AND INFORMATION

Office of Student Affairs and Admissions
College of Nursing
New York University
246 Greene Street, 4th Floor
New York, New York 10003-6677

Phone: 212-998-5317
E-mail: nursing.programs@nyu.edu
Web site: http://www.nyu.edu/info/nursingprogram

THE FACULTY

Carolyn Auerhahn, Clinical Associate Professor; Ed.D., Columbia.
Mary Brennan, Clinical Assistant Professor; M.S., Boston College.
Patricia Burkhardt, Clinical Associate Professor; Dr.P.H., Johns Hopkins.
Elizabeth Capezuti, Associate Professor; Ph.D., Pennsylvania.

Danuta Clemmens, Assistant Professor; Ph.D., Yale.
Babette Cresswell, Instructor; M.S., SUNY at Binghamton.
James DeCarlo, Instructor; M.A., NYU.
May Dobal, Assistant Professor; Ph.D., Texas at Austin.
Caroline Dorsen, Instructor; M.S.N., Yale.
William Fehder, Clinical Associate Professor; Ph.D., Pennsylvania.
Mei Fu, Assistant Professor; Ph.D., Missouri–Columbia.
Terry Fulmer, Erline Perkins McGriff Professor of Nursing and Dean, College of Nursing; Ph.D., Boston College.
Susan Gennaro, Florence and William Downs Professor of Nursing Research; D.S.N., Alabama at Birmingham.
Judith Haber, Ursala Springer Professor of Nursing Leadership and Associate Dean, Graduate Programs, College of Nursing; Ph.D., NYU.
Catherine Hagerty, Instructor; M.A., NYU.
Nancy Jackson, Clinical Associate Professor; Ed.D., Columbia.
Hongsoo Kim, Assistant Professor; Ph.D., NYU.
Rose Knapp, Instructor; M.S., Seton Hall.
Christine Tassone Kovner, Professor; Ph.D., NYU.
Barbara Krainovich-Miller, Clinical Professor; Ed.D., Columbia.
Linda Jane Mayberry, Associate Professor and Director, Doctoral Program, College of Nursing; Ph.D., California, San Francisco.
Diane O. McGivern, Professor; Ph.D., NYU.
Mathy Mezey, Professor; Ed.D., Columbia.
Madeline A. Naegle, Professor; Ph.D., NYU.
Melanie Percy, Assistant Professor; Ph.D., South Carolina.
Hila Richardson, Clinical Professor and Associate Dean, Undergraduate Programs, College of Nursing; Dr.P.H., Columbia.
Deborah Witt Sherman, Associate Professor; Ph.D., NYU.
Lena Sorenson, Assistant Professor; Ph.D., CUNY Graduate Center.
Rebecca Terranova, Instructor; M.A., NYU.
Nancy Van Devanter, Associate Professor; Dr.P.H. Columbia.

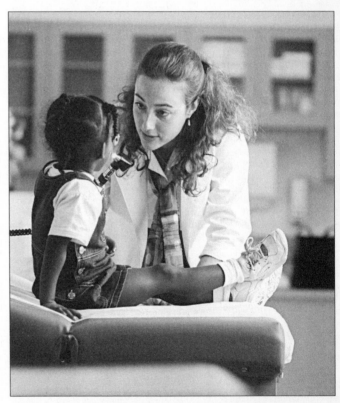

Students in the College of Nursing benefit from clinical and practicum experiences in a wide range of settings.

Northeastern University

School of Nursing
Bouvé College of Health Sciences

Boston, Massachusetts

THE UNIVERSITY

Northeastern University is a private, research-driven, urban university in Boston. The University is committed to achieving excellence through the combination of course work in liberal and professional studies with a variety of practical experiences anchored by the signature co-op program. The University has a distinguished, nationally and internationally known faculty of dedicated teachers, researchers, and scholars. The Bouvé College of Health Sciences at Northeastern University comprises the School of Nursing, the School of Pharmacy, and the School of Health Professions.

THE SCHOOL OF NURSING

The primary mission of the School of Nursing is to prepare nursing leaders for basic and advanced nursing practice that contributes to the health of the nation. Faculty members are actively engaged in nursing practice in a variety of health-care settings and conduct research in their specialty areas. Nursing students spend a substantial portion of their clinical time in the neighborhoods of Boston, working and learning with students from other health disciplines to address the needs of an urban population. Students receive clinical instruction in many of Boston's world-renowned hospitals.

PROGRAMS OF STUDY

The School offers a five-year cooperative education Bachelor of Science in Nursing (B.S.N.) degree program and an upper-division transfer-track into the B.S.N. program for students who meet the requirements for transferable college credit applicable to Northeastern's curriculum. An RN-to-B.S.N. program is also available.

The baccalaureate program is designed to prepare students to become professional nurses for practice in a variety of health-care settings, such as communities, hospitals, neighborhood health centers, schools, and homes. Faculty members focus educational efforts on preparing students to learn management of acute and episodic illnesses and complex chronic diseases of clients. Leadership development, case management, discharge planning, and economics of health care are essential components of the curriculum. The School aims to provide all students—including those with diverse backgrounds and changing career goals—with a broad-based education and the stimulus for ongoing personal and professional growth. The curriculum offers instruction in nursing theory and research, the humanities, and the biological, psychological, physical, and social sciences. More than 50 percent of the course work is in sciences and humanities.

The baccalaureate program alternates academic semesters with paid work experience in health-care settings. This combination of academic study and co-op experience produces an overall learning experience that gives greater meaning to the nursing academic program and direction to a student's career choice and development. Students work with a co-op coordinator to plan paid work experiences that meet their individual needs.

The program is accredited by the Commission on Collegiate Nursing Education and approved by the Board of Registration in Nursing of the Commonwealth of Massachusetts. Successful completion of the baccalaureate program allows graduates to take the National Council Licensing Examination (NCLEX-RN) to become registered nurses.

The School offers two options for individuals who already have a baccalaureate degree in another field who seek a career change into nursing. They can enter the three-year, upper-division transfer-track program and receive a B.S.N. degree, or they can enter the Direct Entry Program to earn a Master of Science degree with a major in nursing. This is a full-time program that combines 64 semester credit hours of RN-preparation course work, one 6- to 8-month cooperative education experience, and completion of one specialization in the Master of Science program (explained below), to prepare graduates as advanced practice nurses.

The School of Nursing offers a Master of Science degree program to prepare graduates as nurse practitioners, clinical specialists, nurse anesthetists, and managers. The master's program offers clinical specializations in acute care nurse practitioner, administration, adult and family primary care nurse practitioner, adult health clinical nurse specialist, anesthesia, pediatric nurse practitioner (acute care or primary care), and psychiatric–mental health nursing. Within the framework of nursing science, the concepts of community-based care, emergent leadership, professional competence, and intra/interdisciplinary collaboration provide the foundation for advanced professional practice. The curriculum varies depending upon the specialization but generally requires 43 semester hours. It is designed so that students can pursue either full-time or part-time study. Full-time students can expect to complete the degree requirements in four semesters over two calendar years. Part-time students may take up to five years to complete the program. Classes are offered in the late afternoon and evening. The B.S.N./M.S. program offers an innovative pathway for nurses holding a diploma or an associate degree in nursing to earn a joint B.S.N./M.S. degree; the program requires at least 67 semester hours for graduation, but may vary based on specialization. The M.S./M.B.A. degree program is an 80-semester-hour program that prepares nurses for executive-level management in health care. The nurse anesthesia program is a full-time, twenty-eight-month, 54-semester-hour program.

Certificates of Advanced Graduate Study are offered in all of the above specialization areas. These postgraduate programs are designed for nurses with a master's degree in nursing who seek further academic preparation to learn advanced practice skills in another specialization or to qualify for national certification.

The Doctor of Philosophy in nursing (Ph.D.) emphasizes clinical research to improve the health care of urban and underserved populations. The degree prepares nurses to become researchers, educators, and scholars in clinical agencies, research centers, or other health-care organizations and in schools of nursing, where they can help to meet the critical need for doctorally prepared nursing faculty members who will shape the upcoming generation of nurses.

Registered nurses may enter the Ph.D. program after completing a baccalaureate or a master's degree in nursing. Entering with a master's, students complete 49 semester hours of course work in research, urban health, and statistics. Students entering with a B.S.N. complete an additional 20 semester hours of course work to broaden their clinical knowledge. All students work closely with their doctoral advisers to select electives and research experiences that support their area of inquiry. The minimum time to complete the degree is three years for postmaster's students and four years for postbaccalaureate students.

AFFILIATIONS WITH HEALTH-CARE FACILITIES

The University's location in Boston enables the School to collaborate with some of the world's premier health-care organizations. Students have supervised clinical experiences in renowned teaching hospitals and co-op opportunities in a range of acute-care, rehabilitation, and community-health facilities. Noted health-care institutions with which the School affiliates include Beth Israel Deaconess Medical Center, Boston Medical Center, Brigham and Women's Hospital, Massachusetts General Hospital, Dana-Farber Cancer Institute, Children's Hospital, and McLean (psychiatric) Hospital as well as Healthcare for the Homeless, Spaulding Rehabilitation Hospital, regional Visiting Nurse associations, and many other highly regarded health-care systems. The School has a partnership with the city and state public health agencies and a mobile outreach van. These allow students unique opportunities to participate in the urban public health initiatives and neighborhood health centers.

ACADEMIC FACILITIES

The George D. Behrakis Health Sciences Center is a seven-story, 117,000-square-foot state-of-the-art building, housing classrooms, laboratories, and clinical facilities that simulate real health-care settings. The nursing laboratory has twelve student-centered practice areas, including fully equipped hospital stations and patient treatment areas. Nursing students practice assessment and procedural skills using simulators and mannequins across the life span.

Northeastern has several interdisciplinary centers and institutes that engage in research in collaboration with academic departments. The Division of Academic Computing provides students with access to computing resources. A high-speed data network links users and facilities on the central campus and three satellite campuses. In addition, the campus network is connected via the Internet to computing resources around the world. University libraries contain more than 893,000 bound volumes, 2.1 million microfilms, 150,000 documents, 8,585 periodical subscriptions, and 18,861 audio, video, and software titles. A central library contains technologically sophisticated services, including online catalog and circulation systems, a gateway to external networked information resources, and a network of CD-ROM optical disk databases.

LOCATION
Northeastern's 67-acre Boston campus is in the heart of the Back Bay section of the city, between the Museum of Fine Arts and Symphony Hall and a short walk from Fenway Park. At Northeastern, students discover that part of the adventure of going to college in Boston is exploring the cultural, educational, historical, and recreational offerings of the city. In addition, Cape Cod and the North Shore of Massachusetts are easily reached by car or public transportation for swimming, surfing, and boating. The scenic areas of northern New England are accessible for skiing, hiking, and mountain climbing.

STUDENT SERVICES
The University has many resources and service offices to meet student needs. These include the University Health and Counseling Services, the Cabot Physical Education Center, the Marino Recreational Center, the campus bookstore, Academic Computing Services, Campus Ministry, housing, dining services, the International Student Office, the English Language Center, the John D. O'Bryant African-American Institute, the Asian-American Center, and the Latino/a Student Cultural Center, among many others. The Bouvé College of Health Sciences Office of Student Services offers academic advising and schedules tutorial sessions and other activities.

THE NURSING STUDENT GROUP
There are more than 700 students enrolled in the School of Nursing: 535 undergraduates and 254 graduate students. They represent a wide variety of academic, professional, and cultural backgrounds. Nursing students come all across the United States as well as from Asia, Europe, and Africa. Approximately 4 percent of the nursing students are men.

COSTS
For 2006–07, tuition was $29,910; room and board cost $10,580. Graduate tuition per semester hour was $825 for full- and part-time students. Full-time mandatory fees ranged from $224 to $2000, depending on the specialty. Books and supplies averaged $800 for the academic year.

FINANCIAL AID
The University operates a substantial aid program designed to make attendance at Northeastern feasible for all qualified students. Approximately 79 percent of the freshman class received some form of financial aid in 2005–06. Financial aid is based on need and academic merit and may consist of grants, loans, work-study employment, or any combination of these three items. To apply, incoming undergraduate students must file a Free Application for Federal Student Aid (FAFSA) and a CSS PROFILE form with the College Scholarship Service by the priority filing date of February 15. Graduate students must file the FAFSA and an Institutional Aid Application.

Northeastern awards need-based financial aid to graduate students through the Nursing Student Loan, Federal Work-Study, and Federal Stafford Student Loan programs. The University also offers a limited number of minority fellowships and Martin Luther King, Jr. Scholarships. In addition, the graduate school offers financial assistance through teaching and research assistantship awards. Assistantship awards vary and can include tuition remission and stipends. Nurse traineeship funds are also available for graduate students in their clinical year.

APPLYING
Admission to Northeastern is selective and competitive. For the 2005–06 academic year, the University received more than 25,000 applications for 2,800 places in the freshman class. In building a diverse and talented class, the University seeks to enroll students who have been successful academically and who have shown a strong commitment to school and community through extracurricular activities. Students who have earned strong grades in a rigorous college-preparatory program, are innovative and creative, and who possess leadership abilities are most successful in the University's admission process. November 15 is the Early Action deadline. This program is an opportunity for students who are applying as freshmen for the fall semester to receive an admission decision early in the application process. Students who have a strong interest in Northeastern University, have succeeded academically in high school, and have demonstrated their involvement with their school and community are encouraged to apply before this deadline. January 15 is the regular deadline for September admission. If accepted for fall admission, freshmen are required to send a tuition deposit by May 1 to secure a place in the class. For transfer students, the priority deadline for the fall is May 1. Campus tours and group information sessions are held daily and are available without an appointment.

Applicants to the graduate program should have earned a baccalaureate degree in nursing from a program accredited by the Commission on Collegiate Nursing Education or by the National League for Nursing Accrediting Commission. The B.S.N./M.S. program, however, allows nurses who have graduated from accredited diploma and associate degree programs to pursue graduate study. The Direct Entry Program allows applicants with a bachelor's degree in a field other than nursing to be admitted as a graduate student in nursing. An elementary statistics course is a prerequisite for all applicants. Graduate level statistics and epidemiology courses are prerequisites for Ph.D. applicants.

Admission requirements include a satisfactory scholastic record, an official copy of all college transcripts, and satisfactory scores on the General Test of the Graduate Record Examinations (GRE), the Miller Analogies Test (MAT), or the Graduate Management Admission Test (GMAT) for M.S./M.B.A. applicants. Three letters of recommendation, a personal goal statement, one to two years of current professional nursing practice, and current registration to practice nursing in the United States are also required. There are some modifications in the requirements for the Direct Entry program, the B.S.N./M.S. program, and for international students, including the submission of TOEFL scores by international students whose native language is not English. The application fee is $50 for the graduate programs.

Students may be admitted in the fall, spring, or summer semesters, depending on the program of study; however, students interested in full-time study should submit their application by March 1 for the fall semester. Applications for the nurse anesthesia specialization are due December 1 and applications for the Direct Entry and Ph.D. programs are due February 1 for admission in the fall semester. Special needs students are welcome.

CORRESPONDENCE AND INFORMATION
Office of Undergraduate Admissions
150 Richards Hall
Northeastern University
360 Huntington Avenue
Boston, Massachusetts 02115
Phone: 617-373-2200
       617-373-3100 (TTY)
Fax: 617-373-8780
E-mail: admissions@neu.edu
Web site: http://www.admissions.neu.edu

Graduate Application Inquiries and Application Requests
Bouvé College of Health Sciences
120 Behrakis Health Science Center
Northeastern University
Boston, Massachusetts 02115-5096
Phone: 617-373-3125
Fax: 617-373-4701
E-mail: bouvegrad@neu.edu
Web site: http://www.bouve.neu.edu

THE DEAN
Nancy Hoffart, Dean and Professor, School of Nursing; Ph.D., RN.

Quinnipiac University
Department of Nursing
Hamden, Connecticut

THE UNIVERSITY

Quinnipiac University, founded in 1929, is an independent, coeducational, nonsectarian institution. It is primarily a residential university on an attractive New England campus. Quinnipiac employs a large undergraduate faculty (286 full-time members) relative to the size of its undergraduate student body (5,422), keeping the University-wide student-faculty ratio at 16:1. The full graduate and undergraduate enrollment is 7,341. The University maintains an extensive network of professional associations with the health, business, and education communities through prominent clinical programs and internship placements.

THE DEPARTMENT OF NURSING

The baccalaureate nursing program at Quinnipiac University was instituted in 1991, with the first class graduating in 1995. The National Council Licensure Examination for Registered Nurses (NCLEX-RN) pass rate is greater than 95 percent. There are currently 12 full-time faculty members and about 25 adjunct faculty members.

The undergraduate curriculum is an upper-division major. Students admitted to the professional component in the junior year must have attained a cumulative grade point average of 3.0. Continued good standing requires that the cumulative as well as the semester grade point average of 3.0 be maintained for the remainder of the program.

The nursing curriculum at Quinnipiac fosters professional socialization for future roles and responsibilities within the profession. Graduates of the program are prepared as generalists to begin the practice of holistic professional nursing with sound theoretical foundations and more than 800 hours of diverse clinical practice experiences. Graduates are also prepared for graduate study. In addition to the generalist perspective, the curriculum provides an introductory specialty focus in which senior students may select a precepted experience during the last semester of their senior year.

PROGRAMS OF STUDY

All programs within the School of Health Sciences are based on a comprehensive foundation in the liberal arts and sciences. Students may attend on a part-time or full-time basis. A state-of-the-art critical care skills laboratory, utilizing resources from other health-related disciplines, is used for teaching advanced skills.

Accredited by the National League for Nursing Accrediting Commission (NLNAC), Quinnipiac's bachelor's degree program in nursing offers the theoretical and clinical education students need to enter professional nursing practice. Graduates of the program are eligible to take the NCLEX-RN exam and are well prepared for graduate study in nursing. In addition to the traditional four-year program, an innovative accelerated option is available to non-nurse college graduates.

Students admitted to the accelerated B.S.N. option earn a second baccalaureate degree in nursing in one calendar year of full-time study that commences in May.

Because nursing involves a wide range of responsibilities, the program takes a holistic approach to the sciences, health-care theory, and the techniques of nursing. Quinnipiac's nursing faculty members also introduce their students to the cultural, social, and economic implications of health-care management.

Beginning with the first nursing course, students benefit from well-equipped labs, detailed simulations of health-care facilities, patient-oriented education, and highly effective field experiences.

The graduate nursing program, also accredited by the NLNAC, seeks to prepare professional nurses at an advanced theoretical and clinical practice level in order to address present and potential societal health needs. Three available tracks are adult nurse practitioner, family nurse practitioner, and forensic nurse clinical specialist. Post-master's certificate tracks in adult and family nurse practice are also available. Quinnipiac's M.S.N. includes core courses that cover advanced concepts and theoretical foundations of nursing, research methods, and health-care policy and economics.

AFFILIATIONS WITH HEALTH-CARE FACILITIES

The school's strong affiliates with health-care providers in the area allow students to complete clinical work at such institutions as Yale–New Haven Hospital, Connecticut Children's Medical Center, the Hospital of St. Raphael, and Veterans Administration Medical Center, Mid-State Medical Center, as well as in private practices, clinics, and other health-care centers.

ACADEMIC FACILITIES

Modern buildings surround 500 acres of rolling fields and streams adjacent to Sleeping Giant State Park on the Mount Carmel (main) campus. Library holdings total 304,857, with 4,291 periodicals and extensive online resources. Quinnipiac is one of the top 10 most-wired campuses in the country (*PC Magazine*, January 2007), and this is reflected in its academic facilities and programs. All incoming students must purchase a University-recommended laptop computer for use in the classroom and in the residence halls. Students can reach all online services from the data network in their dorm rooms or from the wireless network that covers the library and classrooms.

The technologically advanced portion of the nursing curriculum is supported by grants that afford students an opportunity to practice with sophisticated equipment in the clinical skills practice lab prior to actual clinical practice. Innovative software provides computer-assisted learning with a variety of simulated patient-care situations that challenge the student to use critical-thinking skills.

LOCATION

Quinnipiac's campus is located in suburban Hamden, Connecticut, a southern New England town 8 miles from metropolitan New Haven and 25 miles from Hartford. It is easily reached via the New England Turnpike (Interstate 95), Interstate 91, the Wilbur Cross Parkway (Route 15-Merritt Parkway), and Interstate 84. The closest airport is Hartford (BDL), which is within 45 minutes of the campus. Area attractions include the Yale Repertory Theater; the Schubert, Long Wharf, and Chevy (Oakdale) Theaters; the Peabody Museum; dance clubs; museums; and cinemas.

STUDENT SERVICES

Quinnipiac University has a variety of resources and services to meet the needs of students, including a 28,000-square-foot state-of-the-art recreation and fitness center, the Learning Center, the International Student Club, the Office of Multicultural Affairs, and the Counseling Center.

THE NURSING STUDENT GROUP

Students in the nursing program come from a wide variety of backgrounds and geographic locations. The majority are resident full-time students. Quinnipiac's low student-faculty ratio of 16:1 ensures that nursing students receive personal attention from their professors. Graduates are employed in large medical centers, community health centers, primary-care facilities, and small community hospitals.

COSTS

Tuition and fee costs for the 2006–07 academic year were $26,280 for full-time enrollment (16 credit hours per semester). Room and board costs were $10,700. Additional expenses include books, lab fees, immunizations, uniforms, malpractice insurance, CPR certification, and travel to and parking at clinical sites.

FINANCIAL AID

Approximately 70 percent of freshmen receive financial aid, with freshman awards averaging $14,000 through a combination of grants (not to be repaid), student loans, and on-campus jobs. The University offers merit-based scholarships; the admissions application deadline for these is February 1. Students should complete and submit the Free Application for Federal Student Aid (FAFSA) to the federal processor by March 1.

APPLYING

Quinnipiac generally receives between 11,000 and 12,000 applications for the freshman class of 1,300 and admits about 50 percent of those who apply. While February 1 is the stated application deadline, applications are read on a rolling-admission basis, and it is recommended that students file their applications early in the fall of their senior year of high school. The results of the SAT or ACT should be forwarded to Quinnipiac University. For fall 2007, the University continues to use the critical reading and the mathematics section of the SAT and/or the composite score on the ACT for admission and scholarship purposes. The University has a rolling admissions policy and begins notifying students of decisions in mid-December. Freshman students generally have a 3.4 GPA or better average in college-preparatory courses (transfer students have a 3.0 GPA or better), rank in the top 30 percent of their high school class, and have an average combined score of 1120 on the SAT .

CORRESPONDENCE AND INFORMATION

Joan Isaac Mohr, Vice President and Dean
Carla M. Knowlton, Director
Undergraduate Admissions
Quinnipiac University
275 Mount Carmel Avenue
Hamden, Connecticut 06518

Phone: 203-582-8600
       800-462-1944 (toll-free)
Fax: 203-582-8906
E-mail: admissions@quinnipiac.edu
Web site: http://www.quinnipiac.edu

THE FACULTY

Cynthia Barrere, Associate Professor of Nursing; Ph.D., Connecticut.

E. Jane Bower, Associate Professor of Nursing; Ph.D., Adelphi.

Janet Dombroski, Assistant Professor of Nursing; M.S.N., Pace.

Anne Durkin, Associate Professor of Nursing; Ph.D., Connecticut.

Mary Helming, Assistant Professor of Nursing.

Laima Karosas, Associate Professor of Nursing; M.S.N., Yale.

Jeanne LeVasseur, Associate Professor of Nursing; Ph.D., Connecticut.

Elizabeth McGann, Professor of Nursing and Department Chair; D.N.Sc., Yale.

Barbara Moynihan, Associate Professor of Nursing; Ph.D., Connecticut.

Lisa O'Connor, Assistant Professor of Nursing; M.S.N., Hartford.

Lynn Price, Associate Professor of Nursing; J.D., George Washington.

Janice Thompson, Associate Professor of Nursing; Ph.D., Adelphi.

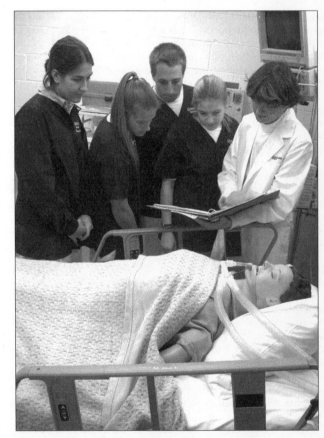

Nursing students utilize the critical-care laboratory.

Regis College
Center for Health Sciences, Nursing Program
Weston, Massachusetts

THE COLLEGE
Regis College is a coeducational, Catholic liberal arts and sciences college with several undergraduate and graduate programs. The College was founded in 1927 by the Congregation of the Sisters of Saint Joseph of Boston; their members desired to put their resources to use for the good of society through education. Regis College offers bachelor's degrees in a wide variety of majors and master's degrees in education, health product regulation, leadership and organizational change, nursing, organizational and professional communication, and public administration.

THE DIVISION OF NURSING
Established in 1983, the Division of Nursing began as a B.S. degree–completion program for registered nurses. A weekend track was started in 1989 and was selected by the Army Nurse Corps as an educational pathway that would fulfill reserve nurses' military obligations while they earned a baccalaureate degree. The first military weekend group graduated in 1992. The programs now include a B.S.N. program and a graduate program with a variety of traditional and accelerated tracks. The nursing programs reflect the mission of Regis College—to educate individuals to attain personal and career goals while also addressing the changing needs of society. The faculty is dedicated to excellence in teaching and is committed to the integration of theory and practice in professional nursing. Students can expect a challenging educational experience in a supportive environment. The nursing programs are fully accredited by the National League for Nursing Accrediting Commission and offer flexible options for study on a full- or part-time basis.

PROGRAMS OF STUDY
The undergraduate program offers a B.S.N., a four-year course of study that prepares individuals for professional practice as registered nurses. This program integrates study in the liberal arts and sciences with professional nursing education. Students gain diverse clinical experiences within the greater Boston area and develop skills that prepare them to provide care to clients in a wide variety of health-care settings.

The graduate program offers a Master of Science, with a focus in nursing leadership for diverse health-care systems or nurse practitioner studies. The nurse practitioner studies track offers three primary-care options: pediatric, family, and psychiatric mental health nurse practitioner studies. An accelerated curriculum track is designed for non-nurses who hold a baccalaureate degree in a field other than nursing. This track requires the completion of certain prerequisite courses and takes three years, including two summers of study. Students take the NCLEX-RN exam after sixteen months, and a B.S.N. is awarded at the end of the second year. Students have the option of exiting the program with the B.S.N. At the completion of the third year, the M.S. is awarded, and students are eligible to take nurse practitioner certification examinations.

The RN to B.S. to M.S. Upward Mobility track allows students with an associate degree or diploma in nursing to earn both the B.S. and M.S. within one curriculum. Students have the option of exiting the program with the B.S.N. Registered nurses who have a baccalaureate degree in a discipline other than nursing may enter this accelerated pathway as well. Classes are offered during the day, in the evening, on weekends, and during the summer. For RNs, post-master's certificates and certificates in nursing leadership and in nursing education are also offered.

AFFILIATIONS WITH HEALTH-CARE FACILITIES
The nursing programs at Regis College offer a wide variety of health-care settings in which students may obtain enriching clinical experiences that are appropriate for their educational and professional goals. Students are placed in ambulatory, acute-, subacute-, and long-term-care facilities; nurse-managed clinics in homeless shelters; elementary and secondary schools; and elderly and low-income housing in both urban and suburban settings. Qualified nurse practitioner studies students have the opportunity to complete a portion of the clinical requirement in approved national or international settings. The Nursing Program also offers on-site workplace courses for the master's degree programs for registered nurses employed in the Boston area, including the Lahey Clinic, St. Elizabeth's Hospital, Hallmark Health Systems, Boston Medical Center, New England Baptist Hospital, Newton Wellesley Hospital, New England Medical Center, and Cambridge Hospital.

ACADEMIC FACILITIES
The Regis College Library provides resources and services to meet the research and study needs of undergraduate and graduate students and faculty members. The library contains 140,000 volumes and 787 current periodical subscriptions in print. Regis College Library has approximately 115 nursing periodicals in paper format plus more than 600 nursing journal titles containing full-text articles that are available through the library's subscriptions to online nursing databases. The library also has thousands of nursing books, including a large reference collection and an extensive collection located in the library stacks.

LOCATION
Regis College is located on a beautiful 132-acre residential campus just 12 miles west of Boston, which is home to some of the world's leading educational, cultural, and health-care facilities. The College is easily accessible via major highways and is linked to metropolitan public transportation by a free campus shuttle bus.

STUDENT SERVICES
Regis College offers a wide range of student services, including the Fine Arts Center, which includes the 650-seat Eleanor Welch Casey Theatre and the Carney Art Gallery. The Athletic Facility features a regulation 75-foot pool with outdoor patio and sun deck plus a fitness center. The Student Union building houses the main dining room and College Café, the campus bookstore, and the post office. On-campus housing is available for undergraduate students. Qualified nursing students are invited to join Sigma Theta Tau, the international nursing honor society.

THE NURSING STUDENT GROUP
There are approximately 250 undergraduate nursing students and 450 graduate nursing students. Master's-prepared nurses have gone on to hold distinguished positions in every area of the health-care industry, including administration, clinical practice, academia, and government.

COSTS

Undergraduate tuition for 2006–07 was $23,680; room and board were $10,560. Summer tuition depends on the number of credits carried. VISA, MasterCard, or Discover may be used for tuition payment. A tuition payment plan is also available. For further information, students should contact the Controller's Office at 781-768-7200. The total cost of the program varies depending upon the number of credits transferred or granted by examination or articulation.

FINANCIAL AID

The Regis College Office of Financial Aid is located in College Hall, Room 121. Students who are interested in applying for financial aid may request information by calling 781-768-7180. Prospective students should investigate sources of financial assistance, including loans, employer tuition remission, and scholarships. The Higher Education Information Center (phone: 617-536-0200; Web site: http://www.heic.org), which is located in the Boston Public Library at Copley Square, houses a national financial aid database.

APPLYING

All undergraduate nursing applicants are processed through the Regis College Office of Admission and are considered on a rolling basis. Applicants must submit a completed application, an essay, two letters of recommendation (one from a teacher and one from a guidance counselor), official transcripts, and SAT or ACT scores.

CORRESPONDENCE AND INFORMATION

Office of Admission
Regis College
235 Wellesley Street
Weston, Massachusetts 02493-1571
Phone: 781-768-7100
        866-GET-REGIS (toll-free)
Fax: 781-768-7071
E-mail: admission@regiscollege.edu
Web site: http://www.regiscollege.edu

THE FACULTY

Roseanne Barrett, Associate Professor of Nursing; Ph.D., Boston College.
Cynthia Bashaw, Assistant Professor of Nursing; M.S., Regis College.
Maureen Beirne-Streff, Associate Professor of Nursing; Ed.D., Boston University.
Michael Bilozur, Assistant Professor of Biology; Ph.D., Boston College.
Nancy Bittner, Associate Professor of Nursing; Ph.D., Rhode Island.
Fran Borger-Klempner, Assistant Professor of Nursing; M.S., Catholic University.
Patricia Ciarleglio, Lecturer in Nursing and Placement Coordinator; M.S., Regis College.
Karen Crowley, Assistant Professor of Nursing; M.S., Simmons; FNP.
Mary Crowley, Nursing Laboratory Coordinator; M.S., Boston University.
Joanne Dalton, Associate Professor of Nursing; Ph.D., Rhode Island.
Patricia Dardano, Associate Professor of Nursing; D.N.Sc., Boston University.
Eda George, Associate Professor of Nursing; Ph.D., Brandeis.
Elisa Giaquinto, Assistant Professor of Nursing; M.S., Brown.
Penelope Glynn, Associate Professor of Nursing; Ph.D., Boston College.
Joanne Haynes, Assistant Professor of Nursing; M.S., Regis College.
Antoinette Hays, Associate Professor and Center Director for Nursing; Ph.D., Brandeis.
Joanne Hyde, Lecturer in Nursing; M.S., Boston University.
Philip Jutras, Associate Professor of Management; Ed.M., Massachusetts Boston; Ph.D., Boston College.
Marylou Kelleher, Lecturer in Nursing; M.S., Regis College.
Mary Lombard, Professor of Biology; Ph.D., Boston College.
Margherite Matteis, Associate Professor of Nursing; Ph.D., NYU.
Luanne Nugent, Lecturer in Nursing; M.S., Boston University.
Marybeth Scanlon, Lecturer in Nursing; M.S., Regis College.
Mary Smalarz, Associate Professor of Nursing; Ed.D., Boston University.
Nancy Street, Assistant Professor of Nursing; M.S., Boston College.

Saint Anthony College of Nursing

Rockford, Illinois

THE COLLEGE

Saint Anthony College of Nursing is an upper-division college, offering the last two years of a four-year program for a Bachelor of Science in Nursing. The College of Nursing educates nurses in the science of nursing and the art of life. Students are encouraged to think freely and creatively and become excellent decision makers. The Bachelor of Science in Nursing degree program balances the study of science and liberal arts so graduates are prepared to face challenges in and out of the workplace.

The Sisters of the Third Order opened the Saint Anthony School of Nursing in 1915. During the early 1990s, the institution became a baccalaureate degree–granting institution and changed its name to Saint Anthony College of Nursing. During the school's history, more than 2,700 of its graduates have joined the nursing profession. In August 2006, the College admitted the first students to the Master of Science in Nursing degree program.

The College is a private, Catholic institution the provides quality undergraduate and graduate nursing education. This education, grounded in the liberal arts and sciences, is provided in an environment that encourages open inquiry and lifelong learning in order to serve persons with the greatest care and love.

PROGRAMS OF STUDY

The College offers the final two years of a four-year Bachelor of Science in Nursing (B.S.N.) degree. These two years consist of nursing theory courses and extensive clinical practice experience. The College provides more than 700 hours of direct clinical experience in a variety of acute-care settings, including a Level 1 trauma center. Students also gain experience working in ambulatory care settings, such as home health care, mental health clinics, community agencies, and clinics. Student gain clinical experience with children, adults, and geriatric patients.

There is also a program with which actively licensed Illinois-registered professional nurses can earn a B.S.N. degree (RN to B.S.N.). RNs should contact the Student Affairs Office for information about earning credits for licensure and certifications. A Student at Large program is available for those who wish to enroll without pursuing a degree or who wish to start nursing courses prior to full acceptance.

The Master of Science in Nursing (M.S.N.) program, designed for the part-time student to complete within three years, leads to an M.S.N. degree for nurse educators, clinical nurse leaders, and clinical nurse specialists in adult health concepts.

ACADEMIC FACILITIES

In addition to the facilities of the OSF Saint Anthony Medical Center, students take advantage of the Sister Mary Linus Learning Resource Center, which provides access to a wide variety of both physical and online research material, as well as the recently built skills lab, where equipment, procedures, and safety are learned prior to patient contact.

LOCATION

Saint Anthony College of Nursing is located in Rockford, Illinois, which is 75 miles northwest of Chicago. Rockford is well-known for its industrial corporations and agriculture. Many recreational and cultural opportunities are available in this community of 160,000. In addition to Saint Anthony College of Nursing, there are three other institutions of higher education, three hospitals, a State of Illinois mental health and developmental center, and numerous health-care agencies located in the greater Rockford area.

COSTS

Tuition for the fall 2006 semester was $8085 per semester for full-time students and $506 per credit hour for part-time students. Also required was a $50 application fee, $200 tuition deposit, $50 computer fee, and other miscellaneous fees. Book prices vary. Each student was also required to pay a $13 annual Professional Liability Insurance Fee. There are several payment options, including cash, check, or credit card. The College reserves the right to revise fees at any time. Graduate tuition was $600 per credit hour.

FINANCIAL AID

The primary purpose of the financial aid program is to assure that students who want to attend but who need monetary assistance have the ability to do so. Students must be enrolled in at least 6 credits during a semester and make satisfactory progress. In addition to federal and state programs, several College, community, and health-agency grants are available. To apply for financial aid, a student must complete the Free Application for Federal Student Aid (FAFSA). For additional information, students should contact the College Financial Aid Officer.

APPLYING

A total of 32 prerequisite credits and one of the nursing prerequisite sciences (anatomy and physiology, microbiology, or organic chemistry) must have been completed with a minimum cumulative grade point average (GPA) of 2.5 on a 4.0 scale and a minimum nursing prerequisite science GPA of 2.7 on a 4.0 scale in order to be considered for provisional acceptance. Courses must have been taken at a regionally accredited college or university for a grade of C or above to be considered for transfer credits. Credit may also be awarded for acceptable scores on AP or CLEP tests (as recommended by the American Council on Education) in appropriate subject areas. A total of 64 prerequisite credits must be completed before starting the nursing program. A written statement of personal, professional, educational, and career goals must be completed on campus at the time of the personal interview. This statement is reviewed for both content and ability to communicate effectively.

Three acceptable professional references must be submitted, including one from a current or recent instructor. The other two references should be from a current or recent employer, another instructor, or a school counselor. For those applicants whose primary language is not English, a minimum TOEFL score of 550 is required. Students must also receive satisfactory scores on admission testing for math, reading, English/composition, sciences, and critical thinking.

Admitted students must be in good physical and mental health and be able to carry out the functions of a nursing student as determined by the College. A physical exam within six months of entrance into the B.S.N. degree program is required. Specific health requirements are determined by the College and/or government and clinical agency mandates, including verification of immunizations (tetanus/diphtheria, polio, measles, and mumps), a statement regarding history of chicken pox, rubella titer (students must prove immunity to rubella and rubeola), and a two-step TB skin test no earlier than three weeks before classes begin (an annual TB skin test thereafter and/or annual TB assessment by the College nurse). Affiliated agencies where students have clinical experience may require additional tests. Students are notified by the College when testing is requested by these agencies. Obtaining necessary examinations and tests is the responsibility of the student.

A completed application for admission to the B.S.N. degree program must be submitted to the Office of Student Affairs with the appropriate application fee. Evidence of successful completion of American Heart Association Healthcare Provider cardiopulmonary resuscitation training (to be updated annually) must be submitted in accordance with the College's CPR policy. Verification of health/accident and auto insurance (if operating a motor vehicle) must be on file in the Student Services Office. Professional liability insurance is required. A Transfer/Withdrawal/Dismissal Form must be completed if an applicant has attended another nursing or professional healthcare program but did not satisfactorily complete it.

CORRESPONDENCE AND INFORMATION

Cheryl Delgado
Admissions Representative
Saint Anthony College of Nursing
5658 East State Street
Rockford, Illinois 61008-2468

Phone: 815-227-2141
Fax: 815-395-2275
E-mail: cheryldelgado@sacn.edu
Web site: http://www.sacn.edu

Seton Hall University
College of Nursing
South Orange, New Jersey

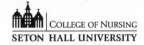

COLLEGE OF NURSING
SETON HALL UNIVERSITY

THE UNIVERSITY

Founded in 1856, Seton Hall is a private coeducational Catholic institution—the nation's oldest diocesan institution of higher education in the United States. It is made up of nine colleges and schools, including SetonWorldWide, the University's online campus. The University enrolls about 10,000 students. Seton Hall University is accredited by the Middle States Association of Colleges and Schools and the Commission on Collegiate Nursing Education, among others.

THE COLLEGE OF NURSING

The College of Nursing has educated many individuals who are in positions of leadership, both locally and throughout the country. The College currently comprises three departments: the Department of Adult Health Nursing, the Department of Family Health Nursing, and the Department of Behavioral Sciences, Community and Health Services. The College's mission is to educate baccalaureate-prepared generalists, master's-prepared advanced practitioners of nursing, and doctorally prepared nurses who aspire to be innovators and leaders in the nursing profession. Both undergraduate and graduate curricula exist within a University community that embraces a student body made rich through cultural, ethnic, and racial diversity—a community where religious commitment and academic freedom are valued. The College of Nursing strives to cultivate values in its students that enable a commitment to lifelong service and compassion to humanity.

PROGRAMS OF STUDY

Undergraduates can pursue a traditional program, the 127-credit Bachelor of Science in Nursing (B.S.N.); an accelerated program for students who have earned a baccalaureate degree in another discipline; or a B.S.N. completion program for registered nurses.

The College of Nursing offers nine 30- to 46-credit majors leading to the Master of Science in Nursing (M.S.N.) degree. Areas of concentration include adult nurse practitioner, pediatric nurse practitioner, gerontological nurse practitioner, health-systems administration, case management/healthcare administration, and school nursing.

The College also offers a 30-credit Master of Arts (M.A.) degree in nursing education for nurses who hold an M.S.N., which can be completed in combination with any of the clinical specialization programs. In conjunction with the Stillman School of Business, the College offers a dual-degree program, the M.S.N. degree in health-systems administration and the Master of Business Administration (M.B.A.) degree.

The College offers a 46-credit Ph.D. program in nursing with a focus in clinical outcomes and evidence-based practice.

The College also offers certificate programs in nursing case management/administration, health-systems administration, Lamaze International childbirth educator, and school nursing as well as a post-master's certification program for nurse practitioners.

The following programs are also offered as online programs through SetonWorldWide: M.S.N. in adult nurse practitioner, pediatric nurse practitioner, gerontological nurse practitioner, health-systems administration, administration/nursing case management; B.S.N. for RNs; and post-master certificates for adult nurse practitioner, pediatric nurse practitioner, and gerontological nurse practitioner.

AFFILIATIONS WITH HEALTH-CARE FACILITIES

The College of Nursing is affiliated with a wide variety of health-care agencies and community resources for clinical practice. These facilities are carefully selected to provide optimal learning experiences for students in all programs.

ACADEMIC FACILITIES

The College of Nursing is the primary site for the students' didactic instruction, with one of the finest physical facilities available to a school of nursing anywhere in the country. The College has its own building, with classrooms designed to accommodate various class sizes and teaching strategies, such as seminar rooms, small-to-large classrooms, and an amphitheater that seats 150 people.

The College has a large media and learning resources center, with extensive audiovisual holdings and a state-of-the-art computer laboratory that has ten IBM desktop computers operating under a Windows XP plat-

form and available printing services from each station. The computer lab is wireless and provides desktop space for laptop computers. The College also has a sophisticated Patient Care Simulation Learning Laboratory that is equipped with several patient-care simulators, a full range of physical examination and treatment equipment, and audiovisual materials. Students use the laboratory to acquire their initial preparation in advanced physical and psychosocial assessment skills. A wide variety of clinical sites are used to prepare students with the advanced nursing knowledge and skills necessary for their roles as educators, administrators, or advanced nurse practitioners.

LOCATION

Seton Hall is located on 58 acres in the village of South Orange, New Jersey, a suburban residential area 14 miles southwest of New York City. The town center is a 10-minute walk from the campus and features bookstores, coffee shops, and restaurants. The heart of midtown Manhattan is about 25 minutes away; students can take advantage of everything this exciting city has to offer while still living in a suburban area.

STUDENT SERVICES

Qualified nursing students are eligible to apply for membership in the Gamma Nu Chapter of Sigma Theta Tau International Honor Society of Nursing. The Gamma Nu Chapter presents scholarly programs throughout the academic year and also sponsors an annual research day. The honor society serves as a positive vehicle for dialogue among nurse scholars.

THE NURSING STUDENT GROUP

Of the 500 undergraduate nursing students, 8 percent are men. There are 175 combined full- and part-time graduate students.

COSTS

The cost for tuition for the 2006–07 academic year was $759 per credit for undergraduate courses and $787 per credit for graduate courses. A University fee is assessed each semester. For undergraduates, room and board cost about $10,160.

FINANCIAL AID

The College of Nursing's Web site offers information on a variety of undergraduate and graduate financial aid and scholarship options. Approximately 68 percent of the baccalaureate students receive some form of aid. In addition to aid available through Enrollment Services, full-time graduate nursing students are eligible to apply for aid through the Division of Graduate Nursing. Federal Nurse Traineeships cover a portion of a student's tuition expenses for full-time matriculated graduate students. The Veterans Administration Health Professional Scholarship Program is available to full-time students pursuing graduate preparation in gerontology. The scholarships are part of a competitive federal program that awards a monthly stipend, tuition, fees, and other reasonable educational expenses, including books and laboratory expenses. In return for each year of the award, scholarship recipients must agree to serve one year as full-time Veteran Administration employees in the Department of Medicine and Surgery, with a minimum service obligation of two years. Full-time graduate students may apply for a graduate assistantship (at the master's level) and teaching assistantships (at the doctoral level), which provide tuition and a monthly stipend.

APPLYING

Undergraduate applicants should have a minimum GPA of 3.0 and should have completed 1 unit each in biology and chemistry. To apply, students must submit the completed application and $45 application fee, official high school transcripts, SAT scores, and a personal statement. The deadline is March 1.

For graduate applicants, undergraduate courses in statistics and basic physical assessment are required. For admission to the nurse practitioner track, it is recommended that applicants have a minimum of at least one year of nursing experience prior to enrolling in practicum courses. Applicants must have a baccalaureate degree with a major in nursing from a program accredited by the National League for Nursing Accrediting Commission (NLNAC) or the Commission on Collegiate Nursing Education (CCNE), a minimum B average overall and in all nursing courses, professional liability insurance, and registered professional nurse licensure in the student's state of practice. Students must submit the completed application, the nonrefundable $50 application fee, a statement of professional goals, scores of the Miller Analogies Test (MAT) or Graduate Record Examinations (GRE), and two letters of reference (one professional, one academic). The College of Nursing processes graduate applications on a rolling basis.

Applicants for the Ph.D. program in nursing must have a master's degree in nursing from a program accredited by the National League for Nursing Accrediting Commission (NLNAC) or the Commission on Collegiate Nursing Education (CCNE) and a minimum 3.0 GPA. Requirements for admission include scores on the Graduate Record Examinations (GRE), a completed application, two letters of recommendation, official transcripts, a statement of career goals, a writing sample, and a resume. Applicants should contact Mary Jo Bugel, Director of Recruitment, directly at 973-761-9285 to apply. The application deadline is June 1 for the fall semester.

CORRESPONDENCE AND INFORMATION:
Mary Jo Bugel, Director of Recruitment
Department of Graduate Nursing
College of Nursing
Seton Hall University
South Orange, New Jersey 07079-2697

Phone: 973-761-9285
Fax: 973-761-9607
E-mail: bugelmar@shu.edu
Web site: http://nursing.shu.edu/

THE FACULTY
Barara Blozen, Instructor; M.A., NYU. Behavioral sciences, community and health.

Kathleen Boreale, Instructor; M.S., Rutgers; APRN, BC, CCRN. Adult health nursing.

Wendy C. Budin, Associate Professor; Ph.D., NYU; RN, BC. Health care of women and the childbearing family; nursing research: social support, breast-cancer adjustment, and education.

Pat Camillo, Associate Professor; Ph.D., Wisconsin–Madison; RNC, ARNP-BC. Women's health across the life span, experience and management of menopause, women's mental health, culture of primary health care.

Jessie Casida, Assistant Professor; M.S., Columbia; RN, CCRN, APN-C. Cardiothoracic surgery/cardiology critical care, heart failure/transplant, implantable LVAD patients' caregivers, organizational culture and leadership.

Catherine Cassidy, Assistant Professor and Director, Graduate Program; Ph.D., NYU; RN. Adult health nursing.

Thomas Cox, Visiting Associate Professor; Ph.D., Virginia Commonwealth; RN. Alternative and complementary health, spirituality, nursing philosophy and theory, research methodology and data analysis, insurance risk transfers to health-care professionals and health-care organizations, ergonomics and human-computer integration, psychiatric nursing, nursing leadership/management.

Linda D'Antoni, Faculty Associate; M.S.N., Rutgers; RN. Adult health nursing.

Jane Cerruti Dellert, Assistant Professor; Ph.D., Rutgers; APRN-BC, CPNP. Parenting, nurse-parent support, children's sports and exercise participation, child-care health consultation.

Josephine De Vito, Associate Professor; Ph.D., NYU; RN. Self-perceptions of parenting among adolescent mothers during the four- to six-week postpartum period.

Gloria Essoka, Distinguished Visiting Professor and Chair, Family Health Nursing; Ph.D., NYU; RN.

Marie Foley, Associate Professor and Director, School Nurse Programs; Ph.D., NYU; RN.

Mary Fortier, Instructor; M.S.N., NYU; RN.

Donna A. Gaffney, Associate Professor; D.N.Sc., Pennsylvania; RN, FAAN. Psychiatric mental-health nursing, forensic nursing, violence prevention and intervention.

Gloria R. Gelmann, Associate Professor; Ed.D., Columbia Teachers College; RN, APN, CPNP/A.

Peggy Greene, Associate Professor; Ed.D., Columbia; RN. Adult health, community health, psychosocial nursing, bioethics, culture and health, leadership and trends, nursing across the life span.

Jamesetta Halley-Boyce, Associate Professor; Ph.D., Walden; RN, FACHE. Program direction, health-systems administration.

Phyllis Shanley Hansell, Professor and Dean; Ed.D., Columbia; RN, FAAN. Stress and coping, social support of families and children with HIV/AIDS.

Susan J. Hart, Assistant Professor; M.S.N., Seton Hall; RN.

Laura Hollywood, Assistant Professor; M.S.N., Columbia; RNC, CNM, FNP.

Gail Herbert Iglesias, Associate Professor; Ph.D., NYU; RN. Depression in elderly, psychiatric nursing in the community.

Margaret Huryk, Assistant Professor; M.S.N., Rutgers; RN. Adult health nursing.

Melinda L. Jenkins, Associate Professor; Ph.D., Pennsylvania; FNP. Family health nursing.

Maria Torchia LoGrippo, Faculty Associate; M.S.N., Pennsylvania; RN. Adult health nursing.

Judith A. Lothian, Associate Professor; Ph.D., NYU; RN. Maternal/child health.

Deborah A. Mandel, Instructor; M.S.N., Pennsylvania; RNC, APN, C. Family health nursing.

Ann Marie Mauro, Assistant Professor; Ph.D., NYU; RN. Cardiovascular nursing, uncertainty in illness, psychosocial adjustment to illness, coping and grieving post–9/11, adult health, nursing research and education.

Denise Nash-Luckenbach, Instructor; M.S.; RN, CCRN. Adult health nursing.

Catherine M. Olsen, Assistant Professor; M.S.N., Akron; APRN, BC. Chronic illness, family therapy.

Brenda Petersen, Instructor; Behavioral Sciences, M.S.N.; RN. Community and health.

Bridget Porta, Instructor; M.S., Rutgers; RN, APN. Adult health nursing.

Patricia Ropis, Instructor; M.S.N., Kean; RN. Critical care, home care and hospice, uses of alternative therapies in nursing practice, effects of stress in nursing, impact of the environment on health.

Mary Carol Rossignol, Assistant Professor; D.N.Sc., Widener; RN. Critical thinking, diabetic women with heart disease, clinical teaching, septic shock.

Jean Rubino, Faculty Associate; Ed.D., Columbia Teachers College; APRN-BC. Mental-health issues across the life span, especially the older adult; anthropology; complimentary modalities.

Jeanne Ruggiero, Associate Professor; Ph.D., Rutgers; RN. Adult health nursing.

Phyllis Russo, Associate Professor and Director, Accelerated Program in Nursing; Ed.D., Seton Hall; RN. Stress and support in older caregivers of children with HIV/AIDS, effect of prayer on terminally ill, concepts of caring in nursing, progression of women in higher education.

Mary Ann Meredith Scharf, Associate Professor; Ed.D., Columbia Teachers College; RN. Community-health nursing, communicable diseases.

Kathleen Walsh Scura, Associate Professor; Ed. D., Sarasota; RN. Adult health nursing.

Maria Serrano, Instructor; M.S.N., Kean; RN. Adult health nursing.

Theodora Sirota, Associate Professor; Ph.D., NYU; RN.

Kathleen Sternas, Associate Professor; Ph.D., Case Western Reserve; RN. Stress, appraisal, coping, resources, and health of individuals experiencing a variety of stressors, including breast cancer, bereavement, and relocation to a nursing home; community-health nursing; community partnerships and service learning; bioterrorism and disaster planning in communities.

Bonnie A. Sturm, Assistant Professor; Ed.D., Columbia Teachers College; RN. Issues involving ethics or conflict (especially in relation to experience of nurses and students), demonstration of the value of nursing interventions in improving health outcomes (in particular, therapeutic interventions in psychiatric nursing), value of the therapeutic relationship in treatment and care of individuals with mental illness in diverse community settings, studies in learning and motivation (related to clients or students).

Sherri Suozzo, Instructor; M.S.N., Pennsylvania; RN, APN-C, AOCN. Adult health nursing.

Linda Ulak, Associate Professor; Chair, Undergraduate Nursing; and Director, RN Program; Ed.D., Seton Hall; RN, CS, CCRN.

Caryle Wolahan, Visiting Professor; Ed.D., Columbia; RN, FAAN. Behavioral sciences, community and health.

Joyce Wright, Assistant Professor and Director, Accelerated Program in Lakewood, NJ; D.N.Sc., Widener; RN, CCRN. Adult health nursing, leadership, critical-care nursing.

Thomas Edison State College
School of Nursing
Trenton, New Jersey

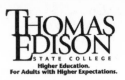

THOMAS EDISON
STATE COLLEGE
Higher Education.
For Adults with Higher Expectations.

THE COLLEGE

Thomas Edison State College provides flexible, high-quality collegiate learning opportunities for self-directed adults. Cited as "one of the brighter stars of higher learning" by the *New York Times* and identified by *Forbes* magazine as one of the top twenty colleges and universities in the nation in the use of technology to create learning opportunities for adults, Thomas Edison State College provides high-quality higher education to adults wherever they live and work. Founded in 1972, Thomas Edison State College enables adult students to complete associate, baccalaureate, and master's degrees through distance learning, using a variety of different methods of credit earning.

THE NURSING PROGRAM

The School of Nursing at Thomas Edison State College offers an RN-B.S.N./M.S.N. Nurse Educator degree program that is designed for experienced RNs who want a high-quality education with the convenience and flexibility that an online program can provide. Admission is open and rolling; RNs can enroll any day of the year. The schedule is self-paced; there is no time limit for degree completion. There is no residency requirement. Maximum credit for prior learning is given, and multiple credit earning options are available. With highly interactive, asynchronous online group discussions, adult independent learners become part of a community of learners where experiences are shared and learning is enhanced. More than 500 RNs are currently enrolled in the School.

In the School of Nursing, experienced and academically qualified nurse educators from throughout the country fulfill the roles traditionally held by faculty members in campus-based programs. Known as mentors, these educators all have a minimum of a master's degree in nursing, with approximately 85 percent prepared at the doctoral level and many tenured at their home institution.

PROGRAMS OF STUDY

The Bachelor of Science in Nursing (B.S.N.) degree includes 9 graduate credits (three courses) that are applied to the School's Master of Science in Nursing (M.S.N.) degree program at no additional per-credit tuition charge if the student continues on for that degree. Initiated in 1983 as an examination-based program to provide for additional educational opportunities for RNs in New Jersey to attain a B.S.N. degree, the program transitioned to an online format in 2001, became the School of Nursing in 2003, and was opened to out-of-state RNs in 2004. The M.S.N. degree program opened in 2006.

The B.S.N. degree requires a minimum of 120 semester hours of credit—60 in general education, 48 in nursing, and 12 in free electives. RN graduates of an associate degree nursing program or a diploma program of nursing may have 20 credits from previous course work applied toward the nursing requirement. A total of 80 credits may be accepted from a community college, and up to 60 credits, including the 20 credits used in the nursing requirement, may be awarded to diploma graduates based on current RN licensure. There is no age restriction on credits transferred to Thomas Edison State College to meet general education requirements or lower-division nursing requirements. All credits transferred to Thomas Edison State College to satisfy upper-division nursing requirements must be from an accredited baccalaureate or higher-degree nursing program or from other Thomas Edison State College–approved credit-earning methods, must be newer than ten years, and must have a grade equivalent of C or better for the B.S.N. degree and B or better for the M.S.N. degree.

In addition to the 20-credit lower-division nursing requirement for the B.S.N. degree, there is a 28-credit upper-division nursing requirement. All eight requirements may be satisfied by twelve-week, online nursing courses offered quarterly by the School. All nursing courses are 3 credits each, with the exception of Community Health Nursing, which is 7 credits.

All nursing courses are independent learning, highly interactive courses that require student participation in asynchronous online group discussions at least three times weekly, in addition to readings and the online submission of written assignments. Assessment of learning by the online course mentors occurs via the online group discussion participation and written assignments; there are no proctored examinations. Graduations are quarterly.

There is no time limit for degree completion; however, students are required to complete a minimum of 3 credits that apply to degree requirements in each twelve-month period to remain on active status in the School. On completion of the B.S.N. degree, graduates who continue on for the M.S.N. degree have only an additional nine courses to complete, or 27 of the required 36 credits to complete the M.S.N. degree. The B.S.N. degree program is accredited by the National League for Nursing Accrediting Commission (NLNAC). A letter of support to develop the RN-B.S.N./M.S.N. degree program is on file from NLNAC; accreditation is being sought in accordance with accreditation guidelines.

ACADEMIC FACILITIES

Thomas Edison State College uses state-of-the-art technology to deliver its academic program via the Intranet. Students have access to the rich library research facilities of the New Jersey State Library, which is an affiliate of Thomas Edison State College. Students also have access to the Virtual Academic Library Environment (VALE), a consortium of fifty-two New Jersey colleges and universities, which provides access to a network of research libraries.

LOCATION

Thomas Edison State College is located in the capital city of Trenton, New Jersey, but its reach is global. Students live and study in all fifty states and more than seventy other countries. The College's campus comprises the Kelsey Building at 101 West State Street and the adjacent Townhouse Complex, the Academic Center at 167 West Hanover Street, the Canal Banks

Building at 221 West Hanover Street, and the Kuser Mansion at 315 West State Street. The College's state-of-the-art facilities, from electronic classrooms and computer labs to a corporate-style education conference room and other amenities, allow Thomas Edison State College to link students and mentors at dozens of colleges throughout the country and around the world.

STUDENT SERVICES

The Thomas Edison State College School of Nursing programs are distinctive in that they are completed entirely at a distance; therefore, students are provided access to the services needed primarily via online format. The College offers all core student services via the Internet through iTESC®, a suite of online services. Also through the Internet, students have access to such services as course and test registration and payment; displaying of registration schedules, course and mentor availability, and grades; displaying and updating of student information; online course and mentor evaluations; and other services.

In addition to technical support provided by the College's Office of Management Information Systems (MIS), a technical support mentor is embedded in the School's online nursing program. This mentor answers questions and provides support for students and other mentors when any technological issue arises. Writing assistance is available in the online courses.

B.S.N. degree students have access to all academic advisement services provided by the College, including the availability of an academic adviser for nursing. Enrolled students may access advisement services by the U.S. Postal Service, fax, e-mail, telephone, or in-person appointments. All College and program publications provided to students may also be accessed on the College Web site.

THE NURSING STUDENT GROUP

Students in the Thomas Edison State College School of Nursing degree program are typically midcareer professionals with a wide variety of nursing practice and management experience. The average student is 41 years old. Of the approximately 500 students enrolled in the 2006–07 academic year, nearly all were actively employed in nursing. Approximately 10 percent of the enrolled students were men, and the program enjoyed a 25 percent diversity rate.

COSTS

The tuition for the 2006–07 academic year was $286 per credit for New Jersey residents and $335 per credit for out-of-state residents for the B.S.N. degree; $433 per credit for the M.S.N. degree. There is a $75 nonrefundable application fee and a one-time nonrefundable $300 B.S.N. credential-review fee. The estimated cost for books and supplies for the online nursing courses is $100 per course.

FINANCIAL AID

Nursing students support their study primarily with employer tuition aid and loans. Unsubsidized loans are available to all accepted applicants. The Thomas Edison State College Office of Financial Aid & Veterans' Affairs is available to assist students.

APPLYING

Applicants to the School of Nursing must be RNs with a current and valid license in the United States and proficiency in using a computer, browsing the Web, and sending and receiving Internet mail, including attachments. They must also have access to, and a familiarity with, PowerPoint and Excel software. Minimum system requirements to access an online course are access to the Internet; Internet browser, such as Netscape 8.1 or newer or Internet Explorer 5.5 or newer; and Windows 98 or higher or equivalent operating system. Applicants must submit the completed School of Nursing application with the nonrefundable application fee, nonrefundable B.S.N. credential review fee, and a notarized copy of RN current license valid in the U.S. to the College's Office of Admissions. Applicants should have all official college transcripts and college-level examination score reports sent to the College's Office of the Registrar.

CORRESPONDENCE AND INFORMATION

Renee San Giacomo
Director of Admissions
Thomas Edison State College
101 West State Street
Trenton, New Jersey 08608-1176

Phone: 888-442-8372 (toll-free)
Fax: 609-984-8447
E-mail: nursinginfo@tesc.edu
Web site: http://www.tesc.edu

Thomas Jefferson University
School of Nursing
Philadelphia, Pennsylvania

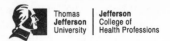

THE UNIVERSITY

Jefferson College of Health Professions (JCHP) is an integral part of one of the nation's oldest academic health centers, Thomas Jefferson University, which also includes Jefferson Medical College and Jefferson College of Graduate Studies. JCHP has three schools: a School of Health Professions (consisting of the Departments of Bioscience Technologies, General Studies, Couple and Family Therapy, Occupational Therapy, Physical Therapy, and Radiologic Sciences), a School of Nursing, and a School of Pharmacy (scheduled to open in fall 2008).

JCHP is part of a campuswide commitment to excellence in educating health-care professionals and discovering knowledge to define the future of clinical care. Scholarship and applied, collaborative, and interdisciplinary research are integral to generating this new health-care knowledge.

JCHP is an upper-division college, meaning that students generally transfer into a program in their junior year. High school students can reserve a seat in a future class by applying to JCHP through the Plan a College Education (PACE) program and attending an affiliated school for two years. Those interested in physical therapy, occupational therapy, or bioscience technologies can take advantage of special agreements with Elizabethtown College, Muhlenberg College, Penn State Abington, Saint Joseph's University, and Villanova University. An associate degree program in nursing for high school graduates is also available.

THE SCHOOL OF NURSING

For more than 100 years, Jefferson has been educating men and women for the nursing profession, first through a diploma program and now with a continuum of professional development opportunities, from associate degree to Master of Science in Nursing. Jefferson awards the Associate to Bachelor of Science in Nursing (A.S.N.-B.S.N.), the Bachelor of Science in Nursing (B.S.N.), the Master of Science in Nursing (M.S.N.), and post-master's certificates. All nursing programs are fully accredited by the American Association of Colleges of Nursing Commission on Collegiate Nursing Education (CCNE) through 2011.

The majority of Jefferson's nursing faculty members are doctorally prepared. All faculty members have a deep commitment to their roles as teachers, and they work hard to develop professionalism within students. Undergraduate and graduate students have the opportunity to participate in faculty research, scholarly activities, and practice, as well as to collaborate in interdisciplinary University projects. The School of Nursing currently enrolls 556 undergraduates, the majority of whom are full-time, and 249 graduate students, the majority of whom enroll on a part-time basis.

PROGRAMS OF STUDY

The first half of the A.S.N.-B.S.N. curriculum offered by the School of Nursing prepares students to serve as generalists in the role of caregiver in a hospital or in-patient setting. Students complete 68 credits of general education and nursing course work, completing the A.S.N. program in two academic years. Graduates may then progress to complete a bachelor's degree in two or more years. This program is offered at the Center City Philadelphia campus and the Geisinger Medical Center campus in Danville, Pennsylvania.

The B.S.N. curriculum is an upper-division program that emphasizes interdisciplinary education among students in the health professions. Students enter the nursing program at Jefferson after completing 59 lower-division credits in the sciences and humanities. The B.S.N. program balances liberal arts, sciences, and humanities with professional nursing preparation. It emphasizes health promotion, maintenance, and disease prevention as well as managing individuals and families coping with acute and chronic illness. Students complete 64 nursing credits at Jefferson. Full-time and part-time options are available. Graduates are prepared to practice professional nursing as generalists in a variety of health-care settings. The undergraduate program is among the most progressive in the United States.

The RN-B.S.N. program is designed to prepare registered nurses who graduated from diploma or associate degree nursing programs for an increased leadership role in nursing. Students complete 60 credits of sciences and humanities in lower-division courses prior to entering the nursing major at Jefferson. Thirty-five upper-division credits are awarded for previous nursing knowledge, and RN students have the unique opportunity to earn 10 of the remaining upper-division credits through a portfolio assessment of previous nursing knowledge. This enables RN students to begin the program in their senior year and complete the program in two semesters of full-time study or two years of part-time study. RNs can earn the B.S.N. completely online.

The RN-B.S.N./M.S.N. option allows RN students who have obtained their basic nursing education through either a diploma or associate degree program to qualify for admission to graduate nursing education through a combined B.S.N./M.S.N. program. With this option, RN students can earn the B.S.N. and M.S.N. degrees in a seamless integrated curriculum. Both degrees can be completed entirely online. An Accelerated Pathway option is available to RN students with a baccalaureate degree in a field other than nursing.

Two programs leading to the B.S.N. and M.S.N. degrees are available to highly motivated, academically talented students who hold a bachelor's degree in a field other than nursing. The Facilitated Academic Coursework Track (FACT) is a very intense program that enables prelicensure students to complete both degrees in two calendar years of full-time study. The Accelerated Pathway to the M.S.N. for Second-Degree Students is slower paced and enables students to earn both degrees in three academic years of full-time study. (A similar program is available for RNs.)

The Master of Science in Nursing program prepares nurses for advanced and sophisticated clinical practice. The graduate program offers nurse practitioner, clinical nurse specialist, and post-master's certificate programs in acute care, adult health, community systems administration, family medicine, neonatal, nursing informatics, nurse anesthesia (CRNA), oncology, and pediatrics.

The curriculum is predicated on the School of Nursing's belief that professional nursing is an art and a science that incorporates theory, research, and clinical practice. The graduate curriculum is organized using a core curriculum concept. Most courses are available both in the classroom and via the Internet. All specialty areas except CRNA require 36 credits and can be completed part-time or full-time. The 74-credit CRNA program requires thirty months of full-time study.

AFFILIATIONS WITH HEALTH-CARE FACILITIES

The University shares its campus with Thomas Jefferson University Hospital, one of the nation's premier health-care facilities. The multi-institutional Jefferson Health System and other leading hospitals and agencies throughout the region offer outstanding learning opportunities in a broad array of health-care settings.

ACADEMIC FACILITIES

Administrative and academic offices, classrooms, laboratories, and a Learning Resource Center, including a computer laboratory, are located in Jefferson's Edison Building. Jefferson Alumni Hall, a basic medical science/student commons building, houses Jefferson College of Graduate Studies, basic science departments, classrooms, and research laboratories. The University library and administrative offices are located in the Scott Building. Clinical experience is acquired at Thomas Jefferson University Hospital or at more than 1,800 clinical affiliate sites.

Professional counseling services are available for all students who need assistance in resolving academic, vocational, and personal concerns.

LOCATION

Jefferson is in the center of Philadelphia, stretching from 8th to 11th Streets and from Chestnut to Locust Streets. In this prime location, a short walk takes students almost anywhere they need to go. Jefferson is four blocks from Independence Hall and the Liberty Bell, three blocks from Chinatown, seven blocks from South Street's funky shops and restaurants, and eight blocks from Rittenhouse Square's popular park and shopping area. Students may also use the bus (several lines run through the campus) or subway (only two blocks away) to get across town. Getting out of town is a breeze; the Market East regional rail station is two blocks away, Amtrak's 30th Street Station is less than a mile, and the Philadelphia International Airport is a 30-minute train ride.

Living on campus means that classes, the hospital, and the library are within easy walking distance. From studios to luxury three-bedroom apartments, Jefferson housing offers something to match almost any budget. The on-campus community includes students from JCHP, Jefferson Medical College, and Jefferson College of Graduate Studies, as well as postdoctoral fellows and medical residents.

STUDENT SERVICES

The University's many resources and services include academic advising, counseling, housing, student health, tutoring, day care, fitness facilities, computing services, student organizations, and career services.

THE NURSING STUDENT GROUP

Students enrolled in the undergraduate and graduate programs represent a diverse group in terms of age, gender, ethnicity, cultural background, socioeconomic status, and religious orientation. In fall 2005, approximately 36 percent of the students indicated that they are members of ethnic minority groups. About 15 percent of the undergraduate students are registered nurses pursuing the B.S.N. Nursing students are active in University-wide student organizations and activities as well as nursing-specific organizations and activities. Jefferson's graduates are highly respected and recruited. The job placement rate for 2005 nursing graduates who pursued employment was 97 percent, with graduates often receiving multiple offers.

COSTS

Tuition for full-time B.S.N. students for the 2006–07 academic year was $23,184. Part-time tuition was $744 per credit. Tuition for full-time M.S.N. students was $25,248. Part-time tuition was $800 per credit. The twelve-month FACT fee was $28,075.

FINANCIAL AID

Jefferson is committed to meeting the financial needs of its students. More than 79 percent of the current students receive financial assistance. Aid can include Federal Pell Grants, National Direct Student Loans, the College Work-Study Program, Air Force ROTC scholarships, nursing scholarships, nursing loans, state grants, work scholarships, state-guaranteed loans, and academic scholarships. Completed applications must be received by the Financial Aid Office no later than May 1 to ensure the maximum award.

APPLYING

Prospective students should apply as soon as possible after September 1 for the following year. Applications are evaluated on a rolling basis. FACT applicants must have all application materials submitted no later than March 1. Along with a completed application and nonrefundable application fee of $50, applicants must submit transcripts for all college work, an essay, and two letters of recommendation. An interview is required for all academically eligible applicants. A high school transcript is required for PACE applicants. An evaluation of international transcripts by the World Education Service (WES) is required. All international students and U.S. permanent residents must demonstrate English language proficiency, as outlined by the Office of Admissions.

Applications to the M.S.N. program are accepted on an ongoing basis. For all programs except CRNA, full-time students begin the program in the summer semester. Part-time students may begin in the fall, spring, or summer semester. Admission requirements include RN licensure, a bachelor's degree in nursing or a nurse doctorate, a minimum GPA of 3.0 on a 4.0 scale, competitive scores on the GRE or MAT if the cumulative GPA from the B.S.N. is less than 3.2, undergraduate courses in statistics and nursing research, a course in basic physical assessment skills, computer literacy, two letters of reference, a resume, and an essay addressing professional goals. CRNA applicants also need current ACLS and PALS certification, a resume that demonstrates a minimum of one year of experience in a critical-care nursing setting, and an interview with the CRNA program director. The CRNA program is a full-time program that begins in January.

CORRESPONDENCE AND INFORMATION

Office of Admissions
Edison Building, Suite 1610
Thomas Jefferson University
130 South 9th Street
Philadelphia, Pennsylvania 19107-5233
Phone: 215-503-8890
      877-JEFF-CHP (toll-free)
Fax: 215-503-7241
Web site: http://www.jefferson.edu/jchp

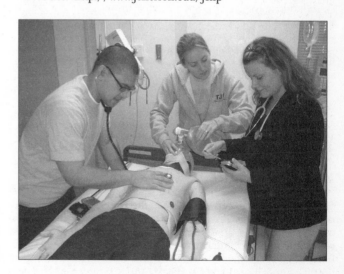

The University of Akron
College of Nursing
Akron, Ohio

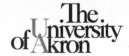

THE UNIVERSITY

The University of Akron (UA) is the public research university for northern Ohio. Founded in 1870, it is the only public university in Ohio with a science/engineering program ranked among the nation's top five by *U.S. News & World Report.* The University of Akron excels in such areas as polymer science, gerontological nursing, global business, and marketing.

The University of Akron is also a world leader in creating new materials for the new economy; a national leader in the development, protection, management, and commercialization of intellectual property; and a regional leader in information technology initiatives.

UA's polymer science and engineering program is ranked second in the nation, serves Ohio's $22-billion polymer industry, and includes NASA-supported nanotechnology initiatives. The University also has strong ties with business leaders, including IT partnerships with IBM, Cisco Systems, and TimeWarner.

Serving more than 23,000 students, the University offers approximately 300 associate, bachelor's, master's, doctoral, and law degree programs and approximately 100 certificate programs through ten degree-granting colleges at its main campus in Akron and its Wayne College branch campus in Orrville and at sites throughout Medina and Summit counties.

Professionals who want to improve their careers can select from a wide range of workshops and courses, including weekend programs offering degrees at an accelerated pace, through The University of Akron's Workforce Development and Continuing Education Division. The New Landscape for Learning, an ongoing, major campus renovation campaign that began in 2000, has added ten new buildings, fifteen major additions and renovations to existing facilities, and 30 acres of new green space to campus. In 2007, the University will open its fifteenth new residence hall. In 2006, the John S. and James L. Knight Foundation gave its largest-ever single grant, $10 million, to support UA's innovative efforts to revitalize a 40-block area surrounding its campus.

For more information about The University of Akron, students should visit the University's Web site (http://www.uakron.edu) or call 800-655-4884 (toll-free).

THE COLLEGE OF NURSING

Founded in 1967, the College has a long tradition of excellence. The College offers multiple educational programs designed to meet the needs of both students aspiring to become professional nurses and practicing professional nurses seeking career advancement.

Located on the campus in Mary Gladwin Hall, the College offers the basic baccalaureate program (B.S.N.), an accelerated B.S.N. for students who hold a bachelor's degree in an area other than nursing, an RN/B.S.N. sequence for registered nurse graduates of associate degree and diploma programs, an LPN/B.S.N. sequence for licensed practical nurses aspiring to become professional nurses, the Master of Science in Nursing (M.S.N.) degree, and the RN/M.S.N. sequence for registered nurse graduates of associate degree and diploma programs who meet graduate standards. The University of Akron and Kent State University offer a Joint Ph.D. in Nursing (JPDN) program, a single doctoral program with a single, unified doctoral nursing faculty and student body. The program prepares scholars in

nursing with balanced preparation to be researchers, educators, administrators, consultants, or entrepreneurs.

There are 48 full-time and 44 part-time faculty members. Twenty-four full-time faculty members (50 percent) hold doctoral degrees. The remainder have master's degrees in nursing, with many having earned certification in advanced practice specialty areas.

The College offers clinical experiences for students in a wide variety of traditional and nontraditional settings and with diverse patient populations, including care of adults in hospitals, community agencies, and homes; care of well and ill elderly; care of newborns and children; care of persons with mental health problems in hospitals and community agencies; critical care; and extended care and rehabilitation.

The College is approved by the Ohio Board of Nursing, and fully accredited by the Commission on Collegiate Nursing Education (CCNE).

International study in nursing through a summer elective course is often available.

PROGRAMS OF STUDY

The basic baccalaureate program leading to the B.S.N. degree and RN licensure is a four-year program that is balanced between nursing courses and University courses. Students enter the program after completing one year of prerequisite University courses. The nursing courses span three years, with clinical experiences in each semester of the program. The senior year features a senior practicum that is designed to give the student greater depth in an area of the student's choosing. A Cooperative Education Program is available to combine work and study.

A fifteen-month accelerated B.S.N. program is open to students who already hold a bachelor's degree and have completed prerequisite courses. All science courses must have been taken within the last five years.

The RN/B.S.N. sequence has been serving the educational needs of registered nurses since 1980. The sequence features learning contracts to allow flexible hours for clinical requirements and classroom time scheduled one day per week. Once students are admitted to the major, they can complete the sequence in one calendar year of full-time study; a part-time option is available. There is no testing required for admission. An outreach RN/B.S.N. sequence is offered at the Lorain County Community College campus and Wayne College.

The LPN/B.S.N. sequence was begun in 1990. The College was one of the first baccalaureate programs in the country to offer a sequence for LPNs. This sequence features testing for advanced placement and credit for prior learning. The LPN can finish the baccalaureate program in four semesters if advanced placement is earned.

The Master of Science in Nursing (M.S.N.) degree program prepares graduates for roles in advanced practice or advanced role preparation in administration. Within the advanced practice options, students may choose adult/gerontological health nursing, behavioral health nursing, child and adolescent health nursing, or nurse anesthesia tracks. Advanced practice options include preparation as a nurse practitioner or clinical nurse specialist. All M.S.N. graduate students take a common core and advanced practice or role options that include advanced clinical experiences.

The RN/M.S.N. sequence is designed for RN graduates of associate degree and diploma programs who meet graduate admission criteria. Students take three years to complete the sequence, which includes baccalaureate and master's course work. Through this program, the student receives both the B.S.N. and M.S.N. degrees.

An M.P.H. consortium program exists with the Northeast Ohio University College of Medicine (NEOUCOM).

ACADEMIC FACILITIES
The College has a state-of-the-art learning resources center that includes simulated patient care areas and a computer laboratory. The College also has a Center for Nursing, which links the College to the community and is used by clients for health-care services and by the faculty and students as a practice and research site. The nursing library holdings are contained in the Science and Technology Library of the University. Nursing students have full access to all the facilities and services of the entire University.

LOCATION
Located in the northeast region of Ohio, Akron offers a wide variety of recreational, business, and cultural activities. The area is perfect for recreational activities that encompass all seasons. The University's presence in northeast Ohio provides numerous opportunities in major collegiate, amateur, and professional sports, concerts, cultural events, and commerce, all within easy driving distance and many accessible via public transportation. On campus, the Ohio Ballet, Emily Davis Art Gallery, University Orchestra, Opera/Musical Theatre, concerts, recitals, choral programs, Touring Arts Program, University Theatre, Repertory Dance Company, and professional artists performing at Edwin J. Thomas Performing Arts Hall contribute to the University's rich cultural environment.

Blossom Music Center, summer home of the Cleveland Orchestra, is located 20 minutes north of the campus. The city of Cleveland with all its fine recreational, sports, and cultural offerings is just 40 minutes from the University.

STUDENT SERVICES
The University has many resource and service offices to meet student needs. Campus resources include the Academic Advisement Center, Adult Resource Center, Sixty Plus Program, Placement Services, Student Employment, Career Placement Services, Student Volunteer Program, Counseling and Testing Center, Financial Aid Office, Student Health Services, Pan-African Culture and Research Center, Office of International Programs, Office of Multicultural Development, Peer Counseling Program, Office of Accessibility, and writing, reading, and math developmental laboratories.

Undergraduate and graduate student organizations exist to involve students in the governance of the College. The Delta Omega chapter of Sigma Theta Tau, the international honor society of nursing, is housed within the College. The Collegiate Nursing Club, which is open to all undergraduate students, is affiliated with the National Student Nurses Association.

A new campus Student Recreation and Wellness Center and the Ocasek Natatorium are open to nursing students.

THE NURSING STUDENT GROUP
Enrollment in the undergraduate program is 595; it is 224 in the graduate program. Full-time and part-time students are represented in both programs. Postbaccalaureate students, RNs, LPNs, transfer students, and new high school graduates are represented in the College. About 10 percent of each entering B.S.N. class in the undergraduate program are men.

COSTS
Undergraduate tuition and fees for the 2006–07 academic year for Ohio residents were $349.29 per credit up to 11.5 credits or a $4191.48 flat fee per semester for 12 to 15 credits. Nonresidents paid a $308.27 per-credit surcharge.

Graduate tuition costs for the 2006–07 academic year were $366.69 per credit for Ohio residents. There was a $245.03 per-credit surcharge for nonresidents.

Additional costs include housing, transportation, books, course laboratory fees, immunizations, CPR certification, uniforms, and liability insurance.

FINANCIAL AID
Financial aid is available through the University as well as the College of Nursing. The University offers a variety of scholarships, grants, loans, student assistantships, work-study opportunities, and graduate assistantships. The College offers a variety of scholarships, graduate assistantships, and Federal Graduate Nurse Traineeships.

APPLYING
Students applying for the baccalaureate program must have completed one year of prerequisite college/university courses and have earned at least a 2.75 grade point average in those prerequisite courses. Applicants must be enrolled at The University of Akron for the spring semester prior to admission and are ranked according to grade point average in science courses after completion of the spring semester. Each year, up to 160 students are admitted into the undergraduate program. Course work begins in the fall.

Students entering the LPN/B.S.N. sequence must hold a current Ohio LPN license and have completed two years of prerequisite college/university courses with a minimum overall college grade point average of 2.75. Course work begins in the spring semester.

Requirements for the RN/B.S.N. sequence include completion of prerequisite courses and current Ohio RN licensure. Course work begins in the summer.

Students applying to the M.S.N. program must hold a baccalaureate degree in nursing from an NLNAC-accredited nursing program; complete prerequisite courses; submit scores from the GRE taken within the last five years (CRNA program only), an essay, and three letters of reference; and hold a current Ohio RN license.

CORRESPONDENCE AND INFORMATION
Office of Student Affairs
College of Nursing
The University of Akron
Akron, Ohio 44325-3701

Phone: 888-477-7887 (toll-free)

Office of Undergraduate Admissions
The University of Akron
Akron, Ohio 44325-2001

Phone: 330-972-7100

Office of Graduate Admissions
The University of Akron
Akron, Ohio 44325-2101

Phone: 330-972-7663

Office of Financial Aid
The University of Akron
Akron, Ohio 44325-6211

Phone: 330-972-7032

Web site: http://www.uakron.edu

The University of Alabama in Huntsville
College of Nursing
Huntsville, Alabama

THE UNIVERSITY

The University of Alabama in Huntsville (UAH), one of the three campuses comprising the University of Alabama System, is accredited by the Commission on Colleges of the Southern Association of Colleges and Schools to award bachelor's, master's, and doctoral degrees. Nestled in the rolling foothills of north-central Alabama, Huntsville is internationally renowned for its high-technology industry and its ties to the U.S. space program. UAH was one of the original groups of colleges and universities to be designated a space-grant college. UAH offers both undergraduate and graduate nursing programs and is the area's center for research activities in nursing.

The modern 350-acre UAH campus has thirty-one major buildings, including the College of Nursing. UAH has more than 7,100 students and more than 300 full-time faculty members, 89 percent with terminal degrees.

THE COLLEGE OF NURSING

The College of Nursing offers the Bachelor of Science in Nursing (B.S.N.) degree and the Master of Science in Nursing (M.S.N.) degree as well as a Post-master's Family Nurse Practitioner Certificate and a Graduate Nursing Education Certificate. The undergraduate and graduate programs are designed to give the student the theoretical and experiential bases for current and future practice. The College of Nursing is accredited by the Collegiate Commission on Nursing Education and is approved by the Alabama Board of Nursing.

Although nursing is becoming highly specialized, it remains, fundamentally, a caring profession. UAH took both of these aspects into consideration when designing its curriculum in nursing. In addition to focusing on essentials of nursing in hospitals, the curriculum also emphasizes community-based practice and primary care. When the revised curriculum for the College of Nursing was submitted for approval, the Alabama Board of Nursing applauded the efforts of the UAH College of Nursing in developing an innovative and forward-looking program for preparing students to function in the rapidly changing nursing field.

The 40 faculty members in the College of Nursing place a high priority on teaching and individual attention to students. The undergraduate student-faculty ratio in clinical areas is less than 10:1. The professors have an ongoing concern with some of the most significant issues in nursing today, including breast cancer research, nursing ethics, health care to underserved rural populations, space research, and health policy.

PROGRAMS OF STUDY

The Bachelor of Science in Nursing (B.S.N.) degree provides the nursing theory, science, humanities, and behavioral science preparation necessary for the full scope of professional nursing responsibilities and provides the knowledge base necessary for advanced education in specialized clinical practice. Building on the foundation provided by 60 semester hours of general education requirements, the baccalaureate curriculum provides extensive clinical opportunities in the context of a holistic, family-centered, community-based approach. Computer technology is integrated throughout the curriculum. A minimum of 129 semester hours are required for the B.S.N.; 69 semester hours must be in nursing.

The UAH College of Nursing also offers a specialized B.S.N. curriculum designed for registered nurses. This program recognizes the unique abilities and needs of registered nurse students and builds on students' existing knowledge and experience. Classes are offered online, with one or two campus visits per semester. This twelve-month program offers both full- and part-time attendance options. The students in the RN/B.S.N. program must also earn 128 semester hours of credit. Registered nurse students receive 32 semester hours of validated nursing credit for previous nursing knowledge and take an additional 37 semester hours of nursing at UAH. The RN-M.S.N. early decision option is available to associate degree–prepared RNs. Nurses who decide early in their course of study that they wish to receive both a B.S.N. and an M.S.N. can complete both in a seven-semester sequence. Students enrolled in this option may have both online and on-campus courses.

The graduate program in nursing leads to the Master of Science in Nursing degree. This program focuses on preparation for advanced nursing practice. It prepares graduates to assume leadership roles in the direct delivery of care as nurse practitioners in primary care (family nurse practitioners) and in acute care (acute-care nurse practitioners or adult health clinicians) or in the administration of health-care delivery systems (leadership in health-care systems or clinical nurse leaders). The M.S.N. program can be completed in four semesters, although other options are also available for students who prefer a slower pace. With the exception of the leadership in health-care systems program, which is offered in an online format, graduate courses are taught one day a week to accommodate the majority of students who continue to practice while pursuing the M.S.N. The length of the program varies by specialty and ranges from 39 to 42 semester hours. Both thesis and nonthesis options are available. Nurse practitioner students complete 588 clinical hours, adult health clinicians and clinical nurse leaders complete 504 clinical hours, and students in the leadership in health-care systems program complete 336 clinical hours.

The Graduate Certificate in Nursing Education is a five-course, 15-semester-hour program offered to graduate and postgraduate nursing students. The Post-M.S.N. Family Nurse Practitioner Certificate Program is designed for individuals who have already earned a master's degree in nursing and who desire additional preparation for family nurse practitioner certification. The program is three semesters in length.

ACADEMIC FACILITIES

Located in the center of the UAH main campus, the Nursing Building is a spacious, four-story structure that houses state-of-the-art equipment, lecture rooms, and laboratories for teaching nursing. The building also contains faculty and administrative offices. A Learning Resource Center (LRC), equipped with a comprehensive selection of audiovisual materials, is available to students for independent study and group learning activities. A well-equipped computer lab in the Learning Resource Center is available for use by all nursing students.

Located adjacent to the Nursing Building, the UAH library has a collection of 412,571 volumes and receives some 2,766 periodicals. The library houses both monographs and journals useful to nursing students. A well-equipped computer lab that duplicates the lab found in the LRC is available for use by all nursing students. Students are also able to use the Medical Library at the University of Alabama School of Medicine–Huntsville Program, which is located in the heart of the city's medical district.

Clinical experiences are arranged in a variety of appropriate settings within the Huntsville area, which serves as a regional center for state-of-the-art health care. With three major hospitals in Huntsville and a wide variety of health-care facilities located close by, adequate resources are available to offer students a broad array of clinical nursing experiences.

LOCATION
The University is located in Huntsville, Alabama, adjacent to Cummings Research Park and close to Redstone Arsenal and NASA's Marshall Space Flight Center. A wonderful mix of modern amenities and old Southern charm, Huntsville is a regional center for arts, entertainment, industry, and medicine. Located in the foothills of the Appalachian Mountain chain, Huntsville is 4 hours from Memphis and Atlanta and approximately 2 hours from Birmingham and Nashville.

STUDENT SERVICES
UAH provides a full-range of student services for all members of the student body. These services include the student counseling center, wellness center, tutorial services, academic advisement center, and office of multicultural affairs.

The College of Nursing funds and supports its own Office of Student Affairs to meet the needs of all students enrolled in the College. Located in the Nursing Building and staffed by student services professionals, the Office of Student Affairs provides assistance with admissions, academic advisement and registration services, information on financial aid, and referral services.

The University also provides a rich and varied extracurricular program. There are more than 100 student clubs and organizations on campus, including dozens of honor societies, preprofessional clubs, and sororities and fraternities. Cabarets, films, dances, concerts, and lectures are offered throughout the year. In addition to a full slate of intramural activities, UAH fields varsity teams in eight sports.

THE NURSING STUDENT GROUP
Approximately 500 undergraduate and 200 graduate students, representing a wide variety of ages, ethnic backgrounds, and experiences, make up the diverse students body in the College of Nursing.

COSTS
Tuition and fees for the 2006–07 academic year were approximately $3600 per semester for in-state baccalaureate students. Graduate tuition and fees were approximately $4300 per semester. For RN/B.S.N. students, additional expenses may include fees for Credit by Validation. Supplementary costs may be incurred for items required at the time of admission, such as fees for uniforms, liability insurance, physical examinations, CPR certification, and hepatitis B immunizations.

FINANCIAL AID
Various types of financial aid are available based on scholastic performance and financial need. While some institutional scholarships are awarded solely on a student's academic record, many require demonstration of financial need. Interested students should contact the Office of Financial Aid and complete both a UAH scholarship application and the Free Application for Federal Student Aid (FAFSA).

Federal Professional Nurse Traineeships are available to eligible graduate students. Applications are provided to students after they accept their offer of admission. Some graduate teaching assistantships are also available each academic year.

APPLYING
All applicants for admission to the B.S.N. degree program of the College of Nursing must complete UAH admission requirements, be admitted as regular degree-seeking students, and declare nursing as their major. Students are admitted to the upper division once a year for fall semester. Admission to the upper-division nursing major is competitive. A separate application for the upper-division nursing major must be completed on forms provided by the College of Nursing and received by March 1 preceding the fall semester for which admission is sought. Each lower-division course requirement for the nursing major must be completed with a minimum grade of C prior to admission to the upper division.

RN/B.S.N. students are admitted once a year. Registered nurse students must submit proof of current and unencumbered licensure. Recent graduates of associate degree or diploma nursing programs who are not yet licensed may be admitted to complete lower-division course work, but they are not admitted to the upper-division clinical component of the program until they are licensed. Each lower-division course requirement must be completed with at least a grade of C prior to admission to the RN/B.S.N. program. The deadline for applications is March 1 preceding the fall semester for which admission is sought.

An RN-M.S.N. early decision option is available to associate degree–prepared RNs so they may complete the B.S.N. and the M.S.N. in a seven-semester sequence. Applicants must complete UAH requirements for the undergraduate and graduate admission offices and submit a separate application to the College of Nursing and proof of a current, unencumbered nursing license. The application deadline for priority consideration is March 1 preceding the fall semester for which admission is sought.

M.S.N. students are admitted once a year for the fall semester. The application deadline for priority consideration is April 15 preceding the fall semester for which admission is sought. Applicants must have a B.S.N. from an accredited program, a minimum GPA of 3.0, current GRE or MAT scores, three recommendations, satisfactory completion of a basic statistics course, and a current, unencumbered nursing license. Admission is competitive.

Post-master's students are admitted once a year for the fall semester. The application deadline is April 15. Applicants must have an M.S.N., credit for graduate-level health assessment and pathophysiology, two recommendations, and a current, unencumbered nursing license.

Prior to admission to any program, students are advised through the College of Nursing Office of Student Affairs. All interested students should contact the Office of Student Affairs for detailed program information, admission requirements, and application deadlines.

CORRESPONDENCE AND INFORMATION
Office of Student Affairs
NB 207
UAH College of Nursing
Huntsville, Alabama 35899

Phone: 256-824-6742
Fax: 256-824-6026
E-mail: nursing@email.uah.edu
Web site: http://onlinenurse.nb.uah.edu
      http://www.uah.edu

University of Cincinnati
College of Nursing
Cincinnati, Ohio

THE UNIVERSITY

The University of Cincinnati offers students a balance of educational excellence and real-world experience. Since its founding in 1819, UC has been the source of many discoveries creating positive change for society, including the first antihistamine, co-op education, the first electronic organ, and the oral polio vaccine. The University also has many prestigious alumni, including the designer of the Golden Gate Bridge.

Each year, this urban, public, research university graduates 5,000 students, adding to more than 200,000 living alumni around the world.

UC is the largest employer in the Cincinnati region, with an economic impact of more than $3 billion.

To learn more about UC, students should visit the University's Web site at http://www.uc.edu.

THE COLLEGE OF NURSING

In 2003, *U.S. News & World Report* ranked the UC College of Nursing in the top 6 percent of baccalaureate and higher degree programs. The College has a long history of excellence in nursing education. In 1916 it became the first baccalaureate program in nursing in the United States. In addition to the Bachelor of Science in Nursing (B.S.N.), the College offers Master of Science in Nursing (M.S.N.) and Doctor of Philosophy (Ph.D.) in nursing programs. The College prepares beginning and advanced practitioners of professional nursing to function in a variety of settings with diverse populations. Opportunities abound for practicing nurses to maintain, improve, and expand their competencies.

The College is fully accredited by the Commission of Collegiate Nursing Education (CCNE). The appropriate graduate programs are fully accredited by the Council on Accreditation of Nurse Anesthesia Educational Programs and the Division of Accreditation of the American College of Nurse Midwives. The Pediatric Nurse Practitioner Program is recognized by the National Certification Board of Pediatric Nurse Practitioners and Nurses.

The College is an integral part of the University and its Medical Center. Cooperative relations among the units of the University, myriad health-care settings, and the diversity of the greater Cincinnati community facilitate creative approaches for leadership and excellence in nursing. The College is a World Health Organization Collaborating Center affiliate.

The faculty members of the College are well prepared to provide excellent classroom and clinical instruction. The College employs 75 full-time faculty members. Many faculty members are nationally certified in a clinical area of specialization. They contribute to the improvement of the profession and health care through their outstanding teaching, research, and service.

The Institute for Nursing Research, which is a collaborative effort with Patient Care Services at University Hospital, fosters health-related research. Major research foci are injury and violence, substance abuse, symptom management, and oncology. Multiple NIH grants have been received to promote research in these areas.

PROGRAMS OF STUDY

The College's B.S.N. program options include a traditional track and an RN/B.S.N. track. The prenursing year for traditional students exposes them to nursing through the course Success in College and Nursing. The B.S.N. curriculum provides a foundation for community-focused professional practice with individuals and families having a variety of health-care needs. Community-focused professional practice includes acute care in hospitals as well as other health-care environments. Emphasis is placed on clinical competence, critical thinking, professional roles, participation in multidisciplinary teams, and a commitment to continued learning. Full- or part-time study is possible.

The master's program prepares nurses for advanced practice nursing and for leadership and management in diverse health-care environments. It offers an accelerated pathway for individuals holding baccalaureate degrees in fields other than nursing who wish to become advanced practice nurses. The master's curriculum consists of core courses plus courses in the student's selected area of clinical focus. A scholarly project is required for degree completion. Upon completion of the program, graduates meet current national specialty certification requirements for advanced practice in their chosen field. Nurse practitioner preparation in acute care and adult, family, pediatric, neonatal, and women's health nursing is offered. Clinical nurse specialist options include acute and ambulatory care, community health, occupational health, and psychiatric nursing. Other options are nurse anesthesia, nurse midwifery, and nursing service administration (including an M.S.N./M.B.A. option). Post-master's certificate programs for practitioners, psychiatric nursing in primary care, occupational health nursing, and nursing education are available.

The doctoral program focuses on the preparation of nurses for positions of leadership in academic and health services institutions and health policy agencies. The curriculum is designed with a core of required courses and a cognate area of the student's choosing to support preparation for research in a defined area. Students may enter the doctoral program upon completion of a B.S.N. or M.S.N. degree. Doctoral students are required to be in residence for full-time study during three of five consecutive quarters, excluding those for a dissertation.

AFFILIATIONS WITH HEALTH-CARE FACILITIES

The Medical Center and main University campuses are contiguous. Units in the Medical Center in addition to the College of Nursing include the Colleges of Allied Health Sciences, Pharmacy, and Medicine. Some affiliated institutions adjacent to the Medical Center are the University Hospital, the Veterans Affairs Medical Center, the Cincinnati Children's Hospital Medical Center, the Shriners Burns Institute, the Cincinnati Center for Developmental Disorders, and the Cincinnati Health Department. The College is affiliated with multiple hospitals, home care services, community agencies, and health service providers. Cooperative relationships provide rich educational, clinical, and research resources.

ACADEMIC FACILITIES

The College has numerous academic resources. The resources include multiple libraries and on-site research and technology support.

The College's Solomon P. Levi Library is one of the best nursing libraries and houses more than 300 journals relevant to nursing. In addition, the library connects to all the University libraries and OhioLINK, the statewide online catalog. These connections provide students, wherever they are, with access to the second-largest library system in the country.

The College's Research Institute provides grant development and project management assistance, statistical consultation, and data management support.

Among the technology resources are an equipped classroom for live interactive distance learning, a learning center incorporating clinical practice laboratories, a twenty-three-station student computer lab, online teaching materials, and faculty support for development of electronic resources and use of the University's online delivery system. All classrooms are equipped with projection and computer systems to assist faculty members in facilitating learning.

LOCATION

The University is only 10 minutes from downtown Cincinnati, so students can easily benefit from city activities. The city is big enough to have nationally renowned arts organizations and major-league sports, yet small enough to take pride in its neighborhood cafés and scenic parks. Cincinnati is known for its restaurants, riverfront recreation areas, and festivals such as Oktoberfest and the Appalachian Fair. Cincinnati is accessible by various modes of transportation and is the hub of a network of interstate highways.

STUDENT SERVICES

Education does not stop at the academic doors. The University is a place where students are continually learning, sharing, and growing. Students may choose to live in residence halls or take part in a variety of clubs. Diversity is an important part of the University community, with a number of ethnic organizations, services, and events. Students take part in intramural sports, attend College Conservatory of Music concerts and plays, or sometimes just hang out.

The College's Office of Student Affairs provides academic counseling and support services for students in every program of the College. The office offers a variety of orientation and career development programs to help students attain their professional goals. Coordinators for each program assist students and make the students' use of general University services easier.

There are many opportunities for student growth outside of the College's classroom and clinical settings. Some students have taken advantage of opportunities for international experiences. Undergraduate and graduate students participate in a variety of student government, philanthropic, and social organizations. Undergraduate students are active in the National Student Nurse Association. Students in all programs who excel in scholarship, research, or clinical practice are recognized through induction into the College's Beta Iota chapter of Sigma Theta Tau, the international honor society for nursing, and through College, University, and national awards.

THE NURSING STUDENT GROUP

The students in all programs in the College of Nursing represent diverse backgrounds in age, gender, ethnicity, nationality, and experience. The undergraduate program enrollment comprises approximately 650 students, about 15 percent of whom are registered nurses returning for baccalaureate degrees. The master's program enrollment averages 200 students, about 60 percent of whom are enrolled full-time. The doctoral program has 30 students, most of whom are enrolled full-time. Graduates of the College are sought by local, state, and national employers.

COSTS

Tuition and fees for the entire three-quarter academic year in 2006–07 were approximately $9400 for undergraduates and $11,660 for graduate students who were full-time students and Ohio residents. Full-time nonresident student tuition was $23,922 for undergraduates and $21,495 for graduate students per year. Tuition per credit hour was $262 (undergraduate, Ohio resident), $665 (undergraduate, nonresident), $389 (graduate, Ohio resident), and $717 (graduate, nonresident). Health insurance and parking, if needed, were additional costs.

University housing costs were approximately $7770 per year for residence hall room and board and $540 to $770 per month for apartments. For those who wish to live off campus, Cincinnati offers reasonable, suitable housing for rent.

FINANCIAL AID

Financial assistance for students derives from a variety of sources such as College and University scholarships, low-interest loans, University Graduate Assistantships, and Professional Nurse Traineeship funds. Scholarships, assistantships, and traineeships are awarded on a competitive basis. The majority of full-time graduate students receive some type of financial assistance.

APPLYING

B.S.N. program applicants should obtain program information and application materials from the University's Office of Admissions. All traditional freshman are admitted to prenursing. Applicants who qualify as Academic Scholars at the time of admission to prenursing are guaranteed admission to the nursing major if they maintain grades of C or better in all required prenursing courses, with a minimum GPA of 2.75 in these courses. For all other applicants and transfer students, admission into the nursing major is on a competitive basis.

The application process for the M.S.N. and Ph.D. programs is handled through the College's Office of Student Affairs. Program and financial aid information as well as application materials are available on the Web at http://www.uc.edu. Graduate Record Examinations (GRE) scores are required as part of the admission process. TOEFL scores are required of all applicants whose native language is not English. Applicants who have completed the application process by January 1 are given priority consideration for fall admission and financial assistance. For individuals seeking admission to the nurse anesthesia major, the application deadline is October 1 for each class that starts the following September.

CORRESPONDENCE AND INFORMATION

Office of Student Affairs
College of Nursing
University of Cincinnati
P.O. Box 210038
Cincinnati, Ohio 45221-0038

Phone: 513-558-3600
Fax: 513-558-7523
E-mail: nursing@uc.edu
Web site: http://www.uc.edu
        http://www.nursing.uc.edu

University of Delaware
School of Nursing
Newark, Delaware

THE UNIVERSITY

The University of Delaware has grown from its founding as a small private academy in 1743 to a major university. As one of the oldest land-grant institutions, as well as a sea-grant, space-grant, and urban-grant institution, Delaware offers an impressive collection of educational resources. Undergraduates may choose to major in one or more of hundreds of majors and minors. The University's distinguished faculty includes internationally known scientists, authors, and teachers who are committed to continuing the University of Delaware's tradition in providing one of the highest-quality undergraduate educations available.

The University comprises seven colleges: Agricultural and Natural Resources; Arts and Sciences; Business and Economics; Engineering; Health Sciences; Human Services, Education, and Public Policy; and Marine Sciences. Enrollment in the fall 2006 semester was 20,380 students, including 15,849 undergraduates, 3,446 graduate students and doctoral students, and 1,085 continuing education students.

THE SCHOOL OF NURSING

The School of Nursing is housed within the College of Health Sciences. It offers undergraduate programs for traditional nursing students, accelerated students, and registered nurses, all leading to the Bachelor of Science in Nursing (B.S.N.) degree. The School also offers a graduate program leading to the Master of Science in Nursing (M.S.N.) degree. All programs are fully accredited by the National League for Nursing Accrediting Commission and the Commission on Collegiate Nursing Education.

PROGRAMS OF STUDY

The traditional undergraduate program is available to beginning students of nursing, including new high school graduates, transfer students, and change-of-major students. This program requires 122 semester credits for completion. In the freshman year, nursing majors are introduced to the profession through course work and lab experiences while developing a firm foundation in the essential science and liberal arts courses. In the sophomore year, students complete all of the essential science courses and most of the liberal arts courses while further developing clinical and decision-making skills in nursing through simulation and laboratory experiences. In the junior year, there is an expansion of nursing knowledge in both essential and specialty clinical nursing domains while completing associated field experiences. Finally, senior-level nursing students enter a residency period in which they are immersed in clinical experiences for the entire year in order to enhance their nursing knowledge and to prepare them for entry into practice. Students may elect to take selected courses during winter or summer sessions. Honors courses and a nursing honors program are available to qualified undergraduate students. In addition, the School of Nursing is actively involved in the University Study Abroad Program.

An accelerated program of study is available for adults who have previously earned a baccalaureate degree. This option allows students to pursue a course of study whereby they complete all of their nursing requirements (62 credits) in sixteen months. To pursue this option, the student must have completed all prerequisite courses and have earned a 3.0 GPA or higher prior to beginning any nursing courses.

The RN to B.S.N. program is for RNs who are graduates of associate degree or diploma programs. The program requires 120 credits for program completion. The program is offered in an online format and is available to RNs nationwide. All students

must, however, attend two 1-credit weekend experiences. This innovative format provides the needed flexibility for busy adult students who pursue degree completion while continuing to work full- or part-time. The program can be completed in fifteen months but must be completed within five years of the first nursing course. The program utilizes a work site model for exam proctoring. Any health-care facility, industry wellness center, or community college can become a participating work site. There are currently 181 work sites spanning multiple states and one other country. Graduates of accredited associate degree and diploma programs who are licensed may directly transfer up to 30 credits in nursing as evidence of their basic nursing knowledge. State-of-the-art technologies are used to facilitate communication, advisement, and course work among and between students and faculty members. Full library access is provided via the Internet.

An online RN-M.S.N. option is also offered to RNs who are graduates of associate degree or diploma programs. Qualified applicants can complete the B.S.N. and M.S.N. requirements concurrently in the RN to M.S.N. program, which requires 134 credits for graduation and prepares graduates as clinical nurse specialists in children's health, adult health, or adult or child psychiatric concentrations.

A health services administration degree program has been added.

The graduate program includes core concepts in advanced nursing practice as well as concepts that are specific to the areas of specialization. The curriculum is built on theories and professional practice that students have obtained at the baccalaureate level of nursing education and provides a foundation for future doctoral study. Research is an area of emphasis in graduate study. Students may elect to complete a thesis, a nonthesis scholarly project, or a 3-credit research application course.

The graduate program prepares clinical nurse specialists (CNS) in children's health, adult health, and adult or child psychiatric specialties. Nurse practitioner (NP) concentrations are available in adult and family primary-care specialties. A concentration is also available in health services administration. Students in the CNS concentrations complete 34 credit hours, with emphasis on the three spheres of influence: clients (patients/families/communities), nursing personnel, and health organizations and networks.

The adult nurse practitioner concentration requires 40 credit hours, while the family nurse practitioner concentration requires 43 credit hours. Nurse practitioner clinical courses are offered on campus only at this time. Health services administration students must complete 37 credit hours and are prepared to assume leadership positions as health-care managers. Students may elect to enroll full-time or part-time.

Post-master's certificate programs are available in all of the concentrations for students who already hold a Master of Science degree in nursing. Clinical nurse specialists and nurse practitioners are eligible to sit for the national certification examinations and have exceptionally high pass rates. The health services administration concentration and CNS concentrations utilize Web-based or Web-enhanced delivery systems. Other core and selected specialty courses may also be offered in a Web-based format.

The Division of Special Programs works collaboratively with all departments within the college to coordinate technology-related learning activities. Continuing professional education programs and credit courses delivered locally and in a distance format are another focus of the division. Online certificate programs available are: Online RN Refresher Course; Clinical Research Monitoring & Coordination; and Injury Prevention. Other certificate programs available in a distance format include Cognitive Therapy: Interventions for Healthcare Providers and Cognitive Therapy: Advanced Applications for Healthcare Providers.

ACADEMIC FACILITIES
The University libraries contain more than 2.7 million volumes of books and bound periodicals, 3.4 million items in microtext, and subscriptions to more than 12,000 periodicals. The libraries provide access to more than 6,800 online full-text journals and to more than 240 networked databases. DELCAT is the library's online catalog, giving information for materials located in the libraries and on the libraries' Web site (http://www.lib.udel. edu). The libraries offer an online reference service, online interlibrary loan forms, and electronic reserves for selected courses. Special library services are available for distance learning students.

The information technology resources available at the University of Delaware are unparalleled. The University's commitment to providing a superior technology environment enables students and faculty members to pursue academic studies and to conduct the business of campus life with ease and efficiency.

Students use a wide range of technology in all disciplines—electronic mail, word processing, and state-of-the-art tools to search the Internet. All University classrooms are connected to the campus network, enabling faculty members to use a wide variety of multimedia services and devices in their teaching. A majority of faculty members in the nursing program use the University's Course Management System to enhance and expand the boundaries of teaching.

Many classrooms have Internet connections at student seats to facilitate the use of laptop computers. Instructional video is broadcast over the University television network, and many classes include special viewings as part of course requirements.

Students on campus can connect their computers directly to the campus network in their residence hall rooms. Off-campus students can dial in to the network from surrounding regions. General-access computing sites are available for student use on campus, and these sites have network ports to connect laptop computers.

Wireless access areas are available across campus, including computing sites, the Morris Library, student centers, classroom buildings, meeting areas in academic buildings, and residence hall lounges. The Morris Library carrels also have network ports for direct connections.

The School of Nursing has two general practice labs, a critical-care lab, and an examination suite for nurse practitioner students. A clinical simulation laboratory and resource center provide students with a safe clinical practice site prior to direct patient care. Students may access a computer laboratory housed in the building. Faculty members are committed to the development and integration of technologies in the teaching/learning process.

LOCATION
Situated in the small, picturesque town of Newark, Delaware, the University's main campus is less than 2½ hours from the metropolitan bustle of New York City, Baltimore, Philadelphia, and Washington, D.C. The campus is convenient to an impressive array of major clinical facilities as well as cultural and recreational resources.

STUDENT SERVICES
The University has many resources and services to meet individual student needs. These include the Student Support Services Program, the University Writing Center, the Center for Counseling and Student Development, the Mathematical Sciences Teaching and Learning Center, the English Language Institute, and the Career Planning and Placement Office.

Undergraduate nursing students are encouraged to participate in the local chapter of the National Student Nurses Organization and/or the Black Student Nurses Association. Registered nurse students have their own electronic support group.

THE NURSING STUDENT GROUP
Approximately 550 students are enrolled in the traditional undergraduate program, including 60 adult students pursuing the accelerated degree option. In addition, 100 matriculated RN students are enrolled in the RN to B.S.N. program. Enrollment in the graduate program is approximately 100.

COSTS
For the 2006–07 academic year, tuition was $6980 for undergraduate Delaware residents and $17,690 for nonresidents. Tuition covers registration for 12 to 17 credits per semester. Students taking fewer than 12 credits were charged $291 per credit hour for Delaware residents and $737 per credit hour for nonresidents. Room rates were $2168 to $3073, depending on dorm choice, and board costs were $1515.

FINANCIAL AID
In most cases, the University awards aid on the basis of need. Financial aid may include grants, loans, and employment opportunities. The University also offers a number of scholarships based on academic proficiency alone. Students have been able to successfully obtain nurse traineeships, National Student Nurses Association scholarships, and other specialty scholarships.

APPLYING
Applicants to the undergraduate degree programs can apply online (http://www.udel.edu/viewbook) or can request an application by contacting the Admission's Office (302-831-8125). Applicants to the graduate program can request an application online (http://www.udel.edu/gradoffice) or by contacting the Office of Graduate Studies (302-831-2129). The application deadlines are January 15 for fall admission and November 1 for spring admission. For information regarding specific requirements, students should contact the appropriate unit in the college.

CORRESPONDENCE AND INFORMATION
For information about the B.S.N. and M.S.N. nursing programs:

School of Nursing
College of Health Sciences
University of Delaware
Newark, Delaware 19716

Phone: 302-831-1253
E-mail: ud-nursing@udel.edu
Web site: http://www.udel.edu/nursing

For information about the online RN Refresher course and certificate programs:

Division of Special Programs
College of Health Sciences
University of Delaware
Newark, Delaware 19716

Phone: 800-UOD-NURS (toll-free)
E-mail: dsp-email@udel.edu
Web site: http://www.udel.edu/DSP

University of Illinois at Chicago
College of Nursing
Chicago, Illinois

THE UNIVERSITY

The University of Illinois at Chicago (UIC) serves approximately 25,000 students, who reflect the ethnic and racial diversity of Chicago itself. Seventy-five percent of these students come from Cook County and 48 percent are residents of Chicago. The Colleges of Nursing, Medicine, Pharmacy, Dentistry, and Health and Human Development Sciences and the School of Public Health are located within the 305-acre west side Medical Center District about 2 miles west of downtown Chicago. The district has the world's largest concentration of public and private health-care facilities and includes the University of Illinois at Chicago Medical Center, Cook County Hospital, Rush-Presbyterian-St. Luke's Medical Center, West Side Veterans Administration Medical Center, Institute for Juvenile Research, Illinois State Psychiatric Institute, and Illinois State Pediatric Institute.

THE COLLEGE OF NURSING

The UIC College of Nursing is consistently recognized as one of the top ten nursing programs in the United States. The mission of the College includes the triad of university functions—teaching, research, and service—providing university education in nursing to meet the present and future needs of society. In 2006, the College was sixth in total NIH research and research training dollars, and in 2004, it was ranked eighth out of 142 schools of nursing by *U.S. News & World Report*. The nurse midwifery program was ranked third among its competitors. Fully accredited by the Commission on Collegiate Nursing Education (CCNE), the College offers programs leading to the degrees of Bachelor of Science in Nursing (B.S.N.), Master of Science (M.S.) in nursing sciences, and Doctor of Philosophy (Ph.D.) in nursing sciences. The College, which has provided high-quality education since 1951, is currently designated as a WHO Collaborating Centre for Nursing and Midwifery. The faculty includes 21 members of the American Academy of Nursing. Worldwide, alumni are a source of leadership in academic, health-system, corporate, and political arenas.

PROGRAMS OF STUDY

Transfer students are admitted to the generic baccalaureate program in Chicago and Urbana-Champaign. The program, which prepares beginning nurses to function in a variety of settings, requires 57 liberal arts and sciences semester hours and 63 nursing semester hours for graduation. Students may complete the program in two years. RN-B.S.N. students applying to the program offered in Chicago, Quad Cities, and Urbana-Champaign must meet the transfer admission requirements, which include 57 semester hours of liberal arts and sciences course work and a cumulative GPA of at least 2.5 (A=4.0). Completion of three NLN Mobility Profile II examinations and three transition courses determine credit by exemption for up to 33 semester hours of nursing course work, leaving 30 semester hours of nursing course work, which may be completed in four semesters.

The master's program for non-nurses (Graduate Entry Program) is designed for those individuals who wish to become nurses and hold a baccalaureate degree in a field other than nursing. The program begins with fifteen months of highly intensive study that provides students with the foundations of nursing practice and prepares them to take the National Council Licensing Examination for registered nurses (NCLEX-RN). The pre-NCLEX portion is only available on a full-time basis. After successful completion of the NCLEX-RN, the student begins the advanced-practice specialty courses in any of the master's programs offered at UIC.

The master's program prepares nurses for advanced practice roles, with emphasis on basic, clinical, and nursing sciences; knowledge of health systems and environment; and understanding of professional issues of advanced practice roles, while a research focus is maintained. The roles are clinical nurse specialist, which utilizes advanced information within a specialty to manage complex health problems, and nurse practitioner, which emphasizes the comprehensive care of patients as well as the ability to manage the complex problems addressed by the specialty.

Within each specialty and option, there are several concentrations of study. These include administrative studies in nursing (alone or combined as a dual-degree option with an M.B.A. or health informatics), medical-surgical nursing (acute care, geriatric, adult), maternal-child nursing (nurse midwifery; women's health; pediatric, including PNP; perinatal), public health nursing (dual-degree option with an M.P.H., school health, community nurse specialist, family nurse practitioner, occupational health nursing), and psychiatric–mental health nursing.

Master's courses are offered at all locations and may use teleconference or videoconferencing. The 36 required semester hours include statistics, nursing inquiry I & II, health environment and systems, and issues of advanced practice in nursing (10 semester hours); advanced nursing courses (23–36 semester hours); electives (2–3 semester hours); a thesis (5 semester hours) or a research project (3 semester hours); and a final examination. More than 36 semester hours are required to complete most of the specialty concentrations.

Post-master's programs are available in most of the study options. This prepares individuals to sit for examinations for certification in these fields.

The Ph.D. program develops leaders in nursing who influence the provision of health care through systematic investigation, education, policy development and implementation, and expert professional practice. Major areas of research include administration, physiological and psychological studies related to the care of the acutely and chronically ill, health promotion and maintenance, stress and coping, narcolepsy, quality of life, community health nursing, women's health, family, and gerontological nursing. The Ph.D. degree requires 96 semester hours, including nursing theory (6 semester hours), statistics (6 semester hours), research methods (6 semester hours), advanced nursing and non-nursing courses (15 semester hours), independent research (31 semester hours), and a previously completed M.S. program (32 semester hours). A preliminary oral examination, dissertation, and final oral examination are required to earn the Ph.D. in nursing sciences.

The B.S.N. to Ph.D. program allows the exceptional student to proceed directly from the B.S.N. to the Ph.D. in nursing science degrees.

Through the CIC, a consortium of the Midwest's "Big Ten" universities and the University of Chicago, doctoral students may register for course work or independent study in the other universities of the CIC and work with experts in their research areas. The Graduate Entry Program is designed for students who hold baccalaureate degrees in other fields and wish to pursue a master's degree in nursing.

ACADEMIC FACILITIES
UIC libraries hold more than 5.7 million items, including more than 6,000 current periodicals and more than 500,000 bound periodical volumes, books, government documents, and audio-visual items housed in the Library of the Health Sciences, which is the regional medical library for 2,700 medical libraries in ten states from Ohio to the Dakotas. The Interlibrary Loan Service is offered to students and faculty and staff members, and the libraries of two other Chicago institutions, the University of Chicago and Northwestern University, are available for use by graduate students. The Academic Computer Center provides computing and network support for instructional and research needs of the University's students and faculty and staff members.

LOCATION
Situated 2 miles west of Chicago's downtown, UIC is surrounded by world-renowned architecture, theater, art, music, and sports activities. Easily accessible from both airports by public transportation and the Eisenhower Expressway, the College is located in a historic neighborhood, currently the center of a new, rapidly growing residential and professional community.

STUDENT SERVICES
The Center for Excellence provides an array of services from career counseling and academic skills courses to personal counseling and assistance for disabled students. Other services include two fitness/recreation centers, a child-care center, the Office of International Studies, and support organizations such as African American Academic Network, Latin American Recruitment and Education Services, and the Native American Support Program for members of minority groups.

THE NURSING STUDENT GROUP
Students reflect the ethnic and racial diversity of Chicago itself. UIC has long provided solid academic training for first-generation college students from the city's numerous ethnic groups and currently provides opportunities to students returning to school following a significant absence due to other career or family responsibilities. About 10 percent of those enrolled in the undergraduate program are men. Even though University housing is available, 85 percent of Chicago students commute or live in apartments near the campus.

COSTS
For 2006–07, full-time tuition and fees per semester for undergraduates were $5671 for Illinois residents and $11,866 for nonresidents. For full-time graduate students, tuition and fees were $8038 for Illinois residents and $14,037 for nonresidents. Part-time undergraduate tuition ranged from $2512 to $4096 for Illinois residents and from $4577 to $8226 for nonresidents; part-time graduate study ranged from $3301 to $5674 for Illinois residents and from $5300 to $9674 for nonresidents. On-campus housing was available in Chicago for approximately $9000 for two semesters; costs may vary depending on location.

FINANCIAL AID
Several financial assistance programs are available through the Office of Student Financial Aid. Applications for financial aid in the form of research or training assistantships, fellowships, traineeships, and tuition waivers are submitted to the College of Nursing. These financial aid awards are made from the College's resources. The College of Nursing makes recommendations to the Graduate College for such awards as University Fellowships and the Abraham Lincoln Graduate Fellowship.

APPLYING
Applicants for the B.S. degree must have completed the following liberal arts and sciences requirements: English composition I and II; microbiology; general and organic chemistry; anatomy; physiology; 6 semester hours of social science; 6 semester hours of humanities, nutrition, and life span, human growth, and development; and a cultural diversity course. A minimum cumulative GPA of 2.5 (A=4.0) and a minimum GPA of 2.0 in natural science courses are required. Applicants must submit two letters of recommendation, a personal statement, a College information form, and a prerequisite evaluation form. The applicant to the RN-B.S.N. program must have a current RN license or be scheduled to take the NCLEX at the first opportunity after graduation from a diploma or associate degree nursing program accredited by the NLNAC.

Graduate Entry applicants must have a minimum GPA of 3.00 in the last 60 hours of the baccalaureate degree. There are no restrictions on field of study, but prior academic work must include introductory research, two semesters of anatomy and physiology, 6 semester hours of English composition, 6 semester hours of humanities, 6 semester hours of social sciences, and general chemistry or biology. All applicants must take the GRE. The GMAT is accepted in lieu of the GRE for students applying to Administrative Nursing, M.S./M.B.A., or M.S./Health Informatics programs. TOEFL scores are required for international students. Applicants must submit a statement of career goals, a curriculum vitae, and three letters of reference. Faculty members interview suitable applicants.

M.S. applicants must have a current RN license (several specialty concentrations require an Illinois license) and either a B.S.N. degree from a CCNE- or NLNAC-accredited program or a B.S. degree from an accredited institution in a field other than nursing; a minimum GPA of 3.0 (A=4.0); introductory courses in statistics and research methods or their equivalent; GRE General Test scores (or GMAT scores for the M.S. dual-degree M.B.A. or health informatics option); TOEFL scores (for international students); a statement of career goals; a curriculum vitae; three letters of reference; and a faculty interview. The GRE requirement may be waived for students holding a 3.25 GPA (A=4.0) in the final 60 hours of their bachelor's degree program.

Ph.D. applicants must meet the requirements for entry into the M.S. program, possess an M.S. degree from a CCNE- or NLNAC-accredited program, and present evidence of potential for advanced scholarship. The applicant who has a B.S. degree from an accredited nursing program and an M.S. degree in a field other than nursing is eligible for consideration for admission. The GRE requirement is not waived for Ph.D. applicants.

Prospective applicants should contact the College of Nursing Office of Academic Programs for specific application deadlines and priority application dates. Applications for the B.S.N., selected M.S., and the Ph.D. programs are accepted for fall only. Admission to several of the M.S. options is for any term.

CORRESPONDENCE AND INFORMATION
Office of Academic Programs
College of Nursing (M/C 802)
University of Illinois at Chicago
845 South Damen Avenue
Chicago, Illinois 60612-7350

Phone: 312-996-7800
Fax: 312-996-8066
E-mail: con@uic.edu
Web site: http://www.uic.edu/nursing

University of Michigan
School of Nursing
Ann Arbor, Michigan

THE UNIVERSITY

The University of Michigan, located in Ann Arbor, Michigan, has more than 445,000 alumni worldwide. Graduates of the University have made substantial contributions to intellectual, scientific, and cultural growth. Its internationally ranked faculty, supported by the most advanced research programs, prepares students to teach, lead, heal, and innovate in the global society of the twenty-first century. The University of Michigan is consistently ranked among the nation's top ten universities.

THE SCHOOL OF NURSING

The University of Michigan School of Nursing has held an unsurpassed reputation of excellence for more than 100 years, because it has kept pace with advances in knowledge and technology and trends in health care. The School of Nursing is also unparalleled in terms of its distinguished faculty, with more than 90 percent of all tenure-track faculty members doctorally prepared. This caliber of faculty preparation enhances the balance between clinical and theoretical experiences for students.

Matching faculty strength with current societal needs has led to the formation of three School-supported, interdisciplinary Centers of Excellence where educational, clinical, and research initiatives are fostered. Results influence nursing science, practice, and public health policy. The centers are focused on three areas: enhancement and restoration of cognitive function, advancing the science of health promotion and risk reduction across the life span, and concepts of frailty and vulnerability as applied to life's later stages. Each center offers periodic forums where members present results of their research. Students in undergraduate and graduate programs can apply to become a Center Scholar in one of the centers. In addition to the Centers of Excellence, the Grants and Research Office works with the program areas to maintain an exciting and productive research environment in the School of Nursing. The center stimulates, coordinates, and facilitates research through a variety of functions such as consulting on research design and data analysis, assisting in the preparation of grant proposals, and identifying reviewers for proposals before submission for external funding.

PROGRAMS OF STUDY

Nursing education is an investment in the future of health care in terms of both the individual nurse and the overall health-care delivery system. The School of Nursing is strongly committed to the concept that nurses must continue to be challenged educationally in order to meet the rigors of a highly complex, diverse profession.

The Bachelor of Science in Nursing (B.S.N.) degree is the basis for a career in nursing. The School of Nursing's four-year B.S.N. program offers applicants direct admission as freshmen. Transfer students may be admitted to the second-year level of the program, depending upon the course work they have already completed and the availability of openings in the second year. The School offers an accelerated B.S.N. program for students with bachelor's degrees in other fields. Students in the accelerated Second Career program will be able to complete a B.S.N. degree and prepare for the registered nurse NCLEX exam and licensing in twelve months. If a student would like to pursue an advanced degree in nursing, a University of Michigan School of Nursing Master of Science or post-baccalaureate Ph.D. degree may be completed.

In addition to the four-year B.S.N. program, the School offers a B.S.N. completion program in Ann Arbor, Traverse City, and Kalamazoo for the A.D.N. or diploma nurse. The School's RN to B.S.N. to M.S. program combines undergraduate and graduate studies for highly motivated RNs. This program may be completed in three to four part-time years, depending on the master's specialty.

At the Master of Science level, the School of Nursing, through the University's Horace H. Rackham School of Graduate Studies, offers advanced practice certification and clinical nurse specialist programs in medical-surgical nursing; adult or pediatric acute-care nurse practitioner; psychiatric–mental health nursing; psychiatric–mental health nurse practitioner; gerontological nursing; gerontological nurse practitioner; adult primary-care adult nurse practitioner (a women's health/childbearing families post-master's certificate option); family nurse practitioner; occupational health nursing; community care/home health nursing; infant, child, and adolescent health primary-care pediatric nurse practitioner; and nurse midwifery (with a concentration in women's health). Program offerings also include nursing business and health systems with a focus in nursing informatics, nursing management/administration, nursing and health-care policy, or entrepreneurial nursing (Web-based format); dual degrees in nursing and business administration, nursing and information, and nursing and health services administration. A post-master's teaching certificate is the newest offering as of fall 2006. Most of the tracks offer post-master's options, and some programs are available through On Job/On Campus.

The On Job/On Campus Program is flexible, offering students an opportunity to learn while maintaining work and family responsibilities. Classes are scheduled for one long weekend two times a semester for twenty to twenty-two months. The emphasis of the program is on home health-care nursing, occupational health nursing, and community care nursing.

The curriculum plan of the master's programs is implemented through four major components: core courses, specialization courses, cognates, and a master's project. Core courses, which are required in all master's-level programs, fall into three subject categories: theory development, leadership, and research. Nursing specialization courses are designed to prepare students for advanced nursing practice in their respective areas of study. Cognate courses related to a student's program are selected from other University of Michigan graduate areas. All master's degree students are required to complete a master's project that involves participation in research or that is practice or policy oriented.

The School's Ph.D. program prepares an exclusive community of nurse-scientists capable of developing new knowledge necessary to support and advance nursing practice. This postbaccalaureate program is predicated on a strong foundation of clinical expertise and framed within a nursing perspective. Graduates of this prestigious and rigorous program have assumed leadership positions in every area of nursing, including health-care policy, academe, professional organizations, and health-care settings.

The School of Nursing has offered postdoctoral study opportunities since 1987. Currently, this training is offered in health promotion and risk reduction, women's health disparities, and neurobehavior, with support from the National Institutes of Health. The goal of the health promotion and risk reduction training program is to develop scientists capable of sustaining independent research careers focused on generating knowledge about health promotion and risk reduction within the theoretical perspective of nursing science. The goal of the women's health disparities training program is to prepare scientists in an interdisciplinary environment to address women's health needs across the lifespan. The goal of the neurobehavior training program is to develop scientists capable of sustaining independent research careers focused on generating knowledge about human responses and behaviors associated with altered brain functioning.

ACADEMIC FACILITIES
There are more than 7 million volumes in the nineteen libraries on the University's campus. Also on campus are nine museums, several hospitals, hundreds of laboratories and institutes, and more than 12,000 microcomputers.

LOCATION
The University of Michigan is located in Ann Arbor, a city well-known for its parks, rivers, and historical heritage. Ann Arbor's designation as an "All-America City" complements its well-earned title, "Research Center of the Midwest."

STUDENT SERVICES
The University of Michigan has many services available to students, including the Affirmative Action Office, Career Planning and Placement, Center for the Education of Women, Services for Students with Disabilities, the International Center, Minority Student Services, Office of Multicultural Affairs, Office of the Ombudsman, Sexual Assault Prevention and Awareness Center, Student Legal Services, Student Organization Development Center, University Health Center, and a multitude of academic and personal counseling services.

THE NURSING STUDENT GROUP
Of the 847 students registered at the School, approximately 625 are undergraduates. The total student body includes students of color (African Americans, Native Americans, Asians, and Hispanics). The University of Michigan School of Nursing is proud of its continued commitment to a diverse student body.

COSTS
For 2006–07, full-time tuition costs per term for resident undergraduate lower-division courses were $4570; for nonresidents, $14,870. For resident graduate students, full-time tuition costs were $8390; for nonresidents, $16,900.

FINANCIAL AID
Financial assistance based on need is available through the Office of Financial Aid. It may consist of a combination of grants, scholarships, and loans, including Nursing Student Loans and work-study opportunities. A limited number of need-based grants and loans are available after enrollment directly through the School of Nursing. Graduate assistance can be obtained from various sources. Some Graduate Student Teaching and Graduate Student Research Assistantships are available within the School of Nursing. Fellowships and scholarships are available through the Horace H. Rackham School of Graduate Studies.

APPLYING
The deadline for applications to the Accelerated Second Career Nursing program is September 15 for the following fall term. The deadline for applications to the generic B.S.N. program (including sophomore transfers) is February 1. The deadline for RN/B.S.N. programs is February 1 for best financial aid consideration, if applicable; otherwise the deadline is July 1. Applications to the Master of Science nursing programs are accepted year-round. Based on a rolling admissions plan, applicants may be admitted for the fall, winter, or spring semester. The deadline for applications to the Ph.D. program is December 1 for the following fall term. To request additional information about University of Michigan School of Nursing programs or to inquire about the application deadline, students should call 734-647-0109 or 800-458-8689 (toll-free).

CORRESPONDENCE AND INFORMATION
All University of Michigan Nursing Programs:
Office of Academic Affairs
School of Nursing
University of Michigan
400 North Ingalls, #1160
Ann Arbor, Michigan 48109-0482

Phone: 734-647-0109
Fax: 734-647-1419
E-mail: umnursing@umich.edu
Web site: http://www.nursing.umich.edu/

University of Michigan Office of Undergraduate Admissions:
Office of Undergraduate Admissions
1220 Student Activities Building
University of Michigan
Ann Arbor, Michigan 48109-1316

Graduate School Admissions:
Horace H. Rackham School of Graduate Studies
University of Michigan
915 East Washington
Ann Arbor, Michigan 48109-1070

Nursing Doctoral and Postdoctoral Programs:
Dr. Richard W. Redman, Director
Doctoral and Postdoctoral Studies
School of Nursing
University of Michigan
400 North Ingalls Building, Room 1154
Ann Arbor, Michigan 48109-0482

Phone: 734-764-9454
Fax: 734-763-6668
E-mail: rwr@umich.edu

University of Minnesota, Twin Cities Campus

School of Nursing

Minneapolis, Minnesota

THE UNIVERSITY

The University of Minnesota, with its four campuses, ranks among the top twenty universities in the United States. It is both a state land-grant university, with a strong tradition of education and public service, and a major research institution with scholars of national and international reputation. The Academic Health Center on the Minneapolis campus comprises the Medical School, School of Dentistry, School of Nursing, School of Public Health, and College of Pharmacy.

THE SCHOOL OF NURSING

Established in 1909, the School of Nursing is ranked among the nation's top nursing schools and is a leader in improving health care through research, education and service. Its scientists, renowned nationally and around the world, discover practical health-care treatments and solutions people use today to improve their daily lives. The oldest continuing university-based school of nursing in the world, it produces 55 percent of the faculty in Minnesota's public and private nursing schools, advanced practice nurses, and nurses who can assume leadership positions.

PROGRAMS OF STUDY

The School of Nursing offers three degrees: the Bachelor of Science in Nursing, the Master of Science with a major in nursing, and the Doctor of Philosophy with a major in nursing. A Post-Baccalaureate Certificate Program is also offered. The baccalaureate, postbaccalaureate, and master's programs are accredited by the Commission on Collegiate Nursing Education (the CCNE does not accredit doctoral programs).

The baccalaureate program is a three-year major admitting approximately 130 students each fall to two campuses: Minneapolis and Rochester, Minnesota.

The Post-Baccalaureate Certificate Program is a graduate-level program that spans sixteen months. The courses overlap those of the M.S. program, and prerequisites must be completed prior to entry. Entry to this program is competitive and is limited to 40 students. Students should contact the School of Nursing for information about the prerequisites.

The Graduate School offers the Master of Science degree with a major in nursing under two plans: Plan A (thesis option) and Plan B (nonthesis option). The M.S. program offers seventeen areas of study through Plan B, some of which are offered as Web-based programs. Areas of study include clinical nurse specialist (adult health, gerontological, pediatric, psych–mental health), nurse practitioner (family, pediatric, gerontological, women's health), nursing administration, children with special health-care needs nursing, public health nursing (adolescent health), nursing education, nurse midwifery, and nurse anesthesia. An M.P.H./M.S. dual degree is also available. The M.S. program can be completed in approximately two years of full-time study.

The Ph.D. program is research oriented and is designed to prepare creative and productive scholars in nursing.

ACADEMIC FACILITIES

The University library system is the seventeenth-largest research library in North America, lending more books and journal articles to other libraries than any other in the nation. Students have access to more than 20,000 computer workstations as well as the clinics and laboratories of the University of Minnesota Medical Center, Fairview.

LOCATION

The Twin Cities area, with more than 2 million people, is the metropolitan and cultural center of the upper Midwest. The Minnesota Orchestra, the Tyrone Guthrie Theater, and a rich array of art galleries, museums, and small theaters provide extensive cultural opportunities. Outdoor recreation is exceptional. Numerous lakes within the metropolitan area offer various sports activities throughout the year.

STUDENT SERVICES

The University provides a host of support services for students, including Boynton Health Service, disability services, International Study and Travel Center, student unions, Minnesota Women's Center, Sexual Violence Program, Student Diversity Institute, University Counseling & Consulting Service, student cultural centers, and more.

THE NURSING STUDENT GROUP

The School of Nursing enrolls about 860 students. The B.S.N. program has approximately 360 students; the master's program, 350 students; and the Ph.D. program, 62 students. There are 88 students in the Post-Baccalaureate Certificate Program.

COSTS

Tuition in 2005–06 for the B.S.N. program was $3570 for 13 or more credits per semester for residents and $9385 for 13 or more credits per semester for nonresidents. For full-time graduate students, tuition (6 to 14 credits) was $4374 per semester for residents and $7924 for nonresidents. Per-semester fees included a University fee, $450; student services fee, $290.82; and technology fee, $110, for a total of $850.82.

FINANCIAL AID

Financial aid resources include graduate fellowships, graduate teaching and research assistantships, scholarships from the School of Nursing Foundation, traineeship grants, and loans from the Office of Student Financial Services.

APPLYING

Requirements for B.S.N. program applicants include applicable prerequisite course work prior to application, a preferred minimum grade point average of 2.8 on a 4.0 scale in the prerequisites and a preferred minimum 2.8 cumulative GPA, and a profile statement. The application deadline is February 1 for the following fall semester.

Applicants to the Post-Baccalaureate Certificate program must have completed a baccalaureate degree in a non-nursing area and have completed applicable prerequisite course work. Successful applicants typically have a cumulative GPA of at least 3.5 from their degree-granting institution. Application requirements include two letters of reference and essay question completion. The application deadline is December 15 for the following fall.

M.S. program applicants must have an RN license and a bachelor's degree with a major in nursing or, if the degree is not in nursing, evidence of ability in health promotion, community health nursing, leadership, and teaching. Application requirements include two letters of reference (more for certain areas) and the completion of profile essays. Some areas of study require registered nursing experience prior to applying. Application deadlines are August 1, November 1, and January 1. For the nurse practitioner, clinical nurse specialist, nurse midwifery, and children with special health-care needs areas of study, priority is given to applicants who submit their applications by the November 1 deadline. For the nurse anesthesia area of study, priority is given to applicants who submit their applications by the August 1 deadline.

Applicants to the Ph.D. program must have a master's degree or a bachelor's degree with an exceptionally strong record in the physical or behavioral sciences. Applicants must submit GRE scores with the analytical writing test, two letters of reference, and a profile statement. Admission and fellowship applications must be received by October 1 for the fall semester.

CORRESPONDENCE AND INFORMATION

UMTC School of Nursing
5-160 Weaver-Densford Hall
308 Harvard Street Southeast
Minneapolis, Minnesota 55455

Phone: 612-625-7980
E-mail: sonstudentinfo@umn.edu
Web site: http://www.nursing.umn.edu

THE FACULTY

Melissa D. Avery, Associate Professor; Ph.D., Minnesota. Exercise as a therapeutic intervention for women with gestational diabetes, maternal nutrition and other antenatal factors influencing infant birth weight, outcomes of nurse midwifery care.

Linda H. Bearinger, Professor; Ph.D., Minnesota. Public health issues and interventions among adolescents, health decision-making among at-risk populations.

Donna Z. Bliss, Associate Professor; Ph.D., Pennsylvania. Effects of dietary fiber on the colon.

Linda Chlan, Assistant Professor; Ph.D., Minnesota. Effects of music on anxiety and discomfort in mechanically ventilated patients.

Connie W. Delaney, Professor and Dean; Ph.D., Iowa. Health informatics, management and international minimum data sets.

Joanne Disch, Professor and Director, Katharine J. Densford International Center for Nursing Leadership; Ph.D., Michigan. Nursing leadership and management.

Laura J. Duckett, Associate Professor; Ph.D., Minnesota. Maternal employment and breast-feeding.

Sandra R. Edwardson, Professor; Ph.D., Minnesota. Cost-quality trade-offs in nursing services, elderly self-care behavior.

Kathy Fagerlund, Assistant Professor, Ph.D. Costs and benefits of nurse anesthesia education, interactions of anesthesia and Parkinson's disease.

Jayne A. Fulkerson, Associate Professor; Ph.D., Minnesota. Risk and the protective factors in the development of eating disorders, obesity, substance use, and mental health among children and adolescents.

Ann Garwick, Associate Professor; Ph.D., Minnesota. Children with chronic disabilities and their families, family health and care giving.

Joseph Gaugler, Assistant Professor; Ph.D., Pennsylvania. Longitudinal implications: care for disabled adults, effects of social integration on outcomes in long-term care.

Linda Gerdner, Assistant Professor; Ph.D., Iowa. Management of agitation in persons with Alzheimer's disease and related disorders (ADRD), culturally sensitive care in persons with ADRD and their family caregivers.

Cynthia Gross, Professor; Ph.D., Yale. Quality of life outcomes of persons after transplantation and during drug therapy; quality of life and health status in patients with lung disorders, diabetes, or renal failure; reliability and validity of quality of life instruments and clinical assessments for research.

Laila Gulzar, Assistant Professor; Ph.D. International and interorganizational collaboration, cross-cultural health and cultural competence, nursing curing Islamic civilization (sixth through twelfth centuries), women's access to primary health care, health-care experiences of immigrants.

Linda Halcón, Assistant Professor; Ph.D., Minnesota. Public health nursing, epidemiology.

Helen E. Hansen, Associate Professor; Ph.D., Kansas. Nursing administration, health-care delivery systems, health team collaboration, leadership.

Susan Henly, Associate Professor; Ph.D., Minnesota. Psychometric methods for nursing research; covariance structures analysis, bonding, and maternal role development; social context for breast-feeding.

Ann Jones, Director of Undergraduate Studies; Ph.D. Transition experiences of new graduate nurses.

Catherine Juve, Associate Education Specialist; Ph.D., Minnesota. Substance abuse in pregnancy.

Merrie J. Kaas, Associate Professor; D.N.Sc., California, San Francisco. Older women's mental health, mental health/illness in long-term care.

Madeleine Kerr, Associate Professor; Ph.D., Michigan. Health promotion interventions with workers, research with Mexican-American and other ethnic/racial groups, occupational health: health protective behaviors.

Mary Jo Kreitzer, Associate Professor; Ph.D., Minnesota. Prayer/spirituality and transplant patients.

Kathleen E. Krichbaum, Associate Professor; Ph.D., Minnesota. Factors contributing to quality of care for the elderly in nursing homes, clinical teaching effectiveness, evaluating clinical learning.

Martha Kubik, Assistant Professor; Ph.D., Minnesota. School- and community-based intervention research; adolescent health: physical activity and eating; youth depression; population-based health care.

Barbara J. Leonard, Professor; Ph.D., Minnesota. Child health care, care of children with special health-care needs.

Marsha L. Lewis, Associate Professor; Ph.D., Minnesota. Clinical and client decision making, quality of life for the chronically mentally ill.

Joan Liaschenko, Associate Professor; Ph.D., California, San Francisco. Ethics, nursing practice, nursing humanities, philosophy of nursing, psychiatric nursing, home-care nursing.

Linda L. Lindeke, Associate Professor; Ph.D., Minnesota. Advanced nursing practice, high-risk infants.

Ruth D. Lindquist, Associate Professor; Ph.D., Minnesota. Risks of and response to cardiovascular disease, personal control and quality of life in health care, alterations in homeostatic function in elderly, critical care.

Wendy S. Looman, Assistant Professor; Ph.D. Social Capital; family-community interactions: special needs children.

Margaret Moss, Assistant Professor; D.S.N., Texas. Gerontology, minority aging, American Indians and aging.

Christine Mueller, Associate Professor; Ph.D., Maryland. Clinical and cost outcomes for nursing home residents using research-based clinical protocols and organizational interventions via advanced practice nurses; staffing in long-term-care facilities.

Carol O'Boyle, Assistant Professor; Ph.D., Minnesota. International health, infectious disease and control, nursing theory and learning.

Susan O'Connor-Von, Assistant Professor; D.N.Sc. Pediatric pain, preparation for surgery, childhood preoperative fears, nonpharmocologic interventions for pain management.

Cynthia Peden-McAlpine, Assistant Professor; Ph.D., Adelphi. Expert thinking in nursing practice, critical care and public health nursing, nurse executive practice, moral aspects of thinking in nursing practice, phenomenological and hermeneutic methodology.

Cheryl Robertson, Assistant Professor; Ph.D., Minnesota. Effects of war, repression, and torture on the health of families and communities, focusing on models that promote resilience and health systems capacity development.

Mary Rowan, Senior Teaching Specialist and Coordinator of Nursing Post-Baccalaureate Program; Ph.D., Minnesota. Ethics, technology-enhanced education.

Renee Sieving, Assistant Professor; Ph.D., Minnesota. Youth-health promotion; prevention of adolescent multiple health-risk behaviors: sexual risks, violence.

Diane Treat-Jacobson, Assistant Professor; Ph.D., Minnesota. Outcomes of exercise training in patients with claudication from peripheral arterial disease (PAD), quality-of-life assessment/measurement.

Cecilia Wachdorf, Senior Teaching Specialist; Ph.D., South Florida. Models of health care and value systems of midwives, comparisons of nurse and direct-entry midwives.

Bonnie Westra, Assistant Professor; Ph.D., Wisconsin. Informatics, business process improvement, systems analysis, quality improvement, public health policy.

Jean Wyman, Professor; Ph.D., Washington (Seattle). Gerontological nursing, urinary incontinence, fall prevention and exercise in the elderly.

Gretchen Zunkel, Assistant Professor; Ph.D., Washington (Seattle). Women's mental health, self-regulation; interventions: depression, PTSD, personality disorders; family mental health promotion.

University of Pennsylvania
School of Nursing
Philadelphia, Pennsylvania

THE UNIVERSITY

The University of Pennsylvania (Penn) is an independent, nonsectarian institution. As one of the finest universities in the country, it offers an outstanding array of resources for both undergraduate and graduate students. The excellence of its twelve graduate and four undergraduate schools offers students the opportunity to take elective courses across the campus in a wide range of subjects, making it one of the major centers for learning and research in the nation. Penn will be graduating the students of the twenty-first century from a unified academic community that provides a framework to foster student and faculty collaboration across the University, enhancing opportunities for a diversified approach to education and research.

THE SCHOOL OF NURSING

Penn is the only Ivy League institution offering a baccalaureate nursing program that begins day one, master's programs in nursing, and doctoral nursing study. The University of Pennsylvania Medical Center began training professional nurses in 1886. Today the School of Nursing at Penn offers one of the most progressive and highly regarded programs in the country.

The University of Pennsylvania School of Nursing is consistently ranked among the nation's top graduate schools of nursing in a major survey conducted by *U.S. News & World Report*. In determining its rankings, the criteria considered were the School's reputation for scholarship, curriculum, research, and the quality of the faculty and students.

The University has virtually all of its undergraduate and graduate facilities—including its hospitals, libraries, and laboratories—on one campus, giving nursing students access to people, ideas, and information on a multitude of subjects. Nursing students have matchless opportunities for clinical experience at the world-renowned University of Pennsylvania Health System, the Children's Hospital of Philadelphia, the Penn Nursing Network (nurse-managed clinical practices), and the Philadelphia VA Medical Center in addition to many other clinical agencies and health-care institutions in the Philadelphia region.

At Penn, nursing students are taught and advised by a faculty that is nationally and internationally recognized for its leadership in education, practice, and research. Undergraduate and graduate students often take advantage of the opportunity to participate in faculty research and scholarly publications. The Penn faculty members have a deep commitment to their role as teachers as well as to the development of professional and personal alliances between students and faculty.

PROGRAMS OF STUDY

The School of Nursing offers a Bachelor of Science in Nursing (B.S.N.) degree with a program that balances the liberal arts, science, and professional nursing preparation. Courses in the nursing major emphasize critical-thinking skills, interpersonal communication, clinical competence, and research. Special opportunities include nursing-specific study-abroad programs; joint- and dual-degree programs, dual-degree options, and minors in Penn's College of Arts and Sciences, Annenberg School for Communication, Wharton School, and School of Engineering and Applied Science; and submatriculation (initiating pursuit of a graduate degree while working toward the completion of the B.S.N.) into Penn's School of Law or one of the School of Nursing's sixteen M.S.N. specialties.

In 1997, the University initiated an undergraduate joint degree program offered by the School of Nursing and the Wharton School. Graduates are awarded a B.S.N. from the School of Nursing and Bachelor of Science in Economics from the Wharton School with a concentration in health-care management and policy. Additional programs include a health communication minor with the Annenberg School for Communication, and a B.S.N./Ph.D. option.

Penn offers an accelerated program allowing students already holding a baccalaureate degree to complete a B.S.N. or B.S.N./M.S.N. degree. These second-degree accelerated programs build on an individual's present level of education so that students need only complete required nursing-specific courses.

The RN Return Program is designed to educate hospital diploma and associate degree RNs for an increased leadership roles in nursing by earning a B.S.N. degree. Previous college and university courses are evaluated for transfer credit, and many clinical nursing courses may be challenged by taking specified Excelsior College examinations.

The School of Nursing offers the Master of Science in Nursing (M.S.N.) degree, including nurse practitioner programs in adult acute care, adult health, adult oncology, family health, gerontology, neonatal, pediatrics, pediatric acute/chronic, pediatric critical-care, pediatric oncology, and women's health. Advanced practice specialist programs include the nurse anesthesia, nurse midwifery, and the psychiatric–mental health advanced practice programs. Administration programs are available in health leadership and nursing and health-care administration. There are also many special options at Penn Nursing, including unique opportunities and minors. There are four unique opportunities: adult home care, clinical nurse specialist, occupational/environmental health, and perinatal. Students enrolled in graduate programs may apply for one of ten minors: adult acute care, adult oncology, behavioral health, forensic science, gerontology, health informatics, health leadership, nursing and health-care administration, palliative care, and women's health studies. An M.S.N. in nursing administration/M.B.A. degree program is offered with the Wharton Business School and a M.S.N./M.P.H. degree program is offered with the Graduate Program in Public Health Studies in the School of Medicine. Penn Nursing also offers a post-master's teacher education program.

The School of Nursing recognizes the evolving nature of health care and the desire on the part of many nurses to expand or alter current roles and responsibilities. Post-master's certificate programs for those who already possess a master's degree in nursing and are interested in either extending their knowledge and skill in their current area of practice or changing to a new area of nursing practice. Students have the option of designing their own curriculum to include two or more programs.

The mission of the doctoral program of the University of Pennsylvania School of Nursing is to prepare nurse scientists for successful careers, particularly in research-intensive environments. Graduates of this program will be leaders who will move the science of nursing forward through the conduct and dissemination of research for the advancement of nursing practice. These nurse scientists will take responsibility to shape and advance health care, with the ultimate goal of improving the public's health through the integration of theory, research, and practice.

The educational experience focuses on the processes of understanding and examining of substantive bodies of knowledge. Development as a researcher is fostered through exposure to the philosophic and methodological aspects of nursing and related basic and applied disciplines.

For students with a special interest, there are also joint programs, such as a Ph.D. in nursing and a master's in bioethics or a Ph.D. in nursing and a Master of Business Administration from the Wharton School. M.S.N./Ph.D. and M.S./Ph.D. options are also available.

ACADEMIC FACILITIES
The Penn Library is made up of fifteen facilities and holds more than 5 million printed volumes, 4 million items in microfilm, 39,426 serial subscriptions and 9,552 e-journals, 9,196 computer files, and 239,537 locally digitized images.

The Mathias J. Brunner Instructional Technology Center, located within the School, is a state-of-the-art facility featuring virtual learning and patient-care simulation.

Specialized centers at the School of Nursing include the Center for Nursing Research; the Center for Biobehavioral Research; the Center for Health Disparities Research; the Center for Health Outcomes and Policy Research; the Barbara Bates Center for the Study of the History of Nursing; and the Center for Gerontologic Nursing Science.

LOCATION
Philadelphia is the fifth-largest metropolitan area in the United States. The four undergraduate schools and twelve graduate schools of the University are located on a 260-acre tract on the west side of the Schuylkill River. Unified by a network of pedestrian walkways and almost entirely closed off to cars, the campus contributes to the sense of community that is characteristic of Penn. Although situated in a major urban setting just across the river and less than 2 miles from the center of Philadelphia, the University is surrounded by a largely residential community known as University City.

STUDENT SERVICES
On Penn's campus there are many resources and services available to meet the needs of its diverse student body. At the University level, Penn's students may take advantage of the cultural centers, religious organizations, academic advising, counseling, housing, dining, student health, tutoring, day-care, athletic facilities, and computing services. Within the School of Nursing, student organizations and the professional staff of student services personnel are available to meet any student needs.

THE NURSING STUDENT GROUP
The School of Nursing populations comprise a diverse group of students. Within the University, the School creates an intimate niche that enables students to receive personalized attention from the faculty and staff members. Each student is paired with a School of Nursing faculty adviser to further enhance student-faculty interaction.

COSTS
Tuition for full-time B.S.N. students for the 2006–07 academic year was $30,598. Part-time tuition was $3908 per course. Tuition for full-time M.S.N. students was $45,146 (twelve-month program); it was $3715 per course part-time. Full-time Ph.D. students are fully funded with a stipend and tuition support for the first four years. Part-time Ph.D. tuition was $4074 per course in 2006–07.

FINANCIAL AID
Penn is committed to meeting the financial need of all of its students. Many different sources of aid are available. Scholarships, grants, low-interest student loans, and teaching and research assistantships are awarded appropriately, based on a student's need and level of study. Financial aid counseling is available for individual consultation and support. Students are encouraged to work directly with the School to assist them in developing the means to support their education.

APPLYING
Freshman applicants to the B.S.N. program should be completing a general college-preparatory program in high school. They must also take the SAT and two SAT Subject Tests or the ACT. If taking the ACT, applicants are required to take the new ACT with writing.

Prospective freshman students can apply under one of two admissions plans. The Early Decision Plan (EDP) is for those applicants who have decided that the University of Pennsylvania School of Nursing is their first-choice college and agree to attend if accepted. Applications are due by November 1, with decisions mailed in mid-December. Regular decision applications to the School of Nursing are due by January 1, and students are notified by the end of February.

Transfer students are admitted for the fall semester only. The application deadline is March 15, with notification beginning early May.

B.S.N./M.S.N. and B.S.N. second degree applicants must apply by October 15 for June or September admission and receive notification by late January. The Graduate Record Examinations (GRE) are required for B.S.N./M.S.N. applicants.

It is important that applicants to all of the baccalaureate options arrange a personal interview with an admissions counselor in the School of Nursing. This interview will afford students an opportunity to learn more about the specific program they are considering and to better understand the course work required to complete the B.S.N. degree. Online applications are available.

All master's and doctoral applicants must have completed an accredited baccalaureate nursing program, have taken a course in basic statistics, and have nursing licensure. Applicants should interview with the appropriate program director and must submit, along with the completed application forms, GRE General Test scores, transcripts, references, and essays. Applicants who have earned a GPA of 3.2 or higher in their baccalaureate nursing program may be eligible for the GRE waiver program. International students must submit results from the TOEFL and GRE and may be asked to have their foreign transcripts evaluated in a Full Educational Course-by-Course Report by the Commission on Graduates of Foreign Nursing Schools or World Education Services. Applications are accepted on a rolling basis for most M.S.N. programs; however, applicants are encouraged to submit applications early to secure clinical placement and maximum financial aid. Applications to the M.S.N./Ph.D. program are due by November 1. Applications for the doctoral program must be submitted by December 15.

For more information, to request written materials, or for access to the online application, prospective students should access the School's Web site.

CORRESPONDENCE AND INFORMATION
Killebrew-Laporte Center for Admissions and Student Affairs
Claire M. Fagan Hall
School of Nursing
University of Pennsylvania
420 Guardian Drive
Philadelphia, Pennsylvania 19104-6096
Phone: 215-898-4271
        866-867-6877 (toll-free)
Fax: 215-573-8439
E-mail: admissions@nursing.upenn.edu
Web site: http://www.nursing.upenn.edu

University of Phoenix Online
School of Nursing
Phoenix, Arizona

THE UNIVERSITY

University of Phoenix was established in Phoenix, Arizona, in 1976 to serve the educational needs of working students and their employers. Today, University of Phoenix is the largest accredited private university in the United States, with more than 20,000 highly qualified instructors, over 190 campuses and learning centers, and Internet delivery worldwide. University of Phoenix helps thousands of working students achieve a higher level of success every year.

In addition to nursing, degree programs in business, management, e-business, technology, criminal justice, and education are also offered. A commitment to educational excellence and unsurpassed student service has made University of Phoenix one of the nation's leading universities for working students.

University of Phoenix is a private institution of higher learning. Its main headquarters are located at 4615 E. Elwood Street, Phoenix, Arizona 85040. The University is accredited by The Higher Learning Commission and is a member of the North Central Association of Colleges and Schools (312-263-0456; http://www.ncahigherlearningcommission.org).

The Bachelor of Science in Nursing and Master of Science in Nursing programs are accredited by the Commission on Collegiate Nursing Education (One Dupont Circle, NW, Washington, D.C. 20036-1120; 202-887-6791). Florida: University of Phoenix is licensed by the Florida Commission for Independent Education, License No. 2308. Georgia: University of Phoenix is authorized under the Nonpublic Postsecondary Educational Institutions Act of 1990. Indiana: University of Phoenix is fully accredited by the Indiana Commission for Postsecondary Proprietary Education, AC-0188. The Indianapolis Campus is located at 7999 Knue Road, Suites 100 and 500, Indianapolis, Indiana 46250; The Northwest Indiana Campus is located at 359 East 81st Avenue, Merrillville, Indiana 46410. Ohio: The registration number is 1154320. The Cleveland Campus is located at 5005 Rockside Road, Suite 130, Independence, Ohio 44131-2194; the Cincinnati Campus is located at 9050 Centre Pointe Drive, Suite 250, West Chester, Ohio 45069-4875; the Columbus Campus is located at 8415 Pulsar Place, Columbus, Ohio 43240-4032. Online: 3157 East Elwood Street, Phoenix, Arizona 85034. South Carolina: University of Phoenix is licensed by the South Carolina Commission on Higher Education. The campus is located at 1001 Pinnacle Point Drive, Columbia, South Carolina 29223. Tennessee: The Memphis Campus is located at 65 Germantown Court, Suite 100, Cordova, Tennessee 38018; The Nashville Campus is located at 616 Marriott Drive, Suite 150, Nashville, Tennessee 37214; The Franklin Campus is located at 377 Riverside Drive, Franklin, Tennessee 37064; The Chattanooga Campus is located at 1208 Pointe Centre Drive, Chattanooga, Tennessee 37421. Virginia: State Council of Higher Education for Virginia has authorized University of Phoenix to offer degree or certificate programs. Any course, degree or certificate program offered has been approved by the University of Phoenix governing board. Credit earned for coursework in Virginia can be transferred to University of Phoenix's principal location outside Virginia as part of the University's existing degree or certificate programs.

THE SCHOOL OF NURSING

University of Phoenix Online offers a comprehensive online nursing program that provides unparalleled convenience and flexibility for the RN who seeks advanced education. A distinguished blend of established academic practices and innovative instructional delivery systems has helped to build the University, with a growing network of campuses and learning centers throughout the United States. The goal is to provide all nursing students with the means to be more effective at their jobs so that they may reap the rewards that follow.

The degree programs are taught by faculty members who work in the fields they teach and who bring academic and experiential insight to every course. Faculty members are carefully chosen both for their success in their own careers and for their ability and desire to effectively facilitate a challenging and rewarding learning environment. They also hold master's or doctoral degrees. Each instructor is skilled in the unique craft of providing course instruction, direction, and feedback to students. This integration of advanced academic preparation, communications expertise, and current professional experience ensures that students learn real-world application.

PROGRAMS OF STUDY

The Bachelor of Science in Nursing (B.S.N.) program is designed to develop the professional knowledge and skills of working registered nurses. The curriculum is built upon a foundation of biological, physical, and social sciences that contribute to the science of nursing. The liberal arts components enhance the development of the intellectual, social, and cultural aspects of the professional nurse. The degree program uses an instructional program with behavioral objectives that concentrate on the development of the nurse's role as caregiver, teacher, and manager of care. Utilizing a self-care framework, working registered nurses are prepared as generalists who are able to apply professional skills and knowledge to nursing, clients, and health-care systems.

The Bachelor of Science in Health Administration (B.S.H.A.) program is designed to integrate a foundation of general education and applied sciences with the expertise that prepares the graduate for professional careers in a variety of health-care or related health settings. The B.S.H.A. curriculum addresses the basic body of knowledge, understanding, and skills identified as relevant to health-care services such as management, finance and accounting, legal and ethical parameters, health and disease factors, and human and information resources.

In addition, University of Phoenix offers two specialty degrees incorporating the B.S.H.A.: B.S.H.A./Health Information Systems and B.S.H.A./Long Term Care.

The Master of Science in Nursing (M.S.N.) program is designed to develop and enhance the knowledge and skills of registered nurses. It is designed for nurses who want to pursue more advanced positions in today's challenging health-care environment. The program blends nursing theory with advanced practice concepts necessary to successfully work within the structure, culture, and mission of any size health-care organization or educational setting. Students complete core courses in advanced nursing content and process as well as on leadership skills. Specializations assist students to concentrate on developing increased knowledge and/or skills in a specific area of content or advanced practice role. In addition, University of Phoenix offers a specialty degree that incorporates the M.S.N.: M.S.N./Nursing/Health Care Education.

The Master of Business Administration/Health Care Management (M.B.A./HCM) degree program is designed for professionals seeking management positions in the health-care field. The program is structured with two primary goals in mind. The first is to provide students with a broad-based understanding of current management tools and techniques with practical application in the health-care industry. The second goal is to prepare students to manage human and material resources effectively and efficiently within the health-care environment. The program emphasizes fundamental curriculum, critical thinking, and decision making that have been positioned for the changing requirements and dynamics of the health-care industry. Students are required to give due consideration to the broader implications of decisions, such as the potential effect on governmental relations, marketing, human resources, and finances and operations.

The Master of Health Administration (M.H.A.) program prepares leaders who can effectively respond to the dynamic and ever-changing health-care industry. These individuals have a capacity to critically examine and evaluate issues and trends and are empowered to influence the destiny of the global health-care system. The curriculum is tailored to the needs of the health-care leader/manager by providing content in finance, policy, research, technology, quality improvement, economics, marketing, and strategic planning.

In addition, the M.S.N./M.H.A. dual degree combines essential elements from both degree programs to provide students with the knowledge and skills needed to effectively examine and evaluate issues and trends impacting health care.

The dual M.S.N./M.B.A./HCM degree program is designed to provide nurses with a unique blend of advanced nursing and business management skills to manage today's innovative health-care delivery systems. The program combines essentials from both degree programs to provide students with the knowledge and skills necessary to enhance and support patient services.

ACADEMIC FACILITIES
The online learning format relies on computer communications to link faculty members and students from around the world into interactive electronic forums. Classes are kept small for maximum interaction, and degrees are completed entirely online for the convenience of working students.

LOCATION
Once enrolled in an online degree program, students log on at least four days each week to participate in class discussions. Students work online, sending and receiving material to and from class groups.

STUDENT SERVICES
University of Phoenix offers its students exceptional customer service. An experienced nursing enrollment representative is available to answer all questions regarding programs, start dates, financing, and the application process. A free pre-evaluation of potential credits for prior education or work experience can also be requested. Once the application and fees have been received, an enrollment representative will process the application, ship the software, and help order textbooks and course materials. During class, students have access to a full range of online research libraries and services. Every instructor provides guidance and feedback on student progress.

THE NURSING STUDENT GROUP
University courses are designed for working adults who have busy work schedules and full personal lives. The average age of entering University of Phoenix students is approximately 36 years, with a household income of $70,000 to $79,000. Nearly 60 percent of entering students have at least eleven years of work experience, and about 60 percent of students receive some tuition assistance from their employers—double the national average for adult students at other institutions.

COSTS
Undergraduate nursing tuition is $430 per credit, and graduate nursing tuition is $485 per credit. There is an application fee of $45 and a degree completion fee of $65. Textbook costs vary by course.

FINANCIAL AID
University of Phoenix participates in many financial aid programs, including the Federal Stafford Student Loan, the Federal PLUS Loan, and the Federal Pell Grant. The University does not charge students for processing financial aid applications. Financial options, including financial aid, are available to those who qualify. For further details about eligibility and to receive application forms, students should speak with a finance representative.

APPLYING
Applicants must be employed in a nursing role or have access to an appropriate health-care environment. Nursing students must have a diploma or an associate degree in nursing, with a cumulative GPA of at least 2.0 and a current RN license. One hallmark of the B.S.N. program is that there is no testing of prior nursing knowledge if the RN is in good standing within the state of practice. Graduate students must have an undergraduate nursing degree or other related health-care degree from a regionally accredited college or university, with a cumulative GPA of 2.5 or better (3.0 for prior graduate work). Students must also be currently employed, with a minimum of three years of work experience as an RN (or two years of work experience as an RN plus one year in a related field). RNs who have a nonnursing bachelor's degree take three bridge courses from the B.S.N. program prior to being eligible for graduate M.S.N. course work. Unless students rely on international transcripts for admission, all that is needed to begin the first course is a completed application, enrollment agreement, and disclosure form. While students are in their first three classes, enrollment representatives work with them to complete transcript requests, the Comprehensive Cognitive Assessment, and any other items necessary for formal registration. To apply for admission, students should visit http://myapply.phoenix.edu/apply.

CORRESPONDENCE AND INFORMATION:
University of Phoenix
4615 East Elwood Street
Phoenix, Arizona 85040

Phone: 877-611-3390 (toll-free in U.S.)
Fax: 602-387-6440
Web site: http://www.uopx.com/petersons

University of Pittsburgh
School of Nursing
Pittsburgh, Pennsylvania

THE UNIVERSITY
Founded in 1787, the University of Pittsburgh is the oldest institution of higher education west of the Allegheny Mountains. It is an independent, state-related, nonsectarian coeducational institution offering a variety of undergraduate and graduate programs. Total enrollment at the Pittsburgh campus is approximately 27,000, including nearly 10,000 graduate and professional students. In recognition of the strength of its graduate programs, the University was elected in 1974 to the Association of American Universities, an organization of the sixty-two leading research universities in the United States and Canada.

THE SCHOOL OF NURSING
Established in 1939 as an independent professional school of the University, the School of Nursing has a positive impact on the quality of health care for all segments of the population through its teaching, research, and service. It offers educational programs that anticipate and reflect the health-care needs of the region, state, and nation, resulting in the awarding of more than 11,000 degrees to nursing students, including 8,151 baccalaureate degrees, 3,076 master's degrees, 184 doctoral degrees, and thirteen master's certificates. The average student nurse population is 1,016. Nursing students benefit from a low student-faculty ratio, small class sizes, and the extensive resources and enrichment opportunities of a research intensive university and a major metropolitan medical center.

The School is nationally known for the strengths of its clinical practice and research programs. Students hone clinical practice skills utilizing the strongest network of health-care providers in the nation, anchored by the University of Pittsburgh Medical Center. Clinical faculty members maintain their own professional clinical practice in order to enhance their skills and knowledge. Faculty members and students are engaged in multidisciplinary clinical and basic science research that aims to provide a scientific basis for the care of individuals across the life span.

PROGRAMS OF STUDY
The School of Nursing has undergraduate and graduate programs. There are three undergraduate programs: the baccalaureate or prelicensure program, the Accelerated 2nd Degree B.S.N. Program, and the RN Options Program. All yield a Bachelor of Science in Nursing degree (B.S.N.) upon completion.

Baccalaureate students typically enter as freshmen unless they have completed all required freshman courses and are accepted into the sophomore class. The 124-credit curriculum emphasizes liberal arts and sciences courses during the first year and introduces clinical study during the second year. The last two years include a variety of clinical experiences culminating in a leadership/transition course where seniors work closely with professional nurse preceptors. Many undergraduates choose to complete an independent study with faculty mentors. Graduates are eligible to take the National Council Licensure Examination (NCLEX) to become registered nurses (RN).

Registered nurses who wish to obtain a B.S.N. or M.S.N. have the RN Options Program to provide quality educational opportunities that will prepare them to advance their careers. Nurses may be full- or part-time students and proceed directly into a master's program after completing the bachelor's program. Each nurse receives individualized guidance to create their academic plan.

The Accelerated 2nd Degree B.S.N. Program is designed to enable students with a previous baccalaureate degree to earn a baccalaureate degree in nursing. This is an intensive, fast-paced program that builds upon a student's previous education while providing science and nursing content to enable students to earn a B.S.N. degree within three terms of full-time study and are eligible to take the RN licensing examination. Admission to this option is highly competitive and is based upon proven academic achievement and grades earned in prerequisite courses. Two of the accelerated courses and one of the prerequisite courses are master's-level courses. Successful completion of this program earns the student 8 credits toward the M.S.N. degree, should the student decide to pursue a master's degree in nursing at the University of Pittsburgh School of Nursing.

Postbaccalaureate certificates include health-care genetics, health-care management, and school nurse certification.

Graduate programs include master's and doctoral degrees. Professional nurses who wish to pursue a graduate degree have several choices at the School. The School of Nursing prepares advanced practice nurses for nurse anesthetist, nurse practitioner, or clinical nurse specialist roles. Nurse practitioner options include acute-care nurse practitioner with a concentration in adult health, cardiopulmonary, critical care, oncology, or a directed option. A primary-care nurse practitioner can specialize in family, pediatrics, psychiatric, or adult roles. Another career path available is the role of the clinical nurse specialist. This program offers a choice of focus in medical/surgical or psychiatric nursing. Advanced specialist roles prepare nurses to become leaders in the areas of administration, education, informatics, research, or clinical nurse leader.

Master's programs vary from 41 to 52 credits. The curriculum consists of core courses, advanced nursing practice specialty courses, role development courses, and electives. Core courses include health promotion, pathophysiology, physical diagnosis, pharmacology, nursing theory and research, and the research practicum. Minors are also available in nursing education, nursing research, nursing informatics, or nursing administration, along with the school nurse certificate and management certificate for health professionals. For those who have a current master's degree, a second master's option is also available, and a thesis is optional. There are post-master's certificate options in administration, education, informatics, and health-care genetics as well as five nurse practitioner options.

The Doctor of Philosophy (Ph.D.) program prepares scholars to extend scientific knowledge that advances the science and practice of nursing and to contribute to the scientific base of other disciplines. The curriculum includes courses in the history and philosophy of science, nursing theory development, the structure of nursing knowledge, issues influencing leadership and public policy in nursing and health, advanced statistics, quantitative research methods, research methodologies, instrumentation, and a research practicum with an experienced researcher. An area of research emphasis, which matches a faculty member's research emphasis, is selected by the student early in the program. Current faculty research initiatives include adolescent health, health-care outcomes, chronic disorders, critical care, health promotion, and mental health. The culminating requirement is a dissertation.

Two options exist for completing the doctoral program. The traditional M.S.N.–Ph.D. option is for students with a nursing master's degree. This option requires the completion of 64 credits. A one-term, full-time residency is required; however, the remainder of the degree requirements may be completed through either full- or part-time study. The B.S.N.-Ph.D. option, for nurses who wish to focus their career in research, does not require a master's degree. This option requires full-time study to complete 95–97 credits.

The Doctor of Nursing Practice (D.N.P.) is another doctoral program that is offered. This practice-focused doctoral program prepares nursing leaders for the highest level of clinical nursing practice beyond the initial preparation in the discipline. Throughout the program students develop the clinical, organizational, economic, and leadership skills to design and implement programs of care delivery that significantly impact health-care outcomes and have the potential to transform health-care delivery. Graduates with this terminal clinical degree are prepared for roles in direct care or indirect, systems-focused care. Advanced practice nurses practicing in today's health-care environment require complex clinical skills and sophisticated knowledge of the evidence-base for practice. Graduates of the D.N.P. program are able to affect the health-care delivery system by evaluating the evidence base for nursing practice, becoming leaders in the clinical arenas, establishing standards and policies, and meeting the needs of today's diverse health-care systems.

ACADEMIC FACILITIES
Nursing students have access to the University Library System, which is the 26th-largest academic research library in all of North America and the 16th-largest among the prestigious public libraries of the Association of American Universities. It provides a large array of innovative, world-class services. The School of Nursing Learning Resources Center (LRC) provides reference services, a nursing skills practice laboratory, a computer laboratory, a small television studio, and a graphics laboratory. The LRC

computer laboratory is open 60 hours per week and provides microcomputer capability and access to the University mainframe computer system and to the Internet. Students also use the University's computer labs, which are located around the campus.

LOCATION
The University's 132-acre campus is situated in Oakland, the heart of Pittsburgh's educational, medical, and cultural center. Within walking distance of the campus are theaters, art galleries, museums, libraries, and concert halls.

Pittsburgh has consistently been named one of the nation's most livable cities in various national surveys. Most students and many faculty members live within walking distance of the University, in Oakland, Squirrel Hill, or Shadyside. These areas abound in ethnic restaurants and in shops of all varieties, reflecting the cosmopolitan background of the residents. Most people find that Pittsburgh is a friendly, warm, active, exciting, and comfortable city in which to live.

STUDENT SERVICES
The University offers students a wide variety of services, including outpatient health care at the Student Health Service; career development, learning skills, and psychological services; veterans and disabled student services; numerous student activities; and child care.

THE NURSING STUDENT GROUP
In 2005–06, the School of Nursing enrolled 623 undergraduate students and 417 graduate students. Of the total student population, more than 50 percent were already registered nurses who were working toward B.S.N., M.S.N., or Ph.D. degrees in order to advance their career by assuming a new role or by changing career direction, or to increase their personal satisfaction.

COSTS
Undergraduate tuition per term in 2006–07 for full-time study was $7154 for in-state and $13,145 for out-of-state students. Tuition per credit for part-time study was $596 for in-state and $1095 for out-of-state students. Full-time student fees were $712 per year. On-campus housing costs ranged from $1655 to $2995 per term. Available meal plan options varied from $300 to $1920 per term.

Graduate tuition per term in 2006–07 for full-time study was $8192 for in-state and $10,640 for out-of-state students. Tuition per credit for part-time study was $671 for in-state and $872 for out-of-state students. Full-time student fees were $629 per year.

FINANCIAL AID
The University awards financial assistance to both undergraduate and graduate students through scholarships, loans, part-time employment, work-study, and School of Nursing awards. Freshman applicants should apply by March 1, continuing students by April 1, and graduate students by June 1.

Master's students receive a variety of financial aid through the School of Nursing, including Professional Nurse Traineeships for full-time study, University tuition aid for part-time study, specified scholarships, and loans.

Doctoral students also receive aid from the School. Out-of-state full-time students who meet specific criteria pay in-state tuition rates due to school-based scholarships. Many full-time doctoral students have graduate assistant, researcher, or teaching fellow positions, which are primarily merit-based, pay a stipend, and include a tuition scholarship and individual health insurance. These students work 10–20 hours per week, and many have excellent experiences on faculty research projects or teaching. Workshops on applying for predoctoral and postdoctoral training grant fellowships are provided. In addition, other scholarships and part-time tuition aid are available. Students should apply for all School-based aid by June 1 and should contact the Student Services Office for further information.

APPLYING
Applicants to all programs should present appropriate transcripts, admission test scores, and other required material by the deadline date. For the latest and most complete admission information, applicants should contact the Student Services Office. High school applicants and those applying for transfer from another college or university should contact the University Office of Admissions and Financial Aid at 412-624-PITT to receive information and an application. Admission decisions are made on a rolling basis, but applicants should apply as early as possible. Registered nurse applicants are admitted on a rolling basis for all terms.

Undergraduate prelicensure applicants are evaluated primarily on the basis of their high school or previous college-level academic work, with an emphasis on performance in science courses. For high school applicants or transfer applicants with fewer than 24 credits, SAT scores as well as the student's high school record are considered.

Master's applicants must have a baccalaureate degree in nursing, a current license to practice, and one to two years of experience (for full-time study). Admission decisions are based upon a faculty interview, professional goals, previous academic performance, and GRE or MAT scores, if required by the program. Applications are due January 5 for the anesthesia program, for full-time and part-time study. Applications for full-time study for all other programs must be made by August 1 for fall term, December 1 for spring term, and April 1 for summer term. Applicants for part-time study may be admitted to any term on a rolling admissions basis as long as spaces are available.

Doctoral applicants must have a baccalaureate degree in nursing, documentation of academic success in an appropriate master's program, evidence of competence in scholarly research and the ability to communicate in writing, and competitive GRE scores. Admission decisions are based upon previous academic performance, faculty interviews, professional and research goals, a match between the applicant's research interest and those of available faculty members, and GRE scores. Applications are accepted on a rolling basis.

CORRESPONDENCE AND INFORMATION
Student Services
School of Nursing
239 Victoria Building
University of Pittsburgh
3500 Victoria Street
Pittsburgh, Pennsylvania 15261
Phone: 412-624-4586
      888-747-0794 (toll-free)
Fax: 412-624-2409
E-mail: sao50@pitt.edu
Web site: http://www.nursing.pitt.edu

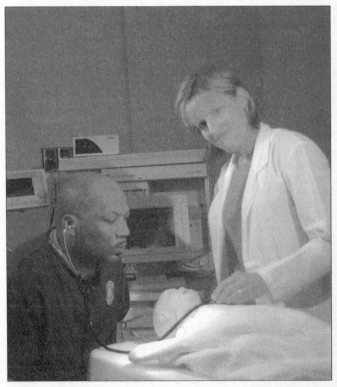

Students gain hands-on experience at the University of Pittsburgh School of Nursing.

University of St. Francis
College of Nursing and Allied Health
Joliet, Illinois

THE UNIVERSITY

The University of St. Francis (USF) is a national leader in offering educational opportunities to health-care professionals. Founded in 1920 by the Sisters of St. Francis of Mary Immaculate, the University's mission includes using high-quality programming to address unmet educational needs.

More than 3,700 students are served in various graduate and undergraduate programs at locations throughout the nation, including nearly 1,500 students at the University's main campus in Joliet, Illinois.

The University of St. Francis faculty is committed to teaching. The University has 83 full-time faculty members. Sixty adjunct faculty members bring a variety of academic and professional experience to the classroom. Faculty advisers are an integral part of the USF experience.

USF faculty members are invested in the success of their students, both academically and personally. Nursing faculty members are strong clinicians. Their intense commitment to health care and to patients ensures that students are challenged academically while still offered a personal, caring support system.

One hundred percent of USF health-care graduates find employment or enter graduate school within six months of graduation.

The University of St. Francis is fully accredited by the Higher Learning Commission and is a member of the North Central Association of Colleges and Schools (Web site: http://www.higherlearningcommission.org; telephone: 312-263-0456). The University also is accredited by the Commission on Collegiate Nursing Education (CCNE).

THE COLLEGE OF NURSING AND ALLIED HEALTH

Founded in 1920, the University of St. Francis' College of Nursing and Allied Health has educated three generations of nurses, who are recognized throughout the regional health-care arena as exceptional clinicians and dedicated professionals.

The University promotes hands-on learning and partners with 208 health-care organizations to provide meaningful clinical experiences for its students. Supervisors at these organizations say that USF students are among the best prepared, most enthusiastic, and most inquiring of the nursing students with whom they work. The many areas of health care—hospitals, home health, managed care, primary-care clinics, public health, hospice care, long-term care, and mental health—are addressed in the curriculum and made available to students through clinical experiences. The nursing program focuses on the development of critical-thinking skills, cultural awareness, and patient advocacy as areas that help students excel in the dynamic health-care field.

The College of Nursing, in keeping with the University's Franciscan tradition, subscribes to the values of respect, compassion, service, and integrity, which are essential to becoming a caring, effective health-care professional.

USF is one of the few schools in the nation to provide its prenursing and premed students with the opportunity to regularly use state-of-the-art learning tools. These include A.D.A.M., revolutionary software that allows students to dissect a virtual cadaver in more detail, as well as a complete cadaver lab. A state-of-the-art nursing-skills simulation laboratory provides students with an opportunity to practice skills on computerized mannequins in a safe environment.

The passing rates of USF nursing graduates on the state licensure examination are above the national average pass rate. The NCLEX passing rate for the past academic year of nursing graduates was 91 percent.

PROGRAMS OF STUDY

The College of Nursing and Allied Health offers the Bachelor of Science in Nursing (B.S.N.) program in the traditional format for incoming freshmen and for transfer students and as a Fast Track option for registered nurses with an ADN or diploma. Course work may be available through traditional classroom study and online.

The four-year and transfer programs are based in a strong liberal arts component of general education that enhances the critical-thinking skills necessary for the scientific inquiry of nursing studies. Once in the upper-division level, course work is intensive and focused. Students learn not only science and nursing proficiencies but also about themselves as people and caregivers.

The RN-B.S.N. Fast Track is an online program designed to provide an educational opportunity for registered nurses to obtain a baccalaureate degree in nursing. Students may attend full- or part-time. Advanced-placement credit is awarded upon submission of transcripts from an associate or diploma nursing program.

The Master of Science in Nursing (M.S.N.) program has two tracks of study: nurse practitioner and clinical nurse specialist, with concentrations in gerontology and/or nursing education. The nurse practitioner track at the Joliet campus prepares the student to provide primary health care in the community setting and in inpatient facilities. The Albuquerque, New Mexico, campus offers the family nurse practitioner program. Both campuses offer on-site and online courses. After completion of their studies, graduate students are eligible to take the adult, family, or gerontology nurse practitioner or the clinical nurse specialist national certification exam and apply for advanced practice licensure.

The Master of Science in physician assistant studies at the University of St. Francis is a nationally focused, graduate-level program in primary-care medicine. The program educates students to provide high-quality diagnostic and therapeutic medical services with physician supervision. Consistent with the mission of the University of St. Francis, physician assistant students are educated to provide health care to a variety of patient populations, with a special emphasis on the underserved. This program, located in Albuquerque, is a full-time, twenty-seven-month professional education program. The program consists of fifteen months of classroom and laboratory instruction followed by twelve months of supervised clinical rotations. Students must complete the entire twenty-seven-month program at the University of St. Francis. Upon successful completion of the program, students are awarded a Master of Science degree in physician assistant studies and are eligible to take the national certifying examination. This program is fully accreditation by ARC-PA. The physician assistant (PA) studies program students recently scored in the top 10 percent of all programs in the country this year, ranking fourteenth in academic performance out of 136 PA programs in the nation.

The College of Nursing and Allied Health at USF also offers Bachelor of Science degrees in medical technology, nuclear medicine technology, radiography, and radiation therapy. USF is one of only two universities in Illinois that offers a B.S. degree in radiation therapy.

AFFILIATIONS WITH HEALTH-CARE FACILITIES
Key to students becoming exceptional, caring nurses are the hands-on learning experiences gained only through clinical settings. USF students may have clinical experiences with any of 208 health-care organizations. The University maintains working relationships with high-quality health-care organizations such as Hope Children's Hospital, Silver Cross Hospital, the Will County Health Department, Provena Saint Joseph Medical Center, and Saint James Hospital. The University's relationship with the nearby Provena Saint Joseph Medical Center offers educational opportunities rich in practical application.

Working relationships extend to the areas of hospitals, home health, managed care, primary clinics, public health, hospice care, long-term care (nursing homes), and public health. Students may even choose to learn about health care in other countries. One student recently studied the health-care system of Norway and spent a summer at the University of Oslo.

ACADEMIC FACILITIES
The College of Nursing and Allied Health recently moved into state-of-the-art facilities on the Joliet campus. Computerized classrooms, the new SIM lab, and cutting-edge equipment and technology are included in this new facility.

The University of St. Francis also has a center in Albuquerque, where the physician assistant studies program and the Master of Science in Nursing family nurse practitioner program are offered.

LOCATION
The University of St. Francis campus is in a historic residential district known as Joliet's Cathedral area. The University is 35 miles southwest (about 45 minutes) of Chicago and is easily accessible by major roadways and trains. The University also offers classes at a variety of health-care facilities throughout the nation.

STUDENT SERVICES
The University of St. Francis is committed to educating students both in the classroom and through activities outside the classroom. A variety of student clubs and organizations are available as well as volunteer activities. Student Affairs sponsors many entertainment events as well as the Student Government Association. Cultural musical events, which bring internationally and nationally acclaimed performers to the University, are sponsored through the Featured Performances series. Exhibits that bring the works of regionally recognized artists to campus also are planned.

THE NURSING STUDENT GROUP
The University of St. Francis has 530 students in its nursing programs. Of the total, 72 are in the RN-B.S.N. Fast Track program, 68 are graduate students, 516 are women, and 198 are members of minority groups. About 122 are part-time students. University of St. Francis nursing program graduates enjoy a 100 percent placement rate.

COSTS
Tuition and fees for full-time students are $19,150; room and board are $7280. Fast Track tuition was $425 per credit hour for the 2006–07 academic year.

FINANCIAL AID
The University of St. Francis is committed to assisting students in obtaining a high-quality, private education. The University spent nearly $9 million in institutional aid and scholarships in addition to nearly $3 million in federal and state assistance to enable students to attend USF. In order to apply for all forms of federal, state, and USF assistance, students must complete a financial aid application form. USF prefers that students complete the Free Application for Federal Student Aid (FAFSA). M.S.N. students can apply for Advanced Nursing Education Traineeship funds awarded to the University. Several students have received scholarships from Johnson & Johnson's The Promise of Nursing Campaign.

APPLYING
Freshmen are admitted in the fall and spring. Students should take the ACT or SAT and visit the campus for an interview by April 1. Entrance exams should be taken in the spring of the junior year or the fall of the senior year in high school. Applications should be filed by July 1 for fall entry and December 1 for spring entry, along with high school transcripts and an application fee of $30. Notification is on a rolling basis.

Transfer students anticipating enrollment as nursing majors should submit applications for admission and have transcripts forwarded to the Admissions Office one year in advance of their projected entry semester.

RN-B.S.N. Fast Track and Master of Science in Nursing students should submit transcripts from previously attended schools. Physician assistant studies students should complete the admissions process through Central Application Service for Physician Assistants (CASPA) at http://www.caspaonline.org.

Informational packet requests may be obtained from the Admissions Office via e-mail.

CORRESPONDENCE AND INFORMATION
University of St. Francis
500 Wilcox Street
Joliet, Illinois 60435
Phone: 815-740-5037
       800-735-7500 (toll-free)
E-mail: admissions@stfrancis.edu
Web site: http://www.stfrancis.edu

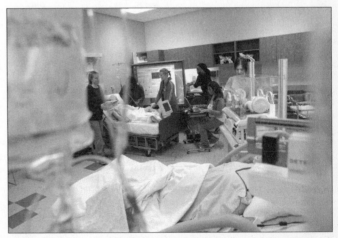

Students receive hands-on instruction with state-of-the-art technology and equipment.

University of San Diego
Hahn School of Nursing and Health Science
San Diego, California

THE UNIVERSITY

Chartered in 1949, the University of San Diego (USD) is an independent, private Catholic institution of higher education known for its commitment to teaching, research, the formation of values, and community involvement. As an independent Catholic school, USD is a nonprofit corporation governed by a Board of Trustees.

U.S. News & World Report ranks USD in the top 100 universities in the United States. The University has active chapters of Phi Beta Kappa and Mortar Board and has obtained Carnegie Research II status. USD comprises a community of scholars committed to teaching and research, both in and out of the classroom. Of the full-time faculty, 97 percent hold the Ph.D. or other terminal degree. Professors, rather than teaching assistants, teach all classes and supervise laboratories.

During the last three decades, enrollment has tripled to 7,500 students, who may choose from more than sixty undergraduate and graduate degree programs. The University's academic units include the College of Arts and Sciences and the Schools of Business Administration, Education and Leadership Science, Law, and Nursing and Health Science and the new School of Peace Studies.

USD offers higher education to individuals of all races, creeds, and cultural backgrounds and aspires to excellence in all that it undertakes. In its holistic approach to education, the University recognizes the physical, spiritual, intellectual, emotional, cultural, and social needs of its students and how those needs are dependent on each other for personal growth.

THE SCHOOL OF NURSING AND HEALTH SCIENCE

Since its inception in 1974, the Hahn School of Nursing and Health Science has provided high-quality education to more than 1,400 alumni and 150 doctorally prepared nurse scientists. The School has consistently placed in the top tier of graduate nursing programs nationally. Characterized as a private school with a public conscience, faculty members prepare nurse scientists and leaders in education and practice in a research-intensive community of progressive scholars. Prominent alumni include the first Nurse Admiral; the former Chief Nurse of the Navy Nurse Corps, who was Deputy to the Surgeon General; and the chief executive officers and research directors of numerous health agencies. Current enrollment consists of 250 registered nurse (B.S.N./M.S.N.), Master's Entry Program in Nursing, advanced practice master's, and Ph.D. students. The School seeks to deepen its commitment to social justice and health care as a human right by influencing health policy and promoting an ethical approach to nursing characterized by compassion and respect for the dignity of the individual.

In addition, the School provides volunteer international clinical, research, and cultural immersion experiences in Mexico, the Dominican Republic, Northern Ireland, and England and African and Pacific Rim countries. Students who elect to participate in these opportunities are accompanied by faculty members who are experts in international health.

PROGRAMS OF STUDY

The School of Nursing offers the Ph.D., master's, and baccalaureate degrees to registered nurses, and a Master's Entry Program in Nursing (MEPN) for those with a baccalaureate or higher degree in a field other than nursing. Programs have received full accreditation from the Commission on Collegiate Nursing Education (CCNE) and the California Board of Registered Nursing. The School specializes in personalized attention and small classes, labs, and clinical practicums that are taught by doctorally prepared and/or clinically certified faculty members. Classes in the nursing programs are offered in traditional fifteen-week semesters in spring and fall and also in concentrated intersession and summer semesters, allowing students to take courses twelve months out of the year.

The master's degree program includes advanced practice nursing programs (nurse practitioner, clinical nurse specialist, and executive nurse leader with an option for a joint M.S.N./M.B.A. degree) and the master clinical nurse program. The nurse practitioner master's and post-master's degree certificate programs offer family, adult, and pediatric nurse practitioner specialties. Gerontological, Latino health care, and mind-body integrative health-care options are available to nurse practitioner students as subspecialties.

The Ph.D. in Nursing Program. The Ph.D. program prepares beginning-level nurse scientists, nursing faculty members, and executive nurse leaders. Numerous scholarships and forgivable federal and California state loans are available to Ph.D. students. The Ph.D. program is based on the belief that nursing is a science, that nursing scholars must receive doctoral preparation to develop as scientists, and that doctoral education is best accomplished in a milieu in which faculty members and students participate in a partnership of inquiry. Successful graduates think critically, conduct research to improve the health status of health consumers, lead the profession and public to policies that promote health, serve as successful collaborators and principal investigators on interdisciplinary research teams, lead health-care agencies, and prepare the next generation of nurse scientists and faculty members. To achieve this expertise, students are educated and socialized for their roles both didactically (through course work, seminars, and tutorials), and experientially (through research assistantships, collaboration with faculty mentors, and independent research). The program of study includes a minimum of 48 units of post-master's course work and a dissertation. These 48 units comprise 9 units of core course work, 18 units of research course work, 9 units in the student's research emphasis area, and a minimum of 12 dissertation units. The School has multiple resources available to faculty members and students that support and enhance their scholarly inquiry.

The Master of Science in Nursing Program. The Master of Science in Nursing curriculum consists of two core courses and additional courses designed to prepare graduates for advanced practice or specialist nursing at the bedside. The specialty tracks range in length from 30 to 42 semester units. Graduates of the Family, Adult (including gerontological subspecialty), Pediatric, and Clinical Nurse Specialist Programs are eligible for certification by the American Nurses Credentialing Center (ANCC). In addition, Pediatric Nurse Practitioner graduates are eligible for certification by the National Certification Board of Pediatric Nurse Practitioners. Graduates of the Executive Nurse Leader Program are eligible for certification by the ANCC.

The Master's Entry Program in Nursing (MEPN) (for non-RNs). The Master's Entry Program in Nursing is designed for students with bachelor's or higher degrees in non-nursing disciplines who are seeking a new career in nursing and have completed prerequisite courses in the physical and behavioral sciences. Following successful completion of five consecutive semesters of course and clinical work, students are eligible to take the National Council Licensure Examination (NCLEX) for registered nurse licensure, and receive the master's degree as a bedside clinical nurse. Students are eligible to continue on toward the Ph.D. or one of the Advanced Practice Nursing Programs.

The Bachelor of Science in Nursing Program (post-RN). The Bachelor of Science in Nursing program is planned specifically for registered nurses. An accelerated RN to master's degree option also is available. The School provides this upper-division professional major for graduates of hospital diploma and associate degree programs who have met the specified prerequisite admission requirements. The program is designed to prepare the nurse to accept increased responsibility within the health-care system.

The Accelerated RN to Master of Science in Nursing Program. The Accelerated RN to Master of Science in Nursing program leads to both the B.S.N. and M.S.N. degrees and eligibility for certification as a public health nurse in the State of California. The student takes graduate courses in nursing research, health-care issues and policy, and health-care systems analysis as part of the B.S.N. degree requirements. The master's degree portion of the program offers the student any of the track and specialization options available in the Master of Science in Nursing program.

AFFILIATIONS WITH HEALTH-CARE FACILITIES

The School is affiliated with a wide variety of clinical resources, including UCSD Medical Center, Sharp Health Care (Hospitals and Clinics), Scripps Health (Hospitals and Clinics), Children's Hospital, Veterans Administration Hospital, Kaiser Permanente, and Balboa Naval Hospital. Because of its focus on health promotion, a large number of community agencies are utilized, including schools, home health agencies, the San Diego Department of Health Services, HMOs, and community clinics.

ACADEMIC FACILITIES

The University provides students access to state-of-the-art computer laboratories and the Helen K. and James C. Copley Library, which houses 500,000 volumes, 351,000 titles, and 2,200 print periodicals subscriptions and provides access to about 18,000 current periodicals in electronic form, including a well-serviced health sciences collection. Students and faculty members have access to the School of Law Legal Research Center as well as additional resources in area medical and health sciences libraries. The San Diego Library Circuit, a collaborative effort among San Diego State University; the University of California, San Diego; California State University, San Marcos; and the University of San Diego, allows access to an additional 2 million titles.

The Hahn School of Nursing and Health Science occupies a well-appointed, recently renovated two-story building with 18,000 square feet of space and the newly renovated and equipped 3,000-square-foot Barcelona Advanced Nursing Skills Laboratory. The main building houses administrative office suites, office space for 62 faculty and administrative personnel, a large auditorium-style classroom, two midsized classrooms, four seminar rooms, a primary computer lab, conference rooms, a library with videoconferencing capabilities, and student, faculty, and staff terraces, patios, kitchens, and lounges. Each classroom is a smart classroom, i.e., equipped with a large whiteboard, electronic screen, overhead projector, ceiling-mounted data projector, speakers, and a media cabinet containing a laptop computer, audio tuner, and VHS playback machine. All faculty members have office space equipped with networked desktop computers with SPSS and printers. Other equipment includes interactive conferencing, software (Access, Excel, PowerPoint, Word, Netscape, Office 97, SPSS, N-Query, QSD, NUD*IST, NVIVO, SPSS, ADAM, Atlas of Clinical Anatomy, 64 Diagnostic Reasoning Cases, Doctor's Dilemma, Human Physiology, Interactive Electrocardiography, Immunology, and FLIPS), Scantron with a Scanbook computer, copiers, color printers, fax machines, and a Wi-Fi system for the building.

The Barcelona Nursing Skills Laboratory contains a hospital area with six fully equipped patient units; four fully equipped exam rooms, including a pediatric examination room; a fifteen-station computer laboratory; three faculty offices; a faculty/student lounge and work area; and a laundry room. A ceiling-mounted data projector and screen also enable this laboratory to be used for computer training sessions.

LOCATION

San Diego offers a wide variety of clinical and biomedical resources and recreational, business, science, art, and cultural activities. With an average temperature of 64°F in February and 76°F in August, the area is perfect for biking, jogging, tennis, softball, and all aquatic sports. San Diego is also noted for a world-famous zoo, museums, Spanish missions, SeaWorld San Diego, and major sports programs.

USD and its beautiful 182-acre campus reflecting Spanish Renaissance architecture, which has attained landmark status, rests on a prominent hilltop in proximity to the scientific, health-care, and business resources of California's birthplace and second-largest city. The campus has commanding views of the Pacific Ocean, Mission Bay, San Diego Bay, and the surrounding mountains.

STUDENT SERVICES

The University has many resources and services designed to meet student needs. These include the Manchester Family Child Development Center (child care and development), Health Center, Sports and Recreation Center, bookstore, post office, Academic Computing Services, Campus Ministry, housing, dining services, and the Hahn University Center and its facilities, including the Multicultural Center. The International Resource Center and International Student Association offer personal and academic advising and activities.

COSTS

Tuition costs for the 2006–07 academic year were $1050 per unit for the B.S.N., $1050 per unit for the M.S.N., and $1065 per unit for the doctoral program. Since most students are registered nurses, they seldom live in campus housing. However, living expenses, including room and board, transportation, and personal expenses, are estimated at approximately $12,000. Other educational expenses, including books, immunizations, instruments, insurance, travel to clinical sites, and student fees, totaled approximately $5000.

FINANCIAL AID

Many financial resources, including merit scholarships, traineeships, federal and state forgivable loans, and other types of loans are available to help students.

APPLYING

Applicants to all nursing degree programs, except the Master's Entry Program, must have California nursing licensure as an RN and professional liability and malpractice insurance. The B.S.N., Accelerated RN to M.S.N., and MEPN programs require completion of all nursing program prerequisites prior to admission and a GPA of at least 3.0 on a 4.0 scale. The master's and post-master's programs further require a bachelor's or a master's degree in nursing respectively, from an approved, accredited institution; a minimum GPA of 3.0 on a 4.0 scale; letters of reference; and a 3-unit course in statistics. GRE scores are encouraged. Additional requirements for the Ph.D. program include a minimum GPA of 3.5 on a 4.0 scale, scores from the Graduate Record Examinations (taken in the past five years), two letters of reference from doctorally prepared faculty members, and a sample of scholarly writing. Applicants with non-nursing baccalaureate or master's degrees may be considered for admission to the M.S.N. and Ph.D. programs, respectively. All applicants must show proof of required immunizations and screening tests, including a recent physical examination. Students should contact the appropriate office at the University for complete information about admission requirements and application deadlines.

CORRESPONDENCE AND INFORMATION

Office of Undergraduate Admissions
University of San Diego
5998 Alcala Park
San Diego, California 92110-2492

Phone: 619-260-4506
Fax: 619-260-6836

Office of Graduate Admissions
University of San Diego
5998 Alcala Park
San Diego, California 92110-2492

Phone: 619-260-4524
Fax: 619-260-4158
Web site: http://www.sandiego.edu/academics/nursing

ADMINISTRATION AND FACULTY

Sally Brosz Hardin, Professor and Dean; Ph.D.; RN, FAAN.
Anita Hunter, Associate Professor and Director, MEPN, CM, and RN/B.S.N./M.S.N. Programs; Ph.D.; RN, CPNP.
Susan Instone, Associate Professor and Director, Advanced Practice Nursing Programs; D.N.Sc.; RN, CPNP.
Patricia Roth, Professor and Director, Ph.D. Program; Ed.D.; RN.
Nancy Gaffrey, Clinical Placement Coordinator; M.S.N.; RN, CNS.

Faculty
Cheryl K. Ahern-Lehmann, Clinical Associate Professor; Ph.D.; RN,C; ANP.
Susan Bonnell, Clinical Instructor; M.S.N.; RN, CPNP.
Mary Jo Clark, Professor; Ph.D.; RN.
Cynthia D. Connelly, Professor; Ph.D.; RN, FAAN.
Connie Curran, Clinical Instructor; M.S.N.; RN, CNS.
Carol Enright, Adjunct Clinical Instructor; M.S.N.; RN.
Anastasia Fisher, Associate Professor; D.N.Sc.; RN.
Michael Gates, Assistant Professor; Ph.D.; RN.
Jane Georges, Associate Professor; Ph.D.; RN.
Dale Glazer, Adjunct Assistant Professor; Ph.D.
Diane Hatton, Professor; D.N.Sc.; CS.
Kathy Shadle James, Associate Professor; D.N.Sc.; RN, CNP.
Nancy Jex Sabin, Clinical Instructor; M.S.; RN, FNP,
Sheryl E. Leary, Clinical Instructor; M.S.N.; RN.
Sharon Ann McGuire, Assistant Professor; Ph.D.; RN, CNP.
Mary-Rose Mueller, Associate Professor; Ph.D.; RN.
Patricia Quinn, Clinical Associate Professor; Ph.D.(c); ANP.
Linda A. Robinson, Associate Professor; Ph.D.; RN, CS.
Linda D. Urden, Clinical Professor; D.N.Sc.; CAN,BC; FAAN.

University of Southern Indiana
College of Nursing and Health Professions
Evansville, Indiana

THE UNIVERSITY

The University of Southern Indiana (USI), established in 1965, is a comprehensive public university offering undergraduate and graduate degrees. The University is composed of five colleges—the Colleges of Nursing and Health Professions, Science and Engineering, Business, Education and Human Services, and Liberal Arts.

The University of Southern Indiana has a strong tradition of commitment to education excellence. In 1996, the University and the School of Nursing began offering Internet-based courses and programs for students. Undergraduate programs in nursing, health services, and imaging sciences and graduate programs in nursing, health administration, and occupational therapy are available online from the College of Nursing and Health Professions.

On-campus facilities include a student fitness and health center, a bookstore, athletic facilities, a computer center, and a comprehensive library that provides online reference materials.

THE SCHOOL OF NURSING

The School of Nursing was founded in 1988 as the first state-supported baccalaureate nursing program in southern Indiana. In 1996, the School initiated a master's degree program in nursing. The School also offers a post-master's nurse practitioner certificate program as well as other programs designed to meet the needs of practicing nurses in today's health-care environment.

Recognizing the complexity of health care, the School of Nursing has developed an undergraduate and graduate nursing curriculum designed to prepare students efficiently and expertly. This curriculum emphasizes clinical nursing competence and uses a wide array of learning resources, including computerized simulation learning mannequins.

The School of Nursing has been a leader in the development of distance education courses and programs. The RN-B.S.N., RN-M.S.N., and M.S.N. nursing programs may be completed through the Internet. In addition to these nursing programs, the College of Nursing and Health Professions offers online programs in health services, health administration, and radiologic and imaging sciences. Additional information may be obtained through the College's Web site at http://health.usi.edu.

PROGRAMS OF STUDY

The baccalaureate nursing program is designed to prepare the professional nurse to plan, implement, and evaluate health care for individuals, families, and groups in institutional and community settings. The nursing program is based on a planned progression of courses arranged to build upon previous knowledge and to develop skills and performance at an increasing level of competence. The 128 credits required for the degree include the University core curriculum courses supportive to the nursing major and 69 hours of nursing courses.

The second degree B.S.N. program is designed for students who already hold a baccalaureate degree in another discipline. Once the prerequisite courses—Chemistry, Anatomy and Physiology, Microbiology, Nutrition, and Statistics—are completed, the student enrolls in nursing courses and completes the baccalaureate degree in nursing in twenty-one months.

Registered nurses with an associate degree or diploma may obtain a baccalaureate degree in nursing through the RN-B.S.N.

completion option. The nursing courses required for this option are provided online. The flexibility of the RN-B.S.N. option provides nurses with the opportunity to complete the course requirements in their own communities and on their own schedule with reasonable costs. The RN-B.S.N. curriculum is built upon a foundation of biological, physical, and social sciences and acknowledgment of previously learned nursing content. No further testing of prior knowledge is required for nurses who hold a valid RN license and are in good standing in their current employment position.

The RN-M.S.N. program is designed for registered nurses with an associate degree or diploma who are interested in graduate nursing education and preparation for an advanced practice nursing role. The program builds on a student's prior learning and requires three years of current practice experience as a registered nurse. Students, in consultation with a faculty adviser, develop a plan of study that is based on prior learning and the student's selected graduate study major. After completion of University core courses, 20–25 hours of undergraduate nursing courses, and successful completion of 12 hours of graduate course credits, a Bachelor of Science in Nursing degree is awarded. At this point in their program of study, students are granted full admission into the graduate program. After completion of the remaining required graduate nursing courses, students are awarded an M.S.N. degree.

The Master of Science in Nursing is offered for nurses seeking advanced education in professional nursing. The graduate program prepares nurses for advanced practice as acute care nurse practitioners, family nurse practitioners, nurse educators, and nurse managers/leaders. The graduate degree is awarded upon the completion of 39 to 42 credits, dependent upon the graduate nursing specialty. Post-master's certificate programs are available for clinical nurse specialist, nurse practitioner, nursing management and leadership, and nursing education.

The baccalaureate and graduate nursing programs are fully accredited by the Commission on Collegiate Nursing Education. The 25 members of the nursing faculty represent diverse areas of teaching, practice, and research. Faculty members have expertise and strong clinical practice backgrounds in their areas of teaching.

AFFILIATIONS WITH HEALTH-CARE FACILITIES

The School of Nursing is affiliated with a variety of clinical facilities, including hospitals, community agencies, physician practice groups, HMOs, schools, clinics, home health agencies, senior centers, and day-care centers that are used throughout the program of study. Written agreements are established with preceptors and health-care facilities located conveniently from a student's home community.

ACADEMIC FACILITIES

The David L. Rice Library houses about 341,000 volumes, 7,800 listening and viewing materials, and 600,000 items in microformat and subscribes to 41 electronic online databases with more than 12,000 full-text online journals. The library is fully automated for literature searches and online full-text journal searches. More than 1,100 online nursing and health-care journals are available for enrolled students.

The Computer Center has campus labs throughout the University and dedicated equipment for online learning.

Technical assistance and a variety of color graphics, database management systems, simulations, and software are available for students. The technology team is also available to assist students enrolled in distance education courses.

The Charles E. Day Learning Resource Center, located in the College of Nursing and Health Professions, includes a learning laboratory with the latest technology. The learning laboratory simulates the hospital and home settings with appropriate supplies and computerized patient models.

LOCATION
Evansville, Indiana, with a population of approximately 135,000, is home to the University of Southern Indiana. Evansville is big enough to provide metropolitan amenities but small enough to have small-town charm and hospitality. Located at a horseshoe bend on the Ohio River, Evansville has a long and colorful history. The campus is conveniently located 7 miles from downtown Evansville.

STUDENT LIFE
A wide variety of organizations and activities contribute to the total education of the on-campus student. More than eighty student organizations provide activities that include student government, leadership academy, career organizations, multicultural center, athletics, student publications, and a student-operated radio station.

The USI Association of Nursing Students and the Omicron Psi chapter of Sigma Theta Tau International Nursing Honor Society provide students with the opportunity to develop leadership skills; to participate in local, regional, and national nursing forums; and to work collaboratively with nursing school faculty members.

THE NURSING STUDENT GROUP
In fall 2006, the School of Nursing enrolled more than 400 undergraduate and 200 graduate nursing students. The diversity of the nursing student population is representative of the general population of the geographic regional area.

COSTS
In 2006–07, undergraduate tuition for in-state students was $145 per credit hour or $2300 per semester for full-time study (15 hours). For graduate students, in-state tuition was $215 per credit or $2000 per semester for full-time study (9 hours). University fees ranged from $150 to $300 per semester. Other fees and housing costs are determined on an individual basis.

FINANCIAL AID
USI offers a wide variety of financial assistance programs through various federal and state programs. Additional scholarships are offered through contributions made to the School by alumni and patrons. The amounts and types of financial assistance that a student receives include full tuition and living expenses as well as other scholarships that are determined by the eligibility of the applicant for the respective nursing program.

APPLYING
Applicants for the B.S.N. program must first be admitted to the University. A second application is then submitted to the nursing program.

Admission to the undergraduate nursing program may occur prior to matriculation to the University for high school students with outstanding high school achievement and high SAT/ACT scores. The larger proportion of students are evaluated and admitted after the fall semester of their second year or when required credit hours are completed.

Criteria for admission to the nursing program (guaranteed admission) for high school students prior to the fall semester of their second year includes admission to the University; completion of the nursing application; a minimum high school GPA of 3.5 on a 4.0 scale and a combined SAT score of at least 1800 or equivalent ACT score. To maintain this guaranteed admission status and begin nursing courses in their second year, students must maintaining a college GPA of at least 3.0 on a 4.0 scale during the first 30 credit hours with a grade of C or better in all science courses, Nutrition 376, English 101, English 201, CMST (Communications) 101/107, Psychology 201, and Sociology 121.

Admission to the program for all other students is competitive and based upon the following criteria: admission to the University; completion of the nursing application; college GPA; a grade of C or better in all science courses, Nutrition 376, English 101, English 201, CMST 101/107, Psychology 201, and Sociology 121; and a combined SAT score of at least 1500 or equivalent ACT score.

All students selected for admission to the nursing program must also meet clinical agency requirements, present evidence of satisfactory health status, be eligible for RN licensure, be capable of fulfilling clinical practice requirements, and submit a satisfactory drug screen and criminal record check.

RN-B.S.N. applicants must hold a current unencumbered registered nurse license in one of the fifty states or territories, meet general University requirements for admission, and have graduated from an accredited nursing program with a minimum GPA of 2.7. RN-M.S.N. applicants must have three years experience as a registered nurse, hold a current, unencumbered RN license, and must have a minimum GPA of 3.0.

Applicants to the master's and post-master's degree programs are required to have a current license as a registered nurse in one of the fifty states or territories, hold an earned B.S. or M.S. degree in nursing from an accredited school, have a minimum GPA of 3.0, have practiced as an RN for 2,000 hours within the last five years, and provide letters of reference.

Admission and enrollment information is available online at the College's Web site (http://health.usi.edu).

CORRESPONDENCE AND INFORMATION
Admissions and Advising Coordinator
College of Nursing and Health Professions
University of Southern Indiana
8600 University Boulevard
Evansville, Indiana 47712

Phone: 812-465-1150
E-mail: cnhpadmissions@usi.edu
Web site: http://health.usi.edu

The University of Tampa
Department of Nursing
Tampa, Florida

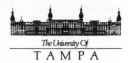

THE UNIVERSITY

The University of Tampa (UT), founded in 1931, is a medium-sized, residential, private university that integrates the richness of the liberal arts tradition with twenty-first-century technology and innovative teaching strategies. The College of Liberal Arts and Sciences and the College of Business offer more than 100 fields of study and preprofessional programs. Graduate programs in business, teaching, and nursing and an Evening College complement the curriculum.

The 209 full-time faculty members include distinguished scholars, authors, artists, and educators who promote student- and community-responsive learning opportunities. The 5,125 currently enrolled students experience classes in small, personalized settings that balance "learning by thinking" with "learning by doing."

In an innovative first-year program, students explore global issues and cultures, examine career possibilities, and refine their critical-thinking and communication skills. Students, representing fifty states and territories and nearly 100 countries, find their academic experience at UT to be an enriching one that encourages a global perspective, provides opportunities to apply their skills and knowledge throughout the curriculum, and prepares them for future career challenges. For qualifying students, the Honors Program offers expanded opportunities for instruction, internships, and study abroad.

Eighty percent of UT's nine residence halls are new since 1998, and 70 percent of all full-time students live on campus. The Vaughn Center and residence hall complex serves as the hub of campus life.

UT has one of the best NCAA Division II sports programs. Spartan athletes compete on fourteen men's and women's varsity teams. The swimming pool, tennis courts, jogging track, outdoor volleyball and basketball courts, crew training facility, and modern fitness center are enjoyed by all, making sunshine, sports, and fitness hallmarks of the UT experience.

The University of Tampa is accredited by the Southern Association of Colleges and Schools to award associate, baccalaureate, and master's degrees. In addition, the University is accredited for teacher education by the Florida State Board of Education. The Florida State Approving Agency for Veterans' Training recognizes the University with approval for veterans' educational benefits. The University is an associate member of the European Council of International Schools (ECIS), a European accrediting association. All nursing programs are accredited by the National League for Nursing Accrediting Commission (NLNAC), and the University is a member of the American Association of Colleges of Nursing and the National Organization of Nurse Practitioner Faculties.

THE DEPARTMENT OF NURSING

The Department of Nursing admitted its first class in 1981 and graduated its charter class in 1984. The B.S.N. completion program gained accreditation from the National League for Nursing Accrediting Commission (NLNAC) in 1986. The Master of Science in Nursing (M.S.N.) degree program was awarded NLNAC accreditation in 1998. Master's degree options include family and adult nurse practitioner studies and nursing education. Post-master's certificates may be earned in each of these concentrations.

PROGRAMS OF STUDY

In 2002, UT began a traditional four-year Bachelor of Science in Nursing (B.S.N.) program (accredited by the NLNAC in 2003), helping to round out a slate of offerings that already included RN to B.S.N. completion and RN/B.S.N./M.S.N. tracks. The RN to B.S.N. program allows RN graduates of diploma and associate degree programs to complete the B.S.N. degree, and it provides a foundation for graduate education. RNs with associate degrees who seek a Master of Science in Nursing (M.S.N.) degree enroll in the RN to B.S.N./M.S.N. option, enabling the qualified RN to complete both the B.S.N. and M.S.N. degrees more rapidly than in traditional programs. Certain undergraduate courses are then replaced by graduate-level courses. Students formally apply to the M.S.N. program and complete the GRE during the progression of the B.S.N. program. In this option, when required undergraduate courses are completed, students are awarded the B.S.N.

The master's degree program offers family nurse practitioner and adult nurse practitioner concentrations. UT's graduate nursing education concentration responds to the critical shortage of nurse educators throughout the nation. It is the only nursing education program in west central Florida.

Many nurses seeking graduate degrees choose one of the nurse practitioner concentrations because of the opportunity to impact patient care decisions and health-care policy with greater autonomy. UT's nursing education concentration is poised to add significantly to the number of nurse educators who will have positive effects on the nursing shortage.

All of these programs recognize that nursing is a very different career than it was prior to the explosion of new information, new technology, new pharmacology, and the demands of a burgeoning health-care consumer population. Along with judgment and critical thinking, UT's nursing programs prepare graduates who are superbly educated, empowered, ethical, and politically articulate. Nurses are educated to have authority—not only when they occupy high-level positions, but at the bedside.

AFFILIATIONS WITH HEALTH-CARE FACILITIES

In keeping with the University's commitment to hands-on, real-world learning, UT's nursing programs enjoy affiliations with more than 120 Tampa Bay–area clinical facilities. There are twenty-five hospitals and nearly 1,000 doctor's offices in Hillsborough County alone. Tampa General Hospital, an 877-bed acute-care facility and level one trauma center, has established a partnership with UT's four-year B.S.N. program. State-of-the-art clinical laboratories utilizing computer-generated simulations as well as simulated human models are available for UT nursing students at Tampa General Hospital and on campus. These laboratories provide students with opportunities to learn and practice their nursing skills with the latest technology available.

The Tampa Bay area is rich in clinical experience opportunities. Specialty facilities and expert health-care professionals enrich the education of UT nursing students through their willingness to precept, mentor, and teach in the University's programs. Myriad opportunities for challenging positions in all aspects of health await those graduates who choose to remain in Florida following graduation.

ACADEMIC FACILITIES

For nursing and all students, the Macdonald-Kelce Library is well-equipped to meet the diversified needs of college students. It has more than 250,000 bound volumes and some 1,600 periodicals. In addition, the library is a member of the Tampa Bay Library Consortium, which provides delivery of books and research materials from a variety of member libraries. UTOPIA, an electronic online catalog, allows patrons to search other libraries and databases, check the status of their accounts, and even read government documents. Students can access UTOPIA from home, residence hall, office, or anywhere an online computer can be found.

Many of UT's classrooms are tech supported, but the Computer Resources Center is the technological center of the University. It offers hands-on experience in a laboratory environment, combining practical application with theoretical instruction. The entire campus is linked by a high-speed campus computer network and many areas are wireless. All members of the UT community have free Internet access and e-mail. All students in every residence hall have their own computer jacks, and they may use one of the many computer labs located in convenient areas on campus.

LOCATION

Surrounding the UT campus is Tampa, a vibrant, ethnically and culturally diverse, modern city located on the west central coast of Florida. Once a sleepy southern town, Tampa's boom began in the 1950s and continues unabated in the 2000s. An imposing skyline continues to burst into bloom over a cityscape that was almost entirely flat just two decades ago. Tampa is just an hour west of Orlando's Disney attractions and 30 minutes from beautiful gulf beaches.

More than a million residents now inhabit the city and surrounding Hillsborough County, with more than 2 million in the four-county Tampa–St. Petersburg–Clearwater metroplex (commonly referred to simply as "Tampa Bay") and 4 million in the eleven-county region. Tampa is the educational, medical, cultural, economic, business, shipping, entertainment, and legal center of it all, and the community is involved with its premier private university. More than 700 Tampa Bay community leaders serve on University boards and advisory groups.

STUDENT SERVICES

Leadership opportunities abound in an atmosphere of individual discovery and development fostered by the University's active campus life, including Greek life, more than 120 student clubs and organizations, and service learning opportunities. A cocurricular transcript option gives UT graduates a resume-enhancing edge with prospective employers and graduate schools. Professionals in the Academic Center for Excellence (ACE), the Saunders Writing Center, and the Academic Advising and Career Services offices help students stay on track academically.

THE NURSING STUDENT GROUP

There are 383 students currently enrolled in UT nursing programs: 44 in the B.S.N. completion program, 90 in the M.S.N. and postgraduate certificate programs, and 249 in the Department's four-year B.S.N program. The B.S.N. completion and graduate programs are designed for adult learners who attend part-time. The majority are already working in various health-care settings in the Tampa Bay community. Applying from many parts of the country, most four-year students are residential and attend full-time during the day. Because of the critical shortage of nurses to serve a growing population of acutely ill and elderly patients, many graduates select employment in Florida, where they receive excellent salaries and benefits.

COSTS

Undergraduate tuition and fee costs for the 2006–07 academic year were $19,628 for full-time study. Room and board charges averaged $7252 for a double room for the academic year. RN to B.S.N. tuition was $398 per credit hour. Graduate tuition (for graduate-level courses only) was $426 per credit hour. Additional fees for books, supplies, lab fees, etc., also apply, and vary by semester.

FINANCIAL AID

Special Florida and federal financial aid incentives are in place to encourage students to pursue nursing degrees. UT awards institutional financial aid based on merit and need to full-time undergraduate students. Some graduate assistantships and federal traineeships are awarded to M.S.N. students each year. Students are encouraged to explore outside funding sources such as employers and health-related agencies. All students pursuing at least half-time study are eligible for loans. Information on financial assistance is available online at http://www.ut.edu or by calling the Financial Aid Office at 813-253-6219.

APPLYING

University admission application forms are available on the University's Web site for downloading or completion online. Applications for admission to the RN to B.S.N. and M.S.N. programs are evaluated on a rolling basis, and students may enter in the fall, spring, or summer terms.

Undergraduate students apply to the four-year baccalaureate nursing program by first applying to the University, completing the regular UT undergraduate admissions application. Official transcripts from all schools attended, SAT or ACT scores, an essay, and a recommendation from a guidance counselor or teacher are required. Acceptance to the University does not constitute admission to the nursing program. Separate application is made to the nursing program once pre-nursing requirements have been met. Meeting minimal requirements does not guarantee admission to this high-demand, limited-enrollment program. Four-year B.S.N. students are admitted to the nursing program each fall for the spring term only.

Admission to the RN to B.S.N. program requires the applicant to be currently licensed in Florida as a registered nurse. Applicants who provide proof of eligibility for licensure may attend the first semester, but they must have obtained a Florida RN license by the end of that semester to continue in the program. Applicants to this program must submit the regular undergraduate admission application and provide official transcripts from each college attended. Admission to the M.S.N. program requires a graduate M.S.N. application, current Florida licensure as an RN, a GPA of 3.0 or higher in the last 60 credit hours of college/university courses, a computer course, a statistics course, and successful completion of the GRE. Two professional letters of reference and a resume are also required. Applicants with a Florida license and a baccalaureate degree in a discipline other than nursing may enroll in the pre-M.S.N. program to complete additional course work prior to full admission to the M.S.N. degree program.

CORRESPONDENCE AND INFORMATION:

Admissions Office
University of Tampa
401 West Kennedy Boulevard
Tampa, Florida 33606

Phone: 813-253-6273
Fax: 813-258-7398
E-mail: nursing@ut.edu
Web site: http://www.ut.edu

University of Wisconsin–Madison
School of Nursing
Madison, Wisconsin

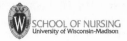
SCHOOL OF NURSING
University of Wisconsin-Madison

THE UNIVERSITY
In achievement and prestige, the University of Wisconsin–Madison (UW–Madison) has long been recognized as one of America's great universities. Founded in 1849, it is today one of the nation's largest public land-grant institutions, with an international reputation as a leading teaching and research university. As stated in the *Vision for the Future,* the University's mission is "to create, integrate, transfer and apply knowledge." The University offers a complete spectrum of liberal arts studies, professional programs, and student activities. With more than 40,000 students, the student body is diverse and cosmopolitan.

THE SCHOOL OF NURSING
The School of Nursing has had a strong commitment to enhancing health care since its beginning in 1924. Consistently ranked among top nursing schools for graduate education and research, the School is an integral part of the UW–Madison health sciences complex. Members of the faculty are academically well prepared and recognized as scholars, researchers, expert clinicians and teachers, and leaders in the profession.

The School offers a Bachelor of Science degree in nursing, a Master of Science degree and a Doctor of Philosophy degree with a major in nursing, and opportunities for postdoctoral research. In fall 2005, the School enrolled 307 students in the baccalaureate nursing major, 55 returning RN students, 143 students in the M.S. program, 12 students in post-master's nurse practitioner options, and 31 students in the Ph.D. and postdoctoral programs.

PROGRAMS OF STUDY
The Bachelor of Science program prepares individuals for entry-level professional practice and provides a basis for leadership roles and graduate study. The 124-credit curriculum comprises course work in general education, nursing practice, and electives. Students are admitted to the nursing major in the junior year. An Honors Program is offered, providing opportunities for high-ability students who seek greater depth and challenge in their educational experience. Students have the opportunity to complete the nursing component of the program either at the UW–Madison campus or the Western Campus for Nursing located at Gundersen Lutheran Medical Center in LaCrosse, Wisconsin. An Early Entry Ph.D. option is designed for undergraduate students who are interested in research careers in nursing.

The BSN@Home Program, of which the UW–Madison School of Nursing is a partner, is offered for registered nurse students seeking a baccalaureate degree. The program is offered to Wisconsin residents via the Internet and the combined resources of five University of Wisconsin System nursing schools.

An RN/B.S./M.S. accelerated track is offered for registered nurses who are highly motivated, who have a high level of academic achievement, and whose educational goal is a master's or a doctoral education. The faculty recognizes that RN students have acquired considerable knowledge and clinical competency through previous education and professional employment and is committed to assisting them in meeting their career goals.

The purpose of the Master of Science degree program is to prepare nurses for leadership roles in advanced clinical practice and education or to provide a basis for further research preparation. A minimum of 36 graduate credits is required, although many of the program options require additional credits in order to meet national credentialing requirements. The master's curriculum is reflective of faculty expertise and scholarship, as well as the standards and guidelines of the profession, and is designed to maintain a high standard of scholarship and prepare individuals with in-depth knowledge and experience in their selected areas of practice. Students select both a clinical and a functional role focus. Clinical population options are adult health and illness, geriatric, medical-surgical, pediatric, psychiatric–mental health, and women's health nursing. The nurse practitioner options include acute care, adult, geriatric, pediatric, psychiatric mental health, and women's health. New program initiatives include the NET option (an online sequence that prepares nurse educators for tomorrow) and a dual-degree M.S./M.P.H. program. Program graduates are eligible for national certification and reimbursable professional practice. In Wisconsin, graduates can apply to become Advanced Practice Nurse Prescribers. Students and alumni consistently evaluate the master's program as strong, and graduates have been highly successful in attaining professional certification and finding positions.

Established in 1984, the Ph.D. program in nursing is characterized by an early and continuous training in research, a strong scientific base in nursing, and a minor in a related discipline. The purpose of the program is to prepare nurses to assume major roles in the development, evaluation, and dissemination of knowledge about phenomena of interest in nursing. Graduates become the scholars and teachers who move the nursing profession forward through systematic inquiry into nursing issues. The curriculum leading to the doctorate includes seven components: existing and evolving knowledge in nursing, methods of nursing inquiry, research ethics, nursing doctoral seminars, course work in a minor field, teaching and learning, and research/dissertation credits. Graduates of the program have assumed faculty positions at major universities in the United States, Canada, and many other countries and have been awarded postdoctoral fellowships to further their research. Doctoral and postdoctoral funding is available as part of an NINR-funded training program in patient-centered interventions. The Bolliger Post Doctoral Fellowship provides funding for nurse researchers to work on their individual research under the direction of a senior faculty member in the School of Nursing.

AFFILIATIONS WITH HEALTH-CARE FACILITIES
Faculty and staff members maintain affiliations with many health, education, and social service agencies throughout urban and rural Wisconsin, including the Wisconsin Department of Health and Family Services and many public health departments, schools, and hospitals. The School is especially committed to performing research and providing student clinical experiences in health professional shortage areas, as exemplified by participation in the Area Health Education Centers (AHEC) of Wisconsin.

ACADEMIC FACILITIES
The Health Sciences Learning Center provides the Schools of Medicine, Nursing, and Pharmacy with state-of-the-art classrooms, computer resources, and distance education facilities as well as a comprehensive health sciences library. Educational

resources for both on-campus and distance students include online access to library journals, Web-based course materials, and videoconferencing technologies. Collaborative arrangements with a number of campus departments expand the practice, education, and research experiences open to students.

LOCATION

Madison, situated on an isthmus between Lakes Mendota and Monona, is a midsize city with a population of about 225,000, known for its natural beauty. With its good economy, low crime rate, and abundance of cultural and recreational activities, Madison ranks consistently among the top cities in the country. Its central location, 90 miles from Milwaukee, 120 miles from Chicago, and 250 miles from Minneapolis, places it within easy driving distance of these major metropolitan areas.

STUDENT SERVICES

Advisers are available in the B.S. program to help students interpret curriculum and academic requirements and plan a balanced program. They also assist with academic problems and acquaint students with campus resources. At the graduate level, students may select, or are assigned, a faculty adviser with whom they plan their program of study. A writing course is taught in the School for graduate students. Career services are also available for students. The campus offers a wide variety of other support services for students, including the International Student Services Office, the McBurney Disability Resource Center, the Multicultural Student Center, and many others.

THE NURSING STUDENT GROUP

The student body comprises students from throughout the U.S. and abroad. The School is committed to recruitment, admission, retention, and graduation of students who are members of minority groups. The student view is welcomed and important. Students serve as voting members on School of Nursing committees.

COSTS

For 2006–07, full-time tuition and fees for resident undergraduate students were $6730; they were $20,730 for nonresidents. Full-time tuition and fees for resident graduate students were $9184; they were $24,454 for nonresidents.

FINANCIAL AID

The campus Office of Student Financial Services awards financial aid based on need. Financial aid packages consist of loans, grants, and work-study assistance. The School of Nursing administers a number of scholarships to qualified nursing students. Scholarships in varying amounts are awarded annually, and some are renewable as long as the recipient is in good academic standing. Several forms of financial aid are available for graduate students. These include traineeships, fellowships, scholarships, research and teaching assistantships, and loans. Advanced Opportunity Fellowships are available for qualified minority or economically disadvantaged students. The School is committed to funding full-time students in the Ph.D. program.

APPLYING

Admission to the nursing major is available in the fall semester only. The deadline for applying is February 1. Individuals may be considered for admission as prenursing students in the fall, spring, and summer sessions, provided they are entering as beginning freshmen or transfer students with more than 24 college credits. The deadline for freshmen and prenursing transfer students is February 1 for summer and fall and October 1 for spring. Admission to the prenursing classification is no guarantee of admission to the nursing major.

Graduate application deadlines depend on the program of interest. Master's and post-master's applications are due March 1 for fall enrollment and October 1 for spring semester enrollment. For the Ph.D. program, applications are due January 15 for fall enrollment and September 15 for spring enrollment.

Prospective students are encouraged to visit the School of Nursing's Web site (http://www.son.wisc.edu) for more detailed information about admission requirements.

CORRESPONDENCE AND INFORMATION

School of Nursing
University of Wisconsin–Madison
600 Highland Avenue
Madison, Wisconsin 53792-2455
Fax: 608-263-5296
Web site: http://www.son.wisc.edu

Undergraduate Admissions, Office K6/146
Phone: 608-263-5202
E-mail: ugadmin@wisc.edu

Graduate Admissions, Office K6/145B
Phone: 608-263-5180
E-mail: gradadmit@son.wisc.edu
Web site: http://www.son.wisc.edu

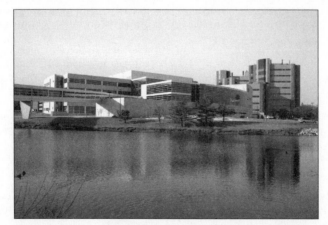

The Health Sciences Learning Center on the UW–Madison campus.

University of Wisconsin–Milwaukee
College of Nursing
Milwaukee, Wisconsin

THE UNIVERSITY
The University of Wisconsin–Milwaukee (UWM) was established in 1956 with the merger of the University of Wisconsin Extension Center in Milwaukee and Wisconsin State College. Since then, UWM has flourished into a major part of the intellectual, cultural, and economic life of southeastern Wisconsin. Ranked by the Carnegie Foundation as a research institution, UWM supports a dynamic academic community of more than 28,000 students, 1,350 faculty and instructional staff members, and 1,900 staff members. As Wisconsin's premier urban research university, UWM offers more than 120 undergraduate majors and sub-majors, forty-eight master's programs, and twenty doctoral programs in thirteen schools and colleges. A recent renaissance exemplified by the Milwaukee Idea, UWM's embodiment of community-university engagement, has resulted in a high level of excitement and productivity campuswide.

THE COLLEGE OF NURSING
Since its inception in 1965, the College of Nursing has been dedicated to providing academic programs of the highest quality that are at the forefront of nursing. The programs are nationally ranked, and the faculty is widely recognized for achievements and innovations.

Reflective of its commitment to the urban community, the College operates the Institute for Urban Health Partnerships, which oversees four Community Nursing Centers that offer the unique ability to integrate the multiple missions of an urban university through outstanding opportunities for student learning, faculty practice, research, and community service.

Bachelor of Science in Nursing and Master of Science and Doctor of Philosophy degrees in nursing are available through programs that provide a solid academic foundation for nursing in a variety of settings. In addition to the pursuit of knowledge, the UWM College of Nursing creates an environment that values and supports personal growth. In fall 2006, the College enrolled 1,373 students in the baccalaureate nursing major, 87 returning RN students, 156 students in master's programs, and 91 students in the doctoral program.

PROGRAMS OF STUDY
The 124-credit baccalaureate curriculum is based on an integrated, nursing-centered model intended to provide optimum preparation for practice as a professional nurse. This curriculum is also offered through consortial programs at the UW–Parkside and UW–Washington County campuses. The program includes course work relevant to professional practice, delivery of nursing care, systems for care delivery, and leadership skill development appropriate to current dynamic and diverse health-care settings.

The College also participates in a unique cooperative arrangement to bring nursing education to students in remote areas, using the latest in distance education technology. This Collaborative Nursing Program (CNP), a cooperative effort of five UW System Colleges of Nursing, enables registered nurse students to complete a baccalaureate degree.

Study in the master's program prepares students to participate in planning and implementing advanced practice nursing to meet the special needs of clients, particularly in urban communities. Within this program, the student may elect a family nurse practitioner option or a clinical nurse specialist option specializing in community health, adult health, maternal-child health, psychiatric–mental health, or systems management. Both options require 46 credits, providing eligibility for graduates to sit for a variety of certification exams.

In addition to these traditional programs, two distinctive options are also in place. A Post-Master's Family Nurse Practitioner Certificate option is available for registered nurses who have completed a master's degree in nursing but who desire preparation as family nurse practitioners. This option requires 21 credits. The second option is a Post–Nurse Practitioner option for baccalaureate-prepared certified nurse practitioners seeking a master's degree. This program requires 25 credits and can be completed in three consecutive semesters of weekend course work and distance learning.

An alternative path to advanced practice nursing is available to students holding a bachelor's degree in another field. Students in the Direct Entry Master's (DEM) Program complete a one-year full-time prelicensure curriculum prior to beginning the advanced practice nursing master's program. Attainment of a Registered Nurse license is required prior to beginning the advanced practice nursing practicum courses. The program is designed to be completed full-time in 2½ years.

Also offered at the graduate level is the Health Professional Educational Certificate, designed to provide health professionals, such as nurses, respiratory therapists, and occupational therapists, with additional preparation in educational principles and theory to support them in their roles as educators of students, staff members, and clients.

The College of Nursing, in collaboration with the UWM School of Business Administration, also offers an M.S. in nursing/M.B.A. degree program. Graduates of this dual program are prepared to assume leadership roles in nursing administration, health-care administration, and management.

Established in 1984, the Ph.D. curriculum includes a required research core that facilitates the development of skills to analyze and generate knowledge in the field of nursing. The historical evolution of nursing science is studied in regard to its philosophical and empirical antecedents, and current nursing science is studied through explorations of the interrelationships among the theory, research, and practice of nursing. Preparation for a role as nurse scientist, responding to and shaping public policy for the health and social needs of the public, also is addressed. Specialty courses enable students to focus on a specific nursing phenomenon and develop a sound theoretical and research base of expertise in this area of interest. Students may elect to pursue their programs of study in a traditional (on-site) format or through online study (Web-based instruction).

A B.S. to Ph.D. option is also offered to nurses who want to pursue research and scholarship goals consistent with doctoral-level education. This track does not include the clinical advanced practice preparation provided through the master's program.

ACADEMIC FACILITIES
The College maintains state-of-the-art resources to support a rich academic environment. The Nursing Learning Resource Center, serving students, faculty members, and the community, is an integral component of both the undergraduate and graduate curriculums. This college laboratory is a mediated and

simulated learning environment in which students perform skills foundational to safe nursing practice. Used as a resource in the development and evaluation of media, the center also houses a modern, well-equipped computer laboratory.

In the Harriet H. Werley Center for Nursing Research and Evaluation, staff members work to develop the research potential of faculty members, students, and the greater nursing community. Personnel offer consultation in design, methodology, data analysis, computer programming, grant proposal writing, and writing for publication.

The Center for Cultural Diversity and Health houses a collection of comprehensive health behavior information for culturally diverse groups in the Milwaukee community. The center provides students, faculty members, and health professionals stimulating learning opportunities in health care for culturally diverse groups through continuing education seminars, clinical practice models, and research, to meet the health needs of culturally diverse groups.

The College's Center for Nursing History includes the Inez G. Hinsvark Historical Gallery, a unique learning resource located on the ground floor of Frances Cunningham Hall. The significant role of nurses in history is brought to life by artifacts, mementos, and photographs as well as borrowed collections.

LOCATION
UWM's 93-acre campus is located on Milwaukee's Upper East Side, one of the city's most attractive residential areas, and is a short walk from historic Lake Park and the beautiful Lake Michigan shoreline. Milwaukee possesses a wealth of cultural and recreational resources. These include the Milwaukee Art Museum, Milwaukee Public Museum, Milwaukee County Zoo, Summerfest, theaters, concert halls, restaurants, parks, professional sports events, and ethnic festivals.

STUDENT SERVICES
Advisers are available to undergraduate students to assist in interpreting curriculum and academic requirements and planning a balanced course of study. A separate adviser is assigned to continuing RN students as well as to the UW-Parkside consortial students. Students may make appointments with their advisers or simply drop in, as time allows, or utilize telephone or e-mail communications. Regular group advising sessions are also offered. Tutorial support in the basic sciences and study groups are among the services offered through the College's Academic Enrichment Center, in addition to the academic support services available to all students on the greater UWM campus.

Graduate students, in addition to their general student services adviser, also may select or are assigned a faculty member with whom they collaborate closely to establish and complete their advanced course of study.

THE NURSING STUDENT GROUP
The student body is a diverse group of individuals pursuing their academic goals in both traditional and nontraditional ways. Students come to UWM from throughout the country and the world, as well as the state of Wisconsin. The College of Nursing maintains a close relationship with two sister schools in South Korea, with exchanges of students and faculty members occurring often.

Graduates of the various programs have found exciting and rewarding positions as nursing professionals, advanced practitioners, researchers, and educators throughout the Metro-Milwaukee area, the Midwest, and beyond.

COSTS
For 2006–07, full-time tuition and fees for resident undergraduate students were $6630, and they were $16,232 for nonresi-

dents. There was a $30-per-credit tuition differential fee applicable to undergraduate nursing students. Full-time tuition and fees for resident graduate students were $8926, and they were $23,292 for nonresidents.

FINANCIAL AID
The campus Financial Aid Office awards financial aid based on need. Financial aid packages consist of loans, grants, and work-study assistance. The College of Nursing administers a number of scholarships to qualified students. Scholarships in varying amounts are awarded annually. Financial aid available to graduate students includes traineeships, fellowships, scholarships, research and teaching assistantships, and loans.

APPLYING
Students who seek to enter the nursing major in September must submit applications by the preceding January 15; for January entrance, the deadline is the preceding July 15. Students who have completed 15 credits or required courses with a cumulative GPA of 3.5 or higher may be eligible for earlier admission. Individuals may be considered for admission as prenursing students in the fall and spring as beginning freshmen or transfer students. Admission to the prenursing classification is no guarantee of admission to the nursing professional program.

Graduate application deadlines depend on the program of interest. Master's applications are due to the UWM Graduate School by January 1 and to the College of Nursing by February 1 for fall enrollment and to the UWM Graduate School by September 1 and to the College of Nursing by October 1 for spring semester enrollment. For the Ph.D. program, applications are due to the UWM Graduate School and to the College of Nursing by February 1 for fall enrollment. Applications received after these dates are reviewed on a rolling basis.

Prospective students are encouraged to visit the College of Nursing Web site for more detailed information about admission requirements.

CORRESPONDENCE AND INFORMATION
College of Nursing
University of Wisconsin–Milwaukee
1921 East Hartford Avenue
P.O. Box 413
Milwaukee, Wisconsin 53211-3060
Fax: 414-229-6474
E-mail: www.asknursing@uwm.edu
Web site: http://www.nursing.uwm.edu

Donna Wier, Senior Advisor
Undergraduate Admissions
Student Affairs Office
Room 129-Cunningham Hall
Phone: 414-229-5481
E-mail: ddw@uwm.edu

Jacqueline Davit, RN Advisor
RN Completion Program Admissions
Student Affairs Office
Room 129, Cunningham Hall
Phone: 414-229-4662
E-mail: jdavit@uwm.edu

Carrie Von Bohlen, Academic Advisor
Graduate Admissions
Student Affairs Office
Room 129, Cunningham Hall
Phone: 414-229-5474
E-mail: cvb@uwm.edu

Ursuline College
The Breen School of Nursing
Pepper Pike, Ohio

THE COLLEGE
Ursuline College is a Catholic liberal arts college offering baccalaureate and graduate programs. Founded as a women's college in 1871, Ursuline's students remain predominantly women. The College is committed to helping both women and men achieve their goals.

Ursuline's nationally recognized core curriculum encourages students to explore their identities and life goals. Ursuline takes a holistic approach to learning, encouraging students to rely on their studies not only as a means for launching a successful career but also for enjoying a happy and meaningful life. This integrated approach is truly reflective of a new generation of students who, along with the faculty, serve as catalysts for the dynamic learning environment at Ursuline. That culture and small classes provide more than 1,400 students with individual attention and special care.

THE SCHOOL OF NURSING
Nursing has been a vital program at Ursuline College since 1975. Today, The Breen School of Nursing has the largest academic program on campus. The School offers B.S.N. and M.S.N. degree programs and post-master's certificates. B.S.N. graduates score exceptionally well on the NCLEX exam, with a 100 percent pass rate two out of the last three years. At the M.S.N. level, the palliative care program is the first of its kind in the country; the case management program is one of the few in the area.

The Breen School of Nursing offers its professional programs within Ursuline's values-based learning environment. An individualized approach enables students to enjoy personal instruction, learn material in greater depth, and gain experience in a wide variety of health-care environments. The Breen School's graduates are sought by employers, who find them to be well prepared and flexible in adapting to new settings. The School has more than 2,000 graduates, many of whom hold leadership positions. In addition to a highly qualified full-time faculty, the M.S.N. program has visiting professors who are nationally recognized leaders in nursing.

PROGRAMS OF STUDY
The Breen School offers programs that prepare nurses for the health-care marketplace of the future, at both the basic (B.S.N.) and advanced practice (M.S.N.) levels.

The B.S.N. program provides a broad foundation by combining Ursuline's liberal studies core with an intensive three-year sequence in the nursing major. Qualified students are admitted directly into nursing. The B.S.N. program (129 credits, 58 of which are in nursing) can be completed in four years. Unique classroom and clinical assignments enable students to develop critical-thinking, communication, technical, and leadership skills. Students complete clinical rotations in renowned health-care institutions in the greater Cleveland area. The School's holistic and values-based nursing program provides a framework for students to learn about the caring and ethical side of health care, pass the NCLEX licensing exam, and adapt to practice in the twenty-first century. There are accelerated tracks for RNs, LPNs, and for those who have earned a bachelor's degree in another discipline. Students may combine traditional, accelerated, and Web courses.

The M.S.N. program prepares advanced practice nurses as clinical nurse specialists (CNS) and nurse practitioners (NP).

The emphasis at the graduate level is on refining analytical skills, developing a clearer ability to connect theory to practice, and enhancing professional skills. All programs have a strong clinical component where caring, communication, and critical thinking are emphasized. There are four tracks: care management, palliative care, adult nurse practitioner, and family nurse practitioner. The number of credit hours required for the M.S.N. degree is 39, with the exception of the family nurse practitioner track, which requires 42 credit hours. Courses are offered in the evenings and on Saturdays in an accelerated model. Students may choose to complete the clinical practicum in the greater Cleveland area or at an alternate location. The palliative care post-M.S.N. track is available via distance learning, and adult/family nurse practitioner post-M.S.N. programs are available on campus. All M.S.N. graduates are eligible to take advanced practice certification exams.

The care management track is a cutting-edge program that prepares students as leaders in outcomes-based practice, quality improvement, and fiscally sound resource management. Students develop a subspecialty area of expertise throughout the program. The palliative care track focuses on care when a cure is no longer possible. Emphasis is on comprehensive care of the mind, body, and spirit through collaborative practice with other health-care providers. The adult nurse practitioner track focuses on health promotion and disease prevention of adults with acute and chronic diseases. The family nurse practitioner track focuses on primary health care across the life cycle with an emphasis on health maintenance, disease prevention, counseling, and education.

AFFILIATIONS WITH HEALTH-CARE FACILITIES
The Breen School of Nursing is affiliated with numerous internationally renowned and community-based health-care agencies throughout the greater Cleveland area. M.S.N. students may elect to do their practicum in another state or country.

ACADEMIC FACILITIES
Ursuline's library, well-known to health professionals in the area, houses more than 125,400 volumes, 369 periodical subscriptions, and 3,641 electronic subscriptions. Membership in OhioLINK and a comprehensive media collection provide access to thousands of additional resources. One of the reference librarians is a liaison with the School of Nursing. Other campus resources include media and computer centers. The College has five dedicated rooms for computers, plus individual computers in numerous locations, including the residence halls. Students enjoy classes in the Bishop Anthony M. Pilla Student Learning Center, which houses a state-of-the-art nursing skills lab.

LOCATION
Ursuline College is located on a beautiful campus in Pepper Pike, a residential suburb approximately 12 miles from downtown Cleveland. The surrounding area has many restaurants and stores, including a large mall just 10 minutes from campus. The Cleveland area offers a multitude of activities such as music, art, science, parks, and sports. Ursuline is easily accessible from Route 271 or via the RTA. For students looking to combine a quiet but serious academic life with the cultural excitement of a major city, Ursuline College provides these unique advantages.

STUDENT SERVICES

In addition to sports, the College provides a fitness center, personal and career counseling, mentoring and cooperative education programs, campus ministry, and an Office for Multicultural Affairs. The Academic Support and Learning Disabilities Center provides academic support services for all students, including assistance with study, testing, and writing skills. Tutoring is available in reading, writing, math, and science. The Program for Academic Success (PAS) was designed to help students who are not prepared for college-level work, especially in math and science.

THE NURSING STUDENT GROUP

Although Ursuline remains a women's college, men are welcome and represent approximately 7 percent of the students who are enrolled in nursing. Most students come from Ohio and surrounding states and represent different ethnic, racial, cultural, religious, and economic backgrounds. Currently, the School of Nursing has approximately 325 undergraduate and 70 graduate students.

COSTS

In 2004–05, undergraduate tuition was $599 per credit hour. Full-time students usually carry 12 to 16 credits. Graduate tuition was $639 per credit hour.

FINANCIAL AID

The Office of Financial Aid administers a number of institutional, state, and federal programs. Financial assistance may include a combination of scholarships, loans, grants, and work-study opportunities. To apply for financial aid, students must complete the Free Application for Federal Student Aid (FAFSA) and the Ursuline College Financial Aid Application. Approximately 85 percent of undergraduates in nursing receive financial aid.

APPLYING

Undergraduate and graduate applications are accepted on a rolling basis. Admission to the B.S.N. program is through the Office of Admission. In addition to criteria for clear admission to the College, applicants seeking admission to the B.S.N. program directly from high school need to have successfully completed algebra, biology (with lab), and chemistry (with lab), each with a grade of 2.5 the first time the courses were taken for credit. High school students must have an overall 2.75 GPA to be admitted to the nursing program. Students may transfer college courses in which they have earned a grade of 2.0.

Admission to the M.S.N. program is through The Breen School of Nursing. Admission criteria include an official transcript verifying completion of an accredited baccalaureate program with a GPA of 3.0. The MAT or GRE may be required of applicants whose GPA is less than 3.0.

CORRESPONDENCE AND INFORMATION

For the Undergraduate Program:
Sarah Carr
Director of Admission
Ursuline College
2550 Lander Road
Pepper Pike, Ohio 44124-4398

Phone: 440-449-4203
       888-URSULINE (toll-free)
Fax: 440-684-6138
Web site: http://www.ursuline.edu

For the Graduate Program:
Carol H. Waggoner, Ph.D., RN
Director, Graduate Program
The Breen School of Nursing
Ursuline College
2550 Lander Road
Pepper Pike, Ohio 44124-4398

Phone: 440-449-3425
Fax: 440-449-4267
E-mail: cwaggoner@ursuline.edu
Web site: http://www.ursuline.edu

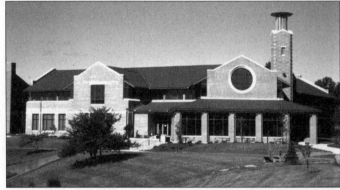

Located on 112 scenic acres in Pepper Pike, Ohio—just 12 miles east of Cleveland—the Breen School of Nursing is a student's pathway to success.

Vanderbilt University
School of Nursing
Nashville, Tennessee

THE UNIVERSITY

Vanderbilt University was established in 1873 through a $1-million donation by Commodore Cornelius Vanderbilt. Vanderbilt University offers a full range of undergraduate programs as well as forty-one master's degree programs and forty Ph.D. programs. There are more than 2,525 full-time faculty members and a diverse student population of almost 11,500.

THE SCHOOL OF NURSING

For more than ninety years, Vanderbilt University School of Nursing (VUSN) has been providing innovative educational opportunities for its students. The School's proudest tradition is educating nurses who are impassioned professionals capable of meeting—and exceeding—the demands of a constantly evolving profession. By 1926, the School had grown from its initiation as the Vanderbilt Hospital Training School (1909) to a school of nursing, offering a diploma in nursing combined with studies in arts and sciences, leading to a B.S. degree. In 1933, VUSN offered the first B.S.N. in Tennessee and became a charter member of the Association of Collegiate Schools of Nursing (ACSN), which later became the National League for Nursing Accrediting Commission (NLNAC), under which the program is currently accredited. The nurse-midwifery program is accredited by the American College of Nurse-Midwives. In 1985, VUSN introduced the Prespecialty Pathway to the master's program, replacing the B.S.N. degree program. The Prespecialty Pathway offers multiple entry options for students seeking to become advanced practice nurses, including those with 78 hours of college credit, an associate degree or diploma in nursing and 78 hours of college credit, or a B.S.N. Recognizing that some nurses who may have earned master's degrees in nursing would like additional or different specialties, VUSN offers a post-master's option. In 1993, the Ph.D. in Nursing Science program was established.

PROGRAMS OF STUDY

Vanderbilt University School of Nursing offers a Master of Science in Nursing (M.S.N.) with multiple entry options. Applicants with a Bachelor of Science in Nursing, an associate degree in nursing and 78 semester hours of college credit, a diploma in nursing and 78 semester hours of college credit, a bachelor's degree in another field, or at least 78 semester hours of college credit are eligible to apply to the program.

The M.S.N. degree is offered with the following specialties: clinical management (clinical nurse leader and clinical nurse specialist roles), family nurse practitioner/acute care nurse practitioner dual certification with a focus in emergency care, women's health nurse practitioner/adult nurse practitioner dual certification, health-systems management, nurse midwifery, nursing informatics, primary-care nurse practitioner (adult, adult/gerontology dual certification, family, pediatric, or women's health), specialty-care nurse practitioner (acute care, neonatal, pediatric acute care, or psychiatric–mental health), and joint degrees combining the Master of Science in Nursing with the Master of Business Administration (M.S.N./M.B.A. dual degree), Master of Divinity (M.S.N./M.Div. dual degree), and Master of Theological Studies (M.S.N./M.T.S. dual degree). The School offers numerous focus areas, including cardiovascular disease management, clinical research management, emergency response management, forensic nursing, oncology, palliative care, transplant services, and trauma. Many of the programs are delivered in a modified distance format to accommodate individuals who work full-time and/or maintain residence outside middle Tennessee. International exchange opportunities are available.

Applicants with a Bachelor of Science in Nursing (B.S.N.) from a CCNE- or an NLNAC-accredited program are admitted directly to the specialty year for a 39-semester-hour program of studies. Nurse-midwifery, dual concentrations, and joint degree programs may require additional semester hours. Admission to the School of Nursing without a B.S.N. degree is possible through the generalist nursing Prespecialty/M.S.N. program. Students with an associate degree in nursing and 78 semester hours of college credit or a diploma in nursing and 78 semester hours of college credit may enter the program and earn the Master of Science in Nursing degree in five semesters of full-time study. Students with a baccalaureate degree in another field or at least 78 semester hours of college credit may enter the program and earn an M.S.N. degree in six semesters of full-time study.

The Ph.D. in Nursing Science Program prepares scholars for research and teaching careers at major universities and for research positions in public or private sectors of health care. Graduates of the program conduct and disseminate research that addresses regional and national needs and extends the knowledge base in the discipline of nursing.

Two tracks of study are available: clinical research and health services research. These areas of study are reflective of the overall research interests and expertise of School of Nursing faculty members and the resources available in the medical center, the University, the School of Nursing nurse-managed and interdisciplinary care delivery centers, and the Veterans Affairs Tennessee Valley Healthcare System (Nashville campus). The Ph.D. in Nursing Science Program offers two entry options: traditional entry and fast-track entry.

The traditional entry option is designed for students with a bachelor's degree in nursing (or B.S.N. equivalent) and a master's in nursing (or a related field).

Fast-track entry is designed for students applying to Vanderbilt's School of Nursing (VUSN) M.S.N. Program and for currently enrolled students. It can provide students with a seamless progression through their graduate studies. Students at the M.S.N. level receive enhanced research opportunities and mentored experiences. Interested applicants may simultaneously apply to the VUSN M.S.N. and Ph.D. programs. Applicants must meet eligibility requirements for both programs and be admitted to both programs.

The faculty of VUSN is committed to the educational preparation of a group of nurse scholars who can lead the nation in demonstrating how well-conceived, theory-based nursing research verifies and extends the body of nursing knowledge. Students work with faculty mentors who guide and oversee their educational programs from admission through the completion of degree requirements. They participate in intensive research experiences connected with faculty research projects and are exposed to a variety of research designs and analysis techniques.

AFFILIATIONS WITH HEALTH-CARE FACILITIES

Vanderbilt University School of Nursing offers its students opportunities to complete clinical courses, conduct inquiry, and learn in diverse settings. The School maintains more than 1,000 contracts with clinical practices in hospitals, communities, health departments, private practices, clinics, outpatient facilities, home-health agencies, skilled-care facilities, nursing homes, schools, and industries. These sites are in urban settings in Nashville, rural areas of Tennessee, and in other areas across the country. The Vanderbilt University Medical Center maintains a reputation for excellence in teaching, practice, and research and provides students with a tertiary academic setting, where patients receive exemplary care from creative health-care teachers and scholars.

ACADEMIC FACILITIES

The Jean and Alexander Heard Library is the collective name for all of the libraries at Vanderbilt, which have a combined collection of more than 3 million volumes. In addition to the Central library, the Biomedical, Divinity, Education, Law, Management, and Science libraries serve their respective schools and disciplines. The state-of-the-art Annette and Irwin Eskind Biomedical Library provides students with access to worldwide information through the very best in informatic retrieval and management technology. Traditional library services, book stacks, and comfortable reading areas are also provided along with technology training assistance.

The focal point of scholarship at the School of Nursing is the Joint Center for Nursing Research (JCNR), which is housed on the fifth floor of Godchaux Hall. Although research and scholarship activities occur throughout the School and are interwoven into all aspects of academic life at Vanderbilt, the center serves as the central resource, repository, and facilitator of faculty member, student, and nursing staff member scholarship. Its mission is to facilitate scholarly activity and thereby promote new knowledge and improved care delivery to the community and the nation. It achieves this mission through the established relationships between the School of Nursing, the University, and affiliated health-care agencies.

LOCATION

Vanderbilt is located on a 333-acre parklike campus approximately 1½ miles from downtown Nashville, providing a peaceful setting within an urban environment. Long known as a center of banking, finance, and publishing, this capital city of Tennessee is a unique blend of Southern hospitality and cosmopolitan diversity that ranks high in the quality-of-life surveys. Nashville has an international airport and is easily accessible from interstate highways.

STUDENT SERVICES

Vanderbilt provides its students with a comprehensive list of services, including the Career Center, Psychological and Counseling Services, Student Health Center, the Office of International Services, the Child Care Center, the Bishop Joseph Johnson Black Cultural Center, and the Margaret Cuninggim Women's Center, as well as security escort services and shuttle bus services.

THE NURSING STUDENT GROUP

Vanderbilt University School of Nursing has been successful in attracting students from diverse educational backgrounds and work experiences. Approximately 45 percent of the M.S.N. class began the program in the 2006 academic year without a background in nursing. These individuals will enter the nursing profession prepared as advanced practice nurses after two full calendar years (six semesters) of study. Ages of class members range from 20 to 60, and 11 percent of the students are men. The School's diverse student body includes Asian Americans, African Americans, American Indians, and Hispanic students, in addition to international students.

COSTS

Tuition for the M.S.N. program for the 2006–07 academic year was $893 per semester hour for all students. Tuition for the Ph.D. in Nursing Science program was $1359 per semester hour. Tuition for both programs is subject to change.

Expenses for books and supplies vary according to specialty. Equipment such as tape recorders and diagnostic tools is required for certain specialties. Other charges include laboratory fees, student activities and recreation fees, liability insurance coverage, and hospitalization insurance.

FINANCIAL AID

Financial aid is available from several sources for full-time M.S.N. students. All students who wish to apply for financial aid and scholarships must apply to the School of Nursing no later than May 1 for the next academic year. Information about financial aid for M.S.N. students can be obtained from the School of Nursing Admissions Office.

Information about financial aid for Ph.D. students can be obtained from the Ph.D. program office, 603 Godchaux Hall, 461 21st Avenue South, Nashville, Tennessee 37240.

APPLYING

Admission requirements for applicants to the M.S.N. program include a minimum 3.0 GPA, three letters of recommendation, a statement of career goals, an interview survey, and minimum GRE scores of 1000 on the verbal and quantitative components and 4.5 on the analytical component. Applications received by December 1 receive priority review. Applications received after December 1 are reviewed until the M.S.N. class is full.

Admission to the Ph.D. in Nursing Science program is through the University's Graduate School, which has oversight responsibility for all doctoral programs in the University. Application materials are returned to the School of Nursing.

Successful applicants to the Ph.D. in Nursing Science program are those whose previous academic performance, letters of reference, Graduate Record Examinations (GRE) scores, and personal statement meet admission standards for the School of Nursing and the University Graduate School. In addition, because of the importance of research oversight in doctoral education, only students whose research and career goals fit with the School's areas of concentration are considered for admission. All applicants are interviewed by the Director of the Doctoral Program and 2 doctoral faculty members.

CORRESPONDENCE AND INFORMATION:

For information on the M.S.N. and Ph.D. in Nursing Science programs:

Admissions Office
Vanderbilt University School of Nursing
Godchaux Hall
461 21st Avenue South
Nashville, Tennessee 37240

Phone: 615-322-3800
Fax: 615-343-0333
E-mail: vusn-admissions@vanderbilt.edu
Web site: http://www.mc.vanderbilt.edu/nursing/

Villanova University
College of Nursing
Villanova, Pennsylvania

College of Nursing
VILLANOVA
UNIVERSITY

THE UNIVERSITY

Villanova University is an independent coeducational institution of higher learning founded by the Augustinians, one of the oldest teaching orders in the Catholic Church. Since its beginning in 1842, the University's Augustinian character has been evident in its devotion to the principles of scholarship, community, and the relationship between mind and heart as well as in its commitment to producing graduates with strong moral values and proficient skills.

Villanova is a comprehensive university with undergraduate academic colleges in the areas of business, engineering, liberal arts and sciences, and nursing. The University offers selected master's and doctoral degrees, including the Master of Science in Nursing (M.S.N.) and Ph.D. in nursing, and maintains a highly regarded School of Law. Villanova's student body of more than 10,000 represents almost every state in the nation as well as forty-four countries. Approximately 50 percent of its undergraduates are men.

THE COLLEGE OF NURSING

The College of Nursing, founded in 1953, has the distinction of being the first collegiate nursing program under Catholic auspices in Pennsylvania, the largest nursing college in the commonwealth within a private university, and the only nursing program in the country under Augustinian sponsorship. All of the programs offered by the College—baccalaureate, master's, doctoral, and continuing education—are fully accredited. There are approximately 5,500 alumni of the degree-granting programs, and the College currently enrolls about 500 undergraduates, the majority of whom are full-time, and 180 graduate students, most of whom enroll on a part-time basis.

The faculty believes that education provides students with opportunities to develop habits of critical, constructive thought so that they may make discriminating judgments in their search for the truth. This type of intellectual development can best be attained in a teaching-learning environment that fosters sharing of knowledge, skills, and attitudes as well as inquiry toward the development of new knowledge. The faculty members and students comprise a community of learners and teacher-scholars. Approximately 80 percent of the full-time faculty members in the College hold an earned doctorate, and many are actively engaged in research. The faculty, however, has teaching as its primary commitment, and most of the teaching is carried out by full-time faculty members.

The College, in conjunction with the University's Office of International Studies, offers a sophomore year abroad in the baccalaureate program at the University of Manchester in Manchester, England. There are a growing number of students sponsored by international organizations who are attending the master's program, and the College is exploring opportunities to expand international experiences for its students. The continuing education program offers a variety of workshops, seminars, conferences, self-study activities, and short courses and a post-master's certificate in nursing administration. All of these options are designed to assist practicing nurses to advance, maintain, and provide high-quality health care.

PROGRAMS OF STUDY

Villanova awards the Bachelor of Science in Nursing (B.S.N.) degree after completion of 136 credits, 75 of which are in nursing; the remaining 61 are in arts and science. The program integrates a liberal education with the ideals, knowledge, and

skills of professional nursing practice under the direction of a qualified faculty. Baccalaureate education prepares individuals for professional nursing practice in a variety of health-care settings and for continuous personal and educational growth, including entrance into graduate education in nursing. The College welcomes applications from adults who wish to begin preparation for a career in nursing. These include individuals who possess undergraduate and/or graduate degrees in other fields as well as adults entering college for the first time. Part-time study is possible during the introductory level of the program. Full-time study is required during the clinical portion of the program. Graduates from diploma and associate degree nursing programs are eligible for admission to the baccalaureate program. Through a series of nursing examinations and clinical validation, a registered nurse student may demonstrate current nursing knowledge, earning 45 credits in nursing. A maximum of 50 percent of the credits from the total curriculum may be transferred by either adult learners or registered nurse students.

The M.S.N. program at Villanova University requires the completion of 45 credits and prepares nurses for roles as nurse practitioners; nurse anesthetists; case management administrators; educators; and health-care administrators. The curriculum includes core courses (including research, theory, and leadership), clinical courses (including a practicum in adult, community, gerontology, parent-child, or psychiatric–mental health nursing), free electives, an independent study course, and role-related courses (including a practicum). No thesis is required; however, students who wish to work with faculty members who are conducting research or who wish to engage in a research-oriented independent study project are encouraged to do so and are assisted in the endeavor.

The Villanova nursing doctoral program leads to the Ph.D. degree and prepares nurses as forward-thinking teacher scholars for academic careers in higher education. Graduates are well-prepared to teach diverse populations of students in a variety of educational and clinical settings using state-of-the-art technology. They provide leadership as the architects of curricula and members of evaluative bodies, are active contributors to the advancement and development of theory and research, and assume the varied roles of faculty members within academic institutions. The doctoral program combines innovative and traditional modalities, offering distance learning opportunities in the fall and spring semesters and on-site experience during summer sessions. The program was designed with a maximum of 51 credits; the length of the program varies depending on previous education, currency of graduate education, and individual needs.

AFFILIATIONS WITH HEALTH-CARE FACILITIES

The College of Nursing is affiliated with more than seventy health-care agencies in the Greater Philadelphia area that provide settings for undergraduate and graduate student clinical experiences. These facilities include hospitals in large medical centers, community hospitals, extended-care facilities, home-health agencies, schools, industrial health settings, senior citizen and community health centers, HMOs, insurance companies, and managed-care agencies.

ACADEMIC FACILITIES

The Falvey Memorial Library provides resources and facilities for study and research by graduate and undergraduate students, faculty members, and visiting scholars. It houses more than 650,000 volumes, of which more than 22,000 are nursing or nursing-related. The library has an extensive periodicals section with 251 nursing and nursing-related holdings. Library services include computerized literature searches with direct access to the National Library of Medicine databases and extensive instructional media services, including a professionally staffed video studio for the production of sophisticated video materials. In addition to the general University library and extensive interlibrary loan access, students in the College of Nursing have access to the Law Library and that of the College of Commerce and Finance. The computing services available to the University community are extensive, with computer stations located throughout the campus. In addition to those available in the primary computing center, the College of Nursing Learning Resource Center houses computers and interactive video systems that are available for the exclusive use of its students and faculty. The Learning Resource Center also maintains extensive holdings of a wide variety of audiovisual materials, training models, computer software programs, and simulations to support the teaching enterprise. Students and faculty members have access to the fully staffed Center during extended weekday and selected weekend hours.

LOCATION

With its more than 250 landscaped acres in one of the most beautiful residential areas in America, the Villanova campus is among the showplaces in the suburban Philadelphia area. Located on the prestigious Main Line, with a station on its campus, Villanova is easily accessible by train from Philadelphia. It also lies in proximity to several major highways that make the Philadelphia airport as well as the New York and Washington, D.C., areas easily accessible. Such a location provides students with safe and easy access to the cultural and recreational opportunities available in Philadelphia and makes those of New York and Washington, D.C., readily available as well.

STUDENT SERVICES

Villanova University offers a wide variety of student services. Campus Ministry promotes a sense of community through the coordination of a variety of programs that are of a religious and human service character with a view to aiding students with their spiritual and personal growth. A full array of student activities, including a theater, Greek system, music activities, intramural and intercollegiate sports, and a fitness center, are available. Such opportunities facilitate the total development of students, promote a spirit of community, provide opportunities for students to interact with other individuals who have varied interests, and provide the supports necessary to succeed academically. In addition, student health services, a counseling center, career planning and placement services, a writing center, and study skills resources are available to all students.

THE NURSING STUDENT GROUP

Most of the individuals enrolled in the undergraduate program are full-time students who began their nursing studies directly after completing high school. Approximately 20 percent of the B.S.N. population are registered nurses or adult learners. Graduates are employed in major health-care facilities, universities, or other settings throughout the country, and approximately 30 percent have completed or are enrolled in graduate programs. Approximately 90 percent of the individuals enrolled in the M.S.N. program are part-time students with several years experience as nurses. Students in the program received their undergraduate education in a wide variety of institutions, and the number of international students enrolled in the master's program is increasing steadily. Graduates of this program hold positions of leadership, such as nurse practitioner, nurse anesthetist, administrator, educator, and case manager, in some of the most prestigious health-care institutions in the country. Approximately 20 percent of the M.S.N. graduates have completed or are enrolled in doctoral programs.

COSTS

Full-time tuition for the undergraduate program in the 2006–07 academic year was $33,000 for freshmen and $29,590 for sopho-

mores, juniors, and seniors. The per-credit rate for undergraduate courses was $1235 ($1375 for freshmen), and general fees were $300. The part-time per-credit undergraduate rate was $410 for evening and $630 for day study. For the 2006–07 academic year, tuition for the master's program was $605 per credit, with a general University fee of $60. For the 2006–07 academic year, tuition for the doctoral program was $755 per credit.

FINANCIAL AID

Undergraduate financial aid is granted on the basis of need and scholastic ability and includes Villanova University scholastic grants, student loans, federal grants, state grants, and scholarships from outside sources such as corporations, unions, charitable trusts, and service clubs. The University financial aid office assists applicants in this process. Financial assistance is available to graduate students in the form of graduate assistantships, professional nurse traineeships, scholarships, and loans.

APPLYING

Admission to the undergraduate program is based on evaluation of high school grade point average, standardized tests (SAT or ACT), rank in class (if available), and student activities resume. Applications must be submitted by January 7, and applicants are notified of their admission decision on an ongoing basis. The deadline for Early Action and Presidential Scholarship consideration is November 1.

For transfer students, adult learners, and registered nurses, applications must be received no later than November 15 (for January entrance) or April 15 (for September entrance). Criteria used to evaluate these applicants include complete transcripts from previous schools, quality point average at previously attended institutions, and evidence of honorable withdrawal from previously attended institutions. Transcripts from a secondary school are required if the applicant has never attended an institution of higher learning. Students interested in the Alternate Curriculum should apply by the deadline of March 1 for entrance into the program in the following August. Eligible students may complete a B.S.N. Express Program application between July 1 and November 1 for the next year's May entering class.

Applications to the M.S.N. program are accepted on an ongoing basis, and students may begin the program in the fall, spring, or summer terms. Admission requirements include the B.S.N., a minimum of one year recent clinical practice in nursing, acceptable scores on the MAT or GRE, undergraduate statistics, physical assessment, three letters of reference from professional nurses, and a personal statement of career goals.

Applicants to the doctoral program should submit all materials by January 15. Materials include the application form, curriculum vitae, application fee, three references, evidence of scholarly writing, essay, official transcripts, GRE scores from the last five years, and TOEFL scores (international students whose first language is not English only). Applicants are notified of acceptance early in the spring semester so that they can plan to attend the summer on-campus orientation and summer session courses.

CORRESPONDENCE AND INFORMATION

Office of Undergraduate Admission
Villanova University
800 East Lancaster Avenue
Villanova, Pennsylvania 19085

Phone: 610-519-4453
Fax: 610-519-6450

Graduate Nursing Program
Office of University Admission
Villanova University
800 East Lancaster Avenue
Villanova, Pennsylvania 19085-1690

Phone: 610-519-4934
Fax: 610-519-7650

Virginia Commonwealth University
School of Nursing
Richmond, Virginia

THE UNIVERSITY

A public, urban university located in the state capital, Virginia Commonwealth University (VCU) was founded in 1838. VCU is ranked by the Carnegie Foundation as one of the nation's top research universities and is one of only three such universities in the state. VCU is composed of two campuses, the Monroe Park Campus and the Medical College of Virginia Campus. More than 29,000 students attend VCU, with 28 percent of the students representing minority groups.

VCU's Medical College of Virginia Campus is home to the Schools of Nursing, Allied Health, Pharmacy, Dentistry, and Medicine. The VCU Medical Center is one of the most comprehensive teaching hospitals in the country, and it is the only hospital in central Virginia to receive Magnet designation for excellence in nursing services.

THE SCHOOL OF NURSING

The School of Nursing originated in 1893 and has evolved from a basic diploma program to a school of more than 800 students, with multiple programs at the baccalaureate, master's, and doctoral degree levels. In addition, the School of Nursing offers post-master's certificate programs. The School of Nursing takes pride in its long history of service to the profession of nursing and continues to be a leader in nursing education in Virginia and the country. Recently the school was ranked fourteenth (out of 200 programs) in National Institutes of Health research funding for schools of nursing.

PROGRAMS OF STUDY

The undergraduate program encompasses the traditional, accelerated B.S., RN-B.S. weekend, and RN-B.S. online programs. Students can enter the traditional undergraduate program as freshmen or may transfer into the nursing program as sophomores after finishing their first year of study in VCU's College of Humanities and Science or at another college or university. Non-nursing college graduates may complete their bachelor's degree in nursing in a year-round, five-semester program. Registered nurses can obtain their bachelor's degree in three semesters by attending class once a month in the RN-B.S. weekend program or through online study. In addition to distance learning, this flexible program is offered in multiple sites across the state of Virginia. Academically talented registered nurses may apply to the RN-M.S. program.

The master's program is designed to prepare graduates for advanced nursing practice as nurse practitioners, clinical nurse specialists, and nurse leaders.

The School offers an entry-level master's program for individuals with bachelor's degrees in disciplines other than nursing. The accelerated second-degree program is a three-year, full-time program that begins in the summer and offers year-round study in adult health–acute (clinical nurse specialist studies (CNS) and nurse practitioner studies (NP) tracks), adult health—primary (NP track), child health (NP track), community health and public health (dual-degree program), family health (NP track), nursing administration and leadership, psychiatric–mental health nursing (CNS and NP), and women's health (NP track). Upon graduation, students are eligible for certification as nurse practitioners or clinical nurse specialists in their chosen specialty area.

The traditional master's program offers full-time and part-time study in adult health–acute (CNS and NP tracks),

adult health–primary (NP track), child health (NP track), community health and public health (dual-degree program), family health (NP track), nursing administration and leadership, integrative psychiatric mental health (CNS and NP), and women's health (NP track). Registered nurses with a bachelor's degree in another discipline may enter the traditional master's program but are also required to complete selected undergraduate upper-division nursing courses.

The goal of the doctoral program in nursing is the preparation of scholars to develop knowledge in the discipline of nursing. The school offers two entry options in the doctoral program—the traditional Ph.D. program for individuals with a master's in nursing and the post-B.S. to Ph.D. option for individuals with a bachelor's degree in nursing.

AFFILIATIONS WITH HEALTH-CARE FACILITIES

The School of Nursing is affiliated with a wide variety of health-care agencies within and outside the metropolitan Richmond area. These include major health-care agencies such as the VCU Medical Center and Hunter Holmes McGuire VA Medical Center as well as other acute- and primary-care settings, ambulatory practice sites, schools, and community health centers.

ACADEMIC FACILITIES

The University library facilities include Cabell and Tompkins-McCaw Libraries. The combined collections in these libraries total more than 1.23 million volumes. The comprehensive collections of Tompkins-McCaw Library are a designated resource library for the Southeastern states in the National Network of Libraries in Medicine. The University Library Services are extensively automated, with almost 900 databases and more than 100 public-access workstations.

LOCATION

The city of Richmond, located on the James River, provides a backdrop for an energetic academic and social life on the Virginia Commonwealth campuses. The University is located 2 hours from the nation's capital, the Blue Ridge Mountains, the Appalachian Trail, and the Atlantic Ocean. The School of Nursing is housed on the Medical Campus, which is located near the state capitol and the government and financial centers of downtown Richmond.

STUDENT SERVICES

The University and School offer a comprehensive array of student services at both the undergraduate and graduate levels. These include academic advising by professional faculty and staff members, academic support services within the School and University, a career and placement center, services for students with disabilities, counseling, and student activities.

THE NURSING STUDENT GROUP

The School of Nursing enrolls approximately 310 traditional undergraduate students and accelerated B.S. students and 270 RN-B.S. (weekend and online) students. In the graduate program, there are approximately 205 accelerated and traditional master's students and 35 doctoral students.

COSTS

The 2006–07 in-state resident, full-time undergraduate tuition and fees were $5765, and out-of-state tuition and fees were

$17,386. In-state graduate tuition and fees were $7731, and out-of-state tuition and fees were $17,386.

FINANCIAL AID

Financial aid is available through the University's Financial Aid Office. The School of Nursing offers scholarships for full-time study. Full-time doctoral students are eligible to receive a stipend and scholarships covering tuition and fees and serve as teaching or research assistants.

APPLYING

All programs use a self-managed application process and require standardized test scores of all applicants except those applying to the RN-B.S. and post-M.S. certificate programs. Suggested application deadlines are as follows: entry-level master's and accelerated B.S. programs, December 1; traditional undergraduate program, January 15; traditional master's program and doctoral program, February 1; RN-B.S. weekend program, March 15. The School of Nursing offers monthly information sessions from September to June.

CORRESPONDENCE AND INFORMATION

Office of Enrollment & Student Services
School of Nursing
Virginia Commonwealth University
P.O. Box 980567
Richmond, Virginia 23298-0567

Phone: 804-828-5171
          800-828-9451 (toll-free)
Fax: 804-828-7743
Web site: http://www.nursing.vcu.edu

THE FACULTY

Sadeeka Al-Majid, Assistant Professor; Ph.D., Wisconsin–Madison.
Jennifer Black, Clinical Instructor; M.S., Virginia Commonwealth.
Anne Boyle, Clinical Assistant Professor; Ph.D., Virginia.

Marie Chapin, Clinical Instructor; M.S.N., Virginia Commonwealth.
Elizabeth Crooks, Clinical Assistant Professor; M.S.N., Case Western Reserve.
Ann Cox, Assistant Professor; Ph.D., Virginia Commonwealth.
Carol Cutler, Clinical Assistant Professor; D.N.Sc., Catholic University.
Anthony DeLellis, Associate Professor and Assistant Dean; Ph.D., Virginia.
Lauren Goodloe, Clinical Associate Professor, Director of Nursing, and Vice President, Patient Care Services; Ph.D., Virginia Commonwealth.
Mary Jo Grap, Professor; Ph.D., Georgia State.
Patricia Gray, Associate Professor and Chair; Ph.D., Utah.
Martha Hart, Clinical Instructor; M.S., Virginia Commonwealth.
Debra Hearington, Assistant Professor; M.S., Virginia Commonwealth.
Robin Hills, Clinical Instructor; M.S., Virginia Commonwealth.
Tanya Huff, Clinical Assistant Professor; M.S.N., Virginia Commonwealth.
Rita Jablonski, Assistant Professor; Ph.D., Virginia.
Nancy Langston, Professor and Dean; Ph.D., Georgia State.
Judith Lewis, Professor; Ph.D., Brandeis.
Susan Lipp, Director of Enrollment and Student Services; M.S.N., North Carolina at Chapel Hill.
Debra Lyon, Associate Professor; Ph.D., Virginia Commonwealth.
Nancy McCain, Professor; Ph.D., Alabama at Birmingham.
Martha Moon, Associate Professor; Ph.D., California, San Francisco.
Cindy Munro, Professor; Ph.D., Virginia Commonwealth.
Rita Pickler, Associate Professor and Chair; Ph.D., Virginia.
Jeanne Salyer, Associate Professor; Ph.D., Virginia Commonwealth.
Inez Tuck, Professor and Chair; Ph.D., North Carolina at Greensboro.
Sandra Voll, Clinical Instructor; M.S., Virginia Commonwealth.
Janet Younger, Professor and Associate Dean; Ph.D., Virginia.

Wayne State University
College of Nursing
Detroit, Michigan

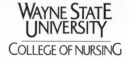

THE UNIVERSITY

Wayne State University (WSU) is among the nation's eighty-eight distinguished public and private universities with the Carnegie Research University I classification. The University is accredited by the North Central Association of Colleges and Schools. High-quality educational programs are offered in more than 600 fields of study leading to more than 300 different degrees at the bachelor's, master's, and doctoral levels. WSU's main campus encompasses 184 acres of landscaped, tree-lined pedestrian malls and ninety-eight research and educational buildings of classic and contemporary design. The multicultural urban context of the University provides a rich environment for student learning.

THE COLLEGE OF NURSING

The College of Nursing is regionally, nationally, and internationally recognized for educating graduate and undergraduate students as practitioners and scholars who provide leadership for the profession and discipline of nursing. The College is committed to research and scholarly activity that contributes to the body of knowledge of care and the human health experience in diverse environmental contexts. Moreover, the College excels in the development, application, and dissemination of knowledge to promote the health and well-being of society through teaching, research, and public service. Wayne State University College of Nursing is consistently ranked among the top graduate schools of nursing in the nation (*U.S. News & World Report*). The College of Nursing, established in 1945 as an autonomous academic unit within the University, is accredited by the National League for Nursing Accrediting Commission and the Commission for Collegiate Nursing Education. Innovative program options at the undergraduate, master's, and doctoral levels are available for learners from diverse backgrounds. The focal areas of research excellence at the College are self-care and caregiving and urban health. The College's undergraduate program is ranked seventh in the nation in Gourman's ratings of leading schools of nursing.

PROGRAMS OF STUDY

The College of Nursing offers programs leading to B.S.N., M.S.N., and Ph.D. in nursing degrees. The College offers graduate certificates in transcultural nursing, nursing education, psychiatric mental health nursing, and nurse midwifery. Interdisciplinary graduate certificates in gerontology and infant mental health are also available. Within the baccalaureate program, options are available for applicants with diverse academic experience, including a traditional option for high school graduates, an accelerated option for college graduates with degrees in disciplines other than nursing, and an option for registered nurses. Graduates of the baccalaureate program are prepared for entry into professional practice. For academically talented registered nurses, an accelerated RN-M.S.N. program is available. The M.S.N. program is designed to prepare nurses for advanced nursing practice in the care of culturally diverse individuals, families, groups, and communities in a variety of health-care settings. The program educates nurses to assume leadership roles as nurse practitioners and clinical nurse specialists. The course experiences are designed to enhance the ability of students to think critically and creatively, engage in scientific inquiry, and use knowledge to direct nursing practice. Within the M.S.N. program, students may study within the following areas of specialization: adult primary-care nursing; gerontological nurse practitioner studies; adult acute-care nursing; adult critical-care nursing; advanced practice

nursing with women, neonates, children, and nurse midwifery; community health nursing; and psychiatric–mental health nurse practitioner studies.

The Ph.D. in nursing program is designed to prepare researchers and scholars who will provide leadership to the profession and discipline of nursing, the program emphasizes the development of the student's capacity to make significant, original contributions to nursing knowledge. The curriculum focuses on scientific inquiry and consists of a series of nursing seminars that address research methods, knowledge development, and the substantive domains of the discipline. The courses are designed to enhance the ability of students to develop and test new or extant nursing theories and acquire skill in the use of both qualitative and quantitative research methods. Three optional paths toward the Ph.D. degree in nursing are offered: two paths for students entering the program with a bachelor's degree in nursing and one path for those entering with a master's degree in nursing.

AFFILIATIONS WITH HEALTH-CARE FACILITIES

The College of Nursing is affiliated with a wide variety of health-care agencies (approximately 100) within and outside metropolitan Detroit. These include major health-care agencies such as the Detroit Medical Center, Henry Ford Health System, St. John's Health System, and the Oakland County Health Department as well as primary-care settings, ambulatory practice sites, schools, and community health centers.

ACADEMIC FACILITIES

The University library facilities include Purdy/Kresge, Science and Engineering, Shiffman Medical, and David Adamany Undergraduate Libraries. Together these campus libraries provide approximately 2.2 million books, with 400,000 covering health topics. Periodical subscriptions number 12,500, of which 2,500 are health-care related. CINAHL and MEDLINE are available.

Through the Learning Resource Center (LRC), the College of Nursing provides computer-assisted instruction programs, interactive video programs, videotapes, and audiotapes for group or individualized student instruction. Auxiliary to the LRC is the Physical Assessment Learning Laboratory, which provides the facilities for students to acquire and master knowledge and skills in assessment and nursing technology. The Center for Health Research provides services to the faculty and graduate students in the form of consultation services and technical assistance.

LOCATION

Wayne State University is located in the cultural center of Detroit, within walking distance of the Detroit Institute of Arts, the Detroit Historical Museum, Science Museum, International Institute, Museum of African American History, Detroit Medical Center, and the main branch of the Detroit Public Library. With easy access to numerous facilities by car or bus, students can enjoy the Detroit Symphony Orchestra, Broadway shows, and performances by well-known entertainers at the Fisher Theatre, the Fox Theatre, and the Masonic Temple Theatre. Historic Bricktown, lively Greektown, and the renowned Renaissance Center are also nearby.

STUDENT SERVICES

The College of Nursing has a full array of student services at both the undergraduate and graduate levels. These include academic advising by professional staff and faculty members, academic support services within the College and within the University, placement services, services for students with disabilities, housing, personal counseling, and student activities.

THE NURSING STUDENT GROUP

The College of Nursing enrolls approximately 425 undergraduates, 150 master's students, and 50 doctoral students. The College's undergraduate student population is predominantly from the greater metropolitan area. The graduate programs represent a culturally diverse student population with representation from throughout North America, South America, Europe, and Africa. Graduates of master's and doctoral programs in nursing are in great demand, and employment opportunities are excellent throughout the nation.

COSTS

Undergraduate tuition during the 2006–07 academic year was $236.30 per credit hour for state residents and $543.30 per credit hour for nonresidents. These rates reflect junior/senior, upper-division status. Graduate tuition was $414.50 per credit hour for state residents and $846.10 per credit hour for nonresidents. A $116.70 registration fee and a per-credit-hour omnibus fee of $16.75 for undergraduates or $25.20 for graduate students (for no more than 12 credit hours for undergraduates) were also required. An undergraduate clinical fee of $75 per clinical hour was required for all undergraduate clinical courses.

FINANCIAL AID

Opportunities for assistance with educational expenses are available to students through the University's Office of Scholarship and Financial Aid and the College of Nursing. Federal, state, and institutional funds are available based on financial need and academic merit. Assistance for both full- and part-time study is available through scholarships and fellowships, teaching and research assistantships, professional nurse traineeships, and nursing loans. Early application is essential.

APPLYING

All students must apply to both the University and the College of Nursing. To be considered for admission, undergraduate applicants must complete a minimum of 30 credits with a minimum honor point average of 2.5 in prerequisite courses. Students must file a B.S.N. application for admission, including transcripts, by March 31 for fall term admission. Applications are reviewed holistically and selection is based on scholarship in prerequisite course work and promise of success in a rigorous science-based curriculum. To qualify for admission, applicants for graduate study must have completed a baccalaureate program in nursing (or the equivalent) accredited by the NLNAC and must have current RN licensure. Selection is based on GRE scores, an autobiographical and goals statement, scholastic achievement, and professional references. A no-GRE option is available for students who meet selective scholastic achievement criteria. Application deadlines for admission to the Master of Science in Nursing program are two months prior to the term of admission. The Ph.D. priority application deadline is four months (six months for international students) prior to the start of the term of admission. Applications received after the priority deadline are considered if space is available.

CORRESPONDENCE AND INFORMATION

Office for Student Affairs
College of Nursing
Wayne State University
Detroit, Michigan 48202
Phone: 313-577-4082
888-837-0847 (toll-free)
Fax: 313-577-6949
Web site: http://www.nursing.wayne.edu

THE FACULTY

Adult Health

Nancy Artinian, Professor; Ph.D., Wayne State, 1988. Stress in spouses and families of coronary bypass surgery patients.

Ramona Benkert, Assistant Professor; Ph.D., Michigan, 2002. Cross-racial health care: Racial identity and cultural mistrust in primary care.

Stephen Cavanagh, Professor and Associate Dean; Ph.D., Texas at Austin, 1987. Stroke, arthritis, and hypertension in the elderly.

M. Kay Cresci, Assistant Professor; Ph.D., Wayne State, 1997. Active aging, cognition and physical activity in older adults, use of World Wide Web with older adults.

Jean E. Davis, Associate Professor and Assistant Dean; Ph.D., Arizona, 1987. Sleep and sleep disorders in vulnerable populations.

Patricia A. Jarosz, Assistant Professor; Ph.D., Michigan, 2001. Obesity and binge eating.

Helene J. Krouse, Professor; Ph.D., Boston College, 1984. Quality of life and sleep problems in allergy and asthma patients.

Marilyn Oermann, Professor; Ph.D., Pittsburgh, 1980. Clinical teaching and evaluation in nursing education.

Rosalind M. Peters, Assistant Professor; Ph.D., Wayne State, 2001. Self-care for hypertension and prevention of kidney disease.

Barbara Pieper, Professor; Ph.D., Wayne State, 1980. Management of pressure ulcers.

Barbara K. Redman, Professor and Dean; Ph.D., Washington (Seattle), 1966. Ethics, patient education, and health policy.

Virginia Rice, Professor; Ph.D., Michigan, 1982. Health promotion and smoking cessation.

April Vallerand, Associate Professor; Ph.D., Pennsylvania, 1995. Pain management and functional status in patients with chronic pain.

Linda Weglicki, Assistant Professor; Ph.D., Michigan, 1999. Adolescent health: Risk behaviors such as adolescent pregnancy; tobacco prevention and cessation.

Family, Community, and Mental Health

Karen Aroian, Professor; Ph.D., Washington (Seattle), 1988. Immigrant and minority health, cross-cultural research methods.

Cynthia A. Danford, Assistant Professor; Ph.D., California, San Francisco, 2002. Child behavior and health outcomes, parent-child interaction cross-culturally.

Judith Floyd, Professor and Associate Dean; Ph.D., Wayne State, 1982. Management of sleep problems across the life span.

Linda Ann Lewandowski, Associate Professor and Interim Assistant Dean; Ph.D., Massachusetts Amherst, 1988. Children and families coping with violence, abuse, and/or trauma.

Judith Fry McComish, Assistant Professor; Ph.D., Wayne State, 1984. Infant mental health, high risk mothers and their infants.

Delbert Martin Raymond III, Assistant Professor; Ph.D., Michigan, 2004. Workers' use of hearing protection.

Stephanie Myers Schim, Assistant Professor; Ph.D., Wayne State, 1997. Community health, leadership, end-of-life care.

Patricia Thornburg, Clinical Assistant Professor; Ph.D., Cincinnati, 1993. Child health promotion, lived experiences of caregivers.

Deborah S. Walker, Associate Professor; D.N.Sc., UCLA, 1994. Models of prenatal care delivery and perinatal outcomes, especially psychosocial outcomes; evidence-based care and innovative uses of information technology in midwifery clinical care and education.

Olivia G. Washington, Associate Professor; Ph.D., Wayne State, 1997. Homelessness, hypertension treatment adherence.

Feleta Wilson, Associate Professor; Ph.D., Wayne State, 1991. Patients' literacy levels and patient education.

Rachel Zachariah, Assistant Professor; D.N.Sc., California, San Francisco, 1985. Pregnancy outcomes of low-income women, health issues of South Asians.

Widener University
School of Nursing
Chester, Pennsylvania

THE UNIVERSITY

Founded in 1821, Widener University is a leading metropolitan university that offers a learning environment in which curricula are connected to societal issues through civic engagement. The University provides a unique combination of liberal arts and professional education. It has a distinct student focus in which dynamic teaching, active scholarship, personal attention, and experiential learning are key components. Located in Pennsylvania and Delaware, Widener is composed of eight schools and colleges offering degree programs at the associate, baccalaureate, master's, doctoral, and first-professional levels. Total enrollment in fall 2006 was 6,460 students, including 2,465 full-time undergraduates, 1,751 graduate students, and 1,489 School of Law students.

THE SCHOOL OF NURSING

Widener's School of Nursing has a long and rich tradition with its origins in the Crozer Foundation of Chester, Pennsylvania. The College of Nursing of the Crozer Foundation was already well established when it became part of Widener in 1970. The School has been continuously accredited by the National League for Nursing Accrediting Commission (NLNAC) since 1972 and continually approved by the Pennsylvania State Board of Nursing. The School maintains two educational sites, one on the Main Campus in Chester and another, for graduate students only, on the Harrisburg Campus. Widener's School of Nursing offers programs for students at the bachelor's, master's, and doctoral level. In addition to the full-time day program, there are a part-time evening/weekend program, a part-time Saturday RN/B.S.N. program, an RN/B.S.N./M.S.N. program, and an RN/M.S.N. accelerated program for RNs with a baccalaureate degree in another discipline. The School's first master's program—in burn, emergency, and trauma—was introduced at Widener in 1980 as the third program of its type nationally and the first in the Northeastern United States. At present, the School offers the Master of Science in Nursing (M.S.N.) and post-master's certificates in the advanced practice specialties of emergency/critical care nursing, adult health nursing, community-based nursing, nurse educator, psychiatric/mental health nursing, and family nurse practitioner. The Doctor of Nursing Science program originated in 1983 and graduated its first student in 1987. An accelerated M.S.N. to Doctor of Nursing Science program, supported by a Department of Health and Human Services Grant, was introduced in fall 2004.

PROGRAMS OF STUDY

The baccalaureate program, leading to licensing as a registered nurse, prepares graduates with a broad education in liberal arts and sciences as well as depth in professional knowledge and skills. In the first two years of the program, undergraduates concentrate on courses in biological and behavioral sciences, humanities, and electives. Upper-level nursing courses build on initial nursing courses as well the integration of knowledge and theories gained from the humanities, social sciences, and natural sciences. Undergraduate students with a cumulative GPA of 3.0 or higher may take up to 6 graduate nursing credits as part of their undergraduate program.

The RN/B.S.N. option, which builds on previous education and experience, is designed for registered nurses employed in the work arena and is scheduled in a part-time Saturday format. Registered nurses are granted 33 credits upon matriculation to the School. Nursing courses prepare registered nurses for an expanded professional role to meet the challenges of changing health-care needs. The RN/B.S.N./M.S.N. option is for students who choose to begin graduate course work as undergraduates.

Options for the Master of Science in Nursing are as follows. Adult health nursing (40 credits) focuses on the advanced practice role by providing a broad foundation in health promotion/disease prevention, concepts of illness care and case management, community and environmental issues, and rehabilitation. Community-based nursing (40 credits) explores the advanced practice role and the health-care needs of individuals, the community, and medically underserved populations. Emergency/critical care nursing (40 credits) provides advanced education to enable professional nurses to plan and implement expert nursing care for critically ill clients or those experiencing a health emergency. Clinical competence, a systems perspective, and the role of the advanced practice nurse as a change agent are emphasized. The nurse educator option (40–43 credits) prepares graduates for faculty roles within the clinical specialty discussed above. Psychiatric/mental health nursing (39 credits) prepares advanced practice nurses for a variety of mental health settings. The family nurse practitioner option (46 credits) prepares the professional nurse to be a provider of primary care to individuals and families across their life spans. A holistic approach to management of family health through interdisciplinary collaboration is a primary emphasis of this advanced practice role.

Post-master's certificates in all M.S.N. disciplines are available for students who wish to continue advancing themselves after obtaining the master's degree.

The RN/M.S.N. accelerated program is designed for RNs with a baccalaureate degree in another discipline. These students take, or transfer from another accredited school of nursing, three undergraduate foundation courses before being admitted to the graduate program.

The primary goal of Widener's doctoral program in nursing is the preparation of nurse scholars for educational leadership roles. Graduates are ready to create and disseminate to the public new knowledge gained from disciplined inquiry related to nursing and nursing education. Students in the program have clinical expertise in nursing at the master's level. Requirements for graduation include completion of at least 48 credits of doctoral course work in nursing beyond the master's degree as well as a minimum of 15 credits of dissertation advisement.

AFFILIATIONS WITH HEALTH-CARE FACILITIES

Widener undergraduate students begin their clinical education in the junior year and complete a total of 680 hours of actual clinical experience in a variety of agencies. Clinical experiences for graduate students take place in various acute and primary practice sites in rural and urban settings. Multiple hospitals, schools, and community health-care agencies in Pennsylvania, New Jersey, and Delaware are used for clinical experiences for both graduate and undergraduate students. Examples include Crozer-Chester Medical Center, Mercy Catholic Medical System, the University of Pennsylvania Health System, Children's Hospital of Philadelphia, and A. I. DuPont Institute.

ACADEMIC FACILITIES

Widener's Wolfgram Memorial Library houses close to 250,000 volumes of books, 175,000 microforms, and 2,000 periodicals as well as audiovisual and other nonprint media. Of these, 12,162 are nursing related and 18,135 are health related. Examples of Web-based resources available to students are CINAHL, MEDLINE, PsychInfo, PsycARTICLES, ERIC, Registry of Nursing Research, and the Online Journal of Knowledge Synthesis for Nursing. Widener's Nursing Learning Resource Center, located in the School of Nursing, gives students practice in simulated clinical settings to prepare them for actual hands-on patient experiences. The Nursing Learning Resource Center houses videotapes, computer-assisted instruction, models, and films. The University also provides state-of-the-art computer labs, and dormitories are wired for Internet use.

LOCATION
Rolling green lawns and an eclectic mixture of architecture characterize Widener's spacious campus in Chester, Pennsylvania. The University is ideally located at the intersection of Route 320 and I-95, near the Philadelphia International Airport, with direct access from I-476. It is just 12 miles southwest of Philadelphia in historic Delaware County. New York City and Washington, D.C., are roughly within a 2-hour drive. The New Jersey beaches and the famous Brandywine River Valley are also nearby. The Harrisburg Campus is located in a suburban setting on 21 acres, 7 miles from downtown Harrisburg.

STUDENT SERVICES
Academic support services include freshman academic advising, tutoring by faculty members and peers, and an early-warning program for incoming freshmen. Individualized writing and reading assistance is provided through the Writing Center and the Reading and Academic Skills Center. A Math Center is also available. The Career Advising and Placement Services (CAPS) Office houses an extensive career library and assists students with career development. Widener has more than sixty student organizations, including the Black Student Union, Commuter Student Organization, Student Government, International Club, and Rotaract Club. In addition, Widener offers NCAA Division III varsity sports and intramural and recreational opportunities for all students.

THE NURSING STUDENT GROUP
Of the more than 680 students in the School of Nursing, 517 are enrolled in the undergraduate program. Undergraduates are expected to be active members of the Widener University Student Nurses' Association (WUSNA), the State Nurses' Association of Pennsylvania (SNAP), and the National Student Nurses' Association (NSNA). These associations provide opportunities for the exchange of ideas and the pursuit of common educational and professional interests. WUSNA officers are elected from the ranks of all classes. Representatives frequently attend the national convention.

All students are eligible for membership in the Eta Beta chapter of the Honor Society of nursing, Sigma Theta Tau International. Candidates for membership are chosen each fall from students enrolled in the baccalaureate and graduate programs.

The School of Nursing Alumni Association (SONAA) actively supports the school with participation in student events and recruitment activities as well as with service and monetary contributions.

COSTS
Tuition costs for the 2006–07 academic year were $26,350 for full-time undergraduate students and $595 per credit for part-time undergraduate nursing students. Graduate nursing tuition was $650 per credit for master's programs and $675 per credit for doctoral study. The cost of room and board ranged from $9200 to $12,740, depending on the accommodations selected. On-campus housing is guaranteed to full-time undergraduates for all four years.

FINANCIAL AID
In 2006, approximately 90 percent of Widener nursing undergraduates received financial aid in the form of grants, loans, scholarships (some specifically for nursing majors), and employment. Eligibility for aid is based on need as well as academic merit.

APPLYING
Admission is competitive. All applicants are evaluated individually to determine their potential for academic success. Widener bases admission decisions on the strength of academic preparation, recommendations, extracurricular activities, personal qualifications, and the pattern of testing on various standardized tests. Since the University has a rolling admissions policy, students are notified of the admission decision soon after their application is completed. Admission into the master's program requires an undergraduate degree, a minimum GPA of 3.0 in the bachelor's program, and a current license as a registered nurse. Admission into the doctoral program requires a minimum GPA of 3.5 from an accredited master's program in nursing, a current license as a registered nurse, a graduate statistics course with a grade of at least C, and graduate courses in nursing theories and conceptional models.

CORRESPONDENCE AND INFORMATION:
Marguerite M. Barbiere, Dean
School of Nursing
Widener University
One University Place
Chester, Pennsylvania 19013-5792
Phone: 610-499-4214
Fax: 610-499-4216
E-mail: Marguerite.M.Barbiere@widener.edu

Cindy Jaskolka, Assistant Dean
Undergraduate Program
Phone: 610-499-4210
E-mail: amjaskolka@widener.edu

Mary Walker, Assistant Dean
Graduate Programs
Phone: 610-499-4208
E-mail: Mary.B.Walker@widener.edu

THE FACULTY
Marguerite M. Barbiere, Ed.D., Dean of Nursing and Professor.
Mary B. Walker, Ed.D., Assistant Dean for Graduate Programs and Associate Professor.
Cindy Jaskolka, M.S.N., Assistant Dean and Lecturer.
Lois R. Allen, Ph.D., Professor.
Mary Baumberger-Henry, D.N.Sc., Associate Professor.
Ellen Boyda, M.S.N., Lecturer.
Lynne C. Borucki, Ph.D., Assistant Professor.
Tammie Calabrese, M.S.N., Lecturer.
Norma Jean Colby, M.S.N., Lecturer.
Donna Callaghan, D.N.Sc., Assistant Professor.
Theresa Decker, M.S.N., Lecturer.
Shirlee Drayton-Brooks, Ph.D., CRNP, Director of the Family Nurse Practitioner Program.
Kristen Evans, M.S.N., Lecturer.
Mary Francis, M.S.N., Lecturer.
Lynn E. Kelly, Ph.D., Associate Professor.
Judith Ann Kilpatrick, D.N.Sc., Assistant Professor.
Anne M. Krouse, Ph.D., Assistant Professor.
Brenda Kucirka, M.S.N., Lecturer.
Susan Mills, M.S.N., Lecturer.
Marye O'Reilly-Knapp, D.N.Sc., Assistant Professor.
Susanne Palmer, Ph.D., Assistant Professor.
Barbara J. Patterson, Ph.D., Associate Professor.
Joyce Rasin, Ph.D., Associate Professor.
Janice L. Reilly, Ed.D., Assistant Professor.
Mary Ellen Santucci, D.N.Sc., Assistant Professor.
Rose Schwartz, M.S.N., Visiting Lecturer.
Doris C. Vallone, Ph.D., Associate Professor.
Pamela Williams, M.S.N., Lecturer.
Joan Webb, M.S.N., Lecturer.
Andrea M. Wolf, N.D., CRNP, Assistant Professor.

Wright State University
College of Nursing and Health
Dayton, Ohio

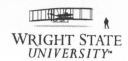

WRIGHT STATE
UNIVERSITY™

THE UNIVERSITY
Wright State University is a comprehensive, state-assisted institution that was founded in 1964 and was granted full university status in 1967. It serves nearly 17,000 students in 100 undergraduate programs and nearly fifty master's, Ph.D., and professional degree programs. The University is composed of eight academic units: Business, Education and Human Services, Engineering and Computer Science, Liberal Arts, Medicine, Nursing and Health, Professional Psychology, and Science and Mathematics.

Wright State is a metropolitan university. It is committed to providing leadership in addressing the educational, social, and cultural needs of the Greater Miami Valley and to promoting the economic and technological development of the region through a strong program of basic and applied research and professional service. Wright State is dedicated to excellence in teaching, research, and service.

Wright State seeks to enroll achievement-oriented traditional and nontraditional students and maintains an open admissions policy for undergraduates.

THE COLLEGE OF NURSING AND HEALTH
The College of Nursing and Health's baccalaureate program began in 1973, and the first students were admitted to the master's program in 1978. The College currently enrolls approximately 600 undergraduate and 200 graduate students.

In 1984, the College entered into a collaborative agreement with the Division of Nursing at Miami Valley Hospital to form a Center for Excellence in Nursing. Through collaboration with nursing staff members, this agreement affords unique opportunities for research, clinical practice, and education for students and the faculty.

The College of Nursing and Health reflects the broader mission of the University by providing excellent educational programs that prepare nurses for a dynamic health-care environment. As part of a metropolitan university, the College accepts the obligation to extend its resources to the surrounding region. It provides leadership to address regional health needs and forms partnerships with other disciplines, institutions, and organizations to cooperatively address health-related community problems. The clinical education programs are structured to provide students with a solid foundation in health assessment, health promotion, community-based practice, and primary health-care concepts.

All of the College's full-time tenure-track faculty members are doctorally prepared. Faculty members teaching in the B.S.N. and M.S. programs have a wealth of clinical expertise. In addition, students gain a breadth and depth of knowledge from nurses serving as preceptors for clinical practicum courses.

PROGRAMS OF STUDY
The College of Nursing and Health offers the B.S.N. degree, the M.S. degree, a joint M.S./M.B.A. degree in conjunction with the Raj Soin College of Business, and a school nurse certificate program in collaboration with the College of Education and Human Services. For RNs with a baccalaureate degree in a traditional discipline area other than nursing, there is a bridge program that allows students to earn the master's degree after completion of a limited number of undergraduate nursing courses. The B.S.N. and M.S. programs are accredited by the Commission on Collegiate Nursing Education (CCNE), and the M.B.A. program is accredited by AACSB International–The Association to Advance Collegiate Schools of Business.

The baccalaureate program emphasizes health and well-being across the life span and prepares graduates for entry into professional practice as generalists. The program provides entry options for prelicensure students, students seeking a second baccalaureate degree in an accelerated format, and RN students who have completed an associate degree or diploma program in nursing. The second degree students can complete the accelerated program in fifteen months. RNs are offered a program that includes transition courses that integrate their previous learning with the new knowledge provided in a baccalaureate program. Courses for RNs are offered on campus and broadcast to the outreach off-campus sites one day a week or online via the Internet. The program may be completed in seven consecutive quarters of full-time study by RNs with an associate degree. The baccalaureate program accommodates both full-time, for prelicensure and BEACON tracks, and part-time students.

The master's program educates nurses for advanced leadership roles in practice and administration as well as for doctoral study in nursing. The curriculum offers students the opportunity to prepare for roles as clinical nurse specialists in adult health or community health; nurse practitioners in the family nurse practitioner, acute-care nurse practitioner, or pediatric nurse practitioner majors, some of which have an option for post-master's study, clinical nurse leaders, school nurses, or nurse administrators in the nurse administrator major or the dual-degree (M.S./M.B.A.) program.

The master's program accommodates both full-time and part-time students, with most classes offered in the late afternoon and evening. The sequence of course offerings is flexible. Students must complete all requirements for the degree within five years.

ACADEMIC FACILITIES
The College of Nursing and Health is housed in University Hall. Clinical instructional facilities are abundant and varied. The College has contracts with more than 200 agencies in the area, including hospitals, rehabilitation centers, county health departments, nursing homes, school systems, senior citizen centers, day-care centers, and other community-based settings, which can be used for clinical experiences and research.

For research, both the Dunbar Library and the Fordham Health Sciences Library provide abundant resources. The Dunbar Library also provides media production services and facilities. The University's Statistical Consulting Center and the College's Center for Nursing and Health Research provide support for research design and data analysis. The College also has a computer laboratory that includes computer-assisted programs for classroom and independent learning.

LOCATION
The campus is located in a rural-suburban setting 10 miles east of Dayton, a business and manufacturing center with a metropolitan population approaching 1 million. The University is adjacent to Wright Patterson Air Force Base, which is a center for Air Force research and procurement. A variety of recreational, cultural, art, science, and business activities are available in the metropolitan area. Transportation to the campus via RTA is available from throughout the Miami Valley. The Dayton International Airport and downtown are less than 25 miles from the campus.

STUDENT SERVICES
The University has many resources and a variety of services for both undergraduate and graduate students. Since Wright State is a leader in providing support and accessibility to students with disabilities, a broad range of physical and academic services are available. In addition, Wright State has an International Student Program, a Child Development Center, an on-campus bookstore, Campus Ministry, six housing communities, dining services, Bolinga Cultural Resources Center, Student Health Services, Counseling Services, and the Nutter Center for sports and recreation.

THE NURSING STUDENT GROUP
There are approximately 600 undergraduate students and 200 graduate students in the College of Nursing and Health. Many of the undergraduate students are employed at least part-time and attend school full-time. Most graduate students are employed full-time in area health-care agencies in a variety of clinical and administrative positions and pursue the part-time plan.

COSTS

Tuition for undergraduate students in 2006–07 was $219 per credit hour (in-state) and $425 per credit hour (out-of-state); full-time tuition for 11 to 18 credit hours was $2426 per quarter (in-state) and $4668 per quarter (out-of-state). Tuition for graduate students was $298 per credit hour (in-state) and $507 per credit hour (out-of-state); full-time tuition for 11 to 18 credit hours was $3240 per quarter (in-state) and $5482 per quarter (out-of-state). Other expenses include books, immunizations, uniforms, insurance, and travel to clinical sites.

FINANCIAL AID

A number of scholarships based on academic excellence, as well as grants based on financial need, are available for undergraduate students. Graduate assistantships and Professional Nurse Traineeships are available for students who meet the criteria. Graduate academic fellowships, awarded on the basis of academic merit, are also available. Need-based Federal Perkins and Federal Stafford Student Loans are available to students who qualify.

APPLYING

To be eligible for admission, undergraduate students must be matriculated at the University, complete all designated prerequisite courses with a grade of C or better, and have a cumulative GPA of at least 2.5.

Graduate applicants must have an overall undergraduate GPA of at least 3.0 or an overall GPA of at least 2.7 with a 3.0 or better in the last 90 quarter hours (60 semester hours); have a B.S.N. degree from a college or university that is accredited by a nationally recognized body for nursing education accreditation or a bachelor's degree in a field other than nursing and be a registered nurse with selected support and professional nursing bridge courses; and have an Ohio RN license. All application materials for fall quarter should be submitted by April 15. Applications received after that date are considered on a space-available basis.

CORRESPONDENCE AND INFORMATION

Office of Admissions
E148 Student Union
Wright State University
3640 Colonel Glenn Highway
Dayton, Ohio 45435
Phone: 937-775-5700

School of Graduate Studies
E344 Student Union
Wright State University
3640 Colonel Glenn Highway
Dayton, Ohio 45435
Phone: 937-775-2976

THE FACULTY

Nezam Al-Nasir, Assistant Professor; M.S.N. (adult health/nursing education), Villanova; Ph.D. (nursing), Cincinnati.

Cheryl Aubin, Clinical Instructor; M.S. (nursing), Andrews.

Janice Belcher, Associate Professor; M.S. (mental health), Ohio State; Ph.D. (nursing administration), Virginia Commonwealth.

Barbara Bogan, Clinical Assistant Professor; M.S. (nursing), Ohio State.

Ann Bowling, Clinical Instructor; M.S.N. (pediatric nurse practitioner), Cincinnati.

S. Jean Budding, Clinical Assistant Professor; M.S. (nursing administration), Wright State.

Beth Cameron, Assistant Professor; M.S. (adult health nursing), Rochester; N.D. (community health), Rush.

Annette Canfield, Clinical Instructor; M.S. (education), Wright State.

Candace Cherrington, Assistant Professor; M.N. (adult health), Kansas; Ph.D. (nursing), Ohio State.

Donna Miles Curry, Associate Professor; M.S.N. (nursing of children), Saint Louis; Ph.D. (family relations and human development), Ohio State.

Jane Doorley, Clinical Assistant Professor; M.S. (rehabilitation/community health nursing), Wright State.

Katherine Enders, Clinical Instructor; M.S.U. (administration), Phoenix.

Barbara Fowler, Professor and Director of Research; M.S.N. (parent/child nursing), Cincinnati; Ed.D. (curriculum and instruction, nursing education), Cincinnati; D.N.Sc. (community nurse practitioner), Rush.

Margaret Clark Graham, Professor; M.S.N. (family nurse practitioner), Vanderbilt; Ph.D. (community health education), Ohio State.

Bobbe Gray, Assistant Professor; M.S.N., (maternal nursing), Ph.D., (nursing), Case Western Reserve.

Carrie Hall, Clinical Instructor; M.S. (family nurse practitioner), Wright State.

Crystal Hammond, Clinical Instructor; M.S.N. (nurse midwifery), Case Western Reserve.

Wajed Hatamleh, Assistant Professor; M.S.N. (nursing), Villanova; Ph.D. (nursing), Cincinnati.

Laura Herbert, Clinical Instructor; M.S., Wright State (community health nursing).

Carol Holdcraft, Assistant Professor and Assistant Dean; M.S.N. (adult psychiatric nursing), Cincinnati; D.N.S. (nursing), Indiana.

Cindra Holland, Assistant Professor; M.S. (adult health), Wright State.

Catherine Johnson, Assistant Professor; M.S. (nursing), Ohio State; M.S. (family nurse practitioner), Wright State; Ph.D. (nursing), Duquesne.

Kathy Keister, Assistant Professor; M.S. (adult health), Illinois; Ph.D. (nursing), Case Western Reserve.

Lynne Kelley, Clinical Assistant Professor; M.P.H. (health policy), Emory; M.S.N. (maternal-child health), Cincinnati.

Kim Lawrence, Clinical Instructor; M.S.N. (nurse midwifery), Cincinnati.

Yi-Hui Lee, Assistant Professor; M.S.N. (pediatrics), National Taiwan; Ph.D. (nursing), Case Western Reserve.

Judie Lincks, Clinical Instructor; M.S. (nursing administration), Wright State.

Mariann Lovell, Assistant Professor; M.S. (community health), Wright State; Ph.D. (nursing), Ohio State.

Mary Lynd, Assistant Professor; M.S.N. (nursing service administration), Cincinnati; Ph.D. (nursing), Texas Woman's.

Patricia Martin, Professor and Dean; M.S. (rehabilitation/community health nursing), Wright State; Ph.D. (nursing), Case Western Reserve.

Gail Moddeman, Assistant Professor; M.S. (nursing administration), Wright State; Ph.D. (nursing), Kentucky.

Carol Nikolai, Clinical Instructor; M.S. (family nurse practitioner), Wright State.

Robin Osterman, Clinical Assistant Professor; M.S.N. (psychiatric nursing), Cincinnati.

Susan Praeger, Professor; M.S. (nursing), New York Medical College; Ed.D. (humanistic nursing education), Northern Colorado.

Christine Riggle, Clinical Instructor; M.S.N. (pediatric nursing), Indiana.

Leatha Ross, Assistant Professor; M.S. (family nurse practitioner), Wright State.

Anne Russell, Clinical Instructor; M.S.N. (adult health/critical care), Pennsylvania.

Kenneth Schmidt, Clinical Instructor; M.S.N. (nursing administration), Phoenix.

Kristine A. Scordo, Professor; M.S. (cardiovascular nursing), Ph.D. (cardiac physiology), Ohio State.

Elizabeth Sorensen, Assistant Professor; M.S. (nursing administration), New Hampshire; Ph.D. (nursing research), Ohio State.

Ann Stalter, Clinical Instructor; M.S. (nursing administration), Wright State.

Kim Stewart, Clinical Instructor; M.S. (adult health nursing), Wright State.

Marianna Sunderlin, Clinical Instructor; M.S.N. (advanced clinical nursing), George Mason.

Alice Teall, Clinical Assistant Professor; M.S. (family nurse practitioner), Wright State.

Patricia Vermeersch, Assistant Professor; M.S. (gerontological nursing), Ph.D. (clinical nursing research), Case Western Reserve.

Joyce Zurmehly, Assistant Professor; M.S.N. (nursing education), Bellarmine; Ph.D. (health services), Walden.

INDEXES

ACCELERATED BACCALAUREATE

Alabama
University of South Alabama, College of Nursing, *Mobile* (BSN)

Arizona
Arizona State University at the Downtown Phoenix Campus, College of Nursing, *Phoenix* (BSN)

Grand Canyon University, College of Nursing, *Phoenix* (BSN)

Northern Arizona University, School of Nursing, *Flagstaff* (BSN)

University of Phoenix Online Campus, College of Health and Human Services, *Phoenix* (BSN)

University of Phoenix-Phoenix Campus, College of Health and Human Services, *Phoenix* (BSN)

University of Phoenix-Southern Arizona Campus, College of Health and Human Services, *Tucson* (BSN)

California
Azusa Pacific University, School of Nursing, *Azusa* (BSN)

Loma Linda University, School of Nursing, *Loma Linda* (BS)

Mount St. Mary's College, Department of Nursing, *Los Angeles* (BSN)

National University, Department of Nursing, *La Jolla* (BSN)

Samuel Merritt College, School of Nursing, *Oakland* (BSN)

University of Phoenix-Bay Area Campus, College of Health and Human Services, *Pleasanton* (BSN)

University of Phoenix-Sacramento Valley Campus, College of Health and Human Services, *Sacramento* (BSN)

University of Phoenix-San Diego Campus, College of Health and Human Services, *San Diego* (BSN)

University of Phoenix-Southern California Campus, College of Health and Human Services, *Costa Mesa* (BSN)

Colorado
Regis University, Department of Nursing, *Denver* (BSN)

University of Northern Colorado, School of Nursing, *Greeley* (BS)

University of Phoenix-Denver Campus, College of Health and Human Services, *Lone Tree* (BSN)

University of Phoenix-Southern Colorado Campus, College of Health and Human Services, *Colorado Springs* (BSN)

Connecticut
Saint Joseph College, Department of Nursing, *West Hartford* (BS)

Florida
Barry University, School of Nursing, *Miami Shores* (BSN)

Florida International University, College of Nursing and Health Sciences, *Miami* (BSN)

Jacksonville University, School of Nursing, *Jacksonville* (BSN)

University of Miami, School of Nursing and Health Studies, *Coral Gables* (BSN)

University of Phoenix-Central Florida Campus, College of Health and Human Services, *Maitland* (BSN)

University of Phoenix-North Florida Campus, College of Health and Human Services, *Jacksonville* (BSN)

University of Phoenix-West Florida Campus, College of Health and Human Services, *Temple Terrace* (BSN)

University of South Florida, College of Nursing, *Tampa* (BS)

Georgia
Georgia State University, School of Nursing, *Atlanta* (BS)

Kennesaw State University, School of Nursing, *Kennesaw* (BSN)

University of Phoenix-Atlanta Campus, College of Health and Human Services, *Atlanta* (BSN)

Hawaii
Hawai'i Pacific University, School of Nursing, *Honolulu* (BSN)

University of Phoenix-Hawaii Campus, College of Health and Human Services, *Honolulu* (BSN)

Illinois
Loyola University Chicago, Marcella Niehoff School of Nursing, *Chicago* (BSN)

Southern Illinois University Edwardsville, School of Nursing, *Edwardsville* (BS)

Indiana
Saint Mary's College, Department of Nursing, *Notre Dame* (BS)

Valparaiso University, College of Nursing, *Valparaiso* (BSN)

Iowa
Allen College, Program in Nursing, *Waterloo* (BSN)

Mercy College of Health Sciences, Division of Nursing, *Des Moines* (BSN)

Kansas
MidAmerica Nazarene University, Division of Nursing, *Olathe* (BSN)

Louisiana
Southeastern Louisiana University, School of Nursing, *Hammond* (BS)

University of Louisiana at Monroe, Nursing, *Monroe* (BS)

University of Phoenix-Louisiana Campus, College of Health and Human Services, *Metairie* (BSN)

Maine
University of Maine at Fort Kent, Department of Nursing, *Fort Kent* (BSN)

Massachusetts
Regis College, Department of Nursing, *Weston* (BSN)

Simmons College, Department of Nursing, *Boston* (BS)

Michigan
Ferris State University, School of Nursing, *Big Rapids* (BSN)

Grand Valley State University, Russell B. Kirkhof College of Nursing, *Allendale* (BSN)

Northern Michigan University, College of Nursing and Allied Health Science, *Marquette* (BSN)

University of Phoenix-Metro Detroit Campus, College of Health and Human Services, *Southfield* (BSN)

University of Phoenix-West Michigan Campus, College of Health and Human Services, *Grand Rapids* (BSN)

Missouri
Cox College of Nursing and Health Sciences, Department of Nursing, *Springfield* (BSN)

Graceland University, School of Nursing, *Independence* (BSN)

Maryville University of Saint Louis, Nursing Program, School of Health Professions, *St. Louis* (BSN)

Research College of Nursing, College of Nursing, *Kansas City* (BSN)

Saint Louis University, School of Nursing, *St. Louis* (BSN)

University of Missouri-St. Louis, College of Nursing, *St. Louis* (BSN)

William Jewell College, Department of Nursing, *Liberty* (BS)

Nebraska
University of Nebraska Medical Center, College of Nursing, *Omaha* (BSN)

Nevada
University of Nevada, Reno, Orvis School of Nursing, *Reno* (BSN)

New Mexico
University of Phoenix-New Mexico Campus, College of Health and Human Services, *Albuquerque* (BSN)

New York
Adelphi University, School of Nursing, *Garden City* (BS)

Hartwick College, Department of Nursing, *Oneonta* (BS)

Mount Saint Mary College, Division of Nursing, *Newburgh* (BSN)

New York University, College of Nursing, *New York* (BS)

Stony Brook University, State University of New York, School of Nursing, *Stony Brook* (BS)

Ohio
Cleveland State University, Department of Nursing, *Cleveland* (BSN)

Kent State University, College of Nursing, *Kent* (BSN)

MedCentral College of Nursing, *Mansfield* (BS)

University of Phoenix-Cleveland Campus, College of Health and Human Services, *Independence* (BSN)

Oklahoma
University of Phoenix-Oklahoma City Campus, College of Health and Human Services, *Oklahoma City* (BSN)

Oregon
Oregon Health & Science University, School of Nursing, *Portland* (BS)

Pennsylvania
College Misericordia, Department of Nursing, *Dallas* (BSN)

DeSales University, Department of Nursing and Health, *Center Valley* (BSN)

Holy Family University, School of Nursing and Allied Health Professions, *Philadelphia* (BSN)

Temple University, Department of Nursing, *Philadelphia* (BSN)

Thomas Jefferson University, Department of Nursing, *Philadelphia* (BSN)

University of Pennsylvania, School of Nursing, *Philadelphia* (BSN)

Puerto Rico
Inter American University of Puerto Rico, Metropolitan Campus, Carmen Torres de Tiburcio School of Nursing, *San Juan* (BSN)

South Carolina
Lander University, School of Nursing, *Greenwood* (BSN)

Medical University of South Carolina, College of Nursing, *Charleston* (BSN)

South Dakota
South Dakota State University, College of Nursing, *Brookings* (BS)

Tennessee
Belmont University, School of Nursing, *Nashville* (BSN)

Carson-Newman College, Department of Nursing, *Jefferson City* (BSN)

Cumberland University, Rudy School of Nursing and Health Professions, *Lebanon* (BSN)

University of Memphis, Loewenberg School of Nursing, *Memphis* (BSN)

The University of Tennessee Health Science Center, College of Nursing, *Memphis* (BSN)

Texas
The University of Texas at El Paso, School of Nursing, *El Paso* (BSN)

Utah
University of Phoenix-Utah Campus, College of Health and Human Services, *Salt Lake City* (BSN)

Virginia
Hampton University, Department of Nursing, *Hampton* (BS)

Marymount University, School of Health Professions, *Arlington* (BSN)

Old Dominion University, Department of Nursing, *Norfolk* (BSN)

Wisconsin
Bellin College of Nursing, Nursing Program, *Green Bay* (BSN)

University of Wisconsin–Oshkosh, College of Nursing, *Oshkosh* (BSN)

CANADA

Alberta
University of Calgary, Faculty of Nursing, *Calgary* (BN)

Nova Scotia
Dalhousie University, School of Nursing, *Halifax* (BScN)

St. Francis Xavier University, Department of Nursing, *Antigonish* (BScN)

Ontario
Queen's University at Kingston, School of Nursing, *Kingston* (BNSc)

Trent University, Nursing Program, *Peterborough* (BScN)

The University of Western Ontario, School of Nursing, *London* (BScN)

Saskatchewan
University of Saskatchewan, College of Nursing, *Saskatoon* (BSN)

ACCELERATED BACCALAUREATE FOR SECOND DEGREE

Alabama
Auburn University, School of Nursing, *Auburn University* (BSN)

Arizona
Arizona State University at the Downtown Phoenix Campus, College of Nursing, *Phoenix* (BSN)

Grand Canyon University, College of Nursing, *Phoenix* (BSN)

Northern Arizona University, School of Nursing, *Flagstaff* (BSN)

The University of Arizona, College of Nursing, *Tucson* (BSN)

Arkansas
University of Arkansas for Medical Sciences, College of Nursing, *Little Rock* (BSN)

California
California State University, Bakersfield, Program in Nursing, *Bakersfield* (BSN)

Loma Linda University, School of Nursing, *Loma Linda* (BS)

Colorado
Colorado State University-Pueblo, Department of Nursing, *Pueblo* (BSN)

University of Colorado at Colorado Springs, Beth-El College of Nursing and Health Sciences, *Colorado Springs* (BSN)

Connecticut
Fairfield University, School of Nursing, *Fairfield* (BS)

Quinnipiac University, Department of Nursing, *Hamden* (BSN)

Saint Joseph College, Department of Nursing, *West Hartford* (BS)

Delaware
University of Delaware, School of Nursing, *Newark* (BSN)

District of Columbia
The Catholic University of America, School of Nursing, *Washington* (BSN)

Georgetown University, School of Nursing and Health Studies, *Washington* (BSN)

Howard University, Division of Nursing, *Washington* (BSN)

Florida
Barry University, School of Nursing, *Miami Shores* (BSN)

Florida Atlantic University, College of Nursing, *Boca Raton* (BSN)

Florida Gulf Coast University, School of Nursing, *Fort Myers* (BSN)

Florida International University, College of Nursing and Health Sciences, *Miami* (BSN)

Jacksonville University, School of Nursing, *Jacksonville* (BSN)

University of Central Florida, School of Nursing, *Orlando* (BSN)

University of Florida, College of Nursing, *Gainesville* (BSN)

University of Miami, School of Nursing and Health Studies, *Coral Gables* (BSN)

University of North Florida, School of Nursing, *Jacksonville* (BSN)

University of South Florida, College of Nursing, *Tampa* (BS)

Georgia
Kennesaw State University, School of Nursing, *Kennesaw* (BSN)

Idaho
Idaho State University, Department of Nursing, *Pocatello* (BSN)

Illinois
Blessing-Rieman College of Nursing, *Quincy* (BSN)

Illinois State University, Mennonite College of Nursing, *Normal* (BSN)

Lewis University, Program in Nursing, *Romeoville* (BSN)

Rush University, College of Nursing, *Chicago* (BSN)

West Suburban College of Nursing, *Oak Park* (BSN)

Indiana
Ball State University, School of Nursing, *Muncie* (BS)

Indiana University–Purdue University Indianapolis, School of Nursing, *Indianapolis* (BSN)

Indiana University South Bend, Division of Nursing and Health Professions, *South Bend* (BSN)

Indiana Wesleyan University, Division of Nursing, *Marion* (BS)

Marian College, Department of Nursing and Nutritional Science, *Indianapolis* (BSN)

Iowa
Allen College, Program in Nursing, *Waterloo* (BSN)

Mercy College of Health Sciences, Division of Nursing, *Des Moines* (BSN)

Kansas
MidAmerica Nazarene University, Division of Nursing, *Olathe* (BSN)

Kentucky
Bellarmine University, Donna and Allan Lansing School of Nursing and Health Sciences, *Louisville* (BSN)

Northern Kentucky University, Department of Nursing, *Highland Heights* (BSN)

Spalding University, School of Nursing, *Louisville* (BSN)

University of Louisville, School of Nursing, *Louisville* (BSN)

Louisiana
University of Louisiana at Lafayette, College of Nursing, *Lafayette* (BSN)

Maine
University of Southern Maine, College of Nursing and Health Professions, *Portland* (BS)

Maryland
The Johns Hopkins University, School of Nursing, *Baltimore* (BS)

Salisbury University, Program in Nursing, *Salisbury* (BS)

Villa Julie College, Nursing Division, *Stevenson* (BS)

Massachusetts
Curry College, Division of Nursing, *Milton* (BS)

Regis College, Department of Nursing, *Weston* (BSN)

Salem State College, Program in Nursing, *Salem* (BSN)

Simmons College, Department of Nursing, *Boston* (BS)

University of Massachusetts Amherst, School of Nursing, *Amherst* (BS)

Michigan
Grand Valley State University, Russell B. Kirkhof College of Nursing, *Allendale* (BSN)

Michigan State University, College of Nursing, *East Lansing* (BSN)

Northern Michigan University, College of Nursing and Allied Health Science, *Marquette* (BSN)

Saginaw Valley State University, Crystal M. Lange College of Nursing and Health Sciences, *University Center* (BSN)

University of Michigan, School of Nursing, *Ann Arbor* (BSN)

Wayne State University, College of Nursing, *Detroit* (BSN)

Minnesota
The College of St. Scholastica, Department of Nursing, *Duluth* (BA)

Concordia College, Department of Nursing, *Moorhead* (BA)

Minnesota State University Mankato, School of Nursing, *Mankato* (BS)

Mississippi
University of Mississippi Medical Center, Program in Nursing, *Jackson* (BSN)

Missouri
Cox College of Nursing and Health Sciences, Department of Nursing, *Springfield* (BSN)

Graceland University, School of Nursing, *Independence* (BSN)

Research College of Nursing, College of Nursing, *Kansas City* (BSN)

Saint Louis University, School of Nursing, *St. Louis* (BSN)

University of Missouri–Columbia, Sinclair School of Nursing, *Columbia* (BSN)

Nebraska

Creighton University, School of Nursing, *Omaha* (BSN)

Nebraska Methodist College, Department of Nursing, *Omaha* (BSN)

University of Nebraska Medical Center, College of Nursing, *Omaha* (BSN)

New Jersey

Fairleigh Dickinson University, Metropolitan Campus, Henry P. Becton School of Nursing and Allied Health, *Teaneck* (BSN)

Rutgers, The State University of New Jersey, College of Nursing, *Newark* (BS)

Seton Hall University, College of Nursing, *South Orange* (BSN)

University of Medicine and Dentistry of New Jersey, School of Nursing, *Newark* (BSN)

William Paterson University of New Jersey, Department of Nursing, *Wayne* (BSN)

New Mexico

New Mexico State University, Department of Nursing, *Las Cruces* (BSN)

University of New Mexico, College of Nursing, *Albuquerque* (BSN)

New York

Adelphi University, School of Nursing, *Garden City* (BS)

The College of New Rochelle, School of Nursing, *New Rochelle* (BSN)

Columbia University, School of Nursing, *New York* (BS)

Dominican College, Department of Nursing, *Orangeburg* (BSN)

Hartwick College, Department of Nursing, *Oneonta* (BS)

New York University, College of Nursing, *New York* (BS)

Pace University, Lienhard School of Nursing, *New York* (BS)

State University of New York Downstate Medical Center, College of Nursing, *Brooklyn* (BS)

University at Buffalo, the State University of New York, School of Nursing, *Buffalo* (BS)

University of Rochester, School of Nursing, *Rochester* (BS)

North Carolina

Duke University, School of Nursing, *Durham* (BSN)

The University of North Carolina at Chapel Hill, School of Nursing, *Chapel Hill* (BSN)

Ohio

Capital University, School of Nursing, *Columbus* (BSN)

Cleveland State University, Department of Nursing, *Cleveland* (BSN)

Kent State University, College of Nursing, *Kent* (BSN)

Mount Carmel College of Nursing, Nursing Programs, *Columbus* (BSN)

The University of Akron, College of Nursing, *Akron* (BSN)

Ursuline College, The Breen School of Nursing, *Pepper Pike* (BSN)

Wright State University, College of Nursing and Health, *Dayton* (BSN)

Oklahoma

Oklahoma City University, Kramer School of Nursing, *Oklahoma City* (BSN)

University of Oklahoma Health Sciences Center, College of Nursing, *Oklahoma City* (BSN)

Oregon

Linfield College, School of Nursing, *McMinnville* (BSN)

Pennsylvania

College Misericordia, Department of Nursing, *Dallas* (BSN)

Drexel University, College of Nursing and Health Professions, *Philadelphia* (BSN)

Duquesne University, School of Nursing, *Pittsburgh* (BSN)

Edinboro University of Pennsylvania, Department of Nursing, *Edinboro* (BS)

Temple University, Department of Nursing, *Philadelphia* (BSN)

Thomas Jefferson University, Department of Nursing, *Philadelphia* (BSN)

University of Pennsylvania, School of Nursing, *Philadelphia* (BSN)

University of Pittsburgh, School of Nursing, *Pittsburgh* (BSN)

Villanova University, College of Nursing, *Villanova* (BSN)

Waynesburg College, Department of Nursing, *Waynesburg* (BSN)

Wilkes University, Department of Nursing, *Wilkes-Barre* (BS)

South Carolina

Lander University, School of Nursing, *Greenwood* (BSN)

Tennessee

Belmont University, School of Nursing, *Nashville* (BSN)

Cumberland University, Rudy School of Nursing and Health Professions, *Lebanon* (BSN)

East Tennessee State University, College of Nursing, *Johnson City* (BSN)

Union University, School of Nursing, *Jackson* (BSN)

University of Memphis, Loewenberg School of Nursing, *Memphis* (BSN)

The University of Tennessee Health Science Center, College of Nursing, *Memphis* (BSN)

Texas

Texas A&M University–Corpus Christi, School of Nursing and Health Sciences, *Corpus Christi* (BSN)

Texas Christian University, Harris School of Nursing, *Fort Worth* (BSN)

Texas Tech University Health Sciences Center, School of Nursing, *Lubbock* (BSN)

The University of Texas Health Science Center at Houston, School of Nursing, *Houston* (BSN)

The University of Texas Medical Branch, School of Nursing, *Galveston* (BSN)

Virginia

George Mason University, College of Nursing and Health Science, *Fairfax* (BSN)

Marymount University, School of Health Professions, *Arlington* (BSN)

Norfolk State University, Department of Nursing, *Norfolk* (BSN)

Shenandoah University, Division of Nursing, *Winchester* (BSN)

Virginia Commonwealth University, School of Nursing, *Richmond* (BS)

West Virginia

West Virginia University, School of Nursing, *Morgantown* (BSN)

Wisconsin

Bellin College of Nursing, Nursing Program, *Green Bay* (BSN)

University of Wisconsin–Eau Claire, College of Nursing and Health Sciences, *Eau Claire* (BSN)

University of Wisconsin–Oshkosh, College of Nursing, *Oshkosh* (BSN)

Wyoming

University of Wyoming, Fay W. Whitney School of Nursing, *Laramie* (BSN)

CANADA

Alberta

University of Calgary, Faculty of Nursing, *Calgary* (BN)

British Columbia

The University of British Columbia, School of Nursing, *Vancouver* (BSN)

Newfoundland and Labrador

Memorial University of Newfoundland, School of Nursing, *St. John's* (BN)

Nova Scotia

Dalhousie University, School of Nursing, *Halifax* (BScN)

St. Francis Xavier University, Department of Nursing, *Antigonish* (BScN)

Ontario

The University of Western Ontario, School of Nursing, *London* (BScN)

ACCELERATED LPN TO BACCALAUREATE

California

Loma Linda University, School of Nursing, *Loma Linda* (BS)

San Francisco State University, School of Nursing, *San Francisco* (BSN)

Kansas

MidAmerica Nazarene University, Division of Nursing, *Olathe* (BSN)

Louisiana

McNeese State University, College of Nursing, *Lake Charles* (BSN)

Michigan

Northern Michigan University, College of Nursing and Allied Health Science, *Marquette* (BSN)

New York

Dominican College, Department of Nursing, *Orangeburg* (BSN)

Ohio

Ursuline College, The Breen School of Nursing, *Pepper Pike* (BSN)

Pennsylvania

The University of Scranton, Department of Nursing, *Scranton* (BS)

Wilkes University, Department of Nursing, *Wilkes-Barre* (BS)

Virginia

George Mason University, College of Nursing and Health Science, *Fairfax* (BSN)

Norfolk State University, Department of Nursing, *Norfolk* (BSN)

CANADA

Nova Scotia

St. Francis Xavier University, Department of Nursing, *Antigonish* (BScN)

ACCELERATED RN BACCALAUREATE

Alabama

The University of Alabama at Birmingham, School of Nursing, *Birmingham* (BSN)

Arizona

Arizona State University at the Downtown Phoenix Campus, College of Nursing, *Phoenix* (BSN)

Arkansas

University of Arkansas for Medical Sciences, College of Nursing, *Little Rock* (BSN)

California

Azusa Pacific University, School of Nursing, *Azusa* (BSN)

Loma Linda University, School of Nursing, *Loma Linda* (BS)

Colorado

Colorado State University-Pueblo, Department of Nursing, *Pueblo* (BSN)

Delaware

Wilmington College, Division of Nursing, *New Castle* (BSN)

District of Columbia

Howard University, Division of Nursing, *Washington* (BSN)

Florida

Florida Gulf Coast University, School of Nursing, *Fort Myers* (BSN)

Jacksonville University, School of Nursing, *Jacksonville* (BSN)

Georgia

Albany State University, College of Health Professions, *Albany* (BSN)

Columbus State University, Nursing Program, *Columbus* (BSN)

Georgia State University, School of Nursing, *Atlanta* (BS)

Illinois

Benedictine University, Department of Nursing, *Lisle* (BSN)

DePaul University, Department of Nursing, *Chicago* (BS)

Lakeview College of Nursing, *Danville* (BSN)

Lewis University, Program in Nursing, *Romeoville* (BSN)

Millikin University, School of Nursing, *Decatur* (BSN)

Olivet Nazarene University, Division of Nursing, *Bourbonnais* (BSN)

University of St. Francis, College of Nursing and Allied Health, *Joliet* (BSN)

Indiana

Indiana University Kokomo, Indiana University School of Nursing, *Kokomo* (BSN)

University of Indianapolis, School of Nursing, *Indianapolis* (BSN)

Iowa

Allen College, Program in Nursing, *Waterloo* (BSN)

Mount Mercy College, Department of Nursing, *Cedar Rapids* (BSN)

Kansas

MidAmerica Nazarene University, Division of Nursing, *Olathe* (BSN)

Tabor College, Department of Nursing, *Hillsboro* (BSN)

Kentucky

Midway College, Program in Nursing (Baccalaureate), *Midway* (BSN)

Spalding University, School of Nursing, *Louisville* (BSN)

University of Louisville, School of Nursing, *Louisville* (BSN)

Louisiana

Southeastern Louisiana University, School of Nursing, *Hammond* (BS)

Maryland

College of Notre Dame of Maryland, Department of Nursing, *Baltimore* (BS)

Columbia Union College, Nursing Department, *Takoma Park* (BS)

Coppin State University, Helene Fuld School of Nursing, *Baltimore* (BSN)

Salisbury University, Program in Nursing, *Salisbury* (BS)

Villa Julie College, Nursing Division, *Stevenson* (BS)

Massachusetts

Regis College, Department of Nursing, *Weston* (BSN)

University of Massachusetts Amherst, School of Nursing, *Amherst* (BS)

Worcester State College, Department of Nursing, *Worcester* (BS)

Minnesota

The College of St. Scholastica, Department of Nursing, *Duluth* (BA)

Missouri

Graceland University, School of Nursing, *Independence* (BSN)

Maryville University of Saint Louis, Nursing Program, School of Health Professions, *St. Louis* (BSN)

Nebraska

Clarkson College, Department of Nursing, *Omaha* (BSN)

Nebraska Wesleyan University, Department of Nursing, *Lincoln* (BSN)

University of Nebraska Medical Center, College of Nursing, *Omaha* (BSN)

New Jersey

College of Saint Elizabeth, Department of Nursing, *Morristown* (BSN)

Felician College, Department of Professional Nursing–BSN, *Lodi* (BSN)

Rutgers, The State University of New Jersey, Camden College of Arts and Sciences, Department of Nursing, *Camden* (BS)

New York

The College of New Rochelle, School of Nursing, *New Rochelle* (BSN)

Daemen College, Department of Nursing, *Amherst* (BS)

Dominican College, Department of Nursing, *Orangeburg* (BSN)

Keuka College, Division of Nursing, *Keuka Park* (BS)

Medgar Evers College of the City University of New York, Department of Nursing, *Brooklyn* (BSN)

Mercy College, Program in Nursing, *Dobbs Ferry* (BS)

Molloy College, Department of Nursing, *Rockville Centre* (BS)

Mount Saint Mary College, Division of Nursing, *Newburgh* (BSN)

Pace University, Lienhard School of Nursing, *New York* (BS)

Roberts Wesleyan College, Division of Nursing, *Rochester* (BScN)

State University of New York at Binghamton, Decker School of Nursing, *Binghamton* (BS)

State University of New York Institute of Technology, School of Nursing and Health Systems, *Utica* (BS)

Stony Brook University, State University of New York, School of Nursing, *Stony Brook* (BS)

University of Rochester, School of Nursing, *Rochester* (BS)

North Carolina

East Carolina University, School of Nursing, *Greenville* (BSN)

Winston-Salem State University, Department of Nursing, *Winston-Salem* (BSN)

Ohio

Ashland University, Department of Nursing, *Ashland* (BSN)

College of Mount St. Joseph, Department of Nursing, *Cincinnati* (BSN)

Kent State University, College of Nursing, *Kent* (BSN)

The Ohio State University, College of Nursing, *Columbus* (BSN)

Otterbein College, Department of Nursing, *Westerville* (BSN)

Ursuline College, The Breen School of Nursing, *Pepper Pike* (BSN)

Walsh University, Department of Nursing, *North Canton* (BSN)

Oklahoma

Bacone College, Department of Nursing, *Muskogee* (BSN)

Northeastern State University, Department of Nursing, *Tahlequah* (BSN)

Oklahoma Wesleyan University, Division of Nursing, *Bartlesville* (BSN)

Pennsylvania

Carlow University, School of Nursing, *Pittsburgh* (BSN)

College Misericordia, Department of Nursing, *Dallas* (BSN)

DeSales University, Department of Nursing and Health, *Center Valley* (BSN)

Duquesne University, School of Nursing, *Pittsburgh* (BSN)

Eastern University, Program in Nursing, *St. Davids* (BSN)

Edinboro University of Pennsylvania, Department of Nursing, *Edinboro* (BS)

Gwynedd-Mercy College, School of Nursing, *Gwynedd Valley* (BSN)

Immaculata University, Department of Nursing, *Immaculata* (BSN)

La Roche College, Department of Nursing and Nursing Management, *Pittsburgh* (BSN)

Mount Aloysius College, Department of Nursing, *Cresson* (BSN)

Thomas Jefferson University, Department of Nursing, *Philadelphia* (BSN)

University of Pennsylvania, School of Nursing, *Philadelphia* (BSN)

Waynesburg College, Department of Nursing, *Waynesburg* (BSN)

West Chester University of Pennsylvania, Department of Nursing, *West Chester* (BSN)

Wilkes University, Department of Nursing, *Wilkes-Barre* (BS)

South Carolina

Lander University, School of Nursing, *Greenwood* (BSN)

Medical University of South Carolina, College of Nursing, *Charleston* (BSN)

University of South Carolina Upstate, Mary Black School of Nursing, *Spartanburg* (BSN)

Tennessee

Cumberland University, Rudy School of Nursing and Health Professions, *Lebanon* (BSN)

East Tennessee State University, College of Nursing, *Johnson City* (BSN)

King College, School of Nursing, *Bristol* (BSN)

University of Memphis, Loewenberg School of Nursing, *Memphis* (BSN)

The University of Tennessee, College of Nursing, *Knoxville* (BSN)

The University of Tennessee at Martin, Department of Nursing, *Martin* (BSN)

The University of Tennessee Health Science Center, College of Nursing, *Memphis* (BSN)

Texas

The University of Texas at Tyler, Program in Nursing, *Tyler* (BSN)

The University of Texas Health Science Center at Houston, School of Nursing, *Houston* (BSN)

Vermont

University of Vermont, Department of Nursing, *Burlington* (BS)

Virginia

George Mason University, College of Nursing and Health Science, *Fairfax* (BSN)

Hampton University, Department of Nursing, *Hampton* (BS)

James Madison University, Department of Nursing, *Harrisonburg* (BSN)

Marymount University, School of Health Professions, *Arlington* (BSN)

Norfolk State University, Department of Nursing, *Norfolk* (BSN)

West Virginia

Marshall University, College of Health Professions, *Huntington* (BSN)

West Liberty State College, Department of Health Sciences, *West Liberty* (BSN)

Wisconsin

Cardinal Stritch University, Ruth S. Coleman College of Nursing, *Milwaukee* (BSN)

University of Wisconsin-Madison, School of Nursing, *Madison* (BS)

University of Wisconsin-Oshkosh, College of Nursing, *Oshkosh* (BSN)

CANADA

Ontario

University of Toronto, Faculty of Nursing, *Toronto* (BScN)

Quebec

Université du Québec à Chicoutimi, Program in Nursing, *Chicoutimi* (BNSc)

Saskatchewan

University of Saskatchewan, College of Nursing, *Saskatoon* (BSN)

ADN TO BACCALAUREATE

Alabama

Troy University, School of Nursing, *Troy* (BSN)

Tuskegee University, Program in Nursing, *Tuskegee* (BSN)

University of South Alabama, College of Nursing, *Mobile* (BSN)

Arizona

Grand Canyon University, College of Nursing, *Phoenix* (BSN)

Northern Arizona University, School of Nursing, *Flagstaff* (BSN)

Arkansas

Arkansas Tech University, Program in Nursing, *Russellville* (BSN)

Harding University, College of Nursing, *Searcy* (BSN)

Henderson State University, Department of Nursing, *Arkadelphia* (BSN)

University of Arkansas at Monticello, Division of Nursing, *Monticello* (BSN)

University of Arkansas for Medical Sciences, College of Nursing, *Little Rock* (BSN)

University of Central Arkansas, Department of Nursing, *Conway* (BSN)

California

Azusa Pacific University, School of Nursing, *Azusa* (BSN)

Biola University, Department of Nursing, *La Mirada* (BSN)

California State University, Chico, School of Nursing, *Chico* (BSN)

California State University, Fresno, Department of Nursing, *Fresno* (BSN)

California State University, Fullerton, Department of Nursing, *Fullerton* (BSN)

California State University, Long Beach, Department of Nursing, *Long Beach* (BSN)

California State University, Northridge, Nursing Program, *Northridge* (BSN)

California State University, Sacramento, Division of Nursing, *Sacramento* (BSN)

California State University, San Bernardino, Department of Nursing, *San Bernardino* (BSN)

California State University, Stanislaus, Department of Nursing, *Turlock* (BSN)

Humboldt State University, Department of Nursing, *Arcata* (BSN)

Loma Linda University, School of Nursing, *Loma Linda* (BS)

Mount St. Mary's College, Department of Nursing, *Los Angeles* (BSN)

Pacific Union College, Department of Nursing, *Angwin* (BSN)

Point Loma Nazarene University, School of Nursing, *San Diego* (BSN)

San Francisco State University, School of Nursing, *San Francisco* (BSN)

Sonoma State University, Department of Nursing, *Rohnert Park* (BSN)

University of California, Los Angeles, School of Nursing, *Los Angeles* (BS)

University of San Diego, Hahn School of Nursing and Health Sciences, *San Diego* (BSN)

Colorado

Colorado State University-Pueblo, Department of Nursing, *Pueblo* (BSN)

Mesa State College, Department of Nursing and Radiologic Sciences, *Grand Junction* (BSN)

Metropolitan State College of Denver, Department of Health Professions, *Denver* (BS)

Connecticut

Sacred Heart University, Program in Nursing, *Fairfield* (BS)

Southern Connecticut State University, Department of Nursing, *New Haven* (BSN)

University of Hartford, College of Education, Nursing, and Health Professions, *West Hartford* (BSN)

District of Columbia

Howard University, Division of Nursing, *Washington* (BSN)

University of the District of Columbia, Nursing Education Program, *Washington* (BSN)

Florida

Barry University, School of Nursing, *Miami Shores* (BSN)

Florida Atlantic University, College of Nursing, *Boca Raton* (BSN)

Florida Gulf Coast University, School of Nursing, *Fort Myers* (BSN)

Florida Southern College, Department of Nursing, *Lakeland* (BSN)

Florida State University, School of Nursing, *Tallahassee* (BSN)

Jacksonville University, School of Nursing, *Jacksonville* (BSN)

St. Petersburg College, Department of Nursing, *St. Petersburg* (BSN)

University of South Florida, College of Nursing, *Tampa* (BS)

The University of Tampa, Department of Nursing, *Tampa* (BSN)

University of West Florida, Department of Nursing, *Pensacola* (BSN)

Georgia

Albany State University, College of Health Professions, *Albany* (BSN)

Armstrong Atlantic State University, Program in Nursing, *Savannah* (BSN)

Brenau University, School of Health and Science, *Gainesville* (BSN)

Georgia Southern University, School of Nursing, *Statesboro* (BSN)

Kennesaw State University, School of Nursing, *Kennesaw* (BSN)

Macon State College, Division of Nursing and Health Sciences, *Macon* (BSN)

Medical College of Georgia, School of Nursing, *Augusta* (BSN)

Thomas University, Division of Nursing, *Thomasville* (BSN)

Guam

University of Guam, College of Nursing and Health Sciences, *Mangilao* (BSN)

Hawaii

University of Hawaii at Hilo, Department in Nursing, *Hilo* (BSN)

University of Hawaii at Manoa, School of Nursing and Dental Hygiene, *Honolulu* (BS)

Idaho

Idaho State University, Department of Nursing, *Pocatello* (BSN)

Lewis-Clark State College, Division of Nursing and Health Sciences, *Lewiston* (BSN)

Illinois

Illinois State University, Mennonite College of Nursing, *Normal* (BSN)

MacMurray College, Department of Nursing, *Jacksonville* (BSN)

McKendree College, Department of Nursing, *Lebanon* (BSN)

Rockford College, Department of Nursing, *Rockford* (BSN)

Rush University, College of Nursing, *Chicago* (BSN)

Trinity College of Nursing and Health Sciences, *Rock Island* (BSN)

West Suburban College of Nursing, *Oak Park* (BSN)

Indiana

Bethel College, Department of Nursing, *Mishawaka* (BSN)

Indiana University East, Division of Nursing, *Richmond* (BSN)

Indiana University–Purdue University Indianapolis, School of Nursing, *Indianapolis* (BSN)

Indiana Wesleyan University, Division of Nursing, *Marion* (BS)

Purdue University, School of Nursing, *West Lafayette* (BS)

University of Saint Francis, Department of Nursing, *Fort Wayne* (BSN)

Iowa

Allen College, Program in Nursing, *Waterloo* (BSN)

Briar Cliff University, Department of Nursing, *Sioux City* (BSN)

Iowa Wesleyan College, Division of Health and Natural Sciences, *Mount Pleasant* (BSN)

Luther College, Department of Nursing, *Decorah* (BA)

Mercy College of Health Sciences, Division of Nursing, *Des Moines* (BSN)

Kansas

Emporia State University, Newman Division of Nursing, *Emporia* (BSN)

Kansas Wesleyan University, Department of Nursing Education, *Salina* (BSN)

MidAmerica Nazarene University, Division of Nursing, *Olathe* (BSN)

University of Kansas, School of Nursing, *Kansas City* (BSN)

Washburn University, School of Nursing, *Topeka* (BSN)

Wichita State University, School of Nursing, *Wichita* (BSN)

Kentucky

Bellarmine University, Donna and Allan Lansing School of Nursing and Health Sciences, *Louisville* (BSN)

Kentucky State University, School of Nursing, *Frankfort* (BSN)

Midway College, Program in Nursing (Baccalaureate), *Midway* (BSN)

Louisiana

McNeese State University, College of Nursing, *Lake Charles* (BSN)

Northwestern State University of Louisiana, College of Nursing, *Shreveport* (BSN)

University of Louisiana at Lafayette, College of Nursing, *Lafayette* (BSN)

University of Louisiana at Monroe, Nursing, *Monroe* (BS)

Maine

University of Southern Maine, College of Nursing and Health Professions, *Portland* (BS)

Maryland

Coppin State University, Helene Fuld School of Nursing, *Baltimore* (BSN)

Salisbury University, Program in Nursing, *Salisbury* (BS)

Villa Julie College, Nursing Division, *Stevenson* (BS)

Massachusetts

Anna Maria College, Department of Nursing, *Paxton* (BSN)

Atlantic Union College, Department of Nursing, *South Lancaster* (BSN)

Fitchburg State College, Department of Nursing, *Fitchburg* (BS)

Framingham State College, Department of Nursing, *Framingham* (BS)

Regis College, Department of Nursing, *Weston* (BSN)

Salem State College, Program in Nursing, *Salem* (BSN)

Simmons College, Department of Nursing, *Boston* (BS)

Michigan

Andrews University, Department of Nursing, *Berrien Springs* (BS)

Grand Valley State University, Russell B. Kirkhof College of Nursing, *Allendale* (BSN)

Lake Superior State University, Department of Nursing, *Sault Sainte Marie* (BSN)

Madonna University, College of Nursing and Health, *Livonia* (BSN)

Northern Michigan University, College of Nursing and Allied Health Science, *Marquette* (BSN)

Spring Arbor University, Program in Nursing, *Spring Arbor* (BSN)

Western Michigan University, College of Health and Human Services, *Kalamazoo* (BSN)

Minnesota

Augsburg College, Program in Nursing, *Minneapolis* (BS)

Mississippi

Delta State University, School of Nursing, *Cleveland* (BSN)

Mississippi University for Women, Division of Nursing, *Columbus* (BSN)

University of Mississippi Medical Center, Program in Nursing, *Jackson* (BSN)

University of Southern Mississippi, School of Nursing, *Hattiesburg* (BSN)

William Carey College, School of Nursing, *Hattiesburg* (BSN)

Missouri

Chamberlain College of Nursing, *St. Louis* (BSN)

Cox College of Nursing and Health Sciences, Department of Nursing, *Springfield* (BSN)

Graceland University, School of Nursing, *Independence* (BSN)

Missouri Southern State University, Department of Nursing, *Joplin* (BSN)

Missouri State University, Department of Nursing, *Springfield* (BSN)

Webster University, Department of Nursing, *St. Louis* (BSN)

Montana

Montana State University–Northern, College of Nursing, *Havre* (BSN)

Nebraska

Clarkson College, Department of Nursing, *Omaha* (BSN)

College of Saint Mary, Division of Health Care Professions, *Omaha* (BSN)

Midland Lutheran College, Department of Nursing, *Fremont* (BSN)

Nebraska Methodist College, Department of Nursing, *Omaha* (BSN)

Nebraska Wesleyan University, Department of Nursing, *Lincoln* (BSN)

Union College, Division of Health Sciences, *Lincoln* (BSN)

University of Nebraska Medical Center, College of Nursing, *Omaha* (BSN)

Nevada

University of Nevada, Reno, Orvis School of Nursing, *Reno* (BSN)

New Hampshire

Rivier College, Department of Nursing and Health Sciences, *Nashua* (BS)

New Jersey

College of Saint Elizabeth, Department of Nursing, *Morristown* (BSN)

Kean University, Department of Nursing, *Union* (BSN)

Monmouth University, Marjorie K. Unterberg School of Nursing, *West Long Branch* (BSN)

Saint Peter's College, Nursing Program, *Jersey City* (BSN)

William Paterson University of New Jersey, Department of Nursing, *Wayne* (BSN)

New York

College of Mount Saint Vincent, Department of Nursing, *Riverdale* (BS)

College of Staten Island of the City University of New York, Department of Nursing, *Staten Island* (BS)

Daemen College, Department of Nursing, *Amherst* (BS)

D'Youville College, Department of Nursing, *Buffalo* (BSN)

Elmira College, Program in Nursing Education, *Elmira* (BS)

Medgar Evers College of the City University of New York, Department of Nursing, *Brooklyn* (BSN)

St. Francis College, Department of Nursing, *Brooklyn Heights* (BS)

St. John Fisher College, Advanced Practice Nursing Program, *Rochester* (BS)

State University of New York at New Paltz, Department of Nursing, *New Paltz* (BSN)

State University of New York at Plattsburgh, Department of Nursing, *Plattsburgh* (BS)

State University of New York College at Brockport, Department of Nursing, *Brockport* (BSN)

State University of New York Institute of Technology, School of Nursing and Health Systems, *Utica* (BS)

State University of New York Upstate Medical University, College of Nursing, *Syracuse* (BS)

University at Buffalo, the State University of New York, School of Nursing, *Buffalo* (BS)

University of Rochester, School of Nursing, *Rochester* (BS)

York College of the City University of New York, Program in Nursing, *Jamaica* (BS)

North Carolina

East Carolina University, School of Nursing, *Greenville* (BSN)

Lees-McRae College, Nursing Program, *Banner Elk* (BSN)

Lenoir-Rhyne College, Program in Nursing, *Hickory* (BS)

Queens University of Charlotte, Division of Nursing, *Charlotte* (BSN)

The University of North Carolina at Chapel Hill, School of Nursing, *Chapel Hill* (BSN)

The University of North Carolina at Charlotte, School of Nursing, *Charlotte* (BSN)

The University of North Carolina at Greensboro, School of Nursing, *Greensboro* (BSN)

Winston-Salem State University, Department of Nursing, *Winston-Salem* (BSN)

North Dakota

Dickinson State University, Department of Nursing, *Dickinson* (BSN)

Medcenter One College of Nursing, Medcenter One College of Nursing, *Bismarck* (BSN)

North Dakota State University, Tri-College University Nursing Consortium, *Fargo* (BSN)

University of North Dakota, College of Nursing, *Grand Forks* (BSN)

Ohio

Ashland University, Department of Nursing, *Ashland* (BSN)

Capital University, School of Nursing, *Columbus* (BSN)

Case Western Reserve University, Frances Payne Bolton School of Nursing, *Cleveland* (BSN)

Cleveland State University, Department of Nursing, *Cleveland* (BSN)

Kent State University, College of Nursing, *Kent* (BSN)

Miami University, Department of Nursing, *Hamilton* (BSN)

Shawnee State University, Department of Nursing, *Portsmouth* (BSN)

The University of Akron, College of Nursing, *Akron* (BSN)

The University of Toledo, College of Nursing, *Toledo* (BSN)

Oklahoma

East Central University, Department of Nursing, *Ada* (BS)

Oklahoma Baptist University, School of Nursing, *Shawnee* (BSN)

Oklahoma City University, Kramer School of Nursing, *Oklahoma City* (BSN)

Oklahoma Panhandle State University, Bachelor of Science in Nursing Program, *Goodwell* (BSN)

Oklahoma Wesleyan University, Division of Nursing, *Bartlesville* (BSN)

Oral Roberts University, Anna Vaughn School of Nursing, *Tulsa* (BSN)

Southern Nazarene University, School of Nursing, *Bethany* (BS)

Southwestern Oklahoma State University, Division of Nursing, *Weatherford* (BSN)

University of Oklahoma Health Sciences Center, College of Nursing, *Oklahoma City* (BSN)

Pennsylvania

Bloomsburg University of Pennsylvania, Department of Nursing, *Bloomsburg* (BSN)

Clarion University of Pennsylvania, School of Nursing, *Oil City* (BSN)

DeSales University, Department of Nursing and Health, *Center Valley* (BSN)

Drexel University, College of Nursing and Health Professions, *Philadelphia* (BSN)

Edinboro University of Pennsylvania, Department of Nursing, *Edinboro* (BS)

Gannon University, Program in Nursing, *Erie* (BSN)

Gwynedd-Mercy College, School of Nursing, *Gwynedd Valley* (BSN)

Holy Family University, School of Nursing and Allied Health Professions, *Philadelphia* (BSN)

Marywood University, Department of Nursing, *Scranton* (BSN)

Mount Aloysius College, Department of Nursing, *Cresson* (BSN)

Penn State University Park, School of Nursing, *State College, University Park* (BS)

Slippery Rock University of Pennsylvania, Department of Nursing, *Slippery Rock* (BSN)

Thomas Jefferson University, Department of Nursing, *Philadelphia* (BSN)

University of Pennsylvania, School of Nursing, *Philadelphia* (BSN)

University of Pittsburgh, School of Nursing, *Pittsburgh* (BSN)

The University of Scranton, Department of Nursing, *Scranton* (BS)

Villanova University, College of Nursing, *Villanova* (BSN)

Widener University, School of Nursing, *Chester* (BSN)

Wilkes University, Department of Nursing, *Wilkes-Barre* (BS)

Puerto Rico

Inter American University of Puerto Rico, Metropolitan Campus, Carmen Torres de Tiburcio School of Nursing, *San Juan* (BSN)

University of Puerto Rico, Medical Sciences Campus, School of Nursing, *San Juan* (BSN)

Rhode Island

University of Rhode Island, College of Nursing, *Kingston* (BS)

South Carolina

Charleston Southern University, Wingo School of Nursing, *Charleston* (BSN)

Medical University of South Carolina, College of Nursing, *Charleston* (BSN)

University of South Carolina Aiken, School of Nursing, *Aiken* (BSN)

South Dakota

Mount Marty College, Nursing Program, *Yankton* (BSc PN)

Presentation College, Department of Nursing, *Aberdeen* (BSN)

Tennessee

Belmont University, School of Nursing, *Nashville* (BSN)

Cumberland University, Rudy School of Nursing and Health Professions, *Lebanon* (BSN)

East Tennessee State University, College of Nursing, *Johnson City* (BSN)

Milligan College, Department of Nursing, *Milligan College* (BSN)

Southern Adventist University, School of Nursing, *Collegedale* (BS)

Tennessee Technological University, School of Nursing, *Cookeville* (BSN)

Tennessee Wesleyan College, Fort Sanders Nursing Department, *Knoxville* (BSN)

University of Memphis, Loewenberg School of Nursing, *Memphis* (BSN)

The University of Tennessee at Chattanooga, School of Nursing, *Chattanooga* (BSN)

The University of Tennessee at Martin, Department of Nursing, *Martin* (BSN)

The University of Tennessee Health Science Center, College of Nursing, *Memphis* (BSN)

Texas

Lamar University, Department of Nursing, *Beaumont* (BSN)

Midwestern State University, Nursing Program, *Wichita Falls* (BSN)

Southwestern Adventist University, Department of Nursing, *Keene* (BS)

Tarleton State University, Department of Nursing, *Stephenville* (BSN)

Texas A&M University-Corpus Christi, School of Nursing and Health Sciences, *Corpus Christi* (BSN)

Texas A&M University-Texarkana, Nursing Department, *Texarkana* (BSN)

Texas Tech University Health Sciences Center, School of Nursing, *Lubbock* (BSN)

The University of Texas at Brownsville, Department of Nursing, *Brownsville* (BSN)

The University of Texas at Tyler, Program in Nursing, *Tyler* (BSN)

The University of Texas Health Science Center at Houston, School of Nursing, *Houston* (BSN)

The University of Texas Health Science Center at San Antonio, School of Nursing, *San Antonio* (BSN)

University of the Incarnate Word, Program in Nursing, *San Antonio* (BSN)

West Texas A&M University, Division of Nursing, *Canyon* (BSN)

Utah

Utah Valley State College, Department of Nursing, *Orem* (BSN)

Weber State University, Program in Nursing, *Ogden* (BSN)

Vermont

Norwich University, Division of Nursing, *Northfield* (BSN)

Southern Vermont College, Department of Nursing, *Bennington* (BSN)

Virginia

Eastern Mennonite University, Department of Nursing, *Harrisonburg* (BSN)

Hampton University, Department of Nursing, *Hampton* (BS)

Jefferson College of Health Sciences, Nursing Education Program, *Roanoke* (BSN)

Marymount University, School of Health Professions, *Arlington* (BSN)

Norfolk State University, Department of Nursing, *Norfolk* (BSN)

Shenandoah University, Division of Nursing, *Winchester* (BSN)

University of Virginia, School of Nursing, *Charlottesville* (BSN)

Virginia Commonwealth University, School of Nursing, *Richmond* (BS)

Washington

Gonzaga University, Department of Nursing, *Spokane* (BSN)

Pacific Lutheran University, School of Nursing, *Tacoma* (BSN)

Walla Walla College, School of Nursing, *College Place* (BS)

West Virginia

Fairmont State University, School of Nursing and Allied Health Administration, *Fairmont* (BSN)

Mountain State University, Program in Nursing, *Beckley* (BSN)

Shepherd University, Department of Nursing Education, *Shepherdstown* (BSN)

Wisconsin

Alverno College, Division of Nursing, *Milwaukee* (BSN)

Columbia College of Nursing/Mount Mary College Nursing Program, *Milwaukee* (BSN)

Concordia University Wisconsin, Program in Nursing, *Mequon* (BSN)

Marian College of Fond du Lac, Nursing Studies Division, *Fond du Lac* (BSN)

Marquette University, College of Nursing, *Milwaukee* (BSN)

University of Wisconsin-Eau Claire, College of Nursing and Health Sciences, *Eau Claire* (BSN)

University of Wisconsin-Madison, School of Nursing, *Madison* (BS)

Wyoming

University of Wyoming, Fay W. Whitney School of Nursing, *Laramie* (BSN)

CANADA

Quebec

Université du Québec en Outaouais, Département des Sciences Infirmières, *Gatineau* (BScN)

BACCALAUREATE FOR SECOND DEGREE

Alabama

Samford University, Ida V. Moffett School of Nursing, *Birmingham* (BSN)

Spring Hill College, Division of Nursing, *Mobile* (BSN)

The University of Alabama, Capstone College of Nursing, *Tuscaloosa* (BSN)

The University of Alabama at Birmingham, School of Nursing, *Birmingham* (BSN)

The University of Alabama in Huntsville, College of Nursing, *Huntsville* (BSN)

Arizona

Arizona State University at the Downtown Phoenix Campus, College of Nursing, *Phoenix* (BSN)

Arkansas

University of Arkansas, Eleanor Mann School of Nursing, *Fayetteville* (BSN)

University of Arkansas for Medical Sciences, College of Nursing, *Little Rock* (BSN)

California

Biola University, Department of Nursing, *La Mirada* (BSN)

California State University, Chico, School of Nursing, *Chico* (BSN)

California State University, Dominguez Hills, Program in Nursing, *Carson* (BSN)

California State University, Fresno, Department of Nursing, *Fresno* (BSN)

California State University, Fullerton, Department of Nursing, *Fullerton* (BSN)

Dominican University of California, Program in Nursing, *San Rafael* (BSN)

Humboldt State University, Department of Nursing, *Arcata* (BSN)

Loma Linda University, School of Nursing, *Loma Linda* (BSN)

Point Loma Nazarene University, School of Nursing, *San Diego* (BSN)

Sonoma State University, Department of Nursing, *Rohnert Park* (BSN)

University of San Francisco, School of Nursing, *San Francisco* (BSN)

Colorado

Colorado State University-Pueblo, Department of Nursing, *Pueblo* (BSN)

Connecticut

Fairfield University, School of Nursing, *Fairfield* (BS)

Saint Joseph College, Department of Nursing, *West Hartford* (BS)

District of Columbia

The Catholic University of America, School of Nursing, *Washington* (BSN)

Howard University, Division of Nursing, *Washington* (BSN)

Florida

Barry University, School of Nursing, *Miami Shores* (BSN)

Florida Southern College, Department of Nursing, *Lakeland* (BSN)

Florida State University, School of Nursing, *Tallahassee* (BSN)

Jacksonville University, School of Nursing, *Jacksonville* (BSN)

University of Miami, School of Nursing and Health Studies, *Coral Gables* (BSN)

University of South Florida, College of Nursing, *Tampa* (BSN)

University of West Florida, Department of Nursing, *Pensacola* (BSN)

Georgia

Albany State University, College of Health Professions, *Albany* (BSN)

Armstrong Atlantic State University, Program in Nursing, *Savannah* (BSN)

Emory University, Nell Hodgson Woodruff School of Nursing, *Atlanta* (BSN)

Georgia Southwestern State University, School of Nursing, *Americus* (BSN)

Kennesaw State University, School of Nursing, *Kennesaw* (BSN)

Illinois

MacMurray College, Department of Nursing, *Jacksonville* (BSN)

Saint Anthony College of Nursing, Saint Anthony College of Nursing, *Rockford* (BSN)

West Suburban College of Nursing, *Oak Park* (BSN)

Indiana

Indiana University Northwest, School of Nursing and Health Professions, *Gary* (BSN)

Purdue University, School of Nursing, *West Lafayette* (BS)

Purdue University Calumet, School of Nursing, *Hammond* (BS)

Iowa

Allen College, Program in Nursing, *Waterloo* (BSN)

Clarke College, Department of Nursing and Health, *Dubuque* (BS)

Morningside College, Department of Nursing Education, *Sioux City* (BSN)

Kansas

Washburn University, School of Nursing, *Topeka* (BSN)

Kentucky

University of Kentucky, Graduate School Programs in the College of Nursing, *Lexington* (BSN)

Maryland

Coppin State University, Helene Fuld School of Nursing, *Baltimore* (BSN)

The Johns Hopkins University, School of Nursing, *Baltimore* (BS)

Massachusetts

Regis College, Department of Nursing, *Weston* (BSN)

Simmons College, Department of Nursing, *Boston* (BS)

Michigan

Eastern Michigan University, School of Nursing, *Ypsilanti* (BSN)

Grand Valley State University, Russell B. Kirkhof College of Nursing, *Allendale* (BSN)

Madonna University, College of Nursing and Health, *Livonia* (BSN)

Saginaw Valley State University, Crystal M. Lange College of Nursing and Health Sciences, *University Center* (BSN)

University of Michigan-Flint, Department of Nursing, *Flint* (BSN)

Western Michigan University, College of Health and Human Services, *Kalamazoo* (BSN)

Minnesota

College of St. Catherine, Department of Nursing, *St. Paul* (BA)

Missouri

Cox College of Nursing and Health Sciences, Department of Nursing, *Springfield* (BSN)

Missouri Southern State University, Department of Nursing, *Joplin* (BSN)

Missouri State University, Department of Nursing, *Springfield* (BSN)

Research College of Nursing, College of Nursing, *Kansas City* (BSN)

Nebraska

University of Nebraska Medical Center, College of Nursing, *Omaha* (BSN)

New Jersey

Rutgers, The State University of New Jersey, Camden College of Arts and Sciences, Department of Nursing, *Camden* (BS)

Rutgers, The State University of New Jersey, College of Nursing, *Newark* (BS)

Seton Hall University, College of Nursing, *South Orange* (BSN)

New York

Adelphi University, School of Nursing, *Garden City* (BS)

College of Mount Saint Vincent, Department of Nursing, *Riverdale* (BS)

The College of New Rochelle, School of Nursing, *New Rochelle* (BSN)

Lehman College of the City University of New York, Department of Nursing, *Bronx* (BS)

Molloy College, Department of Nursing, *Rockville Centre* (BS)

New York University, College of Nursing, *New York* (BS)

St. John Fisher College, Advanced Practice Nursing Program, *Rochester* (BS)

State University of New York College at Brockport, Department of Nursing, *Brockport* (BSN)

University at Buffalo, the State University of New York, School of Nursing, *Buffalo* (BS)

University of Rochester, School of Nursing, *Rochester* (BS)

Wagner College, Department of Nursing, *Staten Island* (BS)

North Carolina

East Carolina University, School of Nursing, *Greenville* (BSN)

Queens University of Charlotte, Division of Nursing, *Charlotte* (BSN)

The University of North Carolina at Greensboro, School of Nursing, *Greensboro* (BSN)

Winston-Salem State University, Department of Nursing, *Winston-Salem* (BSN)

Ohio

Ashland University, Department of Nursing, *Ashland* (BSN)

Kent State University, College of Nursing, *Kent* (BSN)

Wright State University, College of Nursing and Health, *Dayton* (BSN)

Oklahoma

Oklahoma Baptist University, School of Nursing, *Shawnee* (BSN)

Oklahoma Wesleyan University, Division of Nursing, *Bartlesville* (BSN)

Oregon

Linfield College, School of Nursing, *McMinnville* (BSN)

Pennsylvania

Bloomsburg University of Pennsylvania, Department of Nursing, *Bloomsburg* (BSN)

Carlow University, School of Nursing, *Pittsburgh* (BSN)

Cedar Crest College, Department of Nursing, *Allentown* (BS)

College Misericordia, Department of Nursing, *Dallas* (BSN)

Eastern University, Program in Nursing, *St. Davids* (BSN)

Edinboro University of Pennsylvania, Department of Nursing, *Edinboro* (BS)

Gannon University, Program in Nursing, *Erie* (BSN)

Indiana University of Pennsylvania, Department of Nursing and Allied Health, *Indiana* (BSN)

La Salle University, School of Nursing and Health Sciences, *Philadelphia* (BSN)

Neumann College, Program in Nursing and Health Sciences, *Aston* (BS)

Robert Morris University, School of Nursing and Allied Health, *Moon Township* (BSN)

Thomas Jefferson University, Department of Nursing, *Philadelphia* (BSN)

University of Pennsylvania, School of Nursing, *Philadelphia* (BSN)

The University of Scranton, Department of Nursing, *Scranton* (BS)

Villanova University, College of Nursing, *Villanova* (BSN)

Widener University, School of Nursing, *Chester* (BSN)

Rhode Island

Rhode Island College, Department of Nursing, *Providence* (BS)

South Carolina

Lander University, School of Nursing, *Greenwood* (BSN)

South Dakota

Presentation College, Department of Nursing, *Aberdeen* (BSN)

Tennessee

Belmont University, School of Nursing, *Nashville* (BSN)

Cumberland University, Rudy School of Nursing and Health Professions, *Lebanon* (BSN)

University of Memphis, Loewenberg School of Nursing, *Memphis* (BSN)

The University of Tennessee at Chattanooga, School of Nursing, *Chattanooga* (BSN)

The University of Tennessee Health Science Center, College of Nursing, *Memphis* (BSN)

Texas

Texas A&M University–Corpus Christi, School of Nursing and Health Sciences, *Corpus Christi* (BSN)

Texas Woman's University, College of Nursing, *Denton* (BS)

University of Mary Hardin-Baylor, College of Nursing, *Belton* (BSN)

The University of Texas Health Science Center at Houston, School of Nursing, *Houston* (BSN)

Utah

Westminster College, School of Nursing and Health Sciences, *Salt Lake City* (BSN)

Virginia

Eastern Mennonite University, Department of Nursing, *Harrisonburg* (BSN)

Hampton University, Department of Nursing, *Hampton* (BS)

Marymount University, School of Health Professions, *Arlington* (BSN)

Washington

Seattle University, College of Nursing, *Seattle* (BSN)

West Virginia

Mountain State University, Program in Nursing, *Beckley* (BSN)

Wisconsin

Alverno College, Division of Nursing, *Milwaukee* (BSN)

Bellin College of Nursing, Nursing Program, *Green Bay* (BSN)

Edgewood College, Program in Nursing, *Madison* (BS)

Marquette University, College of Nursing, *Milwaukee* (BSN)

University of Wisconsin–Oshkosh, College of Nursing, *Oshkosh* (BSN)

CANADA

Alberta

University of Alberta, Faculty of Nursing, *Edmonton* (BScN)

University of Calgary, Faculty of Nursing, *Calgary* (BN)

Manitoba

Brandon University, School of Health Studies, *Brandon* (BN)

University of Manitoba, Faculty of Nursing, *Winnipeg* (BN)

Nova Scotia

Dalhousie University, School of Nursing, *Halifax* (BScN)

Ontario

McMaster University, School of Nursing, *Hamilton* (BScN)

Saskatchewan

University of Saskatchewan, College of Nursing, *Saskatoon* (BSN)

GENERIC BACCALAUREATE

Alabama

Auburn University, School of Nursing, *Auburn University* (BSN)

Auburn University Montgomery, School of Nursing, *Montgomery* (BSN)

Jacksonville State University, College of Nursing and Health Sciences, *Jacksonville* (BSN)

Oakwood College, Department of Nursing, *Huntsville* (BS)

Samford University, Ida V. Moffett School of Nursing, *Birmingham* (BSN)

Spring Hill College, Division of Nursing, *Mobile* (BSN)

Troy University, School of Nursing, *Troy* (BSN)

Tuskegee University, Program in Nursing, *Tuskegee* (BSN)

The University of Alabama, Capstone College of Nursing, *Tuscaloosa* (BSN)

The University of Alabama at Birmingham, School of Nursing, *Birmingham* (BSN)

The University of Alabama in Huntsville, College of Nursing, *Huntsville* (BSN)

University of Mobile, School of Nursing, *Mobile* (BSN)

University of North Alabama, College of Nursing and Allied Health, *Florence* (BSN)

University of South Alabama, College of Nursing, *Mobile* (BSN)

Alaska

University of Alaska Anchorage, School of Nursing, *Anchorage* (BS)

Arizona

Arizona State University at the Downtown Phoenix Campus, College of Nursing, *Phoenix* (BSN)

Grand Canyon University, College of Nursing, *Phoenix* (BSN)

Northern Arizona University, School of Nursing, *Flagstaff* (BSN)

The University of Arizona, College of Nursing, *Tucson* (BSN)

Arkansas

Arkansas State University, Department of Nursing, *Jonesboro, State University* (BSN)

Arkansas Tech University, Program in Nursing, *Russellville* (BSN)

Harding University, College of Nursing, *Searcy* (BSN)

Henderson State University, Department of Nursing, *Arkadelphia* (BSN)

University of Arkansas, Eleanor Mann School of Nursing, *Fayetteville* (BSN)

University of Arkansas at Fort Smith, Carol McKelvey Moore School of Nursing, *Fort Smith* (BSN)

University of Arkansas at Pine Bluff, Department of Nursing, *Pine Bluff* (BSN)

University of Arkansas for Medical Sciences, College of Nursing, *Little Rock* (BSN)

University of Central Arkansas, Department of Nursing, *Conway* (BSN)

California

Azusa Pacific University, School of Nursing, *Azusa* (BSN)

Biola University, Department of Nursing, *La Mirada* (BSN)

California State University, Bakersfield, Program in Nursing, *Bakersfield* (BSN)

California State University, Chico, School of Nursing, *Chico* (BSN)

California State University, East Bay, Department of Nursing and Health Sciences, *Hayward* (BS)

California State University, Fresno, Department of Nursing, *Fresno* (BSN)

California State University, Long Beach, Department of Nursing, *Long Beach* (BSN)

California State University, Los Angeles, School of Nursing, *Los Angeles* (BS)

California State University, Sacramento, Division of Nursing, *Sacramento* (BSN)

California State University, Stanislaus, Department of Nursing, *Turlock* (BSN)

Dominican University of California, Program in Nursing, *San Rafael* (BSN)

Humboldt State University, Department of Nursing, *Arcata* (BSN)

Loma Linda University, School of Nursing, *Loma Linda* (BS)

Mount St. Mary's College, Department of Nursing, *Los Angeles* (BSN)

National University, Department of Nursing, *La Jolla* (BSN)

Point Loma Nazarene University, School of Nursing, *San Diego* (BSN)

Samuel Merritt College, School of Nursing, *Oakland* (BSN)

San Diego State University, School of Nursing, *San Diego* (BSN)

San Francisco State University, School of Nursing, *San Francisco* (BSN)

San Jose State University, School of Nursing, *San Jose* (BS)

Sonoma State University, Department of Nursing, *Rohnert Park* (BSN)

University of California, Los Angeles, School of Nursing, *Los Angeles* (BS)

University of San Francisco, School of Nursing, *San Francisco* (BSN)

Colorado

Colorado State University-Pueblo, Department of Nursing, *Pueblo* (BSN)

Mesa State College, Department of Nursing and Radiologic Sciences, *Grand Junction* (BSN)

Regis University, Department of Nursing, *Denver* (BSN)

University of Colorado at Colorado Springs, Beth-El College of Nursing and Health Sciences, *Colorado Springs* (BSN)

University of Colorado at Denver and Health Sciences Center, School of Nursing, *Denver* (BS)

University of Northern Colorado, School of Nursing, *Greeley* (BS)

Connecticut

Fairfield University, School of Nursing, *Fairfield* (BS)

Quinnipiac University, Department of Nursing, *Hamden* (BSN)

Sacred Heart University, Program in Nursing, *Fairfield* (BS)

Saint Joseph College, Department of Nursing, *West Hartford* (BS)

Southern Connecticut State University, Department of Nursing, *New Haven* (BSN)

Western Connecticut State University, Department of Nursing, *Danbury* (BS)

Delaware

Delaware State University, Department of Nursing, *Dover* (BSN)

University of Delaware, School of Nursing, *Newark* (BSN)

Wesley College, Nursing Program, *Dover* (BSN)

District of Columbia

The Catholic University of America, School of Nursing, *Washington* (BSN)

Georgetown University, School of Nursing and Health Studies, *Washington* (BSN)

Howard University, Division of Nursing, *Washington* (BSN)

Florida

Barry University, School of Nursing, *Miami Shores* (BSN)

Bethune-Cookman College, School of Nursing, *Daytona Beach* (BSN)

Florida Agricultural and Mechanical University, School of Nursing, *Tallahassee* (BSN)

Florida Atlantic University, College of Nursing, *Boca Raton* (BSN)

Florida Gulf Coast University, School of Nursing, *Fort Myers* (BSN)

Florida Hospital College of Health Sciences, Department of Nursing, *Orlando* (BS)

Florida International University, College of Nursing and Health Sciences, *Miami* (BSN)

Florida Southern College, Department of Nursing, *Lakeland* (BSN)

Florida State University, School of Nursing, *Tallahassee* (BSN)

Jacksonville University, School of Nursing, *Jacksonville* (BSN)

Nova Southeastern University, College of Allied Health and Nursing, *Fort Lauderdale* (BSN)

South University, Nursing Program, *West Palm Beach* (BSN)

University of Central Florida, School of Nursing, *Orlando* (BSN)

University of Florida, College of Nursing, *Gainesville* (BSN)

University of Miami, School of Nursing and Health Studies, *Coral Gables* (BSN)

University of North Florida, School of Nursing, *Jacksonville* (BSN)

University of South Florida, College of Nursing, *Tampa* (BS)

The University of Tampa, Department of Nursing, *Tampa* (BSN)

University of West Florida, Department of Nursing, *Pensacola* (BSN)

Georgia

Albany State University, College of Health Professions, *Albany* (BSN)

Armstrong Atlantic State University, Program in Nursing, *Savannah* (BSN)

Brenau University, School of Health and Science, *Gainesville* (BSN)

Clayton State University, Department of Nursing, *Morrow* (BSN)

Columbus State University, Nursing Program, *Columbus* (BSN)

Emory University, Nell Hodgson Woodruff School of Nursing, *Atlanta* (BSN)

Georgia Baptist College of Nursing of Mercer University, Department of Nursing, *Atlanta* (BSN)

Georgia College & State University, School of Health Sciences, *Milledgeville* (BSN)

Georgia Southern University, School of Nursing, *Statesboro* (BSN)

Georgia Southwestern State University, School of Nursing, *Americus* (BSN)

Georgia State University, School of Nursing, *Atlanta* (BS)

Kennesaw State University, School of Nursing, *Kennesaw* (BSN)

LaGrange College, Department of Nursing, *LaGrange* (BSN)

Medical College of Georgia, School of Nursing, *Augusta* (BSN)

Piedmont College, School of Nursing, *Demorest* (BSN)

University of West Georgia, Department of Nursing, *Carrollton* (BSN)

Valdosta State University, College of Nursing, *Valdosta* (BSN)

Guam

University of Guam, College of Nursing and Health Sciences, *Mangilao* (BSN)

Hawaii

Hawai'i Pacific University, School of Nursing, *Honolulu* (BSN)

University of Hawaii at Hilo, Department in Nursing, *Hilo* (BSN)

University of Hawaii at Manoa, School of Nursing and Dental Hygiene, *Honolulu* (BS)

Idaho

Boise State University, Department of Nursing, *Boise* (BS)

Idaho State University, Department of Nursing, *Pocatello* (BSN)

Lewis-Clark State College, Division of Nursing and Health Sciences, *Lewiston* (BSN)

Northwest Nazarene University, School of Health and Science, *Nampa* (BSN)

Illinois

Aurora University, School of Nursing, *Aurora* (BSN)

Blessing-Rieman College of Nursing, *Quincy* (BSN)

Bradley University, Department of Nursing, *Peoria* (BSN, BSc PN)

Chicago State University, College of Nursing and Allied Health Professions, *Chicago* (BSN)

Elmhurst College, Deicke Center for Nursing Education, *Elmhurst* (BSN)

Illinois State University, Mennonite College of Nursing, *Normal* (BSN)

Illinois Wesleyan University, School of Nursing, *Bloomington* (BSN)

Lakeview College of Nursing, *Danville* (BSN)

Lewis University, Program in Nursing, *Romeoville* (BSN)

Loyola University Chicago, Marcella Niehoff School of Nursing, *Chicago* (BSN)

MacMurray College, Department of Nursing, *Jacksonville* (BSN)

Millikin University, School of Nursing, *Decatur* (BSN)

Northern Illinois University, School of Nursing, *De Kalb* (BS)

North Park University, School of Nursing, *Chicago* (BS)

Olivet Nazarene University, Division of Nursing, *Bourbonnais* (BSN)

Rockford College, Department of Nursing, *Rockford* (BSN)

Rush University, College of Nursing, *Chicago* (BSN)

Saint Anthony College of Nursing, Saint Anthony College of Nursing, *Rockford* (BSN)

Saint Francis Medical Center College of Nursing, Baccalaureate Nursing Program, *Peoria* (BSN)

St. John's College, Department of Nursing, *Springfield* (BSN)

Saint Xavier University, School of Nursing, *Chicago* (BSN)

Southern Illinois University Edwardsville, School of Nursing, *Edwardsville* (BS)

Trinity Christian College, Department of Nursing, *Palos Heights* (BSN)

University of Illinois at Chicago, College of Nursing, *Chicago* (BSN)

University of St. Francis, College of Nursing and Allied Health, *Joliet* (BSN)

West Suburban College of Nursing, *Oak Park* (BSN)

Indiana

Ball State University, School of Nursing, *Muncie* (BS)

Bethel College, Department of Nursing, *Mishawaka* (BSN)

Goshen College, Department of Nursing, *Goshen* (BSN)

Indiana State University, College of Nursing, *Terre Haute* (BS)

Indiana University Bloomington, Department of Nursing-Bloomington Division, *Bloomington* (BSN)

Indiana University East, Division of Nursing, *Richmond* (BSN)

Indiana University Kokomo, Indiana University School of Nursing, *Kokomo* (BSN)

Indiana University Northwest, School of Nursing and Health Professions, *Gary* (BSN)

Indiana University–Purdue University Indianapolis, School of Nursing, *Indianapolis* (BSN)

Indiana University South Bend, Division of Nursing and Health Professions, *South Bend* (BSN)

Indiana University Southeast, Division of Nursing, *New Albany* (BSN)

Indiana Wesleyan University, Division of Nursing, *Marion* (BSN)

Marian College, Department of Nursing and Nutritional Science, *Indianapolis* (BSN)

Purdue University, School of Nursing, *West Lafayette* (BS)

Purdue University Calumet, School of Nursing, *Hammond* (BS)

Saint Mary's College, Department of Nursing, *Notre Dame* (BS)

University of Evansville, Department of Nursing, *Evansville* (BSN)

University of Indianapolis, School of Nursing, *Indianapolis* (BSN)

University of Saint Francis, Department of Nursing, *Fort Wayne* (BSN)

University of Southern Indiana, College of Nursing and Health Professions, *Evansville* (BSN)

Valparaiso University, College of Nursing, *Valparaiso* (BSN)

Iowa

Allen College, Program in Nursing, *Waterloo* (BSN)

Briar Cliff University, Department of Nursing, *Sioux City* (BSN)

Clarke College, Department of Nursing and Health, *Dubuque* (BS)

Coe College, Department of Nursing, *Cedar Rapids* (BSN)

Grand View College, Division of Nursing, *Des Moines* (BSN)

Luther College, Department of Nursing, *Decorah* (BA)

Morningside College, Department of Nursing Education, *Sioux City* (BSN)

Mount Mercy College, Department of Nursing, *Cedar Rapids* (BSN)

St. Ambrose University, Program in Nursing (BSN), *Davenport* (BSN)

The University of Iowa, College of Nursing, *Iowa City* (BSN)

Kansas

Baker University, School of Nursing, *Topeka* (BSN)

Bethel College, Department of Nursing, *North Newton* (BSN)

Emporia State University, Newman Division of Nursing, *Emporia* (BSN)

Fort Hays State University, Department of Nursing, *Hays* (BSN)

Kansas Wesleyan University, Department of Nursing Education, *Salina* (BSN)

MidAmerica Nazarene University, Division of Nursing, *Olathe* (BSN)

Newman University, Division of Nursing, *Wichita* (BSN)

Pittsburg State University, Department of Nursing, *Pittsburg* (BSN)

Southwestern College, Nursing Program, *Winfield* (BSN)

University of Kansas, School of Nursing, *Kansas City* (BSN)

Washburn University, School of Nursing, *Topeka* (BSN)

Wichita State University, School of Nursing, *Wichita* (BSN)

Kentucky

Bellarmine University, Donna and Allan Lansing School of Nursing and Health Sciences, *Louisville* (BSN)

Berea College, Department of Nursing, *Berea* (BS)

Eastern Kentucky University, Department of Baccalaureate and Graduate Nursing, *Richmond* (BSN)

Kentucky Christian University, School of Nursing, *Grayson* (BSN)

Morehead State University, Department of Nursing, *Morehead* (BSN)

Murray State University, Program in Nursing, *Murray* (BSN)

Northern Kentucky University, Department of Nursing, *Highland Heights* (BSN)

Spalding University, School of Nursing, *Louisville* (BSN)

Thomas More College, Program in Nursing, *Crestview Hills* (BSN)

University of Kentucky, Graduate School Programs in the College of Nursing, *Lexington* (BSN)

University of Louisville, School of Nursing, *Louisville* (BSN)

Louisiana

Dillard University, Division of Nursing, *New Orleans* (BSN)

Grambling State University, School of Nursing, *Grambling* (BSN)

Louisiana College, Department of Nursing, *Pineville* (BSN)

Louisiana State University Health Sciences Center, School of Nursing, *New Orleans* (BSN)

McNeese State University, College of Nursing, *Lake Charles* (BSN)

Nicholls State University, Department of Nursing, *Thibodaux* (BSN)

Northwestern State University of Louisiana, College of Nursing, *Shreveport* (BSN)

Our Lady of Holy Cross College, Division of Nursing, *New Orleans* (BSN)

Southeastern Louisiana University, School of Nursing, *Hammond* (BS)

Southern University and Agricultural and Mechanical College, School of Nursing, *Baton Rouge* (BSN)

University of Louisiana at Lafayette, College of Nursing, *Lafayette* (BSN)

University of Louisiana at Monroe, Nursing, *Monroe* (BS)

Maine

Husson College, School of Nursing, *Bangor* (BSN)

BACCALAUREATE PROGRAMS
Generic Baccalaureate

University of Maine, School of Nursing, *Orono* (BSN)

University of Maine at Fort Kent, Department of Nursing, *Fort Kent* (BSN)

University of Southern Maine, College of Nursing and Health Professions, *Portland* (BS)

Maryland

Columbia Union College, Nursing Department, *Takoma Park* (BS)

Coppin State University, Helene Fuld School of Nursing, *Baltimore* (BSN)

The Johns Hopkins University, School of Nursing, *Baltimore* (BS)

Salisbury University, Program in Nursing, *Salisbury* (BS)

Towson University, Department of Nursing, *Towson* (BS)

University of Maryland, Baltimore, Master's Program in Nursing, *Baltimore* (BSN)

Villa Julie College, Nursing Division, *Stevenson* (BS)

Massachusetts

American International College, Division of Nursing, *Springfield* (BSN)

Boston College, William F. Connell School of Nursing, *Chestnut Hill* (BS)

Curry College, Division of Nursing, *Milton* (BS)

Elms College, Division of Nursing, *Chicopee* (BSc PN)

Endicott College, Major in Nursing, *Beverly* (BS)

Fitchburg State College, Department of Nursing, *Fitchburg* (BS)

Northeastern University, School of Nursing, *Boston* (BSN)

Regis College, Department of Nursing, *Weston* (BSN)

Salem State College, Program in Nursing, *Salem* (BSN)

Simmons College, Department of Nursing, *Boston* (BS)

University of Massachusetts Amherst, School of Nursing, *Amherst* (BS)

University of Massachusetts Boston, College of Nursing and Health Sciences, *Boston* (BS)

University of Massachusetts Dartmouth, College of Nursing, *North Dartmouth* (BSN)

University of Massachusetts Lowell, Department of Nursing, *Lowell* (BS)

Worcester State College, Department of Nursing, *Worcester* (BS)

Michigan

Andrews University, Department of Nursing, *Berrien Springs* (BS)

Calvin College, Department of Nursing, *Grand Rapids* (BSN)

Eastern Michigan University, School of Nursing, *Ypsilanti* (BSN)

Ferris State University, School of Nursing, *Big Rapids* (BSN)

Grand Valley State University, Russell B. Kirkhof College of Nursing, *Allendale* (BSN)

Hope College, Department of Nursing, *Holland* (BSN)

Lake Superior State University, Department of Nursing, *Sault Sainte Marie* (BSN)

Madonna University, College of Nursing and Health, *Livonia* (BSN)

Michigan State University, College of Nursing, *East Lansing* (BSN)

Northern Michigan University, College of Nursing and Allied Health Science, *Marquette* (BSN)

Oakland University, School of Nursing, *Rochester* (BSN)

Saginaw Valley State University, Crystal M. Lange College of Nursing and Health Sciences, *University Center* (BSN)

University of Detroit Mercy, McAuley School of Nursing, *Detroit* (BSN)

University of Michigan, School of Nursing, *Ann Arbor* (BSN)

University of Michigan–Flint, Department of Nursing, *Flint* (BSN)

Wayne State University, College of Nursing, *Detroit* (BSN)

Western Michigan University, College of Health and Human Services, *Kalamazoo* (BSN)

Minnesota

Bethel University, Department of Nursing, *St. Paul* (BSN)

College of Saint Benedict, Department of Nursing, *Saint Joseph* (BS)

College of St. Catherine, Department of Nursing, *St. Paul* (BA)

The College of St. Scholastica, Department of Nursing, *Duluth* (BA)

Concordia College, Department of Nursing, *Moorhead* (BA)

Gustavus Adolphus College, Department of Nursing, *St. Peter* (BA)

Minnesota Intercollegiate Nursing Consortium, *Northfield* (BA)

Minnesota State University Mankato, School of Nursing, *Mankato* (BS)

Minnesota State University Moorhead, Tri-College University Nursing Consortium, *Moorhead* (BSN)

St. Cloud State University, Department of Nursing Science, *St. Cloud* (BS)

St. Olaf College, Department of Nursing, *Northfield* (BA)

University of Minnesota, Twin Cities Campus, School of Nursing, *Minneapolis* (BSN)

Winona State University, College of Nursing, *Winona* (BS)

Mississippi

Alcorn State University, School of Nursing, *Natchez* (BSN)

Delta State University, School of Nursing, *Cleveland* (BSN)

Mississippi College, School of Nursing, *Clinton* (BSN)

Mississippi University for Women, Division of Nursing, *Columbus* (BSN)

University of Mississippi Medical Center, Program in Nursing, *Jackson* (BSN)

University of Southern Mississippi, School of Nursing, *Hattiesburg* (BSN)

William Carey College, School of Nursing, *Hattiesburg* (BSN)

Missouri

Avila University, School of Nursing, *Kansas City* (BSN)

Cox College of Nursing and Health Sciences, Department of Nursing, *Springfield* (BSN)

Graceland University, School of Nursing, *Independence* (BSN)

Maryville University of Saint Louis, Nursing Program, School of Health Professions, *St. Louis* (BSN)

Missouri Southern State University, Department of Nursing, *Joplin* (BSN)

Missouri State University, Department of Nursing, *Springfield* (BSN)

Missouri Western State University, Department of Nursing, *St. Joseph* (BSN)

Research College of Nursing, College of Nursing, *Kansas City* (BSN)

Saint Louis University, School of Nursing, *St. Louis* (BSN)

Saint Luke's College, Nursing College, *Kansas City* (BSN)

Southeast Missouri State University, Department of Nursing, *Cape Girardeau* (BSN)

Truman State University, Program in Nursing, *Kirksville* (BSN)

University of Central Missouri, Department of Nursing, *Warrensburg* (BS)

University of Missouri–Columbia, Sinclair School of Nursing, *Columbia* (BSN)

University of Missouri–Kansas City, School of Nursing, *Kansas City* (BSN)

University of Missouri–St. Louis, College of Nursing, *St. Louis* (BSN)

William Jewell College, Department of Nursing, *Liberty* (BS)

Montana

Carroll College, Department of Nursing, *Helena* (BA)

Montana State University, College of Nursing, *Bozeman* (BSN)

Nebraska

College of Saint Mary, Division of Health Care Professions, *Omaha* (BSN)

Creighton University, School of Nursing, *Omaha* (BSN)

Midland Lutheran College, Department of Nursing, *Fremont* (BSN)

Nebraska Methodist College, Department of Nursing, *Omaha* (BSN)

Union College, Division of Health Sciences, *Lincoln* (BSN)

University of Nebraska Medical Center, College of Nursing, *Omaha* (BSN)

Nevada

Nevada State College at Henderson, Nursing Program, *Henderson* (BS)

University of Nevada, Las Vegas, School of Nursing, *Las Vegas* (BSN)

University of Nevada, Reno, Orvis School of Nursing, *Reno* (BSN)

New Hampshire

Colby-Sawyer College, Department of Nursing, *New London* (BS)

University of New Hampshire, Department of Nursing, *Durham* (BS)

New Jersey

Bloomfield College, Division of Nursing, *Bloomfield* (BS)

The College of New Jersey, School of Nursing, *Ewing* (BSN)

Fairleigh Dickinson University, Metropolitan Campus, Henry P. Becton School of Nursing and Allied Health, *Teaneck* (BSN)

Felician College, Department of Professional Nursing-BSN, *Lodi* (BSN)

Rutgers, The State University of New Jersey, Camden College of Arts and Sciences, Department of Nursing, *Camden* (BS)

Rutgers, The State University of New Jersey, College of Nursing, *Newark* (BS)

Saint Peter's College, Nursing Program, *Jersey City* (BSN)

Seton Hall University, College of Nursing, *South Orange* (BSN)

University of Medicine and Dentistry of New Jersey, School of Nursing, *Newark* (BSN)

William Paterson University of New Jersey, Department of Nursing, *Wayne* (BSN)

New Mexico

New Mexico State University, Department of Nursing, *Las Cruces* (BSN)

University of New Mexico, College of Nursing, *Albuquerque* (BSN)

New York

Adelphi University, School of Nursing, *Garden City* (BS)

College of Mount Saint Vincent, Department of Nursing, *Riverdale* (BS)

The College of New Rochelle, School of Nursing, *New Rochelle* (BSN)

Dominican College, Department of Nursing, *Orangeburg* (BSN)

D'Youville College, Department of Nursing, *Buffalo* (BSN)

Elmira College, Program in Nursing Education, *Elmira* (BS)

Hartwick College, Department of Nursing, *Oneonta* (BS)

Hunter College of the City University of New York, Hunter-Bellevue School of Nursing, *New York* (BS)

Lehman College of the City University of New York, Department of Nursing, *Bronx* (BS)

Long Island University, Brooklyn Campus, School of Nursing, *Brooklyn* (BS)

Molloy College, Department of Nursing, *Rockville Centre* (BS)

Mount Saint Mary College, Division of Nursing, *Newburgh* (BSN)

Nazareth College of Rochester, Department of Nursing, *Rochester* (BS)

New York University, College of Nursing, *New York* (BS)

Pace University, Lienhard School of Nursing, *New York* (BS)

Roberts Wesleyan College, Division of Nursing, *Rochester* (BScN)

The Sage Colleges, Division of Nursing, *Troy* (BS)

St. John Fisher College, Advanced Practice Nursing Program, *Rochester* (BS)

State University of New York at Binghamton, Decker School of Nursing, *Binghamton* (BS)

State University of New York at New Paltz, Department of Nursing, *New Paltz* (BSN)

State University of New York at Plattsburgh, Department of Nursing, *Plattsburgh* (BS)

State University of New York College at Brockport, Department of Nursing, *Brockport* (BSN)

University at Buffalo, the State University of New York, School of Nursing, *Buffalo* (BS)

Utica College, Department of Nursing, *Utica* (BS)

Wagner College, Department of Nursing, *Staten Island* (BS)

North Carolina

Barton College, School of Nursing, *Wilson* (BSN)

East Carolina University, School of Nursing, *Greenville* (BSN)

Fayetteville State University, Program in Nursing, *Fayetteville* (BS)

Lenoir-Rhyne College, Program in Nursing, *Hickory* (BS)

North Carolina Agricultural and Technical State University, School of Nursing, *Greensboro* (BSN)

North Carolina Central University, Department of Nursing, *Durham* (BSN)

Queens University of Charlotte, Division of Nursing, *Charlotte* (BSN)

The University of North Carolina at Chapel Hill, School of Nursing, *Chapel Hill* (BSN)

The University of North Carolina at Charlotte, School of Nursing, *Charlotte* (BSN)

The University of North Carolina at Greensboro, School of Nursing, *Greensboro* (BSN)

The University of North Carolina Wilmington, School of Nursing, *Wilmington* (BSN)

Western Carolina University, Department of Nursing, *Cullowhee* (BSN)

Winston-Salem State University, Department of Nursing, *Winston-Salem* (BSN)

North Dakota

Minot State University, Department of Nursing, *Minot* (BSN)

North Dakota State University, Tri-College University Nursing Consortium, *Fargo* (BSN)

University of Mary, Division of Nursing, *Bismarck* (BSN)

University of North Dakota, College of Nursing, *Grand Forks* (BSN)

Ohio

Capital University, School of Nursing, *Columbus* (BSN)

Case Western Reserve University, Frances Payne Bolton School of Nursing, *Cleveland* (BSN)

Cleveland State University, Department of Nursing, *Cleveland* (BSN)

College of Mount St. Joseph, Department of Nursing, *Cincinnati* (BSN)

Franciscan University of Steubenville, Department of Nursing, *Steubenville* (BSN)

Kent State University, College of Nursing, *Kent* (BSN)

Lourdes College, Nursing Department, *Sylvania* (BSN)

Malone College, School of Nursing, *Canton* (BSN)

Mercy College of Northwest Ohio, Division of Nursing, *Toledo* (BSN)

Mount Carmel College of Nursing, Nursing Programs, *Columbus* (BSN)

The Ohio State University, College of Nursing, *Columbus* (BSN)

Otterbein College, Department of Nursing, *Westerville* (BSN)

The University of Akron, College of Nursing, *Akron* (BSN)

University of Cincinnati, College of Nursing, *Cincinnati* (BSN)

The University of Toledo, College of Nursing, *Toledo* (BSN)

Ursuline College, The Breen School of Nursing, *Pepper Pike* (BSN)

Walsh University, Department of Nursing, *North Canton* (BSN)

Wright State University, College of Nursing and Health, *Dayton* (BSN)

Xavier University, Department of Nursing, *Cincinnati* (BSN)

Oklahoma

East Central University, Department of Nursing, *Ada* (BS)

Langston University, School of Nursing and Health Professions, *Langston* (BSN)

Oklahoma Baptist University, School of Nursing, *Shawnee* (BSN)

Oklahoma City University, Kramer School of Nursing, *Oklahoma City* (BSN)

Oklahoma Wesleyan University, Division of Nursing, *Bartlesville* (BSN)

Oral Roberts University, Anna Vaughn School of Nursing, *Tulsa* (BSN)

Southern Nazarene University, School of Nursing, *Bethany* (BS)

Southwestern Oklahoma State University, Division of Nursing, *Weatherford* (BSN)

University of Central Oklahoma, Department of Nursing, *Edmond* (BSN)

University of Oklahoma Health Sciences Center, College of Nursing, *Oklahoma City* (BSN)

University of Tulsa, School of Nursing, *Tulsa* (BSN)

Oregon

Linfield College, School of Nursing, *McMinnville* (BSN)

Oregon Health & Science University, School of Nursing, *Portland* (BS)

University of Portland, School of Nursing, *Portland* (BSN)

Pennsylvania

Alvernia College, Nursing, *Reading* (BSN)

Bloomsburg University of Pennsylvania, Department of Nursing, *Bloomsburg* (BSN)

Carlow University, School of Nursing, *Pittsburgh* (BSN)

Cedar Crest College, Department of Nursing, *Allentown* (BS)

College Misericordia, Department of Nursing, *Dallas* (BSN)

DeSales University, Department of Nursing and Health, *Center Valley* (BSN)

Drexel University, College of Nursing and Health Professions, *Philadelphia* (BSN)

Duquesne University, School of Nursing, *Pittsburgh* (BSN)

East Stroudsburg University of Pennsylvania, Department of Nursing, *East Stroudsburg* (BSN)

Edinboro University of Pennsylvania, Department of Nursing, *Edinboro* (BS)

Gannon University, Program in Nursing, *Erie* (BSN)

Holy Family University, School of Nursing and Allied Health Professions, *Philadelphia* (BSN)

Indiana University of Pennsylvania, Department of Nursing and Allied Health, *Indiana* (BSN)

La Salle University, School of Nursing and Health Sciences, *Philadelphia* (BSN)

Mansfield University of Pennsylvania, Robert Packer Department of Health Sciences, *Mansfield* (BSN)

Marywood University, Department of Nursing, *Scranton* (BSN)

Messiah College, Department of Nursing, *Grantham* (BSN)

Moravian College, St. Luke's School of Nursing, *Bethlehem* (BS)

Neumann College, Program in Nursing and Health Sciences, *Aston* (BS)

Penn State University Park, School of Nursing, *State College, University Park* (BS)

Robert Morris University, School of Nursing and Allied Health, *Moon Township* (BSN)

Saint Francis University, Department of Nursing, *Loretto* (BSN)

Temple University, Department of Nursing, *Philadelphia* (BSN)

Thomas Jefferson University, Department of Nursing, *Philadelphia* (BSN)

University of Pennsylvania, School of Nursing, *Philadelphia* (BSN)

University of Pittsburgh, School of Nursing, *Pittsburgh* (BSN)

The University of Scranton, Department of Nursing, *Scranton* (BS)

Villanova University, College of Nursing, *Villanova* (BSN)

Waynesburg College, Department of Nursing, *Waynesburg* (BSN)

West Chester University of Pennsylvania, Department of Nursing, *West Chester* (BSN)

Widener University, School of Nursing, *Chester* (BSN)

Wilkes University, Department of Nursing, *Wilkes-Barre* (BS)

York College of Pennsylvania, Department of Nursing, *York* (BS)

Puerto Rico

Inter American University of Puerto Rico, Metropolitan Campus, Carmen Torres de Tiburcio School of Nursing, *San Juan* (BSN)

Pontifical Catholic University of Puerto Rico, Department of Nursing, *Ponce* (BSN)

Universidad Adventista de las Antillas, Department of Nursing, *Mayagüez* (BSN)

Universidad del Turabo, Nursing Program, *Gurabo* (BS)

University of Puerto Rico at Arecibo, Department of Nursing, *Arecibo* (BSN)

University of Puerto Rico at Humacao, Department of Nursing, *Humacao* (BS)

University of Puerto Rico, Mayagüez Campus, Department of Nursing, *Mayagüez* (BSN)

University of Puerto Rico, Medical Sciences Campus, School of Nursing, *San Juan* (BSN)

University of the Sacred Heart, Program in Nursing, *San Juan* (BSN)

Rhode Island

Rhode Island College, Department of Nursing, *Providence* (BS)

Salve Regina University, Department of Nursing, *Newport* (BS)

University of Rhode Island, College of Nursing, *Kingston* (BS)

South Carolina

Charleston Southern University, Wingo School of Nursing, *Charleston* (BSN)

Clemson University, School of Nursing, *Clemson* (BS)

Francis Marion University, Department of Nursing, *Florence* (BSN)

Lander University, School of Nursing, *Greenwood* (BSN)

South Carolina State University, Department of Nursing, *Orangeburg* (BSN)

University of South Carolina, College of Nursing, *Columbia* (BSN)

University of South Carolina Aiken, School of Nursing, *Aiken* (BSN)

University of South Carolina Upstate, Mary Black School of Nursing, *Spartanburg* (BSN)

South Dakota

Augustana College, Department of Nursing, *Sioux Falls* (BA)

Mount Marty College, Nursing Program, *Yankton* (BSc PN)

Presentation College, Department of Nursing, *Aberdeen* (BSN)

South Dakota State University, College of Nursing, *Brookings* (BS)

Tennessee

Austin Peay State University, School of Nursing, *Clarksville* (BSN)

Baptist College of Health Sciences, Nursing Division, *Memphis* (BSN)

Belmont University, School of Nursing, *Nashville* (BSN)

Carson-Newman College, Department of Nursing, *Jefferson City* (BSN)

Cumberland University, Rudy School of Nursing and Health Professions, *Lebanon* (BSN)

East Tennessee State University, College of Nursing, *Johnson City* (BSN)

King College, School of Nursing, *Bristol* (BSN)

Middle Tennessee State University, School of Nursing, *Murfreesboro* (BSN)

Milligan College, Department of Nursing, *Milligan College* (BSN)

South College, Department of Nursing, *Knoxville* (BSN)

Tennessee State University, School of Nursing, *Nashville* (BSN)

Tennessee Technological University, School of Nursing, *Cookeville* (BSN)

Tennessee Wesleyan College, Fort Sanders Nursing Department, *Knoxville* (BSN)

Union University, School of Nursing, *Jackson* (BSN)

University of Memphis, Loewenberg School of Nursing, *Memphis* (BSN)

The University of Tennessee, College of Nursing, *Knoxville* (BSN)

The University of Tennessee at Chattanooga, School of Nursing, *Chattanooga* (BSN)

The University of Tennessee at Martin, Department of Nursing, *Martin* (BSN)

The University of Tennessee Health Science Center, College of Nursing, *Memphis* (BSN)

Texas

Baylor University, Louise Herrington School of Nursing, *Dallas* (BSN)

East Texas Baptist University, Department of Nursing, *Marshall* (BSN)

Lamar University, Department of Nursing, *Beaumont* (BSN)

Midwestern State University, Nursing Program, *Wichita Falls* (BSN)

Patty Hanks Shelton School of Nursing, *Abilene* (BSN)

Prairie View A&M University, College of Nursing, *Houston* (BSN)

Southwestern Adventist University, Department of Nursing, *Keene* (BS)

Tarleton State University, Department of Nursing, *Stephenville* (BSN)

Texas A&M International University, Canseco School of Nursing, *Laredo* (BSN)

Texas A&M University–Corpus Christi, School of Nursing and Health Sciences, *Corpus Christi* (BSN)

Texas Christian University, Harris School of Nursing, *Fort Worth* (BSN)

Texas Tech University Health Sciences Center, School of Nursing, *Lubbock* (BSN)

Texas Woman's University, College of Nursing, *Denton* (BS)

University of Mary Hardin-Baylor, College of Nursing, *Belton* (BSN)

The University of Texas at Arlington, School of Nursing, *Arlington* (BSN)

The University of Texas at Austin, School of Nursing, *Austin* (BSN)

The University of Texas at El Paso, School of Nursing, *El Paso* (BSN)

The University of Texas at Tyler, Program in Nursing, *Tyler* (BSN)

The University of Texas Health Science Center at Houston, School of Nursing, *Houston* (BSN)

The University of Texas Health Science Center at San Antonio, School of Nursing, *San Antonio* (BSN)

The University of Texas Medical Branch, School of Nursing, *Galveston* (BSN)

The University of Texas–Pan American, Department of Nursing, *Edinburg* (BSN)

University of the Incarnate Word, Program in Nursing, *San Antonio* (BSN)

West Texas A&M University, Division of Nursing, *Canyon* (BSN)

Utah

Southern Utah University, Department of Nursing, *Cedar City* (BSN)

University of Utah, College of Nursing, *Salt Lake City* (BS)

Westminster College, School of Nursing and Health Sciences, *Salt Lake City* (BSN)

Vermont

Norwich University, Division of Nursing, *Northfield* (BSN)

University of Vermont, Department of Nursing, *Burlington* (BS)

Virgin Islands

University of the Virgin Islands, Division of Nursing, *Saint Thomas* (BS)

Virginia

Eastern Mennonite University, Department of Nursing, *Harrisonburg* (BSN)

George Mason University, College of Nursing and Health Science, *Fairfax* (BSN)

Hampton University, Department of Nursing, *Hampton* (BS)

James Madison University, Department of Nursing, *Harrisonburg* (BSN)

Jefferson College of Health Sciences, Nursing Education Program, *Roanoke* (BSN)

Liberty University, Department of Nursing, *Lynchburg* (BSN)

Lynchburg College, School of Health Sciences and Human Performance, *Lynchburg* (BS)

Marymount University, School of Health Professions, *Arlington* (BSN)

Old Dominion University, Department of Nursing, *Norfolk* (BSN)

Radford University, School of Nursing, *Radford* (BSN)

Shenandoah University, Division of Nursing, *Winchester* (BSN)

University of Virginia, School of Nursing, *Charlottesville* (BSN)

The University of Virginia's College at Wise, Department of Nursing, *Wise* (BSN)

Virginia Commonwealth University, School of Nursing, *Richmond* (BS)

Washington

Intercollegiate College of Nursing/Washington State University, *Spokane* (BSN)

Northwest University, The Mark and Huldah Buntain School of Nursing, *Kirkland* (BS)

Pacific Lutheran University, School of Nursing, *Tacoma* (BSN)

Seattle Pacific University, School of Health Sciences, *Seattle* (BS)

Seattle University, College of Nursing, *Seattle* (BSN)

University of Washington, School of Nursing, *Seattle* (BSN)

Walla Walla College, School of Nursing, *College Place* (BS)

West Virginia

Alderson-Broaddus College, Department of Nursing, *Philippi* (BSN)

Marshall University, College of Health Professions, *Huntington* (BSN)

Mountain State University, Program in Nursing, *Beckley* (BSN)

Shepherd University, Department of Nursing Education, *Shepherdstown* (BSN)

University of Charleston, Department of Nursing, *Charleston* (BSN)

West Liberty State College, Department of Health Sciences, *West Liberty* (BSN)

West Virginia University, School of Nursing, *Morgantown* (BSN)

West Virginia Wesleyan College, Department of Nursing, *Buckhannon* (BSN)

Wisconsin

Alverno College, Division of Nursing, *Milwaukee* (BSN)

Bellin College of Nursing, Nursing Program, *Green Bay* (BSN)

Carroll College, Nursing Program, *Waukesha* (BS)

Columbia College of Nursing/Mount Mary College Nursing Program, *Milwaukee* (BSN)

Edgewood College, Program in Nursing, *Madison* (BS)

Marian College of Fond du Lac, Nursing Studies Division, *Fond du Lac* (BSN)

Marquette University, College of Nursing, *Milwaukee* (BSN)

Milwaukee School of Engineering, School of Nursing, *Milwaukee* (BSN)

University of Wisconsin–Eau Claire, College of Nursing and Health Sciences, *Eau Claire* (BSN)

University of Wisconsin–Madison, School of Nursing, *Madison* (BS)

University of Wisconsin–Milwaukee, College of Nursing, *Milwaukee* (BSN)

University of Wisconsin–Oshkosh, College of Nursing, *Oshkosh* (BSN)

Viterbo University, School of Nursing, *La Crosse* (BSN)

Wyoming

University of Wyoming, Fay W. Whitney School of Nursing, *Laramie* (BSN)

CANADA

Alberta

University of Alberta, Faculty of Nursing, *Edmonton* (BScN)

University of Calgary, Faculty of Nursing, *Calgary* (BN)

University of Lethbridge, School of Health Sciences, *Lethbridge* (BN)

British Columbia

British Columbia Institute of Technology, School of Health Sciences, *Burnaby* (BScN)

Kwantlen University College, Faculty of Community and Health Sciences, *Surrey* (BSN)

Malaspina University-College, Department of Nursing, *Nanaimo* (BScN)

Trinity Western University, Department of Nursing, *Langley* (BScN)

The University of British Columbia–Okanagan, School of Nursing, *Kelowna* (BSN)

University of Northern British Columbia, Nursing Programme, *Prince George* (BSN)

Manitoba

Brandon University, School of Health Studies, *Brandon* (BN)

University of Manitoba, Faculty of Nursing, *Winnipeg* (BN)

New Brunswick

University of New Brunswick Fredericton, Faculty of Nursing, *Fredericton* (BN)

Newfoundland and Labrador

Memorial University of Newfoundland, School of Nursing, *St. John's* (BN)

Nova Scotia

Dalhousie University, School of Nursing, *Halifax* (BScN)

St. Francis Xavier University, Department of Nursing, *Antigonish* (BScN)

Ontario

Brock University, Department of Nursing, *St. Catharines* (BScN)

Lakehead University, School of Nursing, *Thunder Bay* (BSN)

McMaster University, School of Nursing, *Hamilton* (BScN)

Nipissing University, Nursing Department, *North Bay* (BScN)

Queen's University at Kingston, School of Nursing, *Kingston* (BNSc)

Ryerson University, Program in Nursing, *Toronto* (BScN)

University of Ottawa, School of Nursing, *Ottawa* (BScN)

The University of Western Ontario, School of Nursing, *London* (BScN)

University of Windsor, School of Nursing, *Windsor* (BScN)

York University, School of Nursing, Atkinson Faculty of Liberal and Professional Studies, *Toronto* (BScN)

Prince Edward Island

University of Prince Edward Island, School of Nursing, *Charlottetown* (BScN)

Quebec

McGill University, School of Nursing, *Montréal* (BScN)

Université du Québec en Outaouais, Département des Sciences Infirmières, *Gatineau* (BScN)

Saskatchewan

University of Saskatchewan, College of Nursing, *Saskatoon* (BSN)

INTERNATIONAL NURSE TO BACCALAUREATE

California

Humboldt State University, Department of Nursing, *Arcata* (BSN)

Delaware

Wilmington College, Division of Nursing, *New Castle* (BSN)

Hawaii

Hawai'i Pacific University, School of Nursing, *Honolulu* (BSN)

Iowa

Morningside College, Department of Nursing Education, *Sioux City* (BSN)

Massachusetts

Salem State College, Program in Nursing, *Salem* (BSN)

Nebraska

Nebraska Wesleyan University, Department of Nursing, *Lincoln* (BSN)

University of Nebraska Medical Center, College of Nursing, *Omaha* (BSN)

New Jersey

College of Saint Elizabeth, Department of Nursing, *Morristown* (BSN)

New York

Daemen College, Department of Nursing, *Amherst* (BS)

Lehman College of the City University of New York, Department of Nursing, *Bronx* (BS)

Long Island University, Brooklyn Campus, School of Nursing, *Brooklyn* (BS)

St. Francis College, Department of Nursing, *Brooklyn Heights* (BS)

University at Buffalo, the State University of New York, School of Nursing, *Buffalo* (BS)

Oklahoma

Oklahoma Wesleyan University, Division of Nursing, *Bartlesville* (BSN)

Pennsylvania

Duquesne University, School of Nursing, *Pittsburgh* (BSN)

Eastern University, Program in Nursing, *St. Davids* (BSN)

Holy Family University, School of Nursing and Allied Health Professions, *Philadelphia* (BSN)

Marywood University, Department of Nursing, *Scranton* (BSN)

Neumann College, Program in Nursing and Health Sciences, *Aston* (BS)

Villanova University, College of Nursing, *Villanova* (BSN)

South Dakota

Mount Marty College, Nursing Program, *Yankton* (BSc PN)

Tennessee

Milligan College, Department of Nursing, *Milligan College* (BSN)

Texas

The University of Texas at Tyler, Program in Nursing, *Tyler* (BSN)

CANADA

Ontario

Ryerson University, Program in Nursing, *Toronto* (BScN)

University of Ottawa, School of Nursing, *Ottawa* (BScN)

LPN TO BACCALAUREATE

Arizona

University of Phoenix Online Campus, College of Health and Human Services, *Phoenix* (BSN)

University of Phoenix–Phoenix Campus, College of Health and Human Services, *Phoenix* (BSN)

Arkansas

Arkansas State University, Department of Nursing, *Jonesboro, State University* (BSN)

Arkansas Tech University, Program in Nursing, *Russellville* (BSN)

Harding University, College of Nursing, *Searcy* (BSN)

University of Arkansas, Eleanor Mann School of Nursing, *Fayetteville* (BSN)

University of Arkansas at Monticello, Division of Nursing, *Monticello* (BSN)

University of Arkansas for Medical Sciences, College of Nursing, *Little Rock* (BSN)

University of Central Arkansas, Department of Nursing, *Conway* (BSN)

California

Biola University, Department of Nursing, *La Mirada* (BSN)

California State University, Chico, School of Nursing, *Chico* (BSN)

California State University, Long Beach, Department of Nursing, *Long Beach* (BSN)

California State University, Stanislaus, Department of Nursing, *Turlock* (BSN)

Dominican University of California, Program in Nursing, *San Rafael* (BSN)

Humboldt State University, Department of Nursing, *Arcata* (BSN)

Loma Linda University, School of Nursing, *Loma Linda* (BS)

National University, Department of Nursing, *La Jolla* (BSN)

Sonoma State University, Department of Nursing, *Rohnert Park* (BSN)

Colorado

Colorado State University–Pueblo, Department of Nursing, *Pueblo* (BSN)

Mesa State College, Department of Nursing and Radiologic Sciences, *Grand Junction* (BSN)

University of Phoenix–Southern Colorado Campus, College of Health and Human Services, *Colorado Springs* (BSN)

Delaware

Delaware State University, Department of Nursing, *Dover* (BSN)

Wesley College, Nursing Program, *Dover* (BSN)

District of Columbia

Howard University, Division of Nursing, *Washington* (BSN)

Florida

Barry University, School of Nursing, *Miami Shores* (BSN)

Georgia

Armstrong Atlantic State University, Program in Nursing, *Savannah* (BSN)

Hawaii

Hawai'i Pacific University, School of Nursing, *Honolulu* (BSN)

University of Phoenix–Hawaii Campus, College of Health and Human Services, *Honolulu* (BSN)

Idaho

Boise State University, Department of Nursing, *Boise* (BS)

Idaho State University, Department of Nursing, *Pocatello* (BSN)

Lewis-Clark State College, Division of Nursing and Health Sciences, *Lewiston* (BSN)

Illinois

Blessing-Rieman College of Nursing, *Quincy* (BSN)

Bradley University, Department of Nursing, *Peoria* (BSN, BSc PN)

Chicago State University, College of Nursing and Allied Health Professions, *Chicago* (BSN)

Indiana

Ball State University, School of Nursing, *Muncie* (BS)

Bethel College, Department of Nursing, *Mishawaka* (BSN)

Marian College, Department of Nursing and Nutritional Science, *Indianapolis* (BSN)

Iowa

Allen College, Program in Nursing, *Waterloo* (BSN)

Briar Cliff University, Department of Nursing, *Sioux City* (BSN)

Morningside College, Department of Nursing Education, *Sioux City* (BSN)

BACCALAUREATE PROGRAMS
LPN to Baccalaureate

Kansas
Bethel College, Department of Nursing, *North Newton* (BSN)
Emporia State University, Newman Division of Nursing, *Emporia* (BSN)
Newman University, Division of Nursing, *Wichita* (BSN)
Washburn University, School of Nursing, *Topeka* (BSN)

Louisiana
Grambling State University, School of Nursing, *Grambling* (BSN)
McNeese State University, College of Nursing, *Lake Charles* (BSN)
Nicholls State University, Department of Nursing, *Thibodaux* (BSN)
Northwestern State University of Louisiana, College of Nursing, *Shreveport* (BSN)
University of Louisiana at Monroe, Nursing, *Monroe* (BS)

Massachusetts
Salem State College, Program in Nursing, *Salem* (BSN)
Simmons College, Department of Nursing, *Boston* (BS)

Michigan
Madonna University, College of Nursing and Health, *Livonia* (BSN)

Missouri
Cox College of Nursing and Health Sciences, Department of Nursing, *Springfield* (BSN)
Maryville University of Saint Louis, Nursing Program, School of Health Professions, *St. Louis* (BSN)
Missouri State University, Department of Nursing, *Springfield* (BSN)
Missouri Western State University, Department of Nursing, *St. Joseph* (BSN)

Montana
Carroll College, Department of Nursing, *Helena* (BA)
Montana State University, College of Nursing, *Bozeman* (BSN)

Nebraska
Midland Lutheran College, Department of Nursing, *Fremont* (BSN)
Nebraska Methodist College, Department of Nursing, *Omaha* (BSN)
Union College, Division of Health Sciences, *Lincoln* (BSN)
University of Nebraska Medical Center, College of Nursing, *Omaha* (BSN)

New Jersey
William Paterson University of New Jersey, Department of Nursing, *Wayne* (BSN)

New York
Adelphi University, School of Nursing, *Garden City* (BS)
Dominican College, Department of Nursing, *Orangeburg* (BSN)
Molloy College, Department of Nursing, *Rockville Centre* (BS)
Nazareth College of Rochester, Department of Nursing, *Rochester* (BS)
State University of New York College at Brockport, Department of Nursing, *Brockport* (BSN)

North Carolina
North Carolina Agricultural and Technical State University, School of Nursing, *Greensboro* (BSN)
Queens University of Charlotte, Division of Nursing, *Charlotte* (BSN)
The University of North Carolina at Greensboro, School of Nursing, *Greensboro* (BSN)
Winston-Salem State University, Department of Nursing, *Winston-Salem* (BSN)

North Dakota
Dickinson State University, Department of Nursing, *Dickinson* (BSN)
Minot State University, Department of Nursing, *Minot* (BSN)
North Dakota State University, Tri-College University Nursing Consortium, *Fargo* (BSN)
University of Mary, Division of Nursing, *Bismarck* (BSN)
University of North Dakota, College of Nursing, *Grand Forks* (BSN)

Ohio
Kent State University, College of Nursing, *Kent* (BSN)
Lourdes College, Nursing Department, *Sylvania* (BSN)
MedCentral College of Nursing, *Mansfield* (BS)
Miami University, Department of Nursing, *Hamilton* (BSN)
Otterbein College, Department of Nursing, *Westerville* (BSN)
The University of Akron, College of Nursing, *Akron* (BSN)

Oklahoma
Langston University, School of Nursing and Health Professions, *Langston* (BSN)
Oklahoma Baptist University, School of Nursing, *Shawnee* (BSN)
Oklahoma Wesleyan University, Division of Nursing, *Bartlesville* (BSN)
University of Central Oklahoma, Department of Nursing, *Edmond* (BSN)
University of Oklahoma Health Sciences Center, College of Nursing, *Oklahoma City* (BSN)

Pennsylvania
Alvernia College, Nursing, *Reading* (BSN)
East Stroudsburg University of Pennsylvania, Department of Nursing, *East Stroudsburg* (BS)
Edinboro University of Pennsylvania, Department of Nursing, *Edinboro* (BS)
Holy Family University, School of Nursing and Allied Health Professions, *Philadelphia* (BSN)
La Salle University, School of Nursing and Health Sciences, *Philadelphia* (BSN)
Marywood University, Department of Nursing, *Scranton* (BSN)
Waynesburg College, Department of Nursing, *Waynesburg* (BSN)

South Dakota
Mount Marty College, Nursing Program, *Yankton* (BSc PN)
Presentation College, Department of Nursing, *Aberdeen* (BSN)

Tennessee
Baptist College of Health Sciences, Nursing Division, *Memphis* (BSN)
Cumberland University, Rudy School of Nursing and Health Professions, *Lebanon* (BSN)
East Tennessee State University, College of Nursing, *Johnson City* (BSN)
Milligan College, Department of Nursing, *Milligan College* (BSN)
Tennessee State University, School of Nursing, *Nashville* (BSN)
Union University, School of Nursing, *Jackson* (BSN)

Texas
Southwestern Adventist University, Department of Nursing, *Keene* (BS)
Tarleton State University, Department of Nursing, *Stephenville* (BSN)
The University of Texas at Tyler, Program in Nursing, *Tyler* (BSN)
The University of Texas Health Science Center at San Antonio, School of Nursing, *San Antonio* (BSN)
West Texas A&M University, Division of Nursing, *Canyon* (BSN)

Utah
Southern Utah University, Department of Nursing, *Cedar City* (BSN)

Virginia
Eastern Mennonite University, Department of Nursing, *Harrisonburg* (BSN)
Hampton University, Department of Nursing, *Hampton* (BS)
Shenandoah University, Division of Nursing, *Winchester* (BSN)

Washington
Pacific Lutheran University, School of Nursing, *Tacoma* (BSN)
Walla Walla College, School of Nursing, *College Place* (BS)

West Virginia
Mountain State University, Program in Nursing, *Beckley* (BSN)

Wisconsin
Alverno College, Division of Nursing, *Milwaukee* (BSN)

CANADA

Alberta
Athabasca University, Centre for Nursing and Health Studies, *Athabasca* (BN)
University of Alberta, Faculty of Nursing, *Edmonton* (BScN)

British Columbia
Malaspina University-College, Department of Nursing, *Nanaimo* (BScN)

Manitoba
Brandon University, School of Health Studies, *Brandon* (BN)

LPN TO RN
BACCALAUREATE

Arizona
University of Phoenix–Southern Arizona Campus, College of Health and Human Services, *Tucson* (BSN)

Arkansas
Harding University, College of Nursing, *Searcy* (BSN)
University of Arkansas, Eleanor Mann School of Nursing, *Fayetteville* (BSN)
University of Central Arkansas, Department of Nursing, *Conway* (BSN)

California
California State University, Sacramento, Division of Nursing, *Sacramento* (BSN)
Dominican University of California, Program in Nursing, *San Rafael* (BSN)
Loma Linda University, School of Nursing, *Loma Linda* (BS)
Point Loma Nazarene University, School of Nursing, *San Diego* (BSN)
Sonoma State University, Department of Nursing, *Rohnert Park* (BSN)

Colorado
Colorado State University-Pueblo, Department of Nursing, *Pueblo* (BSN)
Mesa State College, Department of Nursing and Radiologic Sciences, *Grand Junction* (BSN)

District of Columbia
Howard University, Division of Nursing, *Washington* (BSN)

Florida
Barry University, School of Nursing, *Miami Shores* (BSN)

Georgia
Georgia Southern University, School of Nursing, *Statesboro* (BSN)

Illinois

Saint Xavier University, School of Nursing, *Chicago* (BSN)

Indiana

Indiana State University, College of Nursing, *Terre Haute* (BS)

Iowa

Iowa Wesleyan College, Division of Health and Natural Sciences, *Mount Pleasant* (BSN)

Kansas

Wichita State University, School of Nursing, *Wichita* (BSN)

Louisiana

McNeese State University, College of Nursing, *Lake Charles* (BSN)

Southeastern Louisiana University, School of Nursing, *Hammond* (BS)

University of Louisiana at Lafayette, College of Nursing, *Lafayette* (BSN)

Massachusetts

Salem State College, Program in Nursing, *Salem* (BSN)

Michigan

Lake Superior State University, Department of Nursing, *Sault Sainte Marie* (BSN)

Northern Michigan University, College of Nursing and Allied Health Science, *Marquette* (BSN)

Missouri

Cox College of Nursing and Health Sciences, Department of Nursing, *Springfield* (BSN)

Missouri Southern State University, Department of Nursing, *Joplin* (BSN)

Nebraska

Clarkson College, Department of Nursing, *Omaha* (BSN)

Midland Lutheran College, Department of Nursing, *Fremont* (BSN)

University of Nebraska Medical Center, College of Nursing, *Omaha* (BSN)

North Carolina

The University of North Carolina at Greensboro, School of Nursing, *Greensboro* (BSN)

North Dakota

University of North Dakota, College of Nursing, *Grand Forks* (BSN)

Ohio

Malone College, School of Nursing, *Canton* (BSN)

Oklahoma

University of Tulsa, School of Nursing, *Tulsa* (BSN)

Pennsylvania

Alvernia College, Nursing, *Reading* (BSN)

Bloomsburg University of Pennsylvania, Department of Nursing, *Bloomsburg* (BSN)

Holy Family University, School of Nursing and Allied Health Professions, *Philadelphia* (BSN)

The University of Scranton, Department of Nursing, *Scranton* (BS)

Waynesburg College, Department of Nursing, *Waynesburg* (BSN)

Wilkes University, Department of Nursing, *Wilkes-Barre* (BS)

York College of Pennsylvania, Department of Nursing, *York* (BS)

South Dakota

Mount Marty College, Nursing Program, *Yankton* (BSc PN)

Tennessee

Belmont University, School of Nursing, *Nashville* (BSN)

Cumberland University, Rudy School of Nursing and Health Professions, *Lebanon* (BSN)

Milligan College, Department of Nursing, *Milligan College* (BSN)

The University of Tennessee at Martin, Department of Nursing, *Martin* (BSN)

Texas

The University of Texas at Tyler, Program in Nursing, *Tyler* (BSN)

The University of Texas Health Science Center at San Antonio, School of Nursing, *San Antonio* (BSN)

Virginia

Hampton University, Department of Nursing, *Hampton* (BS)

Shenandoah University, Division of Nursing, *Winchester* (BSN)

West Virginia

Alderson-Broaddus College, Department of Nursing, *Philippi* (BSN)

Fairmont State University, School of Nursing and Allied Health Administration, *Fairmont* (BSN)

Wisconsin

Concordia University Wisconsin, Program in Nursing, *Mequon* (BSN)

CANADA

British Columbia

The University of British Columbia–Okanagan, School of Nursing, *Kelowna* (BSN)

RN BACCALAUREATE

Alabama

Auburn University Montgomery, School of Nursing, *Montgomery* (BSN)

Jacksonville State University, College of Nursing and Health Sciences, *Jacksonville* (BSN)

Samford University, Ida V. Moffett School of Nursing, *Birmingham* (BSN)

Tuskegee University, Program in Nursing, *Tuskegee* (BSN)

The University of Alabama, Capstone College of Nursing, *Tuscaloosa* (BSN)

The University of Alabama at Birmingham, School of Nursing, *Birmingham* (BSN)

The University of Alabama in Huntsville, College of Nursing, *Huntsville* (BSN)

University of Mobile, School of Nursing, *Mobile* (BSN)

University of North Alabama, College of Nursing and Allied Health, *Florence* (BSN)

University of South Alabama, College of Nursing, *Mobile* (BSN)

Alaska

University of Alaska Anchorage, School of Nursing, *Anchorage* (BS)

Arizona

Grand Canyon University, College of Nursing, *Phoenix* (BSN)

Northern Arizona University, School of Nursing, *Flagstaff* (BSN)

Arkansas

Arkansas State University, Department of Nursing, *Jonesboro, State University* (BSN)

Arkansas Tech University, Program in Nursing, *Russellville* (BSN)

Harding University, College of Nursing, *Searcy* (BSN)

Southern Arkansas University–Magnolia, Department of Nursing, *Magnolia* (BSN)

University of Arkansas, Eleanor Mann School of Nursing, *Fayetteville* (BSN)

University of Arkansas at Fort Smith, Carol McKelvey Moore School of Nursing, *Fort Smith* (BSN)

University of Arkansas at Monticello, Division of Nursing, *Monticello* (BSN)

University of Arkansas for Medical Sciences, College of Nursing, *Little Rock* (BSN)

University of Central Arkansas, Department of Nursing, *Conway* (BSN)

California

Biola University, Department of Nursing, *La Mirada* (BSN)

California State University, Bakersfield, Program in Nursing, *Bakersfield* (BSN)

California State University, Chico, School of Nursing, *Chico* (BSN)

California State University, Dominguez Hills, Program in Nursing, *Carson* (BSN)

California State University, East Bay, Department of Nursing and Health Sciences, *Hayward* (BS)

California State University, Los Angeles, School of Nursing, *Los Angeles* (BS)

California State University, Northridge, Nursing Program, *Northridge* (BSN)

California State University, Sacramento, Division of Nursing, *Sacramento* (BSN)

California State University, San Bernardino, Department of Nursing, *San Bernardino* (BSN)

Dominican University of California, Program in Nursing, *San Rafael* (BSN)

Holy Names University, Department of Nursing, *Oakland* (BSN)

Humboldt State University, Department of Nursing, *Arcata* (BSN)

Loma Linda University, School of Nursing, *Loma Linda* (BS)

National University, Department of Nursing, *La Jolla* (BSN)

Point Loma Nazarene University, School of Nursing, *San Diego* (BSN)

San Diego State University, School of Nursing, *San Diego* (BSN)

San Francisco State University, School of Nursing, *San Francisco* (BSN)

Sonoma State University, Department of Nursing, *Rohnert Park* (BSN)

University of Phoenix–Central Valley Campus, College of Health and Human Services, *Fresno* (BSN)

University of San Diego, Hahn School of Nursing and Health Sciences, *San Diego* (BSN)

Colorado

Colorado State University-Pueblo, Department of Nursing, *Pueblo* (BSN)

Mesa State College, Department of Nursing and Radiologic Sciences, *Grand Junction* (BSN)

Metropolitan State College of Denver, Department of Health Professions, *Denver* (BS)

Regis University, Department of Nursing, *Denver* (BSN)

University of Colorado at Colorado Springs, Beth-El College of Nursing and Health Sciences, *Colorado Springs* (BSN)

University of Colorado at Denver and Health Sciences Center, School of Nursing, *Denver* (BS)

University of Northern Colorado, School of Nursing, *Greeley* (BS)

Connecticut

Central Connecticut State University, Department of Counseling and Family Therapy, *New Britain* (BSN)

Fairfield University, School of Nursing, *Fairfield* (BS)

Sacred Heart University, Program in Nursing, *Fairfield* (BS)

Saint Joseph College, Department of Nursing, *West Hartford* (BS)

Southern Connecticut State University, Department of Nursing, *New Haven* (BSN)

University of Connecticut, School of Nursing, *Storrs* (BS)

University of Hartford, College of Education, Nursing, and Health Professions, *West Hartford* (BSN)

BACCALAUREATE PROGRAMS
RN Baccalaureate

Western Connecticut State University, Department of Nursing, *Danbury* (BS)

Delaware
University of Delaware, School of Nursing, *Newark* (BSN)

Wilmington College, Division of Nursing, *New Castle* (BSN)

District of Columbia
Georgetown University, School of Nursing and Health Studies, *Washington* (BSN)

Howard University, Division of Nursing, *Washington* (BSN)

Florida
Barry University, School of Nursing, *Miami Shores* (BSN)

Bethune-Cookman College, School of Nursing, *Daytona Beach* (BSN)

Florida Atlantic University, College of Nursing, *Boca Raton* (BSN)

Florida Hospital College of Health Sciences, Department of Nursing, *Orlando* (BS)

Florida International University, College of Nursing and Health Sciences, *Miami* (BSN)

Florida State University, School of Nursing, *Tallahassee* (BSN)

Jacksonville University, School of Nursing, *Jacksonville* (BSN)

Nova Southeastern University, College of Allied Health and Nursing, *Fort Lauderdale* (BSN)

St. Petersburg College, Department of Nursing, *St. Petersburg* (BSN)

University of Central Florida, School of Nursing, *Orlando* (BSN)

University of Florida, College of Nursing, *Gainesville* (BSN)

University of Miami, School of Nursing and Health Studies, *Coral Gables* (BSN)

University of North Florida, School of Nursing, *Jacksonville* (BSN)

University of Phoenix-South Florida Campus, College of Health and Human Services, *Fort Lauderdale* (BSN)

University of South Florida, College of Nursing, *Tampa* (BS)

The University of Tampa, Department of Nursing, *Tampa* (BSN)

University of West Florida, Department of Nursing, *Pensacola* (BSN)

Georgia
Albany State University, College of Health Professions, *Albany* (BSN)

Armstrong Atlantic State University, Program in Nursing, *Savannah* (BSN)

Brenau University, School of Health and Science, *Gainesville* (BSN)

Clayton State University, Department of Nursing, *Morrow* (BSN)

Georgia Baptist College of Nursing of Mercer University, Department of Nursing, *Atlanta* (BSN)

Georgia College & State University, School of Health Sciences, *Milledgeville* (BSN)

Georgia Southwestern State University, School of Nursing, *Americus* (BSN)

Georgia State University, School of Nursing, *Atlanta* (BS)

Kennesaw State University, School of Nursing, *Kennesaw* (BSN)

LaGrange College, Department of Nursing, *LaGrange* (BSN)

Medical College of Georgia, School of Nursing, *Augusta* (BSN)

North Georgia College & State University, Department of Nursing, *Dahlonega* (BSN)

Piedmont College, School of Nursing, *Demorest* (BSN)

Thomas University, Division of Nursing, *Thomasville* (BSN)

University of West Georgia, Department of Nursing, *Carrollton* (BSN)

Valdosta State University, College of Nursing, *Valdosta* (BSN)

Guam
University of Guam, College of Nursing and Health Sciences, *Mangilao* (BSN)

Hawaii
Hawai'i Pacific University, School of Nursing, *Honolulu* (BSN)

University of Hawaii at Hilo, Department in Nursing, *Hilo* (BSN)

University of Hawaii at Manoa, School of Nursing and Dental Hygiene, *Honolulu* (BS)

Idaho
Boise State University, Department of Nursing, *Boise* (BS)

Lewis-Clark State College, Division of Nursing and Health Sciences, *Lewiston* (BSN)

Illinois
Aurora University, School of Nursing, *Aurora* (BSN)

Blessing-Rieman College of Nursing, *Quincy* (BSN)

Bradley University, Department of Nursing, *Peoria* (BSN, BSc PN)

Chicago State University, College of Nursing and Allied Health Professions, *Chicago* (BSN)

Elmhurst College, Deicke Center for Nursing Education, *Elmhurst* (BSN)

Governors State University, Division of Nursing, Communication Disorders, Occupational Therapy, and Physical Therapy, *University Park* (BS)

Illinois State University, Mennonite College of Nursing, *Normal* (BSN)

Illinois Wesleyan University, School of Nursing, *Bloomington* (BSN)

Lakeview College of Nursing, *Danville* (BSN)

Loyola University Chicago, Marcella Niehoff School of Nursing, *Chicago* (BSN)

MacMurray College, Department of Nursing, *Jacksonville* (BSN)

Northern Illinois University, School of Nursing, *De Kalb* (BSN)

North Park University, School of Nursing, *Chicago* (BS)

Rockford College, Department of Nursing, *Rockford* (BSN)

Rush University, College of Nursing, *Chicago* (BSN)

Saint Anthony College of Nursing, Saint Anthony College of Nursing, *Rockford* (BSN)

Saint Francis Medical Center College of Nursing, Baccalaureate Nursing Program, *Peoria* (BSN)

Saint Xavier University, School of Nursing, *Chicago* (BSN)

Southern Illinois University Edwardsville, School of Nursing, *Edwardsville* (BS)

Trinity Christian College, Department of Nursing, *Palos Heights* (BSN)

Trinity College of Nursing and Health Sciences, *Rock Island* (BSN)

University of Illinois at Chicago, College of Nursing, *Chicago* (BSN)

West Suburban College of Nursing, *Oak Park* (BSN)

Indiana
Ball State University, School of Nursing, *Muncie* (BS)

Bethel College, Department of Nursing, *Mishawaka* (BSN)

Goshen College, Department of Nursing, *Goshen* (BSN)

Indiana State University, College of Nursing, *Terre Haute* (BS)

Indiana University Bloomington, Department of Nursing-Bloomington Division, *Bloomington* (BSN)

Indiana University East, Division of Nursing, *Richmond* (BSN)

Indiana University Northwest, School of Nursing and Health Professions, *Gary* (BSN)

Indiana University-Purdue University Fort Wayne, Department of Nursing, *Fort Wayne* (BS)

Indiana University-Purdue University Indianapolis, School of Nursing, *Indianapolis* (BSN)

Indiana University South Bend, Division of Nursing and Health Professions, *South Bend* (BSN)

Indiana University Southeast, Division of Nursing, *New Albany* (BSN)

Indiana Wesleyan University, Division of Nursing, *Marion* (BS)

Marian College, Department of Nursing and Nutritional Science, *Indianapolis* (BSN)

Purdue University, School of Nursing, *West Lafayette* (BS)

Purdue University Calumet, School of Nursing, *Hammond* (BS)

Purdue University North Central, Department of Nursing, *Westville* (BS)

University of Saint Francis, Department of Nursing, *Fort Wayne* (BSN)

University of Southern Indiana, College of Nursing and Health Professions, *Evansville* (BSN)

Valparaiso University, College of Nursing, *Valparaiso* (BSN)

Iowa
Allen College, Program in Nursing, *Waterloo* (BSN)

Briar Cliff University, Department of Nursing, *Sioux City* (BSN)

Clarke College, Department of Nursing and Health, *Dubuque* (BS)

Coe College, Department of Nursing, *Cedar Rapids* (BSN)

Grand View College, Division of Nursing, *Des Moines* (BSN)

Iowa Wesleyan College, Division of Health and Natural Sciences, *Mount Pleasant* (BSN)

Mercy College of Health Sciences, Division of Nursing, *Des Moines* (BSN)

Morningside College, Department of Nursing Education, *Sioux City* (BSN)

St. Ambrose University, Program in Nursing (BSN), *Davenport* (BSN)

The University of Iowa, College of Nursing, *Iowa City* (BSN)

Kansas
Baker University, School of Nursing, *Topeka* (BSN)

Bethel College, Department of Nursing, *North Newton* (BSN)

Emporia State University, Newman Division of Nursing, *Emporia* (BSN)

Fort Hays State University, Department of Nursing, *Hays* (BSN)

Kansas Wesleyan University, Department of Nursing Education, *Salina* (BSN)

MidAmerica Nazarene University, Division of Nursing, *Olathe* (BSN)

Newman University, Division of Nursing, *Wichita* (BSN)

Pittsburg State University, Department of Nursing, *Pittsburg* (BSN)

Southwestern College, Nursing Program, *Winfield* (BSN)

University of Kansas, School of Nursing, *Kansas City* (BSN)

Washburn University, School of Nursing, *Topeka* (BSN)

Wichita State University, School of Nursing, *Wichita* (BSN)

Kentucky
Bellarmine University, Donna and Allan Lansing School of Nursing and Health Sciences, *Louisville* (BSN)

Eastern Kentucky University, Department of Baccalaureate and Graduate Nursing, *Richmond* (BSN)

Midway College, Program in Nursing (Baccalaureate), *Midway* (BSN)

Morehead State University, Department of Nursing, *Morehead* (BSN)

Murray State University, Program in Nursing, *Murray* (BSN)

Northern Kentucky University, Department of Nursing, *Highland Heights* (BSN)

University of Kentucky, Graduate School Programs in the College of Nursing, *Lexington* (BSN)

Louisiana

Dillard University, Division of Nursing, *New Orleans* (BSN)

Grambling State University, School of Nursing, *Grambling* (BSN)

Louisiana State University Health Sciences Center, School of Nursing, *New Orleans* (BSN)

Loyola University New Orleans, Program in Nursing, *New Orleans* (BSN)

Nicholls State University, Department of Nursing, *Thibodaux* (BSN)

Northwestern State University of Louisiana, College of Nursing, *Shreveport* (BSN)

Our Lady of the Lake College, Division of Nursing, *Baton Rouge* (BSN)

Southeastern Louisiana University, School of Nursing, *Hammond* (BS)

University of Louisiana at Lafayette, College of Nursing, *Lafayette* (BSN)

University of Louisiana at Monroe, Nursing, *Monroe* (BS)

Maine

Saint Joseph's College of Maine, Department of Nursing, *Standish* (BSN)

University of Maine, School of Nursing, *Orono* (BSN)

University of Maine at Fort Kent, Department of Nursing, *Fort Kent* (BSN)

University of New England, Department of Nursing, *Biddeford* (BSN)

Maryland

Bowie State University, Department of Nursing, *Bowie* (BSN)

College of Notre Dame of Maryland, Department of Nursing, *Baltimore* (BS)

Coppin State University, Helene Fuld School of Nursing, *Baltimore* (BSN)

The Johns Hopkins University, School of Nursing, *Baltimore* (BSN)

Salisbury University, Program in Nursing, *Salisbury* (BS)

Towson University, Department of Nursing, *Towson* (BS)

University of Maryland, Baltimore, Master's Program in Nursing, *Baltimore* (BSN)

Villa Julie College, Nursing Division, *Stevenson* (BS)

Massachusetts

American International College, Division of Nursing, *Springfield* (BSN)

Anna Maria College, Department of Nursing, *Paxton* (BS)

Atlantic Union College, Department of Nursing, *South Lancaster* (BSN)

Curry College, Division of Nursing, *Milton* (BS)

Elms College, Division of Nursing, *Chicopee* (BSc PN)

Emmanuel College, Department of Nursing, *Boston* (BSN)

Endicott College, Major in Nursing, *Beverly* (BS)

Fitchburg State College, Department of Nursing, *Fitchburg* (BS)

Northeastern University, School of Nursing, *Boston* (BSN)

Regis College, Department of Nursing, *Weston* (BSN)

Simmons College, Department of Nursing, *Boston* (BS)

University of Massachusetts Boston, College of Nursing and Health Sciences, *Boston* (BS)

University of Massachusetts Dartmouth, College of Nursing, *North Dartmouth* (BSN)

University of Massachusetts Lowell, Department of Nursing, *Lowell* (BS)

Michigan

Eastern Michigan University, School of Nursing, *Ypsilanti* (BSN)

Ferris State University, School of Nursing, *Big Rapids* (BSN)

Grand Valley State University, Russell B. Kirkhof College of Nursing, *Allendale* (BSN)

Lake Superior State University, Department of Nursing, *Sault Sainte Marie* (BSN)

Madonna University, College of Nursing and Health, *Livonia* (BSN)

Michigan State University, College of Nursing, *East Lansing* (BSN)

Oakland University, School of Nursing, *Rochester* (BSN)

Saginaw Valley State University, Crystal M. Lange College of Nursing and Health Sciences, *University Center* (BSN)

University of Detroit Mercy, McAuley School of Nursing, *Detroit* (BSN)

University of Michigan, School of Nursing, *Ann Arbor* (BSN)

University of Michigan-Flint, Department of Nursing, *Flint* (BSN)

Wayne State University, College of Nursing, *Detroit* (BSN)

Western Michigan University, College of Health and Human Services, *Kalamazoo* (BSN)

Minnesota

Bemidji State University, Department of Nursing, *Bemidji* (BS)

Bethel University, Department of Nursing, *St. Paul* (BSN)

College of St. Catherine, Department of Nursing, *St. Paul* (BA)

Minnesota State University Mankato, School of Nursing, *Mankato* (BS)

Minnesota State University Moorhead, Tri-College University Nursing Consortium, *Moorhead* (BSN)

Winona State University, College of Nursing, *Winona* (BS)

Mississippi

Alcorn State University, School of Nursing, *Natchez* (BSN)

Mississippi College, School of Nursing, *Clinton* (BSN)

Missouri

Barnes-Jewish College of Nursing and Allied Health, Division of Nursing, *St. Louis* (BSN)

Chamberlain College of Nursing, *St. Louis* (BSN)

Cox College of Nursing and Health Sciences, Department of Nursing, *Springfield* (BSN)

Graceland University, School of Nursing, *Independence* (BSN)

Lincoln University, Department of Nursing, *Jefferson City* (BSN)

Maryville University of Saint Louis, Nursing Program, School of Health Professions, *St. Louis* (BSN)

Missouri Southern State University, Department of Nursing, *Joplin* (BSN)

Missouri Western State University, Department of Nursing, *St. Joseph* (BSN)

Saint Louis University, School of Nursing, *St. Louis* (BSN)

Southeast Missouri State University, Department of Nursing, *Cape Girardeau* (BSN)

Southwest Baptist University, College of Nursing, *Bolivar* (BSN)

University of Central Missouri, Department of Nursing, *Warrensburg* (BS)

University of Missouri-Columbia, Sinclair School of Nursing, *Columbia* (BSN)

University of Missouri-Kansas City, School of Nursing, *Kansas City* (BSN)

University of Missouri-St. Louis, College of Nursing, *St. Louis* (BSN)

Webster University, Department of Nursing, *St. Louis* (BSN)

Montana

Montana State University-Northern, College of Nursing, *Havre* (BSN)

Salish Kootenai College, Nursing Department, *Pablo* (BS)

Nebraska

Clarkson College, Department of Nursing, *Omaha* (BSN)

Creighton University, School of Nursing, *Omaha* (BSN)

Midland Lutheran College, Department of Nursing, *Fremont* (BSN)

Nebraska Wesleyan University, Department of Nursing, *Lincoln* (BSN)

University of Nebraska Medical Center, College of Nursing, *Omaha* (BSN)

Nevada

Nevada State College at Henderson, Nursing Program, *Henderson* (BS)

University of Nevada, Reno, Orvis School of Nursing, *Reno* (BSN)

New Hampshire

Rivier College, Department of Nursing and Health Sciences, *Nashua* (BS)

Saint Anselm College, Department of Nursing, *Manchester* (BS)

University of New Hampshire, Department of Nursing, *Durham* (BS)

New Jersey

Bloomfield College, Division of Nursing, *Bloomfield* (BS)

College of Saint Elizabeth, Department of Nursing, *Morristown* (BSN)

Fairleigh Dickinson University, Metropolitan Campus, Henry P. Becton School of Nursing and Allied Health, *Teaneck* (BSN)

Felician College, Department of Professional Nursing-BSN, *Lodi* (BSN)

Kean University, Department of Nursing, *Union* (BSN)

Monmouth University, Marjorie K. Unterberg School of Nursing, *West Long Branch* (BSN)

New Jersey City University, Department of Nursing, *Jersey City* (BSN)

The Richard Stockton College of New Jersey, Program in Nursing, *Pomona* (BSN)

Rutgers, The State University of New Jersey, College of Nursing, *Newark* (BS)

Saint Peter's College, Nursing Program, *Jersey City* (BSN)

Seton Hall University, College of Nursing, *South Orange* (BSN)

Thomas Edison State College, School of Nursing, *Trenton* (BSN)

University of Medicine and Dentistry of New Jersey, School of Nursing, *Newark* (BSN)

William Paterson University of New Jersey, Department of Nursing, *Wayne* (BSN)

New Mexico

Eastern New Mexico University, Department of Allied Health-Nursing, *Portales* (BSN)

New Mexico State University, Department of Nursing, *Las Cruces* (BSN)

University of New Mexico, College of Nursing, *Albuquerque* (BSN)

New York

Adelphi University, School of Nursing, *Garden City* (BS)

College of Mount Saint Vincent, Department of Nursing, *Riverdale* (BS)

The College of New Rochelle, School of Nursing, *New Rochelle* (BSN)

College of Staten Island of the City University of New York, Department of Nursing, *Staten Island* (BS)

Daemen College, Department of Nursing, *Amherst* (BS)

Dominican College, Department of Nursing, *Orangeburg* (BSN)

D'Youville College, Department of Nursing, *Buffalo* (BSN)

Elmira College, Program in Nursing Education, *Elmira* (BS)

Excelsior College, School of Health Sciences, *Albany* (BSN)

Hartwick College, Department of Nursing, *Oneonta* (BS)

Hunter College of the City University of New York, Hunter-Bellevue School of Nursing, *New York* (BS)

Lehman College of the City University of New York, Department of Nursing, *Bronx* (BS)

Long Island University, Brooklyn Campus, School of Nursing, *Brooklyn* (BS)

Long Island University, C.W. Post Campus, Department of Nursing, *Brookville* (BS)

Mercy College, Program in Nursing, *Dobbs Ferry* (BS)

Molloy College, Department of Nursing, *Rockville Centre* (BS)

Mount Saint Mary College, Division of Nursing, *Newburgh* (BSN)

Nazareth College of Rochester, Department of Nursing, *Rochester* (BS)

New York University, College of Nursing, *New York* (BS)

Pace University, Lienhard School of Nursing, *New York* (BS)

Roberts Wesleyan College, Division of Nursing, *Rochester* (BScN)

The Sage Colleges, Division of Nursing, *Troy* (BS)

St. John Fisher College, Advanced Practice Nursing Program, *Rochester* (BS)

St. Joseph's College, New York, Department of Nursing, *Brooklyn* (BSN)

State University of New York at New Paltz, Department of Nursing, *New Paltz* (BSN)

State University of New York at Plattsburgh, Department of Nursing, *Plattsburgh* (BS)

State University of New York College at Brockport, Department of Nursing, *Brockport* (BSN)

State University of New York Downstate Medical Center, College of Nursing, *Brooklyn* (BS)

State University of New York Institute of Technology, School of Nursing and Health Systems, *Utica* (BS)

Stony Brook University, State University of New York, School of Nursing, *Stony Brook* (BS)

University of Rochester, School of Nursing, *Rochester* (BS)

Utica College, Department of Nursing, *Utica* (BS)

York College of the City University of New York, Program in Nursing, *Jamaica* (BS)

North Carolina

Cabarrus College of Health Sciences, Louise Harkey School of Nursing, *Concord* (BSN)

East Carolina University, School of Nursing, *Greenville* (BSN)

Fayetteville State University, Program in Nursing, *Fayetteville* (BS)

Gardner-Webb University, School of Nursing, *Boiling Springs* (BSN)

North Carolina Agricultural and Technical State University, School of Nursing, *Greensboro* (BSN)

Queens University of Charlotte, Division of Nursing, *Charlotte* (BSN)

The University of North Carolina at Chapel Hill, School of Nursing, *Chapel Hill* (BSN)

The University of North Carolina at Charlotte, School of Nursing, *Charlotte* (BSN)

The University of North Carolina at Greensboro, School of Nursing, *Greensboro* (BSN)

The University of North Carolina at Pembroke, Nursing Program, *Pembroke* (BSN)

The University of North Carolina Wilmington, School of Nursing, *Wilmington* (BS)

Western Carolina University, Department of Nursing, *Cullowhee* (BSN)

Winston-Salem State University, Department of Nursing, *Winston-Salem* (BSN)

North Dakota

Dickinson State University, Department of Nursing, *Dickinson* (BSN)

Medcenter One College of Nursing, Medcenter One College of Nursing, *Bismarck* (BSN)

Minot State University, Department of Nursing, *Minot* (BSN)

University of Mary, Division of Nursing, *Bismarck* (BSN)

University of North Dakota, College of Nursing, *Grand Forks* (BSN)

Ohio

Ashland University, Department of Nursing, *Ashland* (BSN)

Capital University, School of Nursing, *Columbus* (BSN)

Case Western Reserve University, Frances Payne Bolton School of Nursing, *Cleveland* (BSN)

Cedarville University, Department of Nursing, *Cedarville* (BSN)

Cleveland State University, Department of Nursing, *Cleveland* (BSN)

Franciscan University of Steubenville, Department of Nursing, *Steubenville* (BSN)

Kent State University, College of Nursing, *Kent* (BSN)

Kettering College of Medical Arts, Division of Nursing, *Kettering* (BSN)

Lourdes College, Nursing Department, *Sylvania* (BSN)

Malone College, School of Nursing, *Canton* (BSN)

MedCentral College of Nursing, *Mansfield* (BS)

Mercy College of Northwest Ohio, Division of Nursing, *Toledo* (BSN)

Miami University, Department of Nursing, *Hamilton* (BSN)

Mount Carmel College of Nursing, Nursing Programs, *Columbus* (BSN)

Ohio University, School of Nursing, *Athens* (BSN)

Otterbein College, Department of Nursing, *Westerville* (BSN)

Shawnee State University, Department of Nursing, *Portsmouth* (BSN)

The University of Akron, College of Nursing, *Akron* (BSN)

University of Cincinnati, College of Nursing, *Cincinnati* (BSN)

Wright State University, College of Nursing and Health, *Dayton* (BSN)

Oklahoma

Langston University, School of Nursing and Health Professions, *Langston* (BSN)

Northeastern State University, Department of Nursing, *Tahlequah* (BSN)

Oklahoma Baptist University, School of Nursing, *Shawnee* (BSN)

Oklahoma Wesleyan University, Division of Nursing, *Bartlesville* (BSN)

University of Central Oklahoma, Department of Nursing, *Edmond* (BSN)

University of Tulsa, School of Nursing, *Tulsa* (BSN)

Oregon

Linfield College, School of Nursing, *McMinnville* (BSN)

Oregon Health & Science University, School of Nursing, *Portland* (BS)

Pennsylvania

Alvernia College, Nursing, *Reading* (BSN)

Bloomsburg University of Pennsylvania, Department of Nursing, *Bloomsburg* (BSN)

California University of Pennsylvania, Department of Nursing, *California* (BSN)

Cedar Crest College, Department of Nursing, *Allentown* (BS)

Clarion University of Pennsylvania, School of Nursing, *Oil City* (BSN)

College Misericordia, Department of Nursing, *Dallas* (BSN)

DeSales University, Department of Nursing and Health, *Center Valley* (BSN)

Drexel University, College of Nursing and Health Professions, *Philadelphia* (BSN)

East Stroudsburg University of Pennsylvania, Department of Nursing, *East Stroudsburg* (BS)

Gannon University, Program in Nursing, *Erie* (BSN)

Gwynedd-Mercy College, School of Nursing, *Gwynedd Valley* (BSN)

Holy Family University, School of Nursing and Allied Health Professions, *Philadelphia* (BSN)

Indiana University of Pennsylvania, Department of Nursing and Allied Health, *Indiana* (BSN)

Kutztown University of Pennsylvania, Department of Nursing, *Kutztown* (BSN)

La Roche College, Department of Nursing and Nursing Management, *Pittsburgh* (BSN)

La Salle University, School of Nursing and Health Sciences, *Philadelphia* (BSN)

Mansfield University of Pennsylvania, Robert Packer Department of Health Sciences, *Mansfield* (BSN)

Marywood University, Department of Nursing, *Scranton* (BSN)

Millersville University of Pennsylvania, Department of Nursing, *Millersville* (BSN)

Moravian College, St. Luke's School of Nursing, *Bethlehem* (BS)

Neumann College, Program in Nursing and Health Sciences, *Aston* (BS)

Penn State University Park, School of Nursing, *State College, University Park* (BS)

Pennsylvania College of Technology, School of Health Sciences, *Williamsport* (BSN)

Robert Morris University, School of Nursing and Allied Health, *Moon Township* (BSN)

Saint Francis University, Department of Nursing, *Loretto* (BSN)

Slippery Rock University of Pennsylvania, Department of Nursing, *Slippery Rock* (BSN)

Temple University, Department of Nursing, *Philadelphia* (BSN)

Thomas Jefferson University, Department of Nursing, *Philadelphia* (BSN)

University of Pennsylvania, School of Nursing, *Philadelphia* (BSN)

University of Pittsburgh, School of Nursing, *Pittsburgh* (BSN)

University of Pittsburgh at Bradford, Department of Nursing, *Bradford* (BSN)

The University of Scranton, Department of Nursing, *Scranton* (BS)

Villanova University, College of Nursing, *Villanova* (BSN)

Widener University, School of Nursing, *Chester* (BSN)

Wilkes University, Department of Nursing, *Wilkes-Barre* (BS)

York College of Pennsylvania, Department of Nursing, *York* (BS)

Puerto Rico

Universidad Adventista de las Antillas, Department of Nursing, *Mayagüez* (BSN)

Rhode Island

Rhode Island College, Department of Nursing, *Providence* (BS)

Salve Regina University, Department of Nursing, *Newport* (BS)

University of Rhode Island, College of Nursing, *Kingston* (BS)

South Carolina

Charleston Southern University, Wingo School of Nursing, *Charleston* (BSN)

Clemson University, School of Nursing, *Clemson* (BS)

Lander University, School of Nursing, *Greenwood* (BSN)

Medical University of South Carolina, College of Nursing, *Charleston* (BSN)

South Carolina State University, Department of Nursing, *Orangeburg* (BSN)

University of South Carolina, College of Nursing, *Columbia* (BSN)

South Dakota

Mount Marty College, Nursing Program, *Yankton* (BSc PN)

Presentation College, Department of Nursing, *Aberdeen* (BSN)

South Dakota State University, College of Nursing, *Brookings* (BS)

Tennessee

Aquinas College, Department of Nursing, *Nashville* (BSN)

Austin Peay State University, School of Nursing, *Clarksville* (BSN)

Baptist College of Health Sciences, Nursing Division, *Memphis* (BSN)

Belmont University, School of Nursing, *Nashville* (BSN)

Carson-Newman College, Department of Nursing, *Jefferson City* (BSN)

Cumberland University, Rudy School of Nursing and Health Professions, *Lebanon* (BSN)

Lincoln Memorial University, Department of Nursing, *Harrogate* (BSN)

Middle Tennessee State University, School of Nursing, *Murfreesboro* (BSN)

Milligan College, Department of Nursing, *Milligan College* (BSN)

Tennessee State University, School of Nursing, *Nashville* (BSN)

Tennessee Technological University, School of Nursing, *Cookeville* (BSN)

Tennessee Wesleyan College, Fort Sanders Nursing Department, *Knoxville* (BSN)

Union University, School of Nursing, *Jackson* (BSN)

University of Memphis, Loewenberg School of Nursing, *Memphis* (BSN)

The University of Tennessee Health Science Center, College of Nursing, *Memphis* (BSN)

Texas

Angelo State University, Department of Nursing, *San Angelo* (BSN)

Lamar University, Department of Nursing, *Beaumont* (BSN)

Lubbock Christian University, Department of Nursing, *Lubbock* (BSN)

Midwestern State University, Nursing Program, *Wichita Falls* (BSN)

Patty Hanks Shelton School of Nursing, *Abilene* (BSN)

Prairie View A&M University, College of Nursing, *Houston* (BSN)

Southwestern Adventist University, Department of Nursing, *Keene* (BS)

Stephen F. Austin State University, Division of Nursing, *Nacogdoches* (BSN)

Texas A&M International University, Canseco School of Nursing, *Laredo* (BSN)

Texas A&M University-Corpus Christi, School of Nursing and Health Sciences, *Corpus Christi* (BSN)

Texas Woman's University, College of Nursing, *Denton* (BS)

University of Mary Hardin-Baylor, College of Nursing, *Belton* (BSN)

The University of Texas at Arlington, School of Nursing, *Arlington* (BSN)

The University of Texas at Austin, School of Nursing, *Austin* (BSN)

The University of Texas at El Paso, School of Nursing, *El Paso* (BSN)

The University of Texas at Tyler, Program in Nursing, *Tyler* (BSN)

The University of Texas Health Science Center at San Antonio, School of Nursing, *San Antonio* (BSN)

The University of Texas Medical Branch, School of Nursing, *Galveston* (BSN)

The University of Texas-Pan American, Department of Nursing, *Edinburg* (BSN)

Utah

Brigham Young University, College of Nursing, *Provo* (BS)

Southern Utah University, Department of Nursing, *Cedar City* (BSN)

University of Utah, College of Nursing, *Salt Lake City* (BS)

Westminster College, School of Nursing and Health Sciences, *Salt Lake City* (BSN)

Vermont

Norwich University, Division of Nursing, *Northfield* (BSN)

Southern Vermont College, Department of Nursing, *Bennington* (BSN)

University of Vermont, Department of Nursing, *Burlington* (BS)

Virgin Islands

University of the Virgin Islands, Division of Nursing, *Saint Thomas* (BS)

Virginia

Hampton University, Department of Nursing, *Hampton* (BS)

Jefferson College of Health Sciences, Nursing Education Program, *Roanoke* (BSN)

Liberty University, Department of Nursing, *Lynchburg* (BSN)

Marymount University, School of Health Professions, *Arlington* (BSN)

Norfolk State University, Department of Nursing, *Norfolk* (BSN)

Old Dominion University, Department of Nursing, *Norfolk* (BSN)

Radford University, School of Nursing, *Radford* (BSN)

Shenandoah University, Division of Nursing, *Winchester* (BSN)

The University of Virginia's College at Wise, Department of Nursing, *Wise* (BSN)

Washington

Gonzaga University, Department of Nursing, *Spokane* (BSN)

Intercollegiate College of Nursing/Washington State University, *Spokane* (BSN)

Seattle Pacific University, School of Health Sciences, *Seattle* (BS)

University of Washington, School of Nursing, *Seattle* (BSN)

Walla Walla College, School of Nursing, *College Place* (BS)

West Virginia

Alderson-Broaddus College, Department of Nursing, *Philippi* (BSN)

Bluefield State College, Program in Nursing, *Bluefield* (BSN)

Fairmont State University, School of Nursing and Allied Health Administration, *Fairmont* (BSN)

Mountain State University, Program in Nursing, *Beckley* (BSN)

Shepherd University, Department of Nursing Education, *Shepherdstown* (BSN)

West Virginia University, School of Nursing, *Morgantown* (BSN)

West Virginia Wesleyan College, Department of Nursing, *Buckhannon* (BSN)

Wisconsin

Alverno College, Division of Nursing, *Milwaukee* (BSN)

Concordia University Wisconsin, Program in Nursing, *Mequon* (BSN)

Marquette University, College of Nursing, *Milwaukee* (BSN)

Milwaukee School of Engineering, School of Nursing, *Milwaukee* (BSN)

University of Wisconsin-Eau Claire, College of Nursing and Health Sciences, *Eau Claire* (BSN)

University of Wisconsin-Green Bay, BSN-LINC Online RN-BSN Program, *Green Bay* (BSN)

University of Wisconsin-Madison, School of Nursing, *Madison* (BS)

University of Wisconsin-Milwaukee, College of Nursing, *Milwaukee* (BSN)

University of Wisconsin-Oshkosh, College of Nursing, *Oshkosh* (BSN)

Viterbo University, School of Nursing, *La Crosse* (BSN)

CANADA

Alberta

Athabasca University, Centre for Nursing and Health Studies, *Athabasca* (BN)

University of Alberta, Faculty of Nursing, *Edmonton* (BScN)

University of Calgary, Faculty of Nursing, *Calgary* (BN)

University of Lethbridge, School of Health Sciences, *Lethbridge* (BN)

British Columbia

Kwantlen University College, Faculty of Community and Health Sciences, *Surrey* (BSN)

Malaspina University-College, Department of Nursing, *Nanaimo* (BScN)

The University of British Columbia, School of Nursing, *Vancouver* (BSN)

The University of British Columbia-Okanagan, School of Nursing, *Kelowna* (BSN)

Manitoba

Brandon University, School of Health Studies, *Brandon* (BN)

University of Manitoba, Faculty of Nursing, *Winnipeg* (BN)

New Brunswick

Université de Moncton, School of Nursing, *Moncton* (BScN)

Newfoundland and Labrador

Memorial University of Newfoundland, School of Nursing, *St. John's* (BN)

Nova Scotia

Dalhousie University, School of Nursing, *Halifax* (BScN)

St. Francis Xavier University, Department of Nursing, *Antigonish* (BScN)

Ontario

Brock University, Department of Nursing, *St. Catharines* (BScN)

Lakehead University, School of Nursing, *Thunder Bay* (BSN)

McMaster University, School of Nursing, *Hamilton* (BScN)

Queen's University at Kingston, School of Nursing, *Kingston* (BNSc)

Ryerson University, Program in Nursing, *Toronto* (BScN)

Trent University, Nursing Program, *Peterborough* (BScN)

University of Ottawa, School of Nursing, *Ottawa* (BScN)

The University of Western Ontario, School of Nursing, *London* (BScN)

University of Windsor, School of Nursing, *Windsor* (BScN)

York University, School of Nursing, Atkinson Faculty of Liberal and Professional Studies, *Toronto* (BScN)

BACCALAUREATE PROGRAMS
RN Baccalaureate

Quebec

McGill University, School of Nursing, *Montréal* (BScN)

Université de Sherbrooke, Department of Nursing, *Sherbrooke* (BScN)

Université du Québec à Chicoutimi, Program in Nursing, *Chicoutimi* (BNSc)

Université du Québec à Rimouski, Program in Nursing, *Rimouski* (BScN)

Université du Québec en Outaouais, Département des Sciences Infirmières, *Gatineau* (BScN)

Saskatchewan

University of Saskatchewan, College of Nursing, *Saskatoon* (BSN)

RPN TO BACCALAUREATE

California

San Jose State University, School of Nursing, *San Jose* (BS)

Maine

Saint Joseph's College of Maine, Department of Nursing, *Standish* (BSN)

Maryland

Towson University, Department of Nursing, *Towson* (BS)

Michigan

Lake Superior State University, Department of Nursing, *Sault Sainte Marie* (BSN)

Missouri

Chamberlain College of Nursing, *St. Louis* (BSN)

Nebraska

University of Nebraska Medical Center, College of Nursing, *Omaha* (BSN)

New York

St. Francis College, Department of Nursing, *Brooklyn Heights* (BS)

Ohio

Franciscan University of Steubenville, Department of Nursing, *Steubenville* (BSN)

West Virginia

Mountain State University, Program in Nursing, *Beckley* (BSN)

CANADA

Alberta

University of Alberta, Faculty of Nursing, *Edmonton* (BScN)

British Columbia

British Columbia Institute of Technology, School of Health Sciences, *Burnaby* (BScN)

Ontario

Ryerson University, Program in Nursing, *Toronto* (BScN)

University of Ottawa, School of Nursing, *Ottawa* (BScN)

Saskatchewan

University of Saskatchewan, College of Nursing, *Saskatoon* (BSN)

MASTER'S DEGREE PROGRAMS

ACCELERATED AD/RN TO MASTER'S

Alabama
Spring Hill College, Division of Nursing, *Mobile* (MSN)

California
California State University, Fullerton, Department of Nursing, *Fullerton* (MSN)
University of San Diego, Hahn School of Nursing and Health Sciences, *San Diego* (MSN, MSN/MBA)

Connecticut
Sacred Heart University, Program in Nursing, *Fairfield* (MSN, MSN/MBA)
Saint Joseph College, Department of Nursing, *West Hartford* (MS)

Delaware
Wesley College, Nursing Program, *Dover* (MSN)

Florida
Florida Gulf Coast University, School of Nursing, *Fort Myers* (MSN)
Florida Southern College, Department of Nursing, *Lakeland* (MS)

Idaho
Idaho State University, Department of Nursing, *Pocatello* (MS)

Illinois
Rush University, College of Nursing, *Chicago* (MSN)
West Suburban College of Nursing, *Oak Park* (MSN)

Kansas
University of Kansas, School of Nursing, *Kansas City* (MS)

Massachusetts
Regis College, Department of Nursing, *Weston* (MSN)
Simmons College, Department of Nursing, *Boston* (MS, MSN/MS)

Michigan
Madonna University, College of Nursing and Health, *Livonia* (MSN, MSN/MBA)
University of Detroit Mercy, McAuley School of Nursing, *Detroit* (MSN)
Wayne State University, College of Nursing, *Detroit* (MSN)

Mississippi
University of Mississippi Medical Center, Program in Nursing, *Jackson* (MSN)

Missouri
Missouri State University, Department of Nursing, *Springfield* (MSN)

New York
Columbia University, School of Nursing, *New York* (MS, MS/MBA, MS/MPH)
Daemen College, Department of Nursing, *Amherst* (MS)
D'Youville College, Department of Nursing, *Buffalo* (MS)
Pace University, Lienhard School of Nursing, *New York* (MS)
State University of New York Institute of Technology, School of Nursing and Health Systems, *Utica* (MS)
University of Rochester, School of Nursing, *Rochester* (MS, MSN/PhD)

Ohio
Case Western Reserve University, Frances Payne Bolton School of Nursing, *Cleveland* (MSN, MSN/MA, MSN/MBA, MSN/MPH, MSN/PhD)
The Ohio State University, College of Nursing, *Columbus* (MS)

Pennsylvania
DeSales University, Department of Nursing and Health, *Center Valley* (MSN, MSN/MBA)
University of Pennsylvania, School of Nursing, *Philadelphia* (MSN, MSN/MBA, MSN/MPH, MSN/PhD)
The University of Scranton, Department of Nursing, *Scranton* (MS)
Wilkes University, Department of Nursing, *Wilkes-Barre* (MS)

Tennessee
Vanderbilt University, School of Nursing, *Nashville* (MSN, MSN/MBA, MSN/MDIV)

Texas
Texas A&M University-Corpus Christi, School of Nursing and Health Sciences, *Corpus Christi* (MSN)
The University of Texas at Tyler, Program in Nursing, *Tyler* (MSN, MSN/MBA)
The University of Texas Health Science Center at Houston, School of Nursing, *Houston* (MSN, MSN/MPH)

Virginia
James Madison University, Department of Nursing, *Harrisonburg* (MSN)

Wisconsin
Marquette University, College of Nursing, *Milwaukee* (MSN, MSN/MBA)

ACCELERATED MASTER'S

Alabama
University of South Alabama, College of Nursing, *Mobile* (MSN)

California
University of San Francisco, School of Nursing, *San Francisco* (MSN, MSN/MS)
Western University of Health Sciences, College of Graduate Nursing, *Pomona* (MSN)

Florida
University of Miami, School of Nursing and Health Studies, *Coral Gables* (MSN)

Georgia
Albany State University, College of Health Professions, *Albany* (MSN)
University of Phoenix-Atlanta Campus, College of Health and Human Services, *Atlanta* (MSN)

Illinois
Lewis University, Program in Nursing, *Romeoville* (MSN, MSN/MBA)

Massachusetts
Regis College, Department of Nursing, *Weston* (MSN)
Simmons College, Department of Nursing, *Boston* (MS, MSN/MS)
University of Massachusetts Lowell, Department of Nursing, *Lowell* (MS)

Nebraska
Nebraska Wesleyan University, Department of Nursing, *Lincoln* (MSN)

New York
Roberts Wesleyan College, Division of Nursing, *Rochester* (M Sc N)

Ohio
College of Mount St. Joseph, Department of Nursing, *Cincinnati* (MN)
The Ohio State University, College of Nursing, *Columbus* (MS)
Ursuline College, The Breen School of Nursing, *Pepper Pike* (MSN)

Oklahoma
Southern Nazarene University, School of Nursing, *Bethany* (MS)

Pennsylvania
Carlow University, School of Nursing, *Pittsburgh* (MSN)
Thomas Jefferson University, Department of Nursing, *Philadelphia* (MSN)
Villanova University, College of Nursing, *Villanova* (MSN)
Waynesburg College, Department of Nursing, *Waynesburg* (MSN, MSN/MBA)
Widener University, School of Nursing, *Chester* (MSN)

South Carolina
Medical University of South Carolina, College of Nursing, *Charleston* (MSN, MSN/PhD)

Tennessee
Vanderbilt University, School of Nursing, *Nashville* (MSN, MSN/MBA, MSN/MDIV)

Washington
Pacific Lutheran University, School of Nursing, *Tacoma* (MSN)

Wisconsin
Cardinal Stritch University, Ruth S. Coleman College of Nursing, *Milwaukee* (MSN)

ACCELERATED MASTER'S FOR NON-NURSING COLLEGE GRADUATES

California
Azusa Pacific University, School of Nursing, *Azusa* (MSN)
California State University, Long Beach, Department of Nursing, *Long Beach* (MSN, MSN/MPH)
San Francisco State University, School of Nursing, *San Francisco* (MSN)
University of San Francisco, School of Nursing, *San Francisco* (MSN, MSN/MS)

Georgia
Medical College of Georgia, School of Nursing, *Augusta* (MSN)

Kentucky
Spalding University, School of Nursing, *Louisville* (MSN)

Maryland
University of Maryland, Baltimore, Master's Program in Nursing, *Baltimore* (MS, MSN/MBA, MSN/MPH, MSN/PhD)

Massachusetts
Boston College, William F. Connell School of Nursing, *Chestnut Hill* (MS, MS/MA, MS/MBA, MSN/PhD)

Regis College, Department of Nursing, *Weston* (MSN)

Salem State College, Program in Nursing, *Salem* (MSN, MSN/MBA)

Simmons College, Department of Nursing, *Boston* (MS, MSN/MS)

New York
Columbia University, School of Nursing, *New York* (MS, MS/MBA, MS/MPH)

Mercy College, Program in Nursing, *Dobbs Ferry* (MS)

University of Rochester, School of Nursing, *Rochester* (MS, MSN/PhD)

Ohio
Case Western Reserve University, Frances Payne Bolton School of Nursing, *Cleveland* (MSN, MSN/MA, MSN/MBA, MSN/MPH, MSN/PhD)

The Ohio State University, College of Nursing, *Columbus* (MS)

University of Cincinnati, College of Nursing, *Cincinnati* (MSN, MSN/MBA)

Oregon
Oregon Health & Science University, School of Nursing, *Portland* (MS, MSN/MPH)

Pennsylvania
University of Pennsylvania, School of Nursing, *Philadelphia* (MSN, MSN/MBA, MSN/MPH, MSN/PhD)

Tennessee
Vanderbilt University, School of Nursing, *Nashville* (MSN, MSN/MBA, MSN/MDIV)

Virginia
University of Virginia, School of Nursing, *Charlottesville* (MSN, MSN/MA, MSN/MBA, MSN/PhD, MSN/HSM)

Virginia Commonwealth University, School of Nursing, *Richmond* (MS, MS/MPH)

Wisconsin
Marquette University, College of Nursing, *Milwaukee* (MSN, MSN/MBA)

ACCELERATED MASTER'S FOR NURSES WITH NON-NURSING DEGREES

California
Azusa Pacific University, School of Nursing, *Azusa* (MSN)

California State University, Los Angeles, School of Nursing, *Los Angeles* (MS)

San Francisco State University, School of Nursing, *San Francisco* (MSN)

University of San Francisco, School of Nursing, *San Francisco* (MSN, MSN/MS)

Connecticut
Sacred Heart University, Program in Nursing, *Fairfield* (MSN, MSN/MBA)

Illinois
Bradley University, Department of Nursing, *Peoria* (MSN)

Massachusetts
Regis College, Department of Nursing, *Weston* (MSN)

Simmons College, Department of Nursing, *Boston* (MS, MSN/MS)

Mississippi
Delta State University, School of Nursing, *Cleveland* (MSN)

New Jersey
Kean University, Department of Nursing, *Union* (MSN, MSN/MPA)

New York
Columbia University, School of Nursing, *New York* (MS, MS/MBA, MS/MPH)

Mercy College, Program in Nursing, *Dobbs Ferry* (MS)

Ohio
Case Western Reserve University, Frances Payne Bolton School of Nursing, *Cleveland* (MSN, MSN/MA, MSN/MBA, MSN/MPH, MSN/PhD)

College of Mount St. Joseph, Department of Nursing, *Cincinnati* (MN)

Pennsylvania
Waynesburg College, Department of Nursing, *Waynesburg* (MSN, MSN/MBA)

South Carolina
Medical University of South Carolina, College of Nursing, *Charleston* (MSN, MSN/PhD)

Tennessee
University of Memphis, Loewenberg School of Nursing, *Memphis* (MSN)

The University of Tennessee, College of Nursing, *Knoxville* (MSN)

Vanderbilt University, School of Nursing, *Nashville* (MSN, MSN/MBA, MSN/MDIV)

Texas
Texas A&M University–Corpus Christi, School of Nursing and Health Sciences, *Corpus Christi* (MSN)

Virginia
University of Virginia, School of Nursing, *Charlottesville* (MSN, MSN/MA, MSN/MBA, MSN/PhD, MSN/HSM)

Virginia Commonwealth University, School of Nursing, *Richmond* (MS, MS/MPH)

Washington
Intercollegiate College of Nursing/Washington State University, *Spokane* (MN)

Seattle University, College of Nursing, *Seattle* (MSN)

Wisconsin
University of Wisconsin–Milwaukee, College of Nursing, *Milwaukee* (MS, MS/MBA)

ACCELERATED RN TO MASTER'S

Alabama
The University of Alabama at Birmingham, School of Nursing, *Birmingham* (MSN, MSN/MPH)

California
California State University, Los Angeles, School of Nursing, *Los Angeles* (MS)

University of San Diego, Hahn School of Nursing and Health Sciences, *San Diego* (MSN, MSN/MBA)

Connecticut
Sacred Heart University, Program in Nursing, *Fairfield* (MSN, MSN/MBA)

Saint Joseph College, Department of Nursing, *West Hartford* (MS)

Delaware
Wesley College, Nursing Program, *Dover* (MSN)

Florida
Florida Gulf Coast University, School of Nursing, *Fort Myers* (MSN)

Jacksonville University, School of Nursing, *Jacksonville* (MSN, MSN/MBA)

The University of Tampa, Department of Nursing, *Tampa* (MSN)

Illinois
West Suburban College of Nursing, *Oak Park* (MSN)

Indiana
Purdue University Calumet, School of Nursing, *Hammond* (MS)

University of Saint Francis, Department of Nursing, *Fort Wayne* (MSN)

Iowa
The University of Iowa, College of Nursing, *Iowa City* (MSN, MSN/MBA, MSN/MPH)

Kentucky
Spalding University, School of Nursing, *Louisville* (MSN)

Massachusetts
Northeastern University, School of Nursing, *Boston* (MS, MSN/MBA)

Regis College, Department of Nursing, *Weston* (MSN)

Simmons College, Department of Nursing, *Boston* (MS, MSN/MS)

University of Massachusetts Lowell, Department of Nursing, *Lowell* (MS)

Michigan
Madonna University, College of Nursing and Health, *Livonia* (MSN, MSN/MBA)

University of Michigan, School of Nursing, *Ann Arbor* (MS, MSN/MBA, MSN/MPH)

Missouri
Maryville University of Saint Louis, Nursing Program, School of Health Professions, *St. Louis* (MSN)

New Jersey
Fairleigh Dickinson University, Metropolitan Campus, Henry P. Becton School of Nursing and Allied Health, *Teaneck* (MSN)

New York
Daemen College, Department of Nursing, *Amherst* (MS)

Pace University, Lienhard School of Nursing, *New York* (MS)

State University of New York Institute of Technology, School of Nursing and Health Systems, *Utica* (MS)

North Carolina
Queens University of Charlotte, Division of Nursing, *Charlotte* (MSN, MSN/MBA)

Ohio
Kent State University, College of Nursing, *Kent* (MSN, MSN/MBA, MSN/MPA)

University of Cincinnati, College of Nursing, *Cincinnati* (MSN, MSN/MBA)

Pennsylvania
Clarion University of Pennsylvania, School of Nursing, *Oil City* (MSN)

College Misericordia, Department of Nursing, *Dallas* (MSN)

DeSales University, Department of Nursing and Health, *Center Valley* (MSN, MSN/MBA)

Thomas Jefferson University, Department of Nursing, *Philadelphia* (MSN)

University of Pennsylvania, School of Nursing, *Philadelphia* (MSN, MSN/MBA, MSN/MPH, MSN/PhD)

The University of Scranton, Department of Nursing, *Scranton* (MS)

Waynesburg College, Department of Nursing, *Waynesburg* (MSN, MSN/MBA)

Wilkes University, Department of Nursing, *Wilkes-Barre* (MS)

South Carolina
Medical University of South Carolina, College of Nursing, *Charleston* (MSN, MSN/PhD)

Tennessee
Southern Adventist University, School of Nursing, *Collegedale* (MSN, MSN/MBA)

The University of Tennessee, College of Nursing, *Knoxville* (MSN)

Vanderbilt University, School of Nursing, *Nashville* (MSN, MSN/MBA, MSN/MDIV)

Texas

The University of Texas at Tyler, Program in Nursing, *Tyler* (MSN, MSN/MBA)

Virginia

James Madison University, Department of Nursing, *Harrisonburg* (MSN)

Radford University, School of Nursing, *Radford* (MSN)

Washington

Gonzaga University, Department of Nursing, *Spokane* (MSN)

Intercollegiate College of Nursing/Washington State University, *Spokane* (MN)

Wisconsin

Marquette University, College of Nursing, *Milwaukee* (MSN, MSN/MBA)

University of Wisconsin–Madison, School of Nursing, *Madison* (MS, MS/MPH)

CANADA

Quebec

Université du Québec à Chicoutimi, Program in Nursing, *Chicoutimi* (MSN)

MASTER'S

Alabama

Auburn University, School of Nursing, *Auburn University* (MSN)

Auburn University Montgomery, School of Nursing, *Montgomery* (MSN)

Jacksonville State University, College of Nursing and Health Sciences, *Jacksonville* (MSN)

Samford University, Ida V. Moffett School of Nursing, *Birmingham* (MSN, MSN/MBA)

Spring Hill College, Division of Nursing, *Mobile* (MSN)

Troy University, School of Nursing, *Troy* (MSN)

The University of Alabama, Capstone College of Nursing, *Tuscaloosa* (MSN, MSN/MA)

The University of Alabama at Birmingham, School of Nursing, *Birmingham* (MSN, MSN/MPH)

The University of Alabama in Huntsville, College of Nursing, *Huntsville* (MSN)

University of Mobile, School of Nursing, *Mobile* (MSN)

University of South Alabama, College of Nursing, *Mobile* (MSN)

Alaska

University of Alaska Anchorage, School of Nursing, *Anchorage* (MS)

Arizona

Arizona State University at the Downtown Phoenix Campus, College of Nursing, *Phoenix* (MS, MS/MPH)

Grand Canyon University, College of Nursing, *Phoenix* (MSN, MSN/MBA)

Northern Arizona University, School of Nursing, *Flagstaff* (MS)

The University of Arizona, College of Nursing, *Tucson* (MS)

University of Phoenix Online Campus, College of Health and Human Services, *Phoenix* (MSN, MSN/MBA)

University of Phoenix–Phoenix Campus, College of Health and Human Services, *Phoenix* (MSN)

University of Phoenix–Southern Arizona Campus, College of Health and Human Services, *Tucson* (MSN)

Arkansas

Arkansas State University, Department of Nursing, *Jonesboro, State University* (MSN)

University of Arkansas, Eleanor Mann School of Nursing, *Fayetteville* (MSN)

University of Arkansas for Medical Sciences, College of Nursing, *Little Rock* (M Sc N)

University of Central Arkansas, Department of Nursing, *Conway* (MSN)

California

Azusa Pacific University, School of Nursing, *Azusa* (MSN)

California State University, Bakersfield, Program in Nursing, *Bakersfield* (MSN)

California State University, Chico, School of Nursing, *Chico* (MSN)

California State University, Dominguez Hills, Program in Nursing, *Carson* (MSN)

California State University, Fresno, Department of Nursing, *Fresno* (MSN)

California State University, Fullerton, Department of Nursing, *Fullerton* (MSN)

California State University, Long Beach, Department of Nursing, *Long Beach* (MSN, MSN/MPH)

California State University, Los Angeles, School of Nursing, *Los Angeles* (MS)

California State University, Sacramento, Division of Nursing, *Sacramento* (MS)

California State University, San Bernardino, Department of Nursing, *San Bernardino* (MSN)

Dominican University of California, Program in Nursing, *San Rafael* (MSN)

Holy Names University, Department of Nursing, *Oakland* (MSN, MSN/MBA)

Loma Linda University, School of Nursing, *Loma Linda* (MS, MSN/MA, MSN/MPH)

Mount St. Mary's College, Department of Nursing, *Los Angeles* (MSN)

Point Loma Nazarene University, School of Nursing, *San Diego* (MSN)

Samuel Merritt College, School of Nursing, *Oakland* (MSN)

San Diego State University, School of Nursing, *San Diego* (MSN)

San Francisco State University, School of Nursing, *San Francisco* (MSN)

San Jose State University, School of Nursing, *San Jose* (MS)

Sonoma State University, Department of Nursing, *Robnert Park* (MSN)

University of California, Los Angeles, School of Nursing, *Los Angeles* (MSN, MSN/MBA)

University of California, San Francisco, School of Nursing, *San Francisco* (MS)

University of Phoenix–Bay Area Campus, College of Health and Human Services, *Pleasanton* (MSN, MSN/MBA, MSN/MHA)

University of Phoenix–Central Valley Campus, College of Health and Human Services, *Fresno* (MSN)

University of Phoenix–Sacramento Valley Campus, College of Health and Human Services, *Sacramento* (MSN)

University of Phoenix–San Diego Campus, College of Health and Human Services, *San Diego* (MSN)

University of Phoenix–Southern California Campus, College of Health and Human Services, *Costa Mesa* (MSN, MSN/MBA)

University of San Diego, Hahn School of Nursing and Health Sciences, *San Diego* (MSN, MSN/MBA)

University of San Francisco, School of Nursing, *San Francisco* (MSN, MSN/MS)

Colorado

Colorado State University–Pueblo, Department of Nursing, *Pueblo* (MS)

Regis University, Department of Nursing, *Denver* (MS)

University of Colorado at Colorado Springs, Beth-El College of Nursing and Health Sciences, *Colorado Springs* (MSN)

University of Colorado at Denver and Health Sciences Center, School of Nursing, *Denver* (MS, MSN/MBA)

University of Phoenix–Denver Campus, College of Health and Human Services, *Lone Tree* (MSN)

University of Phoenix–Southern Colorado Campus, College of Health and Human Services, *Colorado Springs* (MSN)

Connecticut

Fairfield University, School of Nursing, *Fairfield* (MSN)

Quinnipiac University, Department of Nursing, *Hamden* (MSN)

Sacred Heart University, Program in Nursing, *Fairfield* (MSN, MSN/MBA)

Saint Joseph College, Department of Nursing, *West Hartford* (MS)

University of Connecticut, School of Nursing, *Storrs* (MS, MSN/MBA, MSN/MPH)

University of Hartford, College of Education, Nursing, and Health Professions, *West Hartford* (MSN, MSN/MSOB)

Western Connecticut State University, Department of Nursing, *Danbury* (MS)

Yale University, School of Nursing, *New Haven* (MSN, MSN/MPH, MSN/MDIV)

Delaware

University of Delaware, School of Nursing, *Newark* (MSN)

Wesley College, Nursing Program, *Dover* (MSN)

Wilmington College, Division of Nursing, *New Castle* (MSN, MSN/MBA, MSN/MS)

District of Columbia

The Catholic University of America, School of Nursing, *Washington* (MSN, MA/MSM)

Georgetown University, School of Nursing and Health Studies, *Washington* (MS)

Howard University, Division of Nursing, *Washington* (MSN)

Florida

Barry University, School of Nursing, *Miami Shores* (MSN, MSN/MBA)

Florida Agricultural and Mechanical University, School of Nursing, *Tallahassee* (MSN)

Florida Atlantic University, College of Nursing, *Boca Raton* (MS, MS/MBA)

Florida Gulf Coast University, School of Nursing, *Fort Myers* (MSN)

Florida International University, College of Nursing and Health Sciences, *Miami* (MSN)

Florida Southern College, Department of Nursing, *Lakeland* (MS)

Florida State University, School of Nursing, *Tallahassee* (MSN)

Jacksonville University, School of Nursing, *Jacksonville* (MSN, MSN/MBA)

Nova Southeastern University, College of Allied Health and Nursing, *Fort Lauderdale* (MSN, MSN/MBA)

University of Central Florida, School of Nursing, *Orlando* (MSN)

University of Florida, College of Nursing, *Gainesville* (MSN, MSN/PhD)

University of Miami, School of Nursing and Health Studies, *Coral Gables* (MSN)

University of North Florida, School of Nursing, *Jacksonville* (MSN)

University of Phoenix–Central Florida Campus, College of Health and Human Services, *Maitland* (MSN, MSN/MBA, MSN/MHA)

University of Phoenix–North Florida Campus, College of Health and Human Services, *Jacksonville* (MSN)

University of Phoenix–South Florida Campus, College of Health and Human Services, *Fort Lauderdale* (MSN, MSN/MBA, MSN/MHA)

University of Phoenix–West Florida Campus, College of Health and Human Services, *Temple Terrace* (MSN, MSN/MBA, MSN/MHA)

University of South Florida, College of Nursing, *Tampa* (MS, MSN/MPH)

The University of Tampa, Department of Nursing, *Tampa* (MSN)

Georgia

Albany State University, College of Health Professions, *Albany* (MSN)

Armstrong Atlantic State University, Program in Nursing, *Savannah* (MSN, MS/MHSA)

Brenau University, School of Health and Science, *Gainesville* (MSN)

Emory University, Nell Hodgson Woodruff School of Nursing, *Atlanta* (MSN, MSN/MPH)

Georgia Baptist College of Nursing of Mercer University, Department of Nursing, *Atlanta* (MSN)

Georgia College & State University, School of Health Sciences, *Milledgeville* (MSN, MSN/MBA)

Georgia Southern University, School of Nursing, *Statesboro* (MSN)

Georgia State University, School of Nursing, *Atlanta* (MS)

Kennesaw State University, School of Nursing, *Kennesaw* (MSN)

Medical College of Georgia, School of Nursing, *Augusta* (MSN)

North Georgia College & State University, Department of Nursing, *Dahlonega* (MS)

Thomas University, Division of Nursing, *Thomasville* (MSN)

University of West Georgia, Department of Nursing, *Carrollton* (MSN)

Valdosta State University, College of Nursing, *Valdosta* (MSN)

Hawaii

Hawai'i Pacific University, School of Nursing, *Honolulu* (MSN, MSN/MBA)

University of Hawaii at Manoa, School of Nursing and Dental Hygiene, *Honolulu* (MS)

University of Phoenix–Hawaii Campus, College of Health and Human Services, *Honolulu* (MSN)

Idaho

Boise State University, Department of Nursing, *Boise* (MS, MSN/MS)

Idaho State University, Department of Nursing, *Pocatello* (MS)

Illinois

Bradley University, Department of Nursing, *Peoria* (MSN)

DePaul University, Department of Nursing, *Chicago* (MS)

Governors State University, Division of Nursing, Communication Disorders, Occupational Therapy, and Physical Therapy, *University Park* (MS)

Illinois State University, Mennonite College of Nursing, *Normal* (MSN)

Loyola University Chicago, Marcella Niehoff School of Nursing, *Chicago* (MSN, MSN/MBA, MSN/MDIV)

McKendree College, Department of Nursing, *Lebanon* (MSN)

Northern Illinois University, School of Nursing, *De Kalb* (MS, MSN/MPH)

North Park University, School of Nursing, *Chicago* (MS, MSN/MA, MSN/MBA, MSN/MM)

Olivet Nazarene University, Division of Nursing, *Bourbonnais* (MSN)

Rush University, College of Nursing, *Chicago* (MSN)

Saint Anthony College of Nursing, Saint Anthony College of Nursing, *Rockford* (MSN)

Saint Francis Medical Center College of Nursing, Baccalaureate Nursing Program, *Peoria* (MSN)

Saint Xavier University, School of Nursing, *Chicago* (MSN, MSN/MBA)

Southern Illinois University Edwardsville, School of Nursing, *Edwardsville* (MS)

University of Illinois at Chicago, College of Nursing, *Chicago* (MS, MS/MBA, MS/MPH)

West Suburban College of Nursing, *Oak Park* (MSN)

Indiana

Ball State University, School of Nursing, *Muncie* (MS)

Bethel College, Department of Nursing, *Mishawaka* (MSN)

Indiana State University, College of Nursing, *Terre Haute* (MS)

Indiana University–Purdue University Fort Wayne, Department of Nursing, *Fort Wayne* (MS)

Indiana University–Purdue University Indianapolis, School of Nursing, *Indianapolis* (MSN, MSN/MPH)

Indiana Wesleyan University, Division of Nursing, *Marion* (MS)

Purdue University, School of Nursing, *West Lafayette* (MS)

Purdue University Calumet, School of Nursing, *Hammond* (MS)

University of Indianapolis, School of Nursing, *Indianapolis* (MSN, MSN/MBA)

University of Saint Francis, Department of Nursing, *Fort Wayne* (MSN)

University of Southern Indiana, College of Nursing and Health Professions, *Evansville* (MSN)

Valparaiso University, College of Nursing, *Valparaiso* (MSN, MSN/MBA)

Iowa

Allen College, Program in Nursing, *Waterloo* (MSN)

Briar Cliff University, Department of Nursing, *Sioux City* (MSN)

Clarke College, Department of Nursing and Health, *Dubuque* (MSN)

The University of Iowa, College of Nursing, *Iowa City* (MSN, MSN/MBA, MSN/MPH)

Kansas

Fort Hays State University, Department of Nursing, *Hays* (MSN)

University of Kansas, School of Nursing, *Kansas City* (MS)

Washburn University, School of Nursing, *Topeka* (MSN)

Wichita State University, School of Nursing, *Wichita* (MSN, MSN/MBA)

Kentucky

Bellarmine University, Donna and Allan Lansing School of Nursing and Health Sciences, *Louisville* (MSN, MSN/MBA)

Eastern Kentucky University, Department of Baccalaureate and Graduate Nursing, *Richmond* (MSN)

Murray State University, Program in Nursing, *Murray* (M Sc N)

Northern Kentucky University, Department of Nursing, *Highland Heights* (MSN)

Spalding University, School of Nursing, *Louisville* (MSN)

University of Kentucky, Graduate School Programs in the College of Nursing, *Lexington* (MSN)

University of Louisville, School of Nursing, *Louisville* (MSN)

Louisiana

Grambling State University, School of Nursing, *Grambling* (MSN)

Louisiana State University Health Sciences Center, School of Nursing, *New Orleans* (MN)

Loyola University New Orleans, Program in Nursing, *New Orleans* (MSN)

McNeese State University, College of Nursing, *Lake Charles* (MSN)

Northwestern State University of Louisiana, College of Nursing, *Shreveport* (MSN)

Our Lady of the Lake College, Division of Nursing, *Baton Rouge* (MSN)

Southeastern Louisiana University, School of Nursing, *Hammond* (MSN)

Southern University and Agricultural and Mechanical College, School of Nursing, *Baton Rouge* (MSN)

University of Louisiana at Lafayette, College of Nursing, *Lafayette* (MSN)

University of Phoenix–Louisiana Campus, College of Health and Human Services, *Metairie* (MSN, MSN/MBA, MSN/MHA)

Maine

Husson College, School of Nursing, *Bangor* (MSN)

Saint Joseph's College of Maine, Department of Nursing, *Standish* (MSN, MSN/MS)

University of Maine, School of Nursing, *Orono* (MSN)

University of Southern Maine, College of Nursing and Health Professions, *Portland* (MS, MS/MBA)

Maryland

Bowie State University, Department of Nursing, *Bowie* (MSN)

Coppin State University, Helene Fuld School of Nursing, *Baltimore* (MSN)

The Johns Hopkins University, School of Nursing, *Baltimore* (MSN, MSN/MBA, MSN/MPH, MSN/PhD)

Salisbury University, Program in Nursing, *Salisbury* (MS)

Towson University, Department of Nursing, *Towson* (MS)

University of Maryland, Baltimore, Master's Program in Nursing, *Baltimore* (MS, MSN/MBA, MSN/MPH, MSN/PhD)

Massachusetts

American International College, Division of Nursing, *Springfield* (MSN)

Boston College, William F. Connell School of Nursing, *Chestnut Hill* (MS, MS/MA, MS/MBA, MSN/PhD)

Fitchburg State College, Department of Nursing, *Fitchburg* (MS)

MGH Institute of Health Professions, Program in Nursing, *Boston* (MS)

Northeastern University, School of Nursing, *Boston* (MS, MSN/MBA)

Regis College, Department of Nursing, *Weston* (MSN)

Salem State College, Program in Nursing, *Salem* (MSN, MSN/MBA)

Simmons College, Department of Nursing, *Boston* (MS, MSN/MS)

University of Massachusetts Amherst, School of Nursing, *Amherst* (MS)

University of Massachusetts Boston, College of Nursing and Health Sciences, *Boston* (MS)

University of Massachusetts Dartmouth, College of Nursing, *North Dartmouth* (MS)

University of Massachusetts Lowell, Department of Nursing, *Lowell* (MS)

University of Massachusetts Worcester, Graduate School of Nursing, *Worcester* (MS)

Worcester State College, Department of Nursing, *Worcester* (MS)

Michigan

Andrews University, Department of Nursing, *Berrien Springs* (MS)

Eastern Michigan University, School of Nursing, *Ypsilanti* (MSN)

Ferris State University, School of Nursing, *Big Rapids* (MSN, MSN/MBA)

Madonna University, College of Nursing and Health, *Livonia* (MSN, MSN/MBA)

Michigan State University, College of Nursing, *East Lansing* (MSN)

Northern Michigan University, College of Nursing and Allied Health Science, *Marquette* (MSN)

Oakland University, School of Nursing, *Rochester* (MSN)

Saginaw Valley State University, Crystal M. Lange College of Nursing and Health Sciences, *University Center* (MSN)

University of Detroit Mercy, McAuley School of Nursing, *Detroit* (MSN)

University of Michigan, School of Nursing, *Ann Arbor* (MS, MSN/MBA, MSN/MPH)

University of Michigan–Flint, Department of Nursing, *Flint* (MSN)

University of Phoenix–Metro Detroit Campus, College of Health and Human Services, *Southfield* (MSN, MSN/MBA, MSN/MHA)

University of Phoenix–West Michigan Campus, College of Health and Human Services, *Grand Rapids* (MSN)

Wayne State University, College of Nursing, *Detroit* (MSN)

Minnesota

Augsburg College, Program in Nursing, *Minneapolis* (MA)

Bethel University, Department of Nursing, *St. Paul* (MA)

College of St. Catherine, Department of Nursing, *St. Paul* (MA)

The College of St. Scholastica, Department of Nursing, *Duluth* (MA)

Concordia College, Department of Nursing, *Moorhead* (MS)

Minnesota State University Mankato, School of Nursing, *Mankato* (MSN, MSN/MS)

Minnesota State University Moorhead, Tri-College University Nursing Consortium, *Moorhead* (MS)

University of Minnesota, Twin Cities Campus, School of Nursing, *Minneapolis* (MS, MS/MPH)

Winona State University, College of Nursing, *Winona* (MS)

Mississippi

Alcorn State University, School of Nursing, *Natchez* (MSN)

Delta State University, School of Nursing, *Cleveland* (MSN)

Mississippi University for Women, Division of Nursing, *Columbus* (MN)

University of Mississippi Medical Center, Program in Nursing, *Jackson* (MSN)

University of Southern Mississippi, School of Nursing, *Hattiesburg* (MSN)

William Carey College, School of Nursing, *Hattiesburg* (MSN)

Missouri

Barnes-Jewish College of Nursing and Allied Health, Division of Nursing, *St. Louis* (MSN)

Graceland University, School of Nursing, *Independence* (MSN)

Maryville University of Saint Louis, Nursing Program, School of Health Professions, *St. Louis* (MSN)

Missouri State University, Department of Nursing, *Springfield* (MSN)

Research College of Nursing, College of Nursing, *Kansas City* (MSN)

Saint Louis University, School of Nursing, *St. Louis* (MSN, MSN/MPH)

Southeast Missouri State University, Department of Nursing, *Cape Girardeau* (MSN)

University of Central Missouri, Department of Nursing, *Warrensburg* (MS)

University of Missouri–Columbia, Sinclair School of Nursing, *Columbia* (MS)

University of Missouri–Kansas City, School of Nursing, *Kansas City* (MSN)

Webster University, Department of Nursing, *St. Louis* (MSN)

Montana

Montana State University, College of Nursing, *Bozeman* (MN)

Nebraska

Clarkson College, Department of Nursing, *Omaha* (MSN)

Creighton University, School of Nursing, *Omaha* (MS)

Nebraska Methodist College, Department of Nursing, *Omaha* (MSN)

Nebraska Wesleyan University, Department of Nursing, *Lincoln* (MSN)

University of Nebraska Medical Center, College of Nursing, *Omaha* (MSN)

Nevada

University of Nevada, Las Vegas, School of Nursing, *Las Vegas* (MSN)

University of Nevada, Reno, Orvis School of Nursing, *Reno* (MSN, MSN/MPH)

New Hampshire

Rivier College, Department of Nursing and Health Sciences, *Nashua* (MS, MS/MBA)

University of New Hampshire, Department of Nursing, *Durham* (MS)

New Jersey

The College of New Jersey, School of Nursing, *Ewing* (MSN)

Fairleigh Dickinson University, Metropolitan Campus, Henry P. Becton School of Nursing and Allied Health, *Teaneck* (MSN)

Felician College, Department of Professional Nursing–BSN, *Lodi* (MSN, MA/MSM)

Kean University, Department of Nursing, *Union* (MSN, MSN/MPA)

Monmouth University, Marjorie K. Unterberg School of Nursing, *West Long Branch* (MSN)

Rutgers, The State University of New Jersey, Camden College of Arts and Sciences, Department of Nursing, *Camden* (MS)

Rutgers, The State University of New Jersey, College of Nursing, *Newark* (MS, MS/MPH)

Saint Peter's College, Nursing Program, *Jersey City* (MSN)

Seton Hall University, College of Nursing, *South Orange* (MSN, MSN/MA, MSN/MBA)

Thomas Edison State College, School of Nursing, *Trenton* (MSN)

University of Medicine and Dentistry of New Jersey, School of Nursing, *Newark* (MSN)

William Paterson University of New Jersey, Department of Nursing, *Wayne* (MSN)

New Mexico

New Mexico State University, Department of Nursing, *Las Cruces* (MSN)

University of New Mexico, College of Nursing, *Albuquerque* (MSN, MSN/MALAS, MSN/MPA, MSN/MPH)

University of Phoenix–New Mexico Campus, College of Health and Human Services, *Albuquerque* (MSN, MSN/MBA, MSN/MHA)

New York

Adelphi University, School of Nursing, *Garden City* (MS, MS/MBA)

College of Mount Saint Vincent, Department of Nursing, *Riverdale* (MSN)

The College of New Rochelle, School of Nursing, *New Rochelle* (MS)

College of Staten Island of the City University of New York, Department of Nursing, *Staten Island* (MS)

Columbia University, School of Nursing, *New York* (MS, MS/MBA, MS/MPH)

Daemen College, Department of Nursing, *Amherst* (MS)

Dominican College, Department of Nursing, *Orangeburg* (M Sc N)

D'Youville College, Department of Nursing, *Buffalo* (MS)

Excelsior College, School of Health Sciences, *Albany* (MS)

Hunter College of the City University of New York, Hunter-Bellevue School of Nursing, *New York* (MS, MS/MPH)

Lehman College of the City University of New York, Department of Nursing, *Bronx* (MS)

Long Island University, Brooklyn Campus, School of Nursing, *Brooklyn* (MS)

Long Island University, C.W. Post Campus, Department of Nursing, *Brookville* (MS)

Mercy College, Program in Nursing, *Dobbs Ferry* (MS)

Molloy College, Department of Nursing, *Rockville Centre* (MS)

Mount Saint Mary College, Division of Nursing, *Newburgh* (MS)

Nazareth College of Rochester, Department of Nursing, *Rochester* (MS)

New York University, College of Nursing, *New York* (MA, MS/MA)

Pace University, Lienhard School of Nursing, *New York* (MS)

St. John Fisher College, Advanced Practice Nursing Program, *Rochester* (MS)

St. Joseph's College, New York, Department of Nursing, *Brooklyn* (MS)

State University of New York at Binghamton, Decker School of Nursing, *Binghamton* (MS)

State University of New York Downstate Medical Center, College of Nursing, *Brooklyn* (MS, MS/MPH)

State University of New York Institute of Technology, School of Nursing and Health Systems, *Utica* (MS)

State University of New York Upstate Medical University, College of Nursing, *Syracuse* (MS)

Stony Brook University, State University of New York, School of Nursing, *Stony Brook* (MS)

University at Buffalo, the State University of New York, School of Nursing, *Buffalo* (MS)

University of Rochester, School of Nursing, *Rochester* (MS, MSN/PhD)

North Carolina

Duke University, School of Nursing, *Durham* (MSN, MSN/MBA, MSN/MCM)

East Carolina University, School of Nursing, *Greenville* (MSN)

Gardner-Webb University, School of Nursing, *Boiling Springs* (MSN, MSN/MBA)

Queens University of Charlotte, Division of Nursing, *Charlotte* (MSN, MSN/MBA)

The University of North Carolina at Charlotte, School of Nursing, *Charlotte* (MSN, MSN/MHA)

The University of North Carolina at Greensboro, School of Nursing, *Greensboro* (MSN, MSN/MBA)

The University of North Carolina Wilmington, School of Nursing, *Wilmington* (MSN)

Western Carolina University, Department of Nursing, *Cullowhee* (MSN)

Winston-Salem State University, Department of Nursing, *Winston-Salem* (MSN)

North Dakota

North Dakota State University, Tri-College University Nursing Consortium, *Fargo* (MS)

University of Mary, Division of Nursing, *Bismarck* (MSN)

University of North Dakota, College of Nursing, *Grand Forks* (MS)

Ohio

Capital University, School of Nursing, *Columbus* (MSN, MN/MBA, MS/MTS, MSN/JD)

Case Western Reserve University, Frances Payne Bolton School of Nursing, *Cleveland* (MSN, MSN/MA, MSN/MBA, MSN/MPH, MSN/PhD)

Cleveland State University, Department of Nursing, *Cleveland* (MSN, MSN/MBA)

Franciscan University of Steubenville, Department of Nursing, *Steubenville* (MSN)

Kent State University, College of Nursing, *Kent* (MSN, MSN/MBA, MSN/MPA)

Malone College, School of Nursing, *Canton* (MSN)

Mount Carmel College of Nursing, Nursing Programs, *Columbus* (MS)

The Ohio State University, College of Nursing, *Columbus* (MS)

Otterbein College, Department of Nursing, *Westerville* (MSN)

The University of Akron, College of Nursing, *Akron* (MSN)

University of Cincinnati, College of Nursing, *Cincinnati* (MSN, MSN/MBA)

University of Phoenix-Cleveland Campus, College of Health and Human Services, *Independence* (MSN, MSN/MBA)

The University of Toledo, College of Nursing, *Toledo* (MSN)

Ursuline College, The Breen School of Nursing, *Pepper Pike* (MSN)

Wright State University, College of Nursing and Health, *Dayton* (MS, MS/MBA)

Xavier University, Department of Nursing, *Cincinnati* (MSN, MSN/MBA)

Oklahoma

Oklahoma City University, Kramer School of Nursing, *Oklahoma City* (MSN, MSN/MBA)

University of Oklahoma Health Sciences Center, College of Nursing, *Oklahoma City* (MS)

University of Phoenix-Oklahoma City Campus, College of Health and Human Services, *Oklahoma City* (MSN)

Oregon

Oregon Health & Science University, School of Nursing, *Portland* (MS, MSN/MPH)

University of Portland, School of Nursing, *Portland* (MS)

Pennsylvania

Bloomsburg University of Pennsylvania, Department of Nursing, *Bloomsburg* (MSN, MSN/MBA)

Carlow University, School of Nursing, *Pittsburgh* (MSN)

Clarion University of Pennsylvania, School of Nursing, *Oil City* (MSN)

College Misericordia, Department of Nursing, *Dallas* (MSN)

DeSales University, Department of Nursing and Health, *Center Valley* (MSN, MSN/MBA)

Drexel University, College of Nursing and Health Professions, *Philadelphia* (MSN)

Duquesne University, School of Nursing, *Pittsburgh* (MSN)

Gannon University, Program in Nursing, *Erie* (MSN)

Gwynedd-Mercy College, School of Nursing, *Gwynedd Valley* (MSN)

Holy Family University, School of Nursing and Allied Health Professions, *Philadelphia* (MSN)

Immaculata University, Department of Nursing, *Immaculata* (MSN)

Indiana University of Pennsylvania, Department of Nursing and Allied Health, *Indiana* (MSN)

La Roche College, Department of Nursing and Nursing Management, *Pittsburgh* (MSN)

La Salle University, School of Nursing and Health Sciences, *Philadelphia* (MSN, MSN/MBA)

Mansfield University of Pennsylvania, Robert Packer Department of Health Sciences, *Mansfield* (MSN)

Marywood University, Department of Nursing, *Scranton* (MSN, MSN/MPH)

Millersville University of Pennsylvania, Department of Nursing, *Millersville* (MSN)

Neumann College, Program in Nursing and Health Sciences, *Aston* (MSN)

Penn State University Park, School of Nursing, *State College, University Park* (MS, MSN/PhD)

Robert Morris University, School of Nursing and Allied Health, *Moon Township* (MSN)

Temple University, Department of Nursing, *Philadelphia* (MSN)

Thomas Jefferson University, Department of Nursing, *Philadelphia* (MSN)

University of Pennsylvania, School of Nursing, *Philadelphia* (MSN, MSN/MBA, MSN/MPH, MSN/PhD)

University of Pittsburgh, School of Nursing, *Pittsburgh* (MSN)

The University of Scranton, Department of Nursing, *Scranton* (MS)

Villanova University, College of Nursing, *Villanova* (MSN)

West Chester University of Pennsylvania, Department of Nursing, *West Chester* (MSN)

Widener University, School of Nursing, *Chester* (MSN)

Wilkes University, Department of Nursing, *Wilkes-Barre* (MS)

York College of Pennsylvania, Department of Nursing, *York* (MS)

Puerto Rico

University of Puerto Rico, Medical Sciences Campus, School of Nursing, *San Juan* (MSN)

University of the Sacred Heart, Program in Nursing, *San Juan* (MSN)

Rhode Island

University of Rhode Island, College of Nursing, *Kingston* (MS)

South Carolina

Clemson University, School of Nursing, *Clemson* (MS)

Medical University of South Carolina, College of Nursing, *Charleston* (MSN, MSN/PhD)

University of South Carolina, College of Nursing, *Columbia* (MSN, MSN/MPH)

South Dakota

Augustana College, Department of Nursing, *Sioux Falls* (MA)

South Dakota State University, College of Nursing, *Brookings* (MS)

Tennessee

Belmont University, School of Nursing, *Nashville* (MSN)

Carson-Newman College, Department of Nursing, *Jefferson City* (MSN)

East Tennessee State University, College of Nursing, *Johnson City* (MSN)

King College, School of Nursing, *Bristol* (M Sc N, MSN/MBA)

Southern Adventist University, School of Nursing, *Collegedale* (MSN, MSN/MBA)

Tennessee Technological University, School of Nursing, *Cookeville* (MSN, M Sc N)

Union University, School of Nursing, *Jackson* (MSN)

University of Memphis, Loewenberg School of Nursing, *Memphis* (MSN)

The University of Tennessee, College of Nursing, *Knoxville* (MSN)

The University of Tennessee at Chattanooga, School of Nursing, *Chattanooga* (MSN)

The University of Tennessee Health Science Center, College of Nursing, *Memphis* (MSN)

Texas

Angelo State University, Department of Nursing, *San Angelo* (MSN)

Baylor University, Louise Herrington School of Nursing, *Dallas* (MSN)

Lamar University, Department of Nursing, *Beaumont* (MSN, MSN/MBA)

Midwestern State University, Nursing Program, *Wichita Falls* (MSN, MN/MHSA, MSN/MHA)

Patty Hanks Shelton School of Nursing, *Abilene* (MSN)

Prairie View A&M University, College of Nursing, *Houston* (MSN)

Texas A&M International University, Canseco School of Nursing, *Laredo* (MSN)

Texas A&M University-Corpus Christi, School of Nursing and Health Sciences, *Corpus Christi* (MSN)

Texas Christian University, Harris School of Nursing, *Fort Worth* (MSN)

Texas Tech University Health Sciences Center, School of Nursing, *Lubbock* (MSN)

Texas Woman's University, College of Nursing, *Denton* (MS, MSN/MHA)

The University of Texas at Arlington, School of Nursing, *Arlington* (MSN, MSN/MBA, MSN/MHA, MSN/MPH)

The University of Texas at Austin, School of Nursing, *Austin* (MSN, MSN/MBA)

The University of Texas at Brownsville, Department of Nursing, *Brownsville* (MSN)

The University of Texas at El Paso, School of Nursing, *El Paso* (MSN)

The University of Texas at Tyler, Program in Nursing, *Tyler* (MSN, MSN/MBA)

The University of Texas Health Science Center at Houston, School of Nursing, *Houston* (MSN, MSN/MPH)

The University of Texas Health Science Center at San Antonio, School of Nursing, *San Antonio* (MSN, MSN/MPH)

The University of Texas Medical Branch, School of Nursing, *Galveston* (MSN)

The University of Texas-Pan American, Department of Nursing, *Edinburg* (MSN)

University of the Incarnate Word, Program in Nursing, *San Antonio* (MSN, MSN/MBA)

West Texas A&M University, Division of Nursing, *Canyon* (MSN)

Utah

Brigham Young University, College of Nursing, *Provo* (MS)

University of Phoenix-Utah Campus, College of Health and Human Services, *Salt Lake City* (MSN)

Westminster College, School of Nursing and Health Sciences, *Salt Lake City* (MSN)

Vermont

University of Vermont, Department of Nursing, *Burlington* (MS)

Virginia

George Mason University, College of Nursing and Health Science, *Fairfax* (MSN, MSN/MBA)

Hampton University, Department of Nursing, *Hampton* (MS)

James Madison University, Department of Nursing, *Harrisonburg* (MSN)

Jefferson College of Health Sciences, Nursing Education Program, *Roanoke* (MSN)

Liberty University, Department of Nursing, *Lynchburg* (MSN)

Marymount University, School of Health Professions, *Arlington* (MSN)

Old Dominion University, Department of Nursing, *Norfolk* (MSN)

Radford University, School of Nursing, *Radford* (MSN)

Shenandoah University, Division of Nursing, *Winchester* (MSN)

University of Virginia, School of Nursing, *Charlottesville* (MSN, MSN/MA, MSN/MBA, MSN/PhD, MSN/HSM)

Virginia Commonwealth University, School of Nursing, *Richmond* (MS, MS/MPH)

Washington

Intercollegiate College of Nursing/Washington State University, *Spokane* (MN)

Pacific Lutheran University, School of Nursing, *Tacoma* (MSN)

Seattle Pacific University, School of Health Sciences, *Seattle* (MSN)

Seattle University, College of Nursing, *Seattle* (MSN)

University of Washington, School of Nursing, *Seattle* (MN, MN/MPH)

West Virginia

Marshall University, College of Health Professions, *Huntington* (MSN)

Mountain State University, Program in Nursing, *Beckley* (MSN)

West Virginia University, School of Nursing, *Morgantown* (MSN)

Wheeling Jesuit University, Department of Nursing, *Wheeling* (MSN)

Wisconsin

Alverno College, Division of Nursing, *Milwaukee* (MSN)

Bellin College of Nursing, Nursing Program, *Green Bay* (MSN)

Concordia University Wisconsin, Program in Nursing, *Mequon* (MSN)

Edgewood College, Program in Nursing, *Madison* (MS)

Marian College of Fond du Lac, Nursing Studies Division, *Fond du Lac* (MSN)

Marquette University, College of Nursing, *Milwaukee* (MSN, MSN/MBA)

University of Wisconsin–Eau Claire, College of Nursing and Health Sciences, *Eau Claire* (MSN)

University of Wisconsin–Madison, School of Nursing, *Madison* (MS, MS/MPH)

University of Wisconsin–Milwaukee, College of Nursing, *Milwaukee* (MS, MS/MBA)

University of Wisconsin–Oshkosh, College of Nursing, *Oshkosh* (MSN)

Viterbo University, School of Nursing, *La Crosse* (MSN)

Wyoming

University of Wyoming, Fay W. Whitney School of Nursing, *Laramie* (MS)

CANADA

Alberta

Athabasca University, Centre for Nursing and Health Studies, *Athabasca* (MHS)

University of Alberta, Faculty of Nursing, *Edmonton* (MN)

University of Calgary, Faculty of Nursing, *Calgary* (MN)

University of Lethbridge, School of Health Sciences, *Lethbridge* (M Sc)

British Columbia

The University of British Columbia, School of Nursing, *Vancouver* (MSN)

University of Victoria, School of Nursing, *Victoria* (MN)

Manitoba

University of Manitoba, Faculty of Nursing, *Winnipeg* (MN)

New Brunswick

Université de Moncton, School of Nursing, *Moncton* (M Sc N)

University of New Brunswick Fredericton, Faculty of Nursing, *Fredericton* (MN)

Newfoundland and Labrador

Memorial University of Newfoundland, School of Nursing, *St. John's* (M Sc)

Nova Scotia

Dalhousie University, School of Nursing, *Halifax* (MN, MN/MHSA)

Ontario

McMaster University, School of Nursing, *Hamilton* (M Sc, MSN/PhD)

Queen's University at Kingston, School of Nursing, *Kingston* (M Sc)

Ryerson University, Program in Nursing, *Toronto* (MN)

University of Ottawa, School of Nursing, *Ottawa* (M Sc N)

University of Toronto, Faculty of Nursing, *Toronto* (MN)

The University of Western Ontario, School of Nursing, *London* (M Sc N)

University of Windsor, School of Nursing, *Windsor* (M Sc)

Quebec

McGill University, School of Nursing, *Montréal* (M Sc)

Université de Sherbrooke, Department of Nursing, *Sherbrooke* (M Sc)

Université du Québec à Rimouski, Program in Nursing, *Rimouski* (M Sc N)

Université du Québec en Outaouais, Département des Sciences Infirmières, *Gatineau* (M Sc N)

Saskatchewan

University of Saskatchewan, College of Nursing, *Saskatoon* (MN)

MASTER'S FOR NON-NURSING COLLEGE GRADUATES

California

Samuel Merritt College, School of Nursing, *Oakland* (MSN)

San Francisco State University, School of Nursing, *San Francisco* (MSN)

University of California, Los Angeles, School of Nursing, *Los Angeles* (MSN, MSN/MBA)

University of California, San Francisco, School of Nursing, *San Francisco* (MSN)

University of San Diego, Hahn School of Nursing and Health Sciences, *San Diego* (MSN, MSN/MBA)

University of San Francisco, School of Nursing, *San Francisco* (MSN, MSN/MS)

Colorado

University of Phoenix–Denver Campus, College of Health and Human Services, *Lone Tree* (MSN)

Connecticut

Yale University, School of Nursing, *New Haven* (MSN, MSN/MPH, MSN/MDIV)

District of Columbia

Georgetown University, School of Nursing and Health Studies, *Washington* (MS)

Illinois

DePaul University, Department of Nursing, *Chicago* (MS)

University of Illinois at Chicago, College of Nursing, *Chicago* (MS, MS/MBA, MS/MPH)

Maine

University of Southern Maine, College of Nursing and Health Professions, *Portland* (MS, MS/MBA)

Massachusetts

MGH Institute of Health Professions, Program in Nursing, *Boston* (MS)

Northeastern University, School of Nursing, *Boston* (MS, MSN/MBA)

Regis College, Department of Nursing, *Weston* (MSN)

Simmons College, Department of Nursing, *Boston* (MS, MSN/MS)

University of Massachusetts Worcester, Graduate School of Nursing, *Worcester* (MS)

Nebraska

University of Nebraska Medical Center, College of Nursing, *Omaha* (MSN)

New Jersey

Seton Hall University, College of Nursing, *South Orange* (MSN, MSN/MA, MSN/MBA)

New York

Columbia University, School of Nursing, *New York* (MS, MS/MBA, MS/MPH)

Mercy College, Program in Nursing, *Dobbs Ferry* (MS)

Ohio

Case Western Reserve University, Frances Payne Bolton School of Nursing, *Cleveland* (MSN, MSN/MA, MSN/MBA, MSN/MPH, MSN/PhD)

The Ohio State University, College of Nursing, *Columbus* (MS)

University of Phoenix–Cleveland Campus, College of Health and Human Services, *Independence* (MSN, MSN/MBA)

The University of Toledo, College of Nursing, *Toledo* (MSN)

Oklahoma

University of Oklahoma Health Sciences Center, College of Nursing, *Oklahoma City* (MS)

Oregon

Oregon Health & Science University, School of Nursing, *Portland* (MS, MSN/MPH)

University of Portland, School of Nursing, *Portland* (MS)

Pennsylvania

Thomas Jefferson University, Department of Nursing, *Philadelphia* (MSN)

Wilkes University, Department of Nursing, *Wilkes-Barre* (MS)

Tennessee

University of Memphis, Loewenberg School of Nursing, *Memphis* (MSN)

The University of Tennessee, College of Nursing, *Knoxville* (MSN)

Texas

The University of Texas at Austin, School of Nursing, *Austin* (MSN, MSN/MBA)

Vermont

University of Vermont, Department of Nursing, *Burlington* (MS)

Virginia

University of Virginia, School of Nursing, *Charlottesville* (MSN, MSN/MA, MSN/MBA, MSN/PhD, MSN/HSM)

Washington

Pacific Lutheran University, School of Nursing, *Tacoma* (MSN)

University of Washington, School of Nursing, *Seattle* (MN, MN/MPH)

Wisconsin

Marquette University, College of Nursing, *Milwaukee* (MSN, MSN/MBA)

CANADA

Quebec

McGill University, School of Nursing, *Montréal* (M Sc)

MASTER'S FOR NURSES WITH NON-NURSING DEGREES

Alabama

University of South Alabama, College of Nursing, *Mobile* (MSN)

Arizona

University of Phoenix Online Campus, College of Health and Human Services, *Phoenix* (MSN, MSN/MBA)

California

California State University, Dominguez Hills, Program in Nursing, *Carson* (MSN)

California State University, Fresno, Department of Nursing, *Fresno* (MSN)

California State University, Sacramento, Division of Nursing, *Sacramento* (MS)

Dominican University of California, Program in Nursing, *San Rafael* (MSN)

Samuel Merritt College, School of Nursing, *Oakland* (MSN)

San Francisco State University, School of Nursing, *San Francisco* (MSN)

University of California, San Francisco, School of Nursing, *San Francisco* (MS)

University of San Diego, Hahn School of Nursing and Health Sciences, *San Diego* (MSN, MSN/MBA)

University of San Francisco, School of Nursing, *San Francisco* (MSN, MSN/MS)

Western University of Health Sciences, College of Graduate Nursing, *Pomona* (MSN)

Connecticut
Sacred Heart University, Program in Nursing, *Fairfield* (MSN, MSN/MBA)

Saint Joseph College, Department of Nursing, *West Hartford* (MS)

University of Hartford, College of Education, Nursing, and Health Professions, *West Hartford* (MSN, MSN/MSOB)

Delaware
University of Delaware, School of Nursing, *Newark* (MSN)

Florida
Florida Atlantic University, College of Nursing, *Boca Raton* (MS, MS/MBA)

Florida International University, College of Nursing and Health Sciences, *Miami* (MSN)

Florida Southern College, Department of Nursing, *Lakeland* (MS)

University of South Florida, College of Nursing, *Tampa* (MS, MSN/MPH)

Georgia
Thomas University, Division of Nursing, *Thomasville* (MSN)

Illinois
DePaul University, Department of Nursing, *Chicago* (MS)

Rush University, College of Nursing, *Chicago* (MSN)

Saint Francis Medical Center College of Nursing, Baccalaureate Nursing Program, *Peoria* (MSN)

Saint Xavier University, School of Nursing, *Chicago* (MSN, MSN/MBA)

University of Illinois at Chicago, College of Nursing, *Chicago* (MS, MS/MBA, MS/MPH)

University of St. Francis, College of Nursing and Allied Health, *Joliet* (MSN)

West Suburban College of Nursing, *Oak Park* (MSN)

Indiana
University of Saint Francis, Department of Nursing, *Fort Wayne* (MSN)

Iowa
Allen College, Program in Nursing, *Waterloo* (MSN)

The University of Iowa, College of Nursing, *Iowa City* (MSN, MSN/MBA, MSN/MPH)

Kansas
Wichita State University, School of Nursing, *Wichita* (MSN, MSN/MBA)

Kentucky
Bellarmine University, Donna and Allan Lansing School of Nursing and Health Sciences, *Louisville* (MSN, MSN/MBA)

Louisiana
Loyola University New Orleans, Program in Nursing, *New Orleans* (MSN)

Maine
Husson College, School of Nursing, *Bangor* (MSN)

Saint Joseph's College of Maine, Department of Nursing, *Standish* (MSN, MSN/MS)

Maryland
University of Maryland, Baltimore, Master's Program in Nursing, *Baltimore* (MS, MSN/MBA, MSN/MPH, MSN/PhD)

Massachusetts
MGH Institute of Health Professions, Program in Nursing, *Boston* (MS)

Regis College, Department of Nursing, *Weston* (MSN)

Salem State College, Program in Nursing, *Salem* (MSN, MSN/MBA)

Simmons College, Department of Nursing, *Boston* (MS, MSN/MS)

University of Massachusetts Amherst, School of Nursing, *Amherst* (MS)

Worcester State College, Department of Nursing, *Worcester* (MS)

Michigan
Grand Valley State University, Russell B. Kirkhof College of Nursing, *Allendale* (MSN, MSN/MBA)

University of Detroit Mercy, McAuley School of Nursing, *Detroit* (MSN)

Minnesota
Concordia College, Department of Nursing, *Moorhead* (MS)

Metropolitan State University, School of Nursing, *St. Paul* (MSN)

Minnesota State University Mankato, School of Nursing, *Mankato* (MSN, MSN/MS)

Minnesota State University Moorhead, Tri-College University Nursing Consortium, *Moorhead* (MS)

Missouri
Saint Louis University, School of Nursing, *St. Louis* (MSN, MSN/MPH)

New Hampshire
Rivier College, Department of Nursing and Health Sciences, *Nashua* (MS, MS/MBA)

University of New Hampshire, Department of Nursing, *Durham* (MS)

New Jersey
The College of New Jersey, School of Nursing, *Ewing* (MSN)

Fairleigh Dickinson University, Metropolitan Campus, Henry P. Becton School of Nursing and Allied Health, *Teaneck* (MSN)

Kean University, Department of Nursing, *Union* (MSN, MSN/MPA)

Monmouth University, Marjorie K. Unterberg School of Nursing, *West Long Branch* (MSN)

Saint Peter's College, Nursing Program, *Jersey City* (MSN)

Seton Hall University, College of Nursing, *South Orange* (MSN, MSN/MA, MSN/MBA)

William Paterson University of New Jersey, Department of Nursing, *Wayne* (MSN)

New Mexico
University of New Mexico, College of Nursing, *Albuquerque* (MSN, MSN/MALAS, MSN/MPA, MSN/MPH)

New York
Adelphi University, School of Nursing, *Garden City* (MS, MS/MBA)

College of Mount Saint Vincent, Department of Nursing, *Riverdale* (MSN)

Lehman College of the City University of New York, Department of Nursing, *Bronx* (MS)

Long Island University, C.W. Post Campus, Department of Nursing, *Brookville* (MS)

Mercy College, Program in Nursing, *Dobbs Ferry* (MS)

Pace University, Lienhard School of Nursing, *New York* (MS)

Roberts Wesleyan College, Division of Nursing, *Rochester* (M Sc N)

State University of New York Upstate Medical University, College of Nursing, *Syracuse* (MS)

North Carolina
East Carolina University, School of Nursing, *Greenville* (MSN)

The University of North Carolina at Chapel Hill, School of Nursing, *Chapel Hill* (MSN, MSN/MS)

Ohio
Case Western Reserve University, Frances Payne Bolton School of Nursing, *Cleveland* (MSN, MSN/MA, MSN/MBA, MSN/MPH, MSN/PhD)

The University of Toledo, College of Nursing, *Toledo* (MSN)

Wright State University, College of Nursing and Health, *Dayton* (MS, MS/MBA)

Xavier University, Department of Nursing, *Cincinnati* (MSN, MSN/MBA)

Oregon
Oregon Health & Science University, School of Nursing, *Portland* (MS, MSN/MPH)

Pennsylvania
Bloomsburg University of Pennsylvania, Department of Nursing, *Bloomsburg* (MSN, MSN/MBA)

Drexel University, College of Nursing and Health Professions, *Philadelphia* (MSN)

Thomas Jefferson University, Department of Nursing, *Philadelphia* (MSN)

Tennessee
Tennessee Technological University, School of Nursing, *Cookeville* (MSN, M Sc N)

University of Memphis, Loewenberg School of Nursing, *Memphis* (MSN)

The University of Tennessee, College of Nursing, *Knoxville* (MSN)

Texas
Texas A&M International University, Canseco School of Nursing, *Laredo* (MSN)

The University of Texas at Austin, School of Nursing, *Austin* (MSN, MSN/MBA)

Vermont
University of Vermont, Department of Nursing, *Burlington* (MS)

Virginia
Jefferson College of Health Sciences, Nursing Education Program, *Roanoke* (MSN)

University of Virginia, School of Nursing, *Charlottesville* (MSN, MSN/MA, MSN/MBA, MSN/PhD, MSN/HSM)

Washington
Gonzaga University, Department of Nursing, *Spokane* (MSN)

Pacific Lutheran University, School of Nursing, *Tacoma* (MSN)

University of Washington, School of Nursing, *Seattle* (MN, MN/MPH)

Wisconsin
Marquette University, College of Nursing, *Milwaukee* (MSN, MSN/MBA)

University of Wisconsin–Madison, School of Nursing, *Madison* (MS, MS/MPH)

Wyoming
University of Wyoming, Fay W. Whitney School of Nursing, *Laramie* (MS)

CANADA

Alberta
Athabasca University, Centre for Nursing and Health Studies, *Athabasca* (MHS)

RN TO MASTER'S

Alabama
Samford University, Ida V. Moffett School of Nursing, *Birmingham* (MSN, MSN/MBA)

Troy University, School of Nursing, *Troy* (MSN)

The University of Alabama, Capstone College of Nursing, *Tuscaloosa* (MSN, MSN/MA)

The University of Alabama at Birmingham, School of Nursing, *Birmingham* (MSN, MSN/MPH)

The University of Alabama in Huntsville, College of Nursing, *Huntsville* (MSN)

Arizona

Grand Canyon University, College of Nursing, *Phoenix* (MSN, MSN/MBA)

Arkansas

University of Arkansas for Medical Sciences, College of Nursing, *Little Rock* (M Sc N)

University of Central Arkansas, Department of Nursing, *Conway* (MSN)

California

Loma Linda University, School of Nursing, *Loma Linda* (MS, MSN/MA, MSN/MPH)

Colorado

University of Colorado at Denver and Health Sciences Center, School of Nursing, *Denver* (MS, MSN/MBA)

Connecticut

Sacred Heart University, Program in Nursing, *Fairfield* (MSN, MSN/MBA)

Saint Joseph College, Department of Nursing, *West Hartford* (MS)

University of Connecticut, School of Nursing, *Storrs* (MS, MSN/MBA, MSN/MPH)

Yale University, School of Nursing, *New Haven* (MSN, MSN/MPH, MSN/MDIV)

Delaware

University of Delaware, School of Nursing, *Newark* (MSN)

District of Columbia

Georgetown University, School of Nursing and Health Studies, *Washington* (MS)

Florida

Florida Atlantic University, College of Nursing, *Boca Raton* (MS, MS/MBA)

Florida State University, School of Nursing, *Tallahassee* (MSN)

Jacksonville University, School of Nursing, *Jacksonville* (MSN, MSN/MBA)

University of Central Florida, School of Nursing, *Orlando* (MSN)

University of North Florida, School of Nursing, *Jacksonville* (MSN)

University of South Florida, College of Nursing, *Tampa* (MS, MSN/MPH)

Georgia

Albany State University, College of Health Professions, *Albany* (MSN)

Armstrong Atlantic State University, Program in Nursing, *Savannah* (MSN, MS/MHSA)

Emory University, Nell Hodgson Woodruff School of Nursing, *Atlanta* (MSN, MSN/MPH)

Georgia College & State University, School of Health Sciences, *Milledgeville* (MSN, MSN/MBA)

Georgia Southern University, School of Nursing, *Statesboro* (MSN)

Georgia State University, School of Nursing, *Atlanta* (MS)

Medical College of Georgia, School of Nursing, *Augusta* (MSN)

Valdosta State University, College of Nursing, *Valdosta* (MSN)

Illinois

DePaul University, Department of Nursing, *Chicago* (MS)

Lewis University, Program in Nursing, *Romeoville* (MSN, MSN/MBA)

Loyola University Chicago, Marcella Niehoff School of Nursing, *Chicago* (MSN, MSN/MBA, MSN/MDIV)

McKendree College, Department of Nursing, *Lebanon* (MSN)

Rush University, College of Nursing, *Chicago* (MSN)

Saint Francis Medical Center College of Nursing, Baccalaureate Nursing Program, *Peoria* (MSN)

University of St. Francis, College of Nursing and Allied Health, *Joliet* (MSN)

West Suburban College of Nursing, *Oak Park* (MSN)

Indiana

Ball State University, School of Nursing, *Muncie* (MS)

Indiana University–Purdue University Indianapolis, School of Nursing, *Indianapolis* (MSN, MSN/MPH)

University of Southern Indiana, College of Nursing and Health Professions, *Evansville* (MSN)

Valparaiso University, College of Nursing, *Valparaiso* (MSN, MSN/MBA)

Iowa

Allen College, Program in Nursing, *Waterloo* (MSN)

Kansas

Pittsburg State University, Department of Nursing, *Pittsburg* (MSN)

University of Kansas, School of Nursing, *Kansas City* (MS)

Wichita State University, School of Nursing, *Wichita* (MSN, MSN/MBA)

Kentucky

Bellarmine University, Donna and Allan Lansing School of Nursing and Health Sciences, *Louisville* (MSN, MSN/MBA)

University of Kentucky, Graduate School Programs in the College of Nursing, *Lexington* (MSN)

Louisiana

Loyola University New Orleans, Program in Nursing, *New Orleans* (MSN)

Maine

Saint Joseph's College of Maine, Department of Nursing, *Standish* (MSN, MSN/MS)

University of Maine, School of Nursing, *Orono* (MSN)

University of Southern Maine, College of Nursing and Health Professions, *Portland* (MS, MS/MBA)

Maryland

University of Maryland, Baltimore, Master's Program in Nursing, *Baltimore* (MS, MSN/MBA, MSN/MPH, MSN/PhD)

Massachusetts

Boston College, William F. Connell School of Nursing, *Chestnut Hill* (MS, MS/MA, MS/MBA, MSN/PhD)

MGH Institute of Health Professions, Program in Nursing, *Boston* (MS)

Northeastern University, School of Nursing, *Boston* (MS, MSN/MBA)

Regis College, Department of Nursing, *Weston* (MSN)

Salem State College, Program in Nursing, *Salem* (MSN, MSN/MBA)

Simmons College, Department of Nursing, *Boston* (MS, MSN/MS)

Michigan

Saginaw Valley State University, Crystal M. Lange College of Nursing and Health Sciences, *University Center* (MSN)

University of Michigan, School of Nursing, *Ann Arbor* (MS, MSN/MBA, MSN/MPH)

University of Michigan–Flint, Department of Nursing, *Flint* (MSN)

Minnesota

Metropolitan State University, School of Nursing, *St. Paul* (MSN)

Winona State University, College of Nursing, *Winona* (MS)

Mississippi

University of Southern Mississippi, School of Nursing, *Hattiesburg* (MSN)

Missouri

Barnes-Jewish College of Nursing and Allied Health, Division of Nursing, *St. Louis* (MSN)

Graceland University, School of Nursing, *Independence* (MSN)

Maryville University of Saint Louis, Nursing Program, School of Health Professions, *St. Louis* (MSN)

Missouri State University, Department of Nursing, *Springfield* (MSN)

Saint Louis University, School of Nursing, *St. Louis* (MSN, MSN/MPH)

University of Missouri–St. Louis, College of Nursing, *St. Louis* (MSN)

Webster University, Department of Nursing, *St. Louis* (MSN)

Nebraska

Clarkson College, Department of Nursing, *Omaha* (MSN)

University of Nebraska Medical Center, College of Nursing, *Omaha* (MSN)

New Jersey

The College of New Jersey, School of Nursing, *Ewing* (MSN)

Fairleigh Dickinson University, Metropolitan Campus, Henry P. Becton School of Nursing and Allied Health, *Teaneck* (MSN)

Seton Hall University, College of Nursing, *South Orange* (MSN, MSN/MA, MSN/MBA)

Thomas Edison State College, School of Nursing, *Trenton* (MSN)

University of Medicine and Dentistry of New Jersey, School of Nursing, *Newark* (MSN)

New York

The College of New Rochelle, School of Nursing, *New Rochelle* (MS)

Daemen College, Department of Nursing, *Amherst* (MS)

D'Youville College, Department of Nursing, *Buffalo* (MS)

Excelsior College, School of Health Sciences, *Albany* (MS)

Long Island University, Brooklyn Campus, School of Nursing, *Brooklyn* (MS)

New York University, College of Nursing, *New York* (MA, MS/MA)

Pace University, Lienhard School of Nursing, *New York* (MS)

St. John Fisher College, Advanced Practice Nursing Program, *Rochester* (MS)

Stony Brook University, State University of New York, School of Nursing, *Stony Brook* (MS)

North Carolina

Duke University, School of Nursing, *Durham* (MSN, MSN/MBA, MSN/MCM)

East Carolina University, School of Nursing, *Greenville* (MSN)

Gardner-Webb University, School of Nursing, *Boiling Springs* (MSN, MSN/MBA)

Queens University of Charlotte, Division of Nursing, *Charlotte* (MSN, MSN/MBA)

The University of North Carolina at Chapel Hill, School of Nursing, *Chapel Hill* (MSN, MSN/MS)

The University of North Carolina at Charlotte, School of Nursing, *Charlotte* (MSN, MSN/MHA)

The University of North Carolina Wilmington, School of Nursing, *Wilmington* (MSN)

North Dakota

University of Mary, Division of Nursing, *Bismarck* (MSN)

Ohio

Capital University, School of Nursing, *Columbus* (MSN, MN/MBA, MS/MTS, MSN/JD)

Case Western Reserve University, Frances Payne
Bolton School of Nursing, *Cleveland* (MSN,
MSN/MA, MSN/MBA, MSN/MPH, MSN/PhD)
Franciscan University of Steubenville, Department
of Nursing, *Steubenville* (MSN)
The University of Akron, College of Nursing,
Akron (MSN)
Xavier University, Department of Nursing,
Cincinnati (MSN, MSN/MBA)

Pennsylvania
Bloomsburg University of Pennsylvania,
Department of Nursing, *Bloomsburg* (MSN,
MSN/MBA)
Carlow University, School of Nursing, *Pittsburgh*
(MSN)
College Misericordia, Department of Nursing,
Dallas (MSN)
DeSales University, Department of Nursing and
Health, *Center Valley* (MSN, MSN/MBA)
Drexel University, College of Nursing and Health
Professions, *Philadelphia* (MSN)
Duquesne University, School of Nursing,
Pittsburgh (MSN)
Gannon University, Program in Nursing, *Erie*
(MSN)
Gwynedd-Mercy College, School of Nursing,
Gwynedd Valley (MSN)
Indiana University of Pennsylvania, Department of
Nursing and Allied Health, *Indiana* (MSN)
La Roche College, Department of Nursing and
Nursing Management, *Pittsburgh* (MSN)
La Salle University, School of Nursing and Health
Sciences, *Philadelphia* (MSN, MSN/MBA)
Penn State University Park, School of Nursing,
State College, University Park (MSN, MSN/PhD)
Slippery Rock University of Pennsylvania,
Department of Nursing, *Slippery Rock* (MSN)
Thomas Jefferson University, Department of
Nursing, *Philadelphia* (MSN)
University of Pittsburgh, School of Nursing,
Pittsburgh (MSN)
The University of Scranton, Department of
Nursing, *Scranton* (MS)
Widener University, School of Nursing, *Chester*
(MSN)
Wilkes University, Department of Nursing,
Wilkes-Barre (MS)
York College of Pennsylvania, Department of
Nursing, *York* (MS)

Rhode Island
University of Rhode Island, College of Nursing,
Kingston (MS)

South Carolina
Clemson University, School of Nursing, *Clemson*
(MS)
Medical University of South Carolina, College of
Nursing, *Charleston* (MSN, MSN/PhD)

South Dakota
South Dakota State University, College of Nursing,
Brookings (MS)

Tennessee
East Tennessee State University, College of
Nursing, *Johnson City* (MSN)
Tennessee State University, School of Nursing,
Nashville (MSN)
The University of Tennessee, College of Nursing,
Knoxville (MSN)

Texas
Midwestern State University, Nursing Program,
Wichita Falls (MSN, MN/MHSA, MSN/MHA)
Texas Christian University, Harris School of
Nursing, *Fort Worth* (MSN)
Texas Tech University Health Sciences Center,
School of Nursing, *Lubbock* (MSN)
Texas Woman's University, College of Nursing,
Denton (MS, MSN/MHA)
The University of Texas at El Paso, School of
Nursing, *El Paso* (MSN)

The University of Texas at Tyler, Program in
Nursing, *Tyler* (MSN, MSN/MBA)
The University of Texas Health Science Center at
San Antonio, School of Nursing, *San Antonio*
(MSN, MSN/MPH)
The University of Texas Medical Branch, School of
Nursing, *Galveston* (MSN)
West Texas A&M University, Division of Nursing,
Canyon (MSN)

Vermont
University of Vermont, Department of Nursing,
Burlington (MS)

Virginia
George Mason University, College of Nursing and
Health Science, *Fairfax* (MSN, MSN/MBA)
Marymount University, School of Health
Professions, *Arlington* (MSN)
Old Dominion University, Department of Nursing,
Norfolk (MSN)
Shenandoah University, Division of Nursing,
Winchester (MSN)
Virginia Commonwealth University, School of
Nursing, *Richmond* (MS, MS/MPH)

Washington
Gonzaga University, Department of Nursing,
Spokane (MSN)
Pacific Lutheran University, School of Nursing,
Tacoma (MSN)

West Virginia
West Virginia University, School of Nursing,
Morgantown (MSN)

Wisconsin
Marquette University, College of Nursing,
Milwaukee (MSN, MSN/MBA)
University of Wisconsin-Eau Claire, College of
Nursing and Health Sciences, *Eau Claire* (MSN)
University of Wisconsin-Milwaukee, College of
Nursing, *Milwaukee* (MS, MS/MBA)

CANADA

Alberta
University of Calgary, Faculty of Nursing, *Calgary*
(MN)

New Brunswick
Université de Moncton, School of Nursing,
Moncton (M Sc N)

Quebec
Université du Québec à Chicoutimi, Program in
Nursing, *Chicoutimi* (MSN)

JOINT DEGREES

Alabama
Samford University, Ida V. Moffett School of
Nursing, *Birmingham* (MSN, MSN/MBA)
The University of Alabama, Capstone College of
Nursing, *Tuscaloosa* (MSN, MSN/MA)
The University of Alabama at Birmingham, School
of Nursing, *Birmingham* (MSN, MSN/MPH)

Arizona
Arizona State University at the Downtown
Phoenix Campus, College of Nursing, *Phoenix*
(MS, MS/MPH)
Grand Canyon University, College of Nursing,
Phoenix (MSN, MSN/MBA)
University of Phoenix Online Campus, College of
Health and Human Services, *Phoenix* (MSN,
MSN/MBA)

California
California State University, Long Beach,
Department of Nursing, *Long Beach* (MSN,
MSN/MPH)
Holy Names University, Department of Nursing,
Oakland (MSN, MSN/MBA)

Loma Linda University, School of Nursing, *Loma
Linda* (MS, MSN/MA, MSN/MPH)
University of California, Los Angeles, School of
Nursing, *Los Angeles* (MSN, MSN/MBA)
University of Phoenix-Bay Area Campus, College
of Health and Human Services, *Pleasanton*
(MSN, MSN/MBA, MSN/MHA)
University of Phoenix-Southern California
Campus, College of Health and Human Services,
Costa Mesa (MSN, MSN/MBA)
University of San Diego, Hahn School of Nursing
and Health Sciences, *San Diego* (MSN, MSN/
MBA)
University of San Francisco, School of Nursing,
San Francisco (MSN, MSN/MS)

Colorado
University of Colorado at Denver and Health
Sciences Center, School of Nursing, *Denver* (MS,
MSN/MBA)

Connecticut
Sacred Heart University, Program in Nursing,
Fairfield (MSN, MSN/MBA)
University of Connecticut, School of Nursing,
Storrs (MS, MSN/MBA, MSN/MPH)
University of Hartford, College of Education,
Nursing, and Health Professions, *West Hartford*
(MSN, MSN/MSOB)
Yale University, School of Nursing, *New Haven*
(MSN, MSN/MPH, MSN/MDIV)

Delaware
Wilmington College, Division of Nursing, *New
Castle* (MSN, MSN/MBA, MSN/MS)

District of Columbia
The Catholic University of America, School of
Nursing, *Washington* (MSN, MA/MSM)

Florida
Barry University, School of Nursing, *Miami Shores*
(MSN, MSN/MBA)
Florida Atlantic University, College of Nursing,
Boca Raton (MS, MS/MBA)
Jacksonville University, School of Nursing,
Jacksonville (MSN, MSN/MBA)
Nova Southeastern University, College of Allied
Health and Nursing, *Fort Lauderdale* (MSN,
MSN/MBA)
University of Florida, College of Nursing,
Gainesville (MSN, MSN/PhD)
University of Phoenix-Central Florida Campus,
College of Health and Human Services, *Maitland*
(MSN, MSN/MBA, MSN/MHA)
University of Phoenix-South Florida Campus,
College of Health and Human Services, *Fort
Lauderdale* (MSN, MSN/MBA, MSN/MHA)
University of Phoenix-West Florida Campus,
College of Health and Human Services, *Temple
Terrace* (MSN, MSN/MBA, MSN/MHA)
University of South Florida, College of Nursing,
Tampa (MS, MSN/MPH)

Georgia
Armstrong Atlantic State University, Program in
Nursing, *Savannah* (MSN, MS/MHSA)
Emory University, Nell Hodgson Woodruff School
of Nursing, *Atlanta* (MSN, MSN/MPH)
Georgia College & State University, School of
Health Sciences, *Milledgeville* (MSN, MSN/MBA)

Hawaii
Hawai'i Pacific University, School of Nursing,
Honolulu (MSN, MSN/MBA)

Idaho
Boise State University, Department of Nursing,
Boise (MS, MSN/MS)

Illinois
Lewis University, Program in Nursing, *Romeoville*
(MSN, MSN/MBA)
Loyola University Chicago, Marcella Niehoff
School of Nursing, *Chicago* (MSN, MSN/MBA,
MSN/MDIV)

Northern Illinois University, School of Nursing, *De Kalb* (MS, MSN/MPH)

North Park University, School of Nursing, *Chicago* (MS, MSN/MA, MSN/MBA, MSN/MM)

Saint Xavier University, School of Nursing, *Chicago* (MSN, MSN/MBA)

University of Illinois at Chicago, College of Nursing, *Chicago* (MS, MS/MBA, MS/MPH)

Indiana

Indiana University-Purdue University Indianapolis, School of Nursing, *Indianapolis* (MSN, MSN/MPH)

University of Indianapolis, School of Nursing, *Indianapolis* (MSN, MSN/MBA)

Valparaiso University, College of Nursing, *Valparaiso* (MSN, MSN/MBA)

Iowa

The University of Iowa, College of Nursing, *Iowa City* (MSN, MSN/MBA, MSN/MPH)

Kansas

Wichita State University, School of Nursing, *Wichita* (MSN, MSN/MBA)

Kentucky

Bellarmine University, Donna and Allan Lansing School of Nursing and Health Sciences, *Louisville* (MSN, MSN/MBA)

Louisiana

University of Phoenix-Louisiana Campus, College of Health and Human Services, *Metairie* (MSN, MSN/MBA, MSN/MHA)

Maine

Saint Joseph's College of Maine, Department of Nursing, *Standish* (MSN, MSN/MS)

University of Southern Maine, College of Nursing and Health Professions, *Portland* (MS, MS/MBA)

Maryland

The Johns Hopkins University, School of Nursing, *Baltimore* (MSN, MSN/MBA, MSN/MPH, MSN/PhD)

University of Maryland, Baltimore, Master's Program in Nursing, *Baltimore* (MS, MSN/MBA, MSN/MPH, MSN/PhD)

Massachusetts

Boston College, William F. Connell School of Nursing, *Chestnut Hill* (MS, MS/MA, MS/MBA, MSN/PhD)

Northeastern University, School of Nursing, *Boston* (MS, MSN/MBA)

Salem State College, Program in Nursing, *Salem* (MSN, MSN/MBA)

Simmons College, Department of Nursing, *Boston* (MS, MSN/MS)

Michigan

Ferris State University, School of Nursing, *Big Rapids* (MSN, MSN/MBA)

Grand Valley State University, Russell B. Kirkhof College of Nursing, *Allendale* (MSN, MSN/MBA)

Madonna University, College of Nursing and Health, *Livonia* (MSN, MSN/MBA)

University of Michigan, School of Nursing, *Ann Arbor* (MS, MSN/MBA, MSN/MPH)

University of Phoenix-Metro Detroit Campus, College of Health and Human Services, *Southfield* (MSN, MSN/MBA, MSN/MHA)

Minnesota

Minnesota State University Mankato, School of Nursing, *Mankato* (MSN, MSN/MS)

University of Minnesota, Twin Cities Campus, School of Nursing, *Minneapolis* (MS, MS/MPH)

Missouri

Saint Louis University, School of Nursing, *St. Louis* (MSN, MSN/MPH)

Nevada

University of Nevada, Reno, Orvis School of Nursing, *Reno* (MSN, MSN/MPH)

New Hampshire

Rivier College, Department of Nursing and Health Sciences, *Nashua* (MS, MS/MBA)

New Jersey

Felician College, Department of Professional Nursing-BSN, *Lodi* (MSN, MA/MSM)

Kean University, Department of Nursing, *Union* (MSN, MSN/MPA)

Rutgers, The State University of New Jersey, College of Nursing, *Newark* (MS, MS/MPH)

Seton Hall University, College of Nursing, *South Orange* (MSN, MSN/MA, MSN/MBA)

New Mexico

University of New Mexico, College of Nursing, *Albuquerque* (MSN, MSN/MALAS, MSN/MPA, MSN/MPH)

University of Phoenix-New Mexico Campus, College of Health and Human Services, *Albuquerque* (MSN, MSN/MBA, MSN/MHA)

New York

Adelphi University, School of Nursing, *Garden City* (MS, MS/MBA)

Columbia University, School of Nursing, *New York* (MS, MS/MBA, MS/MPH)

Hunter College of the City University of New York, Hunter-Bellevue School of Nursing, *New York* (MS, MS/MPH)

New York University, College of Nursing, *New York* (MA, MS/MA)

The Sage Colleges, Division of Nursing, *Troy* (MS, MS/MBA)

State University of New York Downstate Medical Center, College of Nursing, *Brooklyn* (MS, MS/MPH)

University of Rochester, School of Nursing, *Rochester* (MS, MSN/PhD)

North Carolina

Duke University, School of Nursing, *Durham* (MSN, MSN/MBA, MSN/MCM)

Gardner-Webb University, School of Nursing, *Boiling Springs* (MSN, MSN/MBA)

Queens University of Charlotte, Division of Nursing, *Charlotte* (MSN, MSN/MBA)

The University of North Carolina at Chapel Hill, School of Nursing, *Chapel Hill* (MSN, MSN/MS)

The University of North Carolina at Charlotte, School of Nursing, *Charlotte* (MSN, MSN/MHA)

The University of North Carolina at Greensboro, School of Nursing, *Greensboro* (MSN, MSN/MBA)

Ohio

Capital University, School of Nursing, *Columbus* (MSN, MN/MBA, MSN/JD)

Case Western Reserve University, Frances Payne Bolton School of Nursing, *Cleveland* (MSN, MSN/MA, MSN/MBA, MSN/MPH, MSN/PhD)

Cleveland State University, Department of Nursing, *Cleveland* (MSN, MSN/MBA)

Kent State University, College of Nursing, *Kent* (MSN, MSN/MBA, MSN/MPA)

University of Cincinnati, College of Nursing, *Cincinnati* (MSN, MSN/MBA)

University of Phoenix-Cleveland Campus, College of Health and Human Services, *Independence* (MSN, MSN/MBA)

Wright State University, College of Nursing and Health, *Dayton* (MS, MS/MBA)

Xavier University, Department of Nursing, *Cincinnati* (MSN, MSN/MBA)

Oklahoma

Oklahoma City University, Kramer School of Nursing, *Oklahoma City* (MSN, MSN/MBA)

Oregon

Oregon Health & Science University, School of Nursing, *Portland* (MS, MSN/MPH)

Pennsylvania

Bloomsburg University of Pennsylvania, Department of Nursing, *Bloomsburg* (MSN, MSN/MBA)

DeSales University, Department of Nursing and Health, *Center Valley* (MSN, MSN/MBA)

La Salle University, School of Nursing and Health Sciences, *Philadelphia* (MSN, MSN/MBA)

Marywood University, Department of Nursing, *Scranton* (MSN, MSN/MPH)

Penn State University Park, School of Nursing, *State College, University Park* (MS, MSN/PhD)

University of Pennsylvania, School of Nursing, *Philadelphia* (MSN, MSN/MBA, MSN/MPH, MSN/PhD)

Waynesburg College, Department of Nursing, *Waynesburg* (MSN, MSN/MBA)

South Carolina

Medical University of South Carolina, College of Nursing, *Charleston* (MSN, MSN/PhD)

University of South Carolina, College of Nursing, *Columbia* (MSN, MSN/MPH)

Tennessee

King College, School of Nursing, *Bristol* (M Sc N, MSN/MBA)

Southern Adventist University, School of Nursing, *Collegedale* (MSN, MSN/MBA)

Vanderbilt University, School of Nursing, *Nashville* (MSN, MSN/MBA, MSN/MDIV)

Texas

Lamar University, Department of Nursing, *Beaumont* (MSN, MSN/MBA)

Midwestern State University, Nursing Program, *Wichita Falls* (MSN, MN/MHSA, MSN/MHA)

Texas Woman's University, College of Nursing, *Denton* (MS, MSN/MHA)

The University of Texas at Arlington, School of Nursing, *Arlington* (MSN, MSN/MBA, MSN/MHA, MSN/MPH)

The University of Texas at Austin, School of Nursing, *Austin* (MSN, MSN/MBA)

The University of Texas at Tyler, Program in Nursing, *Tyler* (MSN, MSN/MBA)

The University of Texas Health Science Center at Houston, School of Nursing, *Houston* (MSN, MSN/MPH)

The University of Texas Health Science Center at San Antonio, School of Nursing, *San Antonio* (MSN, MSN/MPH)

University of the Incarnate Word, Program in Nursing, *San Antonio* (MSN, MSN/MBA)

Virginia

George Mason University, College of Nursing and Health Science, *Fairfax* (MSN, MSN/MBA)

University of Virginia, School of Nursing, *Charlottesville* (MSN, MSN/MA, MSN/MBA, MSN/PhD, MSN/HSM)

Virginia Commonwealth University, School of Nursing, *Richmond* (MS, MS/MPH)

Washington

University of Washington, School of Nursing, *Seattle* (MN, MN/MPH)

Wisconsin

Marquette University, College of Nursing, *Milwaukee* (MSN, MSN/MBA)

University of Wisconsin-Madison, School of Nursing, *Madison* (MS, MS/MPH)

University of Wisconsin-Milwaukee, College of Nursing, *Milwaukee* (MS, MS/MBA)

CANADA

Nova Scotia

Dalhousie University, School of Nursing, *Halifax* (MN, MN/MHSA)

Ontario

McMaster University, School of Nursing, *Hamilton* (M Sc, MSN/PhD)

Concentrations within Master's Degree Programs

CASE MANAGEMENT

California State University, Los Angeles, CA
California State University, San Bernardino, CA
Carlow University, PA
DePaul University, IL
Duke University, NC
Florida State University, FL
Gonzaga University, WA
Grand Valley State University, MI
The Johns Hopkins University, MD
Kent State University, OH
Lewis University, IL
Loyola University New Orleans, LA
Northern Arizona University, AZ
Pacific Lutheran University, WA
Saint Peter's College, NJ
Samuel Merritt College, CA
San Francisco State University, CA
Seton Hall University, NJ
Shenandoah University, VA
Université de Moncton, NB
The University of Alabama, AL
The University of Alabama at Birmingham, AL
University of Central Florida, FL
University of Kentucky, KY
University of Maryland, Baltimore, MD
University of Nebraska Medical Center, NE
University of New Brunswick Fredericton, NB
The University of North Carolina at Chapel Hill, NC
University of San Francisco, CA
University of Wisconsin-Madison, WI
Ursuline College, OH
Valdosta State University, GA
Villanova University, PA
Yale University, CT
York College of Pennsylvania, PA

CLINICAL NURSE LEADER

California State University, Bakersfield, CA
Spring Hill College, AL
University of Portland, OR

CLINICAL NURSE SPECIALIST PROGRAMS

Acute Care

Arizona State University at the Downtown Phoenix Campus, AZ
California State University, Fresno, CA
Case Western Reserve University, OH
Colorado State University-Pueblo, CO
Duquesne University, PA
Georgia Baptist College of Nursing of Mercer University, GA
Grand Canyon University, AZ
Indiana University–Purdue University Indianapolis, IN
The Johns Hopkins University, MD
Kent State University, OH
King College, TN
Liberty University, VA
Loyola University Chicago, IL
McGill University, QC
Medical College of Georgia, GA
New York University, NY
Pacific Lutheran University, WA
Regis College, MA
Saint Louis University, MO
Samford University, AL
Seattle Pacific University, WA
Thomas Jefferson University, PA

Université de Sherbrooke, QC
Université du Québec à Chicoutimi, QC
University of Alberta, AB
University of Arkansas, AR
University of Arkansas for Medical Sciences, AR
University of Calgary, AB
University of California, Los Angeles, CA
University of Central Florida, FL
University of Cincinnati, OH
University of Illinois at Chicago, IL
University of Kentucky, KY
University of Manitoba, MB
University of Maryland, Baltimore, MD
University of Massachusetts Boston, MA
University of Miami, FL
University of Nebraska Medical Center, NE
University of New Brunswick Fredericton, NB
University of North Dakota, ND
University of Oklahoma Health Sciences Center, OK
University of Ottawa, ON
University of Pennsylvania, PA
University of San Diego, CA
University of South Alabama, AL
University of South Carolina, SC
The University of Tennessee Health Science Center, TN
The University of Texas Health Science Center at Houston, TX
The University of Texas Health Science Center at San Antonio, TX
University of Utah, UT
University of Virginia, VA
University of Washington, WA
The University of Western Ontario, ON
Virginia Commonwealth University, VA
Wayne State University, MI
Wichita State University, KS
Yale University, CT

Adult Health

Alverno College, WI
Angelo State University, TX
Arizona State University at the Downtown Phoenix Campus, AZ
Arkansas State University, AR
Armstrong Atlantic State University, GA
Auburn University, AL
Auburn University Montgomery, AL
Azusa Pacific University, CA
Ball State University, IN
Bloomsburg University of Pennsylvania, PA
Boston College, MA
California State University, Chico, CA
California State University, Long Beach, CA
California State University, Sacramento, CA
The Catholic University of America, DC
Clemson University, SC
College Misericordia, PA
College of Mount Saint Vincent, NY
The College of New Jersey, NJ
The College of St. Scholastica, MN
College of Staten Island of the City University of New York, NY
Concordia College, MN
Dalhousie University, NS
DeSales University, PA
East Carolina University, NC
Eastern Michigan University, MI
Florida International University, FL
Georgia College & State University, GA
Georgia State University, GA
Gonzaga University, WA
Governors State University, IL
Grand Canyon University, AZ
Grand Valley State University, MI

Hampton University, VA
Idaho State University, ID
Indiana University–Purdue University Indianapolis, IN
The Johns Hopkins University, MD
Kennesaw State University, GA
Kent State University, OH
King College, TN
La Salle University, PA
Lehman College of the City University of New York, NY
Loma Linda University, CA
Long Island University, C.W. Post Campus, NY
Louisiana State University Health Sciences Center, LA
Malone College, OH
Marquette University, WI
McGill University, QC
McNeese State University, LA
Medical College of Georgia, GA
Medical University of South Carolina, SC
Memorial University of Newfoundland, NL
Minnesota State University Moorhead, MN
Molloy College, NY
Mount Carmel College of Nursing, OH
Mount Saint Mary College, NY
Murray State University, KY
New York University, NY
North Dakota State University, ND
Northern Illinois University, IL
Northwestern State University of Louisiana, LA
The Ohio State University, OH
Oregon Health & Science University, OR
Otterbein College, OH
Pacific Lutheran University, WA
Penn State University Park, PA
Purdue University Calumet, IN
Radford University, VA
Ryerson University, ON
Saint Anthony College of Nursing, IL
St. John Fisher College, NY
St. Joseph's College, New York, NY
Saint Louis University, MO
Saint Xavier University, IL
Salem State College, MA
Samford University, AL
San Diego State University, CA
San Francisco State University, CA
Seattle Pacific University, WA
Southeastern Louisiana University, LA
Southeast Missouri State University, MO
State University of New York Downstate Medical Center, NY
Stony Brook University, State University of New York, NY
Texas Christian University, TX
Texas Woman's University, TX
Thomas Jefferson University, PA
Troy University, AL
Union University, TN
Université du Québec à Chicoutimi, QC
University at Buffalo, the State University of New York, NY
The University of Akron, OH
The University of Alabama at Birmingham, AL
The University of Alabama in Huntsville, AL
University of Alberta, AB
University of Arkansas for Medical Sciences, AR
The University of British Columbia, BC
University of Calgary, AB
University of Cincinnati, OH
University of Colorado at Colorado Springs, CO
University of Colorado at Denver and Health Sciences Center, CO
University of Connecticut, CT
University of Delaware, DE

University of Illinois at Chicago, IL
The University of Iowa, IA
University of Kansas, KS
University of Kentucky, KY
University of Louisiana at Lafayette, LA
University of Louisville, KY
University of Massachusetts Dartmouth, MA
University of Miami, FL
University of Minnesota, Twin Cities Campus, MN
University of Missouri–Columbia, MO
University of Missouri–St. Louis, MO
University of Nebraska Medical Center, NE
University of New Brunswick Fredericton, NB
University of New Hampshire, NH
The University of North Carolina at Charlotte, NC
University of North Dakota, ND
University of North Florida, FL
University of Pennsylvania, PA
University of Puerto Rico, Medical Sciences
    Campus, PR
University of St. Francis, IL
University of San Diego, CA
The University of Scranton, PA
University of Southern Mississippi, MS
The University of Tennessee, TN
The University of Texas at Austin, TX
The University of Texas Health Science Center at
    Houston, TX
The University of Texas–Pan American, TX
University of the Incarnate Word, TX
The University of Toledo, OH
University of Toronto, ON
University of Utah, UT
The University of Western Ontario, ON
University of Wisconsin–Eau Claire, WI
University of Wisconsin–Madison, WI
University of Wisconsin–Milwaukee, WI
Ursuline College, OH
Valdosta State University, GA
Valparaiso University, IN
Western Connecticut State University, CT
West Suburban College of Nursing, IL
Widener University, PA
Winona State University, MN
Wright State University, OH
York College of Pennsylvania, PA

Cardiovascular

Case Western Reserve University, OH
Creighton University, NE
Duke University, NC
The Johns Hopkins University, MD
Kent State University, OH
Loyola University Chicago, IL
McGill University, QC
The Ohio State University, OH
Oregon Health & Science University, OR
Samford University, AL
Seattle Pacific University, WA
Université du Québec à Chicoutimi, QC
University of Alberta, AB
University of Calgary, AB
University of California, San Francisco, CA
University of Illinois at Chicago, IL
University of Nebraska Medical Center, NE
University of New Brunswick Fredericton, NB
University of North Florida, FL
University of Washington, WA
Yale University, CT

Community Health

Arizona State University at the Downtown
    Phoenix Campus, AZ
Augsburg College, MN
Augustana College, SD
Bloomsburg University of Pennsylvania, PA
Boston College, MA
California State University, Fresno, CA
California State University, Sacramento, CA
California State University, San Bernardino, CA
Case Western Reserve University, OH
The Catholic University of America, DC

College Misericordia, PA
Creighton University, NE
Dalhousie University, NS
DePaul University, IL
D'Youville College, NY
East Carolina University, NC
Georgia Southern University, GA
Hampton University, VA
Hawai'i Pacific University, HI
Holy Family University, PA
Hunter College of the City University of New
    York, NY
Indiana University of Pennsylvania, PA
Indiana University–Purdue University Indianapolis,
    IN
Intercollegiate College of Nursing/Washington
    State University, WA
Jacksonville State University, AL
The Johns Hopkins University, MD
Kean University, NJ
Lewis University, IL
Liberty University, VA
Louisiana State University Health Sciences Center,
    LA
McGill University, QC
Memorial University of Newfoundland, NL
New Mexico State University, NM
Northern Illinois University, IL
North Park University, IL
The Ohio State University, OH
Oregon Health & Science University, OR
Penn State University Park, PA
Rush University, IL
Rutgers, The State University of New Jersey,
    College of Nursing, NJ
Ryerson University, ON
Salem State College, MA
Samford University, AL
San Diego State University, CA
Seattle Pacific University, WA
Seattle University, WA
Southeastern Louisiana University, LA
State University of New York at Binghamton, NY
Stony Brook University, State University of New
    York, NY
Texas Woman's University, TX
Thomas Jefferson University, PA
Université de Moncton, NB
Université de Sherbrooke, QC
Université du Québec à Chicoutimi, QC
Université du Québec à Rimouski, QC
Université du Québec en Outaouais, QC
University of Alaska Anchorage, AK
University of Alberta, AB
The University of British Columbia, BC
University of Calgary, AB
University of California, San Francisco, CA
University of Central Arkansas, AR
University of Cincinnati, OH
University of Colorado at Colorado Springs, CO
University of Colorado at Denver and Health
    Sciences Center, CO
University of Connecticut, CT
University of Illinois at Chicago, IL
The University of Iowa, IA
University of Kentucky, KY
University of Maryland, Baltimore, MD
University of Massachusetts Dartmouth, MA
University of Miami, FL
University of Michigan, MI
University of Nebraska Medical Center, NE
University of New Brunswick Fredericton, NB
The University of North Carolina at Charlotte, NC
University of North Dakota, ND
University of North Florida, FL
University of Ottawa, ON
University of Puerto Rico, Medical Sciences
    Campus, PR
University of South Alabama, AL
University of South Carolina, SC
University of Southern Mississippi, MS
The University of Texas at Austin, TX

University of Toronto, ON
University of Utah, UT
University of Vermont, VT
University of Virginia, VA
University of Washington, WA
The University of Western Ontario, ON
University of Wisconsin–Milwaukee, WI
Wayne State University, MI
Wesley College, DE
West Chester University of Pennsylvania, PA
Widener University, PA
William Paterson University of New Jersey, NJ
Worcester State College, MA
Wright State University, OH

Critical Care

California State University, Fresno, CA
Case Western Reserve University, OH
Duke University, NC
Georgetown University, DC
Gonzaga University, WA
Indiana University–Purdue University Indianapolis,
    IN
The Johns Hopkins University, MD
Kent State University, OH
King College, TN
McGill University, QC
Medical College of Georgia, GA
Murray State University, KY
New York University, NY
Northwestern State University of Louisiana, LA
Purdue University Calumet, IN
Rush University, IL
Stony Brook University, State University of New
    York, NY
Texas Christian University, TX
Thomas Jefferson University, PA
Université du Québec à Chicoutimi, QC
Université du Québec à Rimouski, QC
Université du Québec en Outaouais, QC
University of Alberta, AB
University of Calgary, AB
University of California, San Francisco, CA
University of Central Florida, FL
University of Kentucky, KY
University of Maryland, Baltimore, MD
University of Massachusetts Boston, MA
University of Nebraska Medical Center, NE
University of New Brunswick Fredericton, NB
University of North Florida, FL
University of Pennsylvania, PA
University of Puerto Rico, Medical Sciences
    Campus, PR
The University of Tennessee Health Science
    Center, TN
The University of Texas Health Science Center at
    San Antonio, TX
University of Toronto, ON
University of Washington, WA
Widener University, PA
Yale University, CT

Family Health

California State University, Sacramento, CA
Dalhousie University, NS
Florida International University, FL
Grand Valley State University, MI
The Johns Hopkins University, MD
Loma Linda University, CA
McGill University, QC
Millersville University of Pennsylvania, PA
Minnesota State University Mankato, MN
Oregon Health & Science University, OR
Pittsburg State University, KS
Point Loma Nazarene University, CA
Ryerson University, ON
Saint Joseph College, CT
Southeastern Louisiana University, LA
Southern University and Agricultural and
    Mechanical College, LA
State University of New York at Binghamton, NY
State University of New York at New Paltz, NY

Stony Brook University, State University of New York, NY
Tennessee State University, TN
Université de Moncton, NB
Université de Sherbrooke, QC
Université du Québec à Chicoutimi, QC
University of Alberta, AB
The University of British Columbia, BC
University of Calgary, AB
University of Central Arkansas, AR
University of Illinois at Chicago, IL
University of Miami, FL
University of Nebraska Medical Center, NE
University of New Brunswick Fredericton, NB
University of North Dakota, ND
University of Pennsylvania, PA
University of San Francisco, CA
University of South Alabama, AL
University of Wisconsin–Eau Claire, WI
Valdosta State University, GA
Webster University, MO

Forensic Nursing
Duquesne University, PA
Fairleigh Dickinson University, Metropolitan Campus, NJ
Fitchburg State College, MA
The Johns Hopkins University, MD
Quinnipiac University, CT
University of Washington, WA

Gerontology
Alverno College, WI
Auburn University, AL
Auburn University Montgomery, AL
Boston College, MA
California State University, Dominguez Hills, CA
California State University, Sacramento, CA
Case Western Reserve University, OH
Clemson University, SC
College of Mount Saint Vincent, NY
The College of St. Scholastica, MN
Creighton University, NE
Dominican University of California, CA
Duke University, NC
Florida Atlantic University, FL
Gonzaga University, WA
Grand Valley State University, MI
Gwynedd-Mercy College, PA
The Johns Hopkins University, MD
Kent State University, OH
Lehman College of the City University of New York, NY
Marquette University, WI
McGill University, QC
Medical University of South Carolina, SC
New York University, NY
Oregon Health & Science University, OR
Penn State University Park, PA
Pittsburg State University, KS
Point Loma Nazarene University, CA
Radford University, VA
Rush University, IL
St. John Fisher College, NY
Saint Louis University, MO
San Diego State University, CA
San Jose State University, CA
Seattle Pacific University, WA
State University of New York at Binghamton, NY
State University of New York at New Paltz, NY
Université de Sherbrooke, QC
Université du Québec à Chicoutimi, QC
Université du Québec à Rimouski, QC
University at Buffalo, the State University of New York, NY
The University of Akron, OH
University of Alberta, AB
University of Calgary, AB
University of California, Los Angeles, CA
University of California, San Francisco, CA
University of Illinois at Chicago, IL
The University of Iowa, IA

University of Kansas, KS
University of Kentucky, KY
University of Manitoba, MB
University of Michigan, MI
University of Minnesota, Twin Cities Campus, MN
University of Missouri–Columbia, MO
University of Nebraska Medical Center, NE
University of New Brunswick Fredericton, NB
University of North Dakota, ND
University of North Florida, FL
University of Oklahoma Health Sciences Center, OK
University of Pennsylvania, PA
University of Puerto Rico, Medical Sciences Campus, PR
University of Rhode Island, RI
University of South Alabama, AL
University of South Florida, FL
The University of Tennessee, TN
The University of Texas Health Science Center at Houston, TX
University of Washington, WA
University of Wisconsin–Madison, WI
Valparaiso University, IN
Washburn University, KS
Wilkes University, PA

Home Health Care
California State University, San Bernardino, CA
Carlow University, PA
McGill University, QC
New York University, NY
Thomas Jefferson University, PA
Université de Moncton, NB
Université du Québec à Chicoutimi, QC
University of Michigan, MI
University of North Dakota, ND
University of Pennsylvania, PA

Maternity-Newborn
Clemson University, SC
College Misericordia, PA
Dalhousie University, NS
Duke University, NC
The Johns Hopkins University, MD
Kent State University, OH
McGill University, QC
Oregon Health & Science University, OR
Seattle Pacific University, WA
State University of New York Downstate Medical Center, NY
Temple University, PA
Troy University, AL
Université du Québec à Chicoutimi, QC
University of Alberta, AB
University of Calgary, AB
University of Illinois at Chicago, IL
University of Nebraska Medical Center, NE
University of New Brunswick Fredericton, NB
The University of North Carolina at Chapel Hill, NC
University of North Florida, FL
University of Pennsylvania, PA
University of Puerto Rico, Medical Sciences Campus, PR
University of South Alabama, AL
The University of Tennessee, TN
University of Washington, WA

Medical-Surgical
Alverno College, WI
Angelo State University, TX
Azusa Pacific University, CA
California State University, Sacramento, CA
Case Western Reserve University, OH
DePaul University, IL
East Carolina University, NC
Florida Southern College, FL
Gannon University, PA
Gonzaga University, WA
Hunter College of the City University of New York, NY

The Johns Hopkins University, MD
Kent State University, OH
Long Island University, C.W. Post Campus, NY
Malone College, OH
McGill University, QC
Montana State University, MT
Murray State University, KY
New Mexico State University, NM
Northern Arizona University, AZ
Oregon Health & Science University, OR
Pacific Lutheran University, WA
Penn State University Park, PA
Point Loma Nazarene University, CA
Rush University, IL
Saint Francis Medical Center College of Nursing, IL
Seattle Pacific University, WA
State University of New York Upstate Medical University, NY
Texas A&M University–Corpus Christi, TX
Texas Christian University, TX
Thomas Jefferson University, PA
Université du Québec à Chicoutimi, QC
University at Buffalo, the State University of New York, NY
University of Alberta, AB
University of Arkansas, AR
University of Calgary, AB
University of Central Arkansas, AR
University of Florida, FL
University of Illinois at Chicago, IL
University of Kentucky, KY
University of Michigan, MI
University of Missouri–Columbia, MO
University of Nebraska Medical Center, NE
University of New Brunswick Fredericton, NB
University of North Florida, FL
University of Pennsylvania, PA
University of Pittsburgh, PA
University of San Diego, CA
University of Southern Maine, ME
The University of Texas at Austin, TX
The University of Texas Health Science Center at San Antonio, TX
University of Virginia, VA
University of Washington, WA
University of Wisconsin–Madison, WI
Vanderbilt University, TN

Occupational Health
Université de Moncton, NB
Université du Québec à Chicoutimi, QC
University of California, San Francisco, CA
University of Cincinnati, OH
University of Illinois at Chicago, IL
The University of Iowa, IA
University of Michigan, MI
University of Washington, WA

Oncology
Case Western Reserve University, OH
Duke University, NC
Gwynedd-Mercy College, PA
Indiana University–Purdue University Indianapolis, IN
The Johns Hopkins University, MD
Kent State University, OH
Loyola University Chicago, IL
McGill University, QC
The Ohio State University, OH
Seattle Pacific University, WA
Thomas Jefferson University, PA
Université du Québec à Chicoutimi, QC
University of Alberta, AB
University of California, Los Angeles, CA
University of California, San Francisco, CA
University of Kentucky, KY
University of Louisville, KY
University of Nebraska Medical Center, NE
University of New Brunswick Fredericton, NB
University of Pennsylvania, PA
University of South Florida, FL

University of Utah, UT
University of Washington, WA
Yale University, CT

Palliative Care
Boston College, MA
Daemen College, NY
The Johns Hopkins University, MD
Seattle Pacific University, WA
Ursuline College, OH

Parent-Child
Azusa Pacific University, CA
California State University, Dominguez Hills, CA
California State University, Sacramento, CA
Clemson University, SC
College Misericordia, PA
Dalhousie University, NS
Hunter College of the City University of New York, NY
The Johns Hopkins University, MD
Kent State University, OH
Lehman College of the City University of New York, NY
Loma Linda University, CA
Long Island University, C.W. Post Campus, NY
Louisiana State University Health Sciences Center, LA
McGill University, QC
Medical University of South Carolina, SC
The Ohio State University, OH
Old Dominion University, VA
Saint Francis Medical Center College of Nursing, IL
Stony Brook University, State University of New York, NY
Université du Québec à Chicoutimi, QC
University of Alberta, AB
University of Calgary, AB
University of Kentucky, KY
University of Nebraska Medical Center, NE
University of New Brunswick Fredericton, NB
University of Washington, WA
University of Wisconsin-Milwaukee, WI

Pediatric
Arizona State University at the Downtown Phoenix Campus, AZ
Auburn University, AL
Auburn University Montgomery, AL
Azusa Pacific University, CA
California State University, Fresno, CA
Case Western Reserve University, OH
The Catholic University of America, DC
Clemson University, SC
Dalhousie University, NS
Duke University, NC
Florida International University, FL
Georgia State University, GA
Grand Valley State University, MI
Gwynedd-Mercy College, PA
Indiana University-Purdue University Indianapolis, IN
The Johns Hopkins University, MD
Kent State University, OH
Marquette University, WI
McGill University, QC
Memorial University of Newfoundland, NL
New York University, NY
Rush University, IL
St. John Fisher College, NY
Saint Louis University, MO
Seattle Pacific University, WA
Stony Brook University, State University of New York, NY
Texas Woman's University, TX
Thomas Jefferson University, PA
Union University, TN
Université de Moncton, NB
Université du Québec à Chicoutimi, QC
The University of Akron, OH
University of Alberta, AB

University of Arkansas for Medical Sciences, AR
University of Calgary, AB
University of California, Los Angeles, CA
University of California, San Francisco, CA
University of Delaware, DE
University of Illinois at Chicago, IL
University of Kentucky, KY
University of Maryland, Baltimore, MD
University of Minnesota, Twin Cities Campus, MN
University of Missouri-Columbia, MO
University of Missouri-Kansas City, MO
University of Missouri-St. Louis, MO
University of Nebraska Medical Center, NE
University of New Brunswick Fredericton, NB
The University of North Carolina at Chapel Hill, NC
University of North Florida, FL
University of Pennsylvania, PA
University of Puerto Rico, Medical Sciences Campus, PR
University of South Alabama, AL
The University of Tennessee, TN
University of Toronto, ON
University of Washington, WA
University of Wisconsin-Madison, WI
Vanderbilt University, TN
Wichita State University, KS
Wright State University, OH

Perinatal
California State University, Sacramento, CA
Georgia State University, GA
The Johns Hopkins University, MD
McGill University, QC
McMaster University, ON
The Ohio State University, OH
Saint Louis University, MO
San Francisco State University, CA
Seattle Pacific University, WA
Stony Brook University, State University of New York, NY
Université du Québec à Chicoutimi, QC
University of Alberta, AB
University of Calgary, AB
University of California, San Francisco, CA
University of Illinois at Chicago, IL
University of Kentucky, KY
University of Manitoba, MB
University of Nebraska Medical Center, NE
University of Pennsylvania, PA
The University of Tennessee, TN
University of Washington, WA
University of Wisconsin-Madison, WI

Psychiatric/Mental Health
Arizona State University at the Downtown Phoenix Campus, AZ
Boston College, MA
California State University, Fresno, CA
California State University, Los Angeles, CA
California State University, Sacramento, CA
Case Western Reserve University, OH
The Catholic University of America, DC
Colorado State University-Pueblo, CO
Creighton University, NE
Dalhousie University, NS
Duquesne University, PA
Florida International University, FL
Georgia State University, GA
Gonzaga University, WA
Grand Valley State University, MI
Hampton University, VA
Hunter College of the City University of New York, NY
Husson College, ME
Indiana University-Purdue University Indianapolis, IN
Kent State University, OH
Louisiana State University Health Sciences Center, LA
McGill University, QC
McNeese State University, LA

Medical University of South Carolina, SC
Memorial University of Newfoundland, NL
MGH Institute of Health Professions, MA
New Mexico State University, NM
New York University, NY
Northeastern University, MA
Northwestern State University of Louisiana, LA
The Ohio State University, OH
Oregon Health & Science University, OR
Point Loma Nazarene University, CA
Rivier College, NH
Rush University, IL
Rutgers, The State University of New Jersey, College of Nursing, NJ
The Sage Colleges, NY
Saint Joseph College, CT
Saint Louis University, MO
Shenandoah University, VA
Stony Brook University, State University of New York, NY
Temple University, PA
Université de Moncton, NB
Université du Québec à Chicoutimi, QC
Université du Québec à Rimouski, QC
Université du Québec en Outaouais, QC
The University of Akron, OH
University of Alaska Anchorage, AK
University of Alberta, AB
The University of British Columbia, BC
University of Calgary, AB
University of California, San Francisco, CA
University of Central Arkansas, AR
University of Colorado at Denver and Health Sciences Center, CO
University of Delaware, DE
University of Florida, FL
University of Hawaii at Manoa, HI
University of Illinois at Chicago, IL
The University of Iowa, IA
University of Kentucky, KY
University of Louisiana at Lafayette, LA
University of Louisville, KY
University of Maryland, Baltimore, MD
University of Massachusetts Amherst, MA
University of Massachusetts Lowell, MA
University of Medicine and Dentistry of New Jersey, NJ
University of Miami, FL
University of Michigan, MI
University of Minnesota, Twin Cities Campus, MN
University of Missouri-Columbia, MO
University of Nebraska Medical Center, NE
University of New Brunswick Fredericton, NB
The University of North Carolina at Chapel Hill, NC
The University of North Carolina at Charlotte, NC
University of North Dakota, ND
University of North Florida, FL
University of Pennsylvania, PA
University of Pittsburgh, PA
University of Puerto Rico, Medical Sciences Campus, PR
University of Rhode Island, RI
University of South Alabama, AL
University of South Carolina, SC
University of Southern Maine, ME
University of Southern Mississippi, MS
University of South Florida, FL
The University of Tennessee, TN
The University of Tennessee Health Science Center, TN
The University of Texas Health Science Center at San Antonio, TX
The University of Toledo, OH
University of Toronto, ON
University of Vermont, VT
University of Virginia, VA
University of Washington, WA
The University of Western Ontario, ON
University of Wisconsin-Madison, WI
University of Wisconsin-Milwaukee, WI
Valdosta State University, GA

CONCENTRATIONS WITHIN MASTER'S DEGREE PROGRAMS
Clinical Nurse Specialist Programs

Vanderbilt University, TN
Virginia Commonwealth University, VA
Wayne State University, MI
Widener University, PA
Wilkes University, PA
Yale University, CT

Public Health

Augustana College, SD
Bloomsburg University of Pennsylvania, PA
California State University, Fresno, CA
Dalhousie University, NS
Emory University, GA
The Johns Hopkins University, MD
La Salle University, PA
Loma Linda University, CA
McGill University, QC
Northern Arizona University, AZ
The Ohio State University, OH
Oregon Health & Science University, OR
Rush University, IL
Ryerson University, ON
San Francisco State University, CA
Seattle Pacific University, WA
Thomas Jefferson University, PA
Université de Moncton, NB
Université du Québec à Chicoutimi, QC
University of Alberta, AB
The University of British Columbia, BC
University of Calgary, AB
University of Colorado at Denver and Health
  Sciences Center, CO
University of Florida, FL
University of Illinois at Chicago, IL
University of Kentucky, KY
University of Massachusetts Amherst, MA
University of Missouri-Columbia, MO
University of Nebraska Medical Center, NE
University of New Brunswick Fredericton, NB
The University of Texas at Austin, TX
The University of Texas at Brownsville, TX
University of Vermont, VT
University of Virginia, VA
The University of Western Ontario, ON
Wright State University, OH

Rehabilitation

McGill University, QC
Salem State College, MA
Seattle Pacific University, WA
Université du Québec à Chicoutimi, QC
Université du Québec en Outaouais, QC
University of Calgary, AB

School Health

Azusa Pacific University, CA
Bloomsburg University of Pennsylvania, PA
California State University, Bakersfield, CA
California State University, Fullerton, CA
California State University, Sacramento, CA
California State University, San Bernardino, CA
Kean University, NJ
Kent State University, OH
San Diego State University, CA
San Jose State University, CA
Seattle Pacific University, WA
Seton Hall University, NJ
Université de Moncton, NB
Université du Québec à Chicoutimi, QC
University of Delaware, DE
University of Illinois at Chicago, IL
University of Nevada, Reno, NV
University of New Brunswick Fredericton, NB
Wright State University, OH

Women's Health

Drexel University, PA
Grand Valley State University, MI
The Johns Hopkins University, MD
Kent State University, OH
McGill University, QC
The Ohio State University, OH
Oregon Health & Science University, OR

St. John Fisher College, NY
Seattle Pacific University, WA
Stony Brook University, State University of New
  York, NY
Texas Woman's University, TX
Université du Québec à Chicoutimi, QC
University of Alberta, AB
University of Calgary, AB
University of Illinois at Chicago, IL
University of Kentucky, KY
University of Massachusetts Amherst, MA
University of Miami, FL
University of Missouri-Columbia, MO
University of Missouri-St. Louis, MO
University of Nebraska Medical Center, NE
University of New Brunswick Fredericton, NB
The University of North Carolina at Chapel Hill,
  NC
University of North Florida, FL
University of Pennsylvania, PA
University of South Alabama, AL
The University of Tennessee, TN
The University of Texas Health Science Center at
  Houston, TX
University of Toronto, ON
University of Washington, WA
The University of Western Ontario, ON
University of Wisconsin-Madison, WI
University of Wisconsin-Milwaukee, WI
Valparaiso University, IN

HEALTH-CARE ADMINISTRATION

Athabasca University, AB
California State University, Long Beach, CA
Capital University, OH
Cleveland State University, OH
The College of New Rochelle, NY
Daemen College, NY
Duke University, NC
Emory University, GA
Excelsior College, NY
Fairfield University, CT
Georgetown University, DC
Gonzaga University, WA
Graceland University, IA
Grand Canyon University, AZ
Holy Family University, PA
Kean University, NJ
Kent State University, OH
Lewis University, IL
Louisiana State University Health Sciences Center,
  LA
Loyola University New Orleans, LA
Mercy College, NY
Midwestern State University, TX
Oregon Health & Science University, OR
Pacific Lutheran University, WA
Quinnipiac University, CT
Regis College, MA
Regis University, CO
Rivier College, NH
Salisbury University, MD
Seton Hall University, NJ
Southern Adventist University, TN
Southern Illinois University Edwardsville, IL
Southern University and Agricultural and
  Mechanical College, LA
Tennessee Technological University, TN
Towson University, MD
Université de Moncton, NB
The University of Alabama at Birmingham, AL
The University of Alabama in Huntsville, AL
University of Alaska Anchorage, AK
University of Colorado at Denver and Health
  Sciences Center, CO
University of Delaware, DE
University of Hawaii at Manoa, HI
University of Illinois at Chicago, IL
University of Kansas, KS

University of Maine, ME
University of Michigan, MI
University of Mississippi Medical Center, MS
University of Nebraska Medical Center, NE
The University of North Carolina at Charlotte, NC
University of Oklahoma Health Sciences Center,
  OK
University of Pennsylvania, PA
University of Phoenix-Bay Area Campus, CA
University of Phoenix-Central Florida Campus, FL
University of Phoenix-Central Valley Campus, CA
University of Phoenix-Hawaii Campus, HI
University of Phoenix-Louisiana Campus, LA
University of Phoenix-Metro Detroit Campus, MI
University of Phoenix-New Mexico Campus, NM
University of Phoenix-North Florida Campus, FL
University of Phoenix Online Campus, AZ
University of Phoenix-Phoenix Campus, AZ
University of Phoenix-Sacramento Valley Campus,
  CA
University of Phoenix-San Diego Campus, CA
University of Phoenix-Southern Arizona Campus,
  AZ
University of Phoenix-Southern California
  Campus, CA
University of Phoenix-Southern Colorado Campus,
  CO
University of Phoenix-South Florida Campus, FL
University of Phoenix-West Florida Campus, FL
University of Phoenix-West Michigan Campus, MI
University of Rochester, NY
University of San Francisco, CA
The University of Tennessee, TN
The University of Texas at Arlington, TX
University of Virginia, VA
The University of Western Ontario, ON
University of Wisconsin-Milwaukee, WI
Vanderbilt University, TN
Villanova University, PA
Viterbo University, WI
Wright State University, OH

NURSING ADMINISTRATION

Adelphi University, NY
Allen College, IA
American International College, MA
Armstrong Atlantic State University, GA
Azusa Pacific University, CA
Ball State University, IN
Barry University, FL
Bellarmine University, KY
Bellin College of Nursing, WI
Bethel College, IN
Bethel University, MN
Bloomsburg University of Pennsylvania, PA
Bowie State University, MD
Bradley University, IL
California State University, Dominguez Hills, CA
California State University, Fullerton, CA
California State University, Los Angeles, CA
California State University, Sacramento, CA
Capital University, OH
Carlow University, PA
Clarke College, IA
Clarkson College, NE
Clemson University, SC
College Misericordia, PA
College of Mount Saint Vincent, NY
The College of New Jersey, NJ
The College of New Rochelle, NY
The College of St. Scholastica, MN
Creighton University, NE
Delta State University, MS
DePaul University, IL
DeSales University, PA
Drexel University, PA
Duke University, NC
Duquesne University, PA
East Carolina University, NC
East Tennessee State University, TN

Edgewood College, WI
Emory University, GA
Fairleigh Dickinson University, Metropolitan
  Campus, NJ
Ferris State University, MI
Florida Atlantic University, FL
Florida International University, FL
Fort Hays State University, KS
Gannon University, PA
Gardner-Webb University, NC
George Mason University, VA
Georgia College & State University, GA
Gonzaga University, WA
Grand Valley State University, MI
Hampton University, VA
Holy Names University, CA
Idaho State University, ID
Illinois State University, IL
Immaculata University, PA
Indiana State University, IN
Indiana University of Pennsylvania, PA
Indiana University-Purdue University Fort Wayne,
  IN
Indiana University-Purdue University Indianapolis,
  IN
Indiana Wesleyan University, IN
Intercollegiate College of Nursing/Washington
  State University, WA
Jacksonville University, FL
Jefferson College of Health Sciences, VA
The Johns Hopkins University, MD
Kean University, NJ
Kent State University, OH
Lamar University, TX
La Roche College, PA
La Salle University, PA
Lehman College of the City University of New
  York, NY
Lewis University, IL
Loma Linda University, CA
Long Island University, Brooklyn Campus, NY
Louisiana State University Health Sciences Center,
  LA
Loyola University Chicago, IL
Madonna University, MI
Marquette University, WI
Marshall University, WV
Marymount University, VA
Marywood University, PA
McKendree College, IL
Medical University of South Carolina, SC
Mercy College, NY
Metropolitan State University, MN
Midwestern State University, TX
Molloy College, NY
Monmouth University, NJ
Mountain State University, WV
Nebraska Wesleyan University, NE
New Mexico State University, NM
New York University, NY
Northeastern University, MA
Northern Kentucky University, KY
North Park University, IL
Northwestern State University of Louisiana, LA
Nova Southeastern University, FL
The Ohio State University, OH
Ohio University, OH
Old Dominion University, VA
Oregon Health & Science University, OR
Otterbein College, OH
Our Lady of the Lake College, LA
Pace University, NY
Pacific Lutheran University, WA
Patty Hanks Shelton School of Nursing, TX
Penn State University Park, PA
Purdue University Calumet, IN
Queens University of Charlotte, NC
Regis College, MA
Regis University, CO
Research College of Nursing, MO
Roberts Wesleyan College, NY
Sacred Heart University, CT

Saginaw Valley State University, MI
Saint Joseph's College of Maine, ME
Saint Peter's College, NJ
Saint Xavier University, IL
Salem State College, MA
Samford University, AL
San Francisco State University, CA
San Jose State University, CA
Seattle Pacific University, WA
Seton Hall University, NJ
Sonoma State University, CA
South Dakota State University, SD
Southeastern Louisiana University, LA
Southern Connecticut State University, CT
Southern Nazarene University, OK
Spalding University, KY
State University of New York at Binghamton, NY
State University of New York Institute of
  Technology, NY
Texas A&M University-Corpus Christi, TX
Texas Tech University Health Sciences Center, TX
Texas Woman's University, TX
Thomas University, GA
Troy University, AL
Union University, TN
Université de Moncton, NB
The University of Akron, OH
The University of Alabama at Birmingham, AL
University of Arkansas for Medical Sciences, AR
The University of British Columbia, BC
University of California, Los Angeles, CA
University of California, San Francisco, CA
University of Central Florida, FL
University of Cincinnati, OH
University of Colorado at Colorado Springs, CO
University of Colorado at Denver and Health
  Sciences Center, CO
University of Connecticut, CT
University of Detroit Mercy, MI
University of Hartford, CT
University of Illinois at Chicago, IL
University of Indianapolis, IN
The University of Iowa, IA
University of Kansas, KS
University of Kentucky, KY
University of Manitoba, MB
University of Mary, ND
University of Maryland, Baltimore, MD
University of Memphis, TN
University of Michigan, MI
University of Minnesota, Twin Cities Campus, MN
University of Mississippi Medical Center, MS
University of Missouri-Columbia, MO
University of Missouri-Kansas City, MO
University of Missouri-St. Louis, MO
University of Mobile, AL
University of Nebraska Medical Center, NE
University of New Brunswick Fredericton, NB
University of New Mexico, NM
The University of North Carolina at Chapel Hill,
  NC
The University of North Carolina at Greensboro,
  NC
University of North Dakota, ND
University of Pennsylvania, PA
University of Phoenix-Bay Area Campus, CA
University of Phoenix-Central Florida Campus, FL
University of Phoenix-Central Valley Campus, CA
University of Phoenix-Cleveland Campus, OH
University of Phoenix-Denver Campus, CO
University of Phoenix-Hawaii Campus, HI
University of Phoenix-Louisiana Campus, LA
University of Phoenix-Metro Detroit Campus, MI
University of Phoenix-New Mexico Campus, NM
University of Phoenix-North Florida Campus, FL
University of Phoenix-Oklahoma City Campus,
  OK
University of Phoenix Online Campus, AZ
University of Phoenix-Phoenix Campus, AZ
University of Phoenix-Sacramento Valley Campus,
  CA
University of Phoenix-San Diego Campus, CA

University of Phoenix-Southern Arizona Campus,
  AZ
University of Phoenix-Southern California
  Campus, CA
University of Phoenix-Southern Colorado Campus,
  CO
University of Phoenix-South Florida Campus, FL
University of Phoenix-Utah Campus, UT
University of Phoenix-West Florida Campus, FL
University of Phoenix-West Michigan Campus, MI
University of Pittsburgh, PA
University of Puerto Rico, Medical Sciences
  Campus, PR
University of Rhode Island, RI
University of San Diego, CA
University of South Alabama, AL
University of South Carolina, SC
University of Southern Indiana, IN
University of Southern Mississippi, MS
The University of Tennessee, TN
The University of Texas at Arlington, TX
The University of Texas at Austin, TX
The University of Texas at Brownsville, TX
The University of Texas at El Paso, TX
The University of Texas at Tyler, TX
The University of Texas Health Science Center at
  Houston, TX
The University of Texas Health Science Center at
  San Antonio, TX
The University of Texas Medical Branch, TX
University of Toronto, ON
University of Utah, UT
University of Vermont, VT
University of Virginia, VA
The University of Western Ontario, ON
University of West Georgia, GA
University of Wisconsin-Eau Claire, WI
Valdosta State University, GA
Vanderbilt University, TN
Virginia Commonwealth University, VA
Washburn University, KS
Waynesburg College, PA
Webster University, MO
Western Kentucky University, KY
Western University of Health Sciences, CA
West Suburban College of Nursing, IL
West Texas A&M University, TX
Wheeling Jesuit University, WV
Wichita State University, KS
Wilkes University, PA
William Paterson University of New Jersey, NJ
Wilmington College, DE
Winona State University, MN
Wright State University, OH
Xavier University, OH
Yale University, CT
York College of Pennsylvania, PA

NURSE ANESTHESIA

Arkansas State University, AR
Barnes-Jewish College of Nursing and Allied
  Health, MO
Boston College, MA
Bradley University, IL
California State University, Fullerton, CA
Case Western Reserve University, OH
Columbia University, NY
DePaul University, IL
Drexel University, PA
Duke University, NC
East Carolina University, NC
Fairfield University, CT
Florida Gulf Coast University, FL
Florida International University, FL
Gannon University, PA
Georgetown University, DC
La Salle University, PA
Louisiana State University Health Sciences Center,
  LA
Medical College of Georgia, GA

Nurse Anesthesia

Mountain State University, WV
Murray State University, KY
Northeastern University, MA
Oakland University, MI
Old Dominion University, VA
Oregon Health & Science University, OR
Our Lady of the Lake College, LA
Rush University, IL
Samford University, AL
Samuel Merritt College, CA
Southern Illinois University Edwardsville, IL
State University of New York Downstate Medical Center, NY
Texas Christian University, TX
Thomas Jefferson University, PA
Union University, TN
University at Buffalo, the State University of New York, NY
The University of Akron, OH
University of Cincinnati, OH
The University of Iowa, IA
University of Maryland, Baltimore, MD
University of Medicine and Dentistry of New Jersey, NJ
University of Miami, FL
University of Minnesota, Twin Cities Campus, MN
The University of North Carolina at Charlotte, NC
The University of North Carolina at Greensboro, NC
University of North Dakota, ND
University of Pennsylvania, PA
University of Pittsburgh, PA
University of Puerto Rico, Medical Sciences Campus, PR
The University of Scranton, PA
University of South Florida, FL
The University of Tennessee, TN
The University of Tennessee at Chattanooga, TN
The University of Tennessee Health Science Center, TN
The University of Texas Health Science Center at Houston, TX
Villanova University, PA
York College of Pennsylvania, PA
Youngstown State University, OH

NURSING EDUCATION

Adelphi University, NY
Albany State University, GA
Alcorn State University, MS
Allen College, IA
Alverno College, WI
American International College, MA
Andrews University, MI
Angelo State University, TX
Arkansas State University, AR
Auburn University, AL
Auburn University Montgomery, AL
Azusa Pacific University, CA
Ball State University, IN
Barnes-Jewish College of Nursing and Allied Health, MO
Barry University, FL
Bellarmine University, KY
Bellin College of Nursing, WI
Bethel College, IN
Bethel University, MN
Bowie State University, MD
Brenau University, GA
Briar Cliff University, IA
California State University, Chico, CA
California State University, Dominguez Hills, CA
California State University, Fresno, CA
California State University, Long Beach, CA
California State University, Los Angeles, CA
California State University, Sacramento, CA
California State University, San Bernardino, CA
Capital University, OH
Cardinal Stritch University, WI
Carlow University, PA

Carson-Newman College, TN
The Catholic University of America, DC
Clarion University of Pennsylvania, PA
Clarke College, IA
Clarkson College, NE
Clemson University, SC
College Misericordia, PA
The College of New Rochelle, NY
College of St. Catherine, MN
Colorado State University-Pueblo, CO
Concordia College, MN
Concordia University Wisconsin, WI
Creighton University, NE
Daemen College, NY
Delta State University, MS
DePaul University, IL
DeSales University, PA
Dominican University of California, CA
Drexel University, PA
Duke University, NC
Duquesne University, PA
D'Youville College, NY
East Carolina University, NC
East Tennessee State University, TN
Edgewood College, WI
Excelsior College, NY
Fairleigh Dickinson University, Metropolitan Campus, NJ
Ferris State University, MI
Florida Atlantic University, FL
Florida Gulf Coast University, FL
Florida Southern College, FL
Florida State University, FL
Fort Hays State University, KS
Franciscan University of Steubenville, OH
Gannon University, PA
Gardner-Webb University, NC
Georgetown University, DC
Georgia Baptist College of Nursing of Mercer University, GA
Georgia College & State University, GA
Gonzaga University, WA
Graceland University, IA
Grambling State University, LA
Grand Canyon University, AZ
Grand Valley State University, MI
Hampton University, VA
Holy Family University, PA
Idaho State University, ID
Immaculata University, PA
Indiana Wesleyan University, IN
Intercollegiate College of Nursing/Washington State University, WA
Jacksonville University, FL
James Madison University, VA
Jefferson College of Health Sciences, VA
Kent State University, OH
Lamar University, TX
Lehman College of the City University of New York, NY
Lewis University, IL
Loma Linda University, CA
Long Island University, Brooklyn Campus, NY
Long Island University, C.W. Post Campus, NY
Louisiana State University Health Sciences Center, LA
Mansfield University of Pennsylvania, PA
Marian College of Fond du Lac, WI
Marshall University, WV
Marymount University, VA
Maryville University of Saint Louis, MO
McKendree College, IL
McNeese State University, LA
Medical University of South Carolina, SC
Mercy College, NY
MGH Institute of Health Professions, MA
Michigan State University, MI
Midwestern State University, TX
Millersville University of Pennsylvania, PA
Minnesota State University Mankato, MN
Minnesota State University Moorhead, MN
Missouri State University, MO

Molloy College, NY
Monmouth University, NJ
Montana State University, MT
Mountain State University, WV
Mount Carmel College of Nursing, OH
Mount St. Mary's College, CA
Nebraska Methodist College, NE
Nebraska Wesleyan University, NE
Neumann College, PA
New York University, NY
North Dakota State University, ND
Northern Arizona University, AZ
Northern Kentucky University, KY
North Georgia College & State University, GA
Northwestern State University of Louisiana, LA
Nova Southeastern University, FL
Oakland University, MI
Ohio University, OH
Old Dominion University, VA
Otterbein College, OH
Our Lady of the Lake College, LA
Pace University, NY
Pacific Lutheran University, WA
Patty Hanks Shelton School of Nursing, TX
Point Loma Nazarene University, CA
Regis University, CO
Research College of Nursing, MO
Rivier College, NH
Saginaw Valley State University, MI
Saint Anthony College of Nursing, IL
Saint Francis Medical Center College of Nursing, IL
St. John Fisher College, NY
St. Joseph's College, New York, NY
Saint Joseph's College of Maine, ME
Saint Louis University, MO
Salem State College, MA
Samford University, AL
San Jose State University, CA
Seattle Pacific University, WA
Seton Hall University, NJ
Simmons College, MA
Slippery Rock University of Pennsylvania, PA
Sonoma State University, CA
South Dakota State University, SD
Southeastern Louisiana University, LA
Southeast Missouri State University, MO
Southern Adventist University, TN
Southern Connecticut State University, CT
Southern Illinois University Edwardsville, IL
Southern Nazarene University, OK
Southern University and Agricultural and Mechanical College, LA
Spalding University, KY
State University of New York at Binghamton, NY
Temple University, PA
Tennessee State University, TN
Tennessee Technological University, TN
Texas Christian University, TX
Texas Tech University Health Sciences Center, TX
Thomas Jefferson University, PA
Thomas University, GA
Towson University, MD
Troy University, AL
Union University, TN
Université de Moncton, NB
University at Buffalo, the State University of New York, NY
University of Alaska Anchorage, AK
University of Arkansas, AR
University of Arkansas for Medical Sciences, AR
The University of British Columbia, BC
University of Central Arkansas, AR
University of Central Florida, FL
University of Central Missouri, MO
University of Hartford, CT
University of Hawaii at Manoa, HI
University of Indianapolis, IN
The University of Iowa, IA
University of Kansas, KS
University of Louisiana at Lafayette, LA
University of Maine, ME

University of Mary, ND
University of Massachusetts Worcester, MA
University of Medicine and Dentistry of New Jersey, NJ
University of Memphis, TN
University of Mississippi Medical Center, MS
University of Missouri-Columbia, MO
University of Missouri-Kansas City, MO
University of Missouri-St. Louis, MO
University of Mobile, AL
University of Nebraska Medical Center, NE
University of Nevada, Las Vegas, NV
University of Nevada, Reno, NV
University of New Brunswick Fredericton, NB
University of New Mexico, NM
The University of North Carolina at Chapel Hill, NC
The University of North Carolina at Greensboro, NC
The University of North Carolina Wilmington, NC
University of North Dakota, ND
University of Northern Colorado, CO
University of Oklahoma Health Sciences Center, OK
University of Phoenix-Bay Area Campus, CA
University of Phoenix-Central Florida Campus, FL
University of Phoenix-Denver Campus, CO
University of Phoenix-Hawaii Campus, HI
University of Phoenix-Louisiana Campus, LA
University of Phoenix-Metro Detroit Campus, MI
University of Phoenix-New Mexico Campus, NM
University of Phoenix-North Florida Campus, FL
University of Phoenix Online Campus, AZ
University of Phoenix-Phoenix Campus, AZ
University of Phoenix-Sacramento Valley Campus, CA
University of Phoenix-San Diego Campus, CA
University of Phoenix-Southern Arizona Campus, AZ
University of Phoenix-Southern California Campus, CA
University of Phoenix-Southern Colorado Campus, CO
University of Phoenix-South Florida Campus, FL
University of Phoenix-Utah Campus, UT
University of Phoenix-West Florida Campus, FL
University of Pittsburgh, PA
University of Puerto Rico, Medical Sciences Campus, PR
University of Rhode Island, RI
University of St. Francis, IL
University of San Diego, CA
University of Saskatchewan, SK
The University of Scranton, PA
University of South Alabama, AL
University of South Carolina, SC
University of Southern Indiana, IN
University of South Florida, FL
The University of Tampa, FL
The University of Texas at Brownsville, TX
The University of Texas at El Paso, TX
The University of Texas at Tyler, TX
The University of Texas Health Science Center at Houston, TX
The University of Texas Health Science Center at San Antonio, TX
The University of Texas Medical Branch, TX
The University of Toledo, OH
University of Utah, UT
University of Washington, WA
The University of Western Ontario, ON
University of West Georgia, GA
University of Wisconsin-Eau Claire, WI
University of Wisconsin-Madison, WI
University of Wisconsin-Milwaukee, WI
University of Wisconsin-Oshkosh, WI
University of Wyoming, WY
Valdosta State University, GA
Villanova University, PA
Viterbo University, WI
Wagner College, NY
Waynesburg College, PA

Webster University, MO
Western Carolina University, NC
Western Kentucky University, KY
Westminster College, UT
West Suburban College of Nursing, IL
West Texas A&M University, TX
Wheeling Jesuit University, WV
Widener University, PA
William Carey College, MS
William Paterson University of New Jersey, NJ
Wilmington College, DE
Winona State University, MN
Xavier University, OH
York College of Pennsylvania, PA
Youngstown State University, OH

NURSING INFORMATICS

Case Western Reserve University, OH
Duke University, NC
Excelsior College, NY
Fairleigh Dickinson University, Metropolitan Campus, NJ
Ferris State University, MI
Georgia College & State University, GA
Molloy College, NY
New York University, NY
Pace University, NY
Pacific Lutheran University, WA
Saginaw Valley State University, MI
Seattle Pacific University, WA
Tennessee State University, TN
Tennessee Technological University, TN
Thomas Jefferson University, PA
Troy University, AL
University at Buffalo, the State University of New York, NY
University of Colorado at Denver and Health Sciences Center, CO
University of Illinois at Chicago, IL
The University of Iowa, IA
University of Kansas, KS
University of Maryland, Baltimore, MD
University of Medicine and Dentistry of New Jersey, NJ
University of Michigan, MI
University of Nebraska Medical Center, NE
University of New Brunswick Fredericton, NB
The University of North Carolina at Chapel Hill, NC
University of Pennsylvania, PA
University of Pittsburgh, PA
University of San Francisco, CA
The University of Texas Health Science Center at San Antonio, TX
University of Utah, UT
University of Washington, WA
Vanderbilt University, TN

NURSE PRACTITIONER PROGRAMS

Acute Care

Arizona State University at the Downtown Phoenix Campus, AZ
Barry University, FL
California State University, Los Angeles, CA
Case Western Reserve University, OH
Colorado State University-Pueblo, CO
Columbia University, NY
Dalhousie University, NS
Drexel University, PA
Duke University, NC
Emory University, GA
Georgetown University, DC
Indiana University-Purdue University Indianapolis, IN
The Johns Hopkins University, MD
Kent State University, OH

Loyola University Chicago, IL
Marquette University, WI
Memorial University of Newfoundland, NL
MGH Institute of Health Professions, MA
New York University, NY
Northeastern University, MA
Northwestern State University of Louisiana, LA
Rush University, IL
Rutgers, The State University of New Jersey, College of Nursing, NJ
The Sage Colleges, NY
Saint Louis University, MO
San Diego State University, CA
Seton Hall University, NJ
Texas Tech University Health Sciences Center, TX
Thomas Jefferson University, PA
The University of Alabama at Birmingham, AL
The University of Alabama in Huntsville, AL
The University of Arizona, AZ
University of Arkansas for Medical Sciences, AR
University of Calgary, AB
University of California, Los Angeles, CA
University of California, San Francisco, CA
University of Cincinnati, OH
University of Connecticut, CT
University of Florida, FL
University of Illinois at Chicago, IL
University of Kentucky, KY
University of Maryland, Baltimore, MD
University of Massachusetts Worcester, MA
University of Medicine and Dentistry of New Jersey, NJ
University of Miami, FL
University of Michigan, MI
University of Mississippi Medical Center, MS
University of Nebraska Medical Center, NE
University of New Brunswick Fredericton, NB
University of New Mexico, NM
University of Pennsylvania, PA
University of Pittsburgh, PA
University of Rochester, NY
University of South Alabama, AL
University of South Carolina, SC
University of Southern Indiana, IN
University of South Florida, FL
The University of Tennessee Health Science Center, TN
The University of Texas at Arlington, TX
The University of Texas at Tyler, TX
The University of Texas Health Science Center at Houston, TX
The University of Texas Medical Branch, TX
University of Toronto, ON
University of Utah, UT
University of Virginia, VA
University of Washington, WA
University of Wisconsin-Madison, WI
Vanderbilt University, TN
Virginia Commonwealth University, VA
Wayne State University, MI
Wichita State University, KS
Wright State University, OH
Yale University, CT

Adult Health

Adelphi University, NY
Arizona State University at the Downtown Phoenix Campus, AZ
Armstrong Atlantic State University, GA
Azusa Pacific University, CA
Ball State University, IN
Barnes-Jewish College of Nursing and Allied Health, MO
Bloomsburg University of Pennsylvania, PA
Boston College, MA
California State University, Long Beach, CA
California State University, Los Angeles, CA
Case Western Reserve University, OH
Clarkson College, NE
Clemson University, SC
College of Mount Saint Vincent, NY
College of St. Catherine, MN

CONCENTRATIONS WITHIN MASTER'S DEGREE PROGRAMS
Nurse Practitioner Programs

The College of St. Scholastica, MN
College of Staten Island of the City University of New York, NY
Columbia University, NY
Creighton University, NE
Daemen College, NY
Dalhousie University, NS
DePaul University, IL
Duke University, NC
East Carolina University, NC
East Tennessee State University, TN
Emory University, GA
Fairleigh Dickinson University, Metropolitan Campus, NJ
Felician College, NJ
Florida Agricultural and Mechanical University, FL
Florida Atlantic University, FL
Florida International University, FL
George Mason University, VA
Grand Valley State University, MI
Gwynedd-Mercy College, PA
Hunter College of the City University of New York, NY
Indiana University–Purdue University Indianapolis, IN
James Madison University, VA
The Johns Hopkins University, MD
Kennesaw State University, GA
Kent State University, OH
La Salle University, PA
Loma Linda University, CA
Long Island University, Brooklyn Campus, NY
Loyola University Chicago, IL
Loyola University New Orleans, LA
Madonna University, MI
Marian College of Fond du Lac, WI
Marquette University, WI
Maryville University of Saint Louis, MO
McNeese State University, LA
Medical University of South Carolina, SC
Metropolitan State University, MN
MGH Institute of Health Professions, MA
Michigan State University, MI
Molloy College, NY
Monmouth University, NJ
Mount Saint Mary College, NY
New York University, NY
Northeastern University, MA
Northern Illinois University, IL
Northern Kentucky University, KY
North Park University, IL
Oakland University, MI
The Ohio State University, OH
Oregon Health & Science University, OR
Otterbein College, OH
Purdue University, IN
Quinnipiac University, CT
Regis College, MA
The Richard Stockton College of New Jersey, NJ
Rush University, IL
Rutgers, The State University of New Jersey, College of Nursing, NJ
The Sage Colleges, NY
Saint Louis University, MO
Saint Peter's College, NJ
San Diego State University, CA
Seattle Pacific University, WA
Seton Hall University, NJ
Simmons College, MA
Southeastern Louisiana University, LA
Southern Adventist University, TN
Spalding University, KY
State University of New York Institute of Technology, NY
State University of New York Upstate Medical University, NY
Stony Brook University, State University of New York, NY
Temple University, PA
Texas Woman's University, TX
Thomas Jefferson University, PA
Université de Moncton, NB

University at Buffalo, the State University of New York, NY
The University of Akron, OH
The University of Alabama at Birmingham, AL
The University of Arizona, AZ
University of Calgary, AB
University of California, San Francisco, CA
University of Central Arkansas, AR
University of Central Florida, FL
University of Cincinnati, OH
University of Colorado at Colorado Springs, CO
University of Colorado at Denver and Health Sciences Center, CO
University of Connecticut, CT
University of Delaware, DE
University of Florida, FL
University of Hawaii at Manoa, HI
University of Illinois at Chicago, IL
The University of Iowa, IA
University of Kansas, KS
University of Kentucky, KY
University of Louisiana at Lafayette, LA
University of Louisville, KY
University of Massachusetts Boston, MA
University of Massachusetts Dartmouth, MA
University of Massachusetts Worcester, MA
University of Medicine and Dentistry of New Jersey, NJ
University of Miami, FL
University of Michigan, MI
University of Michigan–Flint, MI
University of Missouri–Kansas City, MO
University of Missouri–St. Louis, MO
University of Nebraska Medical Center, NE
University of New Brunswick Fredericton, NB
University of New Hampshire, NH
The University of North Carolina at Chapel Hill, NC
The University of North Carolina at Charlotte, NC
The University of North Carolina at Greensboro, NC
University of Oklahoma Health Sciences Center, OK
University of Pennsylvania, PA
University of Pittsburgh, PA
University of Rochester, NY
University of St. Francis, IL
University of San Diego, CA
University of South Carolina, SC
University of Southern Maine, ME
University of South Florida, FL
The University of Tampa, FL
The University of Tennessee, TN
The University of Texas at Arlington, TX
The University of Texas at Tyler, TX
The University of Texas Health Science Center at Houston, TX
The University of Toledo, OH
University of Toronto, ON
University of Utah, UT
University of Vermont, VT
University of Washington, WA
University of Wisconsin–Eau Claire, WI
University of Wisconsin–Madison, WI
University of Wisconsin–Oshkosh, WI
Ursuline College, OH
Vanderbilt University, TN
Villanova University, PA
Virginia Commonwealth University, VA
Viterbo University, WI
Washburn University, KS
Western Connecticut State University, CT
William Paterson University of New Jersey, NJ
Wilmington College, DE
Winona State University, MN
Yale University, CT

Community Health
Athabasca University, AB
DePaul University, IL
Eastern Kentucky University, KY
Hawai'i Pacific University, HI

The Johns Hopkins University, MD
The Sage Colleges, NY
State University of New York at Binghamton, NY
Université de Moncton, NB
Université Laval, QC
University of California, San Francisco, CA
University of Massachusetts Worcester, MA
University of Miami, FL
University of Nebraska Medical Center, NE
University of New Brunswick Fredericton, NB
University of Pennsylvania, PA
The University of Western Ontario, ON
Washburn University, KS

Family Health
Albany State University, GA
Alcorn State University, MS
Allen College, IA
Arizona State University at the Downtown Phoenix Campus, AZ
Azusa Pacific University, CA
Ball State University, IN
Barry University, FL
Baylor University, TX
Belmont University, TN
Boston College, MA
Bowie State University, MD
Brenau University, GA
Briar Cliff University, IA
Brigham Young University, UT
California State University, Bakersfield, CA
California State University, Dominguez Hills, CA
California State University, Fresno, CA
California State University, Fullerton, CA
California State University, Long Beach, CA
California State University, Los Angeles, CA
California State University, Sacramento, CA
Carlow University, PA
Carson-Newman College, TN
Case Western Reserve University, OH
The Catholic University of America, DC
Clarion University of Pennsylvania, PA
Clarke College, IA
Clarkson College, NE
Clemson University, SC
College Misericordia, PA
College of Mount Saint Vincent, NY
The College of New Jersey, NJ
The College of New Rochelle, NY
The College of St. Scholastica, MN
Colorado State University-Pueblo, CO
Columbia University, NY
Concordia College, MN
Concordia University Wisconsin, WI
Coppin State University, MD
Creighton University, NE
Delta State University, MS
DePaul University, IL
DeSales University, PA
Dominican College, NY
Drexel University, PA
Duke University, NC
Duquesne University, PA
D'Youville College, NY
East Carolina University, NC
Eastern Kentucky University, KY
East Tennessee State University, TN
Emory University, GA
Fairfield University, CT
Felician College, NJ
Florida Atlantic University, FL
Florida Gulf Coast University, FL
Florida International University, FL
Florida State University, FL
Fort Hays State University, KS
Franciscan University of Steubenville, OH
Gannon University, PA
George Mason University, VA
Georgetown University, DC
Georgia College & State University, GA
Georgia Southern University, GA
Georgia State University, GA

Gonzaga University, WA
Graceland University, IA
Grambling State University, LA
Grand Canyon University, AZ
Grand Valley State University, MI
Hampton University, VA
Hawai'i Pacific University, HI
Holy Names University, CA
Howard University, DC
Husson College, ME
Idaho State University, ID
Illinois State University, IL
Indiana State University, IN
Indiana University-Purdue University Indianapolis, IN
Indiana Wesleyan University, IN
Intercollegiate College of Nursing/Washington State University, WA
The Johns Hopkins University, MD
Kennesaw State University, GA
Kent State University, OH
La Roche College, PA
La Salle University, PA
Loma Linda University, CA
Long Island University, Brooklyn Campus, NY
Long Island University, C.W. Post Campus, NY
Loyola University Chicago, IL
Loyola University New Orleans, LA
Malone College, OH
Marshall University, WV
Marymount University, VA
Maryville University of Saint Louis, MO
Medical College of Georgia, GA
Medical University of South Carolina, SC
Metropolitan State University, MN
MGH Institute of Health Professions, MA
Michigan State University, MI
Midwestern State University, TX
Millersville University of Pennsylvania, PA
Minnesota State University Mankato, MN
Minnesota State University Moorhead, MN
Mississippi University for Women, MS
Missouri State University, MO
Molloy College, NY
Monmouth University, NJ
Montana State University, MT
Mountain State University, WV
Murray State University, KY
North Dakota State University, ND
Northeastern University, MA
Northern Arizona University, AZ
Northern Illinois University, IL
Northern Kentucky University, KY
Northern Michigan University, MI
North Georgia College & State University, GA
North Park University, IL
Northwestern State University of Louisiana, LA
Oakland University, MI
The Ohio State University, OH
Ohio University, OH
Old Dominion University, VA
Oregon Health & Science University, OR
Otterbein College, OH
Pace University, NY
Pacific Lutheran University, WA
Patty Hanks Shelton School of Nursing, TX
Penn State University Park, PA
Pittsburg State University, KS
Prairie View A&M University, TX
Purdue University Calumet, IN
Quinnipiac University, CT
Radford University, VA
Regis College, MA
Regis University, CO
Research College of Nursing, MO
Rivier College, NH
Rush University, IL
Rutgers, The State University of New Jersey, College of Nursing, NJ
Sacred Heart University, CT
The Sage Colleges, NY
Saginaw Valley State University, MI

St. John Fisher College, NY
Saint Joseph College, CT
Saint Louis University, MO
Saint Xavier University, IL
Salisbury University, MD
Samford University, AL
Samuel Merritt College, CA
San Diego State University, CA
San Francisco State University, CA
San Jose State University, CA
Seattle Pacific University, WA
Seattle University, WA
Shenandoah University, VA
Simmons College, MA
Slippery Rock University of Pennsylvania, PA
Sonoma State University, CA
South Dakota State University, SD
Southeast Missouri State University, MO
Southern Adventist University, TN
Southern Connecticut State University, CT
Southern Illinois University Edwardsville, IL
Southern University and Agricultural and Mechanical College, LA
Spalding University, KY
State University of New York at Binghamton, NY
State University of New York Downstate Medical Center, NY
State University of New York Institute of Technology, NY
State University of New York Upstate Medical University, NY
Stony Brook University, State University of New York, NY
Temple University, PA
Tennessee State University, TN
Tennessee Technological University, TN
Texas A&M International University, TX
Texas A&M University-Corpus Christi, TX
Texas Tech University Health Sciences Center, TX
Texas Woman's University, TX
Thomas Jefferson University, PA
Troy University, AL
Union University, TN
Université de Moncton, NB
University at Buffalo, the State University of New York, NY
The University of Alabama at Birmingham, AL
The University of Alabama in Huntsville, AL
University of Alaska Anchorage, AK
The University of Arizona, AZ
University of Arkansas for Medical Sciences, AR
The University of British Columbia, BC
University of California, Los Angeles, CA
University of California, San Francisco, CA
University of Central Arkansas, AR
University of Central Florida, FL
University of Central Missouri, MO
University of Cincinnati, OH
University of Colorado at Colorado Springs, CO
University of Colorado at Denver and Health Sciences Center, CO
University of Delaware, DE
University of Detroit Mercy, MI
University of Florida, FL
University of Hawaii at Manoa, HI
University of Illinois at Chicago, IL
University of Indianapolis, IN
The University of Iowa, IA
University of Kansas, KS
University of Kentucky, KY
University of Louisville, KY
University of Maine, ME
University of Mary, ND
University of Maryland, Baltimore, MD
University of Massachusetts Boston, MA
University of Massachusetts Lowell, MA
University of Massachusetts Worcester, MA
University of Medicine and Dentistry of New Jersey, NJ
University of Memphis, TN
University of Miami, FL
University of Michigan, MI

University of Michigan-Flint, MI
University of Minnesota, Twin Cities Campus, MN
University of Mississippi Medical Center, MS
University of Missouri-Columbia, MO
University of Missouri-Kansas City, MO
University of Missouri-St. Louis, MO
University of Nebraska Medical Center, NE
University of Nevada, Las Vegas, NV
University of Nevada, Reno, NV
University of New Brunswick Fredericton, NB
University of New Hampshire, NH
University of New Mexico, NM
The University of North Carolina at Chapel Hill, NC
The University of North Carolina at Charlotte, NC
The University of North Carolina Wilmington, NC
University of North Dakota, ND
University of Northern Colorado, CO
University of North Florida, FL
University of Oklahoma Health Sciences Center, OK
University of Pennsylvania, PA
University of Phoenix-Hawaii Campus, HI
University of Phoenix Online Campus, AZ
University of Phoenix-Phoenix Campus, AZ
University of Phoenix-Sacramento Valley Campus, CA
University of Phoenix-Southern Arizona Campus, AZ
University of Phoenix-Southern California Campus, CA
University of Pittsburgh, PA
University of Rhode Island, RI
University of Rochester, NY
University of St. Francis, IL
University of Saint Francis, IN
University of San Diego, CA
University of San Francisco, CA
The University of Scranton, PA
University of South Alabama, AL
University of South Carolina, SC
University of Southern Indiana, IN
University of Southern Maine, ME
University of Southern Mississippi, MS
University of South Florida, FL
The University of Tampa, FL
The University of Tennessee, TN
The University of Tennessee at Chattanooga, TN
The University of Tennessee Health Science Center, TN
The University of Texas at Arlington, TX
The University of Texas at Austin, TX
The University of Texas at El Paso, TX
The University of Texas at Tyler, TX
The University of Texas Health Science Center at Houston, TX
The University of Texas Health Science Center at San Antonio, TX
The University of Texas Medical Branch, TX
The University of Texas-Pan American, TX
The University of Toledo, OH
University of Toronto, ON
University of Utah, UT
University of Vermont, VT
University of Virginia, VA
University of Washington, WA
University of Wisconsin-Eau Claire, WI
University of Wisconsin-Milwaukee, WI
University of Wisconsin-Oshkosh, WI
University of Wyoming, WY
Ursuline College, OH
Vanderbilt University, TN
Virginia Commonwealth University, VA
Wagner College, NY
Western Carolina University, NC
Western University of Health Sciences, CA
Westminster College, UT
West Texas A&M University, TX
West Virginia University, WV
Wheeling Jesuit University, WV
Wichita State University, KS
Widener University, PA

CONCENTRATIONS WITHIN MASTER'S DEGREE PROGRAMS
Nurse Practitioner Programs

Wilmington College, DE
Winona State University, MN
Winston-Salem State University, NC
Wright State University, OH
Yale University, CT

Gerontology

Barnes-Jewish College of Nursing and Allied Health, MO
Boston College, MA
California State University, Long Beach, CA
Case Western Reserve University, OH
The Catholic University of America, DC
Clemson University, SC
College of St. Catherine, MN
The College of St. Scholastica, MN
College of Staten Island of the City University of New York, NY
Columbia University, NY
Concordia University Wisconsin, WI
Dalhousie University, NS
Duke University, NC
East Tennessee State University, TN
Emory University, GA
Florida Agricultural and Mechanical University, FL
Florida Atlantic University, FL
George Mason University, VA
Grand Valley State University, MI
Hampton University, VA
Hunter College of the City University of New York, NY
Indiana Wesleyan University, IN
James Madison University, VA
Kent State University, OH
Long Island University, Brooklyn Campus, NY
Marquette University, WI
Medical University of South Carolina, SC
MGH Institute of Health Professions, MA
Michigan State University, MI
Nazareth College of Rochester, NY
Neumann College, PA
New York University, NY
Northeastern University, MA
Northern Kentucky University, KY
Oakland University, MI
Oregon Health & Science University, OR
Rush University, IL
The Sage Colleges, NY
Saint Louis University, MO
San Diego State University, CA
Seattle Pacific University, WA
Seton Hall University, NJ
Simmons College, MA
State University of New York at Binghamton, NY
Texas Tech University Health Sciences Center, TX
University at Buffalo, the State University of New York, NY
The University of Akron, OH
University of Arkansas for Medical Sciences, AR
University of California, Los Angeles, CA
University of California, San Francisco, CA
University of Cincinnati, OH
University of Colorado at Colorado Springs, CO
University of Colorado at Denver and Health Sciences Center, CO
University of Hawaii at Manoa, HI
University of Illinois at Chicago, IL
University of Indianapolis, IN
The University of Iowa, IA
University of Kansas, KS
University of Kentucky, KY
University of Maryland, Baltimore, MD
University of Massachusetts Boston, MA
University of Massachusetts Lowell, MA
University of Massachusetts Worcester, MA
University of Medicine and Dentistry of New Jersey, NJ
University of Michigan, MI
University of Minnesota, Twin Cities Campus, MN
University of Missouri-Columbia, MO
University of Nebraska Medical Center, NE
University of New Brunswick Fredericton, NB

The University of North Carolina at Greensboro, NC
University of Pennsylvania, PA
University of Rochester, NY
University of San Diego, CA
University of South Alabama, AL
University of South Florida, FL
The University of Tennessee, TN
The University of Texas at Arlington, TX
The University of Texas at Tyler, TX
The University of Texas Health Science Center at Houston, TX
The University of Texas Health Science Center at San Antonio, TX
The University of Texas Medical Branch, TX
University of Utah, UT
University of Virginia, VA
University of Washington, WA
University of Wisconsin–Madison, WI
Vanderbilt University, TN
Villanova University, PA
Wayne State University, MI
Wilmington College, DE
Yale University, CT

Neonatal Health

Arizona State University at the Downtown Phoenix Campus, AZ
Barnes-Jewish College of Nursing and Allied Health, MO
Baylor University, TX
Case Western Reserve University, OH
The College of New Jersey, NJ
College of St. Catherine, MN
Columbia University, NY
Creighton University, NE
Dalhousie University, NS
Duke University, NC
East Carolina University, NC
Indiana University–Purdue University Indianapolis, IN
Loma Linda University, CA
Louisiana State University Health Sciences Center, LA
McGill University, QC
McMaster University, ON
Medical University of South Carolina, SC
Northeastern University, MA
Northwestern State University of Louisiana, LA
The Ohio State University, OH
Regis University, CO
Rush University, IL
South Dakota State University, SD
Stony Brook University, State University of New York, NY
Thomas Jefferson University, PA
University at Buffalo, the State University of New York, NY
The University of Alabama at Birmingham, AL
University of Calgary, AB
University of California, San Francisco, CA
University of Cincinnati, OH
University of Connecticut, CT
University of Florida, FL
The University of Iowa, IA
University of Louisville, KY
University of Mississippi Medical Center, MS
University of Missouri-Kansas City, MO
University of Nebraska Medical Center, NE
University of New Brunswick Fredericton, NB
The University of North Carolina at Chapel Hill, NC
University of Oklahoma Health Sciences Center, OK
University of Pennsylvania, PA
University of Rochester, NY
University of South Alabama, AL
The University of Tennessee, TN
The University of Tennessee Health Science Center, TN
The University of Texas Health Science Center at Houston, TX

The University of Texas Medical Branch, TX
University of Utah, UT
University of Washington, WA
Vanderbilt University, TN
Wayne State University, MI
West Virginia University, WV

Occupational Health

The University of Alabama at Birmingham, AL
University of California, Los Angeles, CA
University of California, San Francisco, CA
University of Illinois at Chicago, IL
University of Pennsylvania, PA
University of South Florida, FL
University of the Sacred Heart, PR

Oncology

Barnes-Jewish College of Nursing and Allied Health, MO
Columbia University, NY
Dalhousie University, NS
Duke University, NC
Emory University, GA
Thomas Jefferson University, PA
Université de Moncton, NB
University of California, Los Angeles, CA
University of California, San Francisco, CA
University of Maryland, Baltimore, MD
University of Massachusetts Worcester, MA
University of Medicine and Dentistry of New Jersey, NJ
University of Nebraska Medical Center, NE
University of Pennsylvania, PA
University of South Florida, FL
University of Utah, UT
Yale University, CT

Pediatric

Arizona State University at the Downtown Phoenix Campus, AZ
Azusa Pacific University, CA
Boston College, MA
California State University, Fresno, CA
California State University, Long Beach, CA
California State University, Los Angeles, CA
Case Western Reserve University, OH
The Catholic University of America, DC
College of St. Catherine, MN
The College of St. Scholastica, MN
Colorado State University-Pueblo, CO
Columbia University, NY
DePaul University, IL
Drexel University, PA
Duke University, NC
Emory University, GA
Florida International University, FL
Florida State University, FL
Georgia State University, GA
Grand Valley State University, MI
Gwynedd-Mercy College, PA
Hampton University, VA
Hunter College of the City University of New York, NY
Indiana University–Purdue University Indianapolis, IN
The Johns Hopkins University, MD
Kent State University, OH
Lehman College of the City University of New York, NY
Loma Linda University, CA
Loyola University Chicago, IL
Marquette University, WI
Medical College of Georgia, GA
Medical University of South Carolina, SC
MGH Institute of Health Professions, MA
Mississippi University for Women, MS
Molloy College, NY
New York University, NY
Northeastern University, MA
Northern Kentucky University, KY
Northwestern State University of Louisiana, LA
The Ohio State University, OH

Old Dominion University, VA
Oregon Health & Science University, OR
Purdue University, IN
Regis College, MA
Rush University, IL
Rutgers, The State University of New Jersey,
    College of Nursing, NJ
Saint Louis University, MO
Seton Hall University, NJ
Simmons College, MA
Spalding University, KY
State University of New York Upstate Medical
    University, NY
Stony Brook University, State University of New
    York, NY
Temple University, PA
Texas Tech University Health Sciences Center, TX
Texas Woman's University, TX
Thomas Jefferson University, PA
University at Buffalo, the State University of New
    York, NY
The University of Akron, OH
The University of Alabama at Birmingham, AL
University of Arkansas for Medical Sciences, AR
University of California, Los Angeles, CA
University of California, San Francisco, CA
University of Central Florida, FL
University of Cincinnati, OH
University of Colorado at Denver and Health
    Sciences Center, CO
University of Florida, FL
University of Illinois at Chicago, IL
The University of Iowa, IA
University of Kentucky, KY
University of Maryland, Baltimore, MD
University of Michigan, MI
University of Minnesota, Twin Cities Campus, MN
University of Missouri–Columbia, MO
University of Missouri–Kansas City, MO
University of Missouri–St. Louis, MO
University of Nebraska Medical Center, NE
University of Nevada, Las Vegas, NV
University of New Brunswick Fredericton, NB
University of New Mexico, NM
The University of North Carolina at Chapel Hill,
    NC
University of Oklahoma Health Sciences Center,
    OK
University of Pennsylvania, PA
University of Pittsburgh, PA
University of Rochester, NY
University of San Diego, CA
University of South Alabama, AL
University of South Carolina, SC
University of South Florida, FL
The University of Tennessee, TN
The University of Texas at Arlington, TX
The University of Texas at Austin, TX
The University of Texas at Tyler, TX
The University of Texas Health Science Center at
    Houston, TX
The University of Texas Health Science Center at
    San Antonio, TX
The University of Texas Medical Branch, TX
The University of Texas–Pan American, TX
The University of Toledo, OH
University of Toronto, ON
University of Utah, UT
University of Virginia, VA
University of Washington, WA
University of Wisconsin–Madison, WI
Vanderbilt University, TN
Villanova University, PA
Virginia Commonwealth University, VA
Wayne State University, MI
West Virginia University, WV
Wichita State University, KS
Wright State University, OH
Yale University, CT

Primary Care

Arkansas State University, AR

Athabasca University, AB
Azusa Pacific University, CA
California State University, Los Angeles, CA
California State University, Sacramento, CA
Duke University, NC
George Mason University, VA
Gonzaga University, WA
Grand Valley State University, MI
Kennesaw State University, GA
Kent State University, OH
Loma Linda University, CA
Louisiana State University Health Sciences Center,
    LA
Madonna University, MI
MGH Institute of Health Professions, MA
New York University, NY
Northeastern University, MA
The Ohio State University, OH
Oregon Health & Science University, OR
Regis College, MA
Samford University, AL
Seton Hall University, NJ
Simmons College, MA
State University of New York at Binghamton, NY
Université de Moncton, NB
The University of Alabama at Birmingham, AL
The University of British Columbia, BC
University of Connecticut, CT
University of Hawaii at Manoa, HI
University of Manitoba, MB
University of Maryland, Baltimore, MD
University of Massachusetts Worcester, MA
University of Miami, FL
University of Michigan, MI
University of Nebraska Medical Center, NE
University of New Brunswick Fredericton, NB
The University of North Carolina at Chapel Hill,
    NC
University of North Florida, FL
University of Ottawa, ON
University of Pennsylvania, PA
University of Saskatchewan, SK
The University of Tennessee Health Science
    Center, TN
University of Toronto, ON
University of Virginia, VA
University of Washington, WA
Virginia Commonwealth University, VA
Wayne State University, MI
Western Kentucky University, KY

Psychiatric/Mental Health

Arizona State University at the Downtown
    Phoenix Campus, AZ
Boston College, MA
California State University, Long Beach, CA
Case Western Reserve University, OH
The College of St. Scholastica, MN
Columbia University, NY
Drexel University, PA
East Tennessee State University, TN
Fairfield University, CT
Fairleigh Dickinson University, Metropolitan
    Campus, NJ
Florida International University, FL
Gonzaga University, WA
Grand Valley State University, MI
Intercollegiate College of Nursing/Washington
    State University, WA
Kent State University, OH
McNeese State University, LA
Medical University of South Carolina, SC
Memorial University of Newfoundland, NL
MGH Institute of Health Professions, MA
Molloy College, NY
Monmouth University, NJ
New Mexico State University, NM
New York University, NY
Northeastern University, MA
Northern Kentucky University, KY
The Ohio State University, OH
Oregon Health & Science University, OR

Regis College, MA
Rivier College, NH
Rush University, IL
The Sage Colleges, NY
Saint Louis University, MO
Seattle University, WA
Shenandoah University, VA
Stony Brook University, State University of New
    York, NY
University at Buffalo, the State University of New
    York, NY
The University of Akron, OH
University of Alaska Anchorage, AK
The University of Arizona, AZ
University of Arkansas for Medical Sciences, AR
University of California, San Francisco, CA
University of Central Arkansas, AR
University of Cincinnati, OH
University of Colorado at Denver and Health
    Sciences Center, CO
University of Florida, FL
University of Illinois at Chicago, IL
The University of Iowa, IA
University of Kansas, KS
University of Kentucky, KY
University of Louisiana at Lafayette, LA
University of Louisville, KY
University of Maryland, Baltimore, MD
University of Massachusetts Amherst, MA
University of Massachusetts Lowell, MA
University of Massachusetts Worcester, MA
University of Medicine and Dentistry of New
    Jersey, NJ
University of Miami, FL
University of Michigan, MI
University of Michigan–Flint, MI
University of Mississippi Medical Center, MS
University of Missouri–Columbia, MO
University of Nebraska Medical Center, NE
University of New Brunswick Fredericton, NB
The University of North Carolina at Chapel Hill,
    NC
University of North Dakota, ND
University of Pittsburgh, PA
University of Rochester, NY
University of South Alabama, AL
University of South Carolina, SC
University of Southern Maine, ME
University of Southern Mississippi, MS
University of South Florida, FL
The University of Tennessee, TN
The University of Tennessee Health Science
    Center, TN
The University of Texas at Arlington, TX
The University of Texas Health Science Center at
    San Antonio, TX
University of Utah, UT
University of Vermont, VT
University of Virginia, VA
University of Washington, WA
University of Wisconsin–Madison, WI
University of Wyoming, WY
Vanderbilt University, TN
Virginia Commonwealth University, VA
Wichita State University, KS
Winston-Salem State University, NC
Yale University, CT

School Health

The Catholic University of America, DC
Monmouth University, NJ
The Ohio State University, OH
Simmons College, MA
University of Illinois at Chicago, IL

Women's Health

Arizona State University at the Downtown
    Phoenix Campus, AZ
Boston College, MA
California State University, Fullerton, CA
California State University, Long Beach, CA
California State University, Los Angeles, CA

Case Western Reserve University, OH
Columbia University, NY
DePaul University, IL
Drexel University, PA
Emory University, GA
Florida Agricultural and Mechanical University, FL
Georgetown University, DC
Georgia Southern University, GA
Georgia State University, GA
Grand Valley State University, MI
Hampton University, VA
Indiana University–Purdue University Indianapolis, IN
Kent State University, OH
Loyola University Chicago, IL
MGH Institute of Health Professions, MA
Northwestern State University of Louisiana, LA
The Ohio State University, OH
Old Dominion University, VA
Oregon Health & Science University, OR
Pace University, NY
Rutgers, The State University of New Jersey, College of Nursing, NJ
Seton Hall University, NJ
Simmons College, MA
State University of New York Downstate Medical Center, NY
Stony Brook University, State University of New York, NY
Texas Woman's University, TX
University at Buffalo, the State University of New York, NY
The University of Alabama at Birmingham, AL
University of Arkansas for Medical Sciences, AR
University of Cincinnati, OH
University of Colorado at Denver and Health Sciences Center, CO
University of Illinois at Chicago, IL

University of Louisville, KY
University of Massachusetts Amherst, MA
University of Medicine and Dentistry of New Jersey, NJ
University of Miami, FL
University of Minnesota, Twin Cities Campus, MN
University of Missouri–Kansas City, MO
University of Missouri–St. Louis, MO
University of Nebraska Medical Center, NE
University of New Brunswick Fredericton, NB
The University of North Carolina at Chapel Hill, NC
University of Pennsylvania, PA
University of South Alabama, AL
University of South Carolina, SC
The University of Tennessee, TN
The University of Texas at El Paso, TX
The University of Texas at Tyler, TX
The University of Texas Health Science Center at Houston, TX
The University of Texas Medical Branch, TX
University of Utah, UT
University of Washington, WA
University of Wisconsin–Madison, WI
Vanderbilt University, TN
Virginia Commonwealth University, VA
Wayne State University, MI
Wilmington College, DE
Yale University, CT

NURSE-MIDWIFERY

California State University, Fullerton, CA
Case Western Reserve University, OH
Columbia University, NY
East Carolina University, NC
Emory University, GA

Georgetown University, DC
The Johns Hopkins University, MD
Loyola University Chicago, IL
Marquette University, WI
Medical University of South Carolina, SC
New York University, NY
The Ohio State University, OH
Old Dominion University, VA
Oregon Health & Science University, OR
Radford University, VA
San Diego State University, CA
Shenandoah University, VA
State University of New York Downstate Medical Center, NY
Stony Brook University, State University of New York, NY
University of California, San Francisco, CA
University of Cincinnati, OH
University of Colorado at Denver and Health Sciences Center, CO
University of Florida, FL
University of Illinois at Chicago, IL
University of Indianapolis, IN
University of Kansas, KS
University of Maryland, Baltimore, MD
University of Massachusetts Amherst, MA
University of Medicine and Dentistry of New Jersey, NJ
University of Miami, FL
University of Michigan, MI
University of Minnesota, Twin Cities Campus, MN
University of New Mexico, NM
University of Pennsylvania, PA
University of Rhode Island, RI
University of Utah, UT
University of Washington, WA
Vanderbilt University, TN
Wayne State University, MI
Yale University, CT
York College of Pennsylvania, PA

DOCTORAL PROGRAMS

Alabama
The University of Alabama, Capstone College of Nursing, *Tuscaloosa* (EdD)
The University of Alabama at Birmingham, School of Nursing, *Birmingham* (PhD)

Arizona
Arizona State University at the Downtown Phoenix Campus, College of Nursing, *Phoenix* (DNS)
The University of Arizona, College of Nursing, *Tucson* (PhD)

Arkansas
University of Arkansas for Medical Sciences, College of Nursing, *Little Rock* (PhD)

California
Azusa Pacific University, School of Nursing, *Azusa* (PhD)
Loma Linda University, School of Nursing, *Loma Linda* (PhD)
University of California, Los Angeles, School of Nursing, *Los Angeles* (PhD)
University of California, San Francisco, School of Nursing, *San Francisco* (PhD)
University of San Diego, Hahn School of Nursing and Health Sciences, *San Diego* (PhD)

Colorado
University of Colorado at Colorado Springs, Beth-El College of Nursing and Health Sciences, *Colorado Springs* (DNP)
University of Colorado at Denver and Health Sciences Center, School of Nursing, *Denver* (PhD)
University of Northern Colorado, School of Nursing, *Greeley* (PhD)

Connecticut
University of Connecticut, School of Nursing, *Storrs* (PhD)
Yale University, School of Nursing, *New Haven* (PhD)

District of Columbia
The Catholic University of America, School of Nursing, *Washington* (DN Sc)

Florida
Barry University, School of Nursing, *Miami Shores* (PhD)
Florida Agricultural and Mechanical University, School of Nursing, *Tallahassee* (PhD)
Florida Atlantic University, College of Nursing, *Boca Raton* (PhD)
Florida International University, College of Nursing and Health Sciences, *Miami* (PhD)
University of Central Florida, School of Nursing, *Orlando* (PhD)
University of Florida, College of Nursing, *Gainesville* (PhD)
University of Miami, School of Nursing and Health Studies, *Coral Gables* (PhD)
University of South Florida, College of Nursing, *Tampa* (PhD)

Georgia
Emory University, Nell Hodgson Woodruff School of Nursing, *Atlanta* (PhD)
Georgia State University, School of Nursing, *Atlanta* (PhD)
Medical College of Georgia, School of Nursing, *Augusta* (PhD)

Hawaii
University of Hawaii at Manoa, School of Nursing and Dental Hygiene, *Honolulu* (PhD)

Illinois
Loyola University Chicago, Marcella Niehoff School of Nursing, *Chicago* (PhD)
Rush University, College of Nursing, *Chicago* (PhD)
University of Illinois at Chicago, College of Nursing, *Chicago* (PhD)

Indiana
Indiana University-Purdue University Indianapolis, School of Nursing, *Indianapolis* (PhD)
Purdue University, School of Nursing, *West Lafayette* (DNP)

Iowa
The University of Iowa, College of Nursing, *Iowa City* (PhD)

Kansas
University of Kansas, School of Nursing, *Kansas City* (PhD)
Wichita State University, School of Nursing, *Wichita* (DNP)

Kentucky
University of Kentucky, Graduate School Programs in the College of Nursing, *Lexington* (PhD)
University of Louisville, School of Nursing, *Louisville* (PhD)

Louisiana
Louisiana State University Health Sciences Center, School of Nursing, *New Orleans* (DNS)
Southern University and Agricultural and Mechanical College, School of Nursing, *Baton Rouge* (PhD)

Maryland
The Johns Hopkins University, School of Nursing, *Baltimore* (PhD)
University of Maryland, Baltimore, Master's Program in Nursing, *Baltimore* (PhD)

Massachusetts
Boston College, William F. Connell School of Nursing, *Chestnut Hill* (PhD)
Regis College, Department of Nursing, *Weston* (DNP)
University of Massachusetts Amherst, School of Nursing, *Amherst* (PhD)
University of Massachusetts Boston, College of Nursing and Health Sciences, *Boston* (PhD)
University of Massachusetts Lowell, Department of Nursing, *Lowell* (PhD)
University of Massachusetts Worcester, Graduate School of Nursing, *Worcester* (PhD)

Michigan
Michigan State University, College of Nursing, *East Lansing* (PhD)
University of Michigan, School of Nursing, *Ann Arbor* (PhD)
Wayne State University, College of Nursing, *Detroit* (PhD)

Minnesota
University of Minnesota, Twin Cities Campus, School of Nursing, *Minneapolis* (PhD)

Mississippi
University of Mississippi Medical Center, Program in Nursing, *Jackson* (PhD)
University of Southern Mississippi, School of Nursing, *Hattiesburg* (PhD)

Missouri
Saint Louis University, School of Nursing, *St. Louis* (PhD)

University of Missouri-Columbia, Sinclair School of Nursing, *Columbia* (PhD)
University of Missouri-Kansas City, School of Nursing, *Kansas City* (PhD)
University of Missouri-St. Louis, College of Nursing, *St. Louis* (PhD)

Nebraska
University of Nebraska Medical Center, College of Nursing, *Omaha* (PhD)

Nevada
University of Nevada, Las Vegas, School of Nursing, *Las Vegas* (PhD)

New Jersey
Fairleigh Dickinson University, Metropolitan Campus, Henry P. Becton School of Nursing and Allied Health, *Teaneck* (DNP)
Rutgers, The State University of New Jersey, Camden College of Arts and Sciences, Department of Nursing, *Camden* (DNP)
Rutgers, The State University of New Jersey, College of Nursing, *Newark* (PhD)
Seton Hall University, College of Nursing, *South Orange* (PhD)
University of Medicine and Dentistry of New Jersey, School of Nursing, *Newark* (DNP)

New Mexico
University of New Mexico, College of Nursing, *Albuquerque* (PhD)

New York
Adelphi University, School of Nursing, *Garden City* (PhD)
Columbia University, School of Nursing, *New York* (DN Sc)
New York University, College of Nursing, *New York* (PhD)
State University of New York at Binghamton, Decker School of Nursing, *Binghamton* (PhD)
Teachers College Columbia University, Department of Health and Behavioral Studies, *New York* (EdD)
University at Buffalo, the State University of New York, School of Nursing, *Buffalo* (PhD)
University of Rochester, School of Nursing, *Rochester* (PhD)

North Carolina
Duke University, School of Nursing, *Durham* (PhD)
East Carolina University, School of Nursing, *Greenville* (PhD)
The University of North Carolina at Chapel Hill, School of Nursing, *Chapel Hill* (PhD)
The University of North Carolina at Greensboro, School of Nursing, *Greensboro* (PhD)

North Dakota
North Dakota State University, Tri-College University Nursing Consortium, *Fargo* (DNP)
University of North Dakota, College of Nursing, *Grand Forks* (PhD)

Ohio
Case Western Reserve University, Frances Payne Bolton School of Nursing, *Cleveland* (PhD)
Kent State University, College of Nursing, *Kent* (PhD)
The Ohio State University, College of Nursing, *Columbus* (PhD)
The University of Akron, College of Nursing, *Akron* (PhD)
University of Cincinnati, College of Nursing, *Cincinnati* (PhD)

Oregon

Oregon Health & Science University, School of Nursing, *Portland* (PhD)

Pennsylvania

Drexel University, College of Nursing and Health Professions, *Philadelphia* (DNP)

Duquesne University, School of Nursing, *Pittsburgh* (PhD)

Penn State University Park, School of Nursing, *State College, University Park* (PhD)

Thomas Jefferson University, Department of Nursing, *Philadelphia* (DNP)

University of Pennsylvania, School of Nursing, *Philadelphia* (PhD)

University of Pittsburgh, School of Nursing, *Pittsburgh* (PhD)

Villanova University, College of Nursing, *Villanova* (PhD)

Waynesburg College, Department of Nursing, *Waynesburg* (DNP)

Widener University, School of Nursing, *Chester* (DN Sc)

Rhode Island

University of Rhode Island, College of Nursing, *Kingston* (PhD)

South Carolina

Medical University of South Carolina, College of Nursing, *Charleston* (PhD)

University of South Carolina, College of Nursing, *Columbia* (PhD)

South Dakota

South Dakota State University, College of Nursing, *Brookings* (PhD)

Tennessee

East Tennessee State University, College of Nursing, *Johnson City* (DSN)

The University of Tennessee, College of Nursing, *Knoxville* (PhD)

The University of Tennessee Health Science Center, College of Nursing, *Memphis* (PhD)

Vanderbilt University, School of Nursing, *Nashville* (PhD)

Texas

Texas Woman's University, College of Nursing, *Denton* (PhD)

The University of Texas at Arlington, School of Nursing, *Arlington* (PhD)

The University of Texas at Austin, School of Nursing, *Austin* (PhD)

The University of Texas at El Paso, School of Nursing, *El Paso* (PhD)

The University of Texas at Tyler, Program in Nursing, *Tyler* (DNS)

The University of Texas Health Science Center at Houston, School of Nursing, *Houston* (DSN)

The University of Texas Health Science Center at San Antonio, School of Nursing, *San Antonio* (PhD)

The University of Texas Medical Branch, School of Nursing, *Galveston* (PhD)

Utah

University of Utah, College of Nursing, *Salt Lake City* (PhD)

Virginia

George Mason University, College of Nursing and Health Science, *Fairfax* (PhD)

Hampton University, Department of Nursing, *Hampton* (PhD)

University of Virginia, School of Nursing, *Charlottesville* (PhD)

Virginia Commonwealth University, School of Nursing, *Richmond* (PhD)

Washington

University of Washington, School of Nursing, *Seattle* (PhD)

West Virginia

West Virginia University, School of Nursing, *Morgantown* (DSN)

Wisconsin

Marquette University, College of Nursing, *Milwaukee* (PhD)

University of Wisconsin–Madison, School of Nursing, *Madison* (PhD)

University of Wisconsin–Milwaukee, College of Nursing, *Milwaukee* (PhD)

CANADA

Alberta

University of Alberta, Faculty of Nursing, *Edmonton* (PhD)

University of Calgary, Faculty of Nursing, *Calgary* (PhD)

British Columbia

The University of British Columbia, School of Nursing, *Vancouver* (PhD)

University of Victoria, School of Nursing, *Victoria* (PhD)

Manitoba

University of Manitoba, Faculty of Nursing, *Winnipeg* (PhD)

Nova Scotia

Dalhousie University, School of Nursing, *Halifax* (PhD)

Ontario

McMaster University, School of Nursing, *Hamilton* (PhD)

University of Ottawa, School of Nursing, *Ottawa* (PhD)

University of Toronto, Faculty of Nursing, *Toronto* (PhD)

The University of Western Ontario, School of Nursing, *London* (PhD)

Quebec

McGill University, School of Nursing, *Montréal* (PhD)

Université de Montréal, Faculty of Nursing, *Montréal* (PhD)

Université de Sherbrooke, Department of Nursing, *Sherbrooke* (PhD)

Université Laval, Faculty of Nursing, *Québec* (PhD)

POSTDOCTORAL PROGRAMS

Alabama
The University of Alabama at Birmingham, School of Nursing, *Birmingham*

Arizona
The University of Arizona, College of Nursing, *Tucson*

Arkansas
University of Arkansas for Medical Sciences, College of Nursing, *Little Rock*

California
University of California, Los Angeles, School of Nursing, *Los Angeles*
University of California, San Francisco, School of Nursing, *San Francisco*

Colorado
University of Colorado at Denver and Health Sciences Center, School of Nursing, *Denver*

Connecticut
Yale University, School of Nursing, *New Haven*

Illinois
Rush University, College of Nursing, *Chicago*
University of Illinois at Chicago, College of Nursing, *Chicago*

Indiana
Indiana University-Purdue University Indianapolis, School of Nursing, *Indianapolis*

Iowa
The University of Iowa, College of Nursing, *Iowa City*

Maryland
The Johns Hopkins University, School of Nursing, *Baltimore*

Michigan
Michigan State University, College of Nursing, *East Lansing*
University of Michigan, School of Nursing, *Ann Arbor*
Wayne State University, College of Nursing, *Detroit*

Nebraska
University of Nebraska Medical Center, College of Nursing, *Omaha*

New York
University of Rochester, School of Nursing, *Rochester*

North Carolina
The University of North Carolina at Chapel Hill, School of Nursing, *Chapel Hill*

Ohio
Case Western Reserve University, Frances Payne Bolton School of Nursing, *Cleveland*

Oregon
Oregon Health & Science University, School of Nursing, *Portland*

Pennsylvania
Penn State University Park, School of Nursing, *State College, University Park*
University of Pennsylvania, School of Nursing, *Philadelphia*

University of Pittsburgh, School of Nursing, *Pittsburgh*

Tennessee
Vanderbilt University, School of Nursing, *Nashville*

Texas
The University of Texas at Austin, School of Nursing, *Austin*

Utah
University of Utah, College of Nursing, *Salt Lake City*

Virginia
University of Virginia, School of Nursing, *Charlottesville*

Wisconsin
University of Wisconsin-Madison, School of Nursing, *Madison*

CANADA

British Columbia
The University of British Columbia, School of Nursing, *Vancouver*

Ontario
University of Ottawa, School of Nursing, *Ottawa*
The University of Western Ontario, School of Nursing, *London*

Quebec
McGill University, School of Nursing, *Montréal*
Université de Sherbrooke, Department of Nursing, *Sherbrooke*

DISTANCE LEARNING PROGRAMS

BACCALAUREATE PROGRAMS

Arkansas Tech University, AR
Armstrong Atlantic State University, GA
Ashland University, OH
Athabasca University, AB
Belmont University, TN
Bemidji State University, MN
Bloomfield College, NJ
Bluefield State College, WV
Boise State University, ID
California State University, Bakersfield, CA
California State University, Dominguez Hills, CA
California State University, Fullerton, CA
California State University, Stanislaus, CA
California University of Pennsylvania, PA
Chicago State University, IL
Clarion University of Pennsylvania, PA
Clemson University, SC
Cox College of Nursing and Health Sciences, MO
Creighton University, NE
Daemen College, NY
Delta State University, MS
Duquesne University, PA
D'Youville College, NY
East Central University, OK
Eastern Kentucky University, KY
Eastern New Mexico University, NM
East Tennessee State University, TN
Excelsior College, NY
Fairleigh Dickinson University, Metropolitan Campus, NJ
Ferris State University, MI
Florida Atlantic University, FL
Florida Gulf Coast University, FL
Florida International University, FL
Florida State University, FL
Fort Hays State University, KS
Gannon University, PA
Graceland University, IA
Grand Canyon University, AZ
Grand Valley State University, MI
Idaho State University, ID
Indiana State University, IN
Intercollegiate College of Nursing/Washington State University, WA
Jacksonville University, FL
Jefferson College of Health Sciences, VA
Kennesaw State University, GA
Kent State University, OH
Keuka College, NY
Kutztown University of Pennsylvania, PA
Lake Superior State University, MI
Lakeview College of Nursing, IL
Lander University, SC
Lewis-Clark State College, ID
Macon State College, GA
Madonna University, MI
Mansfield University of Pennsylvania, PA
Marian College of Fond du Lac, WI
Marshall University, WV
Marymount University, VA
Medical College of Georgia, GA
Mercy College, NY
Mesa State College, CO
Minnesota State University Moorhead, MN
Mississippi University for Women, MS
Missouri State University, MO
Montana State University, MT
Montana State University-Northern, MT
Morehead State University, KY
Mountain State University, WV
Murray State University, KY
Nazareth College of Rochester, NY
Nebraska Methodist College, NE

New Mexico State University, NM
North Carolina Agricultural and Technical State University, NC
North Carolina Central University, NC
Northeastern State University, OK
Northern Arizona University, AZ
Northern Illinois University, IL
Northwestern Oklahoma State University, OK
Northwestern State University of Louisiana, LA
The Ohio State University, OH
Oklahoma Wesleyan University, OK
Old Dominion University, VA
Oregon Health & Science University, OR
Otterbein College, OH
Pace University, NY
Penn State University Park, PA
Pennsylvania College of Technology, PA
Prairie View A&M University, TX
Presentation College, SD
Radford University, VA
The Richard Stockton College of New Jersey, NJ
Rutgers, The State University of New Jersey, College of Nursing, NJ
Sacred Heart University, CT
Saginaw Valley State University, MI
Saint Joseph College, CT
St. Petersburg College, FL
Seattle Pacific University, WA
Seton Hall University, NJ
South Dakota State University, SD
Southeastern Louisiana University, LA
Southeast Missouri State University, MO
Southern Illinois University Edwardsville, IL
State University of New York at Plattsburgh, NY
State University of New York Institute of Technology, NY
Stony Brook University, State University of New York, NY
Tarleton State University, TX
Tennessee State University, TN
Texas A&M University-Corpus Christi, TX
Texas Christian University, TX
Texas Tech University Health Sciences Center, TX
Texas Woman's University, TX
Thomas Jefferson University, PA
Troy University, AL
Université du Québec à Chicoutimi, QC
The University of Akron, OH
University of Arkansas for Medical Sciences, AR
University of Central Florida, FL
University of Central Missouri, MO
University of Colorado at Denver and Health Sciences Center, CO
University of Connecticut, CT
University of Hawaii at Hilo, HI
University of Hawaii at Manoa, HI
University of Illinois at Chicago, IL
The University of Iowa, IA
University of Maine, ME
University of Maryland, Baltimore, MD
University of Medicine and Dentistry of New Jersey, NJ
University of Memphis, TN
University of Michigan-Flint, MI
University of Mississippi Medical Center, MS
University of Missouri-St. Louis, MO
University of Nebraska Medical Center, NE
University of Nevada, Reno, NV
University of New Brunswick Fredericton, NB
The University of North Carolina at Chapel Hill, NC
The University of North Carolina Wilmington, NC
University of North Dakota, ND
University of Northern Colorado, CO
University of Oklahoma Health Sciences Center, OK

University of Ottawa, ON
University of Pittsburgh, PA
University of Saint Francis, IN
University of Saskatchewan, SK
The University of Tennessee Health Science Center, TN
The University of Texas at Arlington, TX
The University of Texas at Brownsville, TX
The University of Texas at Tyler, TX
The University of Texas Health Science Center at Houston, TX
The University of Toledo, OH
University of West Georgia, GA
University of Wisconsin-Eau Claire, WI
University of Wisconsin-Madison, WI
University of Wisconsin-Oshkosh, WI
University of Wyoming, WY
Valdosta State University, GA
Villa Julie College, MD
Villanova University, PA
Virginia Commonwealth University, VA
Wayne State University, MI
Weber State University, UT
Western Carolina University, NC
Western Kentucky University, KY
West Liberty State College, WV
West Virginia University, WV
Winona State University, MN
Winston-Salem State University, NC
Wright State University, OH
York College of Pennsylvania, PA

MASTER'S DEGREE PROGRAMS

Azusa Pacific University, CA
Baylor University, TX
Bethel University, MN
California State University, Chico, CA
California State University, Dominguez Hills, CA
Clarion University of Pennsylvania, PA
Clemson University, SC
Drexel University, PA
Duke University, NC
Duquesne University, PA
Eastern Kentucky University, KY
Excelsior College, NY
Fairleigh Dickinson University, Metropolitan Campus, NJ
Florida Atlantic University, FL
Florida State University, FL
Fort Hays State University, KS
Gannon University, PA
Graceland University, IA
Grand Canyon University, AZ
Grand Valley State University, MI
Husson College, ME
Indiana State University, IN
Intercollegiate College of Nursing/Washington State University, WA
Jefferson College of Health Sciences, VA
Madonna University, MI
Marian College of Fond du Lac, WI
Marshall University, WV
Marymount University, VA
McNeese State University, LA
Medical College of Georgia, GA
Mercy College, NY
MGH Institute of Health Professions, MA
Minnesota State University Moorhead, MN
Montana State University, MT
Mountain State University, WV
Murray State University, KY
Nazareth College of Rochester, NY

Nebraska Methodist College, NE
North Dakota State University, ND
Northern Arizona University, AZ
Northern Illinois University, IL
Northwestern State University of Louisiana, LA
Old Dominion University, VA
Oregon Health & Science University, OR
Otterbein College, OH
Pace University, NY
Penn State University Park, PA
Purdue University Calumet, IN
Rutgers, The State University of New Jersey, College of Nursing, NJ
Sacred Heart University, CT
Saint Joseph College, CT
Saint Louis University, MO
Sonoma State University, CA
South Dakota State University, SD
Southeastern Louisiana University, LA
Southeast Missouri State University, MO
Southern Illinois University Edwardsville, IL
State University of New York Institute of Technology, NY
Stony Brook University, State University of New York, NY
Texas A&M University-Corpus Christi, TX
Texas Christian University, TX
Texas Tech University Health Sciences Center, TX
Texas Woman's University, TX
Thomas Jefferson University, PA
Troy University, AL
Université du Québec à Chicoutimi, QC
University at Buffalo, the State University of New York, NY
The University of Akron, OH
The University of Arizona, AZ

University of Arkansas for Medical Sciences, AR
The University of British Columbia, BC
University of Central Arkansas, AR
University of Central Missouri, MO
University of Cincinnati, OH
University of Colorado at Denver and Health Sciences Center, CO
University of Connecticut, CT
University of Hawaii at Manoa, HI
University of Illinois at Chicago, IL
The University of Iowa, IA
University of Kansas, KS
University of Louisiana at Lafayette, LA
University of Maryland, Baltimore, MD
University of Massachusetts Worcester, MA
University of Medicine and Dentistry of New Jersey, NJ
University of Memphis, TN
University of Michigan-Flint, MI
University of Mississippi Medical Center, MS
University of Missouri-Kansas City, MO
University of Missouri-St. Louis, MO
University of Nebraska Medical Center, NE
University of Nevada, Reno, NV
The University of North Carolina at Charlotte, NC
The University of North Carolina Wilmington, NC
University of North Dakota, ND
University of Northern Colorado, CO
University of Oklahoma Health Sciences Center, OK
University of Pennsylvania, PA
University of Pittsburgh, PA
University of Saskatchewan, SK
The University of Tennessee Health Science Center, TN
The University of Texas at El Paso, TX

University of Wisconsin-Eau Claire, WI
University of Wyoming, WY
Valdosta State University, GA
Vanderbilt University, TN
Villanova University, PA
Wayne State University, MI
Western Carolina University, NC
Western Kentucky University, KY
West Virginia University, WV
Winona State University, MN
York College of Pennsylvania, PA

DOCTORAL PROGRAMS

Duquesne University, PA
Oregon Health & Science University, OR
Penn State University Park, PA
South Dakota State University, SD
Southeastern Louisiana University, LA
Texas Woman's University, TX
The University of Arizona, AZ
University of Colorado at Denver and Health Sciences Center, CO
University of Massachusetts Worcester, MA
University of Nebraska Medical Center, NE
University of North Dakota, ND
University of Saskatchewan, SK
The University of Tennessee Health Science Center, TN
The University of Texas at El Paso, TX
The University of Texas Health Science Center at San Antonio, TX
Villanova University, PA
West Virginia University, WV

Alabama

Jacksonville State University, College of Nursing and Health Sciences, *Jacksonville*

Samford University, Ida V. Moffett School of Nursing, *Birmingham*

The University of Alabama, Capstone College of Nursing, *Tuscaloosa*

The University of Alabama in Huntsville, College of Nursing, *Huntsville*

University of Mobile, School of Nursing, *Mobile*

University of North Alabama, College of Nursing and Allied Health, *Florence*

Arizona

Arizona State University at the Downtown Phoenix Campus, College of Nursing, *Phoenix*

Grand Canyon University, College of Nursing, *Phoenix*

University of Phoenix-Phoenix Campus, College of Health and Human Services, *Phoenix*

Arkansas

Harding University, College of Nursing, *Searcy*

University of Arkansas, Eleanor Mann School of Nursing, *Fayetteville*

University of Arkansas for Medical Sciences, College of Nursing, *Little Rock*

California

Azusa Pacific University, School of Nursing, *Azusa*

Biola University, Department of Nursing, *La Mirada*

California State University, Chico, School of Nursing, *Chico*

California State University, Dominguez Hills, Program in Nursing, *Carson*

California State University, Fresno, Department of Nursing, *Fresno*

California State University, Fullerton, Department of Nursing, *Fullerton*

California State University, Sacramento, Division of Nursing, *Sacramento*

Dominican University of California, Program in Nursing, *San Rafael*

Pacific Union College, Department of Nursing, *Angwin*

Point Loma Nazarene University, School of Nursing, *San Diego*

San Diego State University, School of Nursing, *San Diego*

San Francisco State University, School of Nursing, *San Francisco*

University of California, Los Angeles, School of Nursing, *Los Angeles*

University of San Francisco, School of Nursing, *San Francisco*

Colorado

University of Colorado at Colorado Springs, Beth-El College of Nursing and Health Sciences, *Colorado Springs*

University of Colorado at Denver and Health Sciences Center, School of Nursing, *Denver*

Connecticut

Quinnipiac University, Department of Nursing, *Hamden*

Sacred Heart University, Program in Nursing, *Fairfield*

University of Connecticut, School of Nursing, *Storrs*

University of Hartford, College of Education, Nursing, and Health Professions, *West Hartford*

Delaware

Wesley College, Nursing Program, *Dover*

District of Columbia

Georgetown University, School of Nursing and Health Studies, *Washington*

Florida

Florida Agricultural and Mechanical University, School of Nursing, *Tallahassee*

Florida Atlantic University, College of Nursing, *Boca Raton*

Florida Gulf Coast University, School of Nursing, *Fort Myers*

Florida Southern College, Department of Nursing, *Lakeland*

Florida State University, School of Nursing, *Tallahassee*

St. Petersburg College, Department of Nursing, *St. Petersburg*

University of Miami, School of Nursing and Health Studies, *Coral Gables*

University of South Florida, College of Nursing, *Tampa*

Georgia

Brenau University, School of Health and Science, *Gainesville*

Georgia Baptist College of Nursing of Mercer University, Department of Nursing, *Atlanta*

Georgia Southwestern State University, School of Nursing, *Americus*

Kennesaw State University, School of Nursing, *Kennesaw*

Valdosta State University, College of Nursing, *Valdosta*

Idaho

Lewis-Clark State College, Division of Nursing and Health Sciences, *Lewiston*

Illinois

Lewis University, Program in Nursing, *Romeoville*

Rush University, College of Nursing, *Chicago*

Saint Xavier University, School of Nursing, *Chicago*

Southern Illinois University Edwardsville, School of Nursing, *Edwardsville*

University of Illinois at Chicago, College of Nursing, *Chicago*

Indiana

Indiana State University, College of Nursing, *Terre Haute*

Indiana University Kokomo, Indiana University School of Nursing, *Kokomo*

Indiana University-Purdue University Fort Wayne, Department of Nursing, *Fort Wayne*

Indiana University-Purdue University Indianapolis, School of Nursing, *Indianapolis*

Purdue University, School of Nursing, *West Lafayette*

University of Southern Indiana, College of Nursing and Health Professions, *Evansville*

Valparaiso University, College of Nursing, *Valparaiso*

Iowa

Allen College, Program in Nursing, *Waterloo*

Briar Cliff University, Department of Nursing, *Sioux City*

Clarke College, Department of Nursing and Health, *Dubuque*

Grand View College, Division of Nursing, *Des Moines*

Iowa Wesleyan College, Division of Health and Natural Sciences, *Mount Pleasant*

Luther College, Department of Nursing, *Decorah*

Mount Mercy College, Department of Nursing, *Cedar Rapids*

The University of Iowa, College of Nursing, *Iowa City*

Kansas

MidAmerica Nazarene University, Division of Nursing, *Olathe*

Pittsburg State University, Department of Nursing, *Pittsburg*

University of Kansas, School of Nursing, *Kansas City*

Washburn University, School of Nursing, *Topeka*

Kentucky

Bellarmine University, Donna and Allan Lansing School of Nursing and Health Sciences, *Louisville*

Berea College, Department of Nursing, *Berea*

Kentucky Christian University, School of Nursing, *Grayson*

Midway College, Program in Nursing (Baccalaureate), *Midway*

Murray State University, Program in Nursing, *Murray*

Spalding University, School of Nursing, *Louisville*

University of Kentucky, Graduate School Programs in the College of Nursing, *Lexington*

Western Kentucky University, Department of Nursing, *Bowling Green*

Louisiana

Louisiana State University Health Sciences Center, School of Nursing, *New Orleans*

McNeese State University, College of Nursing, *Lake Charles*

Nicholls State University, Department of Nursing, *Thibodaux*

Northwestern State University of Louisiana, College of Nursing, *Shreveport*

Our Lady of the Lake College, Division of Nursing, *Baton Rouge*

University of Louisiana at Lafayette, College of Nursing, *Lafayette*

University of Louisiana at Monroe, Nursing, *Monroe*

Maine

Saint Joseph's College of Maine, Department of Nursing, *Standish*

University of New England, Department of Nursing, *Biddeford*

University of Southern Maine, College of Nursing and Health Professions, *Portland*

Maryland

The Johns Hopkins University, School of Nursing, *Baltimore*

University of Maryland, Baltimore, Master's Program in Nursing, *Baltimore*

Massachusetts

Boston College, William F. Connell School of Nursing, *Chestnut Hill*

Endicott College, Major in Nursing, *Beverly*

MGH Institute of Health Professions, Program in Nursing, *Boston*

Northeastern University, School of Nursing, *Boston*

Regis College, Department of Nursing, *Weston*

Salem State College, Program in Nursing, *Salem*

Simmons College, Department of Nursing, *Boston*

University of Massachusetts Amherst, School of Nursing, *Amherst*

University of Massachusetts Boston, College of Nursing and Health Sciences, *Boston*

University of Massachusetts Dartmouth, College of Nursing, *North Dartmouth*
University of Massachusetts Worcester, Graduate School of Nursing, *Worcester*

Michigan
Grand Valley State University, Russell B. Kirkhof College of Nursing, *Allendale*
Madonna University, College of Nursing and Health, *Livonia*
Michigan State University, College of Nursing, *East Lansing*
Northern Michigan University, College of Nursing and Allied Health Science, *Marquette*
Oakland University, School of Nursing, *Rochester*
Saginaw Valley State University, Crystal M. Lange College of Nursing and Health Sciences, *University Center*
University of Michigan-Flint, Department of Nursing, *Flint*
Wayne State University, College of Nursing, *Detroit*

Minnesota
Bemidji State University, Department of Nursing, *Bemidji*
Bethel University, Department of Nursing, *St. Paul*
Minnesota State University Mankato, School of Nursing, *Mankato*
University of Minnesota, Twin Cities Campus, School of Nursing, *Minneapolis*

Mississippi
University of Mississippi Medical Center, Program in Nursing, *Jackson*

Missouri
Cox College of Nursing and Health Sciences, Department of Nursing, *Springfield*
Missouri State University, Department of Nursing, *Springfield*
Missouri Western State University, Department of Nursing, *St. Joseph*
Saint Louis University, School of Nursing, *St. Louis*
University of Missouri-Columbia, Sinclair School of Nursing, *Columbia*

Montana
Carroll College, Department of Nursing, *Helena*

Nebraska
Clarkson College, Department of Nursing, *Omaha*
Midland Lutheran College, Department of Nursing, *Fremont*
Nebraska Methodist College, Department of Nursing, *Omaha*
University of Nebraska Medical Center, College of Nursing, *Omaha*

Nevada
University of Nevada, Las Vegas, School of Nursing, *Las Vegas*

New Hampshire
Saint Anselm College, Department of Nursing, *Manchester*

New Jersey
College of Saint Elizabeth, Department of Nursing, *Morristown*
Fairleigh Dickinson University, Metropolitan Campus, Henry P. Becton School of Nursing and Allied Health, *Teaneck*
Kean University, Department of Nursing, *Union*
Monmouth University, Marjorie K. Unterberg School of Nursing, *West Long Branch*
Rutgers, The State University of New Jersey, College of Nursing, *Newark*
Seton Hall University, College of Nursing, *South Orange*
University of Medicine and Dentistry of New Jersey, School of Nursing, *Newark*

New Mexico
New Mexico State University, Department of Nursing, *Las Cruces*

New York
Adelphi University, School of Nursing, *Garden City*
Columbia University, School of Nursing, *New York*
Elmira College, Program in Nursing Education, *Elmira*
Hunter College of the City University of New York, Hunter-Bellevue School of Nursing, *New York*
Mercy College, Program in Nursing, *Dobbs Ferry*
Molloy College, Department of Nursing, *Rockville Centre*
Nazareth College of Rochester, Department of Nursing, *Rochester*
New York University, College of Nursing, *New York*
Pace University, Lienhard School of Nursing, *New York*
Roberts Wesleyan College, Division of Nursing, *Rochester*
State University of New York at Binghamton, Decker School of Nursing, *Binghamton*
State University of New York at Plattsburgh, Department of Nursing, *Plattsburgh*
State University of New York Downstate Medical Center, College of Nursing, *Brooklyn*
State University of New York Institute of Technology, School of Nursing and Health Systems, *Utica*
State University of New York Upstate Medical University, College of Nursing, *Syracuse*
Stony Brook University, State University of New York, School of Nursing, *Stony Brook*
University of Rochester, School of Nursing, *Rochester*
Utica College, Department of Nursing, *Utica*

North Carolina
The University of North Carolina at Chapel Hill, School of Nursing, *Chapel Hill*
The University of North Carolina at Charlotte, School of Nursing, *Charlotte*
Winston-Salem State University, Department of Nursing, *Winston-Salem*

Ohio
Capital University, School of Nursing, *Columbus*
Case Western Reserve University, Frances Payne Bolton School of Nursing, *Cleveland*
Cleveland State University, Department of Nursing, *Cleveland*
Kent State University, College of Nursing, *Kent*
Malone College, School of Nursing, *Canton*
Otterbein College, Department of Nursing, *Westerville*
Shawnee State University, Department of Nursing, *Portsmouth*
The University of Akron, College of Nursing, *Akron*
University of Cincinnati, College of Nursing, *Cincinnati*
The University of Toledo, College of Nursing, *Toledo*
Wright State University, College of Nursing and Health, *Dayton*

Oklahoma
Oklahoma City University, Kramer School of Nursing, *Oklahoma City*
University of Oklahoma Health Sciences Center, College of Nursing, *Oklahoma City*

Oregon
Linfield College, School of Nursing, *McMinnville*
Oregon Health & Science University, School of Nursing, *Portland*

Pennsylvania
Alvernia College, Nursing, *Reading*
Carlow University, School of Nursing, *Pittsburgh*
DeSales University, Department of Nursing and Health, *Center Valley*

Drexel University, College of Nursing and Health Professions, *Philadelphia*
Duquesne University, School of Nursing, *Pittsburgh*
Eastern University, Program in Nursing, *St. Davids*
Holy Family University, School of Nursing and Allied Health Professions, *Philadelphia*
La Roche College, Department of Nursing and Nursing Management, *Pittsburgh*
La Salle University, School of Nursing and Health Sciences, *Philadelphia*
Marywood University, Department of Nursing, *Scranton*
Millersville University of Pennsylvania, Department of Nursing, *Millersville*
Moravian College, St. Luke's School of Nursing, *Bethlehem*
Mount Aloysius College, Department of Nursing, *Cresson*
Penn State University Park, School of Nursing, *State College, University Park*
Thomas Jefferson University, Department of Nursing, *Philadelphia*
University of Pennsylvania, School of Nursing, *Philadelphia*
University of Pittsburgh, School of Nursing, *Pittsburgh*
Villanova University, College of Nursing, *Villanova*
Wilkes University, Department of Nursing, *Wilkes-Barre*

Puerto Rico
Universidad Adventista de las Antillas, Department of Nursing, *Mayagüez*
University of Puerto Rico, Mayagüez Campus, Department of Nursing, *Mayagüez*
University of Puerto Rico, Medical Sciences Campus, School of Nursing, *San Juan*

Rhode Island
Salve Regina University, Department of Nursing, *Newport*

South Carolina
Clemson University, School of Nursing, *Clemson*
Medical University of South Carolina, College of Nursing, *Charleston*
University of South Carolina Aiken, School of Nursing, *Aiken*

South Dakota
South Dakota State University, College of Nursing, *Brookings*

Tennessee
Middle Tennessee State University, School of Nursing, *Murfreesboro*
Southern Adventist University, School of Nursing, *Collegedale*
Union University, School of Nursing, *Jackson*
The University of Tennessee, College of Nursing, *Knoxville*
The University of Tennessee at Chattanooga, School of Nursing, *Chattanooga*
The University of Tennessee at Martin, Department of Nursing, *Martin*
The University of Tennessee Health Science Center, College of Nursing, *Memphis*
Vanderbilt University, School of Nursing, *Nashville*

Texas
Lamar University, Department of Nursing, *Beaumont*
Midwestern State University, Nursing Program, *Wichita Falls*
Patty Hanks Shelton School of Nursing, *Abilene*
Southwestern Adventist University, Department of Nursing, *Keene*
Tarleton State University, Department of Nursing, *Stephenville*
Texas A&M International University, Canseco School of Nursing, *Laredo*

Texas A&M University–Corpus Christi, School of Nursing and Health Sciences, *Corpus Christi*

Texas Christian University, Harris School of Nursing, *Fort Worth*

Texas Tech University Health Sciences Center, School of Nursing, *Lubbock*

University of Mary Hardin-Baylor, College of Nursing, *Belton*

The University of Texas at Arlington, School of Nursing, *Arlington*

The University of Texas at Tyler, Program in Nursing, *Tyler*

The University of Texas Health Science Center at Houston, School of Nursing, *Houston*

The University of Texas Health Science Center at San Antonio, School of Nursing, *San Antonio*

The University of Texas Medical Branch, School of Nursing, *Galveston*

Virgin Islands

University of the Virgin Islands, Division of Nursing, *Saint Thomas*

Virginia

George Mason University, College of Nursing and Health Science, *Fairfax*

Jefferson College of Health Sciences, Nursing Education Program, *Roanoke*

Old Dominion University, Department of Nursing, *Norfolk*

Shenandoah University, Division of Nursing, *Winchester*

Washington

Gonzaga University, Department of Nursing, *Spokane*

Intercollegiate College of Nursing/Washington State University, *Spokane*

Pacific Lutheran University, School of Nursing, *Tacoma*

University of Washington, School of Nursing, *Seattle*

West Virginia

Fairmont State University, School of Nursing and Allied Health Administration, *Fairmont*

Shepherd University, Department of Nursing Education, *Shepherdstown*

West Virginia Wesleyan College, Department of Nursing, *Buckhannon*

Wisconsin

Alverno College, Division of Nursing, *Milwaukee*

Marquette University, College of Nursing, *Milwaukee*

University of Wisconsin-Eau Claire, College of Nursing and Health Sciences, *Eau Claire*

University of Wisconsin-Madison, School of Nursing, *Madison*

University of Wisconsin-Milwaukee, College of Nursing, *Milwaukee*

University of Wisconsin-Oshkosh, College of Nursing, *Oshkosh*

Viterbo University, School of Nursing, *La Crosse*

CANADA

British Columbia

British Columbia Institute of Technology, School of Health Sciences, *Burnaby*

Thompson Rivers University, School of Nursing, *Kamloops*

Manitoba

University of Manitoba, Faculty of Nursing, *Winnipeg*

New Brunswick

Université de Moncton, School of Nursing, *Moncton*

University of New Brunswick Fredericton, Faculty of Nursing, *Fredericton*

Nova Scotia

St. Francis Xavier University, Department of Nursing, *Antigonish*

Ontario

Laurentian University, School of Nursing, *Sudbury*

Ryerson University, Program in Nursing, *Toronto*

University of Windsor, School of Nursing, *Windsor*

York University, School of Nursing, Atkinson Faculty of Liberal and Professional Studies, *Toronto*

Quebec

Université du Québec à Rimouski, Program in Nursing, *Rimouski*

Université Laval, Faculty of Nursing, *Québec*

Saskatchewan

University of Saskatchewan, College of Nursing, *Saskatoon*

ALPHABETICAL LISTING OF INSTITUTIONS

Notes

Notes

Notes

Notes

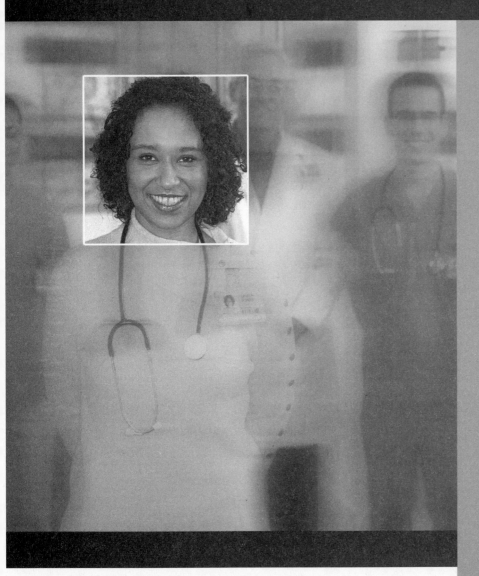

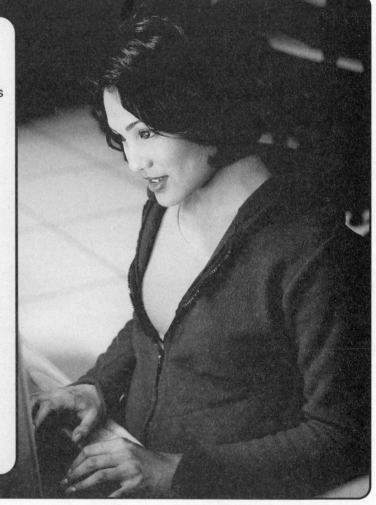
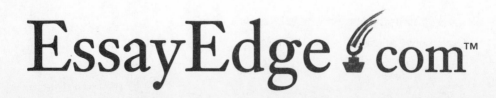

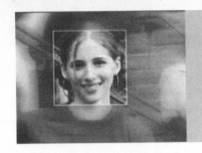

Peterson's
Book Satisfaction Survey

Give Us Your Feedback

Thank you for choosing Peterson's as your source for personalized solutions for your education and career achievement. Please take a few minutes to answer the following questions. Your answers will go a long way in helping us to produce the most user-friendly and comprehensive resources to meet your individual needs.

When completed, please tear out this page and mail it to us at:

Publishing Department
Peterson's, a Nelnet company
2000 Lenox Drive
Lawrenceville, NJ 08648

You can also complete this survey online at **www.petersons.com/booksurvey.**

1. **What is the ISBN of the book you have purchased? (The ISBN can be found on the book's back cover in the lower right-hand corner.)** _____

2. **Where did you purchase this book?**
   ❑ Retailer, such as Barnes & Noble
   ❑ Online reseller, such as Amazon.com
   ❑ Petersons.com
   ❑ Other (please specify) _____

3. **If you purchased this book on Petersons.com, please rate the following aspects of your online purchasing experience on a scale of 4 to 1 (4 = Excellent and 1 = Poor).**

	4	3	2	1
Comprehensiveness of Peterson's Online Bookstore page	❑	❑	❑	❑
Overall online customer experience	❑	❑	❑	❑

4. **Which category best describes you?**
   ❑ High school student
   ❑ Parent of high school student
   ❑ College student
   ❑ Graduate/professional student
   ❑ Returning adult student

   ❑ Teacher
   ❑ Counselor
   ❑ Working professional/military
   ❑ Other (please specify) _____

5. **Rate your overall satisfaction with this book.**

Extremely Satisfied	Satisfied	Not Satisfied
❑	❑	❑

6. Rate each of the following aspects of this book on a scale of 4 to 1 (4 = Excellent and 1 = Poor).

	4	3	2	1
Comprehensiveness of the information	❏	❏	❏	❏
Accuracy of the information	❏	❏	❏	❏
Usability	❏	❏	❏	❏
Cover design	❏	❏	❏	❏
Book layout	❏	❏	❏	❏
Special features (*e.g., CD, flashcards, charts, etc.*)	❏	❏	❏	❏
Value for the money	❏	❏	❏	❏

7. This book was recommended by:
❏ Guidance counselor
❏ Parent/guardian
❏ Family member/relative
❏ Friend
❏ Teacher
❏ Not recommended by anyone—I found the book on my own
❏ Other (please specify) _____

8. Would you recommend this book to others?

Yes	Not Sure	No
❏	❏	❏

9. Please provide any additional comments.

_____

_____

_____

_____

_____

Remember, you can tear out this page and mail it to us at:

Publishing Department
Peterson's, a Nelnet company
2000 Lenox Drive
Lawrenceville, NJ 08648

or you can complete the survey online at **www.petersons.com/booksurvey.**

Your feedback is important to us at Peterson's, and we thank you for your time!

If you would like us to keep in touch with you about new products and services, please include your e-mail address here: _____